Neonatal Nurse Practitioner (NNP-BC®) Certification Review

Amy R. Koehn, PhD, NNP-BC, received her PhD in nursing from Indiana University in 2014. She received her MSN from the University of Colorado at Colorado Springs in 2001 and her BSN from Bethel College in North Newton, Kansas, in 1993. She has over 20 years of experience as a neonatal nurse practitioner (NNP) in a variety of level III and IV NICUs, in roles both at the bedside and as a team member for neonatal air and ground transports. She served as the concentration coordinator for the DNP NNP program at the University of Tennessee Health Science Center from 2015 to 2022. Dr. Koehn has developed continuing education programs for both nursing staff and APRN practitioners. As a mentor for novice practitioners, she developed orientation and education programs for newly graduated NNPs. Her long-standing clinical and academic experiences serve as evidence of the qualification to guide in maintaining the relevance of the ever-evolving NNP role. Dr. Koehn shares her love of learning through lectures at the local, state, and national levels for both academic and commercial purposes. These activities promote continued sharing, learning, and participation in the camaraderie that is the basis to provide the best care for babies and their families!

Neonatal Nurse Practitioner (NNP-BC®) Certification Review

SECOND EDITION

Amy R. Koehn, PhD, NNP-BC

EDITOR

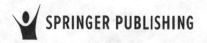 SPRINGER PUBLISHING

Springer Publishing Company, LLC
www.springerpub.com
connect.springerpub.com

Acquisitions Editor: Jaclyn Koshofer
Director, Content Development: Taylor Ball
Production Editor: Ashley Hannen
Compositor: DiacriTech

ISBN: 978-0-8261-6993-8
ebook ISBN: 978-0-8261-6994-5
DOI: 10.1891/9780826169945

23 24 25 26 27 / 5 4 3 2 1

The author and the publisher of this Work have made every effort to use sources believed to be reliable to provide information that is accurate and compatible with the standards generally accepted at the time of publication. Because medical science is continually advancing, our knowledge base continues to expand. Therefore, as new information becomes available, changes in procedures become necessary. We recommend that the reader always consult current research and specific institutional policies before performing any clinical procedure or delivering any medication. The author and publisher shall not be liable for any special, consequential, or exemplary damages resulting, in whole or in part, from the readers' use of, or reliance on, the information contained in this book. The publisher has no responsibility for the persistence or accuracy of URLs for external or third-party Internet websites referred to in this publication and does not guarantee that any content on such websites is, or will remain, accurate or appropriate.

NNP-BC® is a registered trademark of the National Certification Corporation (NCC). NCC does not endorse this resource, nor does it have a proprietary relationship with Springer Publishing Company.

Library of Congress Control Number: 2023938064

Contact sales@springerpub.com to receive discount rates on bulk purchases.

Publisher's Note: **New and used products purchased from third-party sellers are not guaranteed for quality, authenticity, or access to any included digital components.**

Printed in the United States of America.

This book is dedicated to neonatal advanced practice nurses, new and experienced, who devote their time, talents, and hearts to caring for and protecting the tiniest and most fragile of the human population, the babies. It is a calling from the heart that cannot be ignored when heard. At the highest level of nursing, we must remain informed, educated, and knowledgeable about information that impacts our care. This book provides but a stepping stone on your journey in this frequently joyous and occasionally heartbreaking service to infants and their families. May you always continue learning and actively serve by passing on what you have learned to those who come after you. By this legacy, we ensure these precious beings receive care, ensuring their ability to reach the limitless potential in each new life.

Contents

Contributors

Ana I. Arias-Oliveras, MSN, CRNP, NNP-BC
Surgical/Neonatal Advanced Practice Nurse
General, Thoracic, and Fetal Surgery
Newborn/Infant Intensive Care Unit
Children's Hospital of Philadelphia
Philadelphia, Pennsylvania

Debra Armbruster, PhD, APRN, NNP-BC, CPNP-BC
Nationwide Children's Hospital
Columbus, Ohio

Jodi M. Beachy, MSN, NNP-BC
Ohio Health
Dublin, Ohio

Amanda D. Bennett, DNP, NNP-BC, PNP, VA-BC
Adjunct Clinical Assistant Professor
Department of Human Development Nursing Science
University of Illinois Chicago
Chicago, Illinois

Kristin Bindel, MSN, APRN, NNP-BC
Nationwide Children's Hospital
Columbus, Ohio

Elena Bosque, PhD, ARNP, NNP-BC
Department of Neonatology
Seattle Children's Hospital
Seattle, Washington

Cheryl A. Carlson, PhD, APRN, NNP-BC
Clinical Associate Professor
Louise Herrington School of Nursing
Baylor University
Waco, Texas

Vivian Carrasquilla-Lopez, DNP, RN, PNP, NNP-BC
The New York-Presbyterian-Weill Cornell Medical Center
New York, New York
Maimonides Medical Center
Brooklyn, New York
York College of the City University of New York
Jamaica, New York

Rebecca Chuffo Davila, DNP, NNP-BC, FAANP
University of Iowa College of Nursing
University of Iowa Stead Family Children's Hospital
Tiffin, Iowa

Jennifer Fitzgerald, DNP, NNP-BC
University of Maryland School of Nursing
Baltimore, Maryland

Kathryn (Kim) Friddle, PhD, APRN, NNP-BC
Assistant Professor (Clinical)
College of Nursing
University of Utah
Salt Lake City, Utah

Courtney Grassham, MSN, NNP-BC
Pediatrix Medical Group of New Mexico
Albuquerque, New Mexico

Tosha Harris, DNP, APRN, NNP-BC
Assistant Professor
The University of Tennessee Health Science Center
College of Nursing
Memphis, Tennessee

Carolyn J. Herrington, PhD, RN, NNP-BC
Retired Assistant Professor, Clinical
College of Nursing
Wayne State University
Detroit, Michigan

Jacqueline M. Hoffman, DNP, APRN, NNP-BC
Assistant Professor
Department of Women, Children, and Family Nursing
Rush University College of Nursing
Chicago, Illinois

Kimberly Horns, PhD, APRN, NNP-BC, FAANP
Primary Children's Hospital, Intermountain Health Care
Salt Lake City, Utah

Lisa R. Jasin, DNP, NNP-BC
Director, Neonatal Nurse Practitioner Program
College of Nursing and Health
Wright State University Boonshoft School of Medicine
Dayton Children's Hospital
Dayton, Ohio

Allison Z. Kelly, NNP-BC
Nationwide Children's Hospital
Columbus, Ohio

Denise Kirsten, DNP, APRN, NNP-BC
Assistant Professor
Department of Women, Children, and Family Nursing
Nurse Practitioner
Department of Pediatrics
College of Nursing
Rush University
Chicago, Illinois

Marjorie Masten, RN, MSN, CRNP, NNP-BC
Children's Hospital of Philadelphia
Philadelphia, Pennsylvania

Hope McKendree, MSN, CRNP, NNP-BC
The Johns Hopkins Hospital
Baltimore, Maryland

Alexandra Medoro, MD
Nationwide Children's Hospital
Columbus, Ohio

Dawn Mueller-Burke, PhD, NNP-BC
University of Maryland School of Nursing
Baltimore, Maryland

Brooke Murdock, DNP, NNP-BC
Neonatal Nurse Practitioner
Department of Neonatology
University Clinical Health
Le Bonheur Children's Hospital
Regional One Health
Memphis, Tennessee

Leanne M. Nantais-Smith, PhD, RN, NNP-BC
Associate Professor Clinical
Director of Advanced Practice and Graduate Certificate Programs
Graduate Specialty Coordinator, Neonatal Nurse Practitioner Specialty
College of Nursing
Wayne State University
Detroit, Michigan

Yvette Pugh, MS, CRNP, NNP-BC
Holy Cross Hospital
Silver Spring, Maryland

Cheryl B. Robinson, DNS, MS, NNP-BC
Curriculum Design Resources (CDR)
Brunswick, Georgia

Lori Baas Rubarth, PhD, APRN, NNP-BC
Professor and NNP Specialty Track Leader
Creighton University College of Nursing
Omaha, Nebraska

Barbara Snapp, DNP, APRN, NNP-BC
Children's National Hospital
Washington, DC

Karen Stadd, DNP, CRNP, NNP-BC
The Johns Hopkins Hospital
Baltimore, Maryland

Emmeline M. Tate, MSN, CRNP, NNP-BC
The Johns Hopkins Hospital
Bloomberg Children's Center-NICU
Baltimore, Maryland

Patricia E. Thomas, PhD, APRN, NNP-BC, CNE
Clinical Associate Professor
Lead Faculty NNP Program
College of Nursing
University of Texas at Arlington
Arlington, Texas

Ke-Ni Niko Tien, DNP, RN, APRN, NNP-BC
Cleveland Clinic Children's
Cleveland, Ohio

Mary Walters, MSN, NNP-BC
Mercy Medical Center
Baltimore, Maryland

Chandler Williams, DNP, NNP-BC
Neonatal Nurse Practitioner
Children's National Hospital
Washington, DC

Janice Wilson, DNP, NNP-BC, C-ELBW, FAANP
University of Maryland School of Nursing
Baltimore, Maryland

Karen Wright, PhD, APRN, NNP-BC
Assistant Professor
Department of Women, Children, and Family Nursing
Rush University College of Nursing
Chicago, Illinois

List of Reviewers

Tracey Bell, DNP, APRN, NNP-BC
Clinical Assistant Professor
Department of Neonatology
Nell Hodgson Woodruff School of Nursing at
Emory University
Emory University School of Medicine
Atlanta, Georgia

Lauren Casevechia, MSN, APRN, NNP-BC
Department of Neonatology
University Clinical Health
Le Bonheur Children's Medical Center
Regional One Health
St. Francis Hospital
Memphis, Tennessee

Judy Christy, DNP, NNP-BC, CPNP-PC
Neonatal Nurse Practitioner
Le Bonheur Children's Hospital
Memphis, Tennessee

Pamela Harris-Haman, DNP, APRN, NNP-BC
Assistant Professor
Neonatal Nurse Practitioner Track
School of Nursing
University of Texas Medical Branch
Galveston, Texas

Carly Houser, DNP, NNP-BC
Neonatal Nurse Practitioner
Erlanger Health System
Chattanooga, Tennessee

Sura Lee, MSN, CRNP
Surgical Nurse Practitioner
Newborn/Infant Intensive Care Unit
Children's Hospital of Philadelphia
Philadelphia, Pennsylvania

Valerie Moniaci, DNP, APRN, NNP-BC
Director Neonatal Nurse Practitioner Program
College of Nursing
University of Cincinnati
Cincinnati, Ohio

Brooke Murdock, DNP, NNP-BC
Neonatal Nurse Practitioner
Department of Neonatology
University Clinical Health
Le Bonheur Children's Hospital
Regional One Health
Memphis, Tennessee

Jeri Power, NNP-BC, BSN, RN
Neonatal Nurse Practitioner
Department of Neonatology
University Clinical Health
Le Bonheur Children's Hospital
Regional One Health
Memphis, Tennessee

Mary Puchalski, DNP, APRN, CNS, NNP-BC
Clinical Assistant Professor
Neonatal Nurse Practitioner Program
University of Illinois at Chicago
Chicago, Illinois

Megan Schenzel, MSN, NNP-BC
University Clinical Health/Le Bonheur Children's Hospital
Memphis, Tennessee

Patti Scott, DNP, APRN, NNP-BC, C-NPT
TIPQC Infant Quality Improvement Specialist
Assistant Professor of Nursing
Vanderbilt University School of Nursing
Advanced Practitioner Coordinator
Pediatrix Medical Group of Tennessee
Nashville, Tennessee

Angela Warren, BSN, RN, MSN, APRN, NNP-BC
University Clinical Health
University of Tennessee Health Science Center
Memphis, Tennessee

Alyssa B. Weiss, PhD, NNP-BC
Clinical Assistant Professor
Director Neonatal Nurse Practitioner Program
Old Dominion University
College of Health Sciences
School of Nursing
Virginia Beach, Virginia

Chandler Williams, DNP, NNP-BC
Neonatal Nurse Practitioner
Children's National Hospital
Washington, DC

Preface

This book, *Neonatal Nurse Practitioner (NNP-BC®) Certification Review*, is designed as an in-depth study guide for the National Certification Corporation (NCC) certification exam for neonatal nurse practitioners (NNPs). It is appropriate for graduates both at the master of science in nursing (MSN) and doctor of nursing practice (DNP) degree levels. The book may also be used as a comprehensive review for NNPs with existing certification before taking the NCC's continuing competency assessment exam for certification renewal. This book, unique in the market for neonatal content review, synthesizes the knowledge necessary to assist the reader with passing the certification exam for an NNP to become board-certified (i.e., NNP-BC). It follows the outline provided by the NCC of exam content and text references within both the Candidate Guide and Core NP Examination Registration Catalog found on their website. The material is written using the textbook references recommended by the NCC in creating a certification exam. The book is organized in an outline format, highlighting key content information from the reference texts in precise and brief statements. Topics with multiple references are combined into each chapter to provide a broad perspective. References are included so the reader can go directly to the primary textbook source for a more in-depth review. The book does not need to be read sequentially as a whole—rather, the chapters may be read individually, based on an individual's learning needs.

Amy R. Koehn

Acknowledgments

First and foremost, I would like to acknowledge each contributor who donated their time, talent, and energy to make this book come to life a second time. This group project was indeed a demonstration of the best of efforts by all those involved. I am honored and humbled to serve my part, and, from the heart, I thank those who participated.

I want to thank Springer Publishing Company—specifically Jaclyn Koshofer, and Taylor Ball for his tireless work in consistently answering my thousands of emails and keeping me on track.

Finally, I want to acknowledge my husband, Matt. In our 30+ years together, he has supported me through three undergraduate programs, two graduate nursing programs, and the transition from clinician to academic faculty and back again. I say "thank you" for being my partner in life. I would not be who I am today without you.

Pass Guarantee

If you use this resource to prepare for your exam and do not pass, you may return it for a refund of your full purchase price, excluding tax, shipping, and handling. To receive a refund, return your product along with a copy of your exam score report and original receipt showing purchase of new product (not used). Product must be returned and received within 180 days of the original purchase date. Refunds will be issued within 8 weeks from acceptance and approval. One offer per person and address. This offer is valid for U.S. residents only. Void where prohibited. To initiate a refund, please contact Customer Service at csexamprep@springerpub.com.

Part I: Neonatal Nurse Practitioner Certification

Background and Information on Certification

Barbara Snapp

Thank you for choosing *Neonatal Nurse Practitioner (NNP-BC®) Certification Review, Second Edition*, edited by Amy R. Koehn, PhD, NNP-BC, as your study guide. The authors are all knowledgeable educators, nurse practitioners (NPs), and clinical nurse specialists, combining their years of training and experience to help you prepare for the National Certification Corporation (NCC) exam.

At the time of this publication, an introduction would not be complete without a discussion on the impact the coronavirus (COVID-19) has had on the practice of nursing (Kleinpell, 2021). It is simply not possible for anyone to have been unaffected, whether professionally or personally, by this global pandemic. The overall effect has been staggering and has led to a great upheaval in the workforce. One positive outcome of the pandemic has been the focus and recognition on nursing: what we do, how we function, and how nurses are truly the backbone of healthcare. Recognized for the past 19 years by the Gallup Poll as the most trusted profession with the highest ethical standards, the pandemic allowed the public to witness firsthand the bravery, skill, and compassion nurses bring to their work daily. Leadership in ameliorating barriers presented to families due to COVID-19 illustrates the support families can expect from the neonatal nurse practitioner (NNP; Saad, 2020).

▶ THE NURSE PRACTITIONER

The NNP is a registered nurse with a special interest in infants, premature infants, and toddlers through the age of 2, and their families and caretakers (National Association of Neonatal Nurses [NANN] #3059, 2014). NNPs have acquired, at minimum, a graduate-level education in neonatal care and are routinely found in the NICU or newborn care units. The NNP's role encompasses a wide range of activities, including the care of critically ill infants, both term and preterm; delivery room management; discharge planning; developmental follow-up; family care; research; quality improvement (QI); and education (NANN #3058, 2013). Although the role is influenced by individual state practice acts (Barton Associates, 2019), the core competencies and educational requirements to take the certification exam remain the same for all NNPs.

▶ EARLY HISTORY OF PRIMARY CARE NURSE PRACTITIONERS

Recognizing a serious gap in healthcare accessibility, in 1965 a nurse named Loretta Ford and a pediatrician, Henry Silver, created what is credited as the first NP program at the University of Colorado. Following the establishment of these hospital-based programs, within a decade there were 65 pediatric and primary care NP programs operating in the United States (Honeyfield, 2009). Aided by the educational funds made available through the Nurse Training Act of 1984, by the early 1980s there were 15,000 NPs and over 200 NP programs (Honeyfield, 2009).

▶ DEVELOPMENT OF THE NEONATAL NURSE PRACTITIONER ROLE

The NNP role evolved in the early 1970s following the growth of ICUs dedicated to infants. One of the earliest newborn ICUs was created by Dr. Louis Gluck at Yale New Haven Hospital. Found in large, university-affiliated hospitals, these early NICUs were staffed with medical interns and residents. However, the time residents spent in specialty areas was curtailed, and then overall residency hours were limited by graduate medical education (GME) guidelines (Hutter et al., 2006). With a proliferation of NICUs around the country, the promotion of regionalization, and the need for transport teams, additional neonatal specialized personnel were required (Hutter et al., 2006; Samson, 2006).

In 1972, Patricia Johnson created a curriculum for an advanced practitioner but with a focus on neonatal management. Similar to pediatric practitioner programs, neonatal in-hospital programs flourished with little oversight or basic nursing education. Each institution created a curriculum to address its specific hospital needs and then awarded the NNP a certificate upon completion (Honeyfield, 2009).

As a neonatal APRN, you will be the bridge between medicine and nursing, allowing for a robust continuum in patient care services. Leadership in this dual role is unique to NPs and comes with a level of responsibility to improve outcomes through research, QI, advocacy, profession, and self.

1

The importance of research is that it examines current practice, introduces new concepts, generates new knowledge, and improves outcomes. Modest projects are just as important as more complicated ones. As an NP, you will develop an active, inquisitive mind curious about improving current practice or looking at a practice you may wish to adopt. Research is asking questions, working to obtain the answers, then publishing the results so that others may benefit from your work.

QI initiatives will implement or disseminate new knowledge gained from research to improve practice. QI occurs in every unit and may be quite formal with periodic team meetings, frequent plan–do–study–act (PDSA) cycles, and flowcharts, or it may be an informal group having a discussion on how to amend current practice to improve some specific outcome. State collaboratives are experts on QI and can offer insight into comparisons among hospitals with similar patient populations. Larger practices may have their own research teams and data collection abilities. In one recent study, 82.5% of the NNP respondents said they were involved in research and QI, most often in the leadership role (Snapp & Reyna, 2019).

After you pass the NCC exam and are comfortable in your workplace, it will be time to develop your skillset beyond your institution on issues that impact NNP practice. The easiest place to start is volunteering for a national organization. There will be many activities that take very little time but lends support to the project and learning opportunities for you. Other opportunities may be found in the community your hospital system serves.

The ongoing pandemic illustrates the need for self-care for nurses. There is clear evidence of the many stressors that surfaced during COVID-19 (Hossain & Clatty, 2021). Separated families, working long shifts, limited personal protection equipment (PPE), concerns about spreading the infection, and social isolation all increased stress levels exponentially (Haefner, 2021). A 2021 National Association of Pediatric Nurse Practitioners (NAPNAP) survey showed that one-third of the respondents felt professionally burned out, 25% expressed feelings of anxiety, and 15% reported depression (Peck & Sonney, 2021). As the pandemic continues in its many forms, many of these issues may not be immediately remedied.

▶ EDUCATIONAL CHANGES

Neonatal educators recognized the need to shift the NNP educational programs from hospital-based certificates to university-affiliated graduate programs. It is interesting to note this shift was originally met with resistance from the academic leaders as promoting a medical-based education model that required physician involvement but minimal nursing input. Ultimately, the success of the NNP role resulted in a move to graduate education for NPs and acceptance of medical practice knowledge enveloped in a nursing model (Honeyfield, 2009). Curriculum oversight was initially conducted by the American Nurses Association (ANA; 1975–2001), but shifted to the NANN in 2002 when the first Education Standards and Guidelines for NNP Programs was published (Honeyfield, 2009; NANN #3059, 2014).

In 2000, the American Academy of Pediatrics Committee on the Fetus and Newborn endorsed master's-level preparation for NNPs (Samson, 2006). The early part of that decade saw the formation of Licensure, Accreditation, Certification, and Education (LACE), a collaborative group of over 40 key stakeholders representing NPs, nurse midwives, nurse anesthetists, and clinical specialists, created to examine and coordinate LACE for APRNs. The purpose of this collaborative was "to provide a structure for dialogue, debate, and consensus" for an APRN model (Goudreau, 2011).

Although state practice acts vary, most states require board certification and/or a graduate degree and specialty certification for entry into practice. The APRN Consensus Model (National Council of State Boards of Nursing [NCSBN], 2019) allows for more fluidity between states and increased consistency on licensure requirements throughout the United States. An ever-increasing number of states are legislating independent NP practice and NP prescriptive authority (Barton Associates, 2019).

▶ BOARD CERTIFICATION

It was recognized in the early 1970s that neonatal nurses lacked a specialty examination such as those already available for nurse anesthetists and nurse midwives. Originally operating on simultaneous and parallel paths to develop a certification examination, ultimately the ANA and the Nurses' Association of the American College of Obstetricians and Gynecologists (NAACOG) jointly developed a standardized certification examination. Unfortunately, early results revealed widely disparate passing rates. Recognizing that sharing the responsibility was not adequately serving the target nursing population, the NCC was created and is now the board-certifying organization for NNPs (NANN #3059, 2014; Honeyfield, 2009; Hutter et al., 2006; Wohlert, 1979). Dorothy Telega, RN, 1974 NAACOG President, stated: "By achieving formal recognition for superior performance in nursing practice, the certified nurse will serve as a role model and will be identified with excellence in clinical practice" (Wohlert, 1979).

Passing the NCC board certification exam to earn the title of "NNP-BC" is the initial step after graduation toward building a career. Recertification occurs every 3 years and requires an assessment exam that will guide an education plan for tested areas needing improvement (NCC, 2019). Once the areas for improvement are identified, there are many ways to earn continuing nursing education (CNE) to fulfill the NCC educational plan requirements. Conferences paired with an accrediting organization may offer CNE and will often designate the appropriate specific specialty codes: general management, pharmacology, physical assessment, physiology and pathophysiology, or professional practice. Continuing education can also be obtained in other ways, such as precepting students, making continuing education presentations, or authoring a book or journal article (NCC, 2019). The NCC website provides details on maintenance certification: https://www.nccwebsite.org/maintain-your-certification/subspecialty-certification-maintenance (Table 1.1).

Table 1.1 Requirements to Sit for National Certification Corporation Board Certification Examination

Requirements	Time Frame	Additional Requirements	Testing	Maintenance
Current, active, unencumbered U.S. nursing license	Must take the exam within 8 years of graduation from the program	PDF file of diploma for upload to the NCC website PDF file of official transcript which documents successful completion of all coursework and indicates the NNP program;must be issued from the school registrar and uploaded with the application	General assessment: 17%	Completion of the Continuing Competency Assessment at the beginning of the maintenance cycle
Successful completion of an accredited graduate nurse practitioner program that meets the NCC program requirements and prepares neonatal nurse practitioners; program can be a master's DNP or post-master's, and the NCC no longer accepts certificate-prepared applicants		$325, which is composed of a $50 nonrefundable application submission cost and a $275 testing fee Incomplete applications subject to a $30 reprocessing fee	General management: 19%	CE earned based on education plan developed after the assessment is completed CE entered into the maintenance application anytime during the 3-year maintenance cycle
			Pharmacology: 9%	
Minimum of 600 clinical and 200 didactic hours		Complete application checklist	Embryology, physiology, pathophysiology, and systems management: 52%	
			Professional issues: 3%	

CE, continuing education; DNP, Doctor of Nursing Practice; NCC, National Certification Corporation; NNP, neonatal nurse practitioner.
Sources: Data from National Certification Corporation. (2022). *Certification examination core*; National Certification Corporation. (2022). *2022 candidate guide neonatal nurse practitioner NNP-BC.*

▶ SUMMARY

Neonatal Nurse Practitioner (NNP-BC®) Certification Review is intended for use by the new graduate as well as the experienced practitioner. The content is arranged as topic snapshots for a timely review. Should a topic need further investigation, each section and chapter includes references and page numbers to guide the reader to the original sources.

An NNP is a well-respected member of the healthcare team. Achieving board certification is the expectation of a subject matter expert and competent clinician. Dr. Amy R. Koehn and the authors congratulate you on taking this next important and exciting step in your nursing career. Being an NNP is challenging, enjoyable, rewarding, and can lead to many other worthwhile activities. *Neonatal Nurse Practitioner (NNP-BC®) Certification Review* was designed to give you highlights on each topic and provide a quick but thorough resource you can refer to prior to taking the exam and as a guide throughout your NNP career.

Study and Test-Taking Tips

Cheryl B. Robinson

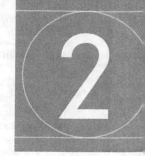

▶ INTRODUCTION

From the moment you decided to accept a position in the NICU, you have been working toward this day. Everything about caring for such a vulnerable population forces each of us to be our best and to understand as much as possible about neonatal-specific development, diseases, and responses to the care we provide. We also become experts at keying in on the wordless cues the most immature of the population scream at us. Certification as a neonatal nurse practitioner (NNP) allows us to demonstrate we have achieved a level of more expert skills and fine-tuned knowledge, and a further enhancing of our ability to care for neonates and their families. The acronym P.A.S.S.—Prepare, Assess, Study, Succeed—has been utilized by veteran NNP educators to help students pass the National Certification Corporation (NCC) NNP exam and is offered here for your benefit.

▶ P.A.S.S.—PREPARE · ASSESS · STUDY · SUCCEED

PREPARE

Overview

The NCC is the certifying body for all NNPs in the United States. Before or during your educational program, be sure to download the latest versions of NCC materials regarding the certification process (www.nccwebsite.org). Each year, the NCC updates exam catalogs, and regardless of your graduation date, the year in which you take the test will be the exam catalog you will need to follow. Download the most current Candidate Guide while still in your educational program. Familiarize yourself with exam fees and eligibility requirements, testing methods (testing center vs. live remote proctoring [LRP]), Americans With Disabilities Act (ADA) requests for testing accommodations, policies and procedures, and certification exam content.

The NCC does not provide any review courses or specific study materials; however, upon acceptance of your application, you will be provided with a detailed outline of the test and suggested study resources (www.nccwebsite.org/ certification-exams/how-to-study). At present, the NCC does provide a preview test that you can purchase on their website, as well as a detailed content test map.

During Your Program

For those who purchase this book during their program— Congratulations! There is a variety of information contained in the chapters that will be helpful as you travel through your academic journey. Once you start the specialized didactic and clinical portion of your studies, every class, every assignment, and every quiz/exam/case study needs to be viewed as part of your preparation for the NCC exam. Required readings will be assigned. Determine the time you can set aside to read, and for that time be intentional. Knowledge retention is increased when dedicated study time becomes part of your study plan (Zakarija-Grkovic et al., 2019). The goal is that you do not return to the same pages twice. The second time you read something, you only retain a fraction of what you ascertained the first time. Even if you get through only several pages per session, get the most out of the reading. You may want to make notecards of the most important points; you may want to draw a figure or a concept map to capture the content. Rereading material will not guarantee retention success (Miyatsu et al., 2018).

Whether your program teaches content from a disease standpoint or from a body system standpoint, you can start to organize your didactic content according to the categories outlined by a certification test map (Figure 2.1). The content areas outlined by the NCC will be fair game for testing, whether or not your program covered the topics. Note, the largest section of the examination (52%) covers embryology, physiology, pathophysiology, and systems management (disease process). You will need to know all aspects of every disease and disease process covered in the test map. The latest test map has separated pharmacology from general management in recognition of the vital nature of the topic impacting all care provided to neonates.

Make your notes now: Do not depend on your memory. You will not remember rationales from the exam or quiz you took last week. Do not memorize specific questions and answers, as you will not see that exact question or the same set of answers again. If you missed a question related to the mechanism of action of Lasix in the kidney,

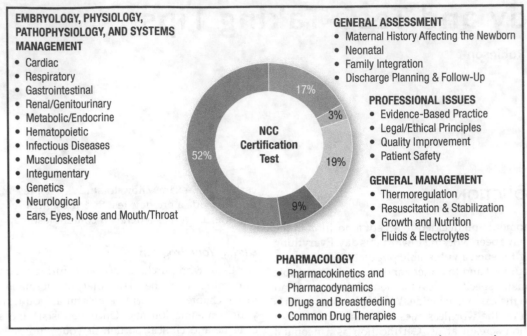

Figure 2.1 National Certification Corporation neonatal nurse practitioner exam question categories.
Source: Adapted from the National Certification Corporation (NCC).

study that concept and not the answer from the test. Knowing the right answer from a certain exam will benefit you less than knowing the correct information pertaining to Lasix and kidney function. For questions to which you have access for review, note the topic of the question: What was the question asking you to consider? As per the NCC outline, place the question topic in either of the following:

- General assessment
- General management
- Pharmacology
- Disease process (embryology/physiology/ pathophysiology/systems management)
- Professional issues

After determining the general topic of the question, decide which part of the NCC's detailed outline the topic matter is addressing. Keep up with what you are covering and what content you are receiving as you progress through the program. Be sure to pay attention to the content you test well on and the content you struggle with. Be honest with yourself and realize you will tend to spend time on the content you already know. Concentrate on the content most difficult for you to test well on. You will want to visit your document later as you begin the concentrated study for the certification exam. Also, keep in mind the percentages allocated to content sections. If the NCC assigns 3% to a topic area, your study time should reflect a similar effort. Hopefully, your program provided you with exam experiences mirroring the NCC exam and percentage content areas.

"When Should I Take the NCC?"

Every student and every certified NNP will have a different answer to this specific question. Most of the available literature, albeit from medicine and not graduate nursing, provides evidence for testing as soon as you are eligible after graduation or after your last didactic/clinical course. (Be aware that if you are completing a bachelor of science in nursing to doctor of nursing practice [BSN-DNP] program, you may need to seek testing eligibility prior to your graduation. The NCC and your school/college of nursing can provide additional information.) For candidates who voluntarily delayed taking the pediatric board certification exam, the result was fewer people successfully passing the exam (Anderson et al., 2021; Nomura et al., 2021). The following conclusions were determined by the authors:

- Essential knowledge weakened with the passage of time between school and the certification exam.
- Candidates who delayed examination were, overall, less confident of their knowledge at the time of graduation.
- Weak clinical students often felt discouraged at graduation so they delayed examination.
- *All candidates, regardless of status at graduation, need to certify as soon as possible to maximize their chance to successfully pass the board examination.*

Studies conducted on other specialties, such as emergency medicine, general surgery, preventive medicine, and internal medicine, also reported that a delay in taking the appropriate certification exam resulted in more failures (Abbott et al., 2021; Nguyen et al., 2021).

"Can I Be Successful?"

Do you possess the qualities and traits to successfully complete your specialty certification exam? If you have successfully completed your program . . . Yes! You do! Qualities and traits outlined in the health sciences literature associated with successful testing include the following:

- energized by learning, able to make connections between new and prior knowledge, increased motivation to succeed, goal-directed, and optimistic perspective (Yatczak et al., 2021)
- naturally ambitious, intellectually curious, intensely interested in the subject material, and enthusiastic about learning (Zakarija-Grkovic et al., 2019)

ASSESS

Quinn et al. (2018) determined from interviews with successful NCLEX-RN® candidates that using practice questions, taking practice tests, making a test review plan, and having appropriate review materials were instrumental to their success. Conversely, Claudette (2014) reported candidates' reasons for their failure on the NCLEX-RN exam, which included "distraction, not knowing what to expect, poor test-taking skills, and overall inadequate preparation" (p. 12). Unsuccessful candidates also falsely concluded that since they had performed better in their program than others who had already been successful on the exam, they should pass as well (Claudette, 2014). You need to judge your performance only against the standard of the course and not fellow students.

Assessment is the starting place for all nursing care and preparing for the NCC exam is no different. There are a few areas of assessment you will need to address:

- What do you know right now?
- How do you manage test anxiety?
- When do you plan on studying?

What Do You Know Right Now?

You need to assess your knowledge base as it stands after completing your program. One way to do this is to take as many practice quizzes or exams as you can find. The book you hold in your hands is an excellent resource, containing end-of-chapter Knowledge Check questions, plus online access to a full practice exam via ExamPrepConnect.com.

Additionally, the NCC website contains a preview test as a detailed content test map you may purchase and take. Again, mark your checklist with the content areas of the questions you do not answer correctly. The point is to develop a study plan concentrating on materials on which you do not already have a firm grasp. Studying what you already know will make you feel smart, but at this point in your preparation know you are smart! Success on the NCC will be determined by taking what you already know well and adding not-so-well-known content at the end of your program.

How Do You Manage Test Anxiety?

First, you must recognize whether or not you have test anxiety. Everyone has some anxiety related to test-taking, and some anxiety is positively correlated with an improved performance (Jerrim, 2022). Test-taking anxiety has been identified by both students and faculty as strongly impacting success rates on the NCELX-RN and other high-stakes exams (Jerrim, 2022; Quinn & Peters, 2017; Silaj et al., 2021). Some students are motivated by the pressure of performing well on an exam, while others experience the pressure as a fear of failure and are overwhelmed (Jerrim, 2022).

Test anxiety may affect cognitive aspects such as forgetfulness, disorganization, or irrelevant thinking (Silaj et al., 2021). Other empirical referents for test anxiety include cognitive impairment, which measures concentration, focus, fear of failure, lack of confidence in skills, feeling unprepared for tests, forgetfulness, or test-irrelevant thinking (Yuguo et al., 2021). In some situations, a student's self-worth may be linked to the outcome of the exam, and fear of failure may result in clinical depression (Anxiety and Depression Association of America [ADAA], 2012). Cognitive test anxiety (CTA) occurs when the student becomes consumed with worry about test-taking and is mentally stressed, in addition to the physiologic or emotional responses such as a pounding heart, sweating, nausea, headache, or crying (Johnson, 2019).

There is a strong positive correlation between high test anxiety and poor test performance (Cassady & Johnson, 2002). Recognizing test anxiety and applying appropriate interventions will improve learning outcomes and in effect increase the chance of success on certification. Students who believe they can be successful (self-efficacy) actually perform better, and controlling test anxiety is one way to add control in the testing environment (Yuguo et al., 2021).

When Do You Plan on Studying?

Urban legends exist concerning the power of cramming before an exam. The academic literature does not support the process. Your entire program has provided you information about when to study for an exam. The NCC exam is just that, an exam. The NCC will notify you of an exam window so that you can realistically identify on a calendar the days you will have available to study. Make an appointment with yourself for a "study date." Put the date on the calendar and do not miss the day!

STUDY

You now have your study exam outline. Studying for the NCC cannot be separated from testing for the NCC. You will be given a maximum of 3 hours to take the exam, and if you take an average of 1 minute per question, you will be sitting for 2 hours and 55 minutes. Therefore, *before* you get to the testing day, you need to structure your study time around 3-hour blocks. Do not let the first time you work intensively be the day of the exam. Think about being in training—you do not run a 10K on the same morning you decide to run a 10K. You must build up your stamina, and in the case of the NCC exam you will need the ability to keep your mind sharp for all 175 questions. Do not consider reading or rereading (mentioned earlier) as study. Reading is what you do prior to studying. You will need to actively engage with the content material. Some examples might include the following:

- Become the teacher and prepare the content to share with someone else.
- Tie the content to a clinical situation or find an example from practice to apply the content.
- Draw a concept map to capture all the areas with associated content (see Figure 2.2).

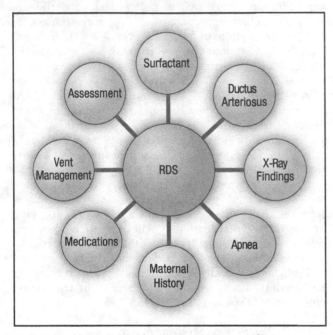

Figure 2.2 Spider concept map example.

RDS, respiratory distress syndrome.

One successful study strategy will be to gather a few texts for *review purposes only*. At this point, learning something new for the first time will not be an efficient use of your time. Put away all your other texts from your program and only choose one or two to review. Some examples of texts for study review might include the following:

- Witt, C. L., & Wallman, C. M. (2023). *Tappero & Honeyfield's physical assessment of the newborn: A comprehensive approach to the art of physical examination* (7th ed.). Springer Publishing Company.
- Gomella, T. L., Eyal, F. G., & Bany-Mohammed, F. (2020). *Gomella's neonatology: Management, procedures, on-call problems, diseases, and drugs* (8th ed.). McGraw Hill/Medical.

Other good resources are question-and-answer texts such as the following:

- Polin, R. A., & Spitzer, A. R. (2014). *Fetal and neonatal secrets* (3rd ed.). Elsevier Saunders.

Successful study habits include taking practice exams, scheduling study time, and spending some time studying with others. Strategies that are not helpful include recopying notes, intensive studying the night before the exam, and making outlines (Zakarija-Grkovic et al., 2019).

We have a tendency to want to study what we already know or what we get right on a quiz. Whatever you do, avoid continuing to study and take exams on your best topics of knowledge. Completing more questions on what you already know will not necessarily correlate with a higher score on the exam. You will get those questions correct on the NCC exam without any further study. Plan to study materials on which you do not already have a firm grasp.

Make sure you build in structure during your study time and avoid multitasking, distractions in the environment, and using your computer (Downs et al., 2015). Research has demonstrated writing by hand to be associated with better retention of materials (Patterson, 2016).

Question Structure

All questions on the NCC certification exam are written to reflect entry-level NNP practice. There are two types of questions: those that have been pretested and statistically analyzed and those that are being pretested to ensure the item meets the statistical threshold set by the NCC for test items.

You should only practice with items that mirror the certification exam. You may have experienced this question format within your program, but if not, that is more reason to avail yourself of one or more of the practice exams previously mentioned.

Questions on the NCC exam contain three parts:

1. Stem . . . (you may think of this as the question)
   - **A.** A key (correct answer)
   - **B.** Distractors (incorrect answer)
   - **C.** Distractors (incorrect answer)
   An example of this is the following:

PRACTICE QUESTION

Aspiration of meconium will:
A. Decrease surface tension
B. Displace natural surfactant
C. Increase pulmonary vasodilation
- Correct Answer: B
Rationale: Meconium displaces surfactant, thereby increasing surface tension and causing pulmonary vasoconstriction.

The Plan of Attack

- Read the stem of the question first and answer the question *before* looking at the distractors.
- Then look at the distractors.
  - If you see a distractor matching your initial answer, choose the distractor and move to the next question.
  - If you do not see your initial answer to the question, return to the stem of the question and reread slowly, followed by reading each of the distractors with the stem. The correct answer should be grammatically correct in line with the stem.
  - If all the distractors match grammatically, then look for keywords in the stem and see if those same keywords appear in one of the distractors.
    - ❑ One technique to determine the answer is to use the answer choices to make a question: In the example: Does aspiration of meconium cause increased pulmonary vasodilation? Does aspiration of meconium cause a decrease in surface tension? Does meconium displace surfactant? The one to which the answer is "yes" is the correct answer.
- *If you are still unsure, mark the question to return to when you finish the remaining questions. Sometimes a later question will contain helpful information to trigger a correct response.*

SUCCEED

Success comes in the form of preparation, and a great way to do this is to prepare checklists.

The following is the first checklist you will need to make:

- You have viewed all the NCC documents regarding certification. Locate the Guide to Testing Methods (www.nccwebsite.org/content/documents/cms/ncc-testing-guide.pdf) *before* you submit your application to the NCC. The comprehensive guide will provide you details about testing.
- You have completed your NNP certification application and mailed the application with fee to the NCC.
- You have received your eligibility letter from the NCC via email.
- You have located an approved testing center and have scheduled a testing day within the 90-day window of the date on the eligibility letter you received from the NCC. *OR*
- You have completed all requirements for LRP. The NCC provides a detailed instruction page to help prepare you and your computer if you decide to test this way.
- You have purchased a basic calculator (battery-operated, noiseless, nonprogrammable, nonprinting). In some instances, the testing center will provide a calculator, but do not leave this item to chance.
- You have learned as much as possible about the exam.
- You have completed at least one trip to the testing center during the same time of day when you will have to arrive for testing.

Drive by the location several times: once to locate and then several times during the time of day you will need to arrive on your testing day. Traffic patterns are important since you will not be able to take your exam if you are 15 minutes late arriving at the site. If late, you will not be able to reschedule, not have your money refunded, and will have to submit a completely new application packet to the NCC. You should determine an alternate route to the testing site in case of traffic problems. Determine, in realistic time, how long the commute will be, what parking entails, the cost either in cash/coin or by credit card, and how long you can park. Once you begin the test, you will not be able to return to your car, so allot yourself a minimum of 4 hours of parking time.

Go into the testing site on one of your visits. Determine the location of the bathroom and whether there are snack or drink machines. Visit the actual testing room if possible. You may need to arrange this opportunity with the testing site prior to your exam date. You want to go into the room and sit at one of the computer terminals. Visualize yourself sitting in the chair and looking at the computer screen. Determine whether there are any smells that are disturbing. You may need to wear a favorite scent on your clothes or place an essential oil on your wrist. Studies have supported the use of aroma therapy to increase concentration when students are testing (Johnson, 2019).

Make a folder that contains all the materials you will need to supply at the testing center.

Next checklist—Be sure you have the following:

- email from the NCC
- two forms of identification: one must be an approved photo identification (ID), and both must have your current name (the *same* as provided to the NCC with your application) and your signature

If you are getting married, think carefully of the logistics of having the same name on your diploma or equivalent, the name on your application packet to the NCC, the name on your eligibility letter from the NCC, and the name on the two IDs you will take to the testing center.

The night before, be sure to be as physically ready as possible. Get a good night's sleep and get hydrated (be sure to go to bathroom before you start the exam).

Certification Test Day

Before you leave your home/hotel:

- Do you have a copy of your NCC eligibility letter?
- Do you have an approved photo ID and another approved ID?

- Do you have proper payment for parking?
- Do you have your preferred snack and/or drink that you will have available to you when you get back to your car after testing?

At the testing center:

- You only have your wallet and keys.
- You only have your eligibility letter.
- You secure your personal items with the test administrator.

Before starting the exam:

- Familiarize yourself with the computer monitor, keyboard, and mouse.
- Determine whether you will want to use the built-in timer on the computer screen.
- Gather the available piece of paper and pencil from the test administrator.
- Take advantage of the practice questions made available by the NCC. You will not lose any time by completing the questions. The questions are meant to help you get familiar with the computer, and exam setup.
- Read over the instructions one more time before you begin.
- Take a few cleansing breaths before you begin.

During the exam:

- Use your scratch paper to write down any equation, lab value, mnemonic, and so on, before you answer the first question. Do not wait until you are in the exam to try and remember.
- Read over each question carefully.
- Answer every question. An unanswered question is considered a wrong answer. Give yourself the benefit of completing all items.

▶ CONCLUSION

As we say to the families of our precious patients, discharge planning begins on the day of admission. So much the same goes for you: Preparation for the NCC certification exam begins on day 1 of your academic program. Every class, every assignment, and every quiz/exam/case study needs to be recorded as part of your preparation in order to develop a study plan concentrating on materials on which you do not already have a firm grasp. You have been working toward this day for years now—you can do it! Just remember to P.A.S.S.!

Exhibit 2.1 P.A.S.S. Checklist: Prepare / Assess / Study / Succeed

NCC Certification Test Map

General Assessment—17% (~30 Qs)

	Passed	Study More
Maternal History Affecting the Neonate	☐	☐
Neonatal Physical Assessment	☐	☐
Family Integration	☐	☐
Discharge Planning and Follow-Up	☐	☐

General Management—19% (~33 Qs)

	Passed	Study More
Thermoregulation	☐	☐
Resuscitation and Stabilization	☐	☐
Growth and Nutrition	☐	☐
Fluids and Electrolytes	☐	☐

Pharmacology—9% (~15 Qs)

	Passed	Study More
Pharmacokinetics and Pharmacodynamics	☐	☐
Drugs and Breastfeeding	☐	☐
Common Drug Therapies	☐	☐

Professional Issues—3% (~5 Qs)

	Passed	Study More
Evidence-Based Practice, Ethical Principles, Professional/ Legal, Patient Safety	☐	☐

Embryology, Physiology, Pathophysiology, and Systems Management—52% (~91 Qs)

	Passed	Study More
Cardiac	☐	☐
Respiratory	☐	☐
Gastrointestinal	☐	☐
Renal/Genitourinary	☐	☐
Metabolic/Endocrine	☐	☐
Hematopoietic	☐	☐
Infectious Diseases	☐	☐
Musculoskeletal	☐	☐
Integumentary	☐	☐
Genetics	☐	☐
Neurologic	☐	☐
Ears, Eyes, Nose, and Mouth/Throat	☐	☐

Copyright by: Cheryl B. Robinson.

Part II: General Assessment

Maternal History Affecting the Newborn in the Antepartum

Courtney Grassham and Lisa R. Jasin

▶ INTRODUCTION

The impact of maternal health history on the outcome of the neonate cannot be overstated. There is a direct correlation between what affects the mother and what affects the neonate. Understanding the links between maternal history and neonatal presentation is key to the initial stabilization of any neonate. This chapter covers maternal hypertension disorders, diabetes, pulmonary conditions, cardiovascular conditions, infectious conditions, hematologic conditions, substance exposure, pharmaceutical exposure, and fetal testing.

▶ HYPERTENSION IN PREGNANCY

- Hypertension is the most common complication in pregnancy and the cause of most of the morbidity /mortality for both maternal and neonatal patients (Table 3.1). Hypertension-related complications are a leading cause of maternal death in the United States (Burgess, 2021; Jeyabalan, 2020; Moore, 2018).

CHRONIC HYPERTENSION

- Chronic hypertension, diagnosed when hypertension is present before pregnancy or recorded before 20 weeks' gestation, affects up to 5% of pregnant patients.
- Most cases of chronic hypertension in pregnancy are idiopathic, also called *essential hypertension*. However, patients should also be evaluated for secondary hypertension, as pregnancy outcomes are worse for patients with secondary hypertension.
- Females with chronic hypertension are at increased risk of slowing fetal growth and superimposed preeclampsia (PE). The severity of maternal and fetal complications depends on the severity of hypertension.
  - When chronic hypertension is secondary to maternal chronic renal disease, there are significantly elevated odds of PE, premature

Table 3.1 Types of Hypertension in Pregnancy

Chronic hypertension	■ Presents before pregnancy ■ Diagnosed before 20 weeks ■ Hypertension that persists more than 12 weeks after delivery
Gestational hypertension	■ New hypertension after 20 weeks with absence of proteinuria ■ If onset before 36 weeks, can progress rapidly to preeclampsia ■ Normalizes after pregnancy

Preeclampsia	■ New hypertension after 20 weeks with new-onset proteinuria (>300 mg in 24 hours) *OR* in the absence of proteinuria, new-onset hypertension with new onset of any of the following (severe features of preeclampsia):
	  ● Thrombocytopenia (<100,000)
	  ● Elevated liver transaminases or severe right upper quadrant pain
	  ● Renal insufficiency/oliguria (a creatinine level >1.1 or one that doubles)
	  ● Pulmonary edema
	  ● New-onset cerebral (headache) or visual disturbances (double vision, floaters, blindness) that do not respond to treatment

Eclampsia	■ Onset of seizures in women with preeclampsia

Sources: Data from Moore, T. (2018). Hypertensive complications of pregnancy. In C. Gleason & S. Juul (Eds.), *Avery's diseases of the newborn* (10th ed., pp. 120–124). Elsevier; Harper, L., Tita, A., & Karumanchi, S. (2019). Pregnancy-related hypertension. In R. Resnik, C. Lockwood, T. Moore, M. Greene, J. Copel, & R. Silver (Eds.), *Creasy and Resnik's maternal-fetal medicine: Principles and practice* (8th ed., p. 810). Elsevier; Jeyabalan, A. (2020). Hypertensive disorders of pregnancy. In R. Martin, A. Fanaroff, & M. Walsh (Eds.), *Fanaroff & Martin's neonatal-perinatal medicine: Diseases of the fetus and infant* (10th ed., p. 251). Elsevier; Burgess, A. (2021). Hypertensive disorders of pregnancy. In K. Simpson & P. Creehan (Eds.), *Perinatal nursing* (5th ed., p. 181). Lippincott Williams & Wilkins; Sibai, B., & Wallace, C. (2017). Preeclampsia and related conditions. In E. C. Eichenwald, A. R. Hansen, C. R. Martin, & A. R. Stark (Eds.), *Cloherty and Stark's manual of neonatal care* (8th ed., pp. 1–14). Lippincott, Williams & Wilkins.

11

delivery, small for gestational age (GA), and pregnancy failure.
- Females with untreated severe chronic hypertension are also at increased risk of stroke and other cardiovascular complications during pregnancy.
■ Monitoring mothers with chronic hypertension includes daily blood pressure checks, routine growth ultrasounds (US), and biophysical profile (BPP) testing, with nonstress testing if there is a concern for fetal status.
■ Treatment of chronic hypertension is often a balancing act between lowering maternal blood pressure and lessening the potential for medications to harm the fetus.
■ The medications most commonly used to manage hypertension include methyldopa, labetalol, hydralazine, and nifedipine.
- Medications avoided during pregnancy due to the risk of fetal damage include angiotensin-converting enzyme (ACE) inhibitors, angiotensin receptor blockers, renin inhibitors, and mineralocorticoid receptor antagonists (Burgess, 2021; Dix, 2016; Harper et al., 2019; Jeyablan, 2020; Moore, 2018).

GESTATIONAL HYPERTENSION

■ *Gestational hypertension* (GH) is defined as new-onset hypertension occurring after 20 weeks of pregnancy without signs of PE (e.g., proteinuria). GH replaces the previous term, *pregnancy-induced hypertension* (PIH). All mothers with a diagnosis of GH should be regarded as being at risk of progression to PE, and the earlier GH is evident the greater the risk of PE.
- GH is a provisional diagnosis during pregnancy. It includes women in three categories: (a) women who will progress to develop PE, (b) women with "transient hypertension of pregnancy" who do not develop PE and revert to normal blood pressures by 12 weeks postdelivery, and (c) women who may have previously unrecognized chronic hypertension.
■ The final diagnosis of GH is applied only if the patient's blood pressure returns to normal at 12 weeks postpartum. GH tends to recur in subsequent pregnancies and predisposes women to hypertension in the future (Burgess, 2021; Dix, 2016; Jeyabalan, 2020; Moore, 2018; Woo et al., 2021).

PREECLAMPSIA–ECLAMPSIA

■ *PE* is defined as a blood pressure >140 mmHg /90 mmHg with proteinuria or severe features. Severe features are described as blood pressure >160 mmHg/110 mmHg, or other criteria as listed in Table 3.1. It is a vasospastic, multisystem, dynamic disorder that is progressive in nature.

■ The etiology of PE is unknown, but theories focus on the stimulation of the inflammatory system by cardiovascular changes in pregnancy, dietary deficiencies, genetic abnormalities, and immunologic response to partially foreign genetic placental and fetal tissue.
■ There is a multitude of risk factors that predispose to the development of PE, including race, age, preexisting diabetes, in vitro fertilization (IVF) pregnancy, history of hypertensive disorders, obesity, and the number of fetus. A combination of any of these factors increases the incidence of PE. Race disparities in African American and Native American women tend to affect severity more than the incidence of PE and may be due to the rates of chronic hypertension in the populations. These populations include African American and Native American women.
- Patients who are obese before pregnancy have a higher risk of developing PE, with an increased risk as obesity worsens.
- Pregnant patients with multiple fetuses tend to develop PE sooner and more severely than those with singleton pregnancy.
■ Pathologic changes are due to disruptions in placental perfusion and endothelial cell dysfunction. Normal vascular remodeling does not occur or only partially develops, resulting in decreased placental perfusion and hypoxia. Placental ischemia stimulates the release of a toxic substance that causes vasospasms and results in hypertension and poor tissue perfusion of all organ systems.
■ Eclampsia, a "severe feature" of PE, is the occurrence of generalized tonic–clonic seizures associated with PE. It affects approximately 1 in 2,500 deliveries in the United States.
■ The usual warning signs of an impending eclampsia are persistent headache, blurred vision, severe epigastric or right upper quadrant abdominal pain, and altered mental status. However, seizures can develop without any warning signs.
■ If eclampsia is left untreated, status epilepticus may develop, which causes repetitive seizures that are more frequent and of longer duration. If the seizures occur while the patient is remote from medical care, maternal and fetal mortality are as high as 50% in severe cases.
- Almost half of the seizures in pregnant women occur before the patient's admission to the labor and delivery department, approximately 30% occur during the intrapartum stage, and the remainder occur postpartum.
- There is a considerable drop in the risk of eclampsia by 48 hours postpartum, with seizures occurring in less than 3% of women beyond this time.
■ The drug of choice for treating eclampsia is IV magnesium sulfate. Secondary treatment with anticonvulsants may be necessary in severe cases.
■ During future pregnancies, women are at higher risk of reoccurrence of PE if delivery is required prior to 28 weeks' gestation. However, emerging evidence exists

that the subsequent cases of PE are not necessarily worse (Dix, 2016; Harper et al., 2019; Jeyabalan, 2020; Moore, 2018; Sibai & Wallace, 2017).

NEONATAL OUTCOMES IN MATERNAL HYPERTENSION

- Severe intrauterine growth restriction (IUGR) is common in the fetus of women who have any form of hypertension in pregnancy secondary to uteroplacental insufficiency. However, the rate and severity do increase if women develop PE superimposed on chronic hypertension.
- Although stillbirth rates associated with PE have declined, neonates born of affected pregnancies maintain a higher risk of neonatal death or morbidities. These risks are inversely related to GA.
- Infants have a higher risk of postnatal complications secondary to frequent hypoxemic insults resulting from uteroplacental insufficiency.
- Neonates born to mothers with PE may also have thrombocytopenia or neutropenia, further complicating the newborn course; however, these conditions usually resolve spontaneously.
- The GA at onset and the severity of maternal symptoms determine the need for intervention. If the infant is less than 28 weeks of age, the effort will be to manage maternal symptoms and allow the infant to mature. If the infant is older than 28 weeks, the course may move to elective delivery after the administration of antenatal cortical steroids (Harper et al., 2019; Jeyabalan, 2020; Moore, 2018).

▶ CARDIAC DISEASE IN PREGNANCY

- The occurrence of cardiac disease in pregnancy includes both congenital and acquired forms of cardiac disease. The number of pregnancies affected by congenital cardiac disease continues to increase as medical advances have resulted in more survivors to adulthood. Understanding the impact of cardiac disease on pregnancy is vital because the maternal cardiovascular system is responsible for meeting the needs of both the mother and the fetus.
- Cardiac adaptations of pregnancy are outlined in Table 3.2.

EFFECT OF CARDIOVASCULAR DISEASE ON PREGNANCY

- The World Health Organization (WHO) has developed a risk classification system for cardiovascular risk that helps define and provide guidelines for treatment of cardiovascular disease in pregnancy. Many congenital heart defects are classified in the system. There are six high-risk cardiac complications: aortic valve stenosis, coarctation of the aorta, Marfan syndrome, peripartum

Table 3.2 Cardiac Adaptations of Pregnancy

Increased	■ Total blood volume ■ Plasma volume ■ Red cell volume ■ Cardiac output ■ Heart rate ■ Uterine blood flow ■ Myocardial contractility
Decreased	■ Diastolic blood pressure ■ Systemic vascular resistance ■ Pulmonary circulation
Unchanged	■ Systolic blood pressure ■ Central venous pressure ■ Pulmonary capillary wedge pressure ■ Ejection fraction ■ Left ventricular stroke work index

Sources: Data from Arafeh, J. (2021). Cardiac disease in pregnancy. In K. Simpson & P. Creehan (Eds.), *Perinatal nursing* (5th ed., p. 335). Lippincott Williams & Wilkins; Blackburn, S. T. (Eds.). (2018). Cardiovascular system. In *Maternal fetal & neonatal physiology: A clinical perspective* (5th ed., p. 253). Elsevier; Blanchard, D., & Daniels, L. (2019). Cardiac disease. In R. Resnik, C. J. Lockwood, T. R. Moore, M. F. Greene, J. A. Copel, & R. M. Silver (Eds.), *Creasy & Resnik's maternal-fetal medicine: Principles and practice* (8th ed.) Elsevier.

cardiomyopathy, severe pulmonary hypertension, and tetralogy of Fallot (TOF). The estimated maternal mortality risk ranges from 5% to 60%.
- A set of cardiovascular disorders fall into the WHO risk classification of II or III, depending on the individual. These defects include any which results in mild left ventricular impairment, hypertrophic cardiomyopathy, Marfan syndrome not associated with aortic root dilation, repaired coarctation of the aorta, and aortic dilation less than 45 mm in individuals with a bicuspid aortic valve (Blanchard & Daniels, 2019).

Acyanotic Congenital Heart Defects
- Atrial septal defect (ASD) is the most common heart defect in pregnancy. The risk category depends on the size of the shunt (a larger defect equals greater risk). There is likely minimal effect on the fetus if there is no maternal pulmonary hypertension.
- The size of the defect dictates the impact of ventricular septal defect (VSD) on pregnancy. Larger defects are associated with an increased risk of congestive heart failure (CHF) and pulmonary hypertension development. If pulmonary hypertension exists, there is a high risk of both maternal and fetal death.
- Pulmonic stenosis leading to a degree of obstruction is more important than the obstruction's location in determining the risk of pregnancy. Moderate pulmonary stenosis usually will not influence the woman or the fetus. Severe pulmonary stenosis will require treatment with a valvuloplasty and typically has minimal effect on the fetus.
- Aortic stenosis may be congenital or acquired. The degree of obstruction is more important than the

location of the obstruction in determining the risk of pregnancy. The presence of a mechanical aortic valve will require continuous anticoagulation (Arafeh, 2021; Blanchard & Daniels, 2019).

Cyanotic Congenital Heart Defects

■ TOF yields minimal maternal risk if the defect has been corrected and there are no subsequent limitations. Pregnancy should be avoided if there is a history of CHF, cardiomegaly, decreased right ventricular pressure, current peripheral hypoxia, or polycythemia. TOF that is uncorrected is associated with a higher rate of maternal morbidity and poor prognosis for infants. Infants born to women with TOF have a 5% to 10% chance of inheriting the defect.

■ Coarctation of the aorta increases maternal risk for PE. The pregnancy will be most affected if it is an uncorrected coarctation. This risk is significantly higher if it is a complicated coarctation.

■ The effects of Marfan syndrome on pregnancy depend on the presence and degree of aortic root involvement, which is determined by the dilation of the aorta. The delivery type depends mainly on the degree of aortic root dilation. Women with no dilation may deliver vaginally; however, women with dilation >4 cm should be delivered via Cesarean section. Increased estrogen lesions in pregnancy put pregnant women at higher risk for aortic dissection (Arafeh, 2021; Blackburn, 2018; Blanchard & Daniels, 2019).

CARDIOMYOPATHIES IN PREGNANCY

■ *Dilated cardiomyopathy* is diffuse dilation of the cardiac muscle that causes a decrease in cardiac output and an increase in cardiac filling pressures, resulting in dyspnea, edema, and fatigue. These patients are at increased risk of pulmonary embolism or stroke. Analysis of serum levels of B-type natriuretic peptide (BNP) may identify those pregnant women with cardiomyopathy at the highest risk for cardiac events. Treatment includes the use of both ACE inhibitors and beta-adrenergic blocking agents to slow the deterioration of left ventricular function.

■ *Peripartum cardiomyopathy* occurs in the last portion of pregnancy or the first months postpartum in patients with no previous cardiac disease. The etiology is unknown but potentially mediated by inflammation, autoimmune processes, endothelial dysfunction, and oxidative stress. There has also been an increased incidence of peripartum cardiomyopathy in pregnant women who are diagnosed with PE. Other identified risk factors include increased maternal age, chronic hypertension, multiple gestation, or multiparity.

  ● The treatment of peripartum cardiomyopathy is like that of other patients with CHF. The vasodilator of choice in pregnancy is hydralazine.

  ● If cardiac dysfunction is severe, anticoagulation may be indicated. Warfarin is not recommended

for anticoagulation in pregnancy. Low-molecular-weight heparin is preferred to unfractionated heparin for anticoagulation.

  ● This cardiomyopathy may reoccur in future pregnancies, even if full recovery is noted as evidenced by a normalized ejection fraction.

■ *Idiopathic hypertrophic cardiomyopathy* is usually inherited in an autosomal dominant fashion; there have been spontaneous mutations identified. Outflow tract obstruction may be increased by physiologic decrease in peripheral vascular resistance in pregnancy, an increase in circulating catecholamines during the labor process, and the use of the Valsalva maneuver in labor.

  ● The goals of treatment include avoiding hypovolemia, maintaining venous return, and avoiding anxiety, excitement, and strenuous activity (Arafeh, 2021; Blackburn, 2018; Blanchard & Daniels, 2019; Kelly, 2018).

▶ PULMONARY DISEASE IN PREGNANCY

■ The cardiorespiratory system must function correctly to achieve proper oxygenation of both maternal and fetal tissues. Pulmonary changes and conditions that may affect maternal oxygenation also affect the fetus (Table 3.3).

PNEUMONIA

■ The most common nonobstetrical infectious cause of morbidity and mortality in the peripartum period is pneumonia. Pneumonia can be associated with poor fetal growth, preterm delivery, and perinatal loss.

■ Pregnant women are at higher risk for bacterial, influenza-associated pneumonia. The two identifiable organisms most commonly causing pneumonia are pneumococcus and *Haemophilus influenzae*. Of the subtypes of influenza, type A is more likely to cause infection.

Table 3.3 Pulmonary Changes in Pregnancy

Increased	■ Minute ventilation ■ Alveolar ventilation ■ Tidal volume ■ Oxygen consumption ■ PaO_2 ■ Arterial pH
Decreased	■ Functional residual capacity ■ Residual volume ■ $PaCO_2$
Unchanged	■ Respiratory rate

$PaCO_2$, partial pressure of carbon dioxide in arterial blood; PaO_2, partial pressure of oxygen in arterial blood.
Source: Data from Whitty, J., & Dombrowski, M. (2019). Respiratory diseases in pregnancy. In R. Resnik, C. Lockwood, T. Moore, M. Greene, J. Copel, & R. Silver (Eds.), *Creasy and Resnik's maternal-fetal medicine: Principles and practice* (8th ed., p. 1043). Elsevier.

- All pregnant women, especially women at high risk for pneumonia, such as those with sickle cell disease, with a splenectomy, or who are immunocompromised, should receive the pneumococcal vaccine to protect them and their fetus. The vaccine helps to confer antibodies on the newborn as well that have detectable levels in cord blood.
- *Viral pneumonia* could be the primary cause or be associated with a secondary bacterial infection. Thus, hospitalized women with viral symptoms should also be treated for the most common organisms that could cause a secondary bacterial infection (Whitty & Dombrowski, 2019).

TUBERCULOSIS

- Pregnancy complicates the multidrug treatment of tuberculosis (TB) because many regimen's drugs are unsafe during pregnancy.
  - Despite concern for treating TB, at-risk women should be screened as it can be vertically and laterally transmitted. Women with a positive purified protein derivative (PPD) can be screened with a chest x-ray after the first trimester.
  - The initial treatment for pregnant women with TB is isoniazid, also known as isonicotinyl hydrazide (INH), and rifampin.
- Neonates born to women taking medications for TB but who have inactive TB need a PPD screen at birth and at 3 months.
- Active TB at the time of delivery is an indication to separate the woman and the child after delivery to prevent transmission to the newborn.
  - Neonates born to women with active TB should receive prophylactic treatment until women have a negative disease screen for 3 months (Whitty & Dombrowski, 2019).

ASTHMA

- Asthma is the most common respiratory complication in pregnancy, and preexisting asthma is worsened by pregnancy.
- Women with preexisting asthma should continue taking control medications and avoiding triggers. They are also at higher risk for PE, premature birth, low birth weight, IUGR, and perinatal mortality. Fetal risks are proportionate to the control of asthma during pregnancy.
- Treatment with any medication during pregnancy is better than hypoxia in the mother. Inhaled corticosteroids are the preferred method of treatment. Oral decongestants used in the first trimester have been associated with gastroschisis development, so inhaled decongestants or inhaled corticosteroids are preferred.

- Labor management should include IV corticosteroids during labor and 24 hours postdelivery if the mother is currently on systemic corticosteroids or has had several short courses of steroids during pregnancy (Whitty & Dombrowski, 2019; Woo et al., 2021).

CYSTIC FIBROSIS

- Increased survival of cystic fibrosis (CF) patients has resulted in more pregnancies affected by CF. Women with CF who have preconception counseling have better maternal and neonatal outcomes.
  - Preconception counseling should include a discussion that pregnancy may shorten the mother's life span and result in a preterm infant. The counseling should also include paternal testing, as all infants will be at least heterozygous carriers for CF.
- Maternal patients with CF are at increased risk of vitamin K deficiency, so prothrombin time should be monitored and women given parenteral vitamin K as indicated (Whitty & Dombrowski, 2019; Woo et al., 2021).

▶ DIABETES MELLITUS IN PREGNANCY

- *Diabetes mellitus* (DM) is defined as a chronic, systemic, endocrine disorder of insulin production or the body's response to insulin. It is characterized by abnormal metabolism of carbohydrates, proteins, fats, and electrolytes, resulting in hyperglycemia and other systemic metabolic disturbances.
  - *Early pregnancy:* There is beta-cell hyperplasia caused by increased insulin production. The relative hyperinsulinism allows for increased fat deposition. The combination of hyperinsulinism and nausea/vomiting associated with early pregnancy increases the risk of hypoglycemia.
  - *Later pregnancy:* During this time, there is accelerated growth and increasing levels of diabetogenic hormones. These hormones include cortisol, estrogen, progesterone, prolactin, and human placental lactogen. Hepatic glucose production also increases during this stage to compensate for periods of maternal fasting (Dysart, 2020; Roth 2021; vanOtterloo, 2016).

CLASSIFICATION OF DIABETES

- Classified according to cause rather than treatment, DM complicates more than 200,000 pregnancies per year in the United States. There are now more women in pregnancy affected by type 2 than type 1 (Dysart, 2020; Roth, 2021; vanOtterloo, 2016).

Type 1 Diabetes

- Type 1 DM (formerly insulin-dependent diabetes mellitus [IDDM]) is a result of absolute insulin deficiency from autoimmune action directed at the pancreas. It usually appears before the age of 30 years.

● Exogenous insulin needs in the first half of pregnancy may decrease, and the risk of hypoglycemic incidents increases, compared with later in pregnancy when the insulin requirement may be as many as two to three times higher than prepregnancy requirements.

● The risk of stillbirth has been demonstrated to be higher in type 1 diabetic women compared with type 2 diabetic women; however, both are significantly higher than in nondiabetic women.

❏ Preexisting diabetes that is poorly controlled can result in a threefold increase in congenital malformations compared with women who do not have diabetes prior to pregnancy.

❏ A prepregnancy hemoglobin A1c (HbA1c) level of greater than 10% puts the embryo at the highest risk. The risk may be compounded if the woman has associated medical conditions that also require medications (Brown & Chang, 2018; Dysart, 2020; Moore et al., 2019; Roth, 2021; vanOtterloo, 2016).

Type 2 Diabetes

■ Type 2 DM (formerly noninsulin-dependent diabetes mellitus [NIDDM]) is caused by a combination of resistance to insulin action and an inadequate compensatory insulin secretory response.

■ It is diagnosed primarily in adults older than 30 years of age but is now seen more frequently in children. It occurs more frequently in women with prior gestational diabetes mellitus (GDM) and individuals with hypertension or dyslipidemia.

■ The disease can be managed with diet and exercise, but almost all need insulin for optimum control during pregnancy (Brown & Chang, 2018; Moore et al., 2019; Roth, 2021; vanOtterloo, 2016).

GESTATIONAL DIABETES MELLITUS

■ *Gestational diabetes mellitus* (*GDM*) is defined as any degree of carbohydrate intolerance with onset or first recognition during pregnancy. GDM accounts for approximately 90% of all diabetes in pregnancy.

■ GD is further categorized into A1 (controlled with diet and exercise) and A2 (controlled with diet and exercise and requires the addition of oral meds and/or insulin).

■ Diagnosis of GDM is based on the results of an oral glucose tolerance test (OGTT). The OGTT is performed in the morning after an overnight fast. A definitive diagnosis is made when any plasma glucose value exceeds 180 mg/dL at 1 hour or greater than 140 mg/dL at 3 hours after the test.

■ Women with GD are at increased risk of GH, PE, and Cesarean delivery, as well as developing diabetes (type 2) later in life. Screening should occur 6 to 12 weeks postpartum (Dysart, 2020; Moore et al., 2019; vanOtterloo, 2016).

■ Table 3.4 outlines the complications of diabetes in pregnancy.
■ Table 3.5 lists the types of fetal congenital anomalies associated with diabetes.

Table 3.4 Complications of Diabetes in Pregnancy

Maternal Complications of Hyperglycemia	Infant Complications of Hyperglycemia
■ Polyhydramnios ■ Hypertension ■ Urinary tract infections ■ Pyelonephritis ■ Monilial vaginitis ■ Retinopathy ■ Nephropathy ■ Increased risk of gestational hypertension, preeclampsia, and vascular disease	■ Increased incidence of respiratory distress syndrome due to inhibiting the release of surfactant ■ Excessive fetal growth and subsequent LGA status ■ Congenital malformations ■ Spontaneous abortion ■ Neonatal metabolic disorders (hypoglycemia, hypocalcemia, hypomagnesemia) ■ Prematurity ■ Hypertrophic and congestive cardiomyopathy ■ Polycythemia ■ Hyperbilirubinemia ■ Birth injury

LGA, large for gestational age.
Sources: Data from Roth, C. K. (2021). Diabetes in pregnancy. In K. Simpson, P. Creehan, N. O'Brien-Abel, C. K. Roth, & A. J. Rohan (Eds.), *Perinatal nursing* (5th ed., p. 207). Lippincott Williams & Wilkins; Woo, C., & Ambia, A. (2021). Prenatal environment: Effect on neonatal outcome. In S. Gardner, B. Carter, M. Enzman-Hines, & S. Niermeyer (Eds.), *Handbook of neonatal intensive care* (9th ed., pp. 18–19). Elsevier; Brown, Z., & Chang, J. (2018). Maternal diabetes. In C. Gleason & S. Juul (Eds.), *Avery's diseases of the newborn* (10th ed., p. 102). Elsevier; Moore, T., Hauguel-De Mouzon, S., & Catalano, P. (2019). Diabetes in pregnancy. In R. Resnik, C. Lockwood, T. Moore, M. Greene, J. Copel, & R. Silver (Eds.), *Creasy and Resnik's maternal-fetal medicine: Principles and practice* (8th ed., pp. 1073–1083). Elsevier.

MEDICAL MANAGEMENT

■ The primary goals of treatment of diabetes in pregnancy are to achieve and maintain normal maternal glucose levels and to promptly identify and manage complications associated with diabetes.

■ Diet and nutrition counseling are always considered the first line of treatment.

■ Insulin has been studied extensively in pregnancy and is known to be safe as it does not cross the placental barrier.

■ Oral medications have become increasingly popular as more studies have been published demonstrating safety. Metformin and glyburide are the most commonly used oral agents. Infants of women treated with glyburide should have frequent monitoring for hyperbilirubinemia.

■ Delivery depends on glycemic control and results of fetal surveillance. It is no longer recommended to deliver automatically before 40 weeks (Blickstein et al., 2020; Brown & Chang, 2018; Roth, 2021; vanOtterloo, 2016; Woo et al., 2021).

Table 3.5 Types of Fetal Congenital Anomalies Associated With Diabetes

Organ System	Anomalies
Central nervous system	■ Spina bifida ■ Anencephaly ■ Hydrocephalus ■ Caudal regression syndrome ■ Holoprosencephaly
Cardiovascular system; these defects account for 40%–50% of congenital anomalies associated with diabetes	■ Ventral septal defect ■ Tetralogy of Fallot ■ Transposition of the great arteries ■ Hypoplastic left heart syndrome ■ Coarctation of the aorta ■ Atrial septal defect ■ Pulmonic stenosis ■ Double outlet right ventricle ■ Truncus arteriosus
Genitourinary tract	■ Hydronephrosis ■ Renal agenesis ■ Ureteral duplication ■ Hypospadias ■ Megaurethra ■ Urogenital malformation sequence
Gastrointestinal tract	■ Intestinal atresias ■ Anal atresia ■ Small left colon syndrome ■ Esophageal atresia ■ Situs anomalies ■ Intestinal malrotation
Skeletal	■ Polydactyly ■ Syndactyly ■ Focal femoral hypoplasia ■ Rib defects ■ Abnormal vertebral segmentation ■ Sacral defects ■ Limb deficiency

Sources: Data from Brown, Z., & Chang, J. (2018). Maternal diabetes. In C. Gleason & S. Juul (Eds.), *Avery's diseases of the newborn* (10th ed., p. 93). Elsevier; Blickstein, I., Perlman, S., Hazan, Y., & Shinwell, E. (2020). Pregnancy complicated by diabetes mellitus. In R. I. Martin, & M. C. Walsh (Eds), *Fanaroff & Martin's neonatal perinatal medicine: Diseases of the fetus and infant* (11th ed., p. 307). Elsevier.

▶ COMMON INFECTIOUS DISEASES IN PREGNANCY

BACTERIAL INFECTIONS

Bacterial Vaginosis

■ The primary symptom of bacterial vaginosis (BV) is a malodorous, thin, gray discharge.

■ Diagnosis is based on having three of the following four symptoms: amine-like or fishy odor after intercourse or administration of a potassium hydroxide (KOH) prep, a thin homogenous gray discharge, noted elevated pH of secretions, and/or presence of clue cells on wet mount.

■ BV is consistently associated with preterm delivery, clinical chorioamnionitis, and endometritis (Duff, 2019).

Gonorrhea

■ Gonorrhea is the oldest known sexually transmitted infection (STI) and is caused by *Neisseria gonorrhoeae*. It may cause disseminated gonococcal infection, preterm premature rupture of membranes, chorioamnionitis, preterm delivery, and fetal/neonatal septicemia.

■ Gonococcal ophthalmia neonatorum usually onsets within 4 days after birth; incubation can be up to 21 days. If the condition is untreated, it can cause corneal ulceration, scarring, and blindness.

■ Gonorrhea is often asymptomatic, and it is estimated that less than half of all cases are detected.

■ All infections should be treated. It is also important for sexual partners to be treated (Duff, 2019; Mooney, 2016).

Chlamydia

■ This is the most common bacterial sexually transmitted disease (STD) infection in the United States and is caused by *Chlamydia trachomatis*.

■ Infection during pregnancy is associated with premature prolonged rupture of membranes, low birth weight, and preterm delivery.

■ *Neonatal conjunctivitis:* 50% of exposed infants develop it in the first 2 weeks of life.

■ *Neonatal pneumonia:* Up to 20% develop pneumonia within 4 months of birth (Duff, 2019; Mooney, 2016).

Syphilis

■ Syphilis is caused by *Treponema pallidum* and is efficiently transmitted sexually and frequently transmitted with only a single encounter.

■ Diagnosis can be made either on microscopic examination or with serologic testing.
  ● There are nonspecific serologic tests, such as the venereal disease research laboratory (VDRL) and rapid plasma reagin (RPR) test, which typically become nonreactive once treatment is completed.
  ● Treponema-specific tests remain positive despite treatment (Duff, 2019).

Urinary Tract Infections

■ Urinary tract infection (UTI) complicates one in five pregnancies and as such is the most common medical complication.

■ UTI is associated with risks to both the fetus and the mother, including pyelonephritis, preterm labor and birth, low birth weight, and increased perinatal mortality.

ASYMPTOMATIC BACTERIURIA

- Multiple meta-analyses confirm the link between asymptomatic bacteriuria (ASB), preterm delivery, and low birth weight infants.
- Diagnosis is by culture of the urine, yielding the presence of 100,000 or more colonies of bacteria per milliliter of urine.
- The bacteria responsible are typically normal flora from the gastrointestinal tract (GIT) and vaginal and periurethral areas. The most common bacteria involved include the following:
  - *Escherichia coli:* resistance present in 30% of strains in the United States
  - *Klebsiella*
  - *Proteus*
  - *Staphylococcus saprophyticus*
  - Group B *Streptococcus* (GBS)
  - *Enterobacter* species
- Short courses of antibiotics are the preferred treatment in pregnancy to minimize the risk to the fetus, increase patient compliance, and minimize the emergence of resistant bacteria and the associated costs.
- Because many cases of UTI predate pregnancy, there is no identified prevention strategy; however, frequent monitoring in identified women with ASB is recommended (Duff, 2019; Mooney, 2016).

VIRAL INFECTIONS

Human Papillomavirus Infection

- Human papillomavirus (HPV) infection is a DNA virus with more than 100 different types and is the most common STI in the United States.
- Neonatal implications include respiratory papillomatosis.
- Treatment is limited to women with multiple lesions near the vaginal introitus (Duff, 2019).

Cytomegalovirus

- Cytomegalovirus (CMV) is a member of the herpes virus family. It is the most common congenital viral infection and may remain dormant in the host for many years. Typical incubation period is 28 to 60 days.
- A woman's first-time or primary exposure in pregnancy is associated with the highest transmission risk and more serious complications for the fetus. In addition, the presence of congenital CMV infection in neonates of previously exposed women may represent reinfection with a different strain of the CMV virus.
  - The risk of congenital infection is highest if the pregnant patient is infected in the third trimester. Conversely, the risk of congenital infection is lowest when the pregnant woman has a recurrent infection.
  - The damage to the fetus in congenital CMV infection may represent infection of the placenta and its sequelae, as opposed to actual infection of the fetus.
- Diagnosis is made by viral culture or polymerase chain reaction (PCR). PCR is the process used in the laboratory to make copies of DNA segments. The highest concentration of the virus is in the plasma, urine, seminal fluid, saliva, and breast milk. Serial monitoring of immunoglobulin titers can distinguish between acute and recurrent infections.
- Testing of the neonate is vital to determine when the infant was exposed. Positive test results before 3 weeks of age represent an in utero infection, while positive test results after 3 weeks of age can represent infection from the birth canal or via the breast milk.
- Maternal treatment may be indicated in primary or recurrent infections and can decrease the incidence of symptomatic infants.
  - Maternal treatments include the use of IV hyperimmune globulin specific for CMV or high-dose valacyclovir.
- CMV prevention includes using safe sex practices, good handwashing when encountering children's diapers or toys, and avoidance of CMV-positive blood products (Duff, 2019; Schleiss & Marsh, 2018).

Herpes Simplex Virus

- Herpes simplex virus (HSV) 1 and HSV 2 can equally cause infection in the oral cavity, skin, and anogenital areas. Diagnosis of primary presentation is evidenced by visible painful vesicles and ulcers. Decreased transmission to an infant is achieved by primary Cesarean section if there are active genital lesions.
- Primary infection late in pregnancy places the fetus at the highest risk of transmission. The risk of neonatal transmission is lower in women experiencing recurrent infections.
- Recurrent presentations have a shorter duration and typically less systemic symptoms.
- The gold standard for testing continues to be viral culture; however, PCR testing is quicker and more sensitive than cultures.
- Acyclovir is the treatment of choice for outbreaks, as well as suppressive therapy (Baley & Gonzalez, 2020; Duff, 2019; Schleiss & Marsh, 2018).

PROTOZOAL INFECTIONS

Trichomoniasis

- Trichomoniasis is a common cause of vaginitis with intense itching, strong odor, and discharge. However, many women will have minimal to no symptoms. The incidence of trichomoniasis may be as high as 50% of pregnancies, depending on the population.
- Cultures are more sensitive than wet prep for diagnostic purposes.

- Premature rupture of membranes occurs more frequently in culture-positive pregnancies.
- The gold standard for treatment is a single dose of metronidazole.
- Routine screening is not recommended in the absence of symptoms (Duff, 2019).

Toxoplasmosis

- Toxoplasmosis is a protozoan dependent on cats and is excreted in the cat's feces.
- Most human infections are asymptomatic unless an immunocompromised human is involved.
  - Congenital infection is most likely to occur when the maternal infection occurs in the third trimester.
- Testing is done by PCR and detection of the antibody to toxoplasmosis.
- Treatment consists of oral sulfadiazine and treatment duration may be as long as 6 weeks.
- As a preventive measure, pregnant women should avoid contact with cat litter. If contact is necessary, litter should be changed daily and gloves always worn (Duff, 2019).

FUNGAL INFECTIONS

Candidiasis

- Vulvovaginal candidiasis is most commonly caused by *Candida albicans*. Increased colonization can occur during pregnancy, in women with diabetes, or in those who have recently taken antibiotics or steroids.
- Diagnosis is made by KOH wet prep/Gram stain or culture of vaginal secretions. If a woman has recurrent infections, the species of *Candida* can be genetically subtyped.
- Congenital infection can manifest within the first 24 hours as superficial skin infections, oral infections, or systemic disease involving multiple organs (Duff, 2019).

▶ COMMON HEMATOLOGIC DISEASES

COAGULATION DISORDERS

Antiphospholipid Syndrome

- Antiphospholipid syndrome (APS) is the most common acquired thrombophilic disorder. Antibodies that promote thrombosis are produced. Women with APS are at increased risk of arterial and venous thrombosis, autoimmune thrombocytopenia, miscarriage, and fetal loss.
- This disorder may be isolated or associated with other autoimmune diseases. The presence of antiphospholipid antibodies (aPL) is found in about 1% to 5% of healthy females. However, these antibodies are found in 15% of females who have recurrent abortions and in 30% to 40% of those with systemic lupus erythematosus (SLE).
- The diagnosis of APS must include clinical criteria (vascular thrombosis, unexplained death of a morphologically normal fetus >10 weeks' gestation, premature birth <34 weeks due to PE or placental insufficiency, or ≥3 otherwise unexplained abortions <10 weeks) as well as the presence of aPL (lupus anticoagulant, anticardiolipin antibody, or anti-beta-2-glycoprotein antibody) on greater than two occasions, at least 12 weeks apart.
- Treatment during pregnancy is with unfractionated or low-molecular-weight heparin with or without low-dose aspirin.
- Of patients with APS who reach viability in pregnancy, 50% develop PE and one-third of pregnancies have IUGR. In addition, abnormal fetal heart rate tracings resulting from Cesarean delivery are common (Blackburn, 2018; Kelly, 2018; Rodger & Silver, 2019).

Inherited Thrombophilias

- Inherited thrombophilias are associated with venous thromboembolism (VTE). VTE includes both deep vein thrombosis (DVT) and pulmonary emboli.
  - The risk of VTE increases up to sixfold in pregnancy. Greater than 80% of DVTs occur on the left because of the right iliac and ovarian veins' compression of the left iliac vein. Three-fourths of DVTs occur during the antepartum period and one-fourth postpartum. Most pulmonary emboli occur postpartum and are associated with Cesarean section.
  - Unfractionated or low-molecular-weight heparin is considered the drug of choice for thromboembolic disorders during pregnancy because the molecular weight of both prevents placental transfer.
    - Coumarin derivatives inhibit vitamin K-dependent coagulation factors due to their ability to cross the placenta, whereas vitamin K-dependent coagulation factors do not. This may impair fetal coagulation and increase the risk of fetal and neonatal hemorrhage.
    - Warfarin, when given during the first 11 to 13 weeks of pregnancy, has been associated with a syndrome involving the face, eyes, bones, and central nervous system (CNS). Warfarin has also been associated with an increased risk of abortion (Blackburn, 2018; Rodger & Silver, 2019).
    - *Factor V Leiden* (FVL) is the most common of the serious inheritable thrombophilias and is the leading cause of activated protein C resistance. It is associated with approximately 40% of VTE events in pregnant women. FVL thrombophilia is associated with early and late pregnancy loss (Rodger & Silver, 2019).

- Antithrombin (AT) gene mutations have been identified. AT deficiency is the least common of the heritable thrombophilias, but can also be acquired secondary to liver impairment, sepsis, disseminated intravascular coagulation, or due to severe nephrotic syndrome.
- Both inherited and acquired AT deficiencies are associated with VTE. AT deficiency is associated with an increased risk of stillbirth after 28 weeks' gestation, fetal growth restriction, abruption, and preterm delivery (Rodger & Silver, 2019).

Acquired Platelet Disorders

- *Primary immune thrombocytopenia* is also known as idiopathic thrombocytopenic purpura (ITP) or autoimmune thrombocytopenia purpura, defined as a platelet count of less than 100,000 cells/dL. Immunoglobulin G (IgG) antibody binds to the platelets and makes them more susceptible to destruction.
- Maternal treatment aims to achieve a platelet count greater than 30,000 during pregnancy and greater than 50,000 at the end of pregnancy. Treatment includes glucocorticoid drugs, IV immune globulin, rhesus immune globulin, platelet transfusion, and splenectomy.
- By definition, ITP is immune-mediated, and the responsible antibody may cross the placenta. The fetus is at risk of thrombocytopenia due to maternal antiplatelet IgG crossing the placenta. This can lead to purpura, ecchymosis, hematuria, and melena, and in rare cases intracranial hemorrhage resulting in severe neurologic impairment or death. There is no clear evidence that Cesarean delivery prevents neonatal intracranial hemorrhage.
- Delivery should be attended by a neonatologist or a pediatrician who can treat possible hemorrhagic complications. Platelets, fresh frozen plasma, and IV immunoglobulin should be readily available (Kelly, 2018; Rodger & Silver, 2019).

Anemia

- The most common anemias in pregnancy are iron deficiency anemia, megaloblastic anemia of pregnancy (folic acid deficiency), and alpha- and beta-thalassemia.
- In early pregnancy, maternal anemia (hemoglobin <8.5 g/dL) is related to preterm birth but not small-for-gestational-age infants. In women with severe anemia (hemoglobin <6–8 mg/dL), maternal arterial oxygen content and oxygen delivery to the fetus are decreased.
  - Elevated hemoglobin (>14.5 g/dL) in early pregnancy is associated with stillbirth and small-for-gestational-age infants (Blackburn, 2018).
- Fetal effects from maternal anemia include the following:

- Increased placental blood flow but a decrease in diffusing distance for oxygen across the placenta
- Redistribution of blood within the fetal organs
- Increased red blood cell (RBC) production (to increase the total oxygen-carrying capacity)
- Decreased growth
- Increased mortality due to an inadequate supply of oxygen and/or nutrients (Blackburn, 2018)

Iron Deficiency Anemia

- Iron deficiency is the most common cause of anemia during pregnancy and is generally preventable or easily treated with iron supplements. When a pregnant woman experiences severe iron deficiency and anemia, the fetus may have decreased RBC volume, hemoglobin, iron stores, and cord ferritin levels. This may carry over to cause a worsening iron deficiency during infancy.
  - Iron deficiency anemia before midpregnancy is associated with an increased risk of low birth weight, preterm birth, and perinatal mortality.
- Folic acid deficiency is the most common cause of megaloblastic anemia in pregnant women. Vitamin B_{12} deficiency is less common in pregnancy. Severe folic acid deficiency has been associated with fetal malformations, including an increased risk of neural tube defects and cleft lip and palate, as well as premature birth and low birth weight infants.
  - Supplementation with folic acid is recommended for women of childbearing age to reduce the risk of neural tube defects. Supplementation should occur before pregnancy because neural tube defects occur early in the first trimester (Blackburn, 2018).

Sickle Cell Disease

- A woman with sickle cell anemia typically has lower hemoglobin levels and oxygen-carrying capacities. As a result, they may become slightly more anemic as plasma volume increases during the pregnancy and may experience an increased risk of sickling attacks.
- Sickled cells can obstruct blood flow in the microvasculature. The areas most susceptible to obstruction are those characterized by slow flow and high oxygen extraction, such as the spleen, bone marrow, and placenta. Obstruction leads to venous stasis, further deoxygenation, platelet aggregation, hypoxia, acidosis, further sickling, and eventually infarction.
- Fetal and neonatal complications secondary to placental infarction and fetal hypoxia include prematurity and fetal growth restriction. Fetal hypoxia results from decreased oxygen transport due to abnormal biochemistry of the maternal hemoglobin and loss of placental tissue for gas and nutrient exchange caused by infarctions (Blackburn, 2018).

▶ FETAL ASSESSMENT

- The goals of fetal assessment are to identify fetuses that are adequately oxygenated or at risk for hypoxia, reduce perinatal morbidity and mortality, and decrease stillbirth and long-term neurologic injury.
- Methods of antenatal testing are either for screening or diagnosis.
  - Antenatal screening methods are tests used for antepartum fetal assessment that will lead to further testing allowing for diagnosis and decision-making. They are not definite, are reported as the ratio of the likelihood the fetus will be abnormal, and include measurements of maternal serum analytes, US evaluations, or both. Screening methods evaluate for risk of structural abnormalities (open neural tube defects or ventral wall defects), fetal aneuploidy (trisomy 21, 13, and 18), and placental abnormalities.
  - In a best-case scenario, the diagnostic testing will determine if the fetus is affected or not. However, no test is 100% effective or correct. Some fetal anomalies can be diagnosed with US. Fetal tissue samples may be required for diagnosis of fetal karyotype abnormalities. Chorionic villous sampling and amniocentesis are used to obtain fetal samples, each with its own limitations and risks.
- Most fetal testing protocols involve a stepwise approach, and the first step is the selection of the appropriate patient. Assessments for low-risk pregnancies include one US examination for dating and one for the basic anatomic survey. High-risk pregnancies are those at greater peril for perinatal morbidity and mortality. These pregnancies often have more justification for targeted or detailed anatomic US examinations and for regular assessment of fetal growth or heart rate assessment (Cypher, 2016; Hackney, 2020; Pettker & Campbell, 2018).

FETAL FIBRONECTIN

- Fetal fibronectin (fFN) is a protein secreted by the trophoblast and is thought to play a role in the placental–uterine attachment. fFN is normally present in the vaginal or cervical fluid prior to 20 weeks. After 20 weeks, fFN may be an indication of imminent labor; therefore, the fFN is used to evaluate women with premature contractions when diagnosis or premature labor is uncertain.
  - A negative fFN test with other reassuring signs, such as no sign of infection, abruption, or progressive cervical change, can be used to avoid more invasive interventions, such as admission, tocolysis, or glucocorticoid administration (Adams, 2021).

NONSTRESS TEST

- The nonstress test (NST) is one of the most common antepartum screens performed after 32 weeks' GA. Fetal heart rate is monitored, as well as uterine activity. Results are given as reactive, nonreactive, or inadequate.
  - A *reactive NST* is a heart rate of between 110 and 160 beats per minute (bpm), normal beat-to-beat variability (5 bpm), and two accelerations of at least 15 bpm lasting at least 15 seconds within 20 minutes.
    - Modifications are made in reference to GA. NSTs for fetuses at less than 32 weeks' gestation are often considered reactive if the acceleration is 10 bpm or more above the baseline and lasts for at least 10 seconds.
  - A *nonreactive NST* is defined as less than two accelerations within a 20-minute time frame within 40 minutes. A nonreactive test is typically repeated later on the same day, or another test of fetal well-being is performed, such as a US, contractions stress test, or BPP.
- The NST is commonly performed weekly, although twice-weekly testing is recommended for high-risk conditions. It is important to note that some abnormal states, such as a fetal CNS abnormality or maternal drug ingestion, may contribute to a nonreactive NST. In these cases, a US examination may provide appropriate information to determine the diagnosis or the required management (Adams, 2021; Berghella & Giraldo-Isaza, 2020; Cypher, 2016; Dukhivny & Wilkins-Haug, 2017; Hackney, 2020; Pettker & Campbell, 2018).

BIOPHYSICAL PROFILE

- The BPP provides an indication of fetal well-being when there is risk for altered oxygenation. The BPP refers to a sonographic scoring system performed over a 30- to 40-minute period designed to assess fetal well-being. The BPP was initially described for testing postterm fetuses but has since been validated for use in both term and preterm fetuses. Notably, the BPP is not validated for use in active labor.
- The individual variables of the BPP become apparent in healthy fetuses in a predictable sequence: fetal tone appears at 7.5 to 8.5 weeks, fetal movement at 9 weeks, fetal breathing at 20 to 22 weeks, and fetal heart rate (FHR) reactivity at 24 to 28 weeks' gestation. Similarly, in the setting of antepartum hypoxia, these characteristics typically disappear in the reverse order in which they appeared (i.e., FHR reactivity is lost first, followed by fetal breathing and fetal movements, and finally fetal tone).
- The BPP combines an NST with amniotic fluid volume (vertical fluid pocket >2 cm), fetal breathing movements, fetal activity, and normal fetal

musculoskeletal tone. Although each of the five features of the BPP is scored equally (2 points if the variable is present or normal and 0 points if absent or abnormal, for a total of 10 points), they are not equally predictive of adverse pregnancy outcomes. For example, amniotic fluid volume is the variable that correlates most strongly with adverse pregnancy events.

- Reassuring tests, with a score of 8 to 10, are repeated weekly.
- Less reassuring results, with a score of 5 to 6, are repeated on the same day.
- Very low scores of 0 to 4 may indicate the need for delivery of the fetus.

■ The likelihood that a fetus will die in utero within 1 week of a reassuring BPP is approximately 0.6 to 0.7 per 1,000. The negative predictive value for a stillbirth within 1 week of a reassuring BPP is >99.9% (Adams, 2021; Berghella & Giraldo-Isaza, 2020; Cypher, 2016; Dukhivny & Wilkins-Haug, 2017; Hackney, 2020; Pettker & Campbell, 2018).

ULTRASOUND

■ US can be used for dating confirmation, early detection of anomalies, and assessment of fetal well-being, as well as a screening tool for detection of aneuploidy in the second trimester. When combined with first-trimester screening for aneuploidy, the use of US has been shown to be valuable in decreasing the risk assessment for trisomy 21.

■ Compared with standard two-dimensional (2D) US, three-dimensional (3D) US allows for the visualization of fetal structures in all three dimensions concurrently for improved characterization of complex fetal structural anomalies. Unlike 2D US, 3D images are greatly influenced by fetal movements and are subject to more interference from structures such as fetal limbs, umbilical cord, and placental tissue. Due to movement interference, visualization of the fetal heart with 3D US is suboptimal.

■ The primary utility of Doppler flow velocimetry is the evaluation of a fetus with possible IUGR. The use of Doppler sonography has not been found to benefit low-risk pregnancies.

■ Doppler flow studies assess maternal–fetal blood flow in the umbilical artery, middle cerebral artery, umbilical vein, and ductus venosus, and provide information regarding fetal adaptation and reserve. Changes in blood flow represent systolic and diastolic shifts during the cardiac cycle. Due to placental capacitance, the umbilical artery is one of the few arteries that normally have forward diastolic flow and is one of the most frequently targeted vessels during pregnancy.

■ Doppler velocimetry of umbilical artery blood flow provides an indirect measure of placental function and fetal status.

- Absent end-diastolic flow (AEDF) indicates elevated placental resistance leading to no blood flow in diastole.
- Reversed diastolic flow (REDF) indicates an AEDF that has continued for a prolonged period and is more indicative of a poor outcome, which includes fetal or neonatal death.
- Severely abnormal umbilical artery Doppler velocimetry (defined as absent or reversed diastolic flow) is an especially ominous observation and is associated with poor perinatal outcome.
- Findings of absent or reversed end-diastolic flow indicate a need to prepare for delivery (Adams, 2021; Berghella & Giraldo-Isaza, 2020; Cypher, 2016; Dukhivny & Wilkins-Haug, 2017; Hackney, 2020; Pettker & Campbell, 2018).

AMNIOTIC FLUID/AMNIOCENTESIS

■ Amniotic fluid serves several important functions for the developing embryo and fetus. It provides cushioning against physical trauma; creates an environment free of restriction and/or distortion, allowing for normal growth and development of the fetus; provides a thermally stable environment; allows the respiratory, gastrointestinal, and musculoskeletal tracts to develop normally; and helps prevent infection.

■ Amniotic fluid removed under US guidance can be analyzed for prenatal diagnosis of karyotypic abnormalities, genetic disorders (for which testing is available), fetal blood type and hemoglobinopathies, and fetal lung maturity; for monitoring of the degree of isoimmunization by measurement of the content of bilirubin in the fluid; and for diagnosis of chorioamnionitis.

- Subjective estimates of the amniotic fluid volume have been validated, but two US measurements, amniotic fluid index (AFI) and maximum vertical pocket (MVP), have been developed to quickly and accurately assess the quantity of amniotic fluid surrounding the fetus.

  ❏ The AFI is a semiquantitative method for assessing the amniotic fluid volume with US. The gravid uterus is divided into four quadrants using the umbilicus, linea nigra, and external landmarks. The deepest amniotic fluid pocket is measured in each quadrant with the US transducer perpendicular to the floor. The four measurements are added together and the sum is regarded as the AFI.

  ❏ The usual range of the AFI most commonly used in clinical practice is greater than 5 to less than 24 cm of fluid. Pregnancies with an AFI of greater than 5 are described as having oligohydramnios, and pregnancies with measurements greater than 24 cm are described as having polyhydramnios.

- Amniocentesis is performed under US guidance and can be performed as early as 10 to 14 weeks gestation. It is typically performed in the second trimester at 15 to 20 weeks.
- Amniotic fluid can be analyzed for alpha-fetoprotein (AFP), acetylcholinesterase (AChE), bilirubin, and pulmonary surfactant. Increased AFP in combination with AChE in the amniotic fluid has a sensitivity of >98% for identification of neural tube defects.
- Fetal cells can be analyzed for chromosomes and genetic makeup. Fluorescence in situ hybridization (FISH) can detect second-trimester karyotype abnormalities of chromosomes 13, 18, 21, X, or Y with approximately 90% sensitivity (Adams, 2021; Berghella & Giraldo-Isaza, 2020; Cypher, 2016; Dukhivny & Wilkins-Haug, 2017; Pettker & Campbell, 2018).

Alpha-Fetoprotein/Triple or Quad Screens

- The quadruple screen (or quad screen) involves analyzing the levels of four maternal circulating factors: maternal serum alpha-fetoprotein (MSAFP), total human chorionic gonadotropin (hCG), unconjugated estriol, and inhibin A between 15 and 22 6/7 weeks' gestation.
  - The triple screen includes MSAFP, hCG, and unconjugated estriol.
  - The penta screen analyzes the hyperglycosylated hCG plus the four quad screen markers and is an alternative for second-trimester screening.
- AFP is a fetal-specific molecule synthesized by the fetal yolk sac, fetal GIT, and fetal liver. The MSAFP is usually significantly lower than the AFP in the fetal plasma or the amniotic fluid.
- MSAFP testing should be offered to all women. MSAFP levels above 2.5 multiples of the median for GA are considered abnormal. Elevated MSAFP occurs in 70% to 85% of fetuses with open spina bifida and 95% of fetuses with anencephaly.
- Clinicians may repeat MASFP testing after the first moderately elevated result. On repeat analysis, one third are below the threshold. A repeat test that is below the threshold after an elevated test has not been associated with an increase in false negative results.
  - In the face of a repeat elevated MSAFP, the next step is a US. In half of patients with elevated levels, ultrasonic examination reveals another cause. This is most commonly an error in the estimate of GA. US that incorporates changes in head shape (lemon sign) or cerebellar deformity (banana sign) increases the sensitivity of US for visual detection of open spinal defects.
- The option of amniocentesis should also be discussed with the patient when an elevated MSAFP is noted.
- In the second trimester, an elevated MSAFP that cannot be explained by a fetal structural abnormality or underlying maternal conditions is associated with poor fetal outcomes, which include increased risk of intrauterine fetal demise (IUFD), placental abruption, and PE (Berghella & Giraldo-Isaza, 2020; Cypher, 2016; Dukhivny & Wilkins-Haug, 2017; Gross & Gheorghe, 2020; Stark, 2017).

▶ FETAL PROCEDURES

- The potential impact of fetal surgery on the mother presents difficult ethical decisions. By undergoing general anesthesia, surgical operation, postoperative recovery, and the remainder of the pregnancy, the mother is subject to a significant risk but can expect no direct health benefit from fetal surgical intervention.
  - Specifically, short-term morbidity after fetal surgery includes preterm labor, the potential risk of anesthesia, the potential need for blood transfusion, premature rupture of membranes, chorioamniotic separation, chorioamnionitis, and placental abruption.
  - Long-term morbidity related to the hysterotomy used in open fetal cases includes infertility, uterine rupture during future pregnancies, and mandatory Cesarean section with future pregnancies.
- Access to the fetus can be considered in three general categories: percutaneous, fetoscopic, and open hysterotomy.
  - Percutaneous procedures are performed through small skin incisions on the mother's abdominal wall, utilizing real-time US to visualize the fetal and maternal anatomy and guide the intervention. Cystic masses, ascites, pleural fluid, or other fluid collections can be aspirated as a diagnostic or therapeutic maneuver. Shunts can be inserted for more definitive drainage of fluid into the amniotic space.
  - Fetoscopic procedures are performed using a 1.2- to 3.0-mm fetoscope with or without a working channel, inserted through a 2.3- to 4.0-mm cannula placed into the uterus. Fetoscopy permits direct visualization of the lesion at the time of intervention, but is still facilitated by the use of fetal US. The growing availability of videoendoscopes has paved the way for the concept of endoscopic fetal surgery.
  - Open fetal procedures are usually performed through a low, transverse maternal skin incision. The fascia can be opened in a vertical or transverse fashion, depending on the exposure needed. Typically, fetal exposure is limited to the site specific to the intervention to avoid hypothermia and unnecessary manipulation of the umbilical cord, which is prone to spasms that can result in fatal fetal ischemia. At the conclusion of the procedure, the amniotic fluid is completely restored and the uterus is closed in multiple layers using absorbable sutures.

▶ ANOMALIES AMENABLE TO FETAL SURGERY

■ Congenital diaphragmatic hernia (CDH) is a defect in the fetal diaphragm that allows herniation of abdominal contents into the thoracic cavity. The exact etiology of the condition is unknown. CDH does not refer to a single clinical entity, and outcomes vary accordingly. Generally, this leads to abnormal development of the lung parenchyma and pulmonary vasculature. Prenatal diagnosis and poor prognosis have made CDH a primary target for effective fetal intervention.

  ● Open fetal surgery was investigated in human fetuses diagnosed with CDH. The first successful case was reported by investigators in 1990. In utero tracheal occlusion was first applied in humans in 1996 with placement of a metallic tracheal clip via maternal laparotomy and open hysterotomy.

  ● Survival has been shown to be dependent on the observed–expected lung-to-head ratio (O/E LHR) measured before the procedure. Despite initially disappointing results, investigators remain optimistic that tracheal occlusion could improve the outcomes for high-risk CDH lesions. International, prospective, randomized trials comparing fetal endoscopic tracheal occlusion (FETO) to expectant management in both moderate and severe lung hypoplasia secondary to CDH are ongoing.

■ Congenital pulmonary airway malformations (CPAMs) are benign cystic pulmonary lesions diagnosed in utero on screening US. Unfortunately, 5% to 30% of prenatally diagnosed CPAMs produce a mediastinal shift, polyhydramnios, and nonimmune hydrops, leading to certain fetal demise without prenatal intervention.

  ● The cyst volume ratio (CVR) is a sonographic marker normalizing lesion volume to head circumference and is a widely used risk stratification tool for the eventual development of nonimmune hydrops. If CVR is less than 1.6 without a dominant cyst, the risk of hydrops is less than 3%.

  ● For a CPAM with a predominant macrocyst or large pleural effusion at less than 32 weeks' gestation, in utero drainage can relieve the mass effect, leading to resolution of hydrops and improved surrounding lung development.

  ● Open fetal thoracotomy for resection of the CPAM is no longer routinely performed due to the success of maternal betamethasone administration and thoracoamniotic shunting.

■ The fetal neck mass poses a significant risk to the fetus, with a nearly 20% risk of IUFD and a 35% risk of death due to airway obstruction immediately after delivery. The primary histologic lesions encountered are cervical teratoma, cystic hygroma, or other vascular malformations. Obstruction of the trachea and esophagus can result in polyhydramnios and preterm labor; local compression can lead to craniofacial defects and cranial nerve injury. Highly vascular lesions can result in high-output cardiac failure with nonimmune fetal hydrops and subsequent IUFD.

  ● The tracheoesophageal displacement index (TEDI) is a useful prognostic measurement defined as the sum of the lateral and ventral displacement of the trachea and esophagus from the ventral most aspect of the cervical spine.

  ● For this reason, the ex utero intrapartum therapy (EXIT) to airway procedure should be considered to permit safe establishment of the airway prior to delivery.
    ❑ The EXIT procedure is a multistaged Cesarean delivery in which the fetus is partially delivered to preserve uteroplacental circulation until a functional fetal airway is established.

■ Fetuses with myelomeningocele (MMC) do not have a high risk of perinatal mortality. However, MMC confers severe long-term morbidity to the child, and up to 30% of patients with MMC die before adulthood, owing to respiratory, urinary, or CNS complications.

  ● The rationale for fetal intervention in MMC is centered on a "two-hit" hypothesis for the development of morbidity, in which the first hit is the original neural tube defect that results in an open spinal canal and the second hit is postulated to be trauma to the exposed neural elements while the fetus is in utero. By minimizing secondary trauma to the exposed neural elements through fetal repair, it was hypothesized that neurologic outcomes for MMC could be improved.

  ● Despite demonstrating a convincing benefit to the fetus regarding neurologic outcomes, the excitement for fetal repair of MMC has been tempered by the incidence of obstetric morbidity demonstrated in trials.

■ Lower urinary tract obstruction (LUTO) is most commonly caused by posterior urethral valves (PUV), but can also result from urethral atresia and Eagle–Barrett syndrome (prune belly). The fetus with LUTO is at high risk for the development of oligohydramnios as a result of mechanical obstruction of urinary flow and dysplastic changes in the kidneys. The bladder outlet obstruction leads to bladder distention, and as this worsens chronic distention results in compensatory hypertrophy and hyperplasia of the bladder wall smooth muscle. Over time, compliance and elasticity decrease and may cause poor postnatal bladder function. Elevated bladder pressure prevents urinary inflow from above, and the ureterovesical angle may change, resulting in reflux hydronephrosis.

  ● Bilateral renal dilation has an increased risk of associated chromosomal anomalies, and therefore an evaluation of fetal chromosomes may be warranted in such cases.

- Fetal interventions employed in the treatment of LUTO include vesicoamniotic shunting (VAS), fetoscopic cystoscopy with PUV ablation, and open fetal vesicostomy. Vesicoamniotic shunt diverts fetal urine into the amniotic space, allowing drainage of the upper urinary tract and preventing pulmonary hypoplasia and physical deformations by restoring amniotic fluid volume.
- The outcome of VAS and the long-term results have not been convincing. Results suggest that irreversible damage to the renal parenchyma occurs prior to diagnosis and that surgical intervention may only provide a small benefit, if any, to

long-term outcome (Moyer et al., 2020; Obican & Odibo, 2019).

▶ CONCLUSION

The healthy development of the fetus is dependent on the health status of the mother. Alterations in the cardiorespiratory, hematologic, or endocrine systems may adversely affect the fetus by either their presence or the treatments needed to correct these alterations. Close monitoring of both maternal and fetal well-being is vital to ensure a positive outcome of the pregnancy.

1. A patient is concerned their current preeclampsia will progress to eclampsia, and the neonatal nurse practitioner (NNP) recognizes that the risk of eclampsia developing is reduced within:

   A. 12 hours after to delivery

   B. 24 hours prior to delivery

   C. 48 hours after delivery

2. A woman in her first pregnancy has developed preeclampsia with severe symptoms at 24 weeks. They are started on medication and routine fetal surveillance. If the fetal surveillance is stable but maternal symptoms worsen, delivery is indicated at a fetal gestational age of:

   A. 26 weeks

   B. 28 weeks

   C. 30 weeks

3. A mother presents in early labor and has a history of chlamydia for which they are currently receiving treatment. The mother states they do not want the infant to have prophylactic antibiotic eye treatment at birth. The neonatal nurse practitioner (NNP) provides information to the mother by discussing that the antibiotic eye treatment will:

   A. Be given at any time and can always be given later if an infection occurs

   B. Decrease the chance of neonatal conjunctivitis and pneumonia infection

   C. Keep the baby from getting an infection and is required for all babies

4. An infant tests positive for cytomegalovirus (CMV) at 5 weeks of age, which indicates an infection related to:

   A. Exposure in utero or during delivery

   B. Maternal passage through breast milk

   C. Nosocomial exposure in the hospital

5. A newborn presents with superficial maculopapular skin lesions scattered on the abdomen, noted at birth. The maternal history is significant for urinary tract infection (UTI) and vulvovaginal candidiasis which was treated with prolonged antibiotics. The neonatal nurse practitioner (NNP) knows to evaluate the neonatal skin lesions as being a result of an infection with:

   A. *Candida albicans*

   B. *Staphylococcus* spp.

   C. *Treponema pallidum*

6. The neonatal nurse practitioner (NNP) recognizes a fetal effect of maternal sickle cell disease includes fetal:

   A. Alkalosis

   B. Anemia

   C. Hypoxia

(See answers next page.)

1. C) 48 hours after delivery

The risk of progression to eclampsia drops significantly after 48 hours. The risks remain the same at 12 to 24 hours after delivery (Harper et al., 2019).

2. B) 28 weeks

Fetal surveillance and maternal symptom management are conservative until 28 weeks. At that point, if maternal symptoms worsen, delivery is considered at 28 weeks after administration of antenatal corticosteroid steroids. Delivery at 26 weeks carries higher neonatal risks than delivery at 28 weeks, and delay until 30 weeks may increase maternal risk (Harper et al., 2019; Moore, 2018).

3. B) Decrease the chance of neonatal conjunctivitis and pneumonia infection

Chlamydia infection is the most common bacterial sexually transmitted disease in the United States and is associated with neonatal infection. Of infants exposed to chlamydia, 50% develop conjunctivitis in the first 2 weeks of life and up to 20% develop pneumonia in the first 4 months of life. Infection from delayed treatment will require systemic antibiotics, and prophylactic treatment is not a guarantee of infection prevention (Duff, 2019).

4. B) Maternal passage through breast milk

The timing of positive test results may help discover when the infant was exposed. Positive results prior to 3 weeks represent an in utero infection, while after 3 weeks of age can represent infection from the birth canal or via the breast milk. Nosocomial infection with CMV is very rare (Duff, 2019; Schleiss & Marsh, 2018).

5. A) *Candida albicans*

Vulvovaginal candidiasis is most commonly caused by *C. albicans*. There can be an increase in colonization in women who are pregnant or who have been treated with antibiotics. The potassium hydroxide (KOH) prep is used for diagnosis. *Staphylococcal* and *T. pallidum* infections do not present with cutaneous lesions (Duff, 2019).

6. C) Hypoxia

Fetal and neonatal complications of prematurity and fetal growth restriction arise secondary to placental infarction and fetal hypoxia. Fetal hypoxia is a result of decreased oxygen transport due to abnormal biochemistry of the maternal hemoglobin and loss of placental tissue for gas and nutrient exchange caused by the infarctions. Infants become polycythemic rather than anemic due to low oxygen availability. Alkalosis is not a considered finding (Blackburn, 2018).

Maternal History in the Intrapartum

Cheryl B. Robinson

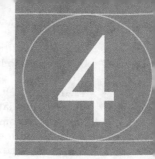

▶ INTRODUCTION

Every pregnancy, whether complicated or not, can be drastically altered during intrapartum. For the fetus, intrapartum places additional physiologic stressors. Depending on the fetus' tolerance to labor and delivery, the neonatal nurse practitioner (NNP) must be ready to intervene as the neonate makes the transition to life outside the womb. An understanding of the intrapartum period and the events that transpire prior to the actual delivery is requisite knowledge for successful resuscitation and stabilization.

- Intrapartum covers the period of time from onset of labor to generally 1 hour after delivery of the neonate. The intrapartum period can be considered high risk based on the medical conditions of the mother, either present prior to pregnancy or as a complication of the pregnancy, or due to events occurring during the labor process placing the mother and/or the fetus at risk of morbidity or mortality.
- The appropriate timing of labor and subsequent birth is strongly associated with positive perinatal outcomes. Infants born prior to 37 0/7 weeks are considered preterm, and those born after 42 0/7 weeks, or 294 days after the first day of the last menstrual cycle, are considered postterm.
- There is no one theory adequately explaining why labor begins. Combined maternal–fetal processes are initiated to decrease uterine quiescence and increase uterine activity. Although the communication pathways between the mother, the fetus, and the placenta require a sequential initiation, redundancy in positive feedforward and negative feedback loops prevents any one single factor to be responsible for the onset of labor (Costantine et al., 2020; Norwitz et al., 2019; Simpson & O'Brien-Abel, 2021).
- Intrapartum has been divided into four stages and is summarized in Table 4.1.

Table 4.1 The Four Stages of Intrapartum

First stage: progression measured by cervical changes, ends with complete cervical dilation	*Latent:* 0–3 cm *Active:* 4–7 or 6 cm for nulliparous women and 5 cm for multiparous women *Transition:* 8–10 cm
Second stage: complete cervical dilation and ends with the birth of the baby	Initial latent phase (passive fetal descent) Active pushing phase
Third stage: begins with the birth of the baby and ends with the delivery of the placenta	
Fourth stage: begins with delivery of the placenta and ends with stabilization of the mother in the immediate postpartum period	

Source: Data from Simpson, K. R., & O'Brien-Abel, N. (2021). Labor and birth. In K. Simpson & P. Creehan (Eds.), *Perinatal nursing* (5th ed., pp. 331–332). Lippincott Williams & Wilkins.

▶ THE PLACENTA

- The placenta has two opposing functions. It is the sole source of sustenance for the fetus and the sole protection against noxious external influences. At the simplest level, the placenta is nothing more than fetal blood vessels and surrounding connective tissue enveloped by a continuous layer of epithelium known as *trophoblast* and sitting in a pool of maternal blood called the *intervillous space* (Redline, 2020).

PLACENTA PREVIA

- The underlying pathogenesis of placenta previa is unknown. It is described as painless third-trimester bleeding. All women presenting with painless vaginal bleeding after 20 weeks' gestation should be assumed to have placenta previa until proven otherwise.

- Vital to the definition is the exact location of the placenta in relation to the internal cervical os. Two terms are recommended: *placenta previa* and *low-lying placenta*. A transvaginal ultrasound (TVUS) after 16 weeks' gestation can have the following results:
  - *Normal:* Placental edge is 2 cm or more from the internal cervical os.
  - *Low-lying:* Placental edge is <2 cm from the internal cervical os.
  - *Placenta previa:* Placental edge covers the internal cervical os.
- Bleeding prior to labor results from the lower uterine segment development, effacement of the cervix with increasing gestational age, prelabor uterine contractions, intercourse, and vaginal examination. Bleeding during labor is due to cervical dilation and the forces separating the placenta from the underlying decidua.
- Low-lying and placenta previa should be delivered by Cesarean section even though there is a risk of intraoperative hemorrhage.
- Risk factors for placenta previa include the following:
  - Prior pregnancy complicated by placenta previa
  - Prior Cesarean section
  - Advanced maternal age (>35 years of age)
  - Multiparity
  - Prior suction curettage
  - Smoking (Hull et al., 2019)

Fetal/Neonatal Complications

- Due to the risk of postpartum hemorrhage, neonatal resuscitation may depend on the amount of maternal blood loss (Hull et al., 2019).

VASA PREVIA

- Although rare, vasa previa occurs with the improper insertion of the umbilical cord into the placenta and can have grave consequences for the fetus. In vasa previa, the insertion of the umbilical cord into the placenta is velamentous, with the umbilical vessels coursing through the fetal membranes before inserting into the placental disc and the unsupported vessels, then overlying the cervix.
  - Unrecognized or overlooked, the fetal mortality rate is almost 60% because at rupture of membranes (ROM) there is tearing of fetal vessels. Because the entire fetal cardiac output passes through the cord, it can take <10 minutes for total fetal exsanguination to occur.
- Risk factors for vasa previa include the following:
  - A low-lying placenta
  - Multiple gestation
  - In vitro fertilization (Hull et al., 2019)

Fetal/Neonatal Complications

- Complications include exsanguination of the fetus, and if born alive the neonate will present with profound hypoxia, acidemia, hypovolemic shock, and severe respiratory and cardiovascular compromise.
- Placental structural anomalies can also predict deformations or disruptions in the fetus (Hull et al., 2019; Redline, 2020).

ABRUPTIO PLACENTAE

- Abruptio placentae is the premature separation of a normally sited placenta before birth, after 20 weeks' gestation. The incidence peaks between 24 and 26 weeks' gestation. The degree of abruption ranges across a broad clinical spectrum, from minor degrees of placental separation, with little effect on maternal or fetal outcome, to major abruption, associated with fetal death and maternal morbidity.
- Abruption results from bleeding between the decidua and the placenta with the hemorrhage dissecting the decidua apart. When this happens, there is loss of the corresponding placental area for gaseous exchange and provision of fetal nutrition.
- Although the process may sometimes be self-limited, there can be ongoing further dissection of the decidua. Dissection can lead to external bleeding if it reaches the placental edge and tracks down between the fetal membranes; circumferential dissection leading to near-total separation of the placenta can occur, particularly with concealed abruption.
- The underlying event in many cases of abruption is thought to be vasospasm of abnormal maternal arterioles; however, abruption may also occur due to trauma, such as a motor vehicle accident. The trauma causes acute shearing forces affecting the placenta–decidua interface. The sudden decompression of an overdistended uterus (such as occurs with membrane rupture in polyhydramnios) or delivery of a multiple gestation pregnancy can also lead to abruption.
- Risk factors for abruption include the following:
  - History of abruption
  - Maternal hypertension
  - Smoking
  - Preeclampsia
  - Substance abuse (cocaine or crack cocaine), causing vasospasm or abrupt increases in blood pressure
  - Multiparity
  - Presence of uterine fibroids (Hull et al., 2019)

Fetal/Neonatal Complications

- Poor infant outcomes of abruptio are associated with increased rates of perinatal asphyxia, intraventricular hemorrhage, periventricular leukomalacia, and cerebral palsy (Redline, 2020; Hull et al., 2019).

▶ **AMNIOTIC FLUID**

AMNIOTIC FLUID VOLUME

- Amniotic fluid volume (AFV) increases progressively between 10 and 30 weeks' gestation.
  - At 12 weeks' gestation, the amount of amniotic fluid (AF) is approximately 50 mL and continues to rise throughout pregnancy to a high of about 1,000 mL between 36 and 38 weeks' gestation. After 30 weeks, the increase slows and the AFV may remain unchanged until 36 to 38 weeks' gestation, when it tends to decrease. After 38 weeks' gestation, the amount of AF starts to decrease. AF contains 98% to 99% water, with its solute composition changing throughout gestation.
- Throughout gestation, AFV is highly regulated, gradually increasing in the first trimester, stabilizing in the second trimester, and decreasing late in the third trimester while remaining in a relatively narrow range of volumes.
- The amniotic fluid index (AFI) is measured by ultrasound. In each quadrant of the uterus, the vertical measures of the fluid pockets that do not include the umbilical cord are added together.
- Sonographic techniques to estimate AFV include subjective (qualitative) estimation, which includes designations of normal, increased, decreased, or absent; and semiquantitative methods: measurement of a two-diameter pocket (2 × 2), maximum vertical or single deepest pocket (SDP), and the AFI (Bahadue & Gecsi, 2020; Ross & Beall, 2019; Simmons & Magann, 2020).

AMNIOTIC FLUID PRODUCTION, COMPOSITION, AND FUNCTION

- AF is necessary for normal human fetal growth and development. The fluid volume cushions the fetus, protecting both the fetus and the umbilical cord from mechanical trauma or external injury, and its bacteriostatic properties may help maintain a sterile intrauterine environment and steady temperature. The space created by the AF allows fetal movement, aids in the normal development of both the lungs and the limbs, and prevents amnion from adhering to the fetus. Finally, AF offers convenient access to fetal cells and metabolic by-products and has been used for fetal diagnosis more often than any other gestational tissue.
- Fetal swallowing, urination, pulmonary secretions, nonkeratinized skin, intramembranous (IM) movement between the fetal blood and the placenta, and transmembranous movement across the amnion and chorion account for the movement of AF and solutes.

- Swallowing in the fetus is demonstrated between 8 and 11 weeks' gestation, with increasing volumes noted as gestational age increases. Near-term fetal swallowed volume is subject to periodic increases as mechanisms for thirst and appetite develop functionality. However, despite the fetal ability to modulate swallowing, this modulation is unlikely to be responsible for AFV regulation.
- Renal nephrons are formed at 9 to 11 weeks, at which time fetal urine is excreted into the AF. The amount of urine produced increases progressively with advancing gestation, and it constitutes a significant proportion of the AF in the second half of pregnancy. Renal agenesis is therefore associated with low AF levels.
- Driven by chloride ion exchange across the pulmonary epithelium, approximately 300 to 400 mL of fluid are excreted from the fetal pulmonary system. Under physiologic conditions, half of the fluid exiting the lungs enters the AF and half is swallowed; therefore, although total lung fluid production approximates one-third that of urine production, the net AF contribution made by lung fluid is only one-sixth that of urine.
- Since fetal skin remains nonkeratinized until weeks 22 to 25, surface exchange is a main factor contributing to fluid dynamics in early pregnancy. Although the actual mechanism is unknown, the prevailing thought is that early AF arises as a transudate of plasma, either from the fetus through nonkeratinized fetal skin or from the mother across the uterine decidua or the placenta surface or both; however, the actual mechanism is unknown.
- Because the volume of AF does not greatly increase during the latter half of pregnancy, another route of fluid absorption is likely. The most likely route is the IM pathway: the route of absorption from the amniotic cavity directly across the amnion into the fetal vessels. Studies have demonstrated a continuous, bidirectional flow of water and solutes from AF to the fetal circulation in vivo.
- Transmembranous movement across the amnion and chorion involves discussion of fluid dynamics and water permeability of the biologic membranes. This process may involve any or all of the following:
  - ❏ Simple diffusion
  - ❏ Diffusion of hydrophilic substances
  - ❏ Facilitated diffusion
  - ❏ Active transport
  - ❏ Receptor-mediated endocytosis (Ross & Beall, 2019; Simmons & Magann, 2020)
- See Figure 4.1.

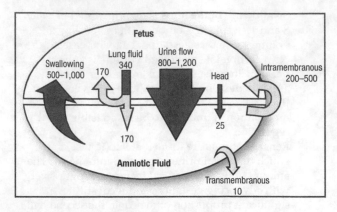

Figure 4.1 Pathways between the fetus and the amniotic fluid (in milliliters).

Source: Reproduced with permission from Gilbert, W. M., Moore, T. R., & Brace, R. A. (1991). Amniotic fluid volume dynamics. *Fetal and Maternal Medicine Review, 3,* 89. Cambridge University Press.

OLIGOHYDRAMNIOS

- *Oligohydramnios* has been defined as an AFV that is <200 mL and occurs in 1% to 2% of pregnancies. A sonograph assessment of an SDP <2 cm and an AFI <5 cm or a qualitative assessment of a low volume can also lead to a diagnosis of oligohydramnios. Additional assessment findings include estimated fetal size less than maternal dates.

- Low AF can be caused by underproduction or loss, or can be idiopathic. Underproduction can be the result of absent or dysfunctional kidneys, urinary tract obstruction, uteroplacental insufficiency, maternal medications, or maternal dehydration. Loss is also caused by ROM.

- If oligohydramnios is prolonged and occurs during the canalicular phase of alveolar proliferation (16–18 weeks' gestation), severe pulmonary hypoplasia associated with high perinatal mortality can occur. Although the exact physiologic cause of pulmonary hypoplasia is unclear, any maternal or fetal complication leading to the inhibition of fetal breathing, any lack of a trophic function of AF within the airways, or any simple mechanical compression of the chest is proposed as a cause.
  - Associated with postmature infants, renal agenesis, polycystic kidneys, and fetal urinary tract obstructions
  - Leakage of AF (Simmons & Magann, 2020)

Fetal/Neonatal Complications

- The NNP should expect with a maternal diagnosis of oligohydramnios for there to be close medical and nursing supervision, with associated fetal monitoring. The labor will likely be induced and there may be presence of amnioinfusion during labor.

- Preparation for an emergent Cesarean section, along with an intensive resuscitation and stabilization, should be anticipated. The neonate will likely have wrinkled, leathery skin, and may have skeletal deformities or experience fetal hypoxia.

- If oligohydramnios is present in a postdate pregnancy, the loss of AF may be from leaking membranes. The possibility of perinatal/fetal infection should be assessed.

POLYHYDRAMNIOS

- The exact cause of polyhydramnios is unknown. Risk factors include multiple gestations, Rh-sensitized pregnancies, and fetal gastrointestinal obstructions and atresias.

- *Polyhydramnios* is generally defined as an AF level >40 or a volume of 2,000 mL of fluid. Fluid pockets can be >8 cm and the condition can have a chronic or rapid onset.

- The etiology of an increased AF level falls into three categories: decreased absorption, overproduction, or idiopathic. Fetal swallowing is the predominant mechanism of AF removal, so congenital abnormalities associated with the gastrointestinal tract (tracheal atresia, duodenal atresia, tracheal or bowel obstruction) or the neurologic system (anencephaly, trisomy 18, trisomy 21) are often present.

- Other factors that can contribute to an overproduction of AF include maternal diabetes; syphilis; Rh isoimmunization, or the presence of atypical antibodies that might lead to hemolytic disease of the newborn; certain fetal or placental (chorioangioma) abnormalities; and a recent history of maternal infection. In the presence of gestational or adult-onset diabetes, increased fetal urination can account for a diagnosis of polyhydramnios, as well as macrosomia.

- Idiopathic causes account for 50% to 60% of cases of polyhydramnios. Only 1% to 2% of all pregnancies are complicated by polyhydramnios. Muscular dystrophies, fetal akinesia, and skeletal dysplasias may also be present when polyhydramnios is diagnosed (Simmons & Magann, 2020).

- In anatomically normal fetuses with otherwise unexplained polyhydramnios, diabetes should be suspected, particularly if there is fetal macrosomia or asymmetrically larger fetal abdominal circumference. These patients should be evaluated with a glucose tolerance test and treated accordingly. Polyhydramnios in diabetes is associated with increased perinatal morbidity and mortality beyond that of the diabetes itself (Simmons & Magann, 2020).

- Uterine overdistention, however, may stimulate preterm uterine contractions and labor may ensue. These patients are at a significantly high risk for premature rupture of membranes (PROM) and cord prolapse (Simmons & Magann, 2020).

Fetal/Neonatal Complications

- Prolapsed umbilical cord at ROM is a concern, as well as an increased incidence of malpresentations.
- Table 4.2 summarizes the comparison between oligohydramnios and polyhydramnios.

Table 4.2 Comparison of Etiologies for Oligohydramnios and Polyhydramnios

Fluid Level	Etiologies

Oligohydramnios	PROM, most common (50%)
	Congenital genitourinary defect (14%):
	■ Renal agenesis, polycystic or multicystic dysplastic kidneys, ureteral or urethral obstruction, including posterior urethral valve syndrome
	Maternal medications:
	■ Prostaglandin synthetase inhibitors (e.g., indomethacin, ibuprofen, sulindac), which reduce fetal glomerular filtration rate
	■ ACE inhibitors contraindicated in pregnancy can cause:
	  ● Twin-to-twin transfusion
	  ● Multiple gestation resulting in placental crowding

Polyhydramnios	Congenital anomalies: ■ Gastrointestinal (duodenal or esophageal atresia, tracheoesophageal fistula, gastroschisis, omphalocele, diaphragmatic hernia) ■ Craniofacial (anencephaly, holoprosencephaly, hydrocephaly, micrognathia, cleft palate) ■ Pulmonary (cystic adenomatoid malformation, chylothorax) ■ Cardiac (malformations, arrhythmias) ■ Skeletal dysplasias ■ Fetal hydrops (immune or nonimmune) ■ Anemia (fetomaternal hemorrhage, parvovirus infection, isoimmunization, thalassemia) ■ Neuromuscular disorders (myotonic dystrophy, Pena–Shokeir) and NTDs ■ Neoplasias (teratomas, hemangiomas)

ACE, angiotensin-converting enzyme; NTD, neural tubular defects; PROM, premature rupture of membranes.
Sources: Data from Blickstein, I., & Shinwell, E. S. (2020). Obstetric management of multiple gestation and birth. In R. Martin, A. Fanaroff, & M. Walsh (Eds.), *Fanaroff & Martin's neonatal-perinatal medicine: Diseases of the fetus and infant* (11th ed., pp. 355–363). Elsevier; Bahadue, F. L., & Gecsi, K. S. (2020). Antenatal and intrapartum care of the high-risk infant. In A. A. Fanaroff & J. M. Fanaroff (Eds.), *Klaus and Fanaroff's care of the high-risk neonate* (7th ed., pp. 9–47). Elsevier; Simmons, P. M., & Magann, E. F. (2020). Amniotic fluid volume. In R. Martin, A. Fanaroff, & M. Walsh (Eds.), *Fanaroff & Martin's neonatal-perinatal medicine: Diseases of the fetus and infant* (11th ed., pp. 368–403). Elsevier.

▶ RUPTURE OF MEMBRANES

IDENTIFYING RUPTURE OF MEMBRANES

- Pooling of fluid in the vaginal vault
- Positive nitrazine testing
- Positive ferning
- Decreased AFI on ultrasound

PREMATURE RUPTURE OF MEMBRANES

- ROM prior to the onset of labor, regardless of gestational age, is the single most common diagnosis with preterm delivery.
- *Preterm premature rupture of membranes* is defined as ROM before 37 weeks' gestation and can be written as PPROM. See Figure 4.2 for the causes of pathologic mechanisms for preterm labor.

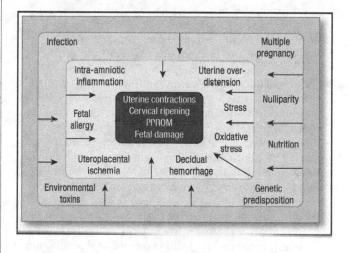

Figure 4.2 Pathologic mechanisms for preterm labor.
PPROM, preterm premature rupture of membranes.
Source: Reproduced with permission from Buhimsch, C. S., Mesiano, S. J., & Muglia, L. J. (2019). Pathogenesis of spontaneous preterm birth. In R. Resnik, C. J. Lockwood, T. R. Moore, M. F. Greene, J. A. Copel, & R. M. Silver (Eds.), *Creasy & Resnik's maternal-fetal medicine: Principles & practice* (9th ed., pp. 92–126e17, p. 98). Elsevier.

Etiology

- Smoking
- Incompetent cervix
- Multiple gestations
- Sexually transmitted diseases (STDs)/sexually transmitted infections (STIs) and other infections

PROLONGED RUPTURE OF MEMBRANES

- ROM exceeding 18 hours
- Associated with prolonged labors
- Labor dystocia or "failure to progress," a leading cause of Cesarean section deliveries

Etiology
- Pregnancies of older women
- Women with increased body mass index (BMI)
- Mothers who receive oxytocin induction and epidurals (Mercer & Chien, 2019)

▶ CHORIOAMNIONITIS

- An intra-amniotic infection, better known as chorioamnionitis, can profoundly impact the morbidity and mortality of a fetus, a neonate, and/or a mother. The choriodecidual space, fetal membranes, placenta, AF, and umbilical cord are all sites for potential microbial (usually polymicrobial) invasion (Costantine et al., 2020; Duff, 2019; Polin & Randis, 2020).
- Clinical chorioamnionitis is usually polymicrobial in origin. The most common organisms contributing to chorioamnionitis are outlined in Table 4.3.
- During the first trimester, the presence of abnormal cervicovaginal flora (e.g., bacterial vaginosis, aerobic vaginitis) is associated with adverse pregnancy outcomes, including early preterm birth and miscarriage and microbial invasion of the amniotic cavity (Costantine et al., 2020; Polin & Randis, 2020).
- Bacterial infection of the amniotic cavity is a major cause of perinatal mortality and maternal morbidity. Significant associations exist between clinical intra-amniotic infection and long-term neurologic development in the newborn, including cerebral palsy. Evidence demonstrates intrauterine infection is associated with increased risk of neonatal respiratory distress syndrome, periventricular leukomalacia, and cerebral palsy.
  - The unifying hypothesis for these varying morbidities is that intra-amniotic infection leads to fetal infection and to an excessive fetal production of cytokines, which leads in turn to pulmonary and central nervous system (CNS) damage.

Table 4.3 Organisms Associated With Chorioamnionitis

Acute Chorioamnionitis	Subclinical Chorioamnionitis
Symptomatic mother	Preterm labor or completely asymptomatic
Group B *Streptococcus* *Escherichia coli* *Streptococcus viridans*	*Ureaplasma urealyticum–* *Mycoplasma hominis* *Gardnerella vaginalis*
Fulminant sepsis at birth Respiratory distress Cardiovascular instability	Variable symptoms at birth Brain injury Chronic lung disease

Sources: Data from Martin, R., Fanaroff, A., & Walsh, M. (Eds.). (2019). *Fanaroff & Martin's neonatal-perinatal medicine: Diseases of the fetus and infant* (11th ed., pp. 404–414). Elsevier; Duff, P. (2019). Maternal and fetal infections. In R. Resnik, C. J. Lockwood, T. R. Moore, M. F. Greene, J. A. Copel, & R. M Silver. (Eds.), *Creasy & Resnik's maternal-fetal medicine: Principles and practice* (8th ed., pp. 862–919.e8). Elsevier.

- Clinical diagnosis is typically based on signs of maternal fever, maternal or fetal tachycardia, uterine tenderness, foul odor of the AF, and peripheral blood leukocytosis. Bacteremia occurs in approximately 10% of women with chorioamnionitis (Duff, 2019).

▶ FETAL HEART RATE MONITORING

- The ability to monitor the fetus during labor has revolutionized the care of pregnant women and their fetus, leading to decreases in maternal, fetal, and neonatal morbidity and mortality. Fetal status is assessed by determining fetal heart rate (FHR) at baseline and the variability of the heart rate, as well as any accelerations or decelerations and the pattern of the heart rate over time.
- FHR analysis is the most common means of evaluating a fetus for adequate oxygenation. The rate and regulation of the fetal heart provide important information for the obstetrician. The average FHR is 155 beats per minute (bpm) at 20 weeks' gestation, 144 bpm at 30 weeks, and 140 bpm at term. This progression is thought to reflect maturation of vagal tone, with consequent slowing of the baseline FHR. Normal fetuses can have variations of 20 bpm faster or slower than these baseline values.
- FHR patterns are the standard language for communicating fetal status and fetal response to labor. The following terminology is recommended:
  - Continuous *electronic fetal monitoring* (EFM) is the preferred method to assess fetal well-being during labor. Generally, EFM requires the use of an external Doppler ultrasound belted around the maternal abdomen and a second pressure transducer.
    - ❏ The Doppler ultrasound plots the FHR and the pressure transducer plots the frequency and duration of uterine contractions.
    - ❏ Rarely, a fetal scalp electrode is placed when there are decelerations in the FHR or the overall rate is difficult to interpret.
  - FHR is reported as either reassuring or nonreassuring in order to guide clinical management (Bahadue & Gecsi, 2020; Nageotte, 2019; Simpson & O'Brien-Abel, 2021).

BASELINE CHANGES

- Accelerations are a visually apparent abrupt increase in FHR above baseline. These are associated with normal FHR variability.
- Decelerations are characterized as early, variable, and late:
  - Early decelerations occur when the FHR decreases concurrently with contractions.

- Variable decelerations demonstrate an abrupt decrease from the FHR baseline lasting not more than 2 minutes. They may or may not be associated with contractions.
- Late decelerations are identified when the FHR slows significantly and does not return to baseline until after the completion of the contraction. These are an ominous sign associated with decreases in uterine blood flow and fetal hypoxia (Nageotte, 2019).

CATEGORIES OF FETAL HEART RATE INTERPRETATION

- Category I is defined as the following: baseline heart rate 110 to 160 bpm; moderate baseline variability, accelerations and/or early decelerations are present or absent; there are no late or variable decelerations.
  - It is interpreted to indicate that all findings are normal and is predictive of normal fetal acid–base balance at the time of observation.
- Category II is defined as tracings that do not meet the criteria for category I or category III.
  - It is an indeterminate interpretation, not predictive of abnormal fetal acid–base status, but cannot be classified as category I or category III.
- Category III is defined by absent baseline variability in the presence of recurrent late or variable decelerations or bradycardia or sinusoidal pattern.
  - It is interpreted to indicate abnormal fetal acid–base balance (O'Brien-Abel & Simpson, 2021).

NORMAL (REASSURING) FETAL HEART RATE

- The baseline features of the FHR are predominant characteristics that can be recognized between uterine contractions. These are the baseline rate and the variability of the FHR:
  - The normal baseline FHR is between 110 and 160 bpm. Rates slower than 110 bpm are called *bradycardia*, while rates faster than 160 bpm are called *tachycardia*.
  - EFM produces an irregular line that represents the slight difference in the time interval and from beat to beat. This demonstrates FHR variability (Nageotte, 2019).

NONREASSURING FETAL HEART RATE

- *Bradycardia* is a baseline FHR of <110 bpm. Some fetuses have a baseline FHR of <110 bpm and are cardiovascularly normal. Others with an FHR <110 bpm may have congenital heart block.
  - Decreases in FHR may be caused by a sudden decrease in oxygenation, such as occurs with placental abruption, maternal apnea, or AF embolus; a decrease or cessation in umbilical blood flow, such as occurs with a prolapsed cord or uterine rupture; and/or a decrease in uterine blood flow, such as occurs with severe maternal hypotension.
- *Tachycardia* is a baseline FHR >160 bpm. With tachycardia, loss of FHR variability is common. Although fetal tachycardia is potentially associated with fetal hypoxia, particularly when it is accompanied by decelerations of the FHR, the more common association is with maternal fever or fetal infection (e.g., chorioamnionitis). Certain drugs also cause tachycardia, such as beta-mimetic agents used for attempted tocolysis, or illicit drugs such as methamphetamine and cocaine.
  - Tachycardia should not be confused with the rare event of fetal cardiac tachyarrhythmia, in which the FHR is >240 bpm. These arrhythmias may be intermittent or persistent, and they are the result of abnormalities of the cardiac electronic conduction system.
- *Absent or minimal baseline variability* may be seen when the fetus experiences progressive hypoxia in cerebral and myocardial tissues. Nonhypoxic causes may be anencephaly, presence of opioids in the maternal system, or a defective cardiac conduction system.
- *Sinusoidal patterns* are extremely regular and smooth with no beat-to-beat or short-term variability. This is commonly seen in Rh-sensitized infants with critical anemia, possibly leading to hydrops. It can also be seen in cases of severe fetal acidemia and as a result of maternal–fetal bleeding (Nageotte, 2019).

▶ MATERNAL INTERVENTIONS AND THE EFFECTS ON THE FETUS

LABOR TOCOLYTICS

- No matter which tocolytic agent the clinician chooses, the evidence supports the use of short-term tocolytic drugs to prolong pregnancy for at least 48 hours to allow for administration of antenatal steroids. This may also allow for transport of the mother to a tertiary care facility and for administration of magnesium sulfate to reduce the risk of cerebral palsy (Costantine et al., 2020).
- Beta-mimetics:
  - Terbutaline is the beta-2-adrenergic agonist that has been most commonly used in obstetrics in the United States, but its use is decreasing (Costantine et al., 2020).
- Calcium channel blockers:
  - Dihydropyridine calcium channel blockers—for example, nifedipine and nicardipine—act on L-type calcium channels to inhibit calcium influx into the

myometrial cells. Reduced intracellular calcium concentrations prevent activation of myosin light chain kinase and thereby myometrium contraction. Adverse events associated with nifedipine are usually mild and related to peripheral vasodilation, for example, flushing. In normotensive women with no underlying heart disease, there is typically minimal effect on blood pressure due to a compensatory rise in heart rate and stroke volume (Costantine et al., 2020).

■ Magnesium sulfate:
- Magnesium sulfate has been one of the most commonly used tocolytic agents, especially since it has been shown to have fetal neuroprotective effects.
- Due to familiarity and its presumed safety, magnesium sulfate has been a mainstay of tocolytic therapy since 1971. Proposed mechanisms of action include competition with calcium at motor end plates and/or at plasma membrane voltage-gated channels. Maternal side effects with magnesium sulfate therapy can range from mild (e.g., flushing and somnolence) to severe (e.g., respiratory depression and cardiac arrhythmias; Costantine et al., 2020; Harper et al., 2019; Mercer & Chien, 2019).
- Although infants born at 34 to 36 weeks' gestation are at a higher risk for complications than term infants, morbidities and mortality are uncommon; therefore, magnesium sulfate for neuroprotection is not typically recommended in this gestational age range (Mercer & Chien, 2019).

LABOR INDUCTION

■ Labor induction involves the stimulation of the uterus to contract before contractions begin on their own. New research suggests that induction for healthy women at 39 weeks in their first full-term pregnancies may reduce the risk of Cesarean birth.
■ There are several methods to start labor, which include ripening the cervix, stripping the membranes, using oxytocin, and rupturing the amniotic sac.
- Ripening of the cervix uses medications that contain prostaglandins. These drugs can be inserted into the vagina or taken by mouth. The cervix can also be expanded by inserting a thin tube that has an inflatable balloon on the end into the cervix and expanded to widen the cervix.
- Stripping of the membranes involves a healthcare professional sweeping a gloved finger over the thin membranes that connect the amniotic sac to the wall of the uterus. This action is done when the cervix is partially dilated. It may cause the body to release natural prostaglandins,

which soften the cervix further and may cause contractions.
- Oxytocin is a hormone that causes contractions of the uterus. It can be used to start labor or to speed up labor that began on its own. Contractions usually start about 30 minutes after oxytocin is given.
- An amniotomy may be done to rupture the amniotic sac. A small hole is made in the membranes with a special tool. This procedure may be done after a woman has been given oxytocin. Amniotomy is done to start labor when the cervix is dilated and thinned and the fetus' head has moved down into the pelvis. Most women go into labor within hours after the amniotic sac breaks (their "water breaks").
■ See Box 4.1 for endogenous and exogenous factors affecting myometrial contractility during labor.

Box 4.1 Factors Affecting Myometrial Contractility During Labor

Uterine Stimulants
■ **Endogenous**
- Oxytocin
- Prostaglandins
- Endothelin
- Epidermal growth factor
■ **Exogenous**
- Oxytocin
- Prostaglandins

Uterine Relaxants
■ **Endogenous**
- Relaxin
- Nitric oxide
- L-arginine
- Magnesium
- Corticotropin-releasing hormone
- Parathyroid hormone-related protein
- Calcitonin gene-related peptide
- Adrenomedullin
- Progesterone
■ **Exogenous**
- Beta-adrenergic agonists (ritodrine hydrochloride, terbutaline sulfate, salbutamol, fenoterol)
- Oxytocin receptor antagonist (atosiban)
- Magnesium sulfate
- Calcium channel blockers (nifedipine, nitrendipine, diltiazem, verapamil)
- Prostaglandin inhibitors (indomethacin)
- Phosphodiesterase inhibitor (aminophylline)
- Nitric oxide donor (nitroglycerin, sodium nitroprusside)

Source: Reproduced with permission from Norwitz, E. R., Mahendroo, M., & Lye, S. J. (2019). Physiology of parturition. In R. Resnik, C. J. Lockwood, T. R. Moore, M. F. Greene, J. A. Copel, & R. M. Silver (Eds.), *Creasy & Resnik's maternal-fetal medicine: Principles & practice* (9th ed., pp. 81–95e6, p. 92). Elsevier.

MATERNAL ANALGESIA

- During labor, a mother's metabolic demand increases. As the metabolic demand increases, so does the increased use of oxygen. When anxiety and pain are added, there is an increased production of catecholamines (epinephrine and norepinephrine), as well as cortisol and glucagon. If placental gas exchange is compromised, the fetus may become hypoxic and acidotic, hence the need to address maternal analgesia.
- The goal of analgesia is pain relief while having the patient remain conscious. This is accomplished by providing partial sensory receptor blockage and not full motor receptor blockage.
- Sedatives and narcotic analgesics are frequently administered alone or in combination in the first stage of labor. There is increasing evidence that opioids given systemically do not relieve the pain of labor but do reduce anxiety and result in sedation. All drugs of this type rapidly appear in the fetal circulation when administered to the mother; therefore, predictably, there will be some sedation of the infant depending on the specific drug given, the amount, the time, and the route of administration (Hoyt, 2020; Thorp & Grantz, 2019).

NEURAXIAL TECHNIQUES

- *Epidural labor analgesia* is a catheter-based technique that provides continuous analgesia during labor through administration of medication into the epidural space. Although it is the most difficult form of anesthesia to administer, it has the advantage of providing excellent pain relief for the first and second stages of labor and for delivery without altering the consciousness of the mother. Analgesia is achieved by administration of local anesthetics, opioids, or both. Drug mixtures of local anesthetics and analgesics result in less motor block; this allows women who have epidural anesthesia to be more mobile during labor, and they are less likely to be confined to the supine position.
- It provides significant relief from the pain of contractions and pressure on the perineum and can be used for vaginal delivery as well as Cesarean section delivery.
  - For patients undergoing Cesarean delivery, opioids can be injected into the epidural space to provide prolonged postoperative analgesia. The rare occurrence of serious respiratory depression is the only major complication, although women may experience transient nausea, urinary retention, and pruritus.
- Both retrospective and prospective controlled trials have demonstrated that epidural analgesia results in longer labors and a higher incidence of operative vaginal delivery and Cesarean delivery than intravenous (IV) analgesia.
- Spinal analgesia can be administered to women without epidural analgesia in the second stage of labor near the time of anticipated delivery. A small dose of a local anesthetic, opioid, or both is injected into the subarachnoid space and has minimal effects on motor nerve function.
  - Spinal anesthesia is associated with the highest incidence of maternal hypotension, and the time from onset of anesthesia to delivery of the infant is directly related to the degree of fetal metabolic acidosis resulting from uteroplacental hypoperfusion.
  - Contractions can be felt, but there is no pain associated with the contraction. The mother can ambulate, has no hypotension, and can have rapid pain relief.
- The *combination of the lumbar epidural technique and spinal analgesia* is a variation of neuraxial analgesia, using an intrathecal dose to initiate analgesia. After placement of the epidural needle, but before insertion of the epidural catheter, a spinal needle is passed through the indwelling epidural needle puncturing the dura, and a small dose of local anesthetic or opioid is administered. This results in a more rapid analgesia than with an epidural. Early studies indicate it to be safe and effective (Hoyt, 2020; Rollins & Rosen, 2018; Simmons & Magann, 2020; Thorp & Grantz, 2019).

REGIONAL TECHNIQUES

- A *paracervical block* is infrequently used to provide pain relief during the first stage of labor. The technique consists of submucosal administration of local anesthetics immediately lateral and posterior to the uterocervical junction, which blocks transmission of pain impulses at the paracervical ganglion. Complications from systemic absorption or transfer of local anesthetic can occur and there is a rare occurrence of direct fetal trauma or injection. Although not advocated with enthusiasm by most authorities, this form of anesthesia is still used, especially in hospitals in which epidural anesthesia is not available.
- A *pudendal block* is a common form of anesthesia used for vaginal delivery. When successful, it provides adequate pain relief for episiotomy, spontaneous delivery, forceps or vacuum extraction delivery from a low pelvic station, and repair of perineal, vaginal, or cervical lacerations.
  - A sheathed needle is guided to the vaginal mucosa and sacrospinous ligament just medial and posterior to the ischial spine. Injection of local anesthetic blocks the sensation of the lower vagina and perineum (Rollins & Rosen, 2018). Because the local anesthetic agent is injected well away from the parauterine vasculature, uteroplacental blood flow and FHR are not

affected (Hoyt, 2020; Rollins & Rosen, 2018; Thorp & Grantz, 2019).

GENERAL ANESTHESIA

- Use of general anesthesia for Cesarean delivery is typically reserved for situations where neuraxial anesthesia is contraindicated or emergent delivery is needed. After denitrogenation of the lungs (i.e., preoxygenation), general anesthesia is induced by rapid-sequence administration of an IV induction agent, followed by a rapidly acting muscle relaxant. The trachea is intubated with a cuffed endotracheal tube, and a surgical incision is made after confirmation of tracheal intubation and adequate ventilation.
  - General anesthesia is characterized by loss of consciousness, analgesia, amnesia, and skeletal muscle relaxation.
  - Benefits of general anesthesia include the establishment of a secure airway and the ability to control ventilation. The process is rapid with reliable onset and there is potential for less hemodynamic instability.
- General anesthesia administration requires prompt delivery of the infant. Delivery of the infant within 90 to 180 seconds after making the uterine incision reduces the risk of fetal hypoxemia from altered uteroplacental and umbilical blood flow (Hoyt, 2020; Rollins & Rosen, 2018; Thorp & Gtrantz, 2019).

▶ POTENTIAL COMPLICATIONS OF THE INTRAPARTUM PERIOD

POSTTERM (POSTDATES): >42 WEEKS' GESTATION

- The problem in defining the end of pregnancy is that the beginning of pregnancy is seldom known; therefore, estimating dates of a spontaneous pregnancy is associated with educated guessing, resulting in accuracies of about +/- 2 to 3 weeks. At the end of gestation, the functioning of the placenta may take one of two paths:
  - If the placenta continues to function well, infants can develop macrosomia.
  - More commonly, the placenta functioning diminishes, resulting in an environment of placental insufficiency. Placental insufficiency generally results in decreased nutrition and decreased oxygen exchange to the fetus, leading not only to a wide range of perinatal morbidities, but also to increased rates of perinatal mortality.

- The benefit of reducing potential fetal risks with induction of labor must be balanced against the morbidity associated with this procedure. Management of an otherwise uncomplicated pregnancy prolonged beyond the estimated date of confinement, when the woman presents with unfavorable cervical conditions, has been the subject of extensive research (Blickstein & Rimon, 2020).

MULTIPLE GESTATIONS

- With multiple gestations, there is an increased risk of preterm birth and a decreased gestational age at birth as the number of fetus increases. PROM is a significant contributor to preterm birth. In about 50% of cases, the timing of delivery of a multiple gestation will be dictated by obvious clinical concerns, such as preterm labor, preeclampsia, or poor fetal growth.
  - Despite these results, the American College of Obstetricians and Gynecologists suggests elective delivery at 38 0/7 to 38 6/7 weeks because rates of neonatal morbidity, including respiratory distress syndrome, septicemia, and NICU admission, were all lower at later gestational ages (Bahadue & Gesci, 2020; Malone & D'Alton, 2019).

SPECIAL CONSIDERATIONS

- Disparity in AFV is a significant finding in twin oligohydramnios-polyhydramnios sequence (TOPS), of which twin–twin transfusion syndrome (TTTS) is the most severe end point. A three- to fivefold increase in morbidity and mortality is associated with TTTS. Discordant fetal weights and AFVs as detected with ultrasound assessment can be found in monochorionic/diamniotic twins, although it has been documented in monochorionic/monoamniotic pregnancies.
- *Monoamniotic twinning* results in a single amniotic sac containing both twins. This setup carries a higher risk of perinatal morbidity and mortality than diamniotic twins.
- Twin reversed arterial perfusion (TRAP) sequence, or acardiac twinning, is a unique abnormality of monochorionic multiple gestations in which one twin has an absent, rudimentary, or nonfunctioning heart. A bizarre range of anomalies can be seen in the acardiac twin, including anencephaly, holoprosencephaly, absent limbs, absent lungs or heart, intestinal atresias, abdominal wall defects, and absent liver, spleen, or kidneys.
- *Asynchronous delivery*, or delayed-interval delivery, refers to delivery of one fetus in a multiple gestation that is not followed promptly by birth of the remaining fetus or fetuses. This an extremely rare event and is usually acceptable as the management of extreme prematurity.

Intrauterine demise of one fetus in a multiple gestation during the first trimester is common and is termed *vanishing twin*. The original thought that the remaining twin was unaffected has now changed as data show the intrauterine demise of one fetus in a monochorionic twin pregnancy at as early as 12 weeks' gestation can result in profound neurologic injury to the surviving fetus. The risk of significant neurologic morbidity is not increased in a dichorionic gestation. Intrauterine demise of one fetus in the second or third trimester is rarer (Malone & D'Alton, 2019; Simmons & Magann, 2020).

MECONIUM-STAINED AMNIOTIC FLUID/MECONIUM ASPIRATION SYNDROME

■ Meconium aspiration syndrome (MAS) is associated with inhalation of meconium and AF during the fetal life or at delivery and is often complicated by significant pulmonary hypertension. It is one of the most common causes of hypoxemic respiratory failure in term newborns who require intensive care.

■ Prevention of MAS has focused on decreasing exposure of the fetal and newborn lung to the noxious effects of inhaled meconium. Infusion of saline into the amniotic cavity (i.e., amnioinfusion) during labor has been studied as a means of both diluting meconium and relieving pressure on the umbilical cord, a potential cause of fetal acidemia.

  ● Fetal acidemia is believed to cause increased intestinal peristaltic activity that results in passage of meconium and fetal gasping, which draws meconium-contaminated AF deep into the lungs.

  ● The presence of meconium-stained fluid may be related to fetal stress as a consequence of chorioamnionitis (Parker & Kinsella, 2018; Polin & Randis, 2020).

PREECLAMPSIA

■ Preeclampsia is a disorder unique to pregnancy characterized by poor perfusion of many vital organs (including the fetoplacental unit) and is completely reversible with termination of pregnancy. Mothers with preeclampsia may present with a variety of signs and symptoms ranging from mild to life-threatening; likewise, the fetus may be minimally to severely affected.

● Preeclampsia is distinguished between two modes: preeclampsia without severe features and preeclampsia with severe features.

  ❏ Preeclampsia without severe features can progress to preeclampsia with severe features over the course of days; therefore, women should be monitored frequently to assess for severe features and deterioration of fetal well-being.

  ❏ Routine administration of parenteral magnesium sulfate for seizure prophylaxis is recommended in women with preeclampsia with severe features. Most seizures occur during the intrapartum and postpartum periods, when the preeclamptic process is most likely to accelerate.

● The presence of a seizure changes the diagnosis of preeclampsia to eclampsia. Several additional criteria are used to differentiate mild from severe preeclampsia:

  ❏ Elevated blood pressure (160 mmHg or higher systolic and 110 mmHg or higher diastolic on two occasions during a 6-hour window while the patient is on bed rest)

  ❏ Proteinuria and/or oliguria (<500 mL in 24 hours)

  ❏ Cerebral or visual disturbances

  ❏ Respiratory distress and/or cyanosis

  ❏ Thrombocytopenia

  ❏ Fetal growth restriction (Bahadue & Gecsi, 2020; Harper et al., 2019)

▶ CONCLUSION

The NNP is dependent on the skill and expertise of the labor and delivery healthcare providers overseeing the care of the fetus prior to delivery. When called to attend a delivery, the NNP needs to ask or seek out the most critical and appropriate information to prepare for a successful resuscitation and stabilization. Most of the maternal history can be reviewed and provide answers to the condition of the neonate after the initial transition period. Having a broad knowledge of the events of intrapartum and the most common complications involved in labor and delivery will situate you well for certification. Always remember: The neonate's history is the maternal history.

1. A velamentous insertion of the umbilical cord is associated with:

   A. Placenta previa
   B. Uterine abruptio
   C. Vasa previa

2. The main contributor to fluid dynamics in early pregnancy is the fetal:

   A. Gastrointestinal system
   B. Integumentary system
   C. Pulmonary system

3. The etiology of increased amniotic fluid may be due to decreased absorption, to overproduction, or to:

   A. Concurrent fetal GI anomaly
   B. Damaged renal physiology
   C. Idiopathic and unknown factors

4. The neonatal nurse practitioner (NNP) asks for information regarding the fetal heart rate (FHR), knowing that a reassuring FHR indicates the fetus is well:

   A. Hydrated
   B. Oxygenated
   C. Positioned

5. The neonatal nurse practitioner (NNP) identifies a fetal heart tracing pattern with notable cardiac decelerations occurring after the onset of the contraction and which does not recover until well after the contraction has stopped as:

   A. Late deceleration
   B. Periodic deceleration
   C. Variable deceleration

6. The neonatal nurse practitioner (NNP) recognizes the parameters used in assessing fetal status with fetal heart rate (FHR) monitoring are:

   A. Baseline rate and variability
   B. Contraction and deceleration
   C. Peak and trough amplitude

7. The neonatal nurse practitioner (NNP) recognizes the first stage of labor ends with:

   A. Complete cervical dilation
   B. Delivery of the fetus and the placenta
   C. Rupture of fetal membrane

1. C) Vasa previa

In vasa previa, the insertion of the umbilical cord into the placenta is velamentous, with the umbilical vessels coursing through the fetal membranes before inserting into the placental disc and the unsupported vessels, then overlying the cervix. Placenta previa denotes the location of insertion over the cervical os. Uterine abruptio describes a tear in the uterine musculature and not in the cord (Hull et al., 2019).

2. B) Integumentary system

Since fetal skin remains nonkeratinized until weeks 22 to 25, surface exchange is a main factor contributing to fluid dynamics in early pregnancy. The gastrointestinal (GI) and pulmonary systems benefit from the presence of amniotic fluid but do not actively contribute to fluid dynamics (Simmons & Magann, 2020).

3. C) Idiopathic and unknown factors

The etiology of an increased amniotic fluid level falls into three categories: decreased absorption, overproduction, or idiopathic. A gastrointestinal (GI) anomaly or damaged renal physiology would contribute to decreased amounts of amniotic fluid (Simmons & Magann, 2020).

4. B) Oxygenated

FHR analysis is the most common means of evaluating a fetus for adequate oxygenation. Maternal hydration and fetal positioning affect FHR but are not referred to in terms of reassuring versus nonreassuring patterns (Nageotte, 2019).

5. A) Late deceleration

Late decelerations are identified when the fetal heart rate (FHR) slows significantly and does not return to baseline until after the completion of the contraction. These are ominous signs associated with decreases in uterine blood flow and fetal hypoxia. Early decelerations occur when the FHR decreases concurrently with contractions. Variable decelerations demonstrate an abrupt decrease from the FHR baseline lasting not more than 2 minutes. They may or may not be associated with contractions. Periodic is not a term used to describe decelerations (Nageotte, 2019).

6. A) Baseline rate and variability

The baseline features of the FHR are predominant characteristics that can be recognized between uterine contractions. They are the baseline rate and the variability of the FHR. Contractions refer to maternal features, while peak and trough amplitude are not clinically measured or useful (Nageotte, 2019).

7. A) Complete cervical dilation

By convention, labor is divided into three stages: (a) first stage: from the onset of labor to full dilation of the cervix; (b) second stage: from full dilation of the cervix to delivery of the infant; and (c) third stage: from delivery of the infant to delivery of the placenta (Thorp & Grantz, 2019).

Maternal History Affecting the Newborn With Intrauterine Drug Exposure

Lisa R. Jasin and Allison Z. Kelly

▶ INTRODUCTION

Prevalence rates of perinatal substance use are difficult to determine due to underreporting, unreliable drug use survey and detection methods, and societal attitudes. However, available data identify that pregnant women use illicit drugs at almost half the rate of the general population. During pregnancy, 16.3% of pregnant patients report tobacco use and 10.8% report alcohol use. Nearly 5.9% of pregnant patients use illicit drugs. It is estimated that 400,000 to 440,000 neonates are affected annually by intrauterine exposure to alcohol or illicit drugs (Prasad & Jones, 2019; Reis & Jnah, 2017; Sullivan, 2016; Wallen & Gleason, 2018).

▶ SUBSTANCE USE DISORDER

- It is important for the neonatal nurse practitioner (NNP) to be aware of and have basic knowledge of the psychology and physiology of dependence to be able to work successfully with the infants' parents, caregivers, and other family members.
- *Substance use disorder* (*SUD*) refers to the compulsive use of drugs despite negative consequences. Cravings and continued use can be triggered by cues derived from the environment that are associated with previous drug use.
- Marijuana has long been noted to be the most common recreational drug used by Americans aged 12 and older, followed by cocaine, hallucinogens, inhalants, methamphetamine, and heroin. Polysubstance use, including alcohol, tobacco, and other drugs, has become more common.
- Pregnant patients may be physically dependent and/or psychologically addicted to a substance. Recently, physical dependence has been termed *dependence*. Physical dependence may occur with multiple classes of nonpsychoactive drugs, such as sympathomimetic vasoconstrictors and bronchodilators, as well as psychoactive drugs. While each drug causes different acute effects, all cause feelings of euphoria and reward. With repeated use, tolerance occurs, requiring escalation of dosing for maintenance. Drug use is less likely among pregnant individuals in the third trimester. This may indicate pregnancy is a motivator of treatment for SUD.

- Preconception education of patients of childbearing age, families, and physicians is key to the prevention of drug effects on the fetus and the newborn. Early education that begins at home and is reinforced in elementary and middle school is optimal. Teenagers who become pregnant are more likely to engage in substance use than their nonpregnant peers.
- An infant of a mother with SUD (formerly referred to as infant of substance-abusing mother) is one whose mother has taken drugs that may potentially cause neonatal withdrawal symptoms. The constellation of signs and symptoms associated with withdrawal, often polysubstance exposure that includes opioids, is called *neonatal abstinence syndrome* (*NAS*; Alpan, 2020; Hudak, 2020; Lüscher, 2021; Patrick, 2017; Sullivan, 2016).

CLASSIFICATION OF SUBSTANCES

- The initial molecular and cellular targets must be identified in order to understand the long-term changes induced by drugs of abuse. Much research has revealed the mesolimbic dopamine system as the prime target of addictive drugs. This system originates in a tiny structure at the tip of the brainstem, the ventral tegmental area (VTA), which projects to the nucleus accumbens, the amygdala, the hippocampus, and the prefrontal cortex. These projection neurons are dopamine-producing neurons. When they begin to fire in large bursts, excessive amounts of dopamine are released.
- Addictive drugs activate the mesolimbic dopamine system with an increased dopamine level. All addictive drugs increase dopamine concentration in the mesolimbic projections. Each addictive drug has a specific molecular target that engages distinct cellular mechanisms to activate the mesolimbic system and can be divided into three classes:

- G_{io} protein-coupled receptors (e.g., opioids, cannabinoids, and gamma-hydroxybutyric acid [GHB])
- Ionotropic receptors or ion channels (e.g., nicotine, alcohol, benzodiazepines, dissociative anesthetics, and some inhalants)
- Monoamine transporters which increase dopamine levels (e.g., cocaine, amphetamines, and ecstasy), with the role of increased level of dopamine still under debate (Alpan, 2020; Lüscher, 2021)

MATERNAL SCREENING

- The American College of Obstetricians and Gynecologists (ACOG) and the American Medical Association endorse universal screening. Every pregnant patient is asked about substance use via the Screening, Brief Intervention, and Referral to Treatment (SBIRT) tool.
- Identification of perinatal substance use is accomplished by obtaining a thorough and accurate history of risk factors for maternal substance use, self-reported use, neonatal history and presentation, and toxicology screens that support maternal substance use (urine screens) or neonatal exposure (urine, meconium, umbilical cord samples).
  - Maternal risk factors include a history of limited, inadequate, or no prenatal care; maternal history of sexually transmitted infections (STIs); perinatal depression; poor nutrition; significant mental illness; and unresolved trauma.
- Brief intervention should include available community resources for education and treatment. These brief interventions may influence patients using substances during pregnancy (Hudak, 2020; Prasad & Jones, 2019; Wallman, 2018).

Biochemical Screening

- In the prenatal and perinatal period, biochemical screening is used to test for drug exposure, including nicotine. Specimens such as hair, cord blood, human milk, and amniotic fluid may be tested. However, the ACOG does not support biochemical screening as the method for detecting substance use in pregnancy. If biochemical testing is performed, maternal consent should be obtained.
- Urine is the most commonly used substance for testing as it is easy to collect. Urine testing may detect threshold levels of drug metabolites only for several days after use.
- Positive results may occur with use of prescribed drugs or secondhand exposure and should be confirmed. False negative can occur even with significant drug exposure (Hudak, 2020; Patrick, 2017; Prasad & Jones, 2019; Wallman, 2018).

▶ INTRAUTERINE EFFECTS OF PERINATAL SUBSTANCE EXPOSURE

- Prenatal exposure to alcohol, tobacco, cannabis, and illicit drugs has the potential to cause harm to the fetus and the neonate. Effects may persist into childhood.
  - All drugs associated with SUD have low molecular weight and are lipid-soluble; thus, they all cross the placenta and cause direct effects on the fetus.
  - Drugs taken orally may have a decreased ability to cross the placenta; intravenous (IV) drugs may cross the placenta readily.
  - The use of IV drugs increases exposure of both the mother and the fetus to HIV and hepatitis.
- Intrauterine exposure to drugs is associated with fetal distress, fetal demise, growth restriction, adverse neurodevelopmental outcomes, lower Apgar scores, and withdrawal in the newborn. Symptoms of drug withdrawal are similar to sepsis, hypoglycemia, and central nervous system (CNS) disorders in the newborn (D'Apolito, 2021; Jackson et al., 2021; Rohan, 2021; Sullivan, 2016).
- Table 5.1 details the direct and indirect effects of substance use on the embryo and the fetus.

Table 5.1 Fetal Direct and Indirect Effects of Substance Use

Direct Effects	Indirect Effects
■ Teratogenic effects ■ Abnormal growth ■ Abnormal maturation ■ Alterations in neurotransmitters ■ Alterations in neural receptors ■ Alterations in brain organization	Vasoconstriction of uterine/placental vessels ■ Placental insufficiency ■ Altered nutrition to the fetus ■ Altered maternal health behaviors ■ Altered nutrition to the fetus

Sources: Data from Hudak, M. (2020). Infants of substance abusing mothers. In R. Martin, A. Fanaroff, & M. Walsh (Eds.), *Fanaroff and Martin's neonatal–perinatal medicine: Diseases of the fetus and infant* (11th ed., pp. 735–736). Elsevier; Reis, P., & Jnah, A. (2017). Perinatal history: Influences on newborn outcome. In B. Snell & S. Gardner (Eds.), *Care of the well newborn* (p. 51). Jones & Bartlett Learning; D'Apolito, K. (2021). Perinatal substance abuse. In T. Verklan, M. Walden, & S. Forest (Eds.), *Core curriculum for neonatal intensive care nursing* (6th ed., pp. 40–41). Elsevier; Wallman, C. (2018). Assessment of the newborn with antenatal exposure to drugs. In E. P. Tappero & M. E. Honeyfield (Eds.), *Physical assessment of the newborn* (6th ed., p. 257). Springer Publishing Company.

NEONATAL SCREENING

- Testing for in utero substance exposure is often based on risk factors; however, using only risk factors fails to identify all substance-exposed neonates. Some institutions advocate for universal testing of all infants (Hudak, 2020).

Urine

- Urine screening may have a high false negative rate. Alcohol may be detected up to 10 hours; opioids, amphetamines, benzodiazepines, and cocaine metabolites may be detected for up to 4 days; and marijuana and barbiturates may be detected up to 6 weeks after the most recent use.
- Urine is easily obtained and is the most common substance used for drug testing. It reflects intake only in the last few days before delivery (Alpan, 2020; D'Apolito, 2021).

Meconium

- Meconium is easily obtained, and drugs may be detected up to 3 days after delivery. It reflects drug use after the first trimester, has a lower rate of false negatives, is a more sensitive test than urine for detecting drug abuse, and reflects usage over a longer period than is detectable by urine testing.
- Drug use during the second and third trimesters can be detected through meconium testing.
- Two to three grams of stool is necessary for testing; therefore, collection of multiple samples is highly recommended (Alpan, 2020; D'Apolito, 2021; Jackson et al., 2021; Patrick, 2017; Prasad & Jones, 2019).

Umbilical Cord

- A 6-in. segment is required for testing and the results are returned more rapidly than meconium.
- Collection and storage may require increased resources.
- Umbilical cord testing may not be as sensitive as meconium testing (D'Apolito, 2021; Jackson, et al., 2021; Patrick, 2017).

Hair

- Hair is by far the most sensitive test available for detection of drug use. Hair grows at 1 to 2 cm per month; hence, maternal hair can be segmented and each segment analyzed for drugs. There is a quantitative relationship between the amount of drug used and the amount incorporated in growing hair.
- The test requires processing before assay, is more expensive, and is currently not as widely available as other test methods (Alpan, 2020).

▶ NEONATAL OUTCOMES

- Substance exposure in utero may have long-term effects on behavior, learning, school performance, and emotional stability.
  - Initially, substance-using mothers and their infants may have difficulty with bonding behaviors. Mothers who are substance users have significantly less positive affect and greater detachment when evaluated with their infant.

- Lower gestational age is correlated with lower risk of withdrawal. This may be due to decreased length and dose of exposure and neurologic immaturity which limits the ability of the premature infant to exhibit signs of withdrawal. Compared with term infants whose mothers were treated with methadone (Dolophine), infants born at less than 35 weeks' gestational age had significantly lower total and CNS abstinence scores.
- Parents of drug-exposed infants may need assistance recognizing infant cues necessary for caregiving and infant symptoms that signal problems (D'Apolito, 2021; Hudak, 2020; Jackson, et al., 2021; Wallman, 2018).

▶ MATERNAL SUBSTANCE USE DISORDER AND BREASTFEEDING

- Breastfeeding of substance-exposed infants can enhance maternal–infant bonding. Breastfeeding may encourage more maternal involvement in the care of one's newborn. The known benefits of breastfeeding and human milk must be weighed against the potential risks to the infant, most of which are not well understood. There are many issues to consider, including lactation pharmacology issues, maternal behaviors that may be dangerous during breastfeeding, coexisting risk factors or conditions, polydrug use/abuse, and infection risks.
- The short-term advantage of breastfeeding is early maternal–infant contact. The en face position of breastfeeding enhances this contact. During the first 1 to 2 hours after birth, the infant's sucking and touching of the mother's areola increases maternal attentiveness to the baby's needs for at least the first week of life.
- When drug safety during lactation is assessed, the benefits of human milk for both the mother and the infant must be made explicit. The evidence of the benefits is generated mostly from cohort studies and epidemiologic analyses, as randomized trials are not possible under most circumstances. However, biologic plausibility and frequently observed associations between breastfeeding and various health benefits support the presence of a causal relationship.
- There are several factors that contribute to a substance passing into the breast milk: drug solubility, protein binding, molecular weight, and degree of ionization. Drugs of larger molecular weight and protein-bound drugs are less likely to pass into the breast milk. Drugs that are lipid-soluble will pass more easily into the breast milk.
- Often, breastfeeding is interrupted or discontinued for maternal therapy even though there are relatively few maternal medications that are not compatible with breastfeeding. Even if the mother is on drugs with potential risks, careful monitoring and strategies to minimize infants' exposure can be often used so that the mother can decide to continue breastfeeding if they choose.

In general, serious side effects in infants are uncommon. Acute toxicity is unlikely for otherwise healthy infants.

■ Breastfeeding is encouraged when the mother is in and plans to continue treatment for SUD and a substance treatment provider endorses that the mother has been able to achieve and maintain sobriety. Breastfeeding is now generally supported in women who are engaged in the treatment for SUDs and who have had a confirmed period of abstinence (from street drugs) prior to delivery, as the benefits of breastfeeding outweigh the small amount of methadone that enters the breast milk.

■ Breastfeeding is contraindicated only if the mother is taking illicit drugs, has polydrug abuse, or is infected with HIV. Breastfeeding may also be discouraged in the following circumstances:
  ● The mother has positive urine toxicology testing for drugs of abuse or misuse of illicit drugs at delivery and has no plans for postpartum substance use treatment.

● For infants whose mothers engage in active, ongoing use of "street" drugs (heroin, cocaine, methamphetamines, marijuana), the risks of breastfeeding outweigh any potential benefits.

■ Maternal use of fluoxetine (Prozac) is not recommended because it produces significant plasma concentrations in some breastfed infants and has a long half-life. A mother on treatment with a selective serotonin reuptake inhibitor (SSRI) who desires to breastfeed their infant should be counseled about the benefits of breastfeeding as well as the potential risk that their infant may continue to be exposed to a measurable level of SSRI with unknown long-term effects.

■ Breastfeeding may need to be temporarily discontinued when mothers are taking medications for diagnostic procedures or are taking drugs with a high potential for toxicity that are given once. In such cases, previously expressed milk or formula may be used. The timing for reinstitution of breastfeeding varies with the

Table 5.2 Recommendations for Breastfeeding With Substance Exposure

Substance	Breastfeeding	Presence in Breast Milk	Additional Information
Nicotine	Equivocal	It is 1.5–3 times greater in breast milk than in maternal blood plasma.	Infants may sleep less and have more ear and respiratory infections associated with an increased incidence of infant respiratory allergy and SIDS.
Alcohol	Contraindicated	It is concentrated in breast milk and can decrease milk production.	Mothers should have no more than one drink and should wait at least 2 hours before breastfeeding.
Marijuana/ tetrahydrocannabinol	Contraindicated	It is concentrated in breast milk compared with maternal blood plasma levels.	
Cocaine	Contraindicated	It may be found in breast milk up to 36 hours after use.	
Methamphetamines	Contraindicated	Concentration in the breast milk is 2.8–7.5 times higher than that in maternal plasma.	High levels of methamphetamine in breast milk may produce an acute neurotoxic syndrome with hypertonia, tremors, apnea, and seizures.
Benzodiazepines	Contraindicated	Metabolites have been found in breast milk and infant blood.	
Opioids	Contraindicated if illicit use Supported if in a MAT program	Buprenorphine (Subutex) appears in breast milk approximately 2 hours after maternal ingestion. Methadone appears in breast milk at low levels, with absolute levels being dependent on maternal dose.	Infants who breastfeed have a reduction in neonatal abstinence symptoms when the mother is on methadone. Breastfed infants who were exposed to methadone (Dolophine) and buprenorphine (Subutex) required pharmacologic treatment for a shorter period of time than infants who did not breastfeed.

MAT, medication-assisted treatment; SIDS, sudden infant death syndrome.
Sources: Data from Prasad. M., & Jones, H (2019) Substance abuse in pregnancy. In R. Resnik, C. Lockwood, T. Moore, M. Greene, J. Copel, & R. Silver (Eds.), *Creasy and Resnik's maternal-fetal medicine: Principles and practice* (8th ed., pp. 1243–1257.e3). Elsevier; D'Apolito, K. (2021). Perinatal substance abuse. In T. Verklan, M. Walden and S. Forest (Eds.), *Core curriculum for neonatal intensive care nursing* (6th ed., pp. 38–53). Elsevier; Sullivan, C. (2016). Substance abuse in pregnancy. In S, Mattson & J. Smith (Eds.), *Core curriculum for maternal—newborn nursing* (5th ed., pp. 564–579). Elsevier; Hudak, M. (2020). Infants with antenatal exposure to drugs. In R. Martin, A Fanaroff, & M. Walsh (Eds.), *Fanaroff and Martin's neonatal-perinatal medicine: Diseases of the fetus and infant* (11th ed., pp. 735–749). Elsevier; Jackson J., Knappen, B., Olsen, S. (2021). Drug withdrawal in the neonate. In S. Gardner, B. Carter, M. Enzman-Hines, & S. Niermeyer (Eds.), *Merenstein & Gardner's handbook of neonatal intensive care* (9th ed., pp. 250–272). Elsevier.; Blackburn, S. T. (2018h). Pharmacology and pharmacokinetics during the perinatal period. In S. T. Blackburn (Ed.), *Maternal, fetal, & neonatal physiology: A clinical perspective* (5th ed., pp. 180–214). Elsevier; Wallman, C. (2018). Assessment of the newborn with antenatal exposure to drugs. In E. P. Tappero & M. E. Honeyfield (Eds.), *Physical assessment of the newborn: A comprehensive approach to the art of physical examination* (6th ed., pp. 255–262). Springer Publishing Company.

toxicity of the agent (Blackburn, 2018; D'Apolito, 2021; Gardner, Lawrence, & Lawrence, 2021; Hudak, 2020; Ito & Verstegen, 2021; Jackson et al., 2021; Partick, 2017; Wallen & Gleason, 2018).

■ Table 5.2 lists recommendations for breastfeeding with substance exposure.

▶ COMMON SUBSTANCES USED IN PREGNANCY

TOBACCO/NICOTINE

■ Nicotine, including traditional and electronic cigarettes, smokeless tobacco, and nicotine replacement patches, is the substance most frequently used in pregnancy. Nicotine has the most adverse effect on perinatal outcomes, in particular preterm birth. Nicotine crosses the placenta and the blood–brain barrier readily during pregnancy and is the most preventable cause of infant morbidity and mortality.

■ Prevalence is difficult to determine secondary to failure to self-report. In 2016, the percentage of pregnant patients from ages 15 to 44 who used cigarettes was 10.1% (a decrease from 13.6% in 2015).
  ● Smoking among opioid-dependent females is common, at almost 90%. Data reveal 24% to 50% of pregnant individuals do not disclose smoking status when questioned (D'Apolito, 2021, Blackburn, 2018; D'Apolito, 2021; Prasad & Jones, 2019; Sullivan, 2016; Wallman, 2018; Wallen & Gleason, 2018).

Pharmacology

■ The addictive properties of nicotine arise from dopaminergic effects on the brain. Cotinine is the metabolite of nicotine that is measured in a urine drug screen. Nicotine rapidly reaches peak levels in the bloodstream and enters the brain, where peak levels are reached within 10 seconds after inhalation. Immediately after nicotine exposure, the adrenal glands are stimulated and epinephrine is released, causing an increase in blood pressure, respiration, and heart rate.
  ● Cotinine levels consistent with smoking can be seen in patients exposed to secondhand smoke.

■ Cigarette smoke contains approximately 4,000 compounds, including cyanide, carbon monoxide, and many toxic hydrocarbons, which affect oxygen transport in the placenta and can cause adverse effects on the fetus. Nicotine crosses the placenta, with levels in the fetal blood and amniotic fluid significantly exceeding maternal levels (Blackburn, 2018; Prasad & Jones, 2019; Sullivan, 2016; Wallen & Gleason, 2018).

Screening

■ The Tobacco Screening Measure has four staged questions. Additional smoking information can be obtained from the Fagerström Test for Nicotine Dependence, which is composed of six multiple-choice queries regarding smoking behavior. Although this screening tool has not been well validated, it has been found to be reliable with regard to consistent outcomes in patients tested and retested (Prasad & Jones, 2019).

Fetal/Neonatal Effects

■ It is possible that vasospasm secondary to smoking leads to decreased intervillous perfusion, hypoxia, and decreased nourishment to the fetus. Carbon monoxide is slow to clear from fetal circulation and a left shift in the oxyhemoglobin dissociation curve occurs.
  ● Low birth weight (LBW) is dose-dependent, with more smoking during pregnancy the lower the birth weight. One study suggested each pack of cigarettes smoked per day caused a reduction in relative fetal weight of 5%.

■ Smoking may also lead to chromosomal instability secondary to genotoxicity. The most common translocation or deletion is in the 11q23 region. This region is implicated in hematologic malignancies. An association with childhood cancers has been suggested.

■ Maternal genotype appears to have an impact on the risk of LBW and pulmonary function in children of smokers. Serum erythropoietin levels are higher in tobacco smoke-exposed infants at delivery, a finding that is presumed to reflect fetal hypoxia (Prasad & Jones, 2019; Sullivan, 2016; Wallman, 2018; Wallen & Gleason, 2018).

■ Box 5.1 lists the effects of nicotine exposure on the fetus and the neonate.

Box 5.1 Effects of Nicotine on the Fetus and the Neonate

Fetal
■ Fetal hypoxia and intrauterine growth restriction
■ Malformations of the lip or palate (clefts), heart, and/or urinary tract
■ Limb reduction defects

Neonatal
■ Small for gestational age/low birth weight
■ Hypertonicity/jitteriness
■ Altered respiratory function, including increased risk of infections

Sources: Data from Blackburn, S. (2018). *Maternal, fetal, & neonatal physiology: A clinical perspective* (5th ed., p. 206). Elsevier; Prasad, M., & Jones, H (2019) Substance abuse in pregnancy. In R. Resnik, C. Lockwood, T. Moore, M. Greene, J. Copel, & R. Silver (Eds.), *Creasy and Resnik's maternal–fetal medicine: Principles and practice* (8th ed., p. 1246). Elsevier; D'Apolito, K. (2021). Perinatal substance abuse. In T. Verklan, M. Walden & Forest S. (Eds.), *Core curriculum for neonatal intensive care nursing* (6th ed., p. 41). Elsevier; Rohan, A. J. (2021). Common neonatal complications. In K. Simpson, P. Creehan, N. O'Brien-Abel, C. K. Roth. & and A. J. Rohan (Eds.), *Perinatal nursing* (5th ed., p. 671). Wolters Kluwer; Sullivan, C. (2016). Substance abuse in pregnancy. In S. Mattson & J. Smith (Eds.), *Core curriculum for maternal-newborn nursing* (5th ed., p. 571). Elsevier; Wallman, C. (2018). Assessment of the newborn with antenatal exposure to drugs. In E. P. Tappero & M. E. Honeyfield (Eds.), *Physical assessment of the newborn* (6th ed., p. 131, 257). Springer Publishing Company.

Childhood Effects

- Potential long-term morbidities related to fetal exposure to nicotine and toxins from cigarette smoke include decreased cognitive functioning, auditory processing deficits, impulsivity, anxiety, depression, attention deficit hyperactivity disorder (ADHD), reduced lung function, and asthma in the offspring.
- Asthma and other chronic conditions are more common in infants who are exposed to passive smoking. Secondhand smoke increases the risk of sudden infant death syndrome (SIDS) and respiratory illnesses.
- It has been reported that smoking during pregnancy may increase childhood obesity by 55%.
- Smoking during pregnancy may result in altered childhood pulmonary functioning through the first years of life, possibly leading to a lifelong reduction in lung function (D'Apolito, 2021; Gardner, Lawrence, & Lawrence, 2021; Sullivan, 2016; Wallen & Gleason, 2018; Wallman, 2018).
- Mothers who smoke during pregnancy commonly continue to smoke during their infants' childhood.
  - Asthma and other chronic conditions are more common in infants who are exposed to passive smoking.

Treatment

- Treatments for nicotine addiction include the nicotine itself in forms that are slowly absorbed and several other drugs. Nicotine that is chewed, inhaled, or transdermally delivered can be substituted for the nicotine in cigarettes, thus slowing the pharmacokinetics and eliminating the many complications associated with the toxic substances found in tobacco smoke.
- Patients who smoke tobacco or use e-cigarettes should be counseled to quit. Patients who are most likely to quit have done so by their first prenatal visit, while those who have not quit by the first prenatal visit are likely to continue smoking throughout pregnancy without effective intervention. A Cochrane review suggested that interventions geared toward smoking cessation have the potential to decrease LBW and preterm births.
- Recommendations for treatment include psychosocial interventions that exceed minimal advice to quit throughout pregnancy, as well as pharmacotherapy (nicotine replacement or bupropion; D'Apolito, 2021; Lüscher, 2021; Prasad & Jones, 2019; Sullivan, 2016; Woo et al., 2021).

ALCOHOL

- Alcohol is one of the most misused substances during pregnancy and the most common teratogen to which the fetus is exposed. Alcohol exposure in utero is the leading cause of preventable birth defects in the United States.

- Among pregnant females aged 15 to 44 years, 10.8% reported current alcohol use, 3.7% reported binge drinking, and 1% reported heavy drinking. Binge drinking in the first trimester of pregnancy was reported by 10.1% of females aged 15 to 44 and has been reported as high as 11.9% of pregnant females.
- The highest use of alcohol use in pregnancy is not determined by socioeconomic status. In some states, alcohol use in pregnancy was highest in females older than 35, non-Hispanic females, females with more than high school education, and females with higher degrees (Blackburn, 2018; Jackson, et al., 2021; Prasad & Jones, 2019; Reis & Jnah, 2017; Sullivan, 2016).

Pharmacology

- Ethanol, the alcohol contained in alcoholic beverages, is absorbed via the digestive tract and into the body fat and bloodstream. Alcohol is metabolized to acetaldehyde by alcohol dehydrogenase, primarily in the liver. Acetaldehyde is short-lived, but can cause significant tissue damage, particularly in the liver where most alcohol is metabolized.
  - When consuming the same amount of alcohol, pregnant individuals clear alcohol more slowly than nonpregnant individuals, likely related to hormonal alterations in alcohol-metabolizing enzymes.
- Ethanol enhances the effects of the inhibitory neurotransmitter gamma-aminobutyric acid and lessens the effect of the excitatory neurotransmitter glutamate. Ethanol acts as a CNS depressant or sedative. Alcohol acts as an antagonist at the N-methyl-D-aspartate (NMDA) receptors and as a facilitator at the gamma-aminobutyrate agonist (GABA) receptors. Dopamine is released in response to alcohol use and provides reinforcement of alcohol use (Prasad & Jones, 2019; Wallen & Gleason, 2018).

Screening

- Screening for alcohol use can be difficult. Barriers include lack of practitioner time, inadequate practitioner assessment and intervention skills, pessimistic healthcare provider attitudes about their contribution to or facilitation of change, and practitioners fearing that patients may view questions about drinking as offensive.
- Unless a pregnant patient is obviously intoxicated, biochemical screening is not endorsed.
- Instruments are available to screen for alcohol use in pregnancy. Screening tools for substance abuse include terminology to elicit feedback about alcohol as well as other drug use. Examples are Ewing's Four Ps Screening Tool and the CRAFFT Substance Abuse Screen for Adolescents and Young Adults.
- The simplest and easiest tool for alcohol screening is the CAGE questionnaire. T-ACE is another questionnaire in use. The T-ACE questions address

Tolerance, Annoyance, the need to Cut down and the use of Eye-openers (Prasad & Jones, 2019; Reis & Jnah, 2017).

Fetal/Neonatal Effects

- Alcohol is a known teratogen, and the American Academy of Pediatrics' (AAP) Committee on Substance Abuse strongly affirmed that there is no known safe level for use in pregnancy. Alcohol at any point in pregnancy can affect the brain or other areas of development. Ethanol easily crosses the placenta and is present in fetal blood at maternal levels within 2 hours of alcohol consumption. Healthcare professionals should counsel all individuals not to drink any alcohol while pregnant.
- There is a dose-related risk, with increased risk of fetal alcohol spectrum disorders (FASDs) with heavy or binge drinking. FASD is estimated to occur in 0.2 to 1.5 of 1,000 births.
- Even small amounts of alcohol, less than one-half drink per day, while pregnant have resulted in harmful outcomes for the infant. Alcohol-related birth defects (ARBDs) are related to the following:
  - Gestational age at exposure and the individual susceptibility of the fetus
  - Amount and pattern of alcohol consumed
  - Maternal metabolism and peak blood alcohol levels
- Decreased birth weight and impact on the fetus correlated with exposure in any trimester. Dysmorphia and growth disturbance were increased in females with first-trimester alcohol use. Birth weight was more significantly affected by second-trimester exposure.
- The characteristics are facial dysmorphia (e.g., smooth philtrum, midface hypoplasia, broad flat nasal bridge, thin vermilion border, short palpebral fissures). Core CNS abnormalities (e.g., dysgenesis of the corpus callosum, cerebellar hypoplasia) may also be noted. Less frequently described are skeletal anomalies, abnormal hand creases, and ophthalmologic, renal, and cardiac anomalies (Blackburn, 2018; D'Apolito, 2021; Prasad & Jones, 2019; Reis & Jnah, 2017; Sullivan, 2016; Wallman, 2018).

Childhood Effects: Fetal Alcohol Spectrum Disorders

- *Fetal alcohol spectrum disorders (FASD)*, the term for the range of effects that may result from prenatal alcohol exposure, is among the most common identifiable causes of developmental delay and intellectual disability, with an average IQ of 67. FASD is not a diagnostic term, rather it refers to specific conditions such as fetal alcohol syndrome (FAS) and alcohol-related neurodevelopmental disorder (ARND). FASD is the result of neuronal damage by alcohol ingestion while pregnant and is preventable.
- Physical characteristics may be noted in the neonate; behavioral problems and learning deficits may be identified after the neonatal period. Collectively, the findings are referred to as FASD and the newborn may have craniofacial deformities, growth problems, and CNS abnormalities.
- It is difficult to obtain exact data on the number of infants exposed to alcohol in utero who subsequently develop FASD; it is estimated that potentially 2 to 5 of every 100 schoolchildren exhibit characteristics of FASD. FASD is diagnosed based on history and physical findings. No laboratory tests are available to determine the extent of fetal alcohol exposure (Alpan, 2020; Jackson, et al., 2021; Reis, & Jnah, 2017; Sullivan, 2016; Wallen & Gleason, 2018; Wallman, 2018).

Treatment

- Consensus guidelines recommend that the safest choice for a patient is to not drink alcohol during pregnancy. It is critical that patients be advised about the risks to their infant as early as possible in the pregnancy. Advice should ideally be given before pregnancy because most pregnant patients do not begin prenatal care until after the first important weeks of pregnancy have passed.
- Treatment for alcoholism is largely psychosocial, with an emphasis on brief interventions. The influence of a nonjudgmental provider cannot be overemphasized. Reduction in alcohol use by heavy drinkers (defined as those having a positive screen on the T-ACE) was greater when a partner chosen by the patient was included in the intervention.
- Treatment of ethanol withdrawal is supportive and relies on benzodiazepines. Heavy reliance is also placed on psychosocial approaches to alcohol addiction (Lüscher, 2021; Prasad & Jones, 2019; Woodward et al., 2018).

MARIJUANA/TETRAHYDROCANNABINOL

- Marijuana is the most common illicit drug implicated in SUD and is the most common illicit substance used in pregnancy. Marijuana is commonly coupled with other exposures. In 2011, there were 18.1 million past-month users. Marijuana use during pregnancy continues to rise in correlation with the legalization of marijuana for both medical and recreational use in some states (D'Apolito, 2021; Prasad & Jones, 2019; Sullivan, 2016; Wallman, 2018).

Pharmacology

- Marijuana is derived from the hemp plant (*Cannabis* species). The active substance in marijuana is delta-9-tetrahydrocannabinol (THC). THC content is 10% to 15%. The dried leaves are most commonly smoked, and in the process 20% to 50% of the THC content is absorbed in the lungs.
- Activation of the CB1 receptors stimulates the mesolimbic dopamine system, which is thought to mediate the rewarding and reinforcing effect of the drug.

■ Marijuana refers to the dried leaves, flowers, stems, and seeds from the hemp plant *Cannabis sativa*, while hashish refers to the resin that the plant produces. The main psychoactive ingredient is delta-9-THC, a small, highly lipophilic molecule that binds to the endogenous cannabinoid receptors (CB1 and CB2) and modifies the release of several neurotransmitters.

■ The half-life of THC is about 4 hours. The onset of effects of THC after smoking marijuana occurs within minutes and reaches a maximum after 1 to 2 hours. THC can be stored in body tissues for as long as 30 days in chronic users, leading to prolonged fetal exposure. THC readily crosses the placenta and collects in the amniotic fluid, while its major metabolite does not (D'Apolito, 2021; Hudak, 2020; Lüscher, 2021; Prasad & Jones, 2019; Wallman, 2018; Wallen & Gleason, 2018).

Screening

■ Methods for screening include the following:
   ● *SBIRT:* a brief intervention approach to treatment of people with SUD or who are at risk of future dependence on alcohol and other substances
   ● *The Four Ps:* asks patients about substance use
   ● *NIDA Quick Screen:* an online screening tool for substance abuse filled out by patients (D'Apolito, 2021)

Fetal/Neonatal Effects

■ Marijuana extract and THC have been studied in many animal models, and no pattern of malformation has emerged as uniquely associated with marijuana exposure.

■ Research in the literature is conflicting, with some studies finding no independent effect on the fetus and others finding decreased fetal growth restriction, prematurity, and stillbirth. Marijuana remains in the body tissues of chronic users for as long as 30 days and can result in prolonged fetal exposure.

■ In a large longitudinal study, the rates of preterm birth, NICU admission, and perinatal mortality were not increased among users. However, sustained weekly use was linked to a trend toward decreased birth weight.

■ Babies may display altered neurobehaviors including response to visual stimuli, increased tremulousness, and high-pitched cry, prolonged startle response, or altered sleep. There is an association between newborns exposed to marijuana prenatally and decreased executive skills, including poor impulse control, visual memory, and attention deficit. Longitudinal studies need to be viewed with the understanding that other licit and illicit substances, as well as social determinants of health, may confound the results (Hudak, 2020; Prasad & Jones, 2019; Jackson et al., 2021; Prasad & Jones, 2019; Sullivan, 2016; Wallman, 2018).

Childhood Effects

■ While some studies show a correlation between prenatal marijuana use and increased hyperactivity, impulsivity, inattention symptoms, and delinquency, other studies have reported minimal effects on cognition, language, and motor development.

■ Prenatal marijuana exposure is reported to be associated with deficiencies in executive function in 9- to 12-year-olds, and recent reports have found that prenatal marijuana exposure has a significant effect on school-age intellectual performance.

■ The amount of abnormality seems to be associated with dose and timing of exposure. No changes in intellectual testing were present in children 3 years of age. Children who were exposed during the first and second trimester of pregnancy demonstrated more hyperactivity, impulsivity, and decreased attention at the age of 10. By the age of 14, children had lower reading, math, and spelling scores (D'Apolito, 2021; Hudak, 2020; Jackson et al., 2021; Sullivan, 2016; Wallen & Gleason, 2018).

Treatment

■ No effective pharmacologic agent is available for treatment of marijuana dependence (Blackburn, 2018h; Hudak, 2020; Prasad & Jones, 2019).

COCAINE

■ The 2010 National Survey on Drug Use and Health (NSDUH) found that 1.5 million Americans were current cocaine users (Prasad & Jones, 2019).

Pharmacology

■ Cocaine is a highly addictive lipophilic alkaloid extracted from the leaves of the plant *Erythroxylum coca*. Rapid tolerance develops and is the basis for the rapid addictive process. It causes blockade of the myocardial fast sodium channels and results in prolongation of the QRS complex and dysrhythmia. Blockade of dopamine reuptake centrally produces a profound euphoria, which is responsible for the high addictive potential. The norepinephrine release related to euphoria augments the norepinephrine reuptake mechanism and contributes further to vasoconstriction and pursuit of the pleasure response.

■ Cocaine has high lipid solubility, low molecular weight, and low ionization at physiologic pH, and thus crosses the placenta by simple diffusion.
   ● There is a low level of plasma esterase in the fetus, and cocaine accumulates secondary to the relatively low pH of fetal blood.

■ Cocaine is metabolized by plasma and hepatic cholinesterases, with renal clearance of the inactive compounds produced. Plasma cholinesterase activity is decreased in pregnant patients, fetuses, and infants, which increases the half-life of cocaine (Hudak, 2020;

Jackson et al., 2021; Prasad & Jones, 2019; Sullivan, 2016; Wallman, 2018).

Screening

■ Cocaine may be detected in neonatal urine for up to 7 days after delivery (Hudak, 2020).

Fetal/Neonatal Effects

■ Cocaine is lipid-soluble and readily crosses the placenta and enters the fetal brain. Cocaine causes significant vasoconstriction and decreases blood flow to the placenta and uterus. This decreases oxygen delivery to the fetus.

■ The vasoconstrictive properties of cocaine can have a wide range of fetal effects. Vasoconstriction related to cocaine use has been correlated with placental abruption, intestinal atresia, and necrotizing enterocolitis in a small series of term and preterm newborns. Cocaine users have an increased risk of giving birth to an infant with urinary tract defects.

■ Cocaine crosses the placenta easily. Cocaine use in pregnancy is associated with preterm birth, small-for-gestational-age (SGA) infants, younger gestational age at birth, and reduced birth weight. Infants who were exposed to tobacco and cocaine or marijuana had less alert responsiveness. Infants with prenatal exposure to cocaine were significantly more likely to require medical support or resuscitation.

■ Acute cocaine use in the third trimester can result in preterm labor, abruptio placenta, increased incidence of premature rupture of membranes, increased meconium staining, precipitous delivery, prematurity, and LBW.

■ The half-life of cocaine is longer in the fetus and neonate than in the adult; thus, cocaine may be present in the neonate for several days after birth. Neurobehavioral abnormalities in infants with in utero cocaine exposure are often seen on day 2 or 3 of life.

■ Neonates exposed to cocaine may be irritable, tremulous, drowsy, and have respiratory distress. These neurobehaviors may reflect the effect of the drug as opposed to withdrawal.

■ Newborns may also present with tachycardia, arrhythmias, hypertension, vasoconstriction, diaphoresis, and mild tremors when cocaine is present in the bloodstream as a result of maternal use. When cocaine use occurs shortly before delivery, there is an association with transient neonatal ventricular tachycardia (Alpan, 2020; Blackburn, 2018; D'Apolito, 2021; Hudak, 2020; Jackson, et al., 2021; Prasad & Jones, 2019; Sullivan, 2016; Wallman, 2018).

Childhood Effects

■ Prenatal cocaine exposure is associated with an increased risk of specific cognitive impairments (visual-spatial skills, general knowledge, and arithmetic skills). Children under the age of 6 who were exposed to cocaine in utero may have growth problems, difficulty controlling inhibitions and paying attention, as well as poor language and motor skills. Large prospective studies have shown relatively subtle cocaine-associated deficits that are dose-dependent. Subtle effects may have a financial impact on schools due to increased numbers of children requiring special services.

■ The home environment is the most important independent predictor of outcome, suggesting the potential to compensate for in utero drug exposure (D'Apolito, 2021; Hudak, 2020; Prasad & Jones, 2019).

Treatment

■ Healthcare providers should offer women accurate and specific information on complications associated with drug use and the increase in morbidity and mortality, including explanation that quitting or decreasing drugs at any time during pregnancy positively impacts maternal and infant outcomes.

■ A strategy to increase feelings of bonding is to encourage the mother and their significant other to listen to fetal heart rate at each visit. Providers can show sonogram pictures to the patient so that they can visualize the fetus. Providers may also promote attachment by recommending attendance at childbirth preparation and parenting classes.

■ Mothers who use cocaine often use other drugs that independently or via drug–drug interactions can affect long-term outcomes of interest. Environmental risk factors (e.g., poverty and exposure to domestic violence or community violence) and caregiver attributes also modulate long-term outcomes. The presence of factors that can confer resiliency to the child may countermand any adverse effects of antenatal exposure. An enriched postnatal environment over the first several years appears crucial in modulating any effects of cocaine on the infant's cognitive and behavioral development. Early intervention should be used in all high-risk infants, particularly those exposed to illicit stimulants prenatally (Hudak, 2020; Sullivan, 2016; Woodward et al., 2018).

METHAMPHETAMINE

■ In the NSDUH, methamphetamine exposure decreased; however, despite the trend, methamphetamine use remains a significant problem in some areas (Prasad & Jones, 2019).

Pharmacology

■ Methamphetamine blocks the reuptake of adrenergic neurotransmitters. Methamphetamine is a sympathomimetic agent that induces euphoria and increases alertness and self-confidence as it produces a massive efflux of dopamine in the CNS. Methamphetamine may be identified in urine drug screens and remains detectable for up to 3 days (Hudak, 2020; Prasad & Jones, 2019; Sullivan, 2016).

Screening

■ There are no well-validated measures that accurately detect stimulant use. Detection depends on accurate self-report. Similar to pregnancies of cocaine users, pregnancies of amphetamine users are characterized by poor prenatal care, sexually transmitted diseases, and cardiovascular problems including placental abruption and postpartum hemorrhage. Other characteristics are "meth mouth," severe tooth decay, dry mouth, and gum disease (Prasad & Jones, 2019; Sullivan, 2016; Wallen & Gleason, 2018).

Fetal/Neonatal Effects

■ Prenatal amphetamine exposure has been shown in some early research to lead to congenital brain lesions, including hemorrhage, infarction, or cavitary lesions.

■ Case reports demonstrate, but do not confirm, cardiovascular, gastrointestinal (GI), and CNS abnormalities; facial clefts; and limb reduction defects, with increased risk of malformation.

■ Due to its vasoconstrictive properties, methamphetamine exposure during pregnancy increases the risk of preterm birth, LBW, and SGA infants. Additionally, small head circumference and increased risk of neonatal death are reported.

■ Neonatal effects mimic those of cocaine. In the neonatal period, neurologic abnormalities, including decreased arousal, poor state control, difficulty with habituation, tremors, hyperactive neonatal reflexes, abnormal cry, increased stress, drowsiness, poor feeding, and seizures, have been reported. Use of methamphetamines may be toxic to the fetal brain and may increase the risk of SIDS (D'Apolito, 2021; Jackson et al., 2021; Prasad & Jones, 2019).

Childhood Effects

■ Long-term adverse neurotoxic effects of in utero methamphetamine exposure on behavior, cognitive skills, and physical dexterity have been reported. Heavy prenatal methamphetamine exposure was associated with anxiety, depression, and attention problems at 3 years of age.

■ Although limited, studies of amphetamine exposure suggest long-term challenges. Prenatal methamphetamine exposure places children at increased risk of anxious/depressive problems and emotional reactivity during the preschool period. By school age, externalizing behaviors (aggressive behavior, rule-breaking) and ADHD symptoms also become more common (D'Apolito, 2021; Hudak, 2020;

Prasad & Jones, 2019; Sullivan, 2016; Woodward et al., 2018).

Treatment

■ There is no pharmacologic treatment for methamphetamine use. Management is psychosocial (Prasad & Jones, 2019). See treatment discussion in the "Cocaine" section.

BENZODIAZEPINES

■ Benzodiazepines are among the most frequently prescribed medications for pregnant women. Diazepam (Valium), alprazolam (Xanax), lorazepam (Ativan), clonazepam (Klonopin), and chlordiazepoxide (Librium) are the most common drugs. Diazepam (Valium) is the only benzodiazepine for which there is sufficient research among pregnant women (Prasad & Jones, 2019).

Pharmacology

■ Benzodiazepines affect the neuroinhibitory neurotransmitter GABA and appear to act on the limbic, thalamic, and hypothalamic level of the CNS to produce sedative and hypnotic effects, reduce anxiety and anticonvulsant effects, and for skeletal relaxation (Prasad & Jones, 2019).

Screening

■ There are no well-validated brief measures to identify benzodiazepine use. Benzodiazepine dependence is very common, and diagnosis of addiction is probably often missed as they are commonly prescribed as anxiolytics and sleep medications. Detection relies on self-report. The self-report of anxiety symptoms during the first trimester of pregnancy is 18% (D'Apolito, 2021; Lüscher, 2021; Prasad & Jones, 2019).

Fetal/Neonatal Effects

■ Diazepam is transferred across the placenta and accumulates in the fetal circulation at about one to three times the level in maternal blood. Presence can lead to preterm delivery, LBW, ventilation at birth, poor muscle tone, poor feeding, drowsiness, poor suck, and hypothermia.

■ Infants who have had a combined exposure to benzodiazepines and opioids demonstrate an increased incidence of NAS. Symptoms may present up to 2 to 3 weeks after birth, complicating the diagnosis and treatment of the problem. Benzodiazepines with longer half-lives are associated with more severe signs and length of withdrawal symptoms. Symptoms may include hypertonia, hypotonia, excessive or poor suck, and vomiting.

● Infants with severe signs are usually treated with phenobarbital (Luminal). Outpatient weaning of phenobarbital has been reported to require weeks to months (D'Apolito, 2021; Hudak, 2020; Prasad & Jones, 2019).

Childhood Effects

- The effects of in utero exposure to benzodiazepines are similar to those of opioids. It has been difficult to differentiate the relative contributions of the drug from those of the child's social environment.
- Children prenatally exposed to benzodiazepines score higher on tests for oppositional-defiant disorder and aggression. Increased internalizing behaviors (anxiousness, emotional reactivity, somatic complaints) and externalizing behaviors (aggression, attention problems) are seen at 1.5 and 3 years of age (D'Apolito, 2021; Prasad & Jones, 2019).

Treatment

- Treatment of benzodiazepine addiction is difficult because the drug is associated with poor psychological functioning and a reduced effect of other interventions for illicit drug use. Successful withdrawal from benzodiazepines is likely to occur only when the taper from benzodiazepine dose is slow and gradual, and in the context of extensive psychological counseling and support (Prasad & Jones, 2019).

OPIOIDS

- The United States is experiencing an epidemic of addiction to prescribed controlled substances, often originally administered for management of chronic pain. More than 116 million Americans receive pharmacologic treatment for chronic pain. Opioid use among pregnant patients increased six times from 2000 to 2009 and continues to increase. Females aged 25 to 34 years are most likely to misuse prescription painkillers. The National Survey on Drug Use and Health (NSDUH) in 2013 found that pregnant females 15 to 17 years of age account for 14.6% of illicit drug users.
- Pregnant patients are uniquely vulnerable to opiate use for many reasons. Opiates are exceedingly addictive and are often obtained by trading sex for drugs. Heroin use in particular is strongly associated with the behaviors of a male partner. Chronic heroin use is estimated to affect 810,000 to 1 million Americans (Prasad & Jones, 2019; Reis, & Jnah, 2017).

Pharmacology

- Opioids are alkaloids derived from the opium poppy and include all opiates plus the semisynthetics, which are derived from alkaloids (hydrocodone, oxycodone, and heroin) plus synthetics (methadone, fentanyl, nalbuphine, and buprenorphine).

- Opiates/opioids are small molecular weight and variably lipophilic compounds that cross both blood–brain and placental barriers. Opiates can be inhaled, injected, snorted, swallowed, or used subcutaneously.
  - 70% of opiate users relapse within 6 weeks of nonmedication rehabilitation efforts (Hudak, 2020; Prasad & Jones, 2019).

Screening

- There are no well-validated screening measures for opioid dependence. A brief interview may uncover opioid abuse. Biologic testing, with the patient's consent, may be warranted.
- Amniotic fluid, cord blood, breast milk, and newborn urine and meconium contain measurable amounts of morphine, the major metabolite of heroin, methadone, and buprenorphine. Urine and meconium can be obtained for toxicology testing. Umbilical cord can be used for toxicology as well. Umbilical cord samples may not be as sensitive as meconium (Jackson et al., 2021; Prasad & Jones, 2019).

Fetal/Neonatal Effects

- Opioid use in pregnancy is associated with intrauterine growth restriction, LBW, placental abruption, preterm labor and birth, fetal death, and in utero passage of meconium. Human and animal studies have shown a direct effect on fetal growth with opioid exposure in pregnancy.
- Common adverse outcomes include preterm delivery, LBW, and perinatal mortality. Other adverse outcomes are attributed to drug-seeking behaviors, concomitant smoking, and inadequate nutrition. An increase in the frequency of SIDS has been noted.
- Between 30% and 80% of infants will develop NAS and require treatment. Signs of withdrawal can occur up to 6 days of life.
- NAS is a risk for all opiate-exposed infants. NAS most often occurs with a mean onset of treatable symptoms at 48 to 72 hours of life and average withdrawal lasting 28 days or more. No studies found a dose–response relationship with maternal use of methadone and NAS. See later discussion for more details (D'Apolito, 2021; Jackson et al., 2021; Prasad & Jones, 2019; Reis & Jnah, 2017; Sullivan, 2016).

Childhood Effects

- Research suggests that school-age children who were exposed to heroin in utero experience developmental delay and may exhibit aggressiveness, hyperactivity, and disinhibition. Variations in parental care may modify the expression of the effects of in utero drug exposure. Exposure to methadone and buprenorphine in utero may result in lower function on tasks requiring short-term memory, inhibition, and lower scores on executive function in children 48 to 57 months of age (D'Apolito, 2021; Prasad & Jones, 2019).

Treatment (Maternal)

- The goal of treatment in pregnancy is maintenance and to provide a dosage of medication-assisted treatment that prevents drug cravings and illicit use and does not create euphoria Opioid detoxification and abstinence during pregnancy are not recommended due to the risk of fetal distress and fetal loss. Detoxification in pregnancy has a relapse rate of more than 50%. Inpatient detoxification may be the only alternative to illicit drug use if the mother does not have access to a supervised opioid maintenance program (Hudak, 2020; Prasad & Jones, 2019).

METHADONE (DOLOPHINE)

- Methadone is a full mu agonist and a weak NMDA receptor agonist. It is well absorbed orally and exhibits a mean half-life of approximately 1 day (vs. only 15–30 minutes for heroin) to produce a sustained effect.
- Benefits of methadone treatment with dosing that sustains opioid concentrations in the mother and the fetus include decreased high-risk behaviors, reduced incarceration, decreased spread of infectious disease, decreased opioid craving, and prevention of fetal stress. Methadone treatment of SUD is associated with decreased maternal complications, decreased prematurity, and improved birth weight (Hudak, 2020; Prasad & Jones, 2019; Sullivan, 2016).

BUPRENORPHINE (SUBUTEX)

- Buprenorphine alone or combined with naloxone (Suboxone) has been used as a primary treatment for heroin addiction and as a replacement for methadone. Buprenorphine is a partial mu agonist and has a very high affinity for the mu opioid receptor. Treatment can be accomplished on an outpatient basis and does not require a daily visit to a maintenance program.
  - One study demonstrated a shorter length of stay for infant treatment of NAS, lower doses of morphine needed for NAS treatment, and shorter duration of treatment as outcomes of maternal treatment with buprenorphine (Hudak, 2020; Prasad & Jones, 2019; Sullivan, 2016).

▶ NEONATAL ABSTINENCE SYNDROME

DEFINITION

- *NAS* is the term that encompasses a constellation of clinical signs associated with opioid withdrawal. The term was introduced into the literature over two decades ago to describe the variable spectrum of signs of neonatal neurologic and behavioral dysregulation that occurs as a result of withdrawal from certain psychoactive drugs, particularly those that cause addiction in adults. The neurobehavioral findings associated specifically with opioid withdrawal at birth, following in utero exposure, have been termed *neonatal abstinence syndrome (NAS)*.
  - NAS is a postnatal drug withdrawal syndrome exhibited by some opioid-exposed infants during pregnancy. It is characterized by hyperactivity of the central and autonomic nervous system and GI system.
  - NAS is the constellation of signs and symptoms associated with withdrawal, often polysubstance exposure including opioids.
  - NAS can result from a variety of opioids, including prescription opioids (e.g., hydrocodone), illicit opioids (e.g., heroin), or medication-assisted treatment (e.g., methadone).
  - Classic NAS occurs secondary to maternal use of morphine, heroin, methadone, buprenorphine, and other prescription opioid analgesics (e.g., oxycodone), and may be combined with withdrawal or effects from antidepressants (particularly SSRIs), anxiolytics, nicotine, and other substances.
- Neonatal abstinence is described as a generalized disorder characterized by CNS hyperirritability, GI dysfunction, respiratory distress, and autonomic dysfunction manifesting as vague symptoms such as yawning, hiccups, sneezing, mottled skin color, and fever.
- The collection of symptoms associated with withdrawal from a dependency-producing substance is called *NAS*. In neonates exposed to opioids in utero, 55% to 94% will develop signs of withdrawal. From 2004 to 2013, the rate of NICU admissions for NAS increased from 7 per 1,000 admissions to 27 cases per 1,000 admissions. In 2014, the rate of NAS was 6.5 per 1,000 hospital deliveries in the United States.
  - Exposure to heroin in utero is associated with intrauterine growth restriction. From 2004 to 2013, the median length of stay of an infant with NAS increased from 13 to 19 days.
- The increase in infants diagnosed with NAS correlates directly with the increase in maternal opioid use in pregnancy. Studies demonstrate inconsistent results when evaluating the relationship between the mother's dose of methadone (Dolophine) and NAS severity; approximately 50% of studies find a relationship and 50% find no relationship (Alpan, 2020; D'Apolito, 2021; Hudak, 2020; Jackson et al., 2021; Partick, 2017; Rohan, 2021; Wallen & Gleason, 2018; Wallman, 2018).

PATHOPHYSIOLOGY

- A neonate can develop dependence secondary to exposure in utero to opiates or opioids used to treat chronic pain, misused by the mother, or for treatment of SUD. A neonate can also develop an iatrogenic dependence due to opioids used for analgesia and sedation after birth. Opiates and opioids that result in dependence include heroin, methadone, morphine, buprenorphine, fentanyl, and other narcotic analgesics.

- Opioid withdrawal is complicated in the newborn due to complex maternal–fetal–placental pharmacokinetics as well as the immaturity of the fetus and newborn neurologic system. The absence of opioids after birth causes an increase in norepinephrine production, which causes most of the clinical symptoms in NAS.
  - Because opioid receptors are located in the CNS and GI tract, NAS causes CNS irritability and GI system dysfunction, in addition to autonomic nervous system overactivity.
- The most severe withdrawal symptoms occur with exposure to opioids, although other drugs can also trigger symptoms.
- Withdrawal in the newborn is physiologic and is not an addiction. Neonates should not be referred to as "addicts" because the practice of addiction involves active, drug-seeking behaviors (D'Apolito, 2021; Jackson et al., 2021; Rohan, 2021; Wallman, 2018).

CLINICAL FEATURES OF NEONATAL ABSTINENCE SYNDROME

- During in utero exposure to addictive substances, the fetus undergoes a biochemical adaptation. At delivery, supply of the substance is discontinued, but newborn metabolism and clearance continue. Withdrawal occurs when critically low levels of the substance in the neonatal system are reached.
- The timing of onset of withdrawal symptoms is dependent on multiple factors, including timing of the most recent exposure, type of opioid exposure, dose of exposure, and level of neurologic maturity in the newborn.
- Most infants exposed to opioids appear physically and behaviorally normal at birth. The presentation of symptoms often begins within 24 to 72 hours of birth.
  - Withdrawal from heroin, which has a short half-life, usually begins within 24 hours of birth.
  - Withdrawal from treatment medications, which have a longer half-life, occurs at 48 to 72 hours after birth.
    - ❏ Methadone withdrawal, which is stored in the fetal lung, liver, and spleen, typically begins at 24 to 72 hours of life.
    - ❏ Buprenorphine (Subutex) withdrawal symptoms peak at 40 hours and are most severe at 70 hours of age.
  - Symptoms of withdrawal may present as late as 7 to 14 days after birth (Hudak, 2020).

- The most common symptoms of NAS primarily occur in the CNS, GI system, and autonomic nervous system.
- Table 5.3 details the symptoms of NAS.
  - Tremors are typically mild and progress from occurring only with stimulation to occurring spontaneously. Disturbed and undisturbed tremors, hyperactive Moro reflex, excess irritability, and failure to thrive are more frequent in infants exposed to methadone in utero. Nasal stuffiness, sneezing, and loose stools are more commonly seen in infants exposed to buprenorphine in utero.
  - In 2% to 11% of infants, seizures may occur in acute withdrawal. These seizures have an unknown etiology and unknown long-term significance. In the absence of seizure activity, abnormal electroencephalograms have been noted in more than 30% of infants exposed to opiates in utero.
- Symptoms usually resolve within 2 weeks, but some mild signs persist for up to 6 months. The severity of NAS does not correlate well with the dose or duration of in utero substance exposure but is affected by the drug or drugs used. Perceived severity of NAS may be affected by the infant's hunger and environmental stimuli (D'Apolito, 2021; Hudak, 2020; Jackson et al., 2021; Rohan, 2021; Wallman, 2018).

Table 5.3 Symptoms of Neonatal Abstinence Syndrome

CNS Symptoms	GI Symptoms	Autonomic Symptoms
■ Tremors (disturbed and undisturbed) ■ Jitteriness ■ Hyperactive Moro reflex ■ Myoclonic jerks ■ Seizures ■ Irritability ■ Poor sleep pattern ■ Excessive/high-pitched crying ■ Increased muscle tone	■ Poor feeding ■ Poor weight gain ■ Hyperphagia (excessive desire to eat) ■ Emesis ■ Diarrhea	■ Sneezing ■ Yawning ■ Mottling ■ Hiccups ■ Nasal stuffiness ■ Fever ■ Sweating

CNS, central nervous system; GI, gastrointestinal.
Sources: Data from Hudak, M. (2020). Infants of substance using mothers. In R. Martin, A. Fanaroff, & M. Walsh (Eds.), *Fanaroff and Martin's neonatal–perinatal medicine: Diseases of the fetus and infant* (11th ed., p. 740). Elsevier; D'Apolito, K. (2021). Perinatal substance abuse. In T. Verklan, M. Walden & Forest, S. (Eds.), *Core curriculum for neonatal intensive care nursing* (6th ed., pp. 45–46). Elsevier; Wallman, C. (2018). Assessment of the newborn with antenatal exposure to drugs. In E. P. Tappero & M. E. Honeyfield (Eds.), *Physical assessment of the newborn* (6th ed., pp. 259–260). Springer Publishing Company; Jackson, J., Knappen, B., & Olsen, S. (2021). Drug withdrawal in the neonate. In S. Gardner, B. Carter, M. Enzman-Hines, & S. Niermeyer (Eds.), *Merenstein & Gardner's handbook of neonatal intensive care* (9th ed., p. 260). Elsevier.

NEONATAL ABSTINENCE SYNDROME SCORING TOOLS

- Objective and ongoing scoring of symptoms of NAS can assist the clinician with decision-making. Multiple tools exist to assist with discrete scoring for NAS. These include the Finnegan Neonatal Abstinence Scoring System, Neonatal Drug Withdrawal Scoring System (the Lipsitz Tool), Neonatal Withdrawal Inventory, Neonatal Narcotic Withdrawal Index, MOTHER NAS Scale, and Neonatal Network Neurobehavioral Scale.
- The Finnegan Neonatal Abstinence Scoring System is the tool used most frequently for scoring neonatal withdrawal in the United States. The Finnegan scoring tool has been studied for validity and reliability.
  - The Finnegan scoring tool uses 21 individual items with a weighted score based on severity. The total score is determined by adding the individual scores together during an assigned scoring interval.
- The Lipsitz Tool is simple to use and has good sensitivity in identifying clinically important withdrawal. The Lipsitz Tool was recommended in the 1998 AAP statement on neonatal drug withdrawal and remains in use.
- Regardless of the choice of scoring tool, one of the most important factors for effective utilization is training and ongoing education for the staff and providers who implement the tool; poor interrater consistency may lead to ineffective medical management (Alpan, 2020; Hudak, 2020; Jackson et al., 2021; Wallman, 2018).

TREATMENT OF NEONATAL ABSTINENCE SYNDROME

Nonpharmacologic Therapy

- Box 5.2 details nonpharmacologic supportive care strategies for infants with NAS.
- The goal of care and treatment is to ensure the infant is able to eat and sleep to ensure adequate weight gain and socialization skills.
  - Regardless of nonpharmacologic or pharmacologic treatment needs, infants with severe signs of withdrawal may require increased calories to achieve growth due to increased metabolic rate, emesis, and loose stools. Infants with NAS may require 150 to 250 cal/kg/d to achieve growth.
  - Infants with severe NAS need careful observation for fever, dehydration, and weight loss. Stabilization with gavage feeding, IV fluids, and electrolytes may be required (Alpan, 2020; Hudak, 2020).

Box 5.2 Nonpharmacologic Strategies for the Infant With Neonatal Abstinence Syndrome

- Small/frequent demand feedings with increased calorie feedings
- Frequent diaper changing and skin care
- Minimizing environmental stimulation (light and noise) and unnecessary handling
- Mittens over the hands (to prevent scratching)
- Pacifier for excessive sucking (nonnutritive)
- Rocking and swaddling
- Soft sheets or sheepskin (decrease excoriation)

Sources: Data from Hudak, M. (2020). Infants of substance-using Mothers. In R. Martin, A. Fanaroff, & M. Walsh (Eds.), *Fanaroff and Martin's neonatal–perinatal medicine: Diseases of the fetus and infant* (11th ed., p. 742). Elsevier; D'Apolito, K. (2021). Perinatal substance abuse. In T. Verklan, M. Walden & Forest, S. (Eds.), *Core curriculum for neonatal intensive care nursing* (6th ed., pp. 47-48). Elsevier; Rohan, A. (2021). Common neonatal complications. In K. Simpson & P. Creehan (Eds.), *Perinatal nursing* (4th ed., p. 673). Wolters Kluwer.

Pharmacologic Therapy

- The goal of medications to treat NAS is to relieve severe signs and symptoms and prevent complications such as fever, weight loss, and seizures if nonpharmacologic care is not able to manage the symptoms. The reduction of symptoms is the only clear benefit of drug therapy. Treatment with drugs may disrupt maternal–infant bonding, as well as guarantees prolongation of hospitalization and increased drug exposure.
- Ideal drug treatment uses a protocol to drive drug titration and control symptoms. The literature does not identify an optimal drug or regimen for NAS treatment. Methadone, morphine, and buprenorphine have been used to relieve the symptoms of NAS (D'Apolito, 2021; Hudak, 2020; Jackson et al., 2021).

OPIOIDS

- An opioid is the primary drug for opioid withdrawal symptoms associated with in utero exposure to opiates. Morphine and methadone are the primary choices. Both drugs bind to opioid receptors in the CNS, causing inhibition of the ascending pain pathways and altering the perception and response to pain. Methadone has a long half-life and provides a steadier level, with the benefit of administration at less frequent intervals. It is a full mu agonist and has approximately 90% oral bioavailability.
- Buprenorphine is a partial mu agonist and kappa agonist, has higher receptor affinity and longer duration of action than methadone, and has approximately 50% oral bioavailability. It is rapidly

absorbed sublingually (D'Apolito, 2021; Jackson et al., 2021; Taketoma, 2021).

ADJUNCT THERAPIES

■ If symptoms of NAS are not controlled despite higher ranges of opioid administration, in utero exposure to other nonopioid drugs should be suspected. This is an indication for secondary drug therapy for treatment of NAS, typically from another drug class.

■ Phenobarbital, a sedative–hypnotic, has been used as a primary treatment medication for NAS, but is also used as an adjunct therapy when symptoms are not resolved with the initial maximum opioid therapy. Phenobarbital is a long-acting barbiturate with sedative, hypnotic, and anticonvulsant properties. It depresses the sensory cortex, decreases motor function, and produces drowsiness. Adjunct treatment with phenobarbital may allow weaning of the primary opioid, but outpatient therapy with phenobarbital may be prolonged as it is weaned.

■ Clonidine stimulates alpha-2-adrenoceptors in the brainstem, activating an inhibitory neuron that results in reduced sympathetic outflow from the CNS and palliation of symptoms of excess autonomic activity via a negative feedback mechanism. It decreases symptoms such as tachycardia, diaphoresis, restlessness, and diarrhea. Clonidine has been used in combination with an opioid to treat withdrawal, with limited case series in newborns (Hudak, 2020; Jackson et al., 2021; Patrick, 2017; Taketomo, 2021).

WEANING FROM PHARMACOLOGIC THERAPY

■ When an infant is stable on a dose that is effective, weaning should begin and proceed slowly.
  ● Weaning regimens vary, with some titrated by Finnegan scores, with a frequent wean or increase based on individual scores. Other regimens wean by 10% to 20% of the total (or initial) dose every other day based on mild signs of withdrawal, weight gain, and ability to sleep.
    ❏ Morphine weans by dose and not interval. Morphine is weaned first by 10% of the maximum dose every 48 hours as long as the average score remains less than 8 until 25% of the maximum dose is reached.
    ❏ Once the baby is stable (scores less than 8) on 25% of the maximum dose for 48 hours, morphine is discontinued.
    ❏ Scoring continues for 48 to 72 hours after the final dose is given. If scores are greater than or equal to 8 after morphine is off, one rescue dose is considered and then the previous

dose level is restarted (Hudak, 2020; Patrick, 2017).

Discharge After Completion of Therapy

■ An infant with NAS is 2.5 times more likely to be readmitted to the hospital within 30 days of discharge than an uncomplicated term infant. Signs of NAS can continue for 6 months; therefore, parents and caregivers should be thoroughly educated about infant behaviors following treatment for NAS.

■ Parents of these infants may need guidance in recognizing behaviors necessitating caregiving and education on substances that should not be used around infants as they are detrimental to the health of the baby (e.g., tobacco).

■ Box 5.3 outlines some possible teaching needs of parents with infants after intrauterine drug exposure.

■ Drug use may remain a factor after families are discharged; therefore, follow-up after discharge by available community services should be part of the discharge plan. Pediatrician follow-up should occur within a few days after discharge. Additionally, home nurse visits and child protective services may become involved if necessary. A referral to early intervention services and other community services may be applicable. Ideally, infant care would occur in conjunction with maternal care.

■ SUD does not occur in isolation. Behaviors associated with substance dependence or addiction lead to adverse pregnancy outcomes. Contributing to the development and maintenance of substance use among pregnant patients, the following factors independently place the family, infant, and child at risk of poor developmental outcomes:
  ● Maternal and neonatal/child malnutrition and/or dehydration
  ● Impoverished housing
  ● Polysubstance use and/or psychiatric comorbidity
  ● Exposure to violence and/or physical abuse

■ When substance-using mothers and their infants were assessed for pattern of interaction, both the mother and the newborn demonstrated poor performance on a measure of social engagement. Mothers demonstrated significantly less positive affect and greater detachment, and infants presented fewer behaviors promoting social involvement. This has wide-reaching implications for bonding and future parent–child interactions. Staff should do what they can to encourage parent–infant contact and interaction while the child is hospitalized in order to maximize feelings of parenthood and lay the foundation for their future interactions (Jackson et al., 2021; Patrick, 2017; Prasad & Jones, 2019).

Box 5.3 Parent Teaching in Caring for an Infant With Intrauterine Opioid Exposure

Symptoms May Persist for 2 to 6 Months

- Infants exposed to narcotics in utero are more irritable, less cuddly, and tremulous, and have increased tone: Parent(s) may interpret these behaviors as signs of rejection; the infant may not want to be held or cuddled as other babies.
- Infants are less responsive to visual stimulation.
- Infants are less likely to maintain a quiet-alert state: Let the parent know symptoms are time-limited.
- Infants have poor feeding habits: They continue to regurgitate yet show vigorous sucking of the fists or pacifier. Constant sucking and exaggerated rooting reflex may lead to overfeeding the infant.
- Loose stools continue: It is important to stress good diaper hygiene to prevent infection from excoriated skin.
- Infants are easily disturbed by sounds: Parent may decrease stimuli in the house.
- Infants sweat more than other newborns: Dress the infant appropriately to avoid overheating.
- Infants have high-pitched cry: They are not easily consoled; parents need someone to share infant care and give them some rest from an irritable infant to prevent neglect or abuse.
- Infants have hypertonia.
- Infants have less eye-to-eye contact, which decreases social interaction.

Source: Reproduced with permission from Jackson, J., Knappen, B., & Olsen, S. (2021). Drug withdrawal in the neonate. In S. Gardner, B. Carter, M. Enzman-Hines, & S. Niermeyer (Eds.), *Merenstein & Gardner's handbook of neonatal intensive care* (9th ed., p. 268). Elsevier.

▶ CONCLUSION

While the NNP will manage primarily the neonate who has experienced intrauterine substance exposure, the importance of treating the whole family cannot be overstated. The NNP must have an appreciation for the toll that SUD takes on the adults of the family as well. Regardless of the medication or protocol used in a specific institution, the overall goals remain the same: to decrease the infant's dependence on the substance by balancing the need for treatment with the desire not to extend the infant's hospital stay. The NNP, as part of the entire neonatology staff, has a duty to promote family integrity and prepare the infant and the family to function successfully post discharge.

1. An infant born at 39 weeks presents at 14 days of age with reports from parents of decreased sleeping associated with irritability, loose stools, and difficulty feeding. Maternal history is significant for chronic diazepam (Valium) use for muscle spasms associated with a previous injury. The neonatal nurse practitioner (NNP) would include in the differential diagnosis withdrawal from:

    A. Benzodiazepines
    B. Hallucinogens
    C. Synthetic opiates

2. An infant is born at 40 weeks' gestation to a patient with history of a substance use disorder who is in a medication-assisted recovery therapy with buprenorphine (Subutex). In monitoring the infant for neonatal abstinence syndrome, the neonatal nurse practitioner (NNP) would expect the onset of symptoms at:

    A. 12 to 24 hours after birth
    B. Less than 12 hours after birth
    C. More than 48 hours after birth

3. The neonatal nurse practitioner (NNP) knows that the most appropriate therapy for an infant experiencing benzodiazepine withdrawal is:

    A. Methadone (Dolophine)
    B. Omeprazole (Prilosec)
    C. Phenobarbital (Luminal)

4. The neonatal nurse practitioner (NNP) addresses medication tolerance during maintenance dosing by:

    A. Decreasing the medication dose
    B. Increasing the medication dose
    C. Withdrawing the medication by no more than 10%

5. A mother has a positive urine drug screen and denies substance use in pregnancy. The mother is visibly upset at being "accused of using drugs." The neonatal nurse practitioner (NNP) bases a discussion with the mother on the fact that positive results:

    A. Indicate substance use disorder regardless of timing
    B. Should be confirmed through a separate sample test
    C. Suggest the infant needs to be started on therapy

6. The neonatal nurse practitioner (NNP) converses with a nurse about appropriate timing to begin therapy for neonatal abstinence syndrome (NAS) and explains that the goal of medication therapy is:

    A. Minimal use to shorten hospital stay
    B. Relief of severe signs and symptoms
    C. Substitution of systemic opioids

7. The SBIRT tool is used to screen patients prenatally for:

    A. Gestational diabetes
    B. Hypertension
    C. Substance use

(See answers next page.)

1. A) Benzodiazepines

Symptoms of withdrawal from benzodiazepines may be delayed for up to 2 to 3 weeks after birth. Symptoms may include poor feeding, altered sleep patterns, and gastrointestinal (GI) disturbances. Symptoms from opiates occur within a few hours to days. A withdrawal pattern for hallucinogens has not been established (Hudak, 2020; Prasad & Jones, 2019).

2. C) More than 48 hours after birth

The mean onset of symptoms that require treatment is 48 to 72 hours of life. The NNP would not expect symptoms related to withdrawal to appear prior to 48 hours of age (Reis & Jnah, 2017).

3. C) Phenobarbital (Luminal)

The most appropriate drug for treatment of benzodiazepine withdrawal is phenobarbital. Methadone (Dolophine) is a therapy indicated for opiate withdrawal. Omeprazole (Prilosec) can be used as an adjunct therapy but is not used as a primary therapy for withdrawal (Hudak, 2020; Prasad & Jones, 2019).

4. B) Increasing the medication dose

With repeated use, tolerance occurs and requires escalation of dosing for maintenance. Decreasing doses will prompt withdrawal and there is no established best practice for the best amount by which to decrease (Lüscher, 2021).

5. B) Should be confirmed through a separate sample test

Positive tests should be confirmed as they can occur due to secondhand exposure or prescribed medications. Results should not be treated as absolutes without confirmatory testing. Decisions about infant therapy should be based on the infant's clinical presentation and need for symptom management rather than maternal test results (Hudak, 2020).

6. B) Relief of severe signs and symptoms

The goal of medication treatment for NAS is to relieve severe signs and symptoms and prevent complications such as fever, weight loss, and seizures if nonpharmacologic care is not able to manage the symptoms. The reduction of symptoms is the only clear benefit of drug therapy. Use of medication therapy should extend for however long the infant requires relief. Similarly, the degree of infant distress should dictate the use of opioids, not the assumption that substitution of medication delivery is necessary (D'Apolito, 2021; Hudak, 2020).

7. C) Substance use

SBIRT stands for Screening, Brief Intervention and Referral to Treatment. Brief intervention may provide influence for women using substances during pregnancy. Screenings for hypertension or gestational diabetes are based on physiologic measurements (Hudak, 2020; Prasad & Jones, 2019).

Neonatal Physical Examination, Gestational Age, and Behavioral Assessments

Vivian Carrasquilla-Lopez and Kristin Bindel

6

▶ INTRODUCTION

The physical examination of a newborn is a comprehensive evaluation. It encompasses a review of maternal and familial health histories, as well as antepartum, intrapartum, and delivery histories; an assessment of gestational age (GA) and fetal growth; and a complete and detailed physical examination of the newborn. It is an essential tool in the assessment of the infant's transition to extrauterine life and in the identification of potential risks or signs of disease processes that may threaten their well-being.

▶ GESTATIONAL AGE ASSESSMENT

GA assessment can be accomplished using several different tools. The accuracy of these varies according to when they are performed. The obstetrical estimate should be considered the most accurate and be used if the infant's physical assessment estimates GA within 2 weeks of the obstetrical estimate (Fanaroff et al., 2020; Tappero, 2021; Walker, 2018).

PRENATAL GESTATIONAL AGE ASSESSMENT TOOLS

- ▪ Last menstrual period (LMP) dating (clinical estimate)
- ▪ Naegele's Rule to determine the estimated date of confinement (EDC); add 7 days to the first day of the last normal menstrual period and count back 3 months
  - ● Accuracy dependent on regular menstrual cycles, with ovulation on day 14 of cycle, as well as accurate maternal memory of the last normal
- ▪ First trimester
  - ● GA determined using crown–rump length
  - ● Most accurate at 7 to 9 weeks' gestation
  - ● Accuracy within 7 days
- ▪ Second trimester
  - ● GA determined using biparietal diameter, head circumference, abdominal circumference, and femur length
    - ● Most accurate at 18 to 20 weeks' gestation
      - ❑ 14 to 20 weeks' gestation accuracy ±11 days
      - ❑ 20 to 28 weeks' gestation accuracy ±14 days
      - ❑ 29 to 40 weeks' gestation accuracy ±21 days (Trotter, 2019; Wilkins-Haug & Heffner, 2017)

POSTNATAL GESTATIONAL AGE ASSESSMENT TOOLS

- ▪ Postnatal assessment of GA is based on the premise that fetal physical and neurologic maturation progresses in an organized, predictable manner. This allows for a reasonably accurate estimate of GA, which is critical to determining infant risk for morbidity and proper counseling to families based on the GA of the infant.
- ▪ Postdelivery, the newborn experiences rapidly changing physiologic, biologic, and physical characteristics. GA instruments have best accuracy if used within the first 48 hours of life, before these changes occur. Neurologic and physical findings may also be altered due to disease processes or extreme prematurity (Smith, 2017; Tappero, 2021; Trotter, 2019).

COMMON NEWBORN GESTATIONAL AGE TOOLS

- ▪ Dubowitz
  - ● 10 neurologic and 10 physical criteria
  - ● Combined score accuracy ±2 weeks
  - ● Overestimates GA in premature infants
- ▪ Ballard
  - ● Six neurologic and six physical criteria
  - ● Revised to New Ballard Tool 1991
- ▪ New Ballard
  - ● Able to assess GA between 20 and 44 weeks
  - ● Accuracy ±2 weeks for well or sick infant
  - ● For infants with estimated GA of 20 to 28 weeks, best timing of exam within the first 12 hours of life

❏ Limitations include the need to perform the assessment when the infant is in a quiet, alert state, and gestational age assessments are not valid when used in infants affected by maternal medications, positional deformities (breech), neurologic disorders, or birth asphyxia (Fanaroff et al., 2020; Tappero, 2021; Trotter, 2019).

❏ See Figure 6.1 and Table 6.1.

Maturational Assessment of Gestational Age (New Ballard Score)

Name_____ Date/time of birth_____ Sex _____

Hospital no._____ Date/time of exam _____ Birth weight _____

Race_____ Age when examined _____ Length_____

Apgar score: 1 minute _____ 5 minutes _____ 10 minutes_____ Head circ. _____

Neuromuscular Maturity

Examiner_____

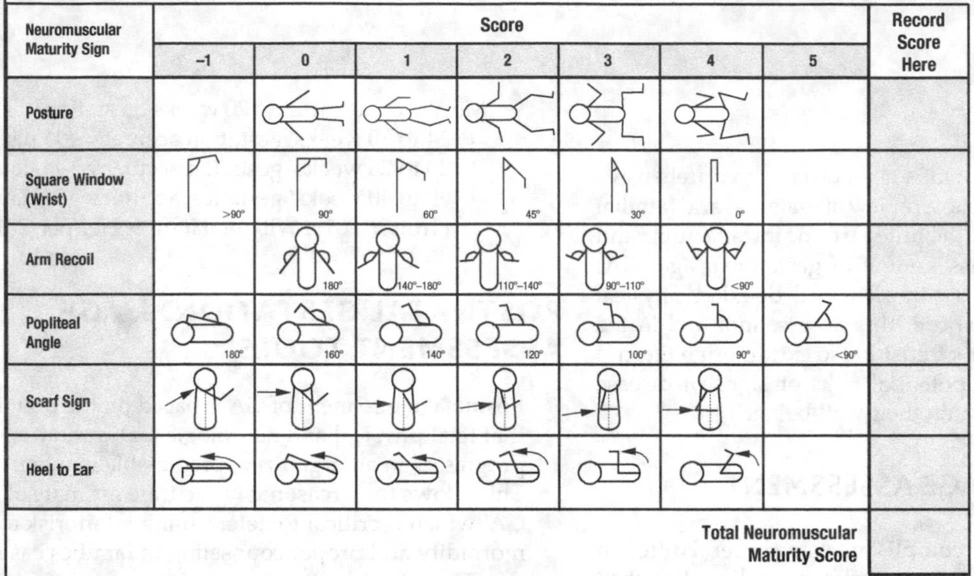

Neuromuscular Maturity Sign	Score							Record Score Here
	−1	0	1	2	3	4	5	
Posture								
Square Window (Wrist)	>90°	90°	60°	45°	30°	0°		
Arm Recoil		180°	140°–180°	110°–140°	90°–110°	<90°		
Popliteal Angle	180°	160°	140°	120°	100°	90°	<90°	
Scarf Sign								
Heel to Ear								

Total Neuromuscular Maturity Score

Physical Maturity

Physical Maturity Sign	Score							Record Score Here
	−1	0	1	2	3	4	5	
Skin	sticky friable transparent	gelatinous red translucent	smooth pink visible veins	superficial peeling and/or rash, few veins	cracking pale area rare veins	parchment deep cracking no vessels	leathery cracked wrinkled	
Lanugo	none	sparse	abundant	thinning	bald areas	mostly bald		
Plantar Surface	heel-toe 40–50 mm:-1 <40 mm:-2	>50 mm no crease	faint red marks	anterior transverse crease only	creases anterior 2/3	creases over entire sole		
Breast	imperceptible	barely perceptible	flat areola no bud	stippled areola 1–2 mm bud	raised areola 3–4 mm bud	full areola 5–10 mm bud		
Eye/Ear	lids fused loosely:- tightly: -21	lids open pinna flat stays folded	sl. curved pinna; soft; slow recoil	well-curved pinna; soft but ready recoil	formed and firm; instant recoil	thick cartilage ear stiff		
Genitals (Male)	scrotum flat, smooth	scrotum empty faint rugae	testes in upper canal rare rugae	testes descending few rugae	testes down and good rugae	testes pendulous deep rugae		
Genitals (Female)	clitoris prominent & labia flat	prominent clitoris & small labia minora	prominent clitoris & enlarging minora	majora & minora equally prominent	majora large minora small	majora cover clitoris and minora		

Total Physical Maturity Score

Score

Neuromuscular_____

Physical_____

Total_____

Maturity Rating

Score	Weeks
−10	20
−5	22
0	24
5	26
10	28
15	30
20	32
25	34
30	36
35	38
40	40
45	42
50	44

Gestational Age (weeks)

By dates_____

By ultrasound_____

By exam_____

Figure 6.1 Ballard exam.

Source: Reprinted with permission from Ballard, J. L., Khoury, J. C., Wedig, K., Wang, L., Eilers-Walsman, B. L., & Lipp, R. (1991). New Ballard score, expanded to include extremely premature infants. *Journal of Pediatrics, 119*(3), 418.

Table 6.1 Summary of the New Ballard Criteria

Neurologic Criteria	Physical Criteria
Posture ■ Hip adduction and flexion increase with increasing GA	**Skin** ■ Transparency decreases with increasing GA ■ Beyond 38 weeks subcutaneous tissue decreases, causing wrinkling and desquamation
Square window ■ Angle decreases with increasing GA ■ Does not change after birth	**Lanugo** ■ Present at 20–28 weeks' GA ■ Decreases with increasing GA
Arm recoil ■ Recoil increases with increasing GA	**Plantar creases** ■ First appear on anterior sole (28–30 weeks) and increase to heel with increasing GA ■ Not an accurate criterion after 12 hours due to drying of skin ■ May be accelerated with oligohydramnios ■ Absence may indicate extreme prematurity or underlying neuromuscular condition
Popliteal angle ■ Angle decreases with increasing GA	**Breast development** ■ Increases with increasing GA ■ No difference between male and female infants
Scarf sign ■ Decreases with increasing GA	**Eyes and ears** ■ Eyes unfused at 26–28 weeks' GA ■ Ear cartilage increases with increasing GA
Heel to ear ■ Decreases with increasing GA	**Genitalia** *Female:* ■ Clitoris becomes less visible with increasing GA ■ Fat deposits in labia majora increase with increasing GA *Male:* ■ Testes descend into the scrotum with increasing GA ■ Rugae of the scrotum increase with increasing GA

GA, gestational age.
Source: Data from Tappero, E. (2021). Physical assessment. In M. T. Verklan, M. Walden, & S. Forest (Eds.), *Core curriculum for neonatal intensive care nursing* (6th ed., pp. 99–130). Elsevier.

▶ EVALUATION OF GROWTH AND MATURITY

DEFINING AGE

■ *GA:* age from the first day of LMP to day of birth
■ *Postmenstrual age (PMA):* age from the first day of LMP to day of assessment

■ *Chronological age:* age from day of birth to day of assessment
■ *Corrected age (CGA):* age from EDC to day of assessment (Trotter, 2019)

GESTATIONAL AGE MATURITY CLASSIFICATIONS

■ *Extremely low gestational age newborn (ELGAN):* 24 to 28 weeks' GA (Fanaroff et al., 2020)
■ *Preterm:* infant born before the end of 37 weeks' GA
■ *Late preterm:* infant born between 34 0/7 and 36 6/7 weeks' GA
■ *Term:* infant born between 38 and 42 weeks' GA
■ *Postterm:* infant born after 42 weeks' GA (Boucher et al., 2017; Smith, 2017; Tappero, 2021)
■ See Table 6.2.

GROWTH CLASSIFICATIONS

■ Normal fetal growth requires contributions from the mother, placenta, and fetus. Intrinsic or extrinsic factors affecting any of these will ultimately affect fetal growth patterns (e.g., race, maternal overall health status, medications during pregnancy, socioeconomic factors, maternal nutrition, altitude, substance abuse, and placental function).
  ● A newborn's growth is assessed using birth measurements of weight, length, and head circumference. These measures should be plotted on recognized acceptable growth curves to determine the infant's growth classification.
    ❏ The U.S. Centers for Disease Control and Prevention (CDC) recommends use of World Health Organization (WHO) curves for 0 to 24 months.
    ❏ The Babson and Benda fetal–infant growth graph extends intrauterine growth from 22 to 10 weeks postterm. Use CDC graphs after 50 weeks.
    ❏ Other recognized, acceptable curves are also available (Smith, 2017; Tappero, 2021; Trotter, 2019).
■ Growth classifications are based on the following growth indices regardless of GA estimation:
  ● *Appropriate for gestational age (AGA):* growth indices between the 10th and 90th percentiles for GA
  ● *Small for gestational age (SGA):* growth indices less than the 10th percentile for GA (Fanaroff et al., 2020)
  ● *Large for gestational age (LGA):* growth indices greater than the 90th percentile for GA
  ● *Occipital frontal circumference (OFC):* should be plotted on growth curve as part of the determination of size—AGA, SGA, or LGA

Table 6.2 Newborn Morbidity and Mortality Risk Based on Maturity Classifications

Maturity Classification	Etiology of Risk	Possible Morbidity
Preterm	■ Immature systems	■ RDS, CLD/BPD ■ NEC ■ ROP ■ Apnea ■ IVH, neurodevelopmental risk ■ Hypotension ■ PDA ■ Nutritional deficiencies, poor growth ■ Fluid and electrolyte imbalances ■ Temperature regulation ■ Immunologic deficiencies, sepsis ■ Anemia ■ Hyperbilirubinemia ■ Perinatal depression
Late preterm	■ Immature systems	■ Respiratory distress ■ Hypoglycemia ■ Hypothermia ■ Apnea ■ Feeding difficulties ■ Hyperbilirubinemia ■ Neurodevelopmental risk ■ Readmission
Term	■ Maternal health history ■ Pre- and intrapartum medications ■ Spontaneous vs. induction of labor ■ *Infection risk:* GBS status/prophylaxis, duration of ROM, maternal fever, chorioamnionitis ■ Fetal presentation ■ *Intrapartum risk factors:* cord prolapse, precipitous delivery, prolonged labor, prolonged head to body delivery interval, signs of fetal distress ■ Delivery mode/assistance	■ *Effects from maternal health conditions:* diabetes, thyroid disease, renal disease, iso- or alloimmunization ■ *Effects from medications:* respiratory depression, hypoglycemia, NAS ■ Immature fetal lungs, retained fetal lung fluid ■ Infection ■ *Birth trauma:* cephalohematoma, subgaleal hemorrhage, shoulder dystocia, brachial plexus injury, facial nerve injury ■ Anemia, perinatal depression, meconium aspiration, pulmonary hypertension, HIE ■ Transient hypoglycemia, hyperbilirubinemia
Postterm	■ Potential placental insufficiency ■ Potential birth complications ■ Occurs in 3%–14% of all pregnancies	■ Nonreassuring fetal HR tracing with labor ■ Meconium aspiration ■ Low Apgar scores ■ Pulmonary hypertension ■ HIE, birth injury ■ Signs of wasting ■ Macrosomia

BPD, bronchopulmonary dysplasia; CLD, chronic lung disease; GBS, group B *Streptococcus*; HIE, hypoxic ischemic encephalopathy; HR, heart rate; IVH, intraventricular hemorrhage; NAS, neonatal abstinence syndrome; NEC, necrotizing enterocolitis; PDA, patent ductus arteriosus; RDS, respiratory distress syndrome; ROM, rupture of membranes; ROP, retinopathy of prematurity.
Source: Data from Abdulhayoglu, E. (2017). Birth trauma. In E. Eichenwald, A. Hansen, C. Martin, & A. Stark (Eds.), *Cloherty and Stark's manual of neonatal care* (8th ed., pp. 64–73). Wolters Kluwer.

■ *Intrauterine growth restriction (IUGR):* This condition occurs when a fetus experiences abnormal, diminished growth velocity, below the expected norms for intrauterine fetal growth patterns over time. The etiology can be intrinsic or extrinsic. Additionally, IUGR is classified into the following:
  ● *Asymmetric IUGR:* also called head sparing; the fetus' head remains relatively normal sized while body growth slows to become disproportionally smaller than anticipated growth indices
  ● *Symmetric IUGR:* proportional decrease in all growth indices (Fanaroff et al., 2020; Johnson, 2019; Smith, 2017; Tappero, 2021; Trotter, 2019; Vargo, 2019; Wilkins-Haug & Heffner, 2017)
■ See Table 6.3.

Table 6.3 Newborn Morbidity and Mortality Risk Based on Growth Classifications

Growth Classification	Etiology	Physical Characteristics	Associated Morbidity
AGA	■ Normal growth of fetus	■ Weight, length, and head circumference within established norms for GA ■ Weight, length, and head circumference plot between the 10th and 90th percentiles for current GA ■ Neuromuscular and physical maturity consistent with GA	■ Normal newborn concerns (birth trauma, transient hypoglycemia or hypothermia, etc.) ■ Morbidities associated with GA (see Table 6.2)

SGA	■ Nonpathologic SGA
	  ● Normal pattern of fetal growth
	  ● Race
	  ● Multiple gestation
	■ Pathologic SGA (see IUGR below)
		■ Nonpathologic SGA:
		  ● Weight and/or length small for established norms for GA
		  ● Weight and/or length <10th percentile for current GA
		  ● Neuromuscular and physical maturity consistent with GA
		■ Pathologic SGA (see IUGR below)
			■ Normal newborn concerns (birth trauma, transient hypoglycemia or hypothermia)
			■ Morbidities associated with GA (see Table 6.2)

Macrosomia/LGA	■ Multiparity ■ Excessive maternal weight gain ■ Abnormal maternal glucose tolerance ■ History of macrosomic infant (incidence 22%) ■ Maternal diabetes (insulin-dependent, noninsulin-dependent, gestational; incidence 20%–40%)	■ Macrosomia (>4,000 g) ■ Large body with AGA head circumference	■ Birth trauma ■ Meconium aspiration ■ RDS ■ Pulmonary hypertension ■ Hypocalcemia ■ Hypoglycemia ■ Hyperinsulinemia ■ Polycythemia ■ Hyperbilirubinemia ■ Poor oral feeding ■ Infrequent congenital heart disease or Beckwith–Wiedemann syndrome
IUGR	■ Maternal age ■ Maternal nutritional status pre- and intrapartum ■ Causes of placental vasoconstriction/insufficiency (maternal smoking) ■ Preeclampsia ■ Chronic hypertension ■ Placental concerns (size, cord anomalies, chronic abruption, choriohemangioma, placental infarction, abnormal cord implantation) ■ Congenital malformations or infections ■ Chromosomal abnormalities (incidence 22%) ■ Multiple gestation (physical space limitations, twin-to-twin transfusion)	■ Wasted appearance of extremities ■ Head disproportionately large for torso ■ Long nails ■ Wizened, old-man face ■ Large anterior fontanel ■ Widened or overlapping cranial sutures ■ Thin umbilical cord with little Wharton jelly ■ Scaphoid abdomen ■ Diminished subcutaneous fat ■ Dry, flaky skin ■ Little vernix ■ Possible meconium staining	■ MAS ■ PPHN ■ Hypotension ■ ATN/renal insufficiency ■ Hypoglycemia ■ Hypothermia ■ Hypoxia ■ Polycythemia/hyperviscosity ■ Neutropenia ■ Thrombocytopenia ■ Sepsis ■ Mortality/morbidity related to underlying etiology ■ Congenital anomaly ■ Perinatal depression ■ Acute renal necrosis/insufficiency

(*continued*)

Table 6.3 Newborn Morbidity and Mortality Risk Based on Growth Classifications (*continued*)

Growth Classification	Etiology	Physical Characteristics	Associated Morbidity
Asymmetric IUGR (head sparing)	■ Etiologic event/process that occurs later in gestation during cellular hypertrophy phase and interferes with oxygen/nutrition delivery to fetus	■ Weight below norm; length and head circumference relatively normal	■ See earlier ■ Potential for postnatal growth and development promising
Symmetric IUGR	■ Etiologic event/process that occurs early in gestation during cellular hyperplasia phase ■ Intrinsic fetal problem (anomaly, chromosomal abnormality, congenital infection)	■ Proportionate below expected growth for weight, length, and head circumference	■ See earlier ■ Potential for growth and development likely limited due to underlying etiology

AGA, appropriate for gestational age; ATN, acute tubular necrosis; GA, gestational age; IUGR, intrauterine growth restriction; LGA, large for gestational age; MAS, meconium aspiration syndrome; PPHN, persistent pulmonary hypertension; RDS, respiratory distress syndrome; SGA, small for gestational age.
Sources: Data from Tappero, E. (2021). Physical assessment. In M. T. Verklan, M. Walden, & S. Forest (Eds.), *Core curriculum for neonatal intensive care nursing* (6th ed., pp. 99–130). Elsevier; Fanaroff, A. A., Lissauer, T., & Fanaroff, J. M. (2020). Physical growth: Physical examination of the newborn infant and the physical environment. In A. A. Fanaroff & J. M. Fanaroff (Eds.), *Klaus and Fanaroff's care of the high-risk neonate* (7th ed., pp. 58–79.e2). Elsevier; Vittner, D. & McGrath, J., (2019). Behavioral assessment. In E. P. Tappero & M. E. Honeyfield (Eds.), *Physical assessment of the newborn: A comprehensive approach to the art of physical examination* (6th ed., p. 193–218). Springer Publishing Company; Smith, V. C. (2017). The high-risk newborn: Anticipation, evaluation, management, and outcome. In E. Eichenwald, A. Hansen, C. Martin, & A. Stark (Eds.), *Cloherty and Stark's manual of neonatal care* (8th ed., pp. 74–90, p. 87). Wolters Kluwer; Trotter, C. W. (2019). Gestational age assessment. In E. P. Tappero & M. E. Honeyfield (Eds.), *Physical assessment of the newborn: A comprehensive approach to the art of physical examination* (6th ed., pp. 23–44). Springer Publishing Company; Wilkins-Haug, L., & Heffner, L. J. (2017). Fetal assessment and prenatal diagnosis. In E. Eichenwald, A. Hansen, C. Martin, & A. Stark (Eds.), *Cloherty and Stark's manual of neonatal care* (8th ed., pp. 5–6). Wolters Kluwer.

WEIGHT-BASED GROWTH CLASSIFICATIONS

■ *Low birth weight (LBW):* birth weight <2,500 g
■ *Very low birth weight (VLBW):* birth weight <1,500 g
■ *Extremely low birth weight (ELBW):* birth weight <1,000 g (Fanaroff et al., 2020; Smith, 2017; Tappero, 2021; Trotter, 2019)

▶ HISTORY: A KEY COMPONENT OF THE NEWBORN PHYSICAL EXAMINATION

■ A comprehensive newborn assessment combines perinatal history, GA assessment, and the neonate's physical exam. These factors assist in the identification of norms and potential risk factors for each individual infant. See Tables 6.4 and 6.5 (Fanaroff et al., 2020; Horns LaBronte, 2019; Johnson & Cochran, 2017; Tappero, 2021; Walker, 2018).

▶ NEONATAL VITAL SIGNS

■ Vital signs will fluctuate based on the infant's state and therefore should ideally be taken when they are quiet. The most accurate assessment is best achieved when the newborn is in a quiet, alert state and without signs of distress.

■ Whenever possible, complete physical examination should occur in a warm and as stress-free environment as possible when the newborn is without signs of distress and vital signs are stable. The examination should be modified based on the response, state, and illness of the infant (Johnson & Cochran, 2017; Tappero, 2021; Trotter, 2019).

TEMPERATURE

■ Normal
  ● Axilla temperature between 36.5°C and 37.4°C (97.7°F and 99.3°F)
■ Abnormal
  ● Hypothermia <36.5°C (97.7°F) for the term neonate and <36.3°C (97.3°F) for the preterm neonate
    ❑ Symptoms include bradycardia, apnea, decreased cardiac output, poor oral feeding, feeding intolerance, hypotension, hypoxia, irritability, respiratory distress, and poor weight gain.
  ● Hyperthermia >37.5°C (99.5°F) for the term neonate and >36.9°C (98.4°F) for the preterm neonate
    ❑ Neonates are at risk because of their inability to dissipate heat. Symptoms include apnea, central nervous system (CNS) depression, hypernatremia, irritability, lethargy, weak cry, poor oral feeding, seizures, and tachycardia (Boucher et al., 2017; Brand & Shippey, 2021).

Table 6.4 Maternal and Perinatal Histories

Maternal History	Perinatal History
Family history ■ Inherited genetic or chromosomal diseases or conditions ■ Chronic disorders or disabilities **Maternal history** ■ General health ■ Gravidity and parity ■ Infertility treatments ■ Prior pregnancy outcomes ■ Blood type and sensitizations ■ Chronic illnesses ■ Infectious disease and inherited disease screenings in pregnancy ■ Pregnancy complications ■ *Age at delivery:* over 40 (chromosomal abnormalities, IUGR, microsomal), under 16 (prematurity, IUGR) ■ Chronic illnesses ■ Surgical procedures or hospitalizations ■ *Medications:* prescribed, illicit, or over-the-counter; nutritional or herbal supplements; alcohol or tobacco use ■ *Obstetric history:* previous pregnancies, issues with infertility, previous fetal or newborn losses or problems ■ Social support and stressors ■ Education and socioeconomic status, religious or cultural considerations, language barriers, or sensory deficits	■ Prenatal care, LMP, EDC, and ultrasound dating ■ Single/multiple gestation ■ Maternal nutrition status and weight gain ■ Blood type/risk for isoimmunization/Rhogam prophylaxis/positive antibody screen ■ *Screening results:* amniocentesis, ultrasounds, triple or quad screen, group B strep culture, congenital infections, and glucose tolerance ■ Maternal diabetes classification and control ■ *Maternal hypertension:* chronic vs. gestational, preeclampsia or eclampsia ■ *Fetal testing results:* serum, ultrasonic, genetic testing, and fetal lung maturity ■ Evidence of placental insufficiency ■ Presence of polyhydramnios, oligohydramnios, and anhydramnios ■ Congenital TORCH infections ■ Abnormal fetal growth ■ Known anomalies (malformation vs. chromosomal)

EDC, estimated date of confinement; IUGR, intrauterine growth restriction; LMP, last menstrual period; TORCH, toxoplasmosis, other agents, rubella (also known as German measles), cytomegalovirus, and herpes simplex.
Sources: Data from Abdulhayoglu, E. (2017). Birth trauma. In E. Eichenwald, A. Hansen, C. Martin, & A. Stark (Eds.), *Cloherty and Stark's manual of neonatal care* (8th ed., pp. 63–73, p. 63). Wolters Kluwer; Tappero, E. (2021). Physical assessment. In M. T. Verklan, M. Walden, & S. Forest (Eds.), *Core curriculum for neonatal intensive care nursing* (6th ed., pp. 99–130). Elsevier; Horns LaBronte, K. (2019). Recording and evaluating the neonatal history. In E. P. Tappero & M. E. Honeyfield (Eds.), *Physical assessment of the newborn: A comprehensive approach to the art of physical examination* (5th ed., pp. 12–20). Springer Publishing Company; Johnson, L., & Cochran, W. D. (2017). Assessment of the newborn history and physical examination of the newborn. In E. Eichenwald, A. Hansen, C. Martin & A. Stark (Eds.), *Cloherty and Stark's manual of neonatal care* (8th ed., pp. 92–93). Wolters Kluwer; Smith, V. C. (2017). The high-risk newborn: Anticipation, evaluation, management, and outcome. In E. Eichenwald, A. Hansen, C. Martin, & A. Stark (Eds.), *Cloherty and Stark's manual of neonatal care* (8th ed., pp. 74–90). Wolters Kluwer.

HEART RATE

■ Normal
  ● Newborn heart rate (HR) between 95 and 160 beats per minute (bpm); at rest 120 to 140 bpm; with activity/crying may be ≥170; and in deep sleep may decrease to 70 to 90 bpm
  ● Preterm HR between 120 and 160 bpm
■ Abnormal
  ● *Bradycardia:* HR ≤80 bpm
  ● *Sinus tachycardia:* HR ≥160 to 180 bpm
    ❑ Usually a physiologic response to anemia, fever, agitation, and infection (Cannon & Synder, 2020; Johnson, 2019; Vargo, 2019)

RESPIRATORY RATE

■ Normal
  ● Respiratory rate between 30 and 60 respirations per minute
  ● Periodic breathing (short pause in breath, between 5 and 10 seconds) common and normal

■ Abnormal
  ● *Tachypnea:* rapid, shallow breathing with rate ≥60 respirations per minute
  ● *Apnea:* pause in breathing of 20 seconds or longer and associated with cyanosis and/or bradycardia (Boucher et al., 2017)
  ● Apnea or bradycardia in term newborn not normal
    ❑ *Etiologic considerations:* metabolic, infectious, neurologic, or hypothermia (Boucher et al., 2017; Johnson, 2019)

BLOOD PRESSURE

■ Blood pressure (BP) values depend on GA and chronological age. It is not routinely measured in otherwise well newborns, but when indicated appropriately sized BP cuff is critical to obtaining an accurate measure (Figure 6.2).
  ● The correct size of BP cuff is determined by measuring the circumference of the extremity. The cuff should be 40% to 50% of the circumference of the extremity (equaling 125%–155% of the diameter

Table 6.5 Intrapartum and Newborn Resuscitation Histories

Intrapartum History	Newborn Birth and Resuscitation
■ Preterm labor ■ Post dates ■ *Bleeding:* placenta previa, placental abruption ■ Hypertension ■ Reason for delivery ■ *Labor/delivery:* spontaneous labor, induction, planned, emergent ■ *Infection risk:* chorioamnionitis, GBS, PROM, fever ■ Infection prophylaxis ■ Fetal lung maturity assessment and biophysical profile ■ Antenatal corticosteroids ■ Cord prolapse ■ Fetal distress/fetal heart monitoring ■ Fetal presentation ■ Mode of delivery ■ *Intrapartum drugs:* magnesium sulfate, analgesia, anesthetic ■ Amniotic fluid color and appearance ■ Prolonged labor ■ *Delivery difficulties:* shoulder dystocia, precipitous delivery, failure to progress, nuchal cord, umbilical cord knot ■ Gestational age at delivery ■ Onset and duration of labor ■ *Rupture of membranes:* spontaneous, artificial, duration ■ Placental findings	**Maternal/delivery history considerations** ■ Known abnormal fetal growth ■ History of SGA/LGA infants ■ Maternal malnutrition ■ History of unexpected losses ■ Use of tobacco or illicit drugs ■ Known placental insufficiency ■ Multiple gestation ■ Twin-to-twin transfusion/treatments/fetal interventions ■ Placental or umbilical abnormalities ■ Presence of diabetes ■ History of congenital infection ■ Known congenital anomalies/malformations ■ Presence of polyhydramnios, oligohydramnios ■ Decreased fetal movement ■ Birth presentation ■ *Delivery assistance:* forceps, vacuum ■ Presence of meconium **Newborn resuscitation** ■ Apgar scores ■ *Required resuscitation measures:* blow by oxygen, PPV, intubation, medications, chest compressions ■ Presence of birth trauma

GBS, group B *Streptococcus*; LGA, large for gestational age; PPV, positive pressure ventilation; PROM, premature rupture of membranes; SGA, small for gestational age.
Source: Data from Abdulhayoglu, E. (2017). Birth trauma. In E. Eichenwald, A. Hansen, C. Martin, & A. Stark (Eds.), *Cloherty and Stark's manual of neonatal care* (8th ed., p. 63). Wolters Kluwer.

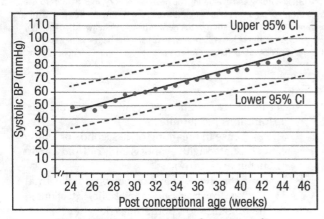

Figure 6.2 Linear regression of mean systolic blood pressures with 95% CIs.

BP, blood pressure; CI, confidence interval.
Source: Reproduced with permission from Gardner, S., Carter, B., Hines, M., & Hernandez, J. (Eds.), *Merenstein & Gardner's handbook of neonatal intensive care* (8th ed.). Elsevier.

of the limb being measured). The cuff should be long enough to entirely encircle the extremity.
■ Normal
  ● *Systolic:* 65 to 95 mmHg
  ● *Diastolic:* 30 to 60 mmHg
■ Abnormal

● A gradient between upper and lower extremity systolic pressure >20 mmHg should be considered suspicious for coarctation or other anomalies of the aorta.
● *Hypertension:* systolic >90 mmHg and diastolic >60 mmHg (Johnson & Cochran, 2017; Tappero, 2021; Vargo, 2019)

CAPILLARY REFILL

■ See "Cardiovascular" section.

PERIPHERAL PULSES

■ See "Cardiovascular" section.

PULSE OXIMETRY

■ See also "Cardiovascular" section.
■ It is generally not part of the initial newborn exam. It is the recommended universal cardiac screening for term infants between 24 and 48 hours of age.
  ● Abnormal results requiring additional evaluation include the following:
  ● Oxygen saturation <90%
  ● Oxygen saturation <95% in the right hand and either foot on three measures separated by 1 hour

- >3% difference in oxygen saturation between the right hand and foot on three measures separated by 1 hour (Johnson, 2019; Vargo, 2019)

▶ HANDS-ON PHYSICAL EXAMINATION

- The physical examination is a systematic head-to-toe approach used to identify congenital anomalies, successful transition from intra- to extrauterine life, effects of antenatal and intrapartum medications (analgesia, anesthetics) on the newborn, and signs and symptoms of life-threatening conditions requiring immediate assessment and intervention. The infant's general appearance should be assessed prior to interacting with them. The infant's state, alertness, movement and tone, signs of wellness or distress (color, respiratory effort, signs of nutritional status), obvious malformation, or anomaly all should be taken into consideration prior to beginning the hands-on assessment (Fanaroff et al., 2020; Horns LaBronte, 2019; Johnson & Cochran, 2017; Tappero, 2021; Walker, 2018).

SKIN

NORMAL FINDINGS

- Normal skin appearance related to GA:
  - *24 to 26 weeks:* translucent—red, many visible blood vessels and scant vernix
  - *35 to 40 weeks:* deep cracks—no visible blood vessels and thick vernix
  - *42 to 44 weeks:* dry, peeling skin—no vernix and loss of subcutaneous fat
- *Acrocyanosis:* bluish discoloration of the palms of the hands and the soles of the feet, often present at birth and may persist for up to 48 hours; should be investigated if acrocyanosis lasts longer than 48 hours (Fanaroff et al., 2020; Walker, 2018; Witt, 2019)
- *Plethora:* ruddy or red appearance of skin which may indicate high hemoglobin or hematocrit level
  - *Polycythemia:* central hematocrit >65%; places infant at risk of hypoglycemia, cyanosis, respiratory distress, or jaundice (Witt, 2019)
- *Jaundice:* yellow color of the skin and/or sclera caused by breakdown of red blood cells which then deposit excess unconjugated bilirubin in the skin (Fanaroff et al., 2020; Walker, 2018; Witt, 2019)
- *Cutis marmorata:* bluish mottling or marbling of the skin; often in response to chilling, stress, or overstimulation caused by constriction of capillaries; usually disappears with warming
  - Common sign in infant with trisomy 18 or trisomy 21
- *Harlequin color change:* sharp, demarcated red color seen on the dependent half of the body when the infant is side-lying; superior half appears pale; seen only in the newborn period; transient phenomenon lasting as long as 30 minutes (Witt, 2019)

- *Erythema toxicum:* also known as "newborn rash"; consists of small, white or yellow papules or vesicles with erythematous bases and eosinophils in sterile fluid under microscopic staining; most often found on the trunk, arms, and perineal areas (Tappero, 2021; Walker, 2018; Witt, 2019)
- *Milia:* small, raised, white epidermal cysts formed by an accumulation of sebaceous gland secretions; may be located on the cheeks and nose, midline palate (called Epstein pearls), and along the lingual or buccal areas of the dental ridges (called Bohn nodules; Walker, 2018; Witt, 2019)
- *Sebaceous gland hyperplasia:* occurs in 50% of newborns; numerous tiny, <0.5 cm, white or yellow papules found on the nose, cheeks, and upper lips
- *Miliaria:* results from obstruction of the sweat ducts due to an excessively warm, humid environment; seen primarily over the forehead, scalp, and skin creases of the neck, thighs, or groin area
- *Café au lait spots:* flat lesion with increased melanin content; regular or irregular borders; no clinical significance if only three or fewer spots present (Witt, 2019)
- *Hyperpigmented macule or congenital dermal melanocytosis:* most common pigmented (gray to blue-green color) lesions in the newborn, caused by melanocytes that infiltrate the dermis; common locations are the buttocks, flanks, and shoulders; generally disappears over the first 3 years of life (Walker, 2018; Witt, 2019)
- *Pustular melanosis:* benign, transient nonerythematous pustules and vesicles that occur as singular or clusters, with their rupture leaving a scaly, white lesion; predominance of neutrophils identified by microscopic staining
- *Congenital melanocytic nevus (pigmented nevus):* generally benign proliferation of melanocytes within the epithelial structures and can extend into the subcutaneous fat; may include hair; range in size from 1 to 20 cm in diameter; at risk of evolving into malignant melanoma; treatment options including laser therapy to reduce size or surgical intervention; repigmentation may occur post laser or surgery due to the remaining nevomelanocytes in the dermis (Witt, 2019)
- *Capillary hemangiomas (also known as "stork bite"):* macular patches with diffuse borders that blanch with pressure; commonly located on the forehead, nape of neck glabella, and eyelids
- *Nevus flammeus (also known as port wine stain):* flat, sharply defined lesion commonly located on the back of the neck; may be abnormal if located on the face following branches of trigeminal nerve (associated with Sturge–Weber syndrome)
- *Strawberry hemangioma:* red, raised, circumscribed, and compressible located anywhere on the body; during the first 6 months of life can increase in size and

then have spontaneous regression, leaving no trace; sometimes several years before complete resolution (Walker, 2018; Witt, 2019)

- *Sucking blisters:* benign findings of skin erosion found on the thumbs, index fingers, wrist, or forearm, caused by intrauterine fetal sucking (Table 6.6)

ABNORMAL FINDINGS

- *Epidermolysis bullosa:* autosomal dominant or recessive genetic disorder characterized by internal and external blistering
- *Staphylococcal scalded skin syndrome:* appears in response to *Staphylococcus aureus* infection, characterized by a "scalded skin" appearance (Witt, 2019)
- *Neurofibromatosis:* an autosomal dominant disorder in which tumors form on the peripheral nerves; cranial nerves may also be affected; characterized by presence of six or more café au lait spots (Walker, 2018; Witt, 2019)

Table 6.6 Common Dermatologic Terminology

Term	Description
Bulla	Vesicle >1 cm in diameter containing serous or seropurulent fluid
Crust	Lesion containing dried serous exudate, blood, or pus on skin surface
Cyst	Raised, palpable fluid or semifluid-filled sac
Ecchymosis	Subepidermal hemorrhage, does not blanch with pressure
Lesion	Any abnormal tissue
Macule	Discolored, flat spot <1 cm in diameter, not palpable
Nodule	Elevated lesion with indistinct border, palpable
Papule	Elevated, solid circumscribed lesion <1 cm, palpable
Petechiae	Pinpoint purplish hemorrhagic spot
Plaque	Elevated lesion with circumscribed borders >1 cm or a fusion of several papules, palpable
Purpura	Elevated, cloudy, purulent fluid-filled lesion
Scale	Area of exfoliation of dead/dying skin, can be caused by excess keratin
Vesicle (blister)	Elevated, serous fluid-filled lesion <1 cm diameter
Wheal	Elevated, reddened, solid fluid-filled lesion in the dermis

Source: Original table created by Pauline D. Graziano APN, MS, NNP-BC and Vivian Lopez RN-NIC, MSN, PNP, NNP-BC 2019 using information from Witt, C. (2019). Skin assessment. In E. P. Tappero & M. E. Honeyfield (Eds.), *Physical assessment of the newborn: A comprehensive approach to the art of physical examination* (6th ed., p. 47). Springer Publishing Company.

HEAD

NORMAL FINDINGS

- *Anterior fontanel (AF):* diamond-shaped, from barely palpable to up to 5 cm across, flat and soft; closure at 6 to 24 months of age
- *Posterior fontanel (PF):* triangular, palpable, and small (<1 cm); closure at 2 to 3 months of age
- *Sutures:* suture lines which may be approximated, separated (up to 1 cm separation within normal limits), or overriding; should be mobile on palpation
- *Molding:* an adaptive mechanism facilitating passage of the head through the birth canal, with the head appearing elongated and asymmetrical and with cranial bones sometimes overlapping; resolves spontaneously
- *Hair:* silky with uniform distribution and pattern of growth; can be straight or curly consistent with ethnicity; one- to two-hair whorls located in the postparietal region (Johnson, 2019)

ABNORMAL FINDINGS

- Can be normal variants or associated with syndromes or chromosomal abnormalities; 90% of all visible anomalies at birth found in this area
- *OFC:* may be affected by cranial molding, scalp edema, or hemorrhage under periosteum; most skull deformities a result of in utero positioning, limited space, or a decrease in amniotic fluid
- *Microcephaly:* OFC <10th percentile; possibly related to poor brain growth or prematurely closed/fused sutures (craniosynostosis)
  - May be an isolated finding but may also have association with genetic syndromes and congenital infections (Goodwin, 2016; Johnson, 2019; Tappero, 2021)
- *Macrocephaly:* OFC >90th percentile on growth chart
  - May be an isolated finding or secondary to hydrocephalus; associated with dwarfism or osteogenesis imperfecta (OI; Johnson, 2019; Tappero, 2021)
- Fontanels (Figure 6.3)
  - AF
    - Very large (>5 cm across), which can be associated with hypothyroidism; may be tense and/or bulging, which can be a sign of increased intracranial pressure
  - PF
    - Large PF (>1 cm), consider hypothyroidism, congenital infection, chromosomal abnormality, or congenital syndrome
    - Palpable third fontanel between AF and PF along the sagittal suture, possible congenital anomaly
    - Closed fontanels (premature closure, craniosynostosis)

❑ Bruit auscultated over the fontanel, possible arteriovenous (AV) malformation (Johnson, 2019; Tappero, 2021; Vargo, 2019)
- Sutures (Figure 6.3)
  - Immobile and rigid (fused), consider craniosynostosis
  - Widely separated, consider hydrocephalus or increased intracranial pressure (Johnson, 2019; Vargo, 2019)
- Shape of skull (Figure 6.4)
  - *Scaphocephaly:* early closure of the sagittal suture
  - *Plagiocephaly:* closure of the suture on one side of the head causing asymmetric, flattened appearance on one side of the head
  - *Brachycephaly:* closure of the coronal suture
  - *Dolichocephaly:* common in preterm infants, head flattened side to side, sutures remain unfused, caused by positioning
  - *Craniosynostosis:* early, abnormal closure of the sutures
    - ❑ *Significance:* primary, isolated finding, metabolic disorders, genetic abnormality, and

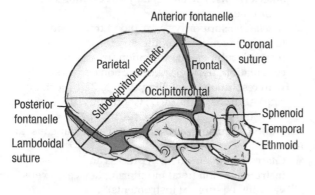

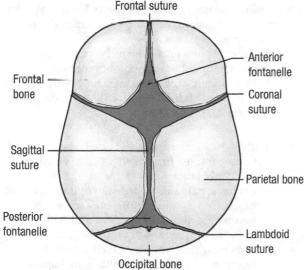

Figure 6.3 Neonatal skull anatomy: bones, sutures, and fontanels.
Source: Reproduced from Chiocca, E. M. (2020). *Advanced pediatric assessment* (3rd ed.). Springer Publishing Company.

hyperthyroidism (Johnson, 2019; Tappero, 2021; Vargo, 2019; Walker, 2018)
- Skull bones
  - Presence of craniotabes
    - ❑ *Causes:* intrauterine fundal pressure on the head with breech positioning; prolonged vertex position in utero; association with hydrocephalus or may just be an incidental finding
    - ❑ *Findings:* snapping sound of soft (demineralized) bones upon palpation; typically found over the parietal and occipital regions along the lambdoid suture; associated with breech presentation
    - ❑ *Resolution:* usually spontaneous within the first weeks of life (Johnson, 2019; Tappero, 2021; Vargo, 2019)
- Skull/scalp malformation
  - Cutis aplasia
    - ❑ *Causes:* most often an isolated finding, but can be associated with trisomy 13
    - ❑ *Findings:* an uncommon, open scalp defect; a circumscribed area that appears shiny and hairless; usual location vertex in front of the lambda
    - ❑ *Resolution:* spontaneous; area scars and remains hairless (Johnson, 2019; Tappero, 2021; Walker, 2018)
  - Encephalocele
    - ❑ *Causes:* incomplete anterior neural tube closure with skull defect (cranium bifidum)
    - ❑ *Findings:* protrusion of meninges and possible cerebral tissue; covered by skin; most commonly found in the occipital region but can be found elsewhere
    - ❑ *Resolution:* severity of findings related to location and size and contents within the sac (Dillon Heaberlin, 2019)
  - Anencephaly
    - ❑ *Causes:* failed closure of the neural tube; results in an underdeveloped cranium due to lack of brain tissue
    - ❑ *Findings:* absent dermal covering; exposed, hemorrhagic, fibrotic cerebral tissue
    - ❑ *Resolution:* death within hours to days of birth (Dillon Heaberlin, 2019; Goodwin, 2016)
- Hair abnormalities
  - Assess for areas of diffuse loss or abundance of hair, abnormal hair texture (brittle, fragile, twisted), and abnormal pattern of hair growth.
  - *White forelock (Waardenburg syndrome):* localized hypopigmentation
  - *Alopecia:* abnormal deficiency of hair
    - ❑ Diffuse loss associated with syndromic or genetic abnormality
    - ❑ Focal loss associated with focal trauma; can indicate underlying scalp lesion
  - Whorls

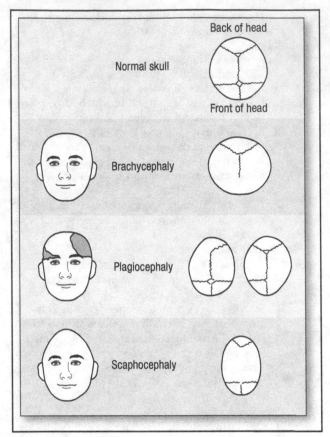

Figure 6.4 Newborn skulls: shapes.

❑ Abnormal position or number may be associated with abnormal brain growth
● Hairline
  ❑ Anterior hairline well onto the forehead
  ❑ *Hirsutism:* excessive hair growth which may be related to metabolic disorder or genetic syndrome, drug-induced, or may be an isolated finding (Johnson, 2019; Tappero, 2021; Walker, 2018)

Birth Trauma

■ Caput succedaneum
  ● *Causes:* edema (subcutaneous, extraperiosteal fluid) from birth process
  ● *Findings:* maximum swelling noted at birth; may include ecchymosis, petechiae, or purpura; poorly defined edges; crosses the suture lines; occurs over the presenting portion of the scalp; usually present with molding
  ● *Resolution:* spontaneous, within days (24–48 hours) of birth (Abdulhayoglu, 2017; Boucher et al., 2017; Johnson, 2019; Tappero, 2021; Vargo, 2019; Walker, 2018)
■ Cephalohematoma
  ● *Causes:* hemorrhage from rupture of the superficial veins between the periosteum and the skull; more frequently associated with instrument-assisted deliveries; incidence about 2.5% of all live births
  ● *Findings:* may be noted at birth or days after; well-demarcated edges; confined by suture lines; most commonly found over the occipital or parietal bones; unilateral
  ● *Resolution:* spontaneous, within weeks to months of age; may result in palpable calcification upon resolution (Abdulhayoglu, 2017; Johnson, 2019; Tappero, 2021; Vargo, 2019; Walker, 2018)
■ Subgaleal hemorrhage—A CLINICAL EMERGENCY
  ● *Causes:* hemorrhage under aponeurosis; subaponeurotic (subgaleal space): the area between the scalp aponeurosis and pericranium, extends from the orbital ridge to the nape of the neck and laterally to the ears, which can allow for massive blood loss
  ● *Findings:* fluctuant, mobile scalp mass; present at birth; crosses the suture lines; poorly defined edges; can develop slowly or rapidly, resulting in shock from massive blood loss; ears may be displaced anteriorly with swelling; may have pallor and poor tone
  ● *Resolution:* supportive care; blood transfusion for hypovolemia; phototherapy for hyperbilirubinemia; evaluation/treatment for coagulation disorder; reabsorption occurs slowly with resolution of swelling; 14% to 22% mortality rate (Abdulhayoglu, 2017; Goodwin, 2016; Johnson, 2019; Tappero, 2021; Walker, 2018)
■ Lacerations, bruising, abrasions, and subcutaneous fat necrosis
  ● *Causes:* trauma from birth process and instrumentation (fetal monitoring device, forceps, vacuum, or surgical instruments)
  ● *Findings:* wounds from birth process—scalp probe puncture, bruising, abrasions, lacerations, and subcutaneous fat necrosis
  ● *Resolution:* spontaneous recovery for most; may require treatment with antibiotic ointment or sterile dressing; occasional need for plastic surgery consultation (Abdulhayoglu, 2017; Johnson, 2019; Tappero, 2021; Witt, 2019)

■ Skull fracture occurring during delivery
  ❑ *Causes:* trauma from birth process/position/instrumentation
  ❑ *Findings:* palpable depression of the skull; most often asymptomatic; may have neurologic depression (associated with increased intracranial hemorrhage presenting with poor tone and decreased activity) requiring neurology consultation; diagnosis confirmed with x-ray (noted fracture of the skull) or head CT (if intracranial injury suspected)

- *Linear:* usually of parietal bone; may be associated with dural tear; can result in herniation of the brain or meninges; may result in lipomeningocele cyst development
- *Depressed:* parietal or frontal bone; often associated with use of forceps
- *Occipital fracture:* occipital bone; most often associated with breech delivery
- *Occipital osteodiastasis:* separation of the basal and squamous portion of the occipital bone; can result in cerebellar contusion with significant hemorrhage and possible death
  - ❏ *Resolution:* no treatment required for uncomplicated fractures (Abdulhayoglu, 2017)

FACE

NORMAL FINDINGS

- Bilateral symmetry of facial shape and organs and bilateral symmetry of facial movement

ABNORMAL FINDINGS

- Asymmetry of facial shape and organs and/or asymmetry of movement; may be caused by birth trauma, prolonged intrauterine compression (multiple gestation, oligohydramnios resulting in flattened features), familial characteristic, or normal variant; or may be associated with congenital malformation, syndrome (often with distinctive facial findings), or chromosomal abnormality
- Facial nerve compression or injury—unilateral
  - *Causes:* intrauterine position or forceps pressure
  - *Findings:* asymmetric facial movement or drooping of one side
  - *Resolution:* most recover spontaneously
- Congenital hypoplasia of the depressor anguli oris (facial muscle associated with frowning)
  - *Causes:* unilateral hypoplasia or agenesis of the depressor anguli oris muscle; may be associated with 22q11.2 deletion syndrome
  - *Findings:* drooping of one corner of the mouth during crying; remainder of facial movement intact
  - *Resolution:* none; cosmetic condition in infancy only
- Facial nerve compression or injury—symmetric, Mobius sequence
  - *Causes:* unknown/random occurrence; sixth (abducens) and seventh (facial) cranial nerve palsy
  - *Findings:* facial paralysis (unilateral or most frequently bilateral); paralysis of sideways (lateral) moving of the eyes; "mask-like" face (limited facial expression during crying/laughing); may have excessive drooling and difficulty with sucking/swallowing; at risk of corneal ulceration (eyelids may remain open during sleep); other malformations/abnormalities may be present

- *Resolution:* multidisciplinary follow-up required (craniofacial surgeons; ears, eyes, nose, and mouth/throat [ENT]; speech; pertussis toxin [PT]; ophthalmologist; Johnson, 2019; Tappero, 2021; Walker, 2018)

EARS

NORMAL FINDINGS

- Bilateral ear shape, placement, and symmetry; complete formation of both internal and external structures
- Placement of ear
  - 30% of the pinna located above an imaginary line between the inner canthus toward the occiput and tragus; helix attached to the scalp horizontal to the inner eye canthus; cranial molding from birth may cause benign distortion (Boucher et al., 2017; Johnson, 2019)
- Rotation of ear
- Less than a 30-degree angle from an imaginary line between the lobule insertion and the helix ear canal
  - Response to auditory stimuli
  - Positive startle or turn toward sound

ABNORMAL FINDINGS

- May be a normal variant/familial finding or an indication of congenital deafness; may also be a result of intrauterine positioning or pressure, associated with renal abnormalities and/or chromosomal or syndromic disorders
- Unilateral or bilateral incomplete formation of internal or external structures
  - *Microtia:* dysplastic ear
  - *Lop ear:* helix folded downward
  - *Cup ear:* small and cup-shaped; associated atresia of the auditory meatus or conductive hearing loss
- Presence of pits, tags, or preauricular sinus
  - Often an isolated finding with no other association; preauricular ear appendages (tags) can be associated with Goldenhar syndrome or other brachial arch abnormalities (cleft lip/palate, mandible hypoplasia)
- Placement of ear
  - *Low-set ears:* >30% of the pinna located below an imaginary line between the inner canthus and tragus; helix attached to the scalp below horizontal to the inner eye canthus; associated with various syndromes or chromosomal abnormalities
- Rotation of ear
  - *Posterior rotation:* >30-degree angle from an imaginary line between the lobule insertion and helix
- Ear canal
  - Visual absence of patent ear canal
- Response to auditory stimuli

- Lack of or diminished response to sound (Johnson, 2019; Walker, 2018)

Universal Hearing Screening

- Recommended for all newborns prior to discharge
- Hearing loss is one of the most common major abnormalities present at birth

EYES

- Dysmorphisms of the eye or ocular region are most frequently cited findings of malformation syndromes.

NORMAL FINDINGS

- Distance between outer canthus can be divided equally in thirds (Figure 6.5).
- Normal palpebral fissure length is 1.5 to 2.5 cm.
- There is no slant between the inner and outer canthus; however, it may be a normal racial determination.
- Eyebrows and eyelashes appear between 20 and 23 weeks' GA and are located in the arc above each eye. They are of equal length to the palpebral fissure.
- Eyes open spontaneously and are symmetric in size and shape.
- Fused eyelids are normal up to 28 weeks' GA.
- Blink reflex should be equal and symmetric.
- Pupils should be symmetric in size, shape, and reactivity to light.
- Lens is clear and intact.
  - *Nearsighted at birth:* By the end of the first week, the infant can clearly see objects 8 to 10 in. from their face.
- Iris color at birth is dark gray, dark blue, or brown. Permanent eye color develops near 6 months of age.
- Sclera is white.
- Retinal red reflex is present.

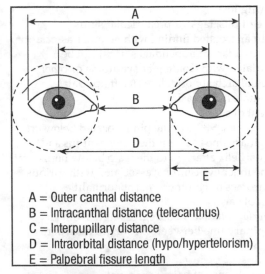

A = Outer canthal distance
B = Intracanthal distance (telecanthus)
C = Interpupillary distance
D = Intraorbital distance (hypo/hypertelorism)
E = Palpebral fissure length

Figure 6.5 Newborn eye.

Source: Reproduced with permission from Zitelli, B. J., & Davis, H. W. (2007). *Atlas of pediatric physical diagnosis* (5th ed.). Mosby.

- Chemical conjunctivitis or edema from routine eye ointment prophylaxis may be a normal finding.
- Normal eye movements:
  - *Nystagmus:* rapid involuntary eyeball movement
    - Normal until 3 to 4 months of age
  - *Strabismus:* appears cross-eyed
    - Caused by weak musculature and muscular incoordination
    - Resolves spontaneously
  - *Pseudostrabismus:* appears cross-eyed due to flattened nasal bridge and epicanthal folds

Common Birth Findings

- *Birth trauma:* eyelid edema or bruising; conjunctival or subconjunctival hemorrhage; spontaneous resolution within 2 weeks of birth
- *Nevus simplex:* common vascular birthmark of the eyelid or glabella
- *Blocked nasolacrimal duct:* causes cloudy drainage without redness or swelling; normal tear production begins at 2 to 3 months age; nasolacrimal ducts fully patent at 5 to 7 months age

ABNORMAL FINDINGS

- Distance between the outer canthus cannot be divided equally in thirds (see Figure 6.5).
- *Hypertelorism:* eyes spaced widely apart; normal variant versus syndromic
- *Hypotelorism:* eyes spaced closer together; normal variant versus syndromic
- Small palpebral fissure
- *Slant:* upward (outer canthus higher than inner canthus) or downward (outer canthus lower than inner) sloping of the eye; may be normal variant of racial determination, but may also be associated with syndromic/chromosomal abnormality
- Eyebrows that meet at the glabella (synophrys) associated with syndromes (Cornelia de Lange)
- Highly arched eyebrows
- Abnormally long-tangled eyelashes associated with syndromes (Cornelia de Lange)
- *Presence of epicanthal folds:* may be normal variant due to racial determination (i.e., with upslanting palpebral fissure in Asians) or a result of in utero compression from oligohydramnios (Potter facies); prominence may be syndromic (trisomy 21)
- Abnormal eye protrusion or enlarged eyeballs
  - Association with hyperthyroidism or congenital glaucoma
  - *Anophthalmos:* absent eyes
  - *Cyclopia:* single eye
- Unable to open eyes spontaneously (after 28 weeks' GA) or asymmetric opening of the eyes
  - *Ptosis:* paralytic drooping of the eyelid
  - *Sunset sign:* lid retraction with downward gaze
    - Associated with hydrocephaly and increased intracranial pressure
- Asymmetry or absence of blink reflex

- *Coloboma:* absence or defect of ocular tissue resulting in keyhole-shaped pupil
  - May be a sporadic finding or may be associated with trisomy 13 or CHARGE syndrome (posterior coloboma, heart disease, choanal atresia, retardation, genital and ear abnormalities)
- *Infantile cataracts:* clouding of normally clear lens
  - *Association:* may be an isolated finding or a result of congenital rubella or cytomegalovirus (CMV) exposure
- *Brushfield spots:* white spots visualized around the iris of the eye
  - *Association:* may be a normal variant; however, 75% association with trisomy 21
- *Blue sclera:* blue-tinted sclera; caused by thinning of sclera tissue
  - Association with OI and other chromosomal abnormalities
- *Absent red (retina) reflex:* possible association with congenital glaucoma, congenital cataract, retinoblastoma, or hemorrhages
- *White reflex (retina), also known as leukocoria:* possible association with congenital cataract, tumor, and chorioretinitis
- Persistence of nystagmus after 4 months
- Congenital glaucoma
  - *Causes:* abnormal development of the eye's drainage system
  - *Findings:* cornea >1 cm in diameter; excessive eye tearing; light sensitivity
  - *Resolution:* requires immediate ophthalmology consult (Johnson, 2019; Walker, 2018)

NOSE

NORMAL FINDINGS

- Neonates are obligate nose breathers until 6 to 12 weeks of age
- Midline position between the eyes
- Bilateral symmetry and patency of nares
- Positional deformities caused by birth process or intrauterine pressure
- Intermittent sneezing

ABNORMAL FINDINGS

- Cyanosis at rest, pink when crying (mouth breathing)
  - *Association:* iatrogenic—excessive suctioning or choanal atresia or stenosis
- Abnormal shape or flattened, broad nasal bridge or nonmidline
  - May be a normal variant, a result of positioning, or may be associated with syndromic abnormality

- Central proboscis with a single nare
- *Nasal flaring:* compensatory sign of respiratory distress
- Excessive, continuous sneezing: potential sign of newborn abstinence syndrome (NAS; Johnson, 2019; Walker, 2018)

MOUTH

NORMAL FINDINGS

- Midline below the philtrum; symmetrical in shape, size, and movement
- Normal reflexes present
- Suck and swallow by 32 to 34 weeks' GA
- Rooting and gag by 36 weeks' GA
- Hard and soft palate intact (upon inspection and palpation)
- Tongue fits within the mouth, with a small singular frenulum
- Mild circumoral cyanosis during newborn period
- *Epstein pearls:* epithelial cell masses that are benign and resolve spontaneously
- *Natal teeth:* benign; often removed in newborn period due to risk of aspiration if dislodged

ABNORMAL FINDINGS

- Offset from midline; philtrum abnormalities; abnormal shape, size, or movement
  - Thin upper lip and flat philtrum, consider fetal alcohol syndrome
  - Microstomia (small mouth), consider trisomy 18
  - Macrostomia (large mouth), consider mucopolysaccharidosis, Beckwith–Wiedemann syndrome, and hypothyroidism
  - Micrognathia (abnormally small jaw with normal-sized tongue), consider Pierre Robin, Treacher Collins, or Cornelia de Lange syndrome
  - Asymmetrical facial movement, observe at rest and crying; consider facial palsy/cranial nerve damage
- Abnormal or absent reflexes
  - Excessive oral secretions, consider esophageal atresia or neurologic issue associated with poor swallow or tone
- Palate
  - Bifid uvula
  - *Cleft of the lip, soft or hard palates:* unilateral, bilateral, incomplete, or complete
  - *Highly arched palate:* caused by decreased activity or sucking in utero; consider neuromuscular disorder
- Abnormalities of the tongue

- Macroglossia (large tongue), consider Beckwith–Wiedemann syndrome, trisomy 21, hypothyroidism, and mucopolysaccharidosis
- *Ankyloglossia:* thick, prominent frenulum; also known as tongue-tied; restricts full movement of the tongue
  - ❏ Severe with persistence of feeding difficulties may consider frenotomy (Boucher et al., 2017; Johnson, 2019; Walker, 2018)

NECK AND THROAT

NORMAL FINDINGS

- Short, thick neck with multiple skin folds; midline trachea; has full rupture of membrane (ROM)

ABNORMAL FINDINGS

- Cystic hygroma—most common neck mass in the newborn
  - *Causes:* sequestered lymph channels that dilate into multiloculated cysts
  - *Findings:* most commonly located on the lateral neck, fluctuant mass with positive transillumination; can result in feeding difficulties or airway compromise with deviation of the trachea
  - *Resolution:* small lesions may regress spontaneously; larger or symptomatic lesions require surgical resection (Johnson, 2019)
- Redundant skin or webbed neck
  - *Causes:* associated with Turner syndrome (46,X), Noonan syndrome, or Down syndrome (trisomy 21)
  - *Findings:* predominant fat pad back of the neck; redundant skin back of the neck; webbed neck: excessive skinfold, usually extending from the mastoid process to the shoulders
  - *Resolution:* benign symptom of a syndrome; cosmetic surgical correction if desired later in life
- Branchial cleft cyst
  - *Causes:* abnormal development of neck tissues, leaving cystic fluid-filled pockets
  - *Findings:* present at birth; palpable small lump located most often near the front edge of the sternocleidomastoid muscle; usually unilateral, painless unless infected, may have opening on the skin through which mucous drains; if large or infected may cause difficulty in swallowing or breathing
  - *Resolution:* may require incision and drainage; antibiotics if infected; surgical removal (Johnson, 2019)
- Sternocleidomastoid injury or congenital muscular torticollis
  - *Causes:* injury to the sternocleidomastoid muscle; may be congenital or caused by birth trauma; usually on the right

- *Findings:* contraction of the neck muscle that pulls the head toward the affected side while the chin points to the opposite side; a palpable small mass at the site of injury
- *Resolution:* physical therapy and stretching exercises; if persists beyond 1 year may require surgical correction (Walker, 2018)
- Torticollis
  - *Causes:* injury sustained to the sternocleidomastoid muscle or to a cervical spine abnormality from birth trauma, intrauterine malposition, muscle fibrosis, or venous abnormality in the muscle
  - *Findings:* spasmodic, unilateral contraction of the neck muscles; usually appears as a firm, fibrous mass or tightness in the sternocleidomastoid muscle at approximately 2 weeks of age; head tilts laterally toward the involved side, with the chin rotated away from the affected shoulder
- Brachial nerve plexus injury
  - *Causes:* stretching and tearing of nerve roots during birth or from pressure from maternal sacral prominence during fetal descent
  - Types:
    - ❏ Erb palsy
      - ○ *Causes:* denervation of the deltoid, supraspinatus, biceps, and brachioradialis involving cervical nerves V and VI
      - ○ *Findings:* intact grasp ("waiter's tip"); results in upper arm paralysis and asymmetric Moro
      - ○ *Resolution:* requires neurology and physical therapy consultations; avoid contractures of joints using passive range of motion exercises; parental education on maintaining normal joint function; reconstructive procedures if needed
    - ❏ Klumpke paralysis
      - ○ *Causes:* involves cervical nerve VIII and thoracic nerve I; denervation of the intrinsic of the hand, flexors of the wrist, fingers, and sympathetics
      - ○ *Findings:* results in lower arm paralysis, absent grasp
      - ○ *Resolution:* requires neurology and physical therapy consultations; avoid contractures of joints using passive range of motion exercises; parental education on maintaining normal joint function; reconstructive procedures if needed
    - ❏ *Total:* combination Erb–Duchenne paralysis and Klumpke paralysis
      - ○ *Causes:* denervation of the entire arm from cervical nerve V to thoracic nerve
      - ○ *Findings:* in entire arm paralysis, arm remains extended and turned inward, hand flaccid ("waiter's tip")
      - ○ *Resolution:* requires neurology and physical therapy consultations; avoid contractures of joints using passive range of motion

exercises; parental education on maintaining normal joint function; reconstructive procedures if needed (Walker, 2018)

CHEST AND LUNGS

NORMAL FINDINGS

- *Acrocyanosis:* cyanosis of hands and feet
  - *Causes:* instability of peripheral circulation
  - *Findings:* normal in the first 24 to 48 hours of life; benign in otherwise asymptomatic infant
- Symmetric chest movement, synchronous movement of abdomen
- Respiratory rate 40 to 60 respirations per minute

Table 6.7 Abnormal Breath Sound Findings

Sound	Finding	Significance
Crackles (rales)	▪ Fine- or low-pitched ▪ Heard on inspiration	▪ Normal finding at birth as fluid clears from lungs ▪ *"Wet" lungs:* edema, congestion ▪ Atelectasis or inflammation
Wheeze	▪ High-pitched, "squeak" ▪ Heard loudest on expiration	▪ Reactive airway (BPD)
Rhonchi	▪ Loud, low-pitched, coarse	▪ Partial obstructed airway by mucous or secretions ▪ May clear with coughing
Stridor	▪ Rough or harsh sound ▪ Worse with inspiration	▪ Reduced airway diameter (edema, mass, vascular ring)
Diminished	▪ Air entry decreased	▪ Atelectasis ▪ Effusion
Pleural friction rub	▪ Dry, rubbing sound ▪ Inspiration or expiration	▪ Inflammation of pleura ▪ Pleural effusion
Peristalsis in chest	▪ Audible bowel sounds	▪ Congenital diaphragmatic hernia

BPD, bronchopulmonary dysplasia.

Sources: Data from Abdulhayoglu, E. (2017). Birth trauma. In E. Eichenwald, A. Hansen, C. Martin, & A. Stark (Eds.), *Cloherty and Stark's manual of neonatal care* (8th ed., pp. 70–71). Wolters Kluwer; Tappero, E. (2021). Physical assessment. In M. T. Verklan, M. Walden, & S. Forest (Eds.), *Core curriculum for neonatal intensive care nursing* (6th ed., pp. 99–130). Elsevier; Fanaroff, A. A., Lissauer, T., & Fanaroff, J. M. (2020). Physical growth: Physical examination of the newborn infant and the physical environment. In A. A. Fanaroff & J. M. Fanaroff (Eds.), *Klaus and Fanaroff's care of the high-risk neonate* (7th ed., pp. 58–79.e2). Elsevier; Vargo, L. (2019). Cardiovascular assessment. In E. P. Tappero & M. E. Honeyfield (2014). *Physical assessment of the newborn: A comprehensive approach to the art of physical examination* (6th ed., pp. 93–110). Springer Publishing Company.

- *Breath sounds* (Table 6.7): symmetrical air entry
- Pattern:
  - Irregular with respirations of varying depths
  - *Periodic breathing:* 5- to 20-second pause in breathing; normal if not associated with change in color, tone, or HR
- *Chest shape:* symmetric, cylindrical shape
- *Nipples:* note placement, pigment, spacing, and amount of palpable breast tissue
  - *Supernumerary or accessory nipples:* normal variant
  - *Secretions:* normal variant—milky white secretions associated with breast tissue hypertrophy caused by maternal hormones
  - *Spacing:* normal distance—less than 25% overall chest circumference

ABNORMAL FINDINGS

- Central cyanosis
  - *Causes:* many possible etiologies, including disease processes or abnormalities that result in insufficient pulmonary oxygen intake, insufficient pulmonary blood flow, or abnormal pulmonary blood flow
  - *Findings:* cyanosis of the mucous membranes; always abnormal
- Asymmetric, asynchronous movement
  - *Causes:* pneumothorax, phrenic nerve injury, diaphragmatic hernia, and congenital heart lesion
- Abnormal breath sounds (see Table 6.7)
- Abnormal breath patterns/presence of work of breathing
  - *Grunting:* compensatory attempt to increase intrathoracic pressure
    - ❏ Allows for increased gas exchange time by trapping air within the alveoli; caused by partially closed glottis
  - *Nasal flaring:* compensatory attempt to open airways
    - ❏ Widens upper airways to decrease resistance
  - *Retractions:* substernal, subcostal, intercostal, and suprasternal
    - ❏ Suprasternal retractions with gasping or stridor, possible airway obstruction
- *Sneezing:* normal, unless excessive or prolonged (consider NAS)
- *Coughing:* always abnormal in newborn
- *Apnea:* pause in respiration lasting 20 seconds or longer
  - Often associated with change in color, bradycardia, or decreased tone; possible causes are apnea of prematurity, infection, respiratory insufficiency, and gastroesophageal reflux
- *Gasping:* respiratory emergency; represents respiratory failure and acidosis
- Chest shape
  - *Pectus excavatum:* deformity caused by excessive growth of the connective tissue (cartilage) that joins the ribs to the breastbone, resulting in an inward defect of the sternum

- Depressed chest wall or funnel shaping
- Paradoxical "seesaw" movement
  - Indicates poor chest wall compliance and loss of volume; chest wall collapses, with stomach bulging on inspiration
- Barrel-shaped
  - Indicates air trapping or hyperinflation; may indicate cardiomegaly
- Short sternum
  - Anterior chest appears short; consider trisomy 18
- Pigeon chest
  - Protrusion of sternum; consider Marfan syndrome
- Abnormal nipple discharge or placement
  - *Purulent discharge:* mastitis; most common organism *Staphylococcal aureus*
  - *Wide-spaced nipples:* >25% overall chest circumference; can be normal variant or associated with chromosomal abnormality of congenital syndrome (Walker, 2018)

CARDIOVASCULAR

NORMAL FINDINGS
- Color
  - *Acrocyanosis:* cyanosis of the hands, feet, and circumoral areas
    - *Causes:* instability of peripheral circulation
    - *Findings:* normal in the first 24 to 48 hours of life
    - Benign in otherwise asymptomatic infant
- *Capillary refill:* normal <3 seconds refill time
- Active precordium
  - *Causes:* hypertrophy of ventricles; congenital heart anomaly and tachycardia; hyperthyroidism; can be present with patent ductus arteriosus (PDA)
  - *Findings:* absence or presence of normal finding shortly after birth of term infant; normal finding in preterm or SGA infant with decreased

subcutaneous tissue; point of maximum impulse (PMI) normally located at the third or fourth intercostal space, just left of the midclavicular line; heartbeat seen or palpated on the chest wall
- EKG
  - *Nonconcerning arrhythmias:* benign, requiring no treatment (Table 6.8)
    - Sinus bradycardia (HR <80 bpm)
      - Common, transient finding in newborn
      - *Causes:* parasympathetic system response to vagal stimulation
      - Normally self-resolving (Cannon & Snyder, 2020)
    - Sinus tachycardia (HR 180–200 bpm)
      - *Causes:* increased activity (crying, movement) with resultant increased demand on the heart
      - Rarely requires treatment (Cannon & Snyder, 2020)
- Auscultation examination (minimally includes assessment over the aortic, pulmonic, tricuspid, and mitral valve sites)
  - Heart sounds (Table 6.9)
  - *Murmurs:* note location, radiation, pitch, loudness/intensity, and timing within cycle
    - *Continuous:* murmur audible beyond the second heart sound into diastole
    - *Systolic ejection murmur:* audible before the first heart sound and ends at or before the second heart sound; indicates flow across pulmonic valve
    - *Innocent/flow murmur:* normal in the first 48 hours of life with transition of fetal to newborn circulation; not caused by cardiovascular disease; EKG normal; grade 1 to 2 (see Table 6.9)
- *Pulses:* represent approximate estimate of cardiac output
  - *Apical pulse:* left ventricle during systole; normal location is at the fourth intercostal space, left of midclavicular line; normally the PMI

Table 6.8 Newborn Cardiac Arrhythmias

Arrhythmia	Cause	EKG Findings	Treatment
Sinus arrhythmia	■ Normal variant	■ Irregular R–R interval	■ None required
Premature atrial beat	■ Early beat from supraventricular focus ■ Normal variant in 30% of term/preterm	■ P-wave occurring earlier than expected in cycle ■ Can be inverted ■ Can occur on previous T-wave ■ PR interval normal	■ Well tolerated ■ Usually requires no treatment ■ Can be seen with CHD, sepsis, hypoxia, and severe RDS ■ If significant, treat underlying cause
Premature ventricular beat	■ Early beat from irritable ventricular focus causing abnormal ventricular conduction ■ *Causes:* hypoxia, irritation from invasive catheter, result of surgical procedure to treat CHD	■ Wide, abnormal QRS	■ Infrequent occurrence ■ No treatment required ■ Adjust tip position of invasive catheter

CHD, congenital heart disease; RDS, respiratory distress syndrome.

Sources: Data from Tappero, E. (2021). Physical assessment. In M. T. Verklan, M. Walden, & S. Forest (Eds.), *Core curriculum for neonatal intensive care nursing* (6th ed., pp. 99–130). Elsevier; Vargo, L. (2019). Cardiovascular assessment. In E. P. Tappero & M. E. Honeyfield (2014). *Physical assessment of the newborn: A comprehensive approach to the art of physical examination* (6th ed., pp. 93–110). Springer Publishing Company.

Table 6.9 Heart Sounds in the Neonate

Sound	Represents	Location	Other
S1	■ First heart sound ■ Closure of the mitral and tricuspid valves	■ Loudest at the heart apex	■ Intensity increas with increas cardiac output ■ Splitting occurs with asynchronous closure of the valves ■ Normal variant
S2	■ Second heart sound ■ Closure of the aortic and pulmonic valves	■ Loudest at the base of the heart	■ Single sound at birth ■ Normally split in 66% by 16 hours of age/80% by 48 hours ■ Wide split—ABNORMAL (may be present with pulmonary stenosis, Ebstein anomaly, total anomalous venous return, tetralogy of Fallot)
S3	■ Increased flow across the atrioventricular valves	■ Heart apex during early diastole	■ Heard with PDA
S4	■ Decreased compliance	■ Heart apex	■ Rare in neonate ■ Always pathologic
Ejection click	■ Normal within the first 24 hours of birth	■ If related to aortic valve—apex ■ If related to pulmonic valve—second to third intercostal space	■ Abnormal finding after 24 hours of life ■ May be present with aortic or pulmonary stenosis, truncus arteriosus, and tetralogy of Fallot

PDA, patent ductus arteriosus.
Source: Data from Tappero, E. (2021). Physical assessment. In M. T. Verklan, M. Walden, & S. Forest (Eds.), *Core curriculum for neonatal intensive care nursing* (6th ed., pp. 99–130). Elsevier.

- *Peripheral pulses:* brachial (palpated at the inner aspect of the elbow); radial (palpated at the inner aspect of the wrist near the base of the thumb); femoral (palpated in the groin, midway between the symphysis pubis and anterior superior iliac spine); dorsalis pedis (palpated in the groove between the first and second toes, slightly medial on the dorsum of the foot); posterior tibial (palpated below and behind the ankle on the inner aspect of the leg)
- Bilateral equal rate and intensity between the upper and lower pulses
  - ❏ Absence or discrepancy in rate/intensity concerning for ductal-dependent cardiac lesion (coarctation of the aorta)
- Pulse grading (Table 6.10)

ABNORMAL FINDINGS
- ■ Color
  - Pallor or mottling
    - ❏ Compensatory peripheral vasoconstriction resulting in shunting of the blood from periphery to central organs; possible causes are sepsis or cardiogenic shock
  - Central cyanosis
    - ❏ If no evidence of respiratory distress and/or worsens with crying, cause is likely congenital heart disease (CHD); assess by the oxygen challenge test (administration of 100% oxygen); if no improvement in saturations, etiology is likely CHD

Table 6.10 Peripheral Pulse Grading

0	Not palpable
+1	Very difficult to palpate; weak, easily obliterated with pressure
+2	Difficult to palpate; can be obliterate with pressure
+3	Easy to palpate; normal pulse; not easy to obliterate
+4	Strong and bounding; not able to obliterate; felt with PDA

PDA, patent ductus arteriosus.

- Capillary refill >3 to 4 seconds
- Precordium
  - ❏ Displaced PMI, consider dextrocardia, tension pneumothorax, and CHD
  - ❏ Presence of heaves, taps, or thrills
    - ○ *Heave:* a palpable lift; PMI that is slow and diffuse; represents ventricular dilation or volume overload
    - ○ *Tap:* a palpable sharp, localized PMI; represents pressure overload and hypertrophy
    - ○ *Thrill:* a palpable murmur (loud, grade 4 murmur); not common in the neonate
- ■ EKG (concerning arrhythmias; see Table 6.8)
  - Bradycardia (not sinus bradycardia)
    - ❏ Consider congenital heart block or cerebral defect.
  - Tachycardia (not sinus tachycardia)

- ❑ Consider respiratory distress, anemia, sepsis, shock, and congestive heart failure.
- Supraventricular tachycardia (HR >200 bpm)
  - ❑ This is a medical emergency and requires immediate intervention.
  - ❑ Causes include abnormal extra electrical pathway. Consider Wolff–Parkinson–White syndrome or Ebstein anomaly.
  - ❑ It results in extreme compromise of cardiac output.
  - ❑ Untreated, prolonged episode can result in congestive heart failure or death within 48 hours.
  - ❑ Treatment includes vagal stimulation (ice to face), drug administration (adenosine), or cardioversion.
- ▪ Pathologic murmurs
  - *Causes:* cardiovascular disease, failed fetal circulation transition, cardiac anomaly
  - *Findings:* may begin or persist after 48 hours of birth; grade 2 or greater (Table 6.11)
- ▪ Pulses
  - Asymmetric or decreased in lower extremities, consider coarctation of the aorta (Vargo, 2019; Walker, 2018)

ABDOMEN

NORMAL FINDINGS

- ▪ *Appearance:* soft, rounded abdomen with synchronous abdominal movement with respirations
- ▪ Umbilical cord
  - Average size 2 cm at the base; normally dries and detaches within 2 weeks of birth
  - Normal color white and gelatinous
    - ❑ Yellow/green color indicating 6 to 12 hours in utero meconium staining
    - ❑ Filled with Wharton jelly protecting one vein and two arteries
    - ❑ Absence of one artery seen in 1% of population; can be an isolated finding or

Table 6.11 Heart Murmur Grading

Grade 1	Soft, barely audible
Grade 2	Soft, easily audible
Grade 3	Moderately loud, no thrill
Grade 4	Loud with thrill (palpable vibration at the site)
Grade 5	Loud, audible with stethoscope lightly on chest
Grade 6	Loud, audible with stethoscope near but off chest

Sources: Data from Tappero, E. (2021). Physical assessment. In M. T. Verklan, M. Walden, & S. Forest (Eds.), *Core curriculum for neonatal intensive care nursing* (6th ed. pp. 99–130). Elsevier; Vargo, L. (2019). Cardiovascular assessment. In E. P. Tappero & M. E. Honeyfield (2014). *Physical assessment of the newborn: A comprehensive approach to the art of physical examination* (6th ed., p. 93–110). Springer Publishing Company; Vargo, L. (2014). Newborn physical assessment. In K. Simpson & P. Creehan (Eds.), *Perinatal nursing* (4th ed., p. 612). Wolters Kluwer/Lippincott, Williams & Wilkins.

an association with abnormal findings of cardiovascular, gastrointestinal, or genitourinary (GU) systems
- Cord length
  - ❑ Normal 30 to 90 cm; length determined by intrauterine space and fetal activity; decreased space or fetal activity resulting in short cord
  - ❑ *Measure of fetal nutritional status:* LGA infant—thick cord; IUGR/postdates/placental insufficiency—small, thin cord
- ▪ *Audible bowel sounds:* audible within the first hours of life (Goodwin, 2016)
- ▪ Patent anus
  - Appears patent; positive anal wink; passage of meconium, normally occurs within the first 48 hours of birth
- ▪ *Muscle tone:* muscles tense with movement, crying, or upon palpation; no evidence of discomfort

ABNORMAL FINDINGS

- ▪ Appearance
  - Asynchrony of abdominal and respiratory movement associated with respiratory distress
  - *Umbilical hernia:* protrusion of abdominal contents at the umbilicus due to weak abdominal musculature or incomplete closure of abdominal muscle wall
    - ❑ Common finding in African Americans, LBW males, and premature infants; closes spontaneously by 2 years of age
  - *Diastasis recti:* midline separation of the rectus abdominal muscles
    - ❑ Midline, elevated ridge from the sternum to the umbilicus; visualized with infant crying; normal variant; resolves spontaneously
  - Sunken, scaphoid abdomen
    - ❑ Diaphragmatic hernia
  - Flaccid skinned, lumpy appearance
    - ❑ Prune belly (Eagle–Barrett syndrome)
  - *Epigastric hernia:* small, firm palpable fat nodule
    - ❑ Location between xyphoid and umbilicus; uncommon; surgical intervention required
  - Marked abdominal distention
    - ❑ May be iatrogenic in infant receiving positive pressure ventilation (PPV); consider bowel obstruction (Goodwin, 2016)
- ▪ Umbilical cord
  - *Omphalitis:* redness encircling the umbilical cord with extension onto the abdomen
    - ❑ Indicative of infection; requires treatment with antibiotic
  - *Patent urachus:* persistence of embryonic connection between the bladder and the umbilicus
    - ❑ Persistent and excessive leak of clear fluid
  - *Omphalomesenteric duct:* persistence of the embryonic tract connecting the ileum to the umbilicus

- ❏ Leakage of ileal content
- *Granuloma/umbilical polyp:* small, red, raw-appearing lesion
  - ❏ Located at the site of separation (Goodwin, 2016; Walker, 2018)
- ◼ Abdominal wall defects
  - *Omphalocele:* herniation of abdominal content into the umbilical cord
    - ❏ *Causes:* disruption of migration of the bowel to reenter the abdomen before the 10th week gestation AND abdominal muscle development defect
    - ❏ *Findings:* clear sac, contiguous with cord
    - ❏ *Associations:* 67% association with cardiac, neurologic, GU, skeletal, or chromosomal abnormalities; Beckwith–Wiedemann syndrome; and trisomy 13, 18, and 21
  - *Gastroschisis:* defect in the abdominal wall allowing the viscera to protrude
    - ❏ *Causes (theories):* in utero rupture of the umbilical cord hernia or possibly a vascular accident interfering with normal formation of the abdominal musculature
    - ❏ *Findings:* no sac; discrete from umbilical cord; usually to the right of midline; exposed abdominal contents appearing edematous, thickened, and matted as a result of in utero exposure to amniotic fluid
    - ❏ *Associations:* usually isolated defect; can be associated with bowel atresia and ischemic enteritis resulting from compromised mesenteric blood flow (Goodwin, 2016)
- ◼ Perianal region
  - Abnormality of bowel patency/stool passage
    - ❏ Not patent or no passage of meconium within the first 48 hours of birth
  - Absence of anal wink/abnormal sphincter tone
    - ❏ Consider CNS abnormality
  - *Fistulas:* anomalous connection between the intestinal and GU tracts
    - ❏ *Rectovaginal fistula:* presence of meconium in the vagina
    - ❏ *Rectourethral fistula:* presence of meconium in the urethral orifice (Goodwin, 2016; Walker, 2018)
- ◼ Muscle tone
  - *Hypertonicity:* possible irritation or pain
  - *Hypotonicity:* possible neuromuscular disease, perinatal depression, neonatal depression secondary to intrapartum drug exposure (Goodwin, 2016)

INTERNAL ORGANS OF THE ABDOMEN

- ◼ Exam progresses from superficial to deeper structures.

LIVER

NORMAL FINDINGS
- ◼ 1 to 2 cm below the right costal margin
- ◼ Firm, smooth, sharp edges

ABNORMAL FINDINGS
- ◼ >2 cm below the right costal margin, possible associations with CHD, infection, hemolytic disease, AV malformation, and right-sided heart failure
- ◼ Palpated on the left (sinus inversus: may be associated with cardiac defects)
- ◼ Boggy, caused by congestion/congestive heart failure
- ◼ Hard or nodular edge (Vargo, 2019)

SPLEEN

NORMAL FINDINGS
- ◼ Left side of the abdomen
- ◼ If palpable felt no lower than 1 cm below the left costal margin

ABNORMAL FINDINGS
- ◼ Edge palpated 1 cm below the left costal margin—enlargement
- ◼ Asplenia
- ◼ Located on the right—situs inversus

KIDNEYS

NORMAL FINDINGS
- ◼ Difficult to palpate, easiest early after birth, before feeding
- ◼ Use deep palpation; 45-degree angle caudal and lateral to umbilicus
- ◼ Normal size 4.5 to 5 cm pole to pole
- ◼ Right kidney slightly lower than the left

ABNORMAL FINDINGS
- ◼ Easily palpated
  - *Enlarged:* >5 cm pole to pole
    - ❏ Consider hydronephrosis or cystic kidney.
- ◼ *Abnormal texture:* not smooth or firm

BLADDER

NORMAL FINDINGS
- ◼ Located 1 to 4 cm above the symphysis pubis
- ◼ Can be percussed (dull sound = urine-filled)

ABNORMAL FINDINGS
- ◼ Continuous distention, consider urinary tract obstruction or CNS abnormality

- Exstrophy of the bladder
  - Herniation of the bladder through the abdominal wall
  - *Causes:* lack of embryologic development of the muscle or connective tissue of the abdominal wall

ABDOMINAL MASSES

- Most abdominal masses palpated at birth are of urinary tract origin (see also "Genitourinary" section).

NORMAL FINDINGS

- Stool palpated in the colon in the lower right/left quadrants
- Gaseous distention

ABNORMAL FINDINGS

- Palpated solid or cystic mass

GROIN/FEMORAL REGION

- Observe at rest and with crying.

NORMAL FINDINGS

- Flat groins
- Equal femoral pulses

ABNORMAL FINDINGS

- Weak or absent femoral pulses, consider coarctation of the aorta or interrupted aortic arch
- Full or bounding pulses, consider PDA
- Inguinal or femoral region bulges (hernia)
  - More common in males or very preterm
  - Evaluate softness and reducibility
  - Surgical repair required; emergent with evidence of strangulation
- Bulge in labia majora, consider hernia or abnormal gonad position (Walker, 2018)

GENITOURINARY

ABNORMAL FINDINGS

- Ambiguous genitalia
  - Presence of a phallic structure that is not discretely female or male
  - Abnormally located ureteral meatus
  - Inability to palpate one or both gonads in males
  - Associated with serious underlying endocrine disorders
  - Evaluation needed with an endocrinologist, genetics, urologist, and social worker (Cavaliere, 2019)

Male

NORMAL FINDINGS

- 2.5 to 3.5 cm in length and 1 cm wide
- Urinary meatus located distal end in the glans
- Noninflamed urethral opening
- Tight foreskin, adhered to the glans (uncircumcised)
- Rugae appear near 36 weeks' GA
- Testes descended into the scrotum by 28 weeks' GA
- Void within the first 24 hours of life
- Rust color stain on diaper caused by presence of uric crystals possible
- Bruising and edema of the genital and buttocks with breech presentation

ABNORMAL FINDINGS

- *Aphallia:* absence of penis
- *Diphallia:* duplicated penis
  - *Two types:* bifid penis and true duplications
- *Chordee:* ventral bowing of the penis
  - Produces a downward curvature on erection; often seen with hypospadias
- *Priapism:* persistent erection of the penis
  - Consider spinal cord lesion.
- *Micropenis:* abnormally small penis that is more than 2.5 *SD* below the mean of the length and width for age using standard charts
- Displaced urethra
- *Epispadias:* urethral meatus located on the dorsal penis
  - Less common than hypospadias
  - Three categories:
    - ❏ *Balanic epispadias:* meatus found at the base of the glans (balanus)
    - ❏ *Penile epispadias:* meatus on the penile shaft
    - ❏ *Penopubic epispadias:* meatus located on the symphysis, not on the penis
- *Hypospadias:* urethral meatus located on the ventral surface of the penis
  - 15% associated with endocrine, chromosomal, or intersex problems
  - Three categories:
    - ❏ *Balanic hypospadias:* meatus found at the base of the glans (balanus)
    - ❏ *Penile hypospadias:* meatus located between the glans and scrotum; often associated with chordee; flattened glans and absence of ventral foreskin
    - ❏ *Penoscrotal hypospadias:* meatus located at the penoscrotal junction; associated with ambiguous genitalia, bifid scrotum, small penis, and undescended testes
- *Cryptorchidism:* undescended testes
  - Most common male genital abnormality; may be unilateral or bilateral
  - Occurrence: 3.7% of term; 21% to 100% of preterm
  - Testes found within normal path of descent, most often below the external inguinal ring

- Usually spontaneously descends by 9 months age
- *Hydrocele:* large scrotal fluid-filled mass
  - Develops during normal fetal development; usually reabsorbed in utero
  - Ability to transilluminate differentiates from solid or blood-filled mass
  - Spontaneous resolution by 3 months of age
- Inguinal hernia (see inguinal or femoral region bulges in the "Groin/Femoral Region" section)
- *Testicular torsion:* twisting of the testes and spermatic cord
  - Small scrotal mass, may be hard and painful; scrotum appears discolored, a red to bluish red
  - May be diagnosed with an ultrasound
  - GU emergency; early identificationcritical to prevent the need for testicular amputation and preserve male fertility

Female

NORMAL FINDINGS

- Symmetric labia majora
- *Term:* labia majora covering the clitoris and the labia minora
- *Preterm:* clitoris exposed
- Presence of vaginal opening (~0.5 cm)
- Hymen tag which may be observed in the vaginal opening
- White to pink-tinged discharge common for 2 to 4 weeks post birth caused by maternal hormone influence

ABNORMAL FINDINGS

- *Periurethral cysts:* most common type of mass, appearing as a whitish epithelial covering next to the unaffected urethral meatus
- Imperforate hymen
  - Suprapubic mass or mass palpated between the labia majora
  - Secretions pooling within the vagina
- *Hydrocolpos:* distention of the vagina
- *Hydrometrocolpos:* distention of the vagina and the uterus
- *Clitoromegaly:* an eight- to tenfold increase in clitoral index (defined as width times length)
  - *Causes:* endocrine abnormalities, congenital adrenal hyperplasia (CAH), maternal factors such as increased androgen production, drugs, and syndromes (Beckwith–Wiedemann, true hermaphroditism)

SPINE

NORMAL FINDINGS

- Spine midline and straight
- No skin disruptions or tufts of hair
- Hyperpigmented blue-gray macule (previously referred to as a "Mongolian spot")
  - Caused by concentrated melanocytes within the dermis; findings benign
  - Most commonly found over the buttocks, flanks, or shoulders
  - Important to document the size and distribution to differentiate these from current or future appearances of bruising (especially if concerns about nonaccidental trauma)
- Simple, blind-ending base dimple, located midline sacrum
- Lateral curvature normal variant (in utero positioning)
- Convex curvature of the lumbar and thoracic spine (best noted in sitting position)
- Extension and lateral bending of spine (noted with passive flexion)

ABNORMAL FINDINGS

- Abnormal-appearing position or curve of the spine
- Skin disruptions or tufts of hair
  - Isolated finding versus hidden spine defect
- Cystic masses
- Hemangioma
  - Isolated finding versus possible abnormality
- Pilonidal dimple, cyst, or sinus tract
  - Isolated finding versus hidden defect (spinal dysraphism)
  - Consider spinal lipoma, dermoid tumor, tethered cord, and split cord
- Winged, elevated scapula (Sprengel deformity)
- Asymmetric gluteal folds
  - Congenital hip dislocation
- Abnormal curvatures
  - *Scoliosis:* abnormal sideway curve of the spine
  - *Kyphosis:* abnormal outward rounded curve of the upper back
  - *Lordosis:* abnormal inward curve of the lower back
  - *Sacrococcygeal teratoma:* most common tumor of the newborn
    - *Causes:* unknown; arises from fetal germ cells
    - *Findings:* usual location base of the coccyx; more common in females; usually benign; can be very large and result in polyhydramnios, fetal urinary obstruction (hydronephrosis), hydrops, tumor bleeding, or rupture
    - *Resolution:* requires surgical resection
- Spinal deformities
  - Congenital scoliosis
    - *Causes:* embryonic defect—failure of vertebral formation, segmentation, or both
    - *Findings:* can occur in any area of the vertebral body
    - *Associations:* 20% to 30% incidence of associated GU tract anomalies; Klippel–Feil syndrome and Sprengel deformity
- *Neural tube defects:* abnormal closure of the posterior neural tube
- Spina bifida occulta

- *Causes:* abnormal closure of the posterior neural tube
- *Findings:* usually asymptomatic (no cord or meninges involvement); most common location lower lumbar or lumbosacral area; covered by skin; often an incidental finding with examination of hair tuft, dimple, sinus, or lipoma; can be associated with tethered cord
- *Resolution:* often asymptomatic requiring no treatment; surgical intervention for tethered cord if present
- Meningocele
  - *Causes:* abnormal closure of the posterior neural tube; meninges protrude through bony defect; usually involve several vertebrae
  - *Findings:* skin covered; spinal roots and nerves normal
  - *Resolution:* surgical closure of defect
- Myelomeningocele
  - *Causes:* abnormal closure of the posterior neural tube; bilateral broadened vertebrae or absent vertebral arches
  - *Findings:* bilateral broadened vertebrae or absent vertebral arches; nerves, spinal roots, and meninges protrude into the sac; spinal cord fused; neural tube exposed; most often occur in lumbar spine; >70% with associated hydrocephalus (may be associated with Arnold–Chiari malformation)
  - *Resolution:* surgical intervention (neurosurgery, plastics) required, as well as neurology, orthopedics, and urology consultation; functional deficits of the lower extremities and neurogenic bladder related to level of involvement (Goodwin, 2016)

Birth Trauma

- Spinal cord injury
  - *Causes:* hyperextension of the head or neck; associated with breech vaginal delivery or severe shoulder dystocia; rate 0.14/10,000 live births; includes spinal epidural hematoma, vertebral artery injury, traumatic cervical hematomyelia, spinal arterial occlusion, and transection of spinal cord
  - *Findings:* depends on the level of the injury
    - ❑ *High cervical injury or brainstem injury:* stillbirth or death within hours; severe respiratory depression, shock, and hypothermia
    - ❑ *Upper, midcervical injury:* central respiratory depression, lower extremity paralysis, absent deep tendon reflexes, urinary retention, and constipation
    - ❑ Below seventh cervical spine injury, may be reversible
    - ❑ *Resolution:* cervical spine x-ray, CT, and/or MRI; neurology and neurosurgery; focus on prevention of additional injury

EXTREMITIES: UPPER

- Fracture of the clavicles
  - *Cause:* It is the most common bone injury of birth (incidence 30% of all live births). fractured clavicle should be suspected when there is a history of difficult delivery. 40% are undiagnosed until after hospital discharge.
  - *Findings:* It may be asymptomatic, with the first clinical sign a palpable callus found at 7 to 10 days of life, swelling or bone irregularity palpated over the clavicle, and crepitus over the clavicles. It may cause spasm of the sternocleidomastoid muscle or pseudoparalysis of the affected extremity caused by pain on movement; asymmetric arm movement or Moro reflex; and pain noted with movement of the arm or shoulder. Visible fracture is confirmed by x-ray.
  - *Resolution:* Although they generally require no treatment, fractures of the clavicle are sufficiently common that the clavicles should be specifically examined in every newborn. Treatment is supportive care and analgesia as needed. Limit arm and shoulder movement. Spontaneous, complete healing is expected.

HUMERUS

NORMAL FINDINGS

- Bilateral symmetry of form, length, and movement

ABNORMAL FINDINGS

- Weakness, paralysis, injury, fracture, or infection, may indicate asymmetry
- Pain on palpation or movement
- Palpated mass
  - Likely hematoma formation at the site of fracture
- Polydactyly
  - *Causes:* congenital anomaly; isolated finding; inherited—autosomal dominant trait; more common in African Americans
  - *Findings:* one or more extra digits on the hands or feet; extra digit can appear as a skin tag or floppy appendage (most common)
- *Macrodactyly:* an enlarged finger or toe
  - *Causes:* normal finding, neurofibromatosis, lymphedema, hemangioma, arterial vascular fistulas, fibrous dysplasia, and lipomas
- *Syndactyly:* congenital webbing of the fingers or toes
  - Males twice as often as females; more common among Caucasians
  - *Causes:* failure of the normal necrosis of the skin that separates the fingers during sixth to eighth week of fetal gestation
  - *Findings:* isolated finding versus association with other congenital anomalies, such as Apert and Streeter dysplasia; the more severe the webbing the more likely of underlying bony abnormalities

Absent Bones

- Congenital absence of the radius (radial dysplasia)

- *Causes:* sporadic inheritance versus association with other congenital sequence/syndrome, VACTERL sequence (vertebral defects, anal atresia, cardiac abnormalities, tracheoesophageal abnormalities, renal and/or limb abnormalities), Fanconi anemia, and Holt–Oram syndrome
- *Findings:* hand and wrist deviated 90 degrees or more; forearm shortened with bowing of the ulna; thumb usually absent or hypoplastic

Disruption Abnormalities

- Amniotic band syndrome
  - *Causes:* Amniotic band encircles the arms, legs, fingers, or toes. There are no gender or ethnic predispositions.
  - *Findings:* Findings vary from mild indentation of the soft tissue to severe amputation.
  - *Resolution:* It depends on the anatomic position and/or associated abnormalities; if vascular, lymphatic, or nerve integrity is compromised, it requires immediate surgical release of band; nonemergent may require staged surgical repairs. It is not life-threatening unless associated with brain malformation or deep facial clefts.

ELBOW, FOREARM, AND WRIST

NORMAL FINDINGS

- Symmetry of size, shape, number of bones, and movement
- Wrist flexion increases with increasing GA

ABNORMAL FINDINGS

- See discussion on amniotic bands, neurologic birth injuries, and congenital absence of radius.

HAND

NORMAL FINDINGS

- Symmetry of size, shape, length, and movement
- Five digits per hand

ABNORMAL FINDINGS

- Single palm crease (Simian crease), can be associated with trisomy 21 (Down syndrome)
- Polydactyly, macrodactyly, syndactyly, and absent bones (see above)
- Flexed fingers with index finger overlapping the third finger, consider trisomy 18
- Puffy hands, normal finding caused by lymphedema from birth positioning; characteristic finding of some syndromes; consider Turner and Noonan syndromes
- See discussion on amniotic bands.

EXTREMITIES: LOWER

Hips

NORMAL FINDINGS

- 20- to 30-degree flexion contraction normal; resolves by 4 to 6 months age
- Normal hip abduction almost 90 degrees

ABNORMAL FINDINGS

- Developmental dysplasia of the hip (DDH)
  - Positive Barlow maneuver
    - Hip is adducted while pushing the thigh posteriorly.
    - Palpable, sometimes audible "clunk" indicates dislocation of the hip.
    - Hip will be relocated by performing the Ortolani maneuver.
  - Positive Ortolani maneuver
    - Thigh of the hip being tested is abducted and gently pulled anteriorly.
    - Palpable, sometimes audible "clunk" will be detected as the femoral head moves over the posterior rim of the acetabulum and back into position, indicating dislocation of the hip.
  - Treatment
    - Treatment includes Pavlik harness or closed reduction surgery (Boucher et al., 2017; Fanaroff et al., 2020; Walker, 2018).
- See discussion on amniotic bands.

Legs

NORMAL FINDINGS

- Symmetry of size, shape, number of bones, and movement
- Mild bowing and internal rotation common due to intrauterine space and fetal positioning

ABNORMAL FINDINGS

- Irregularities in contour, masses, or crepitation
- Pain on movement
- Discrepancy in knee height (Galeazzi or Allis sign)
  - Consider DDH
- *Internal tibial torsion:* inward twisting of the tibia resulting in intoeing of the foot
- Congenital absence of the tibia or fibula
  - *Findings:* Mild to marked shortening of the lower leg; may be partial or complete; knee is unstable with flexion contracture; absence of fibula presentation is shortening of the involved leg with bowing of the tibia anteriorly and medially
- See discussion on amniotic bands.

Ankles and Feet

NORMAL FINDINGS
■ Symmetry of size, shape, length, and movement
■ Five digits per foot

ABNORMAL FINDINGS
■ Clubfoot (talipes equinovarus)
  ● *Findings:* adduction of the forefoot (points medially); pronounced varus of the heel; downward pointing of the foot and toes; lacks full range of motion, resists dorsiflexion
  ● *Resolution:* based on severity; exercises and serial casting, or surgical correction
■ Talipes equinovarus (clubfoot)
  ● *Causes:* positional or structural
  ● *Findings:* inversion of the heel resulting in medial pointing of the soles; forefoot curves inward; ankle in "equinus posture" (toes pointed down; heel points up)
  ● *Resolution:* treatment determined by severity of clubfoot, which varies; some treatments are conservative, such as exercises and serial casting; some require surgical correction when nonoperative treatments are unsuccessful
■ *Metatarsus adductus:* most common congenital foot abnormality
  ● *Causes:* positional deformity as a result of intrauterine positioning; structural deformity
  ● *Findings:* deformity of forefoot; metatarsal bones deviated medially
  ● *Resolution:* spontaneous correction with stretching exercises; casting or surgery if rigid deformity
■ *Rocker bottom feet:* also known as congenital vertical talus
  ● *Findings:* prominence of calcaneus (heel bone); convex rounded bottom of the foot (resembles bottom of rocking chair)
■ See discussion on amniotic bands.

▶ MUSCLE MOVEMENT/TONE/REFLEXES

Evaluation of muscle tone involves resting posture, passive tone, and active tone and should be done when in an awake and alert state.

NORMAL MUSCLE TONE FINDINGS

■ *Phasic:* Brief, forceful contraction results in response to a short-duration, high-amplitude stretch. Tests resistance of the upper and lower extremities to movement.
  ● Examples of resistance are scarf sign and arm/leg recoil.
  ● Minimal resistance is normal at 28 weeks.
  ● Resistance increases with maturity.

■ The biceps reflex and the patellar reflex can be tested in the newborn and the patellar is the most frequently demonstrated after birth. The normal response of the patellar reflex is extension at the knee and visible contraction of the quadriceps.
■ Asymmetric deep tendon reflexes may be due to central or peripheral nervous system impairment.
■ Clonus is rapid movement of a particular joint by sudden stretching of a tendon. Sustained clonus may indicate cerebral irritation (Dillon Heaberlin, 2019).

POSTURAL TONE

■ Test the ability to resist the pull to gravity by grasping the neonate's hands and pulling slowly from the supine to a sitting position. It is best tested by traction response (pull-to-sit maneuver).
  ● During traction, flexion occurs in the elbows, knees, and ankles.
  ● In term neonates, more than minimum head lag is abnormal and may indicate hypotonia.
  ● Neck flexion is absent in preterm infants less than 33 weeks' GA.
■ Strength of the lower extremities is evaluated by observing the infant's stepping reflex and is noted by 37 weeks' GA (Dillon Heaberlin, 2019; Fanaroff et al., 2020; Goodwin, 2016).

ABNORMALITIES OF MUSCLE TONE

Hypotonia

■ Focal injury to the cerebellum can result in contralateral hemiparesis of the face and upper extremities.
■ Neuromuscular diseases such as myasthenia gravis and infantile botulism can cause generalized weakness and hypotonia.
■ Werdnig–Hoffmann disease is a disorder of the lower motor neurons.
  ● Flaccid weakness of the extremities
  ● Continuous and rapid twitching movements of the tongue (Goodwin, 2016)

Hypertonia

■ Less common in the newborn period
■ *Opisthotonos (hypertonia with arching of back):* seen in bacterial meningitis, severe neonatal encephalopathy and massive intraventricular hemorrhage (IVH), and tetanus (Dillon Heaberlin, 2019; Goodwin, 2016)

DEVELOPMENTAL REFLEXES

■ Assessment of developmental reflexes is used to determine the overall well-being of the brain and nervous system. Reflexes are involuntary movements or actions and may be spontaneous and observed with normal newborn activity or in response to an outside action. Some reflexes are only observed during certain periods of development (Goodwin, 2016).

- See Table 6.12 for complete description of developmental reflexes.

BEHAVIORAL ASSESSMENT

- Behavioral assessment provides information about the infant's neurobehavioral functioning and the newborn's capability to control their behavior and to adapt to an environment as seen in different subsystems, such as habituation, orientation, motor behavior, behavioral states, and autonomic system.

- The evaluation of the autonomic nervous system includes evaluation of vital sign stability, neurocutaneous stability, gastrointestinal stability, and the presence or absence of jitteriness or myoclonic jerks (Table 6.13).

- Motor behavior is a comprehensive system that incorporates autonomic, involuntary movement into the objective, purposeful, coordinated movement of the entire body from head to toe. It includes both physical and social activity and behavior (Table 6.14).

Table 6.12 Developmental Reflexes in the Neonate

Reflex	Test	Response
Palmar grasp	■ Stroke palm with finger	■ Grasps finger ■ Stronger in preterm ■ Onset by 28 weeks' GA; well established by 32–34 weeks ■ Response fades at 2–3 months ■ *Absent reflex:* CNS deficit or muscle injury
Rooting reflex	■ Stroke side of cheek	■ Turns head toward direction of touch ■ Onset by 28 weeks' GA; well established by 32–34 weeks ■ *Unilateral absence:* facial paralysis ■ *Bilateral absence:* neurologic depression
Sucking reflex	■ Finger into mouth	■ Sucking ■ Present in utero by ~26 weeks' GA ■ Onset ~28 weeks' GA; well established by 32–34 weeks ■ Disappears by 12 months
Moro (startle) reflex	■ Loud noise or gentle jolt	■ Extends arms, legs, and neck, then pulls back arms and legs ■ Onset 28–32 weeks' GA; well established by 37 weeks ■ Disappears at 5–6 months ■ *Asymmetric response:* brachial plexus injury or fractured clavicle ■ *Absent:* severe brainstem problem
Tonic neck (fencing position)	■ Supine; turn head to one side; hold position 15 seconds	■ Arm and leg extend on facial side; flex on opposite side ■ Onset at 35 weeks' GA; well established by 4 weeks ■ Disappears by 6 months ■ *Absent:* abnormal
Babinski reflex	■ Stroke lateral aspect of sole from heel to ball of foot	■ Hyperextension of all toes ■ Onset at 34–36 weeks' GA; well established by 38 weeks ■ Positive response normal until 2 years of age ■ *Persistent absence:* CNS depression or spinal nerve injury
Galant reflex	■ Prone; stroke down one side of spine	■ Pelvis turns toward stimulated side ■ Present at birth ■ Disappears by 2 months ■ *Asymmetric response:* neurologic abnormality
Stepping reflex	■ Hold upright with soles of feet touching flat surface	■ Alternate stepping movements

CNS, central nervous system; GA, gestational age.

Sources: Data from Tappero, E. (2021). Physical assessment. In M. T. Verklan, M. Walden, & S. Forest (Eds.), *Core curriculum for neonatal intensive care nursing* (6th ed. pp. 99–130). Elsevier; Boucher, N., Marvicsin, D., & Gardner, S. (2017). Physical examination, interventions, and referrals. In B. Snell & S. Gardner (Eds.), *Care of the well newborn* (pp. 130–131, 125). Jones and Bartlett Learning; Dillon Heaberlin, P. (2019). Neurologic assessment. In E. P. Tappero & M. E. Honeyfield (Eds.), *Physical assessment of the newborn: A comprehensive approach to the art of physical examination* (5th ed., p. 173). Springer Publishing Company; Walker, V. P. (2018). Newborn evaluation. In C. A. Gleason, & S. E. Juul, (Eds.),*Avery's diseases of the newborn* (10th ed. pp. 289–311.e1). Elsevier; Goodwin, M. (2016). Abdomen assessment. In E. P. Tappero & M. E. Honeyfield (Eds.), *Physical assessment of the newborn: A comprehensive approach to the art of physical examination* (5th ed., pp. 111–120). Springer Publishing Company.

Table 6.13 Evaluation of the Autonomic System in the Neonate

System	Unstressed	Stressed	Intervention to Correct
Respiratory	■ Smooth, unlabored breathing	■ Tachypnea ■ Irregular breathing pattern ■ Very slow respirations ■ Apnea	■ Reducing environmental stimulation (light, noise, activity)
Color	■ Pink color	■ Pale or mottled ■ Red ■ Dusky or cyanotic	■ Gentle hand containment ■ Offering pacifier during procedures/exams ■ Soft voice ■ Slow movement transitions
Visceral	■ Feeding tolerance ■ Smooth digestion	■ Hiccups or yawns ■ Coughs or sneezes ■ Gagging or spitting up ■ Grunting and straining with defecation	■ Pacing feedings by ability and cues
Autonomic-related motor patterns	■ No tremors or twitching	■ Startles ■ Tremors ■ Twitching of face or extremities	■ Cluster care ■ Gentle repositioning while containing extremities ■ Using nesting or boundaries ■ Managing pain

Source: Data from Spruill, C. T. (2021). Developmental support. In M. T. Verklan, M. Walden, & S. Forest (Eds.), *Core curriculum for neonatal intensive care nursing* (6th ed., pp. 172–190). Elsevier.

Table 6.14 Evaluation of Motor Systems

System	Unstressed	Stressed	Intervention to Correct
Tone	■ Consistent, normal tone for GA ■ Control of movement, activity, and posture	■ Hypertonia or hypotonia ■ Limp ■ Hyperflexion	■ Support rest periods and reduce sleep disruption. ■ Minimize stress. ■ Use containment and swaddling.
Posture	■ Improved, well-maintained posture	■ Unable to maintain flexed, aligned posture	■ Use boundaries, swaddling, and positioning aids to maintain flexion, containment, and alignment.
Movement	■ Control of movements ■ Midline flexion of hands/legs ■ Hands together or to mouth	■ Stiff, extension of extremities/fingers ■ Neck hyperextension ■ Flailing movements	■ Use swaddling, boundaries, nesting, or gentle hand containment. ■ Support overall calming.
Level of activity	■ Activity consistent with environment and GA	■ Frequent squirming ■ Frantic flailing activity ■ Lack of activity/movement	■ Manage pain. ■ Modify environment and reduce stimulation. ■ Encourage skin to skin.

GA, gestational age.

Source: Data from Spruill, C. T. (2021). Developmental support. In M. T. Verklan, M. Walden, & S. Forest (Eds.), *Core curriculum for neonatal intensive care nursing* (6th ed., pp. 172–190). Elsevier.

■ *State* refers to the level of consciousness exhibited by the infant and is determined by the level of arousal and ability to respond to stimuli (Vittner & McGrath, 2019).
  ● The six behavioral states of the newborn are deep sleep, light sleep, drowsiness, quiet alertness, active alertness, and crying (Boucher et al., 2017; Vittner & McGrath, 2019).
  ● The neonate's state should be noted both before and during the examination, optimally with the neonate in the quiet, alert state (Table 6.15).
■ It reflects the infant's ability to integrate in the environment physiologically without disruption in state or physiologic functions (Vittner & McGrath, 2019). Clustering care to allow for uninterrupted sleep, arousing the infant slowly, and introducing one stimulus at a time aid in organization for the infant (Tables 6.16 and 6.17).

Table 6.15 Assessment of Behavior and State of the Neonate

State	Behavior
Deep sleep	■ Closed eyes ■ No spontaneous eye activity ■ Regular breathing
Light sleep	■ Low levels of activity ■ Rapid eye movement possible ■ May startle ■ May make brief fussing noises ■ *Preterm:* may have irregular respirations
Drowsiness	■ Variable activity (mild startles, smooth movement) ■ Some facial movement ■ Eyes open and close ■ Breathing irregular ■ Response to stimuli may be delayed ■ May startle easily
Quiet alert	■ Rarely moves ■ Breathing regular ■ Focuses intently on individuals/objects/stimuli within focal range; widens eyes ■ Face bright and alert
Active alert	■ Moves frequently ■ Abundant facial movement ■ Appears slightly less bright and alert ■ Breathing irregular ■ Periods of fussiness ■ *Preterm:* distressed/unable to organize
Crying	■ Grimacing ■ Eyes shut ■ Breathing irregular ■ Increased movement with color changes ■ Marked response to internal and external stimuli

Source: Data from Vittner, D. & McGrath, J., (2019). Behavioral assessment. In E. P. Tappero & M. E. Honeyfield (Eds.), *Physical assessment of the newborn: A comprehensive approach to the art of physical examination* (6th ed., p. 193–218). Springer Publishing Company.

Table 6.17 The Disorganized Infant

General State	Sensory Threshold Cues and Signs
■ Sudden change in state ■ Sudden change in vital signs ■ Frantic, jittery movements	Overstimulated with signs of stress and fatigue: ■ Gaze aversion ■ Frowning ■ Sneezing, yawning, hiccupping ■ Vomiting ■ Mottling ■ Irregular respirations, apnea, increased oxygen needs ■ Changes in HR ■ Arching or stiffness ■ Finger splaying ■ Fussing, crying

HR, heart rate.
Source: Data from Vittner, D. & McGrath, J., (2019). Behavioral assessment. In E. P. Tappero & M. E. Honeyfield (Eds.), *Physical assessment of the newborn: A comprehensive approach to the art of physical examination* (6th ed., p. 193–218). Springer Publishing Company.

HABITUATION

■ *Habituation* is the infant's ability to decrease a response to a repeat stimulus. When a stimulus is repeated, the initial response will gradually disappear. Habituation provides a defense mechanism for shutting out overwhelming or uncomfortable stimuli (Vittner & McGrath, 2019).

Testing Visual Habituation

■ Shine a bright light when the infant is sleeping and repeat every 5 to 10 seconds. An appropriate response is a grimace. When habituation occurs, responses will become delayed until it disappears (Vittner & McGrath, 2019).

Testing Auditory Habituation

■ Use an object that makes noise and hold the object 10 to 15 in. from the baby and shake the object for

Table 6.16 The Organized Infant

General State	Behavioral Cues	Signs of Approach
■ Stable vital signs ■ Smooth state transition with environmental interaction ■ Easily consoled ■ Able to block out overwhelming stimuli	■ Quiet alert state ■ Focused gaze ■ Dilated pupils ■ Respirations and HR regular ■ Rhythmic sucking ■ Reaching or grasping ■ Hand-to-mouth movement	■ Quiet alert state ■ Focused gaze ■ Dilated pupils ■ Respirations and HR regular ■ Rhythmic sucking ■ Reaching or grasping ■ Hand-to-mouth movement

HR, heart rate.
Source: Data from Vittner, D. & McGrath, J., (2019). Behavioral assessment. In E. P. Tappero & M. E. Honeyfield (Eds.), *Physical assessment of the newborn: A comprehensive approach to the art of physical examination* (6th ed., p. 193–218). Springer Publishing Company.

1 second. Responses include startles, squirming movements, facial grimaces, and respiratory changes. When habituation occurs, infants decrease responses to the stimulus (Vittner & McGrath, 2019).

Testing Tactile Habituation

- This can be determined by stimulating the sole of the foot with a smooth object. A normal response

Summary of Physical Examination of the Neonate

History	Inspection	Auscultation	Palpation	Other
Skin				
■ N/A	■ Color, turgor, texture ■ Birthmarks, lesions, petechiae, rashes, bruising ■ Presence of vernix ■ Presence of birth trauma	■ N/A	■ Presence of masses ■ Abnormal textures	■ Lab work (bilirubin, hematocrit, platelet count, culture, etc.)
Head				
■ Known fetal abnormalities	■ Overall shape and size of skull ■ Presence of molding ■ Presence of birth trauma: scalp probe puncture, lacerations, bruises, abrasions, subcutaneous fat necrosis ■ Hair texture, quantity, distribution ■ Hair whorls: number and position ■ Hairline ■ Shape, integrity, movement, and symmetry of facial organs and ears ■ Note abnormalities of skull or scalp: cutis aplasia, encephalocele	■ Auscultation of head/fontanel for bruit	■ Presence and size of fontanels ■ Cranial sutures: approximated, separated, overriding, mobility ■ Presence of craniotabes ■ Assessment of scalp edema and bruising: caput succedaneum, cephalohematoma, subgaleal hemorrhage	■ Ophthalmoscopic exam ■ Universal hearing screening
Neck				
■ Known fetal abnormality	■ Shape and symmetry ■ Presence of redundant skin or webbed neck ■ Presence of birth trauma ■ Tone, range of motion, and symmetry of movement	■ N/A	■ Range of motion ■ Reflexes ■ Clavicles ■ Masses	■ Transillumination ■ Ultrasound
Chest/Lungs				
■ Gestational age ■ Known fetal anomalies ■ Results of fetal lung maturity ■ Maternal steroids ■ Birth history	■ Note landmark structures ■ General color, tone, activity ■ Assess mucous membranes ■ Note chest shape, movement, symmetry, and synchrony ■ Note respiratory rate and work of breathing ■ Presence of sneezing or coughing ■ Nipple placement, spacing, pigment, secretions	■ Bilateral breath sounds; note pitch, intensity, duration, and symmetry ■ Note presence of crackles, wheezes, rubs, or stridor	■ Palpate clavicles for presence of crepitus or tenderness	■ Transillumination ■ Chest x-ray

History	Inspection	Auscultation	Palpation	Other
Cardiovascular				
■ *Maternal risk factors:* maternal diabetes, lupus erythematous, maternal congenital heart disease (three to four times risk of general population) ■ Presence of other fetal anomalies with 25% association with CHD	■ General color, tone, and activity ■ Assess precordium: quiet, active ■ Capillary refill ■ Presence of systemic cyanosis (key indices of CHD) ■ Presence of edema	■ Heart rate and rhythm ■ Heart sounds ■ Presence of murmurs	■ Peripheral pulses: rate, rhythm, volume, character, symmetry ■ Location of apical pulse/PMI ■ Presence of heaves, taps, or thrills ■ Liver edge	■ Universal oximetry test: CCHD screening ■ Oxygen challenge test ■ Pre- and postductal oximeter saturation comparison ■ Four-limb blood pressure measurement ■ Echocardiogram
Abdomen				
■ Fetal ultrasound with evidence of abnormal size/shape of kidneys, distended bowel, or other masses ■ Presence of polyhydramnios (20%–30%) association with structural abnormalities; most common esophageal or duodenal atresia	■ Abdominal shape, movement, and skin texture ■ Umbilical cord characteristics: color, size, number of vessels, noted abnormalities ■ Presence of abdominal wall defect ■ Perianal region: location of organs, patency, sphincter tone, other noted abnormalities	■ Perform prior to palpation ■ Assess four quadrants for presence and quality of bowel sounds	■ Perform palpation from superficial to deep organs ■ Assess muscle tone ■ Note ability to palpate; shape and size of organs ■ Presence of masses	■ Abdominal ultrasound ■ Abdominal x-ray
Genitourinary				
■ Known fetal anomalies	■ Evaluate external structures ■ Presence of urine ■ Presence of birth trauma	■ N/A	■ Palpable bladder ■ Presence of testes within the canal or scrotum	■ Transillumination ■ Abdominal ultrasound ■ VCUG
Musculoskeletal				
■ Presentation ■ Birth history ■ Abnormal/decreased fetal movement	■ Observe at rest and with movement ■ Note symmetry or abnormalities of movement ■ Number of digits ■ Presence of nails ■ Presence of positional deformities	■ N/A	■ ROM of all extremities ■ Evaluation for hip dysplasia/congenital hip dislocation ■ Positional vs. structural abnormalities	■ x-rays

History	Inspection	Auscultation	Palpation	Other
Spine				
■ Any detected fetal abnormalities	■ Base of skull to coccyx ■ Presence of dimples, cysts, sinus tracts, tufts of hair ■ Skin disruption or discoloration ■ Symmetry of scapula and sides ■ Curvature of spine ■ Visible spinal deformities	■ N/A	■ Dorsal spine processes ■ Curvature of spine	■ Spinal ultrasound
Neurologic/Behavioral				
■ Birth history ■ Abnormal/ diminished fetal movement ■ Known fetal anomaly	■ Evaluated throughout PE ■ Posture, muscle tone, movement, reflexes ■ Evaluation of cranial nerves	■ N/A	■ Evaluated throughout PE	■ Neurology ■ Ultrasound ■ CT/MRI ■ Neurodevelopmental

CCHD, critical congenital heart disease; CHD, congenital heart disease; N/A, not applicable; PE, physical examination; PMI, point of maximum impulse; ROM, rupture of membranes; VCUG, voiding cystourethrogram.

is the infant responding by pulling their foot back. When habituation occurs, the response will gradually disappear (Vittner & McGrath, 2019).

▶ CONCLUSION

Despite the many advances in our medical technology, physical assessment remains one of the most important skills to have as a neonatal practitioner. There is no replacement for our senses in recognizing the subtle signs and symptoms that can be crucial in the timely identification of life-threatening conditions of the newborn requiring immediate intervention or transfer to a higher level of care, or in the identification of potential life-altering conditions (newborn malformation/ anomaly, extreme prematurity) that require timely discussion and support of the newborn's family. Expertise in the art of physical assessment should be the goal of every provider as it remains a critical skill required to ensure good outcomes for all newborns and their families.

1. Postmenstrual age (PMA) is defined as the age from the first day of the last menstrual period (LMP) to the day of:

   A. Assessment
   B. Confinement
   C. Parturition

2. The majority of notable, visible anomalies discovered on physical examination of a newborn are found in the:

   A. Feet
   B. Genitalia
   C. Head

3. The neonatal nurse practitioner (NNP) recognizes that a clinical presentation suggestive of congenital heart disease is one in which cyanosis increases when an infant is:

   A. Crying
   B. Stooling
   C. Tremoring

4. A pregnant patient is preparing to deliver vaginally an infant at 40 5/7 weeks' gestation who is large for gestational age (LGA). This infant is identified as at high risk for intrapartum:

   A. Hypoextension of the neck
   B. Severe shoulder dystocia
   C. Umbilical cord trauma

5. Rugae begin to form on the neonatal scrotum at:

   A. 28 weeks
   B. 34 weeks
   C. 36 weeks

1. A) Assessment

PMA is the age from the first day of LMP to the day of assessment. Estimated date of confinement (EDC) is used to determine the mother's anticipated date of delivery, while parturition is not a commonly used term (Trotter, 2016, 2019).

2. C) Head

Findings can be normal variants or associated with syndromes or chromosomal abnormalities. Ninety percent of all visible anomalies at birth are found in the head area. The head encompasses multiple systems that may be affected by anomalies (e.g., eyes, ears, mouth, palate, nares). The other two systems offered do not contain as main potential anomalies and are more limited (Johnson, 2019; Tappero, 2021).

3. A) Crying

If central cyanosis is present and there is no evidence of respiratory distress and/or it worsens with crying, the cause is likely congenital heart disease (CHD). It can be assessed by the oxygen challenge test (administration of 100% oxygen). If there is no improvement in saturations, etiology is likely CHD. Transient, brief episodes of stooling and tremoring do not result in cardiorespiratory compromise (Tappero, 2021; Vargo, 2019).

4. B) Severe shoulder dystocia

LGA denotes growth indices greater than the 90th percentile for gestational age (GA), which increases the risk for difficult vaginal delivery. An LGA infant may be at risk for hyperextension of the neck (not hypoextension). Umbilical cord trauma can occur at any gestational age regardless of size (Abdulhayoglu, 2017; Tappero, 2019, 2021; Vargo, 2019).

5. C) 36 weeks

Rugae are ridges, wrinkles, or folds. Developmentally, rugae first appear on the front of the scrotal sac at about 36 weeks' gestation, covering the sac by about 40 weeks (Tappero & Honeyfield, 2019).

Clinical Laboratory Tests and Diagnostic Procedures, Techniques, and Equipment

Ke-Ni Niko Tien

▶ INTRODUCTION

Infants in the NICU frequently require laboratory testing or diagnostic procedures to assess their clinical status. It is important to understand physiology to properly provide integral accuracy, precision, sensitivity, specificity, and reference range of laboratory interpretation to provide comprehensive patient care. Common laboratory tests obtained in the NICU include chemistry analysis, hematologic tests, microbiology tests, microscopy tests, blood bank tests (immunohematology tests), immunoassays, cytogenetic tests, and immunology tests. This chapter covers diagnostic studies, procedures, and equipment common to patient care management in the NICU.

▶ CLINICAL LABORATORY TESTS

JUDICIOUS USE OF LABORATORY TESTING

- Judicious use of laboratory testing is critical in any high-acuity setting, particularly in the NICU. It is essential that a neonatal nurse practitioner (NNP) is familiar with the laboratory test collection methods, test interpretation principles, and test utilization in the NICU. There are questions the NNP should consider prior to ordering or obtaining a laboratory sample. These questions will assist in refining critical thinking skills and aid in the selective use of lab work.
  - Does the patient require the laboratory test?
    - ❑ Are the patient examination results abnormal, whereby a laboratory test will help diagnose?
    - ❑ Is the medical history helpful in directing which laboratory test to order?
    - ❑ Does the laboratory test require too much blood volume?
    - ❑ Is the laboratory test the "best" test to answer the clinical question?
  - Will the laboratory test result answer the "so what" question?
    - ❑ Is the laboratory result contributing to the infant's diagnosis?
    - ❑ Is the laboratory result integral to the immediate clinical management of the infant?
    - ❑ Does the potential benefit of the laboratory test outweigh the risk of sequelae in the patient?
  - Is the laboratory test requested still applicable to the current clinical status?
    - ❑ Is the timing of the laboratory test appropriate?
    - ❑ Has the infant's clinical status changed?
  - If the laboratory sample is inadequate, faulty, or "lost," is it necessary to redraw it? (Scheans, 2022)

BIOCHEMICAL TESTS

- Measurements of chemical substances in the body reflect metabolic processes, disease states, and chemical activity or state. These measurements are useful in the diagnosis, planning of care, monitoring of therapy, screening, and determining the severity of disease and the response to treatment. Biochemical testing also provides information for assessing nutritional adequacy or medication toxicity.
- Biochemical substances present in the circulation include sodium (Na^+), potassium (K^+), calcium (Ca^+), magnesium (Mg^+), phosphorus (PO_4^-), chloride (Cl^-), and bicarbonate (HCO_3^-).
  - *Sodium:* The normal range is between 135 and 145 mEq/L. Sodium is the major *extracellular cation* and is involved in water balance. It is recommended to maintain serum sodium in the high-normal range (145–150 mEq/L) during the first 24 to 72 hours of life.
    - ❑ Hyponatremia is a serum sodium concentration of <130 mEq/L.
    - ❑ Hypernatremia is a serum sodium concentration of >150 mEq/L.
  - *Potassium:* The normal range is 3.5 to 5.5 mEq/L. Potassium is the major cation in the intracellular fluid (ICF) and plays an essential role along with sodium in regulating cell membrane potential.
    - ❑ Hypokalemia is a serum potassium concentration of <3.5 mEq/L.

- ❏ Hyperkalemia is a serum potassium concentration of >6 mEq/L (some define the level as >6.5 mEq/L or >7 mEq/L). A level of 6.4 to 7 mEq/L can be life-threatening.
- *Calcium:* The normal range for serum calcium is between 8.5 and 10.2 mg/dL. Serum Ca⁺ is transported in the form of protein-bound Ca, inactivated Ca, and free ionized calcium (iCa; 4.4–5.3 mg/dL or 1.1–1.45 mmol/L; Bell, 2022). Decreased levels from the use of furosemide (Lasix), caffeine citrate (Cafcit), or glucocorticosteroids may negatively impact calcium storage and result in bone demineralization.
  - ❏ Hypocalcemia is a serum calcium concentration of <7 mg/dL or iCa of <4.4 mg/dL (1.1 mmol/L).
  - ❏ Hypercalcemia is a serum calcium concentration of >11 mg/dL or iCa of >5.8 mg/dL (1.45 mmol/L).
- *Magnesium:* The normal range is 1.5 to 2.5 mg/dL. Magnesium is involved in many intracellular enzyme reactions and is primarily regulated by the kidneys.
  - ❏ Hypomagnesemia is a serum magnesium concentration of <1.5 mg/dL.
  - ❏ Hypermagnesemia is a serum magnesium level of >2.5 mg/dL.
- *Phosphorus:* The normal range is 6.5 to 7 mg/dL. A level of <4 mg/dL indicates decreased bone mineralization.
- *Bicarbonate:* The normal range is 22 to 26 mEq/L for neonates.
- *Metabolites:* These are nonfunctioning waste products in the process of being cleared. Examples include bilirubin, ammonia, blood urea nitrogen (BUN), creatinine (Cr), and uric acid.
  - Bilirubin is a by-product of heme breakdown. In the presence of reduced liver function, the organ is unable to excrete conjugated bilirubin into the bile ducts or biliary tract, or excessive load of unconjugated bilirubin (hemolysis) increases indirect bilirubin level.
  - Ammonia is a by-product of colonic bacteria protein breakdown. When the liver is in failure, the ammonia level elevates.
  - BUN is an indirect measurement of kidney function. Elevated values may indicate increased production of urea nitrogen in catabolic states (e.g., tissue breakdown). There is little to no association between BUN levels and protein intake, even when changes in renal function are considered. If BUN is <20 mg/dL, renal insufficiency due to intrinsic acute kidney injury (AKI) should be suspected.
  - Cr is a valid biochemical marker of renal function in newborns, especially for very low birth weight (VLBW) infants. In term infants, the serum Cr level gradually decreases to a stable level of approximately 0.4 mg/dL within the first 2 weeks of age. In preterm infants, the plasma Cr level rises in the first 48 hours before falling.
  - Uric acid may be elevated in the newborn due to increased nucleotide breakdown. High urinary uric acid concentrations may leave pink or red uric acid crystals in the diaper.
- Substances are released from cells as a result of cell damage and abnormal permeability or cellular proliferation. Examples are alkaline phosphatase (ALP), alanine aminotransferase (ALT), aspartate aminotransferase (AST), and creatinine kinase.
  - ALP is derived from the epithelium of the intrahepatic bile cells and can also be found in the bone, kidney, and small intestine. The markers are for managing metabolic bone disease and assessing bone mineralization status. Elevated ALP levels indicate obstructive liver disease, hepatitis, and bone disease. An increase in serum ALP concentration of >500 to 700 mg/dL indicates a decrease in bone mineralization. The infant is at risk of rickets when the level is >500 to 700 mg/dL.
  - ALT is a pyridoxal enzyme that catalyzes the reversible interconversion of alpha-amino group of aspartic acid to the alpha-ketoglutaric acid, and then to the formation of pyruvic acid. It will be elevated in the presence of disseminated herpes simplex virus (HSV). This laboratory test was formerly known as serum glutamic–pyruvic transaminase (SGPT).
  - AST is a pyridoxal phosphate (PLP)-dependent transaminase enzyme that catalyzes the reversible transfer of the alpha-amino group of aspartic acid to the alpha-keto group of alpha-ketoglutaric acid, and then to the formation of oxaloacetic acid. This laboratory test was formerly known as serum glutamic–oxaloacetic transaminase (SGOT).
    - ❏ ALT and AST are the most sensitive tests of hepatocyte necrosis, and the ALT-to-AST ratio can facilitate differentiation of types of liver disease.
  - Creatinine kinase is the most useful enzyme for evaluating muscle disease and damage; however, it does not necessarily correlate with muscle weakness. Interpretation must be with the awareness that levels are usually elevated in the first several days after a vaginal delivery.
- Examples of drugs and toxic substances tested for in laboratory sampling are antibiotics, caffeine citrate, digoxin, phenobarbital, and substances of abuse.
  - Antibiotic levels are gauged through therapeutic drug monitoring (TDM) using plasma medication concentrations to determine and optimize medication therapy.
    - ❏ There are three types of medication levels: peak, trough, and random levels.
  - *Caffeine:* The half-life is approximately 100 hours and its therapeutic level is 5 to 20 mcg/mL.
  - *Phenobarbital:* The therapeutic range for treatment of seizures is 15 to 40 mcg/mL.

- Screening tests for fetal exposure to maternal substance use disorder (SUD) can occur through multiple biological samples including urine, blood, meconium, neonatal hair, and the umbilical cord. Urine drug screen is the most frequently used method; however, the limitation is that it can only detect recent substance use. In contrast, meconium accumulates throughout the pregnancy, which provides higher sensitivity and detects a longer period of drug exposure. Umbilical cord tissue is the most frequently used biologic medium for substance exposure screening (Bell, 2022; Bradshaw, 2022; Cadnapaphornchai et al., 2021; Churchman, 2020; D'Apolito, 2022; Darras & Volpe, 2018; Ditzenberger, 2022; Domonoske, 2022; Jackson et al., 2021; Maguire, 2022; McCandless & Kripps, 2020; Nyp et al., 2021; Parker, 2022; Scheans, 2022; Wright et al., 2018).

HEMATOLOGIC TESTS

- Hematologic tests are done to study the blood and blood-forming tissues of the body, such as the bone marrow and reticuloendothelial system. Testing also includes the study of hemoglobin (Hgb) structure, red cell membrane, and red cell enzyme activity.
  - Whole blood is composed of blood cells suspended in plasma fluid.
  - Plasma is unclotted blood that has been centrifuged to remove any cells and contains the protein *fibrinogen*.
- *Blood cells:* erythrocytes (red blood cells [RBCs]), leukocytes (white blood cells [WBCs]), and thrombocytes (platelets [Plts])
  - *Hematocrit (Hct):* Hct is the percentage of RBCs. Like Hgb, Hct levels are higher after birth and then decrease to cord values by the end of the first week of life. It should be checked along with Hgb or complete blood count (CBC) in infants at high risk, such as twins; infants of a diabetic mother (IDM); those with signs of plethora or hyperviscosity, hypovolemia, or hypotension; history of maternal bleeding; fetal or neonatal blood loss; suspected sepsis; or pathologic jaundice. It ranges between 48% and 60% in term infants.
  - *Hgb:* Hgb is the major iron-containing component of RBCs. It is composed of alpha- and beta-type globin. The binding of oxygen to Hgb is influenced by temperature, pH, carbon dioxide pressure (PCO_2), and the concentration of RBC organic phosphates. RBCs contain 70% to 90% fetal hemoglobin (HbF) at birth and transition to adult hemoglobin (HbA) at the end of fetal life; the range is 16 to 20 g/dL in term infants. The level is higher at birth depending on gestational age (GA) or volume of placental transfusion, such as from delayed cord clamping, decreases by the end of the first week of life, and then reaches a physiologic nadir at 8 to 12 weeks of life.

- *Reticulocyte (retic) count:* Retic count indicates the ability of the bone marrow to adequately produce RBCs. It is also inversely proportional to GA at birth and falls rapidly to less than 2% by 7 days. The retic count is persistently elevated with ongoing RBC destruction, and persistent reticulocytosis may indicate chronic blood loss or hemolysis.
- *Plt count:* Plts are among the agents responsible for hemostasis, coagulation, and thrombus formation. It normally ranges between 150,000 and 400,000/mm^3. Thrombocytopenia (Plt <100,000/mm^3) is most likely associated with bacterial sepsis or viral infection.
- *Peripheral blood smear:* This is used for initial evaluation of anemia to identify abnormal RBC shapes and provide clues to the etiology of the anemia.
- *CBC:* CBC evaluates RBCs, WBCs, and Plts.
- *WBC count:* Maturation occurs in the bone marrow and lymphatic tissues. The normal range is between 5,000 and 30,000 cells/mm^3 at birth. It is optimal to obtain WBC after 4 hours of age and it is recommended to collect the first sample at 6 to 12 hours of age.
- Leukocytosis (WBC >20,000/mm^3) may be normal in a newborn infant.
- Leukopenia (WBC <1,750/mm^3) is an abnormal finding and may indicate sepsis, pregnancy-induced hypertension, asphyxia, or hemolytic disease.
  - WBC differential cell count:
    - Absolute neutrophil count (ANC) = WBC × (% immature neutrophils + % mature neutrophils) × 0.01
    - *Neutropenia (<1,500/mm^3):* This is the most accurate predictor of infection. It is also associated with maternal hypertension, confirmed periventricular hemorrhage, severe asphyxia, and reticulocytosis.
    - Neutrophilia may result from birth or other clinical conditions, such as hemolytic disease, asymptomatic hypoglycemia, trisomy 21, use of oxytocin during labor, maternal fever, stress during labor and birth, exogenous steroid administration, pneumothorax, and meconium aspiration.
- Immature-to-total neutrophil (I:T) ratio:

$$\text{I:T ratio} = (\% \text{ bands} + \% \text{ immature forms}) \div (\% \text{ mature} + \% \text{ bands} + \% \text{ immature forms})$$

- The sensitivity is greater than 90%.
- The value is maximum at birth and then declines to 0.12 after 72 hours of age.
- Eosinophils and basophils are important in allergic response.
- *Plasma:* plasma proteins and coagulation factors I through XIII:
  - Plasma proteins interact with the endothelium, subendothelium, Plts, and circulating cells to promote homeostasis. A drug's affinity for plasma proteins affects the medication's volume of distribution.

- *Albumin:* Albumin is synthesized in the liver. It is the most abundant protein in the plasma. It is also a major component of the anion. It normally ranges between 2.8 and 4.4 g/dL in term neonates. When hepatocellular injury occurs, the level decreases.
- *Fibrinogen (factor I):* Soluble protein in plasma measures the circulating level of protein substrate that is required for clot formation. Low level is seen in disseminated intravascular coagulation (DIC).
- *Prothrombin time (PT; factor II):* Measurement of extrinsic (triggered by tissue injury) and common portions of the coagulation cascade. It measures the time needed for factor II to be converted to thrombin. Decreased vitamin K-dependent clotting factors, hepatocellular injury, and biliary obstruction demonstrate a prolonged PT.
- *Activated partial thromboplastin time (aPTT; factor III):* Measurement of intrinsic (triggered by vascular endothelial injury) and common portions of the coagulation cascade. Both PT and aPTT are prolonged in neonates, especially in preterm neonates. Prolonged value indicates a decrease in both vitamin K-dependent factors and contact factors (XI, XII, prekallikrein).
- *International normalized ratio (INR):* INR is the ratio of sample PT to a normal PT.
- *Plasma:* factors IV through XIII assays:
  - *Factor IV:* Calcium ions serve as a factor in blood coagulation.
  - *Factor V:* Level is low on day 1 of life and then increases to adult value within days. Factor V Leiden (FVL) mutation is the most common of the serious inheritable prothrombotic disorders in neonates.
  - *Factor VII:* Extrinsic pathway and vitamin-K dependent. A prolonged PT with a normal Plt count is seen in neonatal bleeding disorders.
  - *Factor VIII:* Hemophilia A with prolonged aPTT and normal Plt; intrinsic pathway. This is the most common inherited coagulation disorder in the neonatal period.
  - *Factor IX:* Hemophilia B; intrinsic pathway; vitamin K-dependent. It is a less common inherited bleeding disorder. Levels reduce at birth and it is necessary to repeat testing at 6 months of age in mildly affected infants to confirm the diagnosis.
  - *Factors X to XIII:* There are varying combinations of normal and abnormal PT and aPTT levels (Barry et al., 2022; Bradshaw, 2022; Diehl-Jones & Fraser, 2022; Domonoske, 2022; Ferrieri & Wallen, 2018; Ku et al., 2021; Letterio & Ahuja, 2020; Letterio et al., 2020; McClary, 2020; McKinney et al., 2021; Rodger & Silver, 2019; Rudd, 2022; Saxonhouse, 2018).

MICROBIOLOGY TESTS

- Microbiology tests are used in the identification of infectious microorganisms causing disease. Tests include diagnostic bacteriology, mycology, virology, parasitology, and serology.
- Culture of body fluid:
  - Isolation of a pathogen. Cultures can be obtained from blood, cerebrospinal fluid (CSF), and urine. It is the most valid method to establish the diagnosis of bacterial sepsis.
    - ❏ At least 1 mL of blood should be collected for improved recovery of microorganisms in culture and to improve the chance of detection of bacterial presence in the blood (Esper, 2020; Pammi et al., 2021; Rudd, 2022).

MICROSCOPY TESTS

- Examination of body fluids and tissues under a microscope
- Cell counts or testing for fecal blood
- Apt test (alkali denaturation test), based on the alkali resistance of HbF to differentiate swallowed maternal blood from neonatal blood
- Urinalysis, including urine specific gravity, urine electrolytes, and pH to monitor urine output and metabolic derangement (Barry et al., 2021; Cadnapaphornchai et al., 2021; McKinney et al., 2021; Vogt & Springer, 2020).

IMMUNOHEMATOLOGY (BLOOD BANK AND TRANSFUSION MEDICINE)

- Area of blood component preparation, blood donor screening and testing, blood compatibility testing, and blood and stem cell banking
- Blood typing and crossmatching to identify common ABO blood group antigens and antibodies, and Rh factor
- Direct antiglobulin test (DAT)/Coombs; positive result indicates the presence of maternal immunoglobulin G (IgG) antibodies in the infant's RBCs.
- Erythrocyte rosette test and Kleihauer–Betke test both screen for fetomaternal hemorrhage through identification of HbF in maternal blood circulation (Diehl-Jones & Fraser, 2022; McKinney et al., 2021)

IMMUNOASSAYS

- Laboratory method based on antigen–antibody reactions employed in TDM, toxicology screening, detection of plasma proteins, and certain endocrine testing

- Immunology tests for evaluation of immune system activity to diagnose inflammatory responses, immunodeficiency, and autoimmune disorders
- Urine and meconium toxicology test used for detecting possible illicit drugs; due to rapid drug metabolism and elimination, urine sample should be collected as soon as possible after birth
- Latex agglutination test and many drug levels measured by immunoassays (Hudak, 2020; Scheans, 2022)

CYTOGENETIC TESTS

- These tests are used to determine genetic composition by chromosome analysis.
- *Simple karyotype (blood, amniotic fluid, tissue, bone marrow, buccal swab):* Karyotype is a "pictorial presentation of the chromosomal characteristics of an individual or species" (Schiefelbein, 2022). Staining techniques are used that cause dark and light bands to show up on the chromosome. Chromosomes are identified by their distance from the centromere. Normal karyotype includes 46 chromosomes, 22 pairs of autosomes, and one set of sex chromosomes.
- *Fluorescent in situ hybridization (FISH):* FISH combines chromosome analysis with the use of the segments of fluorescence-labeled molecular markers (probes) in order to follow the hybridization of complementary pieces of DNA. FISH is powerful in diagnosing common microdeletions or microduplications and in identifying extra sets of chromosomes.
- *Comparative genomic hybridization (CGh):* CGh is microarray testing. It detects genetic imbalances that are too small to be picked up by routine analysis (Gross & Gheorghe, 2020; Lubbers, 2022; Mitchell, 2020; Schiefelbein, 2022).

IMMUNOLOGY TESTS

- Laboratory evaluation of immune system activity consists of complement activity and its cascade of activation, humoral, and cell-mediated immunity. These tests are used to diagnose inflammatory responses, immunodeficiency, and autoimmune disorders.
- *C-reactive protein (CRP):* CRP is a nonspecific acute-phase reactant synthesized in the liver. Levels elevate within the first 6 to 8 hours of the infective or inflammatory process, with the lowest sensitivity (60%) and peak after 24 hours. Its sensitivity, specificity, and positive predictive values increase over the next 10 to 12 hours after infection.
  - It is most useful in determining the effectiveness of treatment, resolution of disease, and duration of antibiotic therapy. CRP response is found to be more useful in gram-negative infections than infections with coagulase-negative *Staphylococcus* spp. Serial CRP measurements can be used to facilitate monitoring for resolution of infection and response to treatment.
- *Procalcitonin (PCT):* PCT is an acute-phase reactant. It is induced by systemic inflammation and bacterial sepsis. Levels rise much faster than CRP. It rises at 4 hours and peaks at 6 hours, with higher sensitivity and specificity than those of CRP, ranging from 83% to 100%, and then plateaus 8 to 24 hours after a stimulus.
- *Cytokine measurement:* Cytokines' receptors are produced by the placenta and uterine endothelial cells, as well as invading macrophages. Increased levels of interleukin (IL)-1β, IL-6, IL-8, tumor necrosis factor-α, IL-2-soluble receptor (sIL2R), and granulocyte, colony-stimulating factor present during the onset of bacterial infection. The balance of cytokines and proinflammatory or anti-inflammatory factors may be the key trigger for preterm labor caused by intrauterine infection or other forms of inflammation.
- *Complement system:* The complement system is important and central to innate immune response. Complement system activation cascade includes activation of both the classic pathway and the alternative pathway. Examples of C3 can be detected as early as 5 to 6 weeks' GA, increasing to 66% of adult level by 26 to 28 weeks.
- *IgG, immunoglobulin M (IgM), and immunoglobulin A (IgA):* B-lymphocytes characterized by the presence of cell surface immunoglobulin (Ig).
  - *IgG:* IgG is the predominant Ig isotype at all ages. It is the only immunoglobulin that freely crosses the placenta. In a disease state, maternal IgG antibodies can cause hemolysis of RBCs.
  - *IgA:* IgA does not cross the placenta. It can be detected in the saliva of neonates as early as 3 days of life. Increased umbilical cord blood (UCB) IgA concentration may suggest congenital infection such as toxoplasmosis and HIV.
  - *IgM:* IgM is another isotype besides IgG that binds and activates the complement system pathway. Postnatal IgM concentrations rise rapidly for the first month in response to antigenic stimulation. Its level may elevate in the presence of bacterial and/or viral infections (Benjamin & Maheshwari, 2020; Blickstein et al., 2020; Esper, 2020; Ferrieri & Wallen, 2018; Jacquot et al., 2020; Letterio et al., 2020; Pammi et al., 2021; Rudd, 2022; Scheans, 2022; Simhan et al., 2019; Weitkamp et al., 2018).

▶ DIAGNOSTIC STUDIES

RADIOGRAPHY/X-RAY

- Radiography utilizes the natural contrast between air (dark or black presentation) and fluid or tissue (white or gray) on a standard radiograph.
- It is critical to place an infant in an appropriate position to produce a high-quality and accurate

image. A rotated image may lead to a false diagnosis or abnormal central line location. The infant's arms should be extended away from the chest to prevent the scapulae from obscuring the upper lung fields (Jensen et al., 2022; Trotter, 2022; Weinman et al., 2021).

Terms Associated With Radiography

- An *artifact* is a silhouette or shadow on the radiograph that is not part of the patient.
  - *Skinfold:* Skinfold is the most common artifact seen in the neonate. It is visible as a straight line crossing the diaphragm or outside the body (Trotter, 2022).
  - Artifacts present within the radiography can make interpretation difficult.
- Radiographic *density* varies depending on the composition of an organ or tissue. For example, a fluid-filled heart is seen as white versus black for air-filled lungs on an x-ray film.
  - Air, fat, water (including all solid viscera: liver, spleen, kidney, pancreas, and heart), bone, and metal are the only five densities that can be distinguished routinely from x-ray (Trotter, 2022; Weinman et al., 2021; Figure 7.1).

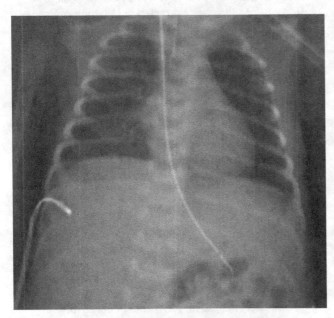

Figure 7.1 Radiograph demonstrating the difference in densities between the air-filled lungs and the more solid organs of the abdomen.

- Radiographic *exposure* denotes the amount of radiation used.
  - *Underexposure/underpenetration:* Images appear light and hazy. It is particularly difficult to view the vertebral bodies and/or any line placement due to the radiograph's brightness (Figure 7.2).

- *Overexposure/overpenetration:* Images are dark and lack contrast (Figure 7.3; Trotter, 2022).
- *Radiolucency* indicates various degrees of transparency of items being radiographed (Trotter, 2022).

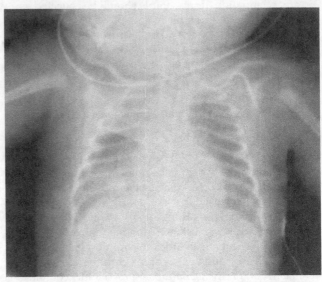

Figure 7.2 Example of an underexposed radiograph.

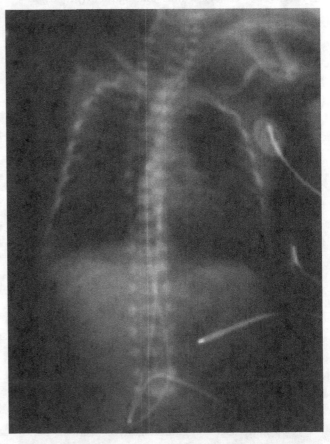

Figure 7.3 Example of an overexposed radiograph image.

- *Radiopaque* indicates a dense and nonpenetrable substance that cannot be radiographed (Trotter, 2022).
- Degree of *rotation* on a radiograph denotes how the neonate's body is turned from the midline. This can make shadows appear larger and distorted (Figure 7.4).
  - A rotated radiograph image may mislead and result in a false diagnosis of cardiomegaly, atelectasis, or abnormal central line location (Jensen et al., 2022; Trotter, 2022).

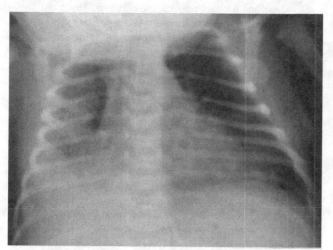

Figure 7.4 Rotation on an anteroposterior radiograph. Note the differences in width of the chest wall. The ribs on the left side are longer, indicating the infant is turned toward to right.

- There are three main *views* used in the NICU.
  - *Anteroposterior (AP) view:* Images are usually captured from above, with the infant lying on the back and their chest upward.
  - *Cross-table lateral view:* Images are captured with the infant lying supine. The x-ray beam passes horizontally from the infant's side through the body (Figure 7.5). It is generally used for assessment of free air and for verifying line placement.
  - *Lateral decubitus view:* Images are obtained by positioning the infant on the side and filming from the back. A right or left lateral decubitus indicates the side on which the infant is lying. The most

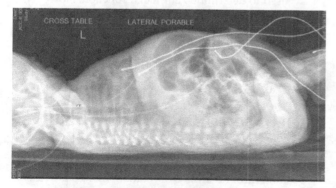

Figure 7.5 Cross-table lateral view of an infant.

common example in the NICU is to obtain a left lateral decubitus (LLD; the infant is lying on their left side with the right side up) view to assess for free abdominal air, which will layer out over the liver (Crisci, 2020; Jensen et al., 2022; Trotter, 2022; Figure 7.6).

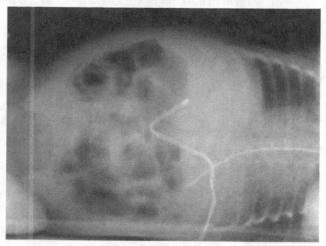

Figure 7.6 Lateral decubitus (left) view of an infant.

Interpretation of Radiographs

- It is important to develop a systematic approach and order, as well as identify any anatomic and pathologic changes when assessing a film, including the lung fields, mediastinum, skeletal system, and catheters.
- Use the alphabetic approach: airway, bones, cardiac structures, diaphragm, effusions, fields and fissures, gastric fundus, and hilum and mediastinum (Jensen et al., 2022; Trotter, 2022).

ENDOTRACHEAL TUBE

- Endotracheal tube (ETT) position can be confirmed on an AP x-ray with midline/neutral head position and not flexed. ETT placement should be in the midtrachea between the second and fourth thoracic vertebral bodies (T2–T4) and at least 1 to 2 cm below the vocal cords or above the carina (Ades & Johnston, 2020; Bailey & Maltsberger, 2021; Crisci, 2020; Diblasi, 2022; Jensen et al., 2022; Trotter, 2022).

UMBILICAL ARTERY CATHETERS AND UMBILICAL VENOUS CATHETERS

- An *umbilical artery catheter (UAC)* is inserted from the umbilicus down toward the pelvis, turning into the internal iliac artery and common iliac artery, and then advancing into the aorta.
  - A high position should be between the sixth and ninth thoracic vertebrae (T6–T10) or T7 to T9 ("7 is heaven, 8 is great, 9 is fine").
  - In low position, the catheter tip is placed between the third and fourth lumbar vertebrae (L3–L4).

■ An *umbilical venous catheter (UVC)* is inserted from the umbilicus cephalad to join the left portal vein. On a lateral radiograph view, the catheter is directly distal to the abdominal wall until it passes through the ductus venosus.

● The correct placement is 0.5 to 2 cm above the diaphragm in the inferior vena cava (IVC) with the catheter tip at T8 to T9. This should equate to just below the junction of the IVC and the right atrium (Bailey & Maltsberger, 2021; Coe et al., 2021; Crisci, 2020; Jensen et al., 2022; Seo, 2020a; Trotter, 2022).

CHEST TUBE

■ An ideal chest tube placement on an AP chest film will be in the midclavicular line (MCL) with the chest tube's distal hole inside the thoracic space (pleural space).

■ A lateral chest x-ray film will determine the anterior or posterior placement. For air evacuation, an anterior placement is desirable. For fluid evacuation, posterior placement is more effective (Gupta & Dirnberger, 2020; Trotter, 2022).

PERCUTANEOUSLY INSERTED CENTRAL CATHETER OR PERCUTANEOUS CENTRAL VENOUS CATHETER

■ Percutaneously inserted central catheters (PICCs) are preferably placed in an upper or lower extremity and terminated in a major vein near the heart.

● If a PICC is placed in an upper extremity, the arm should be extended and at a 45-degree angle from the body for optimal evaluation, while the tip of the catheter should be in the superior vena cava (SVC). It is considered central if the tip of the catheter crosses the MCL and is above the right atrium of the heart.

● If the line is placed in the lower extremities, the legs should be extended and held in place. The appropriate central position should be in the IVC (ideal), or the tip of the catheter crosses the pelvic cavity and rests below the right atrium of the heart (Trotter, 2022).

ULTRASOUND

■ Ultrasound (US) uses an oscillating sound wave with a frequency outside the human hearing range to evaluate the density and movement of tissue and blood flow. It is also used to evaluate internal anatomic structures and function.

■ It is the most commonly used method for evaluation of brain parenchyma and ventricular size, myocardial function and structure, urinary tract anatomy and pathology, masses in the pelvic and abdominal cavities, liver anatomy, and blood flow in major vessels. It provides real-time, dynamic options by using rapid, sequential images.

■ *Benefits:* US is easy to use, has the ability to obtain real-time imaging, and there is no radiation involved. US also provides digital images that can be easily transferred; the device is portable and no sedation is required.

■ *Cautions/Limitations:* The necessity of skilled technicians to obtain good images and the mobility of the patient during the procedure are ongoing challenges.

■ Ultrasonography is the ideal tool to evaluate a neonate's brain and is often the first step in imaging evaluations for any neurologic concern. The most common approach is through the anterior fontanel in order to obtain coronal and parasagittal views.

● Although US is sensitive in noting intracranial hemorrhages and areas of increased echogenicity, it is less sensitive than a CT or MRI in defining subtle areas of anomalies.

■ A two-dimensional echocardiogram (2D ECHO) with Doppler and color Doppler is the primary mode used to identify cardiac size, structure, and function, as well as to diagnose congenital heart diseases. High-frequency sound waves send vibrations through the heart and are then transmitted into a visual image.

■ A limitation to the ECHO is that lesions that are more distal will require other imaging modalities, such as MRI or cardiac catheterization.

■ There are three types of ECHOs:

● *Noninvasive transthoracic ECHO:* This is the most commonly used method. It offers real-time three-dimensional (3D) images that have improved significantly and are clinically useful for evaluating cardiac valve anatomy and function.

● *Transesophageal echocardiography (TEE):* TEE is mainly used in the operating room. It is routinely used for cardiac evaluation in the operating room immediately before and after surgical repair.

● *Fetal echocardiography:* This is used for assessment of the fetal heart and major blood vessel structural defects, cardiac anomaly, and arrhythmias prior to birth.

● *M-mode echocardiography:* This is one of the earliest single dimensional techniques for evaluation of anatomic relationships of the heart and vessels and the motion of the cardiac valves, and for detection of pericardial fluid. It is most commonly used to determine ventricular function. However, 2D ECHO has greater versatility, providing more specific information (Berlin & Meyers, 2020; Crisci, 2020; Jensen et al., 2022; Phelps et al., 2020; Sadowski & Verklan, 2022; Scholz & Reinking, 2018; Swanson & Erickson, 2021; Trotter, 2022; Weinman et al., 2021).

COMPUTED TOMOGRAPHY

■ CT obtains high-quality cross-sectional images of the body by combining a series of x-rays from various positions around an axis of rotation. Images provide

a 2D visualization of the anatomy and can be further enhanced by using a radiographic contrast agent to facilitate the evaluation of blood flow and assist in defining pathologic abnormalities.
■ For identification and diagnosis of space-occupying lesions such as congenital pulmonary airway malformation (CPAM), bronchopulmonary sequestration (BPS), and congenital lobar emphysema, chest CT is more useful (Crisci, 2020; Jensen et al., 2022; Trotter, 2022; Weinman et al., 2021).

MAGNETIC RESONANCE IMAGING

■ MRI uses magnets producing magnetized hydrogen protons to capture images of the body. Its increased sensitivity allows for more precise imaging of the smallest of structures.
■ MRI is used for early diagnosis of intracranial pathologies and/or more accurate definition of tissue structures and fluid collections, and is an adjuvant to clarify fetal US findings.
■ *Benefits:* MRI is a noninvasive method and there is no ionized radiation exposure.
■ *Limitations/cautions:* MRI is expensive and requires anesthesia to obtain high-quality images. It is also time-consuming to obtain an image. Motion-free is necessary for optimal image quality (Berlin & Meyers, 2020; Crisci, 2020; Jensen et al., 2022; Trotter, 2022; Weinman et al., 2021).

FLUOROSCOPY

■ Fluoroscopy is the most commonly used tool in neonates and infants due to its real-time, dynamic images using rapid, sequential x-rays to image the gastrointestinal (GI) and genitourinary tracts.
■ *Benefits:* It allows for real-time evaluation of motion, such as swallowing function, GI peristalsis, and diaphragmatic motion.
■ *Cautions:* Fluoroscopy can result in substantial radiation exposure if appropriate precautions are not used.
■ Neonatal fluoroscopy may be used to help diagnose infants with respiratory distress of unclear etiology, and if there is concern for tracheoesophageal fistula, occult aspiration, diaphragmatic excursion, or airway diseases such as tracheobronchomalacia.
■ A diagnosis of phrenic nerve injury can be confirmed by a fluoroscopy showing paradoxical (upward) movement of the diaphragm with inspiration (Abdulhayoglu, 2017; Crisci, 2020; Jensen, et al., 2022; Weinman et al., 2021).

Upper Gastrointestinal

■ If there are any concerns for malrotation and/or possible volvulus, the upper GI series is the examination of choice.

■ Upper GI series with small-bowel follow-through is one of the most common methods used to evaluate the structure and function of the upper GI tract, including the esophagus, stomach, and small intestine. A series of follow-up x-rays are obtained under fluoroscopy intermittently after a water-soluble contrast is ingested to evaluate the emptying ability of the stomach, intestinal motility, and potential obstruction.

Barium Enema/Contrast Enema

■ Barium enema is the first diagnostic study used to evaluate possible obstruction of the large intestine and to diagnose disorders such as Hirschsprung disease. A series of follow-up x-rays may be taken at timed intervals to evaluate the evacuation of the solution from the bowel. It can also be used for either diagnostic or therapeutic purposes in infants with meconium plug syndrome or meconium ileus (Trotter, 2022; Weinman et al., 2021).

Voiding Cystourethrogram

■ Voiding cystourethrogram (VCUG) is used to evaluate the structure and function of the kidneys, bladder, and lower urinary tract. It is also used to assess possible vesicoureteral reflux (Trotter, 2022; Weinman et al., 2021).

ELECTROENCEPHALOGRAM

■ EEG provides continuous background activity, the synchrony of the activity, and the appearance and disappearance of specific waveforms and patterns of the brain.
  ● It is common to see depression of background activity on EEG in infants with generalized insults, especially hypoxic–ischemic insults.
  ● A very common feature that EEG presents is the development of continuous or intermittent discontinuity and burst-suppression patterns in term infants with neonatal encephalopathies, which are associated with a very high likelihood of an unfavorable outcome.
■ There are two common types of EEG:
  ● *Conventional EEG (cEEG):* cEEG is the gold standard for neonatal seizure detection. It measures the impact of neurologic insult and detects the presence of seizure activity. It is recommended to continuously monitor high-risk neonates with EEG, including suspected neonatal seizures following acute brain injury or when neonatal epilepsy is suspected.
    ❑ *Limitation:* The procedure requires skilled technicians and experienced interpreters of the tracing.
  ● *Amplitude EEG (aEEG):* aEEG is used for continuous monitoring of cerebral electrical activity in critically ill newborns. The signal is rectified and further processed to create a simplified pattern that is easy to interpret by a nonneurologist. It is possible to

display the corresponding, expanded raw EEG trace, which is useful for confirming possible seizure activity.

- ❏ *Benefits:* aEEG is easy to apply at the bedside as no technician is needed to place the sensor. It is also low-cost compared with cEEG monitoring.
- ❏ *Caution:* aEEG may potentially miss some focal abnormalities because the device does not cover the entire brain. aEEG is prone to artifactual signals from movement, high-frequency oscillator ventilation, or extracorporeal membrane oxygenation (ECMO).

■ EEG is indicated for assessment of asphyxiated term infants. The aEEG background tracings have been most useful, particularly on the burst-suppression, continuous low-voltage, and flat trace patterns in neonates receiving neuroprotective therapies, such as therapeutic hypothermia.

■ It is also used in the detection of seizures. Detection of seizures from aEEG has been used primarily in asphyxiated term infants.

■ aEEG has also been used for identifying the effect of anticonvulsant drugs, predicting postneonatal epilepsy, and predicting outcomes in premature infants with large intraventricular hemorrhages (Arensman et al., 2022; Ditzenberger, 2022; Natarajan & Gospe, 2018; Neil & Volpe, 2018).

ELECTROCARDIOGRAPHY

■ EKG is used to measure and display the heart rate and rhythm by calculating body surface electrical potentials generated by the heart. Typically, three electrodes are placed on the upper left chest, the upper right chest, and the lower left abdomen. It is most useful for evaluating cardiac arrhythmia but not structural heart diseases.

■ EKG is the recommended measurement method for obtaining heart rate immediately after birth in the delivery room during resuscitation.

■ *Caution:* Inaccurate measurements may be caused by motion artifacts and little or no cardiac output. Therefore, it should be used with other methods, especially during resuscitation in the delivery room.

■ EKG is indicated for identification of abnormal hemodynamic burdens of the heart.
- It is used for evaluation of arrhythmias and the impact of electrolyte imbalances on electrical conductivity. For example, changes in ST segments or T-waves may suggest myocardial ischemia.
- It is also used to determine the severity of disease by assessing the degree of atrial or ventricular hypertrophy (Owen et al., 2022; Sadowski & Verklan, 2022; Smallwood, 2019; Swanson & Erickson, 2021).

▶ TECHNIQUES/PROCEDURES IN THE NEONATAL INTENSIVE CARE UNIT

BAG AND MASK VENTILATION

■ This is initiated when there is apnea or gasping respirations, the heart rate is less than 100 beats per minute (bpm), and the infant is cyanotic despite supplemental oxygen, respiratory support, or need for continued ventilation. It is also used in response to apnea unresponsive to stimulation or gasping respirations.

■ *Face mask:* Appropriate sizing of a face mask should have the mask covering the chin, mouth, and nose, but not the eyes. A properly sized face mask is required to obtain an adequate seal.

■ *Self-inflating bags (SIBs):* SIBs re-expand after compression. They are the only devices that can be used without a gas supply. They do not provide reliable free-flow oxygen, nor do they deliver consistent tidal volumes (V_T) or inflation pressures.

■ *Flow-inflating bags (FIBs):* FIBs require a continuous gas supply to inflate the bag. High-peak pressures can be achieved with FIBs and deliver continuous positive airway pressure (CPAP) as well as free-flow oxygen.

■ *T-piece resuscitator:* This is a flow-controlled and pressure-limited device. It provides a preset level of positive pressure and positive end expiratory pressure (PEEP) and delivers more accurate and consistent pressure.

■ *Laryngeal mask airway (LMA):* LMA is the most commonly used device for managing difficult airways or craniofacial abnormalities, such as Pierre Robin sequence or micrognathia. LMA does not require visualization of the vocal cords and an instrument for insertion. The deflated mask is manually inserted into the patient's mouth along the hard palate, and then advanced until resistance is felt. Once the mask is inserted completely, the balloon is inflated to form a seal in the pharynx. There is lack of small sizes, as size 1 LMA is designed for infants weighing >2,000 g. Other limitations include the inability to suction secretions from the airway, air leaks with high pressure, and interference with chest compression. A potential complication is the aspiration of gastric contents since the LMA does not provide an occluded airway (Ades & Johnston, 2020; Diblasi, 2022; Fraser & Diehl-Jones, 2022; Heiderich & Leone, 2020; Niermeyer & Clark, 2021; Owen et al., 2022; Pappas & Robey, 2022; Watters & Mancuso, 2019).

ENDOTRACHEAL INTUBATION

■ *Oral endotracheal intubation* is indicated when bag and mask ventilation is ineffective or undesirable to perform resuscitation, need for mechanical ventilation, in infants with diaphragmatic hernia or upper airway obstruction, and heart rate <100 bpm after 30 seconds of effective positive pressure ventilation (PPV).

- The need for administering surfactant or epinephrine
- The need of tracheal suction to clear the airway or to obtain sterile tracheal aspirate culture (Ades & Johnston, 2020; Bailey & Maltsberger, 2021; Niermeyer & Clark, 2021; Owen et al., 2022)
- *Nasal (nasotracheal) intubation* minimizes the chance of accidental dislodgment and decreases tube movement due to excessive secretion burden or oral anomaly.
  - *Cautions:* Nasal intubation has greater difficulty in insertion of the tube; therefore, it should be an elective procedure in a nonemergency situation.
- Complications include pressure necrosis of the nares and nasal septum, potential development of sinusitis, and bleeding (Ades & Johnston, 2020; Carlo & Ambalavanan, 2020).

Oral/Nasal Intubation Technique

- Premedication should be considered prior to the nonemergent intubation per institutional protocol. Medications include vagolytics and analgesic sedation, followed by neuromuscular blockers if applicable.
- Miller (straight) blades are the preferred choice over Macintosh (curved) blades for intubation in neonates.
- Laryngoscope blade size 00 is recommended for extremely preterm infants; blade 0 is for preterm infants and blade 1 is appropriate for term infants (Table 7.1).
- Appropriate uncuffed and uniform-diameter (internal diameter; ID) ETT size should be selected based on the infant's weight or GA (Table 7.2).
- There are a variety of methods used to determine ETT insertion depth. For example:
  - *Nasotragal or nasal tragus length (NTL):* the distance between the infant's nasal septum and ear tragus + 1 cm

Table 7.1 Laryngoscope Size Based on Infant's Weight

Laryngoscope Blade	Weight (g)
00	<1,000
0	1,000–4,000
1	>4,000

Table 7.2 Endotracheal Tube Size by Infant's Gestational Age and Weight

ETT Size (mm; ID)	GA (wk)	Weight (g)	Insertion Depth (cm)
2.5	<28	<1,000	6.5 or <7
3.0	28–34	1,000–2,000	7
3.5	34–38	2,000–3,000	8
4.0	>38	>3,000	9

ETT, endotracheal tube; GA, gestational age; ID, internal diameter.

- *Based on infant's weight and/or GA:* weight in kilograms + 6 cm, which equates to the 7-8-9 rule advocated in the Neonatal Resuscitation Program (NRP)
  - *Caution:* This method may overestimate the insertion depth in infants weighing <750 g.
- The ETT should be inserted to the level of vocal cord marker. If inserting a cuffed ETT, the tube is advanced until the cuff is distal to the vocal cords (Figure 7.7).
- Intubation attempts should be limited to 20 to 30 seconds to prevent hypoxia during the procedure.
- Use an exhaled carbon dioxide (CO_2) detector/end-tidal carbon dioxide ($EtCO_2$) detector, auscultation, and chest radiography to confirm ETT placement. The presence of vapor in the tube is not a reliable indicator.
  - Color change of the CO_2 detector may be delayed in extremely preterm infants, especially if cardiac output is low, as during bradycardia or when the neonate has little to no perfusion (Ades & Johnston, 2020; Bailey & Maltsberger, 2021; Carlo & Ambalavanan, 2020; Niermeyer & Clark, 2021; Owen et al., 2022; Watters & Mancuso, 2019).

Potential Complications of Intubation

- Complications of intubation may include hypoxia, bradycardia, damage of the airway lining, vocal cord injury, misplacement of the tube into the esophagus, bronchus pain, agitation or discomfort, infection, and perforation of the esophagus or trachea (Ades & Johnston, 2020; Bailey & Maltsberger, 2021; Niermeyer & Clark, 2021).

THORACENTESIS

- Thoracocentesis is used for emergency relief of life-threatening pneumothorax or pleural fluid collection from the thoracic cavity. It may also be used for extrapleural drainage after surgical repair of esophageal atresia and/or tracheoesophageal fistula (Bailey & Maltsberger, 2021; Gardner, Enzman, & Nyp, 2021; Gupta & Dirnberger, 2020; Vergales, 2020).

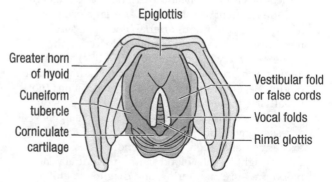

Figure 7.7 Anatomic illustration showing the neonatal upper airway structures.

Needle Aspiration

■ Insert an 18- to 24-gauge angiocatheter at a 45-degree angle in the second intercostal space (ICS) in the MCL or fourth ICS in the anterior axillary line (AAL), and then advance the catheter at a 90-degree angle into the pleural space to avoid blood vessels and nerves (Bailey & Maltsberger, 2021; Gardner, Enzman, & Nyp, 2021; Gupta & Dirnberger, 2020; Vergales, 2020).

Chest Tube Placement

■ Types of thoracostomy include pigtail catheter with suture locks; pigtail catheter with natural coil, nonlocking; chest tube with safety color change indicator, such as Argyle Turkel; and straight chest tube.

■ Elevate the affected site at 45 to 60 degrees, allowing air, with shoulder internally rotated and abducted for easy aspiration.

■ Landmarks for insertion site include the nipple and the fourth or fifth ICS, and anterior and midaxillary lines.
  ● *Lateral approach:* fourth to sixth ICS on lateral or to the AAL
  ● *Superior approach:* second or third ICS on or lateral to the MCL
  ● *Multiple pneumothoraxes:* 4 to 5 cm inferior to the nipple and inserted through the fifth or sixth ICS

■ Provide appropriate nonpharmacologic and pharmacologic pain management and monitor closely (Gardner, Enzman, & Nyp, 2021; Gupta & Dirnberger, 2020; Rodriguez, 2020; Vergales, 2020).

■ Potential complications of procedures involving thoracentesis include mispositioning the tube, hemorrhage, infection, perforation of the lung or adjacent structures, damage to breast tissue, pain, chylothorax, nerve damage (Horner syndrome, diaphragmatic paralysis or eventration), and tip across the anterior mediastinum (Bailey & Maltsberger, 2021; Gardner, Enzman, & Nyp, 2021; Gupta & Dirnberger, 2020; Markham, 2017; Vergales, 2020).

UMBILICAL VESSEL CATHETERIZATION

■ Indications for an *umbilical artery catheter* placement include frequent or continuous arterial blood gas monitoring, continuous arterial blood pressure monitoring, an access of frequent blood sampling in the extremely low birth weight (ELBW) neonates, angiography, resuscitation, continuous administration of glucose/electrolyte solutions or medications (not usually recommended), and exchange transfusion.

■ Indications for *UVC* placement include emergency access for medication and fluid administration, exchange transfusion, central venous access in low birth weight infants, blood sampling, central venous blood pressure monitoring, and diagnosis of total anomalous pulmonary venous drainage below the diaphragm.

■ Contraindications to umbilical line placement include abdominal wall defects, necrotizing enterocolitis (NEC), vascular compromise below the level of umbilicus, and peritonitis (Bailey & Maltsberger, 2021; Coe et al., 2021; Seo, 2020a, 2002b; Travers & Ambalavanan, 2022).

Technique for Placing Umbilical Arterial Catheter/ Umbilical Venous Catheter

■ Choice of catheter size depends on the policy and protocol in each institution.
  ● Size 3.5 Fr is for infants weighing less than 1,250, 1,500, or 2,000 g.
  ● Size 5 Fr is for infants weighing more than 1,250, 1,500, or 2,000 g.
  ● Size 2.5 Fr catheter can be used in ELBW infants and size 8 Fr catheter may occasionally be used for infants weighing more than 3,500 g.

■ Identify cord vessels.
  ● The singular vein is large with 4 to 5 mm in diameter, thin-walled vessel, and is often situated at the 12 o'clock position.
  ● The two umbilical arteries are the continuation of the internal iliac arteries with 2 to 3 mm diameters at their origins and then become small and thickened and white constricted vessels as they approach the umbilicus. They are typically located at the 4 and 8 o'clock position.

■ If the inserted catheter meets any obstruction prior to the desired distance, do not force the catheter past the obstruction.

■ High position: There are several methods to estimate the distance.
  ● *UAC:* The tip of the catheter should terminate below the ductus arteriosus and above or below the visceral arteries. It is at the level of thoracic vertebrae between T6 and T10.
  ● *UVC:* The desired location is T9 to T10, just above the right diaphragm or at the junction of the IVC and the right atrium. However, it is acceptable if the placement is in the ductus venosus for all purposes except pressure monitoring.

■ Low position:
  ● *UAC:* The low position should be at the level of the lumbar vertebrae, L3 to L4, and avoid the tip at the origin of the renal mesenteric or celiac vessels.

■ Never advance the catheter once in place and secured to avoid contaminated catheter into the vessel.

■ Potential complications of umbilical line placements include infections; perforation of vessels, colon, and peritoneum; knot in the catheter or breaking of the catheter; cardiac arrhythmia; hepatic necrosis; portal hypertension; death; as well as microemboli or vasospasm (dusky or purple toes) and compromised arterial blood flow (blanching of the foot or part of the leg; Bailey & Maltsberger, 2021; Berlin & Meyers, 2020; Coe et al., 2021; Seo, 2020a, 2020b; Travers & Ambalavanan, 2022).

PERIPHERAL ARTERY CATHETERIZATION/ PERIPHERAL ARTERY LINE

■ Peripheral artery catheters are indicated when frequent blood sampling is needed and the UAC is not available, when continuous blood pressure monitoring is necessary, or when preductal measurement is needed.

■ The line may be contraindicated in an uncorrected bleeding disorder, limb malformation, inadequate collateral blood flow, and skin infection (Bailey & Maltsberger, 2021; Kaushal & Ramasethu, 2020).

Technique for Placing a Peripheral Artery Line

■ An Allen test is performed to ensure ulnar artery patency. A modified Allen test should be performed when dorsalis pedis or posterior tibial cannulation is attempted.

■ Common sites for catheterization include the radial (most common), ulnar, and posterior tibial arteries. The dorsalis pedis artery can be used as an alternative site. The temporal artery should be avoided due to the potential for neurologic sequelae.

■ For small premature neonates, cannulate the artery by inserting at a 10- to 15-degree angle to the skin with the needle bevel down. Another method is to pass the needle stylet with the bevel up through the artery at a 30- to 40-degree angle. Once blood return is noted, advance the catheter and remove the stylet simultaneously.

■ Potential complications of peripheral artery line (PAL) placement include infection; extravasation of fluids; hematoma or hemorrhage; thromboembolism/ vasospasm/thrombosis; damage to the surrounding tissues, nerves, or structures; necrosis of the forearm, hand, and toe; and air embolism (Bailey & Maltsberger, 2021; Kaushal & Ramasethu, 2020).

PERCUTANEOUSLY INSERTED CENTRAL CATHETER OR PERCUTANEOUS CENTRAL VENOUS CATHETER

■ Indications for a PICC/percutaneous central venous catheter (PCVC) include an intermediate or long-term IV therapy, total parenteral nutrition, long-term antibiotic and IV medicinal therapy, difficult venous access, irritating drug therapy or hyperosmolar IV fluid administration, or VLBW.

● Frequent blood draws only apply to larger lumen catheters due to the risk of clotting (Bailey & Maltsberger, 2021; Choi et al., 2020; Coe et al., 2021).

Technique for Placing Peripherally Inserted Central Catheters/Percutaneous Central Venous Catheter

■ The ideal position of the catheter tip should be in as large a vein as possible, such as outside the heart but not within the right atrium due to the risk of focal myocardial injury, leading to pericardial effusion and cardiac tamponade.

● *Upper extremity:* The catheter tip should be in the SVC or at the junction of the SVC and right atrium.

● *Lower extremity:* The catheter tip should be in the IVC, above the L4 to L5 or the iliac crest below the right atrium.

■ AP and lateral radiographic views are preferred to confirm that the catheter is in a central vein, especially for a catheter placed in a lower extremity.

■ The most common sites of PICC for neonates are the antecubital veins (basilic and cephalic veins) and the greater saphenous veins. Other sites include scalp veins (temporal and posterior auricular veins), popliteal vein, axillary vein, and external jugular vein.

■ Potential complications of PICC/PCVC placement include phlebitis, which is the most common significant complication secondary to infiltration/ extravasation, hemorrhage, or vascular perforation. Catheter complications include shearing or rupture of the catheter and embolization of a catheter fragment. Catheter migration is also possible. Hematologic complications include sepsis, thrombus formation, and embolization of clot. Venipuncture for placement may cause nerve damage or hematoma, and skin disinfectants may result in chemical burns.

● Malpositioning of the catheter may lead to cardiac arrhythmias, pericardial effusion with cardiac tamponade, and even atrial perforation with cardiac tamponade (Bailey & Maltsberger, 2021; Choi et al., 2020; Coe et al., 2021).

LUMBAR PUNCTURE

■ Lumbar puncture (LP) is indicated to diagnose central nervous system (CNS) infection or certain metabolic disorders and to monitor the efficacy of CNS infection treatment. It may also be indicated to drain CSF in communicating hydrocephalus associated with intraventricular hemorrhage.

■ Contraindications may include increased intracranial pressure (ICP) and uncorrected bleeding disorders.

■ There may also be skin or tissue infection near the puncture site, lumbosacral anomalies, and clinical/ cardiorespiratory instability (Bailey & Maltsberger, 2021; Culjat, 2020; Hall & Reavey, 2021).

Technique for Lumbar Puncture

■ Strict aseptic technique must be applied during the procedure. Avoid flexion of the neck to decrease the risk of airway obstruction.

■ Always use a needle with a stylet to avoid the development of intraspinal epidermoid tumor.

■ Insert the needle slowly to prevent a traumatic tap caused by overpenetration.

- Never aspirate CSF with a syringe to avoid potential risk of subdural hemorrhage or herniation.
- The L3 to L4 and the L4 to -L5 interspaces are the desired landmarks (lower interspace should be used for premature infants).
- Provide appropriate pain control prior to and during the procedure.
- Possible complications of an LP procedure include inducing an infection due to nonsterile conditions, epidural abscess, or vertebral osteomyelitis. Persistent bleeding is also possible (Bailey & Maltsberger, 2021; Culjat, 2020; Hall & Reavey, 2021).

▶ TECHNIQUES/EQUIPMENT IN THE NEONATAL INTENSIVE CARE UNIT

CARDIORESPIRATORY MONITORS

- Cardiorespiratory monitors provide reliable and accurate data of infants' cardiac and respiratory activities and identify apnea/bradycardia in infants at risk, as well as early warnings of potential significant changes.
- Cardiorespiratory monitors are indicated in order to continuously monitor for bradycardia (<100 bpm), tachycardia (>180 bpm), apnea, and tachypnea.
  - Multiple probe applications should be avoided because this can compromise EKG signal integrity, and multiple applications of patches may increase the chance of skin damage.
  - Prompt patient assessment and appropriate correction should be followed immediately after the monitor alarm is activated (Abubakar, 2020a; Coe et al., 2021; di Fiore, 2020).

OXYGEN MONITORING

Pulse Oximetry

- Pulse oximetry is the most common, noninvasive, and continuous method of measuring artery oxygen (O_2) saturation by using red and infrared light. Advantages include a short response time in determining O_2 saturation and reducing the number of invasive blood gas measurements.
- Pulse oximetry is indicated for noninvasive continuous monitoring of desaturation events in infants, or intermittent arterial oxygen saturation and heart rate monitoring. Monitor oxygen in infants with hypoxia, apnea/hypoventilation, cardiorespiratory disease, and bronchopulmonary dysplasia (BPD).
  - Titrate oxygen concentration during delivery room resuscitation and in infants receiving supplemental oxygen in the NICU and during transport
  - Diagnose persistent pulmonary hypertension (PPHN) with a persistent ductal shunt

- Screening tool for critical congenital heart disease (CCHD) and performing car seat testing prior to discharge in infants with risk factors
- The use of pulse oximetry does not replace the need for blood gas analysis with clinical sign change and evaluation. Poor perfusion, ambient light such as phototherapy, motion, shock, and severe edema will interfere with accurate reading and decrease the reliability of the pulse oximeter.
- Assess the sensor site to ensure proper circulation and skin integrity. A mispositioned sensor will produce falsely low readings (Abubakar, 2020b; Coe et al., 2021; Eyal, 2020; di Fiore, 2020; Fraser & Diehl-Jones, 2022; Gomella, 2020; Lee & Oh, 2017; Travers & Ambalavanan, 2022).

Near-Infrared Spectroscopy

- Near-infrared spectroscopy (NIRS) relies on light absorption of oxygenated and deoxygenated Hgb to estimate tissue oxygenation and is analogous to the pulse oximetry that is commonly used in clinical practice to monitor arterial oxygen saturation. Both pulse oximetry and NIRS use similar wavelengths of light.
  - The parameters available from NIRS include oxyhemoglobin and deoxyhemoglobin levels, cerebral oxygen saturation, and the fraction of tissue oxygen extraction (this last parameter is calculated in conjunction with arterial oxygen saturation levels obtained with pulse oximetry).
- NIRS is indicated in infants who undergo therapeutic hypothermia management. In neonates with hypoxic–ischemic encephalopathy (HIE) treated with hypothermia, regional cerebral blood flow measured by MRI strongly correlates with mixed venous saturation values measured by NIRS.
- Advances in NIRS have increasingly allowed such assessments in different tissues, including the brain, kidneys, intestine, and muscle, and gained evidence-based application in neonatal intensive care.
- Precaution should guide the use of NIRS as the true value remains unknown and the correlation of cerebral oxygen saturation measured by NIRS and via pulse oximetry decreases in premature infants with respiratory disease (di Fiore, 2020; Neil & Inder, 2018; Neil & Volpe, 2018; Noori et al., 2018; Travers & Ambalavanan, 2022).

CARBON DIOXIDE MONITORING

Transcutaneous Carbon Dioxide Monitoring

- Transcutaneous carbon dioxide monitoring (tcPCO₂/ P_{tcco2}/TCOM) provides continuous indirect estimation of partial pressure of carbon dioxide in arterial blood (PaCO₂) by heated sensor.

■ Use of TCOM is indicated for noninvasive blood gas monitoring of PCO_2 and trending $PaCO_2$, especially when initiating high-frequency ventilation (HFV).
■ Precautions should be taken when used in infants with BPD as $TcPCO_2$ measures greater than $PaCO_2$ in infants with chronic lung disease.
■ Frequent change of electrodes prevents skin damage.

End-Tidal Carbon Dioxide Monitoring

■ $EtCO_2$ monitoring (end-tidal CO_2, capnography, $P_{et}CO_2$) is a noninvasive measurement to continuously estimate and monitor CO_2 through exhaled gas during the respiratory cycle.
  ● *Mainstream:* Sensor is in line with the ETT and the ventilator circuit.
  ● *Sidestream:* Sensor is placed away from the ETT with a low dead space adapter.
■ It provides useful information on CO_2 production, pulmonary perfusion, alveolar ventilation, respiratory patterns, and elimination of CO_2 from the lungs.
■ Indications include confirmation of ETT placement and for continuous monitoring and evaluation of exhaled CO_2 in ventilated infants and to guide management. It can also serve to monitor rate, rhythm, and effectiveness of respiration, as well as systemic perfusion and metabolism, and for monitoring in the operating room. Finally, the device can monitor and evaluate response to therapy of infants with severe pulmonary diseases.
■ Precautions should be taken during interpretation as it provides less accurate data on $PaCO_2$ in infants with significant lung disease.
  ● When the $P_{et}CO_2$ adapter is placed between the ETT and the ventilator flow sensor, V_T measurements may be affected.
  ● Sidestream measurements tend to be less accurate when high respiratory rates occur.
  ● $EtCO_2$ cannot be used in infants with HFV (Abubakar, 2020c; di Fiore, 2020; Fraser & Dihel-Jones, 2022).

INVASIVE BLOOD GAS MONITORING

■ The sample can be drawn from UAC, peripheral artery cannulation (PAC), or heel.
■ Blood gas measurement is the standard method for monitoring oxygenation, ventilation, and acid–base. It also provides measurement of Hgb, electrolytes, and metabolites.
  ● $PaCO_2$ and PaO_2 values are measured and calculated from other derived variables, such as base excess (BE)/deficit, bicarbonate, and oxygen saturation of Hgb from the pH.
■ Invasive blood gas monitoring is indicated for frequent monitoring and evaluation of the response to therapy of infants with respiratory diseases. It may be applied after delivery room resuscitation and for continuous monitoring during surgery.

■ Caution should be exercised as invasively obtaining blood gases is a painful and time-consuming procedure. Recognition that derived values are calculated, which may not be accurate compared with the measured value, should guide practice (di Fiore, 2020; Travers & Ambalavanan, 2022).

▶ INCUBATORS/RADIANT WARMERS

■ Radiant warmers provide heat to an infant's skin via infrared energy. These are controlled and enclosed environments that provide heated and warm air to maintain a neutral thermal environment (NTE).
  ● Double-walled incubators have less radiant heat loss.
  ● Increase the humidity within incubators to prevent evaporative heat loss and decrease the infant's metabolic rate as well as the incidence of electrolyte imbalances.
■ Incubators are indicated for premature ELBW, VLBW, or LBW infants or any infant who is unstable and unable to self-thermoregulate.
■ Caution should be taken against dehydration as increased insensible water loss occurs when infants are under radiant warmers. Manual control on a radiant warmer increases the risk of overheating or overcooling. Maintain the infant 80 to 90 cm from radiant heat to avoid burns.
  ● Incubators limit access to sick infants when extensive procedures are necessary. They may also present as a barrier to mothers and prolong feelings of fear and insecurity in the parents.
  ● High noise levels within incubators cause a negative impact on the hearing development of preterm infants.
  ● High humidity within an incubator may increase the risk of infection (Agren, 2020; Brand & Shippey, 2021; Gardner & Cammock, 2021; Rao & Scala, 2020).

▶ PHOTOTHERAPY

■ Phototherapy is the most common intervention to treat unconjugated hyperbilirubinemia in neonates. Phototherapy uses light energy to alter the shape of bilirubin into a form that does not need conjugation and to be excreted in the bile.
  ● It is also used to reduce the risk of acute bilirubin encephalopathy and toxicity caused by high serum bilirubin levels and to reduce the need for exchange transfusion.
■ Phototherapy is indicated for clinically significant hyperbilirubinemia secondary to increased production (accelerated RBC breakdown) from either hemolytic disease of the newborn, hereditary hemolytic anemias, polycythemia, or extravascular blood (e.g., cephalohematoma, bruising from delivery).

- Significant hyperbilirubinemia may also be secondary to increased reabsorption (enterohepatic circulation) due to delayed passage of meconium (e.g., bowel obstruction) or delayed enteral feedings.
- Contraindications include congenital erythropoietic porphyria or a family history of porphyria, current or history of photosensitive drug/agent use, use of metalloporphyrin heme oxygenase inhibitors, and infants with cholestatic jaundice (Bradshaw, 2022; Kamath-Rayne et al., 2021; Kaplan et al., 2020; Kaushal & Ramasethu, 2020; Watchko & Maisels, 2020).

TECHNIQUES FOR PHOTOTHERAPY USE

- Standard phototherapy delivers irradiance of 10 μW/cm^2/nm in the 430- to 490-nm band at the surface of the infant's body.
- Intensive phototherapy uses special blue fluorescent tubes and light-emitting diode (LED) to provide the most effective phototherapy. It delivers irradiance of 30 μW/cm^2/nm or higher in the 430- to 490-nm band to the greatest possible body surface area in the infant.
- Special blue fluorescent tubes provide greater irradiance than regular blue tubes because the fluorescent tubes omit light in wavelengths that penetrate the skin well and are maximally absorbed by bilirubin in order to convert it to a water-soluble form.
- Devices used include:
  - *Halogen lamps:* provide high irradiance over a small surface area
  - *Fiberoptic systems:* UV-filtered light and with the advantages of minimal "infant–parent separation" during therapy and no eye shields needed
  - *Gallium nitride LEDs:* a cost-effective device for use in phototherapy due to its long lifetime feature

- *Fluorescent tubes:* "special blue" tubes
- *Filtered sunlight:* widely used in resource-poor countries
- Precautions should be taken with the use of occlusive dressings, bandages, topical skin ointments, and plastic, which should not be used while the infant is receiving phototherapy in order to prevent burns.
  - Observe for rebound, which can occur after phototherapy is discontinued. Bilirubin levels should be followed for at least 24 hours to assess for rebound.
  - Short-term side effects of phototherapy include increased insensible water loss and stooling (diarrhea or loose stool), temperature instability, and rash. Eye damage may occur if coverings are not secure. Increased mortality in ELBW infants following continuous intensive phototherapy is noted.

▶ VENTILATORS

For discussions on invasive and noninvasive ventilator techniques and management, please see Chapter 17.

▶ CONCLUSION

It is important to be familiar with the applications and limitations of laboratory data and diagnostic testing methods when determining appropriate care for a vulnerable neonate. This includes choosing the laboratory test which provides the most information for the necessary plan of sampling, ordering the correct diagnostic test to determine the neonate's needs, and being aware of the potential side effects of all interventions performed in the NICU.

1. The neonatal nurse practitioner (NNP) should evaluate laboratory results for both analytic correctness and:

    A. Clinical significance
    B. Normal-range value
    C. Routine necessity

2. The neonatal nurse practitioner (NNP) recognizes that the laboratory value most commonly used as an indicator of neonatal kidney function is serum:

    A. Bicarbonate
    B. Creatinine
    C. Urea nitrogen

3. The neonatal nurse practitioner (NNP) understands that the fundamental method in which phototherapy reduces bilirubin load is by:

    A. Degradation of isomers which are then filtered by the liver
    B. Oxidations of heme into a form able to pass through the spleen
    C. Photoisomerization of bilirubin to a water-soluble form

4. The neonatal nurse practitioner (NNP) is concerned about the appearance of possible free gas on an infant's anterior–posterior (AP) abdominal x-ray. Options for other views with which to evaluate for free gas are the left lateral decubitus view and:

    A. Cross-table lateral view
    B. Posterior–anterior view
    C. Upright view

5. The neonatal nurse practitioner (NNP) reviews an infant's x-ray that is overall very dark, making it difficult for the NNP to identify any specific findings and leading the NNP to recognize that the x-ray has low:

    A. Density
    B. Radiolucency
    C. Thickness

6. Once the neonatal nurse practitioner (NNP) becomes concerned an infant has experienced an intraventricular hemorrhage, the most appropriate next step for the NNP to include in the plan of care is a/an:

    A. Assessment by cranial ultrasound
    B. Daily head circumference measure
    C. MRI scan

7. The preferred site of medication administration during a delivery room resuscitation is a/an:

    A. Endotracheal tube
    B. Laryngeal mask airway
    C. Umbilical venous catheter

1. A) Clinical significance

Laboratory results must undergo a two-step postanalytic review for analytic correctness (using delta checks, linearity ranges, etc.) and clinical significance to the patient (applying critical values, reference ranges, pretest, posttest probability, etc.).

2. B) Creatinine

Creatinine (Cr) is a valid biochemical marker of renal function in newborns, especially in very low birth weight (VLBW) infants. In term infants, the serum Cr level gradually decreases to a stable level of approximately 0.4 mg/dL within the first 2 weeks of age. In preterm infants, the plasma Cr level rises in the first 48 hours before falling.

3. C) Photoisomerization of bilirubin to a water-soluble form

Special blue fluorescent tubes provide greater irradiance than regular blue tubes because the fluorescent tubes omit light in wavelengths that penetrate the skin well and are maximally absorbed by bilirubin in order to convert it to a water-soluble form (Bradshaw, 2022; Kamath-Rayne et al., 2021; Kaplan et al., 2020; Kaushal & Ramasethu, 2020; Watchko & Maisels, 2020).

4. A) Cross-table lateral view

In a cross-table lateral view, images are captured with the infant lying supine and the x-ray beam passes horizontally from the infant's side through the body. It is generally used for assessment of free air and to verify line placement (Crisci, 2020; Jensen et al., 2022; Trotter, 2022).

5. A) Density

Radiographic density varies depending on the composition of an organ or tissue. For example, a fluid-filled heart is seen as white versus black for air-filled lungs on an x-ray film. Air, fat, water (including all solid viscera: liver, spleen, kidney, pancreas, and heart), bone, and metal are the only five densities that can be distinguished routinely from an x-ray (Trotter, 2022; Weinman et al., 2021).

6. A) Assessment by cranial ultrasound

Ultrasonography is the ideal tool to evaluate the neonate's brain and is often the first step in imaging evaluations for any neurologic concern. The most common approach is through the anterior fontanel in order to obtain coronal and parasagittal views (Berlin & Meyers, 2020; Crisci, 2020; Jensen et al., 2022; Phelps et al., 2020; Sadowski & Verklan, 2022; Scholz & Reinking, 2018; Swanson & Erickson, 2021; Trotter, 2022; Weinman et al., 2021).

7. C) Umbilical venous catheter

Indications for umbilical venous catheter placement include emergency access for medication and fluid administration, exchange transfusion, central venous access in low birth weight infants, blood sampling, central venous blood pressure monitoring, and diagnosis of total anomalous pulmonary venous drainage below the diaphragm (Bailey & Maltsberger, 2021; Coe et al., 2021; Seo, 2022a, 2022b; Travers & Ambalavanan, 2022).

Family Integration, Communication, and the Grieving Process

Ana I. Arias-Oliveras and Marjorie Masten

▶ INTRODUCTION

Parenting and parental attachment begin during pregnancy. The increase in maternal hormones during pregnancy stimulates the formation of maternal bonding. After birth, interactions with the baby build strong parental attachment and bonding. A pregnancy that fails to produce a healthy infant is a life-altering event for the family involved. Newborns who are born premature, have congenital issues, or ultimately die represent loss of a "perfect child."

Pregnancy, birth, and parenthood are almost universally defined as a life transition and crisis. Significant adjustments to roles, lifestyles, and relationships are required when becoming a parent. These adjustments cause considerable stress in the individual and may be heightened if the newborn is critically ill at birth or a perinatal loss is experienced. For some parents, this may be the first time they are coping with a significant life challenge, creating the possibility of developing depression, impaired recall, dysfunctional parenting patterns, and poor developmental outcomes for their child.

This chapter reviews several factors that may inhibit bonding between the infant and the parents. Neonatal circumstances such as prematurity, congenital problems, pregnancy or maternal delivery complications, and mood disorders are some of the possible compounding factors that may negatively affect the parent–infant bonding process (Friedman et al., 2020; Gardner & Carter, 2021; Gardner & Voos, 2021; Voos & Fanaroff, 2020).

▶ FAMILY INTEGRATION

BONDING AND ATTACHMENT

■ The beginnings of parent–infant interactions are founded in autonomic, neurologic, and endocrinologic systems. The emotional connection to an infant begins during pregnancy, with increasing levels of oxytocin throughout pregnancy. This hormone reduces anxiety and encourages formation of an emotional bond between the mother and the fetus.
  ● Oxytocin levels in early pregnancy and the postpartum period are significantly correlated with a clearly defined set of maternal bonding behaviors, including gaze, vocalizations, positive affect, affectionate touch, attachment-related thoughts, and frequent checking of the infant.
■ Bonding is a continuous and reciprocal process unique to two people. Bonding occurs on a different timetable for mothers and fathers; mothers experience an intensifying feeling of bonding throughout the pregnancy, while fathers' feelings develop and become congruent after birth.
■ Attachment is the quality of the bond, or affectional tie, between the parents and their infant and is an individualized process. Attachment is characterized by the same qualities used to describe love. Parental love and romantic love activate the same areas of the human brain and result in brain processing of infant cues which elevate oxytocin, the "bonding" hormone (Friedman et al., 2020; Gardner & Voos, 2021; Link, 2016).
■ Table 8.1 outlines Klaus and Kennell's nine steps in the process of attachment. It is worth noting that six of the nine steps of attachment occur *prior to* the infant's birth.

BECOMING A PARENT

■ Becoming a parent requires significant adjustments to roles, lifestyles, and relationships. Previous coping strategies may not be helpful; these situations challenge the individual to develop new problem-solving responses and solutions, resulting in personal growth.
  ● The ability to parent is influenced by many factors that occur before, during, and after the infant's birth. Previous life events, including the degree of life stress and usual coping patterns, genetic factors, previous pregnancies, distress about the parenting role, and interpersonal relationships affect the experience of pregnancy and parenthood.
  ● Cultural differences influence several factors, such as (a) parental emotional responses and perceptions of their infant's illness and disability, (b) parental usage of services, and (c) parental interaction with healthcare providers. Viewing parental attachment behavior through one's personal cultural filter may result in an incorrect assessment of the parent–infant attachment.

Table 8.1 Klaus and Kennell's Nine Steps in the Process of Attachment

Step 1. Planning the pregnancy	Planning is the first step, showing investment and commitment of the parents.
Step 2. Confirming the pregnancy	Confirmation of the pregnancy begins the psychological acceptance of the pregnancy.
Step 3. Accepting the pregnancy	Parents experience a normal feeling of ambivalence. Although the mother does not yet perceive the fetus as separate from themselves, they undergo emotional changes leading toward attachment.
Step 4. Fetal movement	Feeling fetal movement leads to happy thoughts and the mother starts to think of the baby as a separate person.
Step 5. Accepting the fetus	Parents begin to think of the fetus as an individual and start to imagine what the baby will be like, resulting in the establishment of a relationship.
Step 6. Labor and birth	Parental attitudes toward the labor and delivery process may affect their reactions. For example, studies show that those who attend the birth are more attached to the infant than those who do not.
Step 7. Seeing	Studies have shown that immediate attachment is facilitated when the mother can see the baby immediately after birth.
Step 8. Touching	Nurturing maternal touch is associated with more secure attachments.
Step 9. Caregiving	It is crucial for psychic closure of bonding.

Source: Data from Gardner, S. & Voos, K. (2021). Families in crisis: Theoretical and practical considerations. In S. Gardner, B. Carter, & M. Hines (Eds.), *Merenstein & Gardner's handbook of neonatal intensive care* (9th ed., pp. 1039–1045). Elsevier.

- Infant characteristics such as their ability to respond to parent cues and their vulnerability due to illness, as well as overall appearance, parental feelings of loyalty and hope, the behavior of health professionals, separation from the infant, an inability to protect their newborn from pain, and hospital practices, all influence parenting patterns (Gardner & Voos, 2021).

▶ THE INITIAL FAMILY DYNAMICS AND THE "SENSITIVE PERIOD"

BIRTH

- For a term, healthy newborn, all five senses are operational at birth and the infant is ready to cue and shape their environment; likewise, healthy mothers are physiologically and psychologically prepared for reciprocal interaction.
- The maternal cues of voice, touch, and body rhythm begin bonding and create a synchronized "dance" between the mother and the infant. The sensory stimuli of touch, warmth, and odor between the mother and the infant are powerful stimulants, resulting in the release of maternal oxytocin, which aids in breastfeeding and mother–infant attachment.
  - The period of labor and birth and the following days has been called the "sensitive period," and it is during this time that parents are most strongly influenced by the quality of care they receive. Positive effects of early and extended contact, rather than initial separation, have shown significant differences in caregiving behaviors that persist over time.
  - During a period referred to as *primary maternal preoccupation*, the mother develops a great sensitivity to and is focused on the infant's needs. This period begins toward the end of the pregnancy and continues for a few weeks after delivery. Reciprocation of needs and responses from the infant to the mother reinforce synchronized and rewarding interactions for the dyad.
  - Studies have demonstrated that when fathers are allowed to be alone with their newborn, they spend an equal amount of time interacting, holding, touching, and bonding with their baby.
  - The first feelings of love for the infant may not be instantaneous. Many mothers express distress and disappointment when they do not experience feelings of love for their infant in the first minutes or hours after birth. However, studies confirm that normal, healthy mothers may not first feel love for their baby until after a week or longer.
- The birth of a newborn initiates a series of interactions with the parents (particularly the mother) designed to initiate attachment and ensure survival. The high level of positive arousal that infants co-construct with their parents during their face-to-face interactions accelerates the maturation of the infant's relational skills and provides essential environmental inputs for the development of self-regulation and the process of attachment. Parental attachment and appropriate caregiving behaviors are crucial to the infant's physical, psychological, and emotional health and survival.
- Early parent–infant contact facilitates parent–infant attachment and contributes to regulating the newborn's physiology and behavior. Positive effects of early and extended contact, rather than initial separation, have shown significant differences in caregiving behaviors that persist over time (Friedman et al., 2020; Gardner & Voos, 2021).

BARRIERS TO ATTACHMENT

- Early attachment can be easily disturbed and may be permanently altered during the immediate postpartum period if a newborn requires separation from the mother for care. These would include routine procedures such as weighing, measuring, bathing, blood tests, vaccines, and eye prophylaxis. Whenever possible, nonurgent care should be delayed until after the first feeding is completed.

- During medically necessary interventions, it is important to give parents as much interaction (or at least visual contact) with their infant as possible (Friedman et al., 2020; Gardner & Voos, 2021).

▶ FAMILY-CENTERED CARE

- The family-centered care (FCC) principles stress that parents are the most important person in their infant's life and that they have expertise in caring for their infant. Parental values and beliefs should be central during NICU care. Adherence to the FCC principles has been shown to have a significant positive influence on the family's ability to cope with NICU stress. The use of FCC has been shown to enhance the likelihood of successful parent–child relationships (Gardner & Voos, 2021).

BABY-FRIENDLY INITIATIVE

- The Baby-Friendly Hospital Initiative (BFHI) is a global effort launched by the World Health Organization (WHO) and UNICEF in 1991 to implement practices that protect, promote, and support breastfeeding in low-resource settings. Although the initial steps were intended for full-term healthy newborns and their families, a revised version is now intended to be applied to sick and premature neonates.
  - Among the 10 steps for a hospital to achieve a Baby-Friendly designation are to "help mother initiate breastfeeding within one hour of birth and to practice 'rooming in'—allow mothers and infants to remain together 24 hours a day" (Gardner et al., 2021).
- Following the introduction of the Baby-Friendly initiative in maternity units in several countries throughout the world, an unexpected observation was made: The use of "rooming in" and early contact with suckling significantly reduced the frequency of abandonment.
- There is evidence of a "dose–response" relationship between the number of BFHI steps that women are exposed to and improved breastfeeding outcomes (Friedman et al., 2020; Gardner, Lawrence, & Lawrence, 2021; Gardner & Voos, 2021; Snell & Gardner, 2017; Taylor et al., 2018).

SKIN-TO-SKIN CARE OR KANGAROO CARE

- Researchers have discovered that infants who are placed on their mother's chest, skin-to-skin and

covered by a blanket, for the first 90 minutes after birth cried less than babies who were not. An additional review found that early skin-to-skin interactions between mothers and babies reduced crying, improved mother–infant interactions, kept the baby warm, and helped the mothers breastfeed successfully (Voos & Fanaroff, 2020).

▶ FAMILIES IN CRISIS

- When a much-anticipated full-term infant whose mother had an uncomplicated pregnancy is birthed in a manner not expected, the parents can feel an overwhelming sense of shock and disappointment. The infant's healthcare concern can cause a lowering of parental self-esteem and the parents may view this as a failure. Guilt is one of the overwhelming emotions that plague these parents. They frequently experience lowered self-esteem and think of this as a failure of their capacity for reproduction. Parents of infants requiring NICU care often experience high levels of stress, and consequently their ability to interact optimally with their infant is impaired.
  - Stresses that precipitate concern for the health and survival of either the mother or the infant or both may delay the mother's preparation for interactions with the infant and interrupt bond formation.
- Parental perception of support by the medical team has been shown to be inversely correlated with maternal depressive symptoms. The more support the parents feel from the medical team, the fewer depressive symptoms are manifested. The medical health team cannot underestimate its ability to influence how the mother and the family adapt through the behavior of physicians, nurses, and hospital personnel. Early comments by staff, family, and friends *often cement* a lasting impression in the parent's minds.
- Perceived poor care or lack of support during labor and the first days after birth, separation of the mother and the infant, and rules of the hospital may serve as barriers to feeling supported (Gardner & Carter, 2021; Gardner & Voos, 2021; Kenner & Boykova, 2021; Voos & Fanaroff, 2020).

INFLUENCES ON PARENTAL BEHAVIOR

- A schematic diagram of the influences on paternal behavior and the hypothesized resultant disturbances is shown in Figure 8.1.
- Parents' responses to stress can be influenced by parental background and care practices.
  - Included under parental background is the care a parent received from their own parents, as well as cultural patterns and practices, relationships within the family, and events during pregnancy.

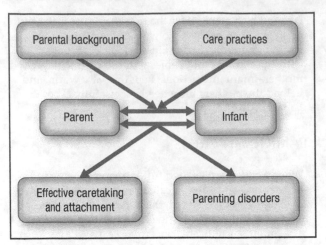

Figure 8.1 Schematic diagram of the major influences on paternal and maternal behavior and the resulting disturbances that we hypothesize may arise from them.

Source: Reproduced with permission from Klaus, M., Kennell, J. H., & Fanaroff, J. (2020). Care of the parents. In A. Fanaroff & J. Fanaroff (Eds.), *Klaus and Fanaroff's care of the high-risk neonate* (7th ed., pp. 148–170.e3). Elsevier.

- Emotional reactions parents may exhibit when their child requires NICU care may include shock, panic, fright, anxiety, isolation, and helplessness.
  - Hospital care practices that reduce anxiety, such as avoiding unnecessary separation of an infant from their parents during the "sensitive period," can contribute greatly to early attachment.
  - Researchers have found that parents are best able to develop a secure attachment with the premature/sick newborn when they are able to see the infant within 3 hours of delivery.
- Outcomes from altered interactions between the parent and the infant result in the chance for negative (parenting disorders) and positive (effective caretaking and attachment) conclusions.
- Contributing factors that impair the parent–infant bond attachment are summarized in Box 8.1.
- Included under parenting disorders are the vulnerable child syndrome, child abuse, failure to thrive, and some developmental and emotional problems in high-risk infants.
- Other maladaptive parenting examples are being overprotective, or emotional disengagement and deprivation, and low adherence to follow-up recommendations, which may affect infant development and growth.
- The most easily manipulated variables in this scheme are the separation of the infant from the mother and the practices in the hospital during the first hours and days of life. It is here, during this period, that studies have in part clarified some of the steps in parent–infant attachment.
  - Parents who miss out on this early interaction experience should be assured that their future

relationship with their baby can still be developed. It is important that parents be given as much contact, physical or visual, as possible (Friedman et al., 2020; Gardner & Voos, 2021; Kenner & Boykova, 2021; Voos & Fanaroff, 2020).

Box 8.1 Six Major Sources of Parental Stress in the NICU

- Preexisting and concurrent personal as well as family factors
- Prenatal, perinatal, and labor and delivery experiences
- Accepting and understanding the infant's illness and the treatment required; also accepting the appearance of the infant during the treatment and of those with congenital anomalies
- Concerns for the outcome of the infant, long term as well as immediate
- Their perceived loss of parental role, as well as loss of personal control of the situation
- Their trust and experience with the healthcare providers

Source: Data from Gardner, S., & Voos, K. (2021). Families in crisis: Theoretical and practical considerations. In S. Gardner, B. Carter, & M. Hines (Eds.), *Merenstein & Gardner's handbook of neonatal intensive care* (9th ed., pp. 1039–1045). Elsevier.

FACILITATING POSITIVE PARENTING IN THE NEONATAL INTENSIVE CARE UNIT

- The healthcare team can help make the NICU experience more positive in multiple ways.
  - Whenever discussing the infant with the parent, make sure to refer to the baby by name and the correct gender. These actions help the parents personalize the infant as theirs.
  - Facilitate opportunities for parents to be involved in their baby's care and advocate for parent–child interactions. Provide opportunities for parent–child physical closeness and intimacy.
  - Allow parents to verbalize feelings of fear and grief while letting them know these are normal feelings.
  - Provide ongoing, optimistic (but realistic), and consistent feedback to parents. Keep parents updated about their baby's medical condition and be free to answer questions.
  - Parents have stated that when a healthcare professional gives information regarding their baby, they want accurate, current, and comprehensive information that is not necessarily pessimistic.
  - Many times, parents may misperceive the information that they are given, so it is essential to find out their understanding of what they have been told and to clarify misinformation when necessary.
  - Pictures can be beneficial when giving detailed information. Remember not to overload the parent with too much information at one time and

continually assess their understanding (Gardner & Voos, 2021; Kenner & Boykova, 2021; Schiefelbein, 2021; Spruill, 2021).

▶ SOCIAL DETERMINANTS OF HEALTH AND NEONATAL OUTCOMES

- Healthcare disparities are differences in healthcare quality, access, and outcomes adversely affecting members of racial and ethnic minority groups and other socially disadvantaged populations. WHO defines *social determinants of health (SDoH)* as the conditions in which people are born, grow, live, work, and age. Another definition identifies SDoH as those nonmedical factors that influence health, including health-related knowledge, attitudes, beliefs, or behaviors.
  - Social determinants greatly impact perinatal outcomes and are largely responsible for preventable health inequities. Poverty limits access to healthy foods and safe neighborhoods and education resources, a known predictor of better health. Social determinants such as insurance status, availability of social support in the form of childcare and adequate housing, neighborhood, and transportation likely play some role in prenatal care utilization and ultimately neonatal outcomes.
- It is unlikely that improving care in the NICU alone will have a dramatic impact on reducing the U.S. neonatal and infant mortality rates. Social determinants of women's health also play a role in birth outcome. For example, low socioeconomic status is a long-known risk factor for preterm birth. Research has demonstrated the areas of greatest impact that will result in improved neonatal health. First, all women, but especially those at highest risk, such as non-Hispanic Black women and Native American/ Alaskan women, must have improved health status even before conception. Discussions and interventions around issues of maternal health, such as obesity, chronic health conditions, and drug use, will have resultant improvements in neonatal health and long-term outcomes.
- It is now well established that major contributors to infant mortality rates in the United States are the significant health disparities. The major health disparity is related to racial and ethnic differences of perinatal health outcomes in all states in the United States, with a wide variation from state to state. In the United States, non-Hispanic Black infants have the highest rates of infant mortality and prematurity compared with other races and ethnic groups. Non-Hispanic Black mothers also have extremely high rates of maternal mortality and morbidity, as well as obesity, leading to other poor outcomes. Native American/Alaska Natives also suffer from a disproportionate share of infant mortality and prematurity, as well as higher rates of sudden unexpected death of infancy.

- The State Perinatal Quality Collaboratives have been an extremely successful model for healthcare providers and families interested in improving prenatal and postnatal outcomes, primarily using quality improvement methodology. Areas successfully addressed have been increased administration of antenatal corticosteroids to mothers at risk of preterm delivery, decrease in elective late preterm deliveries, and antibiotic stewardship. State collaboratives identify best practices within each state and work together to improve maternal and neonatal outcomes through quality improvement processes (Adams, 2021; Savich & Famuyide, 2020; Trembath, 2020).

▶ GRIEF

- Grief is an individualized process influenced by cultural, environmental, spiritual, and religious experiences. Grief is the characteristic response to the loss of a valued "object," be that a person or situation. For grief to occur, the individual must have valued the item lost, which indicates that the loss is perceived as significant and meaningful.
  - Loss, whether real or imagined, actual or possible, is traumatic. The individual is no longer confident in themselves or their surroundings. Healing from the loss will take time, as the individual will adapt into the phase of acceptance on their own accord to minimize the degree of pain and suffering.
- The acceptance of the perceived "loss" (e.g., the discrepancy between the idealized and the physical infant) is vital to the resolution of parental grief (Gardner & Carter, 2021; Kenner & Boykova, 2021; Voos & Fanaroff, 2020).

STAGES OF GRIEF

- Grief is differentiated into three categories: anticipatory grief, chronic grief, and chronic sorrow (Kenner & Boykova, 2021). These categories are summarized in Table 8.2.

Kübler-Ross Stages of Grief

- The experience of grief is a staged process that occurs over time. Each stage of grief represents a psychological defense mechanism used to help the individual adapt to the crisis. The process of grief is dynamic and fluid rather than static and rigid.
- This process is individualized, asynchronous, and progressive at a pace manageable by the individual. Cultural and individual experiences will influence the trajectory. Risk factors for pathologic grief include a history of psychiatric illness, childlessness, and poor social support.
- Knowledge of each stage is necessary to assess where an individual family member, the family as a unit, and

Table 8.2 Categories of Grief

Category	Key Characteristics	Example
Anticipatory grief	Grieving prior to the loss	Parents of a preterm infant in the NICU; guarded bonding due to the potential death or impaired neurodevelopmental outcomes
Chronic grief	Unresolved grief	Parents of an infant born at 23 weeks' gestation who later develops spastic cerebral palsy as a child
Chronic sorrow	Cyclical, permanent grieving without resolution	A mother diagnosed with infertility who experiences multiple spontaneous abortions

Source: Data from Kenner, C., & Boykova, M. (2021). Families in crisis. In M.T. Verklan, M. Walden, & S. Forest. (Eds), *Core curriculum for neonatal intensive care nursing.* (6th ed., pp. 287–299). Elsevier-Saunders.

the staff are in their grieving process (Friedman et al., 2020; Gardner & Carter, 2021).
■ The stages of grief according to Kübler-Ross are summarized in Table 8.3.

COMMON BEHAVIORS OF GRIEF

■ The signs and symptoms of acute grief have been well described and include both somatic and behavioral manifestations of the emotional experience of the loss. The behavior of the bereaved is characterized as ambivalent.
■ Mothers and fathers can have the same reactions to grief reactions but express them very differently. Mothers are more likely than fathers to express symptoms such as crying, sadness, anger, and guilt. This difference in symptomatology does not represent a different experience of grief, but merely a different expression of it.
■ Maternal grief may begin with a period of shock, numbness, confusion, irritability, or anxiety, followed by intense sadness, longing, guilt, and somatic complaints.
■ Paternal grief may be affected by the degree of investment in the pregnancy, impending parenthood, and the circumstances of birth; all affect their feelings of loss. Many men have difficulty dealing with irrational behaviors, as well as with the normal ambiguity and conflict of life.
■ Dealing with more than one grief or loss situation compounds the intensity of mourning and may prolong the grief reaction (Friedman et al., 2020; Gardner & Carter, 2021).

Table 8.3 Kübler-Ross Stages of Grief

Stage	Key Characteristics
Denial	■ This stage may take a few hours to a few weeks. ■ It is characterized by feelings of disbelief after receiving bad news. ■ The individual may compartmentalize the loss. ■ The individual may express anger intermittently.
Anger	■ Prolongation of this stage may inhibit continuation into the subsequent stages. ■ Once the individual is aware of the significance of the loss, they can move onward. ■ Social prohibition of expressing anger is prominent in some cultures and religions. ■ This may lead to depression and a sense of guilt: "Why me?" "Is this my fault?" ■ This stage may last a few months or even a few years. ■ It can be observed concomitantly with the stage of denial. ■ The individual may bargain with God or another spiritual/religious deity.
Depression	■ There is significant variability in the duration of this stage. ■ The acceptance of the loss may trigger depressive episodes. ■ Social interactions with friends and family may cease or be limited.
Acceptance	■ This completes the grieving process.

FACTORS INFLUENCING THE GRIEF PROCESS

■ Risk factors for pathologic grief include a history of psychiatric illness, childlessness, and poor social support. One parameter for differentiating normal from pathologic grief has been the length of time for grief to be resolved. Grief work may still be categorized as normal/uncomplicated even if it lasts longer than a year.
■ Social prohibitions against the expression of anger, especially for women, encourage this powerful emotion to be turned inward toward the self. Those exhibiting maladaptive or destructive behaviors, dominant somatic symptoms, or lack of improvement over the course of months should be referred for evaluation (Friedman et al., 2020; Gardner & Carter, 2021; Voos & Fanaroff, 2021).

▶ MATERNAL POSTPARTUM MOOD DISORDERS

■ It is estimated that maternal mood disorders affect more than 500,000 pregnancies per year. Anxiety is one of the most common mental health disorders during pregnancy, followed by depression. Antepartum depression is a strong risk factor for postpartum disorders. Depression may be affected by the cortisol levels and corticotropin-releasing hormone (CRH). Elevated levels of these hormones can lead to reduction in size of the hippocampus and other areas of the brain.

- Assessment and identification of a maternal mental health disorder will lead to early intervention, thus inhibiting the progression of the disorder to a more severe manifestation, such as postpartum psychosis (Friedman et al., 2020; Whitmer, 2016; Yonkers, 2018).

POSTPARTUM ANXIETY

- Anxiety often coexists with other mood disorders, most commonly with postpartum depression (PPD). Increased rates of anxiety among NICU mothers exist. It disrupts completion of daily activities and with parent–child attachment.
- Interventions which may alleviate the degree of anxiety of mothers in the NICU include holding their infant when medically appropriate and performing common routine cares, such as diapering, bathing, feeding, and so on.
- Early diagnosis and/or antenatal interventions aimed to reduce anxiety may enhance the mother–infant bonding in the postnatal period (Friedman et al., 2020; Whitmer, 2016).

PATERNAL POSTPARTUM DEPRESSION

- The incidence of paternal PPD is estimated at 4% to 12%. The strongest risk factor and predictor of paternal PPD is maternal PPD (see later).
- Paternal depression usually presents after the onset of maternal depression. It may worsen 3 to 6 months after the birth of their child. Symptoms in fathers are similar to those in mothers, although the signs may be more subtle as men can feel less secure about outwardly showing emotions.
- If untreated, paternal depression can impact compliance with medical care and bonding with the infant and affect the interpersonal relationship with the infant's mother. Early treatment will minimize the potential to progress to a more severe psychiatric disorder (Gardner & Voos, 2021).

MATERNAL POSTPARTUM DEPRESSION

- The incidence of depression is variable, but can be seen up to 20% of women. PPD can be seen up to 70% in NICU mothers. Preexisting mental health conditions increase a mother's risk of developing PPD. Other risk factors include familial history, lack of partner support, and low socioeconomic status.
- Symptoms of depression usually present within the first month after delivery. Symptoms include decrease in usual activities, appetite suppression, mood swings, sleep disturbance, and suicidal ideation.
- PPD is a complex, biologic, and psychological phenomenon which presents along a continuum. Severity of symptoms and the degree of impairment of the individual guide interventions (Gardner & Voos, 2021; Whitmer, 2016).

ASSESSMENT TOOLS FOR MATERNAL POSTPARTUM DEPRESSION

- Several assessment tools are available to identify patients at risk of developing PPD. Current recommendation is to utilize these assessment tools at each trimester of pregnancy and intermittently in the postpartum period because most symptoms present post discharge from the hospital.
- The Postpartum Depression Screening Scale (PDSS) is the most reliable tool for NICU mothers. It can be completed in the postpartum area and measures depression symptomatology through a 35-item, self-report, Likert-type scale. The total score ranges from 13 to 175 and a positive screen is a score of 80 or greater.
- The Postpartum Depression Predictors Inventory-Revised (PDPI-Revised) is a checklist that assesses 13 risk factors. It is also completed postpartum, completed by the clinician and the mother, and provides detailed information on symptoms.
- The Edinburgh Postnatal Depression Scale (EPDS) is a 10-item questionnaire to be used by either the mother or the father. A positive score indicates the likelihood of depression but not severity (Gardner & Voos, 2021; Whitmer, 2016).

INTERVENTION AND RESOURCES

- A comprehensive approach is needed, consisting of reassurance and support, nursing home visits, problem-solving education, psychoeducation, psychotherapy, and psychopharmacology.
- Assistance is imperative to provide guidance and reassurance in caring for the infant and each other as partners in childraising. Parenting classes may be offered to enhance parenting competence, and to help parents feel confident, in control, and less frustrated.
- Psychopharmacology may be necessary as the depression becomes more severe and debilitating. Classes of medication often prescribed are selective serotonin reuptake inhibitors (SSRIs), mood stabilizers, antidepressants, and antipsychotics. SSRIs are currently the most prescribed medication to treat depression during and after pregnancy. If the mother is breastfeeding, special considerations should be taken because all psychotropic medications enter the breast milk.
- There is a risk for mothers to be noncompliant with prescribed medications due to concerns of neonatal exposure. Discontinuation of medication will increase

the risk of relapse by more than 60% in comparison with women who remain compliant.

■ Psychiatric treatment may become necessary if, based on the severity of symptoms, concerns for the parent's or the infant's health arise.

■ Support groups specific to PPD are available at the local and national level. The most often used are Depression After Delivery (DAD) Inc., Postpartum Support International (PSI), and the Online PPD Support Group.

■ Education on depression, symptoms, assessment, and interventions should be addressed with the parents in the prenatal period to provide anticipatory guidance for the potential development and trajectory of PPD (Friedman et al., 2020; Gardner & Voos, 2021).

▶ PALLIATIVE CARE

■ WHO defines *palliative care* as an approach that improves the quality of life of patients and their families facing problems associated with life-threatening illness, through prevention and relief of suffering by means of early identification and assessment and treatment of pain and other problems of physical, psychosocial, or spiritual nature (Sturtz, 2020).

■ Current trends in healthcare advocate that palliative care be included with cure-oriented approaches for all patients who have a serious illness. Curative and palliative care can be complementary and concurrent with treatment goals of care guiding life-sustaining interventions while improving the infant's and the parent's quality of life.

■ The National Association of Neonatal Nurses (NANN) considers palliative and end-of-life care as integral aspects of care of the terminally ill infant. End-of-life care supports a peaceful, dignified death for the infant and the provision of support to the family and healthcare providers.

■ Treatment goals should be developed to maintain clear communication between the family, the medical team, and the nursing team. Parents must be fully informed in order to determine an overall treatment goal and to consent to or refuse treatment for their child. The family's values will affect decisions made for the infant.

■ The more complex the medical situation, the more crucial it is that parents receive consistent information, perhaps from a single designated person on the healthcare team.

■ Palliative care should be considered in any of the following circumstances:
  ● Life-limiting diagnosis, poor prognosis, or uncertainty of death after birth
  ● Redirection of treatment goals and intense support for the family
  ● Pain management during the transition period from curative to palliative care or at the end of life
  ● Certainty of death despite life-sustaining interventions (Crotezzo & Carter, 2018; Kenner & Boykova, 2021; NANN, 2015; Sturtz, 2020; Swaney et al., 2021)

PALLIATIVE CARE IN THE NEONATAL INTENSIVE CARE UNIT

■ Pediatric palliative care (PPC) includes a team of pediatric providers who focus on the palliative care needs of infants and children in conjunction with cure-oriented approaches.

■ The overall goals with these conversations are to assess and develop goals of care for the infant. Use of consistent information from all healthcare providers is important to minimize anxiety.

■ End-of-life discussions should be family-centered and involve an interdisciplinary team to promote clear communication, identify goals, and assess cultural, spiritual, and religious concerns.

■ Creation of an environment that will facilitate these discussions is vital. The parents should have a clear understanding of who is present from the medical team and their respective role. A facilitator should state the purpose of the meeting and then prompt discussions with the family as to their understanding of the infant's issue(s). Provide moments of silence intermittently to allow the family to process the information discussed. Review relevant data, decisions (if determined by the end of the meeting), and options with the family and the team. Offer another meeting to the family if needed (Cortezzo & Carter, 2018; Kenner & Boykova, 2021; Swaney et al., 2021).

PARADIGMS OF CARE/END-OF-LIFE CARE

■ End-of-life care is an integral component of palliative care where families are supported in redirecting goals of care to ensure a holistic, dignified death for their infant.

■ The transition from curative care to palliative care occurs once it had been determined that life-sustaining medical treatment is futile. Criteria for considering withholding or withdrawing life-sustaining medical treatment are inevitability of death, ineffective treatment, and poor quality of life.

■ Palliative care milestones are very different from what was anticipated and hoped. Instead of preparing to take an infant home, the focus of care shifts to pain management, grief support, preparing for the dying process, and bereavement support (Cortezzo & Carter, 2018; NANN, 2015; Sudia & Catlin, 2021).

INTEGRATIVE MODEL OF PALLIATIVE CARE

- The following framework is suggested to enhance concurrent care in the NICU:
  - *Admission to the NICU:* Establish a care plan, review with the family, and establish goals of care with the understanding that the goals may be modified based on the infant's medical needs.
  - *Ongoing assessment and decision-making:* Update the family on the infant's current status, modify the care plan when necessary, and consult pediatric subspecialists when needed. The family may be routinely offered a family meeting to discuss complex information. If warranted, consider involving an ethics specialist. Most importantly, support the family during this transition and encourage them to take advantage of services readily available to them, such as chaplain and psychosocial counseling.
  - *Transitional period:* The family decides to either continue with curative care or withdraw life-sustaining interventions. Throughout and until this time, supportive measures remain in place with maintaining open communication with the family.
  - *Bereavement:* Following an infant death, a designated team member should follow up with the family within 1 week to assess their status. Intermittent communication within the first year after an infant's death is acceptable if the family agrees (Cortezzo & Carter, 2018).

▶ CONCLUSION

Pregnancy is most often associated with joyful emotions, expectations, wishes, and goals. At times, the pregnancy may be affected by a change in the maternal health, antenatal fetal diagnosis that may be life-limiting, or a change in the fetal well-being. Having a sick or premature infant who requires neonatal intensive care can initiate many different emotions in parents. These include but are not limited to stress, guilt, anxiety, and fear. Healthcare professionals can help parents with these emotions by listening; giving honest, accurate, and consistent information; and continually assessing parents' understanding of their infant's condition. Families may experience anticipatory grief while they process the information given, weigh the options available, await the birth of their child, and potentially await the death of their child. Understanding the process of grief as an individualized continuum influenced by culture, experiences, and values will enhance the support provided to families.

1. Interdisciplinary collaboration with a family in the NICU requires establishment of trust in conjunction with:

   A. Frequent changes to the medical plan
   B. Recurrent meetings with the ethics team
   C. Transparency with all medical cares

2. The neonatal nurse practitioner (NNP) cares for an infant with multiple, significant congenital anomalies and counsels the parents that one of the criteria for withdrawal of life-sustaining support is the:

   A. Chance of operative correction
   B. Inevitability of neonatal death
   C. Limitation of physical resources

3. The primary goal of implementing family-centered care (FCC) in the NICU is to allow families to:

   A. Cope with the stressors in the NICU
   B. Leave the infant at night to go home
   C. Understand the baby's plan of care

4. Based on recent data, the rate of postpartum depression in mothers whose infant is in the NICU is approximately:

   A. 70%
   B. 80%
   C. 90%

5. The neonatal nurse practitioner (NNP) explains the concepts of social determinants of health (SDoH) as the environments in which an infant and family:

   A. Earn, spend, and live
   B. Grow, educate, and die
   C. Live, work, and play

(See answers next page.)

1. C) Transparency with all medical cares

Treatment goals should be developed to maintain clear communication between the family, the medical team, and the nursing team. For parents to be involved in determining overall treatment goals and the decision-making process, they must be fully informed to consent to or refuse treatment for their child. The family's values will also affect decisions made for the infant. Frequent changes to the medical plan can be frustrating for families in the NICU. Establishing communication between the medical team and the family will minimize mistrust and miscommunication. Involvement of an ethics team often results in a confrontational relationship between the medical team and the parents (NANN, 2015; Swaney et al., 2021).

2. B) Inevitability of neonatal death

Inevitability of death is a criterion for considering withholding or withdrawing life-sustaining medical treatment. Reversible congenital anomalies which may be corrected or managed by operative interventions do not meet the criteria for withdrawal of life-sustaining medical treatment. Physical resources should not play a role in determining whether to sustain or withdraw neonatal care (Fanaroff, 2020).

3. A) Cope with the stressors in the NICU

The FCC principles stress that the parents are the most important person in their infant's life. Adherence to these principles has been shown to have a significant positive influence on the family's ability to cope with NICU stress. There is stress in leaving the infant overnight or having questions about the plan of care; however, the overarching goal of FCC is to help parents deal with all the stressors rather than individual ones (Gardner & Voos, 2021).

4. A) 70%

The incidence of depression is variable, but can be seen up to 20% of mothers. Postpartum depression can be seen up to 70% of NICU mothers (Gardner & Voos, 2021).

5. C) Live, work, and play

The World Health Organization (WHO) defines social determinants of health as the conditions in which people are born, grow, live, work, and age. They consist of policies, programs, and other aspects of societal structure, including government and private sectors, as well as community factors (Savich & Famuyide, 2020).

Discharge Planning and Follow-Up

Amanda D. Bennett and Denise Kirsten

▶ INTRODUCTION

Discharge planning should be an ongoing process between infant caregivers and the multidisciplinary team of the NICU that should facilitate a safe and seamless transition to home. This chapter reviews the concepts and strategies needed for discharge planning and follow-up of the NICU patient. Standards for infants with unique and complex needs after discharge will be addressed.

▶ DISCHARGE PLANNING

- Utilization of a family-centered, multidisciplinary team approach to discharge planning throughout the entire hospitalization will optimize transition to home and the well-being of the infant and the caregiver.
- Families should be active participants of the care team, participating in medical rounds as well as regularly scheduled discharge planning rounds/care conferences throughout the entire hospitalization.
- There should be ongoing discussions between infant caregivers and the NICU team, including the establishment of a clear criteria for discharge readiness (Boxes 9.1 and 9.2).
- The discharge teaching plan should be tailored to meet each family's specific needs. Cultural and language needs must be assessed and incorporated in the plan.
- Families should be offered the opportunity to room-in and care for their infant prior to discharge home to gain and demonstrate confidence and competence. Any home equipment should be delivered to the hospital prior to discharge to allow caregivers to use them (Carter & Carter, 2021; Hummel & Naber, 2021; Smith & Andrews, 2017).

ANTICIPATORY GUIDANCE

- Anticipatory guidance describes the provision of information about what to expect from themselves and others. This term is often used involving conversations on grief after the death of an infant, but the concept may be applied to the situation of a family taking their less-than-perfect infant home from the NICU.

Box 9.1 Suggested Discharge Criteria for the NICU Infant

- Ability to maintain temperature in an open crib
- Ability to breastfeed or bottle-feed without cardiopulmonary compromise
- Demonstrates steady weight gain pattern
- Demonstrates cardiopulmonary stability for a sufficient time frame prior to discharge
- Completion of routine screening tests and immunizations for all infants
- Normal metabolic screening (newborn screening)
- Hearing screening
- Congenital heart disease screening
- Hepatitis B vaccination
- Completion of specialized screening tests and immunizations for infants with specialized needs
- Radiologic studies as indicated (ultrasound, CT scan, MRI)
- Car seat screening
- Ophthalmologic examination
- Palivizumab RSV prophylaxis
- Routine immunizations are up to date per the AAP guidelines
- A comprehensive review of the hospital course, including resolved and ongoing problems, completed with established follow-up plans, made available to the infant's caregivers and all postdischarge healthcare providers

AAP, American Academy of Pediatrics; RSV, respiratory syncytial virus.

Knowledge of potential issues once at home can give parents confidence and aid in the transition (e.g., where they are in the grief process, issues with attachment, the risk of postpartum depression).

- Once transitioned to a primary care setting, anticipatory guidance should be part of all office visits with the healthcare provider. Anticipatory guidance is crucial to the continued success of the family unit and may include topics such as the following:
  - Family support, family resources, and maternal wellness
  - Infant behaviors, parent–child relationship, and safe sleep practices
  - Patterns of feedings, any new or recurring difficulties with oral feedings (breast or bottle), amount the infant should be feeding, and spitting versus vomiting
  - Safety issues such as car seats and smoking within the home

Box 9.2 Suggested Discharge Criteria for the NICU Parent/Caregiver

- Identification of at least two primary caregivers
- Emotional and psychosocial stability, with caregivers demonstrating confidence with infant care at the time of discharge
  - Identification of support system
  - Importance of self-care
  - Completed teaching on the dangers of shaking a baby
- Home environment acceptable to meet the needs of the infant after discharge from the NICU
- Resource availability in place (e.g., financial, utilities, transportation)
- Identification of follow-up primary care provider with an appointment scheduled within 1 week of NICU discharge
- Subspecialty appointments scheduled as appropriate (e.g., ophthalmology, cardiology, developmental follow-up)
- Caregivers have completed teaching and demonstrate competency in the following:
  - rovision of basic infant care
  - Maintaining infant's thermal stability
  - Circumcision care
  - Infant feeding (includes specialized feeding methods as well as specialized formula preparation)
  - Management of home feeding devices (feeding tubes, infusion pumps, stoma care, etc.)
  - Management of cardiopulmonary monitoring and equipment (e.g., apnea monitors, oxygen, ventilators, tracheostomy care)
  - Medication preparation and administration (includes knowledge of adverse effects)
  - Emergency plan (includes CPR training completed, emergency interventions reviewed, and contact numbers identified)
- Provision of safe environment (e.g., back to sleep/safe sleep practices, car seat use, smoke-free, heat, electricity, phone)
- Knowledge of when to call primary care provider or seek emergency services
- Influenza vaccine obtained for all caregivers and members of the home

Sources: Data from Carter, A., & Carter, B. S. (2021). Discharge planning and follow-up of the neonatal intensive care unit infant. In S. Gardner, B. Carter, M. Enzman-Hines, & S. Niermeyer (Eds.), *Merenstein & Gardner's handbook of neonatal intensive care* (9th ed., pp. 1141–1166). Elsevier; Hummel, P., & Naber, M. (2021). Discharge planning and transition to home. In M. T. Verklan, M. Walden, & S. Forest (Eds.), *Core curriculum for neonatal intensive care nursing* (6th ed., pp. 329–345). Elsevier; Smith, V. C., & Andrews, T. M. (2017). Neonatal intensive care unit discharge planning. In E. Eichenwald, A. Hansen, C. Martin, & A. Stark (Eds.), *Cloherty and Stark's manual of neonatal care* (8th ed., pp. 215–234). Wolters Kluwer.

- Routine infant care supplies, illness prevention, and introduction to early intervention (EI) services if appropriate (Gardner & Carter, 2021; Reinhart & Gardner, 2017)

▶ PREDISCHARGE SCREENINGS

HEARING

- Preterm infants are at risk of both conductive (problems with transmission of sound to the cochlea)

Box 9.3 Conditions Associated With Increased Risk of Hearing Loss

- NICU admission for >5 days or any of the following regardless of length of stay:
  - ECMO
  - Assisted ventilation
  - Exposure to ototoxic medications
  - Exposure to loop diuretics
  - Hyperbilirubinemia requiring exchange transfusion
- Family history of permanent childhood hearing loss
- In utero infections such as CMV, herpes, rubella, syphilis, and toxoplasmosis
- Craniofacial anomalies, including those that involve the pinna, ear canal, ear tags, ear pits, and temporal bone anomalies
- Physical findings, such as a white forelock, that are associated with a syndrome known to include a sensorineural or permanent conductive hearing loss
- Syndromes associated with progressive or late-onset hearing loss: neurofibromatosis, osteopetrosis, Usher syndrome, Waardenburg syndrome, Alport syndrome, Pendred syndrome, and Jervell and Lange-Neilsen syndrome
- Neurodegenerative disorders
  - Hunter syndrome
  - Sensory motor neuropathies (i.e., Friedreich ataxia and Charcot–Marie–Tooth syndrome)
- Culture-positive postnatal infections associated with sensorineural hearing loss
  - Bacterial
  - Viral (especially herpes and varicella) meningitis
- Head trauma, especially basal skull/temporal bone fractures that require hospitalization

CMV, cytomegalovirus; ECMO, extracorporeal membrane oxygenation.
Sources: Data from Carter, A., & Carter, B. S. (2021). Discharge planning and follow-up of the neonatal intensive care unit infant. In S. Gardner, B. Carter, M. Enzman-Hines, & S. Niermeyer (Eds.), *Merenstein & Gardner's handbook of neonatal intensive care* (9th ed., pp. 1141–1166). Elsevier; Stewart, J. E., Bentley, J., & Knorr, A. (2017). Hearing loss in neonatal intensive care unit graduates. In E. Eichenwald, A. Hansen, C. Martin, & A. Stark (Eds.), *Cloherty and Stark's manual of neonatal care* (8th ed., pp. 983–1068). Wolters Kluwer; Vohr, B. (2020). Hearing loss in the newborn infant. In R. Martin, A. Fanaroff, & M. Walsh (Eds.), *Fanaroff & Martin's neonatal-perinatal medicine: Diseases of the fetus and infant* (11th ed., pp. 1081–1090). Elsevier.

and sensorineural (damage to the inner ear and auditory nerve) hearing loss, as well as auditory processing deficits.
- NICU graduates have an increased risk of developing hearing loss. When undetected, hearing loss can delay language, communication, and cognitive development. This may affect academic achievement, literacy, and social and emotional development (Carter & Carter, 2021; Vohr, 2018, 2020).
- Box 9.3 lists the conditions associated with increased risk of hearing loss.

Types of Hearing Loss
- *Sensorineural hearing loss* occurs secondary to abnormal development or damage to the outer hair cells and

cochlear hair cells or cranial nerve VIII and impairs neuroconduction of sound energy to the brainstem.

- *Conductive hearing loss* occurs when there is interference in the transmission of sound from the external auditory canal to the inner ear.
  - *Permanent conductive hearing loss* occurs when there is an anatomic obstruction of the outer ear (atresia) or middle ear (fusion of ossicles) that blocks transmission of sound.
  - *Transient conductive hearing loss* occurs when debris in the ear canal or fluid in the middle ear blocks the passage of sound waves to the inner ear.
- *Auditory dyssynchrony or auditory neuropathy* accounts for 10% of all infants diagnosed with severe permanent hearing loss. The function of the outer hair cells remains intact; however, a pathology of the inner hair cells or the myelinated fibers of cranial nerve VIII impairs neuroconduction of sound energy to the brainstem. The electric signals to the brain have responses that are dyssynchronous, so information is not relayed in a consistent manner.
  - Risk factors for dyssynchrony include extreme prematurity, severe hyperbilirubinemia, hypoxia, and immune disorders. There is a genetic basis in approximately 40% of all cases.
- *Central hearing loss* occurs due to an abnormal auditory processing at higher levels of the central nervous system, despite an intact auditory canal and inner ear and normal neurosensory pathways.
- *Mixed hearing loss* occurs when there is a combination of sensorineural or neural hearing loss with transient or permanent conductive hearing loss (Vohr, 2018, 2020).

Screening

- The primary objective of universal newborn hearing screening during hospital birth admission is to detect permanent hearing loss as early as possible in order to maximize language, cognitive, literacy, and social development.
- The two currently acceptable methods for physiologic hearing screening in newborns are the auditory brainstem response (ABR) and the evoked otoacoustic emission (EOAE).
  - The ABR evaluates hearing via surface electrodes placed on the scalp which record neural activity in the cochlea, outer and inner hair cells, auditory nerve (VIII), and brainstem to a series of click sounds. It is reliable after 34 weeks' postnatal age.
  - The EOAE evaluates hearing through inserting a probe which contains a microphone into the ear canal. It records the sound produced by the outer hair cells of a normal cochlea. This method is more likely to be affected by debris or fluid in the external and middle ear, resulting in higher referral rates (Carter & Carter, 2021; Stewart et al., 2017; Vohr, 2018, 2020).
- Table 9.1 shows a comparison of physiologic screening methods for newborn hearing loss.

Table 9.1 Comparison of Physiologic Screening Methods for Newborn Hearing Loss

	EOAE	ABR
Method of measurement	Microphone in a probe inserted into the ear canal	Surface electrodes
What the test measures in response to stimulus	Records the sound produced by the outer hair cells of a normal cochlea Stimulus = sound	Record neural activity in the cochlea, outer and inner hair cells, auditory nerve (VIII), and brainstem Stimulus = click
Detects sensorineural hearing loss	Yes	Yes
Detects auditory neuropathy	No	Yes
Detects transient and permanent conductive hearing loss	Yes	Yes
Threshold for fail	30–35 dB HL	40–45 dB HL
Recommended for NICU screening	No	Yes
Recommended for well-baby screening	Yes	Yes

ABR, auditory brainstem response; dB HL, degree of hearing loss in decibels; EOAE, evoked otoacoustic emission.
Sources: Data from Stewart, J. E., Bentley, J., & Knorr, A. (2017). Hearing loss in neonatal intensive care unit graduates. In E. Eichenwald, A. Hansen, C. Martin, & A. Stark (Eds.), *Cloherty and Stark's manual of neonatal care* (8th ed., pp. 983–1008). Wolters Kluwer; Vohr, D. (2020). Hearing loss in the newborn infant. In R. Martin, A. Fanaroff, & M. Walsh (Eds.), *Fanaroff & Martin's neonatal-perinatal medicine: Diseases of the fetus and infant* (11th ed., pp. 1081–1978). Elsevier; Vohr, B. (2018). Ear and hearing disorders. In C. Gleason & S. Juul (Eds.), *Avery's diseases of the newborn* (10th ed., pp. 1558–1566.e2). Elsevier.

Failed Hearing Screens

- Neonatal intensive care infants have higher false positive rates and higher failure rates than well-baby nursery infants.
- Infants who fail their initial screening should be rescreened before 1 month of age. If the infant is "referred" (failed the screening) after this secondary screening, the infant should have a full-scale auditory diagnostic evaluation by 3 months of age.
  - This guideline is consistent with the Joint Committee on Infant Hearing *1-3-6 recommendation* that all infants should be screened for hearing loss no later than 1 month of age, and that infants who do not pass the screen should have a comprehensive evaluation by an audiologist no later than 3 months of age for confirmation of hearing status.

- Infants with confirmed hearing loss should receive appropriate intervention no later than 6 months of age from professionals with expertise in hearing loss and deafness in infants and young children.
- A portion of infants who fail their initial screen are lost to follow-up. Family issues associated with poor follow-up include age of the mother, insurance status, poverty level, lack of family education regarding screening, and geographic variation (Carter & Carter, 2021; Stewart et al., 2017; Vohr, 2018, 2020).
- All families of infants with hearing loss will benefit from a genetic consultation and counseling, as 50% of congenital hearing loss are hereditary.
  - Of genetic hearing loss, 30% are syndromic and 70% nonsyndromic (50% cases linked to a single gene *GJB2*). Patterns may be autosomal recessive, autosomal dominant, or X-linked.
- Every infant with confirmed hearing loss should be evaluated by an otolaryngologist with knowledge of pediatric hearing loss.
- There are varying degrees of stress when parents are informed that their infant has failed an initial hearing screen, with a continuum of increasing stress for families whose infants progress through the screening, diagnosis, and intervention phases of permanent hearing loss.
- Prompt sharing of diagnostic test results with the family and referral to EI services may facilitate the provision of needed information and support to parents to mediate stress.
- Half of the children identified with congenital hearing loss have been in NICU and about 40% of children with permanent hearing loss have other disabilities, causing the potential for both financial as well as emotional stressors. It becomes important for EI case managers and other members of the infant's care team to coordinate various support resources for the family (Vohr, 2020).

VISION

- The American Academy of Pediatrics (AAP) recommends a red reflex examination prior to discharge from the hospital and all subsequent routine health supervision visits (De Alba Campomanes & Binenbaum, 2018).
  - Discussion regarding the implications for a present, absent, or abnormal red reflex is further discussed in Chapter 16.

Retinopathy of Prematurity

- For an in-depth discussion of the physiology and pathophysiology of retinopathy of prematurity (ROP), please see Chapter 16.
- ROP is diagnosed by retinal examination with indirect ophthalmoscopy and should be performed by an ophthalmologist with expertise in ROP screening.

- While direct examination is standard of care, ROP telemedicine, or retinal digital imaging, is a reasonable alternative.
- All infants with a birth weight <1,500 g or gestational age <30 weeks should be screened for ROP.
- Infants who are born after 30 weeks' gestational age or born at 1,500 to 2,000 g may be considered for screening if they have had a medically unstable course (e.g., severe respiratory distress syndrome, hypotension requiring pressor support, or surgery in the first several weeks of life).
- The first examination should occur at 31 weeks' postmenstrual age (PMA) or at chronological age of 4 weeks, whichever occurs later. However, it is recommended to have the first examination before discharge from the hospital.
  - Some recommend infants who are born at <26 weeks' gestation are examined at the postnatal age of 6 to 8 weeks, those born at 27 to 28 weeks at the postnatal age of 5 weeks, those born at 29 to 30 weeks at the postnatal age of 4 weeks, and those >30 weeks at the postnatal age of 3 weeks.
- Long-term follow-up is determined by the degree of ROP. Infants needing laser or cryotherapy for ROP require ongoing assessment of retina, as well as evaluations for refractive errors, strabismus, and amblyopia.
- It is the NICU medical team's clinical and medicolegal responsibility to schedule needed ROP examinations prior to discharge from the NICU, as well as stressing to caregivers the absolute necessity of keeping these appointments postdischarge (Campomanes & Binenbaum, 2018; Carter & Carter, 2021; Crowley & Martin, 2020; De Alba Campomanes & Binenbaum, 2018; Leeman & VanderVeen, 2017; Sun et al., 2020).

▶ FOLLOW-UP CARE

- A comprehensive discharge summary should be completed and given to primary care providers, subspecialty providers, and the infant's caregivers. The summary should include resolved and ongoing problems, completed screening results and future screening needs (including scheduled vision and hearing follow-up), medications, and primary and specialty follow-up appointments (subspecialists, developmental follow-up, EI, etc.; Carter & Carter, 2021; Hummel & Naber, 2020).

GOALS FOR PRIMARY CARE

- Continuum of care after discharge from the NICU
- Family education about the child's development so they are empowered to optimize their child's health, growth, and development

- Prompt diagnosis and recognition of significant medical and neurodevelopmental conditions, prompting appropriate referral to community services to reduce future medical, social, and economic costs
- Anticipation of future needs to avoid or minimize secondary complications so that optimal development is promoted
- Promotion of the child's integration into the family, school, and community
- Table 9.2 lists the timing and expectations for post-NICU follow-up.

Postdischarge Hearing Screenings

- If a family history of hearing loss is reported for an infant who passes the initial hearing screen, ongoing surveillance is indicated, with at least one follow-up audiologic assessment by 24 to 30 months of age.
- Any caregiver concern regarding hearing, speech, language, or developmental delay in the first 2 to 3 years of age should prompt a referral for further hearing evaluation due to association with an increased risk of late-onset or progressive hearing loss not detected in a newborn screen.

- All infants should have an objective standardized screen of global development with a validated screening tool at 9, 18, and 24 to 30 months of age, or at any time the healthcare professional or the family has concerns. Infants who do not pass the speech–language portion of a global screening or for whom there is a concern regarding hearing or language should be referred for speech–language evaluation and audiology assessment (Vohr, 2020).

Postdischarge Vision Screenings

- The neonatal healthcare teams should provide ongoing eye-related education and support, especially toward reducing the risk of pediatric acute head trauma (shaken baby syndrome). This should be discussed with all parents and caregivers.
  - Viewing of educational videos on shaken baby syndrome (if available)
  - Discussion about crying and parental stress during the first few months of age
- The neonatal healthcare team may also provide support for the families of children with visual impairment, ensuring early, anticipatory referral

Table 9.2 Timing and Expectations for Post-NICU Follow-Up Visits and Timing and Focus of Visit by Age

Age	Focus and/or Findings	Developmental Skills	Services
1–3 months	- Adaptation to home - Accuracy of home medications - Oxygen administration - Formula preparation - Parental concerns	- Adjusting to the environment	- Primary care coordinated services - Early intervention and therapies - NICU follow-up
4–6 months	- Inadequate catch-up growth - Identification of severe neurologic abnormality requiring intervention, occupational therapy, and/or physical therapy	- Coordination - Hearing - Vision	
8–12 months	- Identification of suspected or confirmed cerebral palsy or other neurologic abnormality	- Movements - Language - Interaction	
18–24 months	- Most transient neurologic findings resolved - Neurologically abnormal child will show adaptation and improved functional abilities - Potential catch-up growth should have occurred - Administration of BSID-III to provide assessment of cognitive functioning	- Speech - Increased physical ability	
3 years	- Administration of tests to measure cognitive function - Language may be measured	- Language - Thinking	- Primary care coordinated services - School-related services - Special therapy programs
4–5 years	- Measure of subtle neurologic, visuomotor, and behavioral difficulties, which may affect school performance	- Learning - Physical activity	

BSID-III, Bayley Scales of Infant Development.
Sources: Data from Carter, A., & Carter, B. S. (2021). Discharge planning and follow-up of the neonatal intensive care unit infant. In S. Gardner, B. Carter, M. Enzman-Hines, & S. Niermeyer (Eds.), *Merenstein & Gardner's handbook of neonatal intensive care* (9th ed., pp. 1141–1166). Elsevier; Demauro, S. B., & Hintz, S. R. (2018). Risk assessment and neurodevelopmental outcomes. In C. Gleason & S. Juul (Eds.), *Avery's diseases of the newborn* (10th ed., pp. 971–990. e7). Elsevier; Wilson-Costello, D. & Payne, A. (2020b). The outcome of neonatal intensive care. In A. Fanaroff & J. Fanaroff (Eds.), *Klaus and Fanaroff's care of the high-risk neonate* (7th ed., pp. 437–446). Elsevier; Wilson-Costello, D. E., & Payne, A. H. (2020a). Early childhood neurodevelopmental outcomes of high-risk neonates. In R. Martin, A. Fanaroff, & M. Walsh (Eds.), *Fanaroff & Martin's neonatal-perinatal medicine: Diseases of the fetus and infant* (11th ed., pp. 1090–1109). Elsevier.

to state commissions for the blind, EI services, and ongoing encouragement for parents to maximally utilize such resources when they are available.

■ Children should have an eye examination at every well-child visit. Primary care eye examinations and vision assessments continue to be vital for the detection of conditions that may result in visual impairment or blindness, lead to problems with school or social performance, signal the presence of a serious systemic disease, or threaten the child's life (De Alba Campomanes & Binenbaum, 2018; Hummel & Naber, 2021; Örge & Grigorian, 2020,).

Immunizations

■ The AAP recommends that all preterm infants receive routine immunizations at their chronological age (i.e., birth date), rather than their corrected age.

■ Influenza immunization is recommended yearly for children and caregivers. Infants should be more than 6 months old, and two doses are given in the fall, usually 1 month apart.

■ Respiratory syncytial virus (RSV) prophylaxis, palivizumab (Synagis), is recommended by the AAP for all high-risk infants and young children.
  ● Criteria for RSV prophylaxis have not changed since 2014 and include but are not limited to:
    ❏ Infants born before 29 0/7 weeks' gestation
    ❏ Infants born before 32 0/7 weeks' gestation with chronic lung disease
    ❏ Infants with a persistent need for respiratory medical intervention into the second year of age
    ❏ Other infants with compromised cardiopulmonary, neuromuscular, or respiratory system

■ Shots should begin before discharge into the community setting during the RSV season. These shots are administered monthly from November through March (Carter & Carter, 2021; Demauro & Hintz, 2018; Hummel & Naber, 2021).

Growth and Nutrition

■ Many extremely low birth weight (ELBW), very low birth weight (VLBW), and intrauterine growth restriction (IUGR) infants experience delayed growth and require catch-up after discharge.
  ● *Postnatal growth failure* or *extrauterine growth restriction* is a weight less than the 10th percentile for corrected gestational age (CGA).

■ Optimal growth after discharge is a good measure of physical, neurologic, and environmental well-being.

■ Catch-up of head circumference occurs only during the first 6 to 12 months after the expected date of delivery.

■ Specialized feedings for the first 6 to 9 months postdischarge are needed in infants with ongoing and catch-up requirements not met by term infant formulas.

● Increased calorie postdischarge formulas with increased protein, minerals, and long-chain polyunsaturated fatty acids

● Continued fortification of breast milk or exclusive breast milk feedings, with two to three bottles per day of increased calorie postdischarge formulas

■ Vitamin and iron supplementation:
  ● *Vitamin D:* 400 IU/d is the minimal requirement, which may be achieved by a combination of formula and/or supplement
  ● *Iron:* 2 to 4 mg/kg/d, which may be achieved by a combination of formula and/or supplement, to start at 1 month of age and continue to 12 months (Abrams & Tiosano, 2020; Poindexter & Martin, 2020)

NEUROSENSORY AND DEVELOPMENTAL ASSESSMENT

Correction for Gestational Age

■ Noting the age when an infant achieves milestones, such as gross-motor, fine-motor, language, and adaptive skills, helps determine if delays are present. However, controversy exists regarding the need to correct for degrees of prematurity, that is, whether to use the child's chronological age or to use the corrected age for degree of prematurity.
  ● Corrected age is the chronological age minus the number of weeks born before 40 weeks' gestation and is the preferred term to describe the age of preterm infants after the perinatal period. It is expressed in weeks or months.

■ The best evidence supports the use of correction for prematurity. By convention, most healthcare providers correct through 2 years of age, although reports exist describing the use of correction until 3 years of age.

■ For the extremely low gestational age newborn (ELGAN) infant, those born at 23 to 25 weeks, some literature suggests continued correction through 5 years of age. Although no overall consensus exists, whatever standard is set should be followed consistently by all team members involved in the infant's care (Carter & Carter, 2021; Demauro & Hintz, 2018; Gomella, 2020; Stewart et al., 2017; Wilson-Costello & Payne, 2020b).

Definition of Terms

■ *Neurodevelopmental handicap* has been defined in children who have a neurologic abnormality or a developmental quotient or IQ of less than 70 or 80, depending on the researcher. Children with an IQ of 70 to 85 are considered to have borderline intelligence rather than a classification of cognitive impairment. The World Health Organization (WHO) categorizes the effect a child's handicap/disability has on their ability to function physically and socially within their home and community (International Classification of Functioning, Disability and Health [ICF]).

- *Neurologic abnormality* is usually classified by neurologic diagnosis, which can include hypotonia or hypertonia, cerebral palsy (CP; spastic diplegia or quadriplegia), hydrocephalus, blindness, or deafness.
- *Developmental delay* is used to describe a deficit in any one of the five development domains: cognition, motor, language, adaptive, and social–emotional skills.
- *Global developmental delay* is used to define deficits in two or more areas of development, with scores of more than 2 *SD* below the referenced standards.
- Neurologic examination during infancy is best based on changes in muscle tone that occur within the first year. A detailed, structured neurologic examination as early as full-term corrected age in high-risk infants is highly correlated with neuromotor outcomes at least until 1 year of age.
- The scale developed by Claudine Amiel-Tison provides a qualitative method to assess neurologic integrity, which leads to the categorization of *normal, suspect,* or *abnormal* during the first year after term.
  - It measures the decrease in passive muscle tone (head control, back support, sitting, standing, and walking) contrasted with the progressive increase in active muscle tone that occur together during infancy. It also documents visual and auditory responses and some primitive reflexes (Carter & Carter, 2021; Demauro & Hintz, 2018; Wilson-Costello & Payne, 2020a, 2020b).

DEVELOPMENTAL ASSESSMENT

- The Bayley Scales of Infant Development is the most commonly used tool for monitoring early cognitive and motor development in high-risk infants.
  - The 2006 (newest) version contains five scales: cognitive, language, motor, social–emotional, and adaptive behavior, the latter two in the form of parent questionnaires. This edition of the Bayley Scales does not generate a "mental developmental index," but rather separates cognitive and language scores (Wilson-Costello & Payne, 2020a).
- Multiple tools are available to use for developmental assessment of both the infant and the child. Examples are listed in Table 9.3.

Early Intervention

- Complex disorders of brain development increase with decreasing birth weight and gestational age. Early identification of infants at high risk allows for timely referrals to EI therapies.
  - EI has been shown to improve neurobehavioral development with improved cognitive outcomes and parent–child interactions.

- Referral can be made by the neonatal medical team at the time of NICU discharge, the primary care provider, follow-up clinic specialists, or by the family itself.
- Each child receives a multidisciplinary assessment and service coordinator. Based on the child's assessment, various services with various focus intensities may include occupational therapy, physical therapy, speech therapy, audiology services, vision services, family education with focus on infant growth and development, family counseling, social work services, and transportation for therapies outside the home.
  - *Individuals With Disabilities Education Act* is a federal mandate that each state provides services up to 3 years of age for children with developmental delays or conditions that lead to developmental delay. Each state establishes criteria for referral to EI and services provided within the parameters set by the government (Carter & Carter, 2021; Hummel & Naber, 2021; Wilson-Costello & Payne, 2020a).

▶ OUTCOMES

SCHOOL-AGE OUTCOMES

- Infants who have severe cognitive, motor, or neurosensory impairments in early years (2–3 years of age) are nearly always found to have moderate or severe impairments at school age.
- Few studies have compared school-age outcomes among premature infants over time. Most of the school-age outcome studies of very premature children have compared these survivors with children of normal birth weight. Findings demonstrate former preterm infants have neurologic dysfunction, lower intelligence, and poorer performance on tests of language and academic achievement.
  - These lower scores may be related to difficulties with memory, visuomotor, and fine and gross motor function, and spatial concepts and executive function.
  - Deficits include mild cognitive impairment (IQ 1–2 *SD* below the mean or 70–84); learning, emotional, behavior, motor coordination, and executive function disorders; and poor academic achievement. The most immature infants have the highest risk for poor cognitive outcome.
  - Although most children with VLBW remain in the regular school system, many have difficulty coping with the demands of classroom learning and require individualized education and remedial resources.
- Children with social advantages (two-parent household, educated parents, employed parents) demonstrate more cognitive gains through early childhood than those without social advantages (Demauro & Hintz, 2018; Wilson-Costello & Payne, 2020a).

Table 9.3 Psychomotor and Cognitive Assessment Tools

Test	Age Range	Components	IQ	Most Popular

BSID-III (2006)	1–42 months (first administer at 8–12 months)	■ Cognitive composite score
		■ Language composite score
		  ● Receptive
		  ● Expressive
		■ Motor composite score
		  ● Gross
		  ● Fine
		■ Social–emotional score (per parent report)
		■ Adaptive behavior score (per parent report)
			No	x

Griffiths-III (2016)	2 versions: 0–2 years and 2–8 years		No	
Ages and Stages Questionnaire	3 months to 5 years	■ Qualitative only; parents provide information about child development	No	
WPPSI-IV (2012)	2 years 6 months to 7 years 7 months	■ Verbal, performance, and full-scale scores with means of 100	Yes	x
WISC-V (2014)	6 years 0 months to 16 years 11 months	■ Verbal, performance, and full-scale scores with means of 100	Yes	
WIAT-III (2009)	4 years 0 months to 50 years 11 months	■ Identifies academic strengths and weaknesses ■ Used in clinical, research, and educational settings	Yes	
DAS-III (2007)	2 years 6 months to 17 years 11 months		Yes	
Stanford–Binet Intelligence Scale (2003)	2 years to elementary school years	■ Measure of intelligence highly correlated with school performance	Yes	
K-ABC II (2004)	3 years to 10 years	■ Subscales to assess various components of intelligence	Yes	

BSID-III, Bayley Scales of Infant Development; DAS-III, Differential Ability Scales; K-ABC II, Kaufman Assessment Battery for Children; WIAT-III, Wechsler Individual Achievement Test; WISC-V, Wechsler Intelligence Scale for Children; WPPSI-IV, Wechsler Preschool and Primary Scale of Intelligence.
Sources: Data from Carter, A., & Carter, B. S. (2021). Discharge planning and follow-up of the neonatal intensive care unit infant. In S. Gardner, B. Carter, M. Enzman-Hines, & S. Niermeyer (Eds.), *Merenstein & Gardner's handbook of neonatal intensive care* (9th ed., pp. 1141–1166). Elsevier; Demauro, S. B., & Hintz, S. R. (2018). Risk assessment and neurodevelopmental outcomes. In C. Gleason & S. Juul (Eds.), *Avery's diseases of the newborn* (10th ed., pp. 971–990. e7). Elsevier; Wilson-Costello, D., & Payne, A. (2020b) The outcome of neonatal intensive care. In A. Fanaroff & J. Fanaroff (Eds.), *Klaus and Fanaroff's care of the high-risk neonate* (7th ed., pp. 437–446). Elsevier; Wilson-Costello, D. E., & Payne, A. H. (2020a). Early childhood neurodevelopmental outcomes of high-risk neonates. In R. Martin, A. Fanaroff, & M. Walsh (Eds.), *Fanaroff & Martin's neonatal-perinatal medicine: Diseases of the fetus and infant* (11th ed., pp. 1091–1109). Elsevier.

Behavioral Problems

■ The most commonly reported childhood behavioral problems of prematurity are disorders of attention and hyperactivity, emotional difficulties, and socialization issues. Rates of attention deficit hyperactivity disorder (ADHD) range from 20% to 30% for preterm children versus 5% to 10% for term-born children. Neurobehavioral or psychiatric problems, including autism spectrum disorders (ASDs), are reported with higher frequency in school-age, former preterm children than in the general population.

■ Internalizing problems, such as depression, anxiety, and poor adaptive skills, have all been associated with prematurity, resulting in socialization and peer relationship difficulties. Internalizing symptoms manifest as shyness, social maladaptation, anxiety, and withdrawn behavior.

● Furthermore, motor delays due to prematurity may compromise playground skills, causing peer victimization and rejection (Demauro & Hintz, 2018; Wilson-Costello & Payne, 2020b; Wilson-Costello & Payne, 2020a).

■ Table 9.4 identifies school-age outcomes related to prematurity.

Table 9.4 School-Age Outcomes of Prematurity Neurodevelopmental Impairment

Cognitive	Motor	Sensory	Behavioral	Other

■ Cognitive delay
  ● Most common NDI in children born prematurely
■ Global developmental delay
■ Learning disabilities
  ● Variable cognitive abilities
	■ CP
	■ DCD
	  ● Fine motor incoordination
	  ● Sensorimotor integration problems
		■ Hearing impairment
		■ Visual impairment
			■ ADHD
			■ ASD
			■ Internalizing symptoms
			  ● Shyness
			  ● Depression
			  ● Anxiety
			  ● Poor adaptive skills
				■ Language delay
				  ● Receptive and expressive language
				  ● Visual–perceptual problems
				■ Executive functioning problems

ADHD, attention deficit hyperactivity disorder; ASD, autism spectrum disorder; CP, cerebral palsy; DCD, developmental coordination disorder; NDI, neurodevelopmental impairment.

Sources: Data from Carter, A., & Carter, B. S. (2021). Discharge planning and follow-up of the neonatal intensive care unit infant. In S. Gardner, B. Carter, M. Enzman-Hines, & S. Niermeyer (Eds.), *Merenstein & Gardner's handbook of neonatal intensive care* (9th ed., pp. 1141–1166). Elsevier; Demauro, S. B., & Hintz, S. R. (2018). Risk assessment and neurodevelopmental outcomes. In C. Gleason & S. Juul (Eds.), *Avery's diseases of the newborn* (10th ed., pp. 971–990. e7). Elsevier; Wilson-Costello, D., & Payne, A. (2020). The outcome of neonatal intensive care. In A. Fanaroff & J. Fanaroff (Eds.), *Klaus and Fanaroff's care of the high-risk neonate* (7th ed., pp. 437–446). Elsevier; Hummel, P., & Naber, M. (2020). Discharge planning and transition to home. In M. T. Verklan, M. Walden, & S. Forest (Eds.), *Core curriculum for neonatal intensive care nursing* (6th ed., pp. 329–345). Elsevier; Stewart, J. E., Bentley, J., & Knorr, A. (2017). Hearing loss in neonatal intensive care unit graduates. In E. Eichenwald, A. Hansen, C. Martin, & A. Stark (Eds.), *Cloherty and Stark's manual of neonatal care* (8th ed., pp. 983–1068). Wolters Kluwer; Wilson-Costello, D. E., & Payne, A. H. (2020). Early childhood neurodevelopmental outcomes of high-risk neonates. In R. Martin, A. Fanaroff, & M. Walsh (Eds.), *Fanaroff & Martin's neonatal-perinatal medicine: Diseases of the fetus and infant* (11th ed., pp. 1091–1109). Elsevier.

YOUNG ADULT OUTCOMES

■ Overall, results suggest that neurodevelopmental and growth sequelae of prematurity persist into young adulthood. Traditionally, educational attainment, employment, independent living, marriage, and parenthood have been considered as markers of successful transition to adulthood.
- When compared with controls of normal birth weight, young adults with VLBW have poorer educational achievement. Preterm infants as adults have significantly lower income and are less likely to get married and become parents.

■ Even in adults without neurosensory or cognitive impairment, impairments in learning or executive function may interfere with educational and vocational achievement. Executive function refers to a collection of processes that are responsible for purposeful, goal-directed behavior, such as planning, setting goals, initiating, using problem-solving strategies, and monitoring thoughts and behavior. Executive function deficits primarily involve impairments in response inhibition and mental flexibility.

■ Adolescents and young adults who were born preterm are found to show deficits in executive function on tasks of verbal fluency, inhibition, cognitive flexibility, planning and organization, and working memory, as well as verbal and visuospatial memory. These individuals may have lower IQ on formal testing and fewer attend college than normal birth weight, term-born controls.

■ Medical sequelae of prematurity include chronic illnesses such as asthma or CP, and less physical activity, which impact on respiratory, cardiovascular, and renal function. There is a higher incidence of hypertension, visceral obesity, asthma, neurodevelopmental problems, and perturbations in glucose–insulin homeostasis. Surviving ELBW infants are far more likely to have CP, blindness, and deafness compared with term-born matched controls.
- Overall, 23 to 27 weeks' gestation-born adults are 7.5 times more likely to have a medical disability affecting their ability to work, as compared with term-born adults.
- In adulthood, preterm survivors are more likely to receive disability pensions than term-born controls (Demauro & Hintz, 2018; Wilson-Costello & Payne, 2020a).

▶ CONCLUSION

A stay in the NICU is but a short time frame of a preterm or ill infant's life experience. Infants are not "healed" upon leaving the NICU; on the contrary, the effects of their initial condition and the care they received in the NICU can have lifelong implications. It is because of these implications that preparing the infant and family for discharge is important and impactful toward the successful transition to home and a stable family unit. Family involvement, planning, and coordination are all crucial to the safe transition home and the ongoing well-being of the infant and the family.

1. National recommendations state that all preterm infants receive routine immunizations at their:

   A. Chronological age
   B. Corrected age
   C. Postmenstrual age

2. The type of hearing loss which accounts for a large portion of infants diagnosed with permanent hearing loss is:

   A. Auditory dyssynchrony
   B. Conductive hearing loss
   C. Sensorineural hearing loss

3. When compared with the evoked optoacoustic emissions (EOAE) auditory test, the auditory brainstem response (ABR):

   A. Is affected by debris in the canal
   B. Uses a microphone in the ear
   C. Uses surface electrodes on the scalp

4. The neonatal nurse practitioner (NNP) is arranging follow-up appointments for a patient who was born at 35 weeks' gestation and had a complex hospital course including surgical intervention for a bowel perforation. With regard to the need for a screening exam for retinopathy of prematurity (ROP), the NNP recognizes an exam is necessary:

   A. As an outpatient in 3 weeks
   B. Following 6 months of age
   C. Within 2 days prior to discharge

5. An infant born at 25 weeks' gestation is going home on a preterm formula and the mother wants to know how long they should feed the infant the preterm formula. The neonatal nurse practitioner (NNP) answers based on the knowledge that extremely low gestation age newborn (ELGAN) neonates require preterm formula for at least:

   A. 3 to 5 months
   B. 6 to 9 months
   C. 12 to 15 months

1. A) Chronological age

The American Academy of Pediatrics (AAP) recommends that all preterm infants receive routine immunizations at their chronological age, rather than their corrected age. Immunizations may be significantly delayed if not given until the corrected or postmenstrual age (Blackburn, 2018; Demauro & Hintz, 2018; Smith & Andrews, 2017; Stewart et al., 2017)

2. A) Auditory dyssynchrony

Auditory dyssynchrony or auditory neuropathy accounts for 10% of all infants diagnosed with severe permanent hearing loss. The function of the outer hair cells remains intact; however, a pathology of the inner hair cells or the myelinated fibers of cranial nerve VIII impairs neuroconduction of sound energy to the brainstem. The electric signals to the brain have responses that are dyssynchronous, so information is not relayed in a consistent manner. Conductive hearing loss stems from deformities in the small bones of the ear. Sensorineural hearing loss occurs as a result of damage to the structures or auditory nerve (Stewart et al., 2017; Vohr, 2018, 2020).

3. C) Uses surface electrodes on the scalp

The ABR uses surface electrodes to record neural activity in the auditory nerve (VIII) and brainstem to detect auditory neuropathy. The EOAE records sounds produced by the outer hair cells of a normal cochlea via a microphone. This method is affected by debris or fluid in the ear canal (Stewart et al., 2017; Vohr, 2018, 2020).

4. A) As an outpatient in 3 weeks

Infants who are born after 30 weeks' gestational age or born at 1,500 to 2,000 g may be considered for screening if they have had a medically unstable course (e.g., severe respiratory distress syndrome, hypotension requiring pressor support, or surgery in the first several weeks of age). Some recommend infants who are born at >30 weeks are screened at the postnatal age of 3 weeks. Exams prior to this time may be inconclusive due to clearing of the vitreous fluids, and disease processes may develop unchecked if an exam is delayed months (Carter & Carter, 2021; De Alba Campomanes & Binenbaum, 2018; Leeman & VanderVeen, 2017; Martin & Crowley, 2020; Sun et al., 2020).

5. B) 6 to 9 months

Specialized feedings for the first 6 to 9 months postdischarge are needed in infants with ongoing and catch-up requirements not met by term infant formulas. Increased calorie postdischarge formulas with increased protein, minerals, and long-chain polyunsaturated fatty acids are necessary to aid catch-up growth. Growth may not be achieved in less than 5 months. The use may extend to 12 months, but the infant should receive for at least 6 months (Abrams, 2017; Adamkin & Radmacher, 2020; Anderson et al., 2017; Carter & Carter, 2021; Colaizy et al., 2018; Demauro & Hintz, 2018; Poindexter & Martin, 2020; Stark et al., 2017; Stewart et al., 2017; Wilson-Costello & Payne, 2020b).

Thermoregulation

Amy R. Koehn

▶ INTRODUCTION

Thermoregulation is the foundation of neonatal care. Neonates, specifically the very low birth weight (VLBW) infant, are challenged from birth to interact and function within an environment that is starkly different from that of the protective womb; this is both physiologically and developmentally taxing. Years of research have culminated in a body of knowledge and advanced technology dedicated to thermoregulation. The importance of temperature regulation has been supported by the recommendations of the World Health Organization (WHO) and the Neonatal Resuscitation Program and by the practice guidelines of the Golden Hour protocol. NICU clinicians must make use of available equipment appropriately in order to avoid or minimize thermal irregularities. Clinician interventions, or lack thereof, provided in the delivery suite and daily in the NICU can have lasting effects on neonatal development. This chapter discusses the principles, both physiologic and pathophysiologic, of thermoregulation and interventions to minimize heat loss, and provides a brief overview of the utilization of equipment to assist in the maintenance of a neutral thermal environment (NTE).

▶ PRINCIPLES OF THERMOREGULATION

- Neonatal hypothermia after delivery is a worldwide issue, occurring in all climates. Thermal management of the newborn during the first few hours of life is critical to prevent the detrimental effects of cold stress and hypothermia. Adverse consequences associated with cold stress remain an important contributor to neonatal mortality and morbidity, and the potential impact of optimal thermal care provision on infant health is huge. Even modest long-term exposure to cold will increase thermogenesis, consume oxygen and substrate stores, and impact negatively on growth (Agren, 2020; Brand & Shippey, 2021; Chatson, 2017; Fraser, 2021).
- These risks have prompted organizations such as the Neonatal Resuscitation Program and WHO to stress the importance of normal body temperatures in the delivery room and preventing early postnatal hypothermia (Hodson, 2018).

- The neonate is most vulnerable to heat loss during the first minutes following birth. The primary challenge in thermal management of newborns is the prevention of hypothermia because the neonate is expected to transition from a warm, moist environment to a much colder, drier environment. The newborn's ability to maintain temperature control after birth is determined by external environmental factors and internal physiologic processes (Brand & Shippey, 2021; Fraser, 2021; Hodson, 2018).
- The infant's core temperature decreases rapidly, owing mainly to evaporation from their moist body. These losses may result in a fall of 2°C to 3°C within the first 30 to 60 minutes after birth if the newborn is extremely premature or no wrapping, drying, or clothing is applied in a larger newborn. In addition to evaporative losses from amniotic fluid, losses to cooler room air and cooler structures in the room such as walls also result in large radiant and convective heat losses (Brand & Shippey, 2021; Hodson, 2018).

PHYSIOLOGY OF THERMOREGULATION

- *Thermoregulation* is defined as the means by which the neonate's body temperature is maintained by balancing heat generation and heat loss in a changing environment. It is a critical component in the physiologic adaptation to extrauterine life (Cheffer & Rannalli, 2016).
- The exposure to cold, clamping of the umbilical cord, and the general "stress of being born" induce a thermal response. This response is part of a homeostatic system with input (detectors) and output (effectors) that is aimed at preserving body temperature. Thermal receptors in the skin affect the infant's response to cold stimuli. The most prominent and sensitive skin receptors are in the trigeminal area of the face (Agren, 2020; Brand & Shippey, 2021).
- If environmental cooling exceeds the infant's thermoregulatory response of energy output, the core temperature will drop along with a decrease in oxygen consumption. This "Q10 effect" of decreased metabolism when the environmental temperature falls below a critical point is the basis for the use of

induced hypothermia in other clinical situations. The increase in oxygen consumption and the increase in metabolic output are considered important contributors to increased morbidity and mortality especially in extremely low birth weight (ELBW) infants (Hodson, 2018).

ASSESSING TEMPERATURE IN THE NEONATE

■ The neonate's temperature at birth will be reflective of the intrauterine temperature. If the mother has a fever, it is common for the neonate's temperature to be elevated. It is important to distinguish between environmental, iatrogenic, and infectious causes of elevations in neonatal temperatures (Brand & Shippey, 2021).

■ The optimal temperature for a specific infant cannot be defined by a single central temperature; rather, it is defined by the range of measurable skin temperatures that are associated with minimal heat production. This implies an optimal central or core temperature. The control range refers to the range of environmental temperatures at which body temperature can be kept constant (Hodson, 2018).

■ Early detection and management of hypothermia and hyperthermia is essential to the well-being of neonates. Frequent temperature measurements and observation are key to early detection until the infant's temperature is stable. A drop in skin temperature may be the first sign of hypothermia. The core temperature may not fall until the infant can no longer compensate (Brand & Shippey, 2021; Gardner & Cammack, 2021).

■ In critically ill infants, the skin temperature is usually routinely monitored in addition to axillary temperature readings. A skin probe is secured to the right upper quadrant of the abdomen. The temperature probe should not be placed under the axilla or any other position except as recommended by the manufacturer (Gardner & Cammack, 2021).

■ The use of low-reading thermometers (from 29.4°C/85°F) is recommended because temperature readings <34.4°C (94.0°F) can go undetected with routine thermometers (Chatson, 2017).

■ Rectal temperatures should not be used due to the risk of intestinal perforation and because the core temperature may not decrease until the neonate has totally decompensated (Brand & Shippey, 2021; Gardner & Cammack, 2021).

GOALS FOR ENVIRONMENTAL AND NEONATAL TEMPERATURES

■ The *control range* refers to the range of environmental temperatures at which body temperature can be kept constant by means of regulation. The environmental range of the infant is more limited than that of the adult because of less insulation. The control range for an adult is 0°C (32°F), but for the full-term infant it is 20°C to 23°C (68°F–73.4°F; Blackburn, 2018).

■ For the healthy term infant, standard thermal care guidelines include maintaining the delivery room temperature at 25°C (72°F).
  ● The chilled environment of the surgical suite poses extra challenges to the newborn for thermoregulation. Coordination between neonatal and surgical staff is necessary to prevent heat loss during transport to and while in the surgical suite (Chatson, 2017; Gardner & Cammack, 2021).

■ WHO advocated a 10-step "warm chain," which includes the following elements: environmental modification such as warming the delivery room and examination or transport areas; skin-to-skin holding, mother–baby care, and breastfeeding; delayed bathing and weighing; immediate drying and clothing/blanketing; and adequate staff training in the recognition and management of cold stress (Shaw-Battista & Gardner, 2017).

■ Axillary temperatures are commonly used as they are easy to obtain, are minimally invasive, and correlate well with core temperature. When taken properly, axillary temperatures provide readings as accurate as the rectal and core temperature methods (Brand & Shippey, 2021; Gardner & Cammack, 2021; Hardy et al., 2016). Recommended neonatal temperature ranges are presented in Table 10.1.

NEONATES AT RISK

■ The neonate born before 28 weeks' gestation presents a major challenge in the prevention of heat loss. Hypothermia is reported to occur in most ELBW neonates on their admission to NICU and is especially hard to prevent in neonates born at less than 25 weeks' gestation (Hodson, 2018).

■ Infants at high risk for hypothermia at delivery are listed in Box 10.1.

Table 10.1 Recommended Neonatal Temperatures

Infant	Recommended Temperature Range
Full term	36.5°C–37.5°C (97.7°F–99.5°F)
Preterm	35.6°C–37.3°C (96.0°F–99°F) OR 36.3°C and 36.9°C (97.3°F and 98.4°F)
VLBW	36.7°C–37.3°C (98.0°F–99.0°F)

VLBW, very low birth weight.
Sources: Data from Brand, M. C., & Shippey, A. A. (2021). Thermoregulation. In M. T. Verklan, M. Walden, & S. Forest (Eds.), *Core curriculum for neonatal intensive care nursing* (6th ed. pp. 86–98). Elsevier; Gardner, S. L. & Cammack, B. H. (2021). Heat balance. In S. L. Gardner, B. S. Carter, M. Enzman-Hines, & S. Niermeyer (Eds.), *Merenstein & Gardner's handbook of neonatal intensive care nursing: An interprofessional approach* (9th ed., pp. 137–164). Elsevier; Hodson, A. (2018). Temperature regulation. In C. Gleason & S. Juul (Eds.), *Avery's diseases of the newborn* (10th ed., pp. 361–367). Elsevier.

Box 10.1 Infants at Greatest Risk for Hypothermia

- Less than 28 weeks' gestation
- Birth weight less than 1,500 g
- Intrauterine growth restriction
- Affected by maternal sedation
- Neurologic complications (e.g., asphyxia)
- Abdominal wall, neural tube, or other open skin defects

Sources: Data from Brand, M. C., & Shippey, A. A. (2021). Thermoregulation. In M. T. Verklan, M. Walden, & S. Forest (Eds.), *Core curriculum for neonatal intensive care nursing* (6th ed., pp. 86–98). Elsevier; Chatson, K. (2017). Temperature control. In E. Eichenwald, A. Hansen, C. Martin, & A. Stark (Eds.), *Cloherty and Stark's manual of neonatal care* (8th ed., pp. 185–191). Wolters Kluwer; Hodson, A. (2018). Temperatures regulation. In C. Gleason & S. Juul (Eds.), *Avery's diseases of the newborn* (10th ed., pp. 361–367). Elsevier.

- Neonatal physiology plays a significant role in the rapid development of hypothermia and hyperthermia. The physiologic characteristics of the neonate that lend to thermal irregularities are listed in Box 10.2.

COLD STRESS

- When heat loss is greater than the infant's ability to conserve and produce heat, the newborn is no longer in thermal neutrality; in such a case, the body temperature drops and the newborn is cold-stressed and becomes hypothermic.
  - Hypothermia in a newborn is defined as body temperature below 36.3°C to 36.5°C (97.3°F–97.7°F), measured as an axillary temperature (Agren, 2020; Brand & Shippey, 2021; Gardner & Cammack, 2021; Shaw-Battista & Gardner, 2017).
- WHO developed a classification system to underscore the importance of intervention. Three levels are defined in Table 10.2.
- Consequences of cold stress include a cycle of peripheral vasoconstriction, increased oxygen and glucose consumption, depletion of glycogen, pulmonary vasoconstriction, hypoglycemia, hypoxia, anaerobic metabolism, and metabolic acidosis (Chatson, 2017; Shaw-Battista & Gardner, 2017).
- VLBW infants' limited ability to produce heat, their increased evaporative water loss at birth secondary to extremely thin skin, as well as their small heat capacity (the result of their large surface-to-volume ratio) make them unusually susceptible to cold stress.
- After the immediate newborn period, the more common and chronic problem facing premature infants than actual hypothermia is caloric loss from unrecognized chronic cold stress that results in excess oxygen consumption and slow weight gain (Chatson, 2017).

Box 10.2 Physiologic Reasons for Hypothermia in Neonates

- The infant has a small amount or veritable absence of subcutaneous fat for insulation, along with decreased levels of brown fats and decreased glycogen stores. Thermoregulation in neonates is affected by the type and amount of accumulated fat, which in turn is affected by both gestational age and birth weight.
- Neonates also have a large surface area-to-mass ratio compared with adults. Even healthy term newborns are at risk of heat loss due to their relatively large body surface area.
- In term neonates, the surface area-to-body mass ratio is three times greater than that of an adult.
- There is a lower capacity for heat storage because of the higher temperature of the body shell in relation to the environment and the larger surface-to-volume ratio.
- Preterm infants often have poor vasoconstrictor control.
- The hypothalamus, which regulates temperature, is immature.
- Neonates have decreased spontaneous muscle activity and poorly developed shivering thermogenesis. Term newborns have the ability to maintain this flexed posture, whereas preterm and compromised newborns may lack the muscle tone for this posturing, making them more vulnerable to cold stress.
- There are increased evaporative losses and transepidermal insensible water loss due to their thin permeable skin, allowing water to evaporate from the skin surface. Heat lost by evaporation is known as *TEWL*.

TEWL, transepidermal water loss.
Sources: Data from Brand, M. C., & Shippey, A. A. (2021). Thermoregulation. In M. T. Verklan, M. Walden, & S. Forest (Eds.), *Core curriculum for neonatal intensive care nursing* (6th ed., pp. 86–98). Elsevier, Inc.; Chatson, K. (2017). Temperature control. In E. Eichenwald, A. Hansen, C. Martin, & A. Stark (Eds.), *Cloherty and Stark's manual of neonatal care* (8th ed., pp. 185–191). Wolters Kluwer; Fraser, D. (2021). Newborn adaptation to extrauterine life. In K. Simpson & P. Creehan, N. O'Brien-Able, C. Roth, & A. J. Rohan. (Eds.), *Awhonn's perinatal nursing* (5th ed., pp. 564–578). Wolters Kluwer/Lippincott Williams & Wilkins; Hodson, A. (2018). Temperature regulation. In C. Gleason & S. Juul (Eds.), *Avery's diseases of the newborn* (10th ed., pp. 361–367). Elsevier; Shaw-Battista, J., & Gardner, S. (2017). Newborn transition: The journey from fetal to extrauterine life. In B. J. Snell & S. Gardner (Eds.), *Care of the well newborn* (pp. 69–100). Jones & Bartlett Learning.

Table 10.2 The World Health Organization's Classification of Hypothermia

Cold stress or mild hypothermia	Temperature of 36.0°C–36.4°C
Moderate hypothermia	Temperature of 32.0°C–35.9°C
Severe hypothermia	Temperature below 32°C

Sources: Data from Brand, M. C., & Shippey, A. A. (2021). Thermoregulation. In M. T. Verklan, M. Walden, & S. Forest (Eds.), *Core curriculum for neonatal intensive care nursing* (6th ed. pp. 86–98). Elsevier; Hodson, A. (2018). Temperature regulation. In C. Gleason & S. Juul (Eds.), *Avery's diseases of the newborn* (10th ed., pp. 361–367). Elsevier.

NEONATAL COLD INJURY

- This is a rare, extreme form of hypothermia that may be seen in low birth weight (LBW) infants and term infants with central nervous system (CNS) disorders. Core temperature can fall below 32.2°C (90°F) and infants may have a bright red color due to failure of oxyhemoglobin to dissociate at low temperature. They may also have central pallor or cyanosis. The skin may show edema and sclerema, and occasionally there is generalized bleeding, including pulmonary hemorrhage (Chatson, 2017).

REWARMING TECHNIQUES

- It is controversial whether warming should be rapid or slow, but it is established that rewarming too rapidly may further compromise the already cold-stressed infant and result in apnea. Setting the abdominal skin temperature to 1°C higher than the core temperature or setting it to 36.5°C on a radiant warmer will produce slow rewarming. Another practice is to set the difference between the skin and the ambient air temperature at less than 1.5°C (2.7°F), which results in minimal oxygen consumption. Efforts to block heat loss by convection, radiation, evaporation, and conduction should be initiated (Chatson, 2017; Gardner & Cammack, 2021).
- If hypothermia is mild, slow rewarming is preferred. External heat sources should be slightly warmer than the skin temperature and gradually increased until the NTE temperature range is attained.
- For more extreme hypothermia (i.e., core temperatures less than 35°C [95°F]), a more rapid rewarming with radiant heaters (servo control 37°C [98.6°F]) or heated water mattresses prevents prolonged metabolic acidosis or hypoglycemia and decreases mortality risk.
- Skin, axillary, and environmental temperatures should be measured and recorded every 30 minutes during the rewarming period. During the rewarming process, the hypothermic infant should be observed for hypotension as vasodilation occurs (Gardner & Cammack, 2021).

▶ MECHANISMS OF HEAT PRODUCTION

- After birth, newborns must adapt to their relatively cold environment through the metabolic production of heat because they are not able to generate an adequate shivering response (Chatson, 2017).
- Oxidative glucose, fat, and protein metabolism; nonshivering thermogenesis (NST) of brown fat; and muscle activity are all mechanisms to generate heat in the term newborn. Peripheral vasoconstriction helps prevent heat loss, as does normal newborn flexion (decreased body surface area exposed to air; Shaw-Battista & Gardner, 2017).
- Temperature receptors sensing a low temperature stimulate increased sympathetic output from the CNS, resulting in norepinephrine release, which in turn stimulates beta-adrenergic receptors in brown fat, increasing cyclic adenosine monophosphate (AMP) production. Thus, the thermoregulatory system of the homeothermic infant adjusts and balances heat production, skin blood flow, sweating, and respiration in such a way that the body temperature remains constant within a control range of environmental temperatures.
  - Different thresholds of the effector response for nonshivering and shivering thermogenesis explain the differences observed between hypothermic adults and neonates. In the range of normal to near-normal body temperature (≥36°C), shivering thermogenesis will be nonoperative in the neonate and chemical thermogenesis dominates (Agren, 2020; Hodson, 2018).
- When exposed to cold stress, thermal receptors in the skin transmit messages to the CNS, activating the sympathetic nervous system and triggering metabolism of brown fat, a process that utilizes glucose and oxygen and produces acids as a by-product. Once utilized, brown fat stores are not replaced (Fraser, 2021).

BROWN ADIPOSE TISSUE

- A cold-exposed infant depends primarily on chemical thermogenesis to avoid hypothermia. Exposure to cold induces a sympathetic surge that acts on receptors in brown fat stores. Brown adipose tissue (BAT) is highly vascularized and innervated by sympathetic neurons and generates more energy than any other tissue in the body, hence its importance in thermoregulation. Brown fat comprises most of the fat content of the newborn.
  - The metabolic rate of a newborn has been observed to increase up to threefold when maximally stimulated by cold. However, in the preterm infant, fat stores are scarce and nutritional provision often suboptimal, limiting their thermogenic capacity (Agren, 2020; Brand & Shippey, 2021; Chatson, 2017).
- NST produces energy output and hence heat production through oxidation of fatty acids. The presence of the protein thermogen in brown fat uncouples beta-oxidation, resulting in metabolic production of heat. Glucose or glycerol appears to be an alternative fuel utilized for this purpose.
  - Norepinephrine acts in the brown fat tissue to stimulate lipolysis. Most of the free fatty acids are re-esterified or oxidized; both reactions produce heat (Brand & Shippey, 2021; Chatson, 2017).

- A heavy concentration of blood vessels gives BAT its characteristic brown color and serves to conduct heat into the circulation. BAT is located in the interscapular, paraspinal spaces as well as around the kidneys and adrenal glands; at the nape of the neck, the scapula, and axilla; and in the mediastinum, and around the trachea, heart, lungs, liver, and abdominal aorta kidneys, and adrenal glands (Brand & Shippey, 2021; Fraser, 2021).
- The amount of available BAT is dependent on gestational age. It begins to appear at 25 to 26 weeks in the fetus but is probably not an efficient participant in thermogenesis at this stage of development, so only a minimal amount is available in VLBW infants. Production of brown fat begins around 26 to 28 weeks' gestation and continues for 3 to 5 weeks after birth (Fraser, 2021; Hodson, 2018).

NONSHIVERING THERMOGENESIS

- NST is the major method of heat production in the neonate. NST is triggered when skin temperature decreases to less than 35°C to 36°C (95°F–96.8°F). NST produces energy output and hence heat production through oxidation of fatty acids, largely from brown fat (Hodson, 2018).
  - The initiation of NST at birth depends on cutaneous cooling, separation from the placenta, and the euthyroid state.
  - NST relies on the availability of BAT and therefore is limited in ELBW infants. Infants less than 32 weeks' gestation do not have enough BAT to produce significant amounts of heat by NST (Brand & Shippey, 2021).

▶ MECHANISMS OF AND INTERVENTIONS TO MINIMIZE HEAT TRANSFER

- The term *golden hour* is used in reference to strategies implemented in the delivery room to improve the outcome of neonates. A major focus during the golden hour is prevention of heat loss (Brand & Shippey, 2021).
- The mechanisms of heat transfers are complex, and the contribution of each component involves four means of loss: (a) by radiation, (b) by conduction, (c) by convection, and (d) by evaporation (Agren, 2020; Blackburn, 2018; Brand & Shippey, 2021; Chatson, 2017; Cheffer & Rannalli, 2016; Gardner & Cammack, 2021).
  - All modes of heat transfer influence thermal balance, and the relative contribution of each mode changes with maturity, postnatal age, disease state, and care environment (Agren, 2020; Brand & Shippey, 2021).

- The physiologic control mechanisms of the infant may alter the internal gradient (i.e., vasomotor) to change skin blood flow. The external gradient is of a purely physical nature. The large surface-to-volume ratio of the infant (especially those weighing less than 2 kg) in relation to the adult and the thin layer of subcutaneous fat increase the heat transfer in the internal gradient (Gardner & Cammack, 2021).

RADIANT HEAT LOSS

- *Radiation* is the transfer of heat through infrared energy transfer from a warm object to a cooler object that is not in direct contact. Heat transfer is affected by the temperature gradient and the distance and angle between the heat source and the skin surface. This mechanism of heat loss is influenced by the mean temperature of the skin and the mean temperatures of the surrounding walls, as well as the temperature gradient to nearby objects of lesser temperature (the newborn loses heat by radiation to nearby cooler surfaces such as crib, isolette, windows, or other objects; Brand & Shippey, 2021; Fraser, 2021; Hodson, 2018; Shaw-Battista & Gardner, 2017).
  - Radiation can be responsible for 40% or more of heat loss, so it has been the focus of most research studies (Hodson, 2018).
  - Radiant heat loss is related to the temperature of the surrounding surfaces, not air temperature. Many variables can influence the degree of heat loss, including body surface area, environmental temperature, the type of external heat source, clothing, blankets, caps, heat shields, and swaddling (Hodson, 2018).

Interventions to Minimize

- Standard thermal care guidelines include maintaining the delivery room at an ambient air temperature of 25°C (72°F). A radiant warmer should be used during resuscitation and stabilization.
  - Preterm newborns need additional protection from heat losses, including higher ambient temperature and the use of plastic wraps without drying.
    - ❏ To avoid hypothermia, it is recommended that LBW infants be placed directly in a sterile-food or medical-grade plastic bag or wrapped with occlusive wrap after delivery.
  - Heat loss from the head is clinically important and can be significantly reduced with a three-layered hat, and the neonate's head should remain covered (Brand & Shippey, 2021; Chatson, 2017; Hardy et al., 2016; Hodson, 2018).

EVAPORATIVE HEAT LOSS

- *Evaporation* is heat transfer due to water vaporizing from the large surface area of wet skin and to the duration of exposure into the drier surrounding air as when a newborn wet with amniotic fluid is subjected to dry and cooler surrounding air. In the case of premature infants with thin permeable skin, evaporative heat loss occurs through transepidermal water loss (TEWL). The more immature the newborn, the larger the relative surface area (Hodson, 2018; Shaw-Battista & Gardner, 2017).
  - Evaporative heat losses are inversely related to ambient humidity, and measures to increase the vapor pressure close to the skin simplify fluid and thermal management of extremely preterm infants (Agren, 2020).
- The amount of insensible water loss (IWL) from the skin is inversely related to gestational age. At 25 weeks' gestation, premature infants can lose 15 times more water through their skin than term neonates. This water loss is inversely proportional to gestational age until about 33 weeks' gestation, when TEWL is similar to that of a term infant (Brand & Shippey, 2021).
- The magnitude of water loss through the skin is related to maturity at birth, where the tiniest infants have evaporative heat losses that are many times higher than those of term infants when cared for under similar environmental conditions.
  - In very small infants (<1,500 g), high total body water, very thin skin that is unusually permeable because the keratin layer of the skin has not matured, and relatively large body surface area result in increased evaporative losses in premature infants. This is even more significant in VLBW and especially in ELBW infants (Agren, 2020; Brand & Shippey, 2021; Fraser, 2021).

Interventions to Minimize

- Drying the infant immediately after birth in the delivery room reduces evaporative heat loss.
  - Do not bathe the neonate without first evaluating the consequences of cold stress on the neonate's clinical condition (Agren, 2020; Hardy et al., 2016).
- Ideally, a preheated gel mattress, with a warm bassinet, warm blankets, and a radiant heat source, should be in place. Immediate drying, swaddling (once stabilized), and placement of a cap will reduce evaporative heat loss (Hodson, 2018).
- IWL through the skin continues to contribute to evaporative heat loss and decreases over the first few days after birth. The rate of evaporative water loss depends on the ambient humidity and increases at humidity levels below 50%.
  - Because evaporative loss is related to ambient relative humidity, incubator humidification will decrease heat loss; the higher the humidity, the lower the evaporation. However, in most situations, a higher evaporative loss can be compensated for by a higher air temperature convective gain (Agren, 2020; Hodson, 2018).

CONVECTION HEAT LOSS

- Convection is heat transfer due to air currents or drafts that transfer heat from a solid object to the surrounding air. Heat loss due to convection is determined by the airflow around the infant, the mean temperature of the ambient air, the mean temperature of the skin, the exposed surface area of the infant's (the amount of exposed) skin, and the amount of air turbulence created by drafts (Brand & Shippey, 2021; Chatson, 2017; Fraser, 2021; Hodson, 2018; Shaw-Battista & Gardner, 2017).

Interventions to Minimize

- Remain vigilant to the presence of radiant heat loss to cold walls or windows and convection heat loss in the path of air-conditioning vents (Hardy et al., 2016).
- The relatively larger brain of the newborn is a major heat source, the largest surface area of the body. The brain of the infant is 12% of body weight compared with 2% in the adult, and heat loss from the head is clinically important and can be significantly reduced with a three-layered hat made of wool and gauze when not under the radiant warmer greatly conserves heat (Fraser, 2021).

CONDUCTIVE HEAT LOSS

- *Conduction* is the transfer of heat via direct contact, when two solid objects of different temperatures come in contact, such as from the infant's warm body to a cold table or cold blankets (Chatson, 2017; Fraser, 2021; Shaw-Battista & Gardner, 2017).
- The rate of heat transfer varies with the temperature gradient and the amount of skin in contact with the surface. Heat is transferred more readily from the skin to a metal object than from the skin to a cloth surface.
  - Conductive heat losses contribute minimally to energy expenditure and depend on the thermal conductivity of the mattress, which is low in incubators and under radiant warmers (Brand & Shippey, 2021; Hodson, 2018).

Interventions to Minimize

- Mechanisms for preventing conductive heat loss immediately after birth include using a preheated radiant warmer, warm blankets for drying, and covering scales and x-ray plates with warm blankets (Fraser, 2021).
  - External heat sources, including skin-to-skin care (SSC) and transwarmer mattresses, have demonstrated a reduction in the risk of hypothermia (Chatson, 2017).

- Prewarm linens and equipment that will come into contact with the neonate (Hardy et al., 2016).
- The term and near-term vigorous infants may preferably be placed skin-to-skin on their mother' chest and covered by dry blankets, enabling conductive transfer of maternal heat to the infants and minimizing any ongoing heat loss. Alternatively, the infants may be dried and wrapped with dry blankets (Agren, 2020).
- Figure 10.1 summarizes the methods of heat loss and interventions to minimize.

▶ NEUTRAL THERMAL ENVIRONMENTS

- Minimizing heat loss and maintaining the newborn in a thermally neutral environment are important steps in facilitating a normal neonatal transition (Shaw-Battista & Gardner, 2017).
- The concept of an optimum thermal environment for newborn infants evolved during the 1960s. This "thermoneutral zone" or the thermal neutral environment (TNE) refers to the range of temperature within which the infant can maintain a normal body temperature at minimal metabolic rate (as measured by oxygen consumption) with use of nonevaporative processes only (vasoconstriction, vasodilation, and/ or changes in posture; Agren, 2020; Cheffer & Rannalli, 2016; Hodson, 2018).
- In the NICU, infants require a thermoneutral environment to minimize energy expenditure and optimize growth. Caregivers strive to maintain the infant in a warm environment (the NTE, or the so-called "zone of thermal comfort").
  - Thermoneutral conditions exist when heat production measured by oxygen consumption is minimal and core temperature is within the normal range.
  - A number of factors affect the temperature needed to maintain thermal stability, including gestational age, birth weight, chronological age, humidity, proximity to outside walls and windows, and use of positioning devices, clothing, or swaddling (Brand & Shippey, 2021; Chatson, 2017).

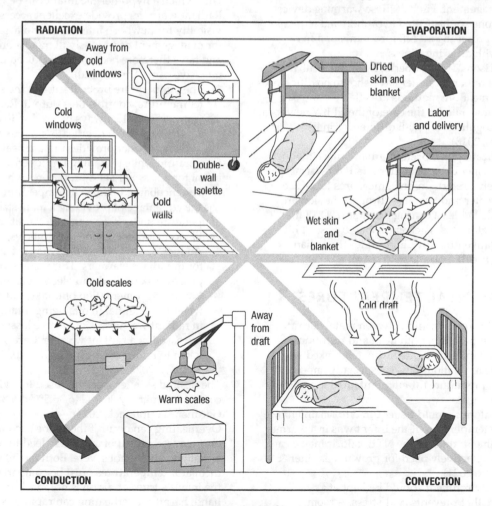

Figure 10.1 Methods of heat loss.

Source: Reproduced with permission from Gardner, S., & Hernandez, J. (2016). Heat balance. In S. Gardner, B. Carter, E. Hines, & J. Hernandez (Eds.), *Merenstein & Gardner's handbook of neonatal intensive care* (8th ed., pp. 105–125). Elsevier.

■ Thermal management relies on simple principles and requires frequent individual evaluation and adjustment. Thermal care benefits from a protocol-driven approach based on guidelines that minimize variation in practice (Agren, 2020).

■ There are three options to achieve a stable and desirable skin temperature of 36.0°C to 36.5°C:
  ● Manual control of incubator temperature
  ● Servo control of incubator air temperature
  ● Servo control of abdominal skin temperature (using an abdominal skin probe)
    ❏ Whether a heat panel or incubator is used, a probe is placed on the infant's abdomen to measure skin temperature. If the infant's skin temperature decreases, the warming device increases its heat output.
      ○ An anterior abdominal temperature of 37.0°C is generally recommended for servo control of radiant heat output, at least as a starting point (Agren, 2020; Hodson, 2018).

■ Both incubators and radiant warmers have been in use in NICUs for several decades and remain the focus of heat management. Each of these warming devices has undergone sophisticated evolution and remains effective in providing a TNE for infants of differing sizes and with differing illnesses.
  ● Comparisons of the superiority of the incubator over the radiant warmer have shown no differences in outcome. Both methods are effective and safe and appropriate for the care of the ELBW newborn, with recognition of small differences in IWL (Hodson, 2018).

■ After stabilization, the preterm infant may either be nursed in an incubator or under a radiant warmer. For extremely preterm infants, measures to reduce insensible water and heat loss through the skin are recommended at least during the first week of life. In the incubator, this is accomplished by use of high ambient relative humidity, and under the radiant warmer by use of a plastic wrap (Agren, 2020).

ENVIRONMENTAL TEMPERATURES

■ Because of the relationship between metabolic rate and body temperature, both fluid and nutritional requirements for growth are intimately linked with temperature regulation. This is especially important to the small premature infant maintained in a slightly cool environment.
  ● Fewer calories would be required for maintenance of body temperature if the infant was in a warmer environment; thus, in the NTE, caloric intake can be more effectively used for growth (Gardner & Cammack, 2021).

■ The home environment should be kept at a temperature that prevents cold stress. A room temperature that is comfortable for the parent usually is suitable for the infant. The infant should be in clothing appropriate for the room temperature. For example, if the parent requires a sweater to be comfortable, the infant probably also requires a sweater.
  ● Parents often overdress the infant or overheat the home and this may cause hyperthermia. Parents should be given written instructions before discharge on how and when to take an axillary temperature, when to call the physician, and how to maintain a comfortable environment for their infant (Gardner & Cammack, 2021).

SERVO CONTROL RADIANT WARMERS

■ This device and the primitive delivery room heaters led to the development of the current radiant warmers now in common use in NICUs. They produce overhead heat in the infrared range distributed in a uniform fashion to the infant and controlled by an abdominal skin thermistor. The high-power output of the device explains the effectiveness and speed with which a hypothermic infant can be warmed. Radiant warmers provide excellent accessibility and visibility for newborn infant care and assessment and for management of seriously ill infants on admission, and have therefore become widely used in neonatal intensive care (Agren, 2020).
  ● The temperature probe itself, not the skin temperature, controls heat output. Radiant warmers should always be used with a servo control to prevent overheating (Hodson, 2018).

■ The radiant warmer provides radiant heat to maintain temperature while providing improved access to the infant for assessment and procedures when compared with an incubator. Infant skin temperature servo control has the advantage of providing a more stable body temperature under changing care conditions, different ventilation modes, opening of port holes, and so on.
  ● An increase in IWL occurs when infants are cared for in radiant warmers. This increased fluid loss poses a risk of fluid and electrolyte imbalance. Careful documentation of intake, output, and weight is essential in managing infants cared for in radiant warmers. Convective losses are also increased in a radiant warmer. Care should be taken to minimize drafts (Agren, 2020; Brand & Shippey, 2021).

■ The desired skin temperature used for skin servo control is generally 36.0°C to 36.5°C (96.8°F–97.7°F; Gardner & Cammack, 2021).

■ Overheating can occur if the probe becomes detached, or if covered with a blanket may lead to overwarming, although usually not severe. Both the infant and incubator temperatures must be compared together, so the infant's true condition is not masked. On the other hand, harmful overheating can rapidly occur unless careful monitoring (preferably continuous) of infant temperature is instituted (Agren, 2020; Hodson, 2018).

- Conductive thermal support may also be provided by the use of a heated mattress. The mattress should always be prewarmed and the temperature never set lower than the desired body temperature because this will lead to significant conductive heat loss and impact negatively on body temperature and weight gain.
  - A transparent heat shield positioned over the infant may influence the heat exchange (occurring through convection, evaporation, and radiation) and result in reduced losses of heat (Agren, 2020).

SERVO CONTROL INCUBATORS

- Incubators are designed to decrease all four forms of heat loss, namely evaporation, conduction, radiation, and convection. Double-walled incubators further decrease heat loss primarily due to radiation and to a lesser degree conduction.
  - Incubator covers can be used to decrease radiant heat loss from incubator walls, to decrease radiant loss in cold climates, and to decrease radiant gain in hot climates, especially on sunny days (Chatson, 2017).
- Skin mode or servo control can be set so that the incubator's internal thermostat responds to changes in the infant's skin temperature to ensure a normal temperature despite any environmental fluctuations (Chatson, 2017).
  - Safety features to prevent overheating include the setting of upper limits of air temperature and alarms to alert the nurse to a detached probe.
  - In this mode, the nurse must document the neonate's axillary temperature, the incubator set point, the skin temperature, and the air temperature.
  - When incubators are in cool surroundings (e.g., during transfer), the inner surface temperature of the single-walled incubator declines to well below that of the air temperature in the incubator (Brand & Shippey, 2021).
- The incubator is controlled either thermostatically by air or infant temperature. Both modes are capable of providing a stable thermoneutral environment. However, their respective advantages and disadvantages need to be understood to properly conduct incubator care.
  - Air temperature servo control usually provides a more stable environment, but makes it necessary to frequently determine infant temperature, thus adding further to the load of procedures disturbing the infants.
  - For both modes, it is essential that procedures such as intravenous (IV) line insertion and intubation are performed through the portholes, and not through the large access panel at the front of the incubator (Agren, 2020).
- An anterior abdominal skin temperature of 36.5°C has been widely used for servo control of incubator air temperature but may be too low to ensure

thermoneutrality. An abdominal skin (or back-to-mattress) temperature setting of 37.0°C may be preferable (Agren, 2020).
- Humidity should be used with VLBW infants to reduce evaporative heat loss through TEWL. Evaporative heat loss is the major source of thermal instability in the first few weeks of life due to increased body surface area, increased skin permeability, and increased extracellular fluid.
- Because evaporative loss is related to ambient relative humidity, incubator humidification will decrease heat loss; the higher the humidity, the lower the evaporation. However, in most situations, a higher evaporative loss can be compensated for by a higher air temperature (convective gain), and a too low incubator humidity will only increase metabolic demand if the infant is nursed below thermoneutral temperature (Brand & Shippey, 2021).
- There is less need for humidity after the first week of life due to maturation of the infant's skin and decreased IWL from TEWL. Barrier maturation usually develops in 2 to 4 weeks. This may take longer in extremely premature infants. Continuing high humidity beyond the first week may slow skin maturation.
  - High incubator ambient humidity (70%–90%) is only vital in situations wherein high IWL per se complicates fluid management, that is, in extremely preterm infants during the first postnatal week(s).
  - An increased risk of *Pseudomonas* infections has been demonstrated with use of incubator humidification when condensation of vapor on the inner incubator walls occurs, which therefore should be avoided (Agren, 2020; Brand & Shippey, 2021).

WEANING FROM SERVO CONTROL

- Premature infants in relatively stable condition can be dressed in clothes and caps and covered with a blanket. The intervention offers a broader range of safe environmental temperatures. Heart rate and respiration should be continuously monitored because the clothing may limit observation (Chatson, 2017).
- Weaning from the incubator can typically be started when the infant is physiologically stable, at least 32 weeks' corrected gestational age, weighs at least 1,500 g, and takes 100 kcal/kg/d, and provided there is no medical indication for continuing incubator/warmer care, such as the need for close observation.
  - Body weight attainment serves as a useful indicator as the infant approaches a weight of at least 1,500 g and takes 100 kcal/kg/d (Brand & Shippey, 2021).
- Crib nursing of full-term infants requires a room temperature of at least 24°C (75°F), while infants of 1,500 g should be in an environment of 26°C to 28°C (79°F–82°F). Smaller infants should be fully dressed,

including a head covering, and may require a room temperature of 30°C (86°F; Hodson, 2018).

SKIN-TO-SKIN PRACTICES

- SSC has been practiced long before the concept of "kangaroo mother care" for preterm infants was introduced. "Kangaroo mother care" was originally used as an effective way for mothers to keep their full-term babies warm while breastfeeding, and subsequently as an alternative method of caring for LBW babies in resource-limited countries.
  - In their original versions, the infant is placed skin-to-skin in a vertical position between the mother's breasts and under their clothes and is exclusively (or almost exclusively) breastfed (Agren, 2020; Hodson, 2018).
- Skin-to-skin contact conserves infant heat through tucked positioning and covering, and positively contributes to thermal gain from continuous adult body heat. It has been shown to be more effective in the prevention and treatment of newborn hypothermia than either an incubator or a radiant warmer (Shaw-Battista & Gardner, 2017).
- During kangaroo care, the parent's clothing around the sides and back of the infant forms a "pouch" that provides insulation and reduces nonevaporative losses (and possibly evaporation losses). ELBW infants, in particular, require careful temperature monitoring during kangaroo care to avoid both heat stress and cooling.
- With skin-to-skin (or kangaroo care), appropriate-for-gestational age (AGA) and small-for-gestational-age (SGA) infants experience beneficial warming effects and a stable skin and core temperatures.
  - Mothers exhibit thermal synchrony with the infants so that their body temperature increases or decreases to maintain their infant's thermal neutrality.
  - Skin-to-skin contact between the mother and the infant reduces conductive and radiant heat loss and is an excellent way to maintain a neutral thermal condition for the healthy newborn.
  - Studies in more immature infants have shown that SSC can be safely applied, and without an increase in metabolic rate, as early as during the first week after birth in stable 28- to 30-week infants, and from the second week in infants born at gestational age of 25 to 27 weeks (Agren, 2020; Blackburn, 2018).
  - During SSC, extremely preterm infants were able to both maintain and increase their body temperature after the drop that occurred during transfer from the incubator (Gardner & Cammack, 2021; Hodson, 2018).
- SSC, provided by the mother or the father, has been introduced for babies requiring neonatal intensive care—even extremely premature infants and those on ventilators (Hodson, 2018). The infants were studied early (first week) after birth and during intensive care, including mechanical ventilation. The study shows that ambient air temperature and humidity are lower during SSC compared with incubator care.
- Several guidelines regarding SSC in the NICU have been published; however, since it requires intensive staffing support, resources, and parent participation, the development of individualized unit guidelines has been recommended (Hodson, 2018)
- Studies have been performed mainly in countries with limited availability to neonatal intensive care, with increasingly known effects and benefits in the moderately preterm and LBW infants.
- At birth, term infants placed skin-to-skin against their mother or who experience skin-to-skin contact later maintain their temperature, as well as infants cared for in standard heating units.
- Studies of skin-to-skin (kangaroo) care with stable preterm infants demonstrate that most infants maintain adequate thermal control during this type of holding (Blackburn, 2018).

HYPERTHERMIA

- The fetus is incapable of independent thermoregulation; heat production and heat loss are controlled by the maternal–fetal thermal gradient.
  - Maternal hyperthermia results in fetal hyperthermia and can lead to compromised fetal oxygen uptake, lower Apgar scores, hypotonia, and increased incidence of advanced resuscitation and oxygen support following delivery.
  - Maternal fever related to infection early in pregnancy has been associated with increased risk of anencephaly, neural tube defects, microcephaly, cleft lip, facial dysmorphosis, and altered growth patterns (Blackburn, 2018).
- Neonatal hyperthermia (37.5°C–38.0°C or 99.5°F–100.4°F) may be caused by maternal fever secondary to epidural anesthesia or infection, environmental factors, cardiac defects, drug withdrawal, infection, dehydration, CNS dysfunction related to birth trauma or malformations, or medications (Blackburn, 2018; Brand & Shippey, 2021).
- The most common causes of neonatal hyperthermia are iatrogenic and environmental in nature. High room temperatures, improperly set heating controls (i.e., radiant warmer left in manual control mode or excessive servo control temperature setting), malpositioned temperature probes, excessive swaddling, and conditions that alter heat control, such as phototherapy use and incubator sun exposure, have been linked to neonatal hyperthermia (Chatson, 2017; Gardner & Cammack, 2021).

The neonate is more susceptible to heat stress due to their larger surface-to-volume ratio, lower heat storage capacity, and narrower temperature control range (Blackburn, 2018).

PRESENTATION

- Hyperthermia causes an increase in metabolic demands, resulting in an increase in oxygen consumption (Blackburn, 2018).
- While environmental conditions may be the primary causation of neonatal hyperthermia, it is important to also assess for signs of infection (Table 10.3). Servo-controlled incubators will have decreased heater output in response to increasing infant skin temperatures, thus keeping the infant's temperature within a normal range (Gardner & Cammack, 2021).
  - Clinicians should closely monitor infants requiring decreased incubator heat support.
  - Sepsis in infants may present with hypothermia or hyperthermia. Hypothermia is more likely to occur in premature infants with bacterial sepsis. Term infants are more likely to present with hyperthermia as a sign of infection (Gardner & Cammack, 2021; Rudd, 2021).
- Sweating is usually not present in infants <36 weeks but may occur in term infants.
- Hyperthermic infants may be irritable, restless, lethargic, hypotonic, apneic, tachypneic, tachycardic, or have a weak or absent cry. Vasodilation to increase heat loss may cause hypotension and dehydration as a result of increased IWLs. Seizures and apnea may also occur as a result of high internal temperatures (Blackburn, 2018; Gardner & Cammack, 2021; Hodson, 2018).
- Infants with temperature irregularities should be monitored closely for any changes in their behavioral, feeding, and respiratory patterns. Axillary temperatures should be evaluated frequently in any infant exhibiting these changes or who feel cool or warm to touch (Gardner & Cammack, 2021).

TREATMENT

- The primary approach to treating hyperthermia is to remove any external sources of heat and to promote heat loss (e.g., removing extra blankets or clothes). Environmental temperature should be lowered approximately every 30 minutes by 0.5°C (Gardner & Cammack, 2021; Hodson, 2018).
- Fluid status should be monitored by assessing the infant's intake and output, serum electrolyte assays, serum and urine osmolality, skin turgor, and mucous membranes. Total intake volume should be adjusted as needed to replace IWL. Blood pressure measurements should be assessed frequently to monitor for hypotension; volume resuscitation should be provided as needed. Assisted ventilation should be provided for persistent apnea or apnea that does not respond to stimulation. Infants with significant hyperthermia should be assessed for subtle seizure signs such as facial grimacing, horizontal eye deviation, nystagmus, eye blinking or fluttering, or staring; tremors, apnea, decorticate posturing, rowing, stepping, or pedaling movements; and tongue thrusting, nonnutritive sucking, lip smacking, or drooling (Ditzenberger, 2021; Gardner & Hernandez, 2016).
- Discharge education related to thermal regulation should focus on proper axillary temperature-taking technique, newborn care, and signs and symptoms of illness (Box 10.3).

Table 10.3 Neonatal Hyperthermia: Environmental Versus Infection Presentation

Environmental	Infection
Generally warm to touch, with trunk and extremities of the same temperature	Cool to touch, with extremities significantly cooler than the trunk
Skin appears flushed or ruddy in color	Skin appears pale blue, hypoperfused
Vasodilation	Vasoconstricted

Sources: Data from Agren, J. (2020). The thermal environment of the intensive care nursery. In R. Martin, A. Fanaroff, & M. Walsh (Eds.), *Fanaroff and Martin's neonatal-perinatal medicine: Diseases of the fetus and infant* (11th ed., pp. 566–576). Elsevier; Chatson, K. (2017). Temperature control. In E. Eichenwald, A. Hansen, C. Martin, & A. Stark (Eds.), *Cloherty and Stark's manual of neonatal care* (8th ed., pp. 185–191). Wolters Kluwer; Gardner, S. L., & Cammack, B. H. (2021). Heat balance. In S. L. Gardner, B. S. Carter, M. Enzman-Hines, & S. Niermeyer (Eds.), *Merenstein & Gardner's handbook of neonatal intensive care nursing: An interprofessional approach* (9th ed., pp. 137–164). Elsevier.

Box 10.3 Parent Teaching and Temperature Regulation

- Teach parents how to take an axillary temperature on their newborn and maintain an axillary temperature of 36.5°C and 37.4°C (97.7°F and 99.3°F).
- Teach parents how to dress their infant with clothes and blankets and use an appropriate environmental temperature to maintain the baby's temperature in the above range.
- Teach parents appropriate safety precautions, which include verbal and written information about recognizing the signs and symptoms of a sick infant, as well as how the infant acts, including temperatures either higher than or more commonly lower than the range of 36.5°C to 37.4°C (97.7°F–99.3°F).
- Teach parents to notify their infant's primary health care provider immediately or to take the infant to the nearest ED for temperatures out of the above range, especially if the baby's feeding pattern changes.

Source: Reproduced with permission from Gardner, S. L. & Cammack, B. H. (2021). Heat balance. In S. L. Gardner, B. S. Carter, M. Enzman-Hines, & S. Niermeyer (Eds.), *Merenstein & Gardner's handbook of neonatal intensive care nursing: An interprofessional approach* (9th ed., pp. 137–164). Elsevier.

▶ CONCLUSION

The significance of thermal regulation in the neonatal population cannot be overstated. An understanding of the physiology and mechanics of thermoregulation is a basic requirement of neonatal care. Beginning at delivery and continuing throughout the neonatal period, infants require a thermally neutral environment to facilitate transition to the extrauterine life, to lower energy expenditure in order to utilize caloric intake to optimize growth, and to lower oxygen consumption. Evidence-based practice guidelines and protocols focusing on thermal management minimize practice variations and promote an environment in which the infant can grow and thrive.

1. The neonatal nurse practitioner (NNP) advocates for interventions to promote neonatal thermoregulation based on knowledge that the infant's admission temperature is a strong indicator of overall neonatal:

   A. Acidosis
   B. Apgar score
   C. Mortality

2. Preterm infants are most vulnerable to hypothermia following delivery during the:

   A. First minutes following birth
   B. Time spent on NICU admission
   C. Transport en route to the NICU

3. The neonatal nurse practitioner (NNP) prepares for the delivery of an infant at 29 weeks' gestational age and places prewarmed linens on the radiant warmer to minimize the infant's heat loss from:

   A. Conduction
   B. Convection
   C. Evaporation

4. A newly born neonate at 24 3/7 weeks' gestation is placed in an isolette and provided with 85% humidity. The neonatal nurse practitioner (NNP) instructs the bedside nurse to keep the isolette walls as dry as possible due to concerns of the infant developing:

   A. Hyperthermia
   B. Polyuria
   C. Septicemia

5. The neonatal nurse practitioner (NNP) attends a Cesarean delivery of an infant at 33 weeks' gestation and is told the mother, who has an epidural in place for the last 8 hours, developed a fever of 38.3°C (101°F). There are no indications of chorioamnionitis. Immediately after birth, the infant's temperature becomes 37.6°C (99.8°F), and the NNP theorizes the infant's hyperthermia is related to the:

   A. Elevated room temperature
   B. Infant's agitation from birth
   C. Maternal epidural anesthesia

6. The neonatal nurse practitioner (NNP) understands that nonshivering thermogenesis (NST) releases heat caused by:

   A. Epinephrine release from adrenal glands
   B. Gluconeogenesis occurring in the liver
   C. Norepinephrine stimulating lipolysis

7. The bedside RN pages the neonatal nurse practitioner (NNP) to alert them to an infant at 29 weeks and 2 days' gestation who has a rectal temperature of 37.9°C (100.2°F). The first step the NNP should direct the bedside RN to perform is to:

   A. Add a cooling blanket to the infant's incubator
   B. Perform an evaluation for sepsis on the infant's blood
   C. Remove external heat sources from the infant

1. C) Mortality

Adverse consequences associated with cold stress remain an important contributor to neonatal mortality and morbidity, and the potential impact of optimal thermal care provision on infant health is huge. Acidosis may occur for reasons other than poor thermoregulation, while temperature is not included in the Apgar scoring matrix (Agren, 2020; Brand & Shippey, 2021; Chatson, 2017; Fraser, 2021).

2. A) First minutes following birth

The neonate is most vulnerable to heat loss during the first minutes following birth because the neonate is expected to transition from a warm, moist environment to a much colder, drier environment. Transport incubators and radiant warmers used during admission to NICU help maintain thermoregulation (Brand & Shippey, 2021; Fraser, 2021; Hodson, 2018).

3. A) Conduction

Conduction is the transfer of heat via direct contact, when two solid objects of different temperatures come in contact, such as from the infant's warm body to a cold table or cold blankets. Convection deals with airflow over the infants, while evaporation is influenced by the amount of moisture on the infant (Chatson, 2017; Fraser, 2021; Shaw-Battista & Gardner, 2017).

4. C) Septicemia

An increased risk of *Pseudomonas* infections has been demonstrated with the use of incubator humidification when condensation of vapor on the inner incubator walls occurs, which therefore should be avoided. Hyperthermia is not a consequence of humidity, and humidity does not affect the infant's urinary output (Agren, 2020; Brand & Shippey, 2021).

5. C) Maternal epidural anesthesia

In this scenario, the infant's hyperthermia is most likely related to maternal sedation. Room temperature may prevent hypothermia but does not cause hyperthermia, nor does agitation.

6. A) Epinephrine release from adrenal glands

NST produces energy output and hence heat production through oxidation of fatty acids. The presence of the protein thermogen in brown fat uncouples beta-oxidation, resulting in the metabolic production of heat. Glucose or glycerol appears to be an alternative fuel utilized for this purpose. Norepinephrine acts in the brown fat tissue to stimulate lipolysis. Most of the free fatty acids are re-esterified or oxidized; both reactions produce heat. Neither gluconeogenesis nor adrenal hormone release produces epinephrine as part of their reaction (Chatson, 2017; Brand & Shippey, 2021).

7. C) Remove external heat sources from the infant

The most common causes of neonatal hyperthermia are iatrogenic and environmental in nature. High room temperatures, improperly set heating controls (e.g., radiant warmer left in manual control mode or excessive servo control temperature setting), malpositioned temperature probes, excessive swaddling, and conditions that alter heat control, such as phototherapy use and incubator sun exposure, have been linked to neonatal hyperthermia. Active cooling is not indicated in nonneurologically related conditions, and an evaluation for sepsis should be undertaken only after environmental causes have been ruled out (Chatson, 2017; Gardner & Cammack, 2021; Gardner & Snell).

Resuscitation and Delivery Room Stabilization

Jodi M. Beachy and Barbara Snapp

▶ INTRODUCTION

A successful resuscitation and stabilization requires good communication, teamwork, and a thorough understanding of neonatal transitional physiology. This chapter discusses transition, resuscitation, and preparation for transport to another healthcare facility if needed.

The American Academy of Pediatrics (AAP) provides the Neonatal Resuscitation Program (NRP), which is considered the gold standard for neonatal resuscitation, and issues a completion certificate which many hospitals require for all nursing staff in women's and children's services (Katheria & Finer, 2018; Ringer, 2017). Although there is an NRP algorithm on the specific steps of resuscitation, this chapter outlines the key components that contribute to understanding normal and abnormal transitional physiology and the science behind proper neonatal resuscitation.

▶ TRANSITION TO EXTRAUTERINE LIFE

- Transition from a fetus to a neonate requires significant physiologic adaptation.
  - Key elements in the birth transition are:
    - ❏ Pulmonary shift from maternally dependent oxygenation to continuous respiration
    - ❏ Cardiovascular change from fetal circulation to mature circulation with increase in pulmonary blood flow
    - ❏ Commencement of independent glucose homeostasis
    - ❏ Independent thermoregulation
    - ❏ Gastrointestinal tract performs digestive and excretory functions
- About 10% of newborns require some form of resuscitative assistance during transition.
- Approximately 5% of newborns will need assistance after delivery to transition successfully. Less than 1% will need advanced resuscitation.
- Immediately after birth, the infant should cry vigorously.
- If the infant experiences asphyxia, either in utero or postnatally, a series of respiratory events follow.

- Primary apnea occurs when the infant ceases respiratory movements after a brief period of rapid breathing.
  - ❏ Stimulation will induce respirations.
- Secondary apnea is the result of respirations progressing to gasping efforts and then ceasing.
  - ❏ Stimulation will not resume respirations; resuscitation must be initiated.
- Since the exact timing of asphyxia cannot be determined, apnea can be either primary or secondary. This is the basis for recommending stimulation first, then quickly progressing to assisted ventilation.
- The need for intervention is determined by heart rate (HR) and respiratory effort.
  - Low HR and poor respiratory effort are the primary indicators for resuscitation.
- Auscultation of the heart is preferred over digital palpation of the cord.
- Cardiac monitoring provides the most accurate HR assessment.
- The Apgar score is not a reliable indicator of the need for resuscitation; rather it quantifies an infant's response to the extrauterine environment and resuscitative measures.
- Pulse oximetry is more reliable than a visual assessment of the infant's color. Color alone is an unreliable assessment of oxygenation.
- The newborn may have bradycardia or HR averaging less than 100 beats per minute (bpm) in the first minute postdelivery, but should rise to 140 to 160 bpm by 2 minutes of life.
  - The infant may also experience tachycardia (HR greater than 160 bpm) for the first few minutes after delivery.
- After birth, it is normal for respirations to be somewhat irregular, with mild grunting and nasal flaring. Fine rales are normal and may be heard throughout the lungs as the lung fluid is cleared.
- Successful transition includes the ability to maintain temperature, sustain respiratory effort, and support systemic perfusion throughout the body (Cheffer & Rannalli, 2016; Goldsmith, 2020; Heideric & Leone, 2020; Katheria & Finer, 2018; Niermeyer & Clarke, 2021; Owen et al., 2022; Pappas & Robey, 2021; Ringer, 2017).

PHYSIOLOGY OF ADAPTATIONS AFTER DELIVERY

Pulmonary

- Several days prior to delivery, there is a biochemical dehydration of the lungs as fluid is actively moved to the interstitial and then drained through the pulmonary and lymphatic systems.
- To adapt to extrauterine life, the infant's lungs must fill with air and begin to exchange gases without the placenta.
- When the low-resistance placental circulation is removed after birth, the infant's systemic vascular resistance increases, while the pulmonary vascular resistance (PVR) begins to fall as a result of pulmonary inflation. A rapid decrease in PVR and an increase in pulmonary blood flow occur after expansion of the lungs with air and filling the pulmonary circuit with blood.
- As the lungs aerate and the PVR falls, blood flow changes from right-to-left through the ductus arteriosus to left-to-right. Pulmonary venous return then begins to provide ventricular preload. Cardiac output increases, as do the HR and blood pressure.
- The increase in systemic pressure, in addition to the decrease in PVR, stimulates functional closure of the ductus arteriosus. The decrease in ductal shunting results in increased venous return to the left atrium, and when the left atrial pressure exceeds the right atrial pressure the foramen ovale functionally closes.
- In some situations, the normal reduction in PVR may not fully occur, resulting in persisting pulmonary hypertension and decreased effective pulmonary blood flow.
  - The infant's normal opening breath generates 20 to 70 or up to 100 cm water (H_2O) pressure, the amount required to replace lung fluid with air and drive the lung fluid into the interstitial tissues.
  - Changes in partial pressure of oxygen in arterial blood (PaO_2) and carbon dioxide ($PaCO_2$) during delivery affect chemoreceptors, which control the depth and rhythm of respirations.
  - A vigorous newborn can generate an adequate functional residual capacity (FRC) with the initial breath. Naturally occurring surfactant reduces surface tension, maintaining FRC.
- Lung compliance improves with the help of catecholamines, especially circulating epinephrine.
- The change in the environment from in utero temperature to external environmental temperature, plus touch and noise, can stimulate initial respirations (Cheffer & Rannalli, 2016; Goldsmith, 2020; Heideric & Leone, 2020; Katheria & Finer, 2018; Niermeyer & Clarke, 2021; Owen et al., 2022; Ringer, 2017).

Cardiovascular

- When the umbilical cord is clamped, the low-pressure placenta is removed and systemic vascular resistance increases.
- PVR falls drastically, while systemic blood pressure increases.
- The end of fetal circulation involves closure of three shunts:
  - *Ductus venosus:* This refers to a right-to-left shunt that closes within minutes of birth due to a cessation of blood flow. Normally gone by 2 weeks of age in most full-term infants, some will remain open longer in premature infants. It becomes the ligamentum venosum.
  - *Foramen ovale:* This is an opening separating the two atria, allowing for left-to-right blood flow. The foramen ovale usually closes functionally after birth with the rising left-sided blood pressure but may remain anatomically open through childhood.
  - *Ductus arteriosus:* This closes within days after birth but may remain patent for several days. By 96 hours, the ductus should be functionally closed in full-term infants; it may occur later in premature infants. Anatomic closure normally occurs by 3 months of age (Heiderich & Leone, 2021; Niemeyer & Clarke, 2021).

Hematologic

- The transition from fetal hemoglobin (HgF) with a high affinity for oxygen to adult hemoglobin (HgA) is accomplished through increased interaction with 2,3-diphosphoglycerate. This increases the hemoglobin's ability to release the oxygen and therefore sends more oxygen to the tissues.
- Hemoglobin levels increase after birth and then decrease by the seventh day of life (McKinney et al., 2021).
- Delayed cord clamping (DCC):
  - Delayed umbilical cord clamping is defined as a 30- to 120-second pause before clamping the cord to allow for placental transfusion of blood to the infant.
  - The benefits of DCC for both the term and preterm infants include:
    - ❑ Increases blood volume by 15% to 20%, with an additional 30 to 150 mL of blood from the placenta
    - ❑ Improves physiologic stability
    - ❑ Increases lung fluid absorption
    - ❑ Increases oxygen-carrying capacity to the tissues
    - ❑ Decreases intraventricular hemorrhage for all grades
    - ❑ Decreases necrotizing enterocolitis (NEC)
    - ❑ Has shown no increased morbidities, but is shown to decrease mortality
    - ❑ Especially beneficial to premature infants
    - ❑ Decreases the need for transfusions
    - ❑ Increases hemoglobin and iron stores in early infancy
    - ❑ Reduces anemia during the first 6 months of life
    - ❑ Increases cardiac output

❑ Increases circulatory stability
- Potential risks of DCC in the normal newborn were initially identified as increased hyperbilirubinemia, polycythemia, and transient tachypnea of the newborn; however, subsequent meta-analyses have not demonstrated an increase of these morbidities in preterm infants associated with DCC. DCC has also been proven not to increase maternal hemorrhage or blood loss.
- DCC is contraindicated in the following situations:
  ❑ Monochorionic placentation due to a theoretical risk of acute twin–twin transfusion
  ❑ Complete placental abruption due to concern about accompanying neonatal blood loss
  ❑ Umbilical cord prolapse and bleeding placenta accreta; in both cases, the infant is at risk of hypovolemia and hypoxia due to compression of the umbilical vein (Goldsmith, 2020; Heideric & Leone, 2020; Katheria et al., 2020; Katheria & Finer, 2018; Niermeyer & Clarke, 2021; Pappas & Robey, 2021)

Metabolic

■ *Asphyxia* is defined as inadequate tissue perfusion that fails to meet the metabolic demands of the tissues for oxygen uptake and waste removal. Asphyxia is characterized by progressive hypoxemia ($\downarrow PaO_2$), hypercarbia ($\uparrow PaCO_2$), and acidosis ($\downarrow pH$).
  - Sodium bicarbonate is no longer recommended for use during resuscitation immediately after birth. Although acidosis frequently persists after a prolonged resuscitation, many infants correct an acidosis spontaneously once the asphyxiating circumstances are relieved and adequate ventilation is established. Metabolic correction of pH is a slow process that takes several hours, and treatment with sodium bicarbonate is not necessary.
■ Infants must transition from transplacental glucose to producing their own energy. Compromised infants who may experience difficulty include those with:
  - Decreased glucose stores
  - Decreased ability to convert stored glucose
  - Inefficient energy production from stored glucose
  - Increased utilization of glucose leading to hypoglycemia
■ Management of hypoglycemia is based on the clinical situation and the particular characteristics of the infant. After birth, the infant must begin producing heat through lipolysis of brown adipose tissue (Cheffer & Rannalli, 2016; Goldsmith, 2020; Heideric & Leone, 2020; Katheria & Finer, 2018; Niermeyer & Clarke, 2021; Pappas & Robey, 2021; Ringer, 2017; Rozance et al., 2021).
■ See Chapter 10 for more information.

▶ NEONATAL RESUSCITATION EDUCATION

■ Follow current NRP guidelines and review competency at least annually.
■ Offer mock codes and simulations for knowledge, practice, and quality improvement.
■ Debrief following all neonatal codes for quality improvement.

PREPARATION

■ Preparation is one of the most important factors for successful neonatal resuscitation.
■ Test team-alert system for an appropriate response time.
■ Anticipate the needs of the neonate by gestational age, if fluid is clear, and other fetal/maternal risk factors, and plan for timing of cord clamping.
  - Very low birth weight (VLBW) and extremely low birth weight (ELBW) infants require additional special care in the delivery room, including the use of plastic wraps or bags and/or use of exothermic mattresses to prevent heat loss due to their thinner skin and increased surface-area-to-body ratio.
■ Have a checklist to evaluate and update equipment as needed (Table 11.1).
  - Identify all resources available for anticipated resuscitation.
  - Gather equipment and ensure proper function.
  - Formulate a plan for correct endotracheal tube size, medications, fluids, and equipment.
■ Assemble the team and have clear role assignments.
■ Develop a system of effective teamwork. Effective teams have clear communication and good leadership. Poor communication and lack of teamwork lead to poor outcomes.
■ Behavioral skills for effective teamwork:
  - Know your environment.
  - Anticipate needs and formulate a plan.
  - Assign leadership role.
  - Use effective and open communication.
  - Delegate the workload.
  - Use all available information to plan the resuscitation.
  - Call for extra help if needed.
  - Remain professional.
■ Prewarm the room to prevent hypothermia. Avoid drafts.
  - Obtain plastic wrap and chemically activated warming pad as needed for gestational age of 32 weeks or less.
■ Have the current NRP algorithm available and visible.

Table 11.1 List of Equipment for Neonatal Resuscitation

Thermal regulation	■ Radiant warmer ■ Temperature sensor ■ Blankets ■ Warming mattress/plastic bag <32 weeks
Suction equipment	■ Bulb syringe ■ Mechanical suction device with tubing ■ Suction catheters (8-, 10-, 12-Fr) ■ Shoulder roll
Ventilation	■ Self-inflating bag with reservoir (cannot give free-flow oxygen or CPAP) ■ Flow-inflating bag (needs gas source, can give blended oxygen 21%–100% oxygen and CPAP) ■ T-piece (needs gas source, PIP/PEEP can be set, can deliver 21%–100% oxygen) ■ Appropriate neonatal-sized mask (covers the mouth and nose but not the eyes) ■ Oxygen ■ Compressed air, oxygen blender, flow meter ■ 8-Fr feeding tube and syringe ■ Stethoscope
Intubation	■ Laryngoscope with blades (00, 0, 1) ■ Batteries, bulbs ■ Endotracheal tubes (2.5, 3.0, 3.5) ■ Tube securing device/tape/scissors ■ Colorimetric end-tidal CO_2 detectors ■ Laryngeal mask ■ Pulse oximeter ■ Oral airway
Medications	■ Epinephrine (0.1 mg/mL concentration) ■ 0.5–1 mL/kg via ETT ■ 0.1–0.03 mL/kg via UVC ■ Normal saline/lactated Ringer's ■ 10 mL/kg ■ UVC insertion supplies
Monitors	■ Pulse oximeter/sensor, place on the right hand/wrist ■ EKG monitor/leads

CO_2, carbon dioxide; CPAP, continuous positive airway pressure; ETT, endotracheal tube; Fr, French; PEEP, positive end-expiratory pressure; PIP, peak inspiratory pressure; UVC, umbilical venous catheter.

Sources: Data from Heideric, A. E., & Leone, T. A. (2020). Resuscitation and initial stabilization. In A. Fanaroff & J. Fanaroff (Eds.), *Klaus and Fanaroff's care of the high-risk neonate* (7th ed., pp. 44–57.e3). Elsevier; Katheria, A., & Finer, N. (2018). Newborn resuscitation. In C. Gleason & S. Juul (Eds.), *Avery's diseases of the newborn* (20th ed., pp. 273–288). Elsevier; Niermeyer, S., & Clarke, S. B. (2021). Care at birth. In S. L. Gardner, B. S. Carter, M. Enzman-Hines, & S. Niemeyer (Eds.), *Merenstein & Gardner's handbook of neonatal intensive care an interprofessional approach* (9th ed., pp. 67–92). Elsevier; Owen, L. S., Weiner, G. M., & Davis, P. G. (2022). Delivery room stabilization and respiratory support. In M. Keszler, G. Suresh, & J. Goldsmith (Eds.), *Goldsmith's assisted ventilation of the neonate: An evidence-based approach to respiratory care* (7th ed., pp. 151–171). Elsevier; Papps, B. E., & Robey, D. L. (2021). Neonatal delivery room resuscitation. In M. T. Verklan, M. Walden, & S. Forest (Eds.), *Core curriculum of neonatal intensive care nursing* (6th ed., pp. 69–85). Elsevier; Ringer, S. A. (2017). Resuscitation in the delivery room. In E. Eichenwald, A. Hansen, C. Martin, & A. Stark (Eds.), *Cloherty and Starks manual of neonatal care* (8th ed., pp. 33–63). Lippincott Williams & Wilkins.

■ Communicate clearly with the family as to the expected resuscitation and possible outcomes (Ali & Sawyer, 2020; Heideric & Leone, 2020; Katheria & Finer, 2018; Niermeyer & Clarke, 2021; Owen et al., 2022; Pappas & Robey, 2021; Ringer, 2017).

RESUSCITATION GOALS

■ Prevent morbidity and mortality
■ Provide effective ventilation, which is the most important task
■ A neutral thermal environment as hypothermia increases the risk of hypoglycemia, acidosis, and respiratory distress, which may contribute to greater morbidity/mortality
■ Effective ventilation, which leads to reduced PVR, which increases blood flow to the lungs and pumps oxygenated blood through the coronary arteries, thus perfusing the heart and increasing the HR
■ Good lung expansion and normal breathing to increase oxygen levels to the targeted range by clearing the airway, and bag and mask if needed
■ Adequate cardiac output (Heideric & Leone, 2020; Katheria & Finer, 2018; Niermeyer & Clarke, 2021; Ringer, 2017).

INITIAL RESUSCITATION STEPS

■ Dry infants greater than 32 weeks' gestational age with dry, warm blankets and remove wet blankets.
■ Infants less than 32 weeks' gestation require no drying but immediate placement in a plastic wrap from shoulders to toes and optional thermal mattress.
■ Stimulate term infants by gently rubbing the back, trunk, extremities, or head.
■ Quick assessment (3 Ts) after delivery includes:
  ● *Is the baby term?* (Term)
  ● *Is the baby breathing and crying?* (Taking a breath)
  ● *Is there good tone?* (Tone normal)
  ● *If the answer is "no" to any of these questions, move the infant to a preheated warmer for further evaluation.*
■ Position and clear the airway (only if needed).
■ Place the infant on their back, head in midline with the neck slightly extended; a shoulder pad (towel or blanket) may be needed for infants with large occiput.
■ Clear the airway as gently as possible, when needed, with the least invasive method possible. Wipe the nose and mouth with a dry towel.
■ Use bulb syringe (preferable) or wall suction catheter.
  ● Suction the mouth, then the nose, to prevent aspiration.
  ● Set the suction pressure to 80 to 100 mmHg.

● Avoid deep suction that is prolonged or vigorous, especially during the first few minutes, due to risk of trauma, edema, bradycardia, and desaturations, which will cause a delay in PaO_2 rise (Ali & Sawyer, 2020; Goldsmith, 2020; Heideric & Leone, 2020; Katheria & Finer, 2018; Niermeyer & Clarke, 2021; Owen et al., 2022; Pappas & Robey, 2021; Ringer, 2017).

PHYSIOLOGIC MONITORING AND EVALUATION

Cardiac Monitoring

■ HR may be evaluated by palpation of a peripheral pulse or the umbilical cord. However, studies have shown that these measurements are not reliable.
■ Cardiac monitoring is more accurate than pulse oximetry in determining the infant's response to resuscitation. Pulse oximetry relies on circulation, which may be poor, while the cardiac monitor measures the heart's electrical activity.
■ EKG leads should be placed when compressions are anticipated/begun (Goldsmith, 2020; Katheria & Finer, 2018; Niermeyer & Clarke, 2021; Owen et al., 2022).

Respiratory Monitoring/Pulse Oximetry

■ The pulse oximeter can be used as a more accurate measure of oxygenation than evaluation of color alone and can be used to guide the titration of supplemental oxygen. Color alone is an unreliable measure to accurately assess the infant's oxygen saturation especially where the room lighting is suboptimal.
■ A pulse oximeter or electronic cardiac monitor should be available for all deliveries and used to confirm cyanosis, to provide supplemental oxygen, or if positive pressure ventilation (PPV) is required.
  ● The pulse oximeter, while helpful, does not provide a reliable HR in the first few minutes of life.
  ● There may be a delay of 1 to 2 minutes after attaching the pulse oximeter until accurate readings of both HR and oxygen saturation are obtained.
■ Place the probe on the preductal right upper extremity. Preductal readings are preferred after birth because they are more reliable than postductal readings. This site avoids the potentially confounding effect of shunting during the transition to an adult-type circulation.
■ Preductal oxygen levels generally should be above 85% to 95% after 10 minutes. Avoid hyperoxia by using the targeted oxygen saturation (SpO_2) range (Table 11.2).
■ Newborns should become pink by 2 to 5 minutes of age (Heideric & Leone, 2020; Katheria & Finer, 2018; Niermeyer & Clarke, 2021; Owen et al., 2022; Pappas & Robey, 2021; Ringer, 2017).

Table 11.2 Target Preductal Saturation Goals After Birth (by Minutes of Age)

1 min	60%–65%
2 min	65%–70%
3 min	70%–75%
4 min	75%–80%
5 min	80%–85%
10 min	85%–95%

Source: Data from Niermeyer, S., & Clarke, S. B. (2021). Care at birth. In S. L. Gardner, B. S. Carter, M. Enzman-Hines, & S. Niemeyer (Eds.), *Merenstein & Gardner's handbook of neonatal intensive care an interprofessional approach* (9th ed., pp. 67–92). Elsevier.

OXYGEN USE AND DELIVERY

■ Oxygen is perhaps the most widely used drug in neonatology but until recently remained poorly evaluated. An appreciation of its life-sustaining properties is now balanced by an understanding of its potential toxicity, even from a relatively short period of resuscitation.
■ Oxygen use in the first few minutes of life could impact survival and common neonatal morbidities associated with prematurity and free-radical diseases, such as neurodevelopmental impairment, retinopathy of prematurity, bronchopulmonary dysplasia (BPD), and NEC.
  ● Current recommendations advise against the routine use of oxygen for transient cyanosis and the avoidance of high concentrations of oxygen whenever possible.
■ Either insufficient or excessive oxygenation can be harmful to the newborn.
  ● The exclusive use of 100% oxygen for postnatal resuscitation, as previously recommended, can result in hyperoxia and changes induced by the generation of oxygen free radicals.
  ● The toxicity of oxygen is anticipated when the cellular antioxidant capacity is impaired, as occurs during the reperfusion phase.
  ● The best concentration with which to initiate resuscitation for preterm infants is not the same as for term infants. Preterm infants have decreased antioxidant enzyme capacity and may therefore be more susceptible to the harmful effects of excessive oxygen exposure. Preterm newborns may be more susceptible to any harmful effects of excessive oxygen exposure due to their decreased antioxidant enzyme capacity.
■ The use of air or a minimally increased concentration of blended air–oxygen mixture as the initial gas results in an appropriate increase in oxygen saturation levels, and trials have shown that survival is improved when resuscitation is initiated with room air compared with 100% oxygen.

- The concentration and duration of supplemental oxygen administration should be individualized to patient needs.
  - Oxygen concentration should be increased to 100% if bradycardia does not improve after 90 seconds of resuscitation while employing a lower oxygen concentration.
- The goal of oxygen administration is to achieve adequate tissue oxygenation.
  - The need to correct hypoxemia (low oxygen content in the blood) is the most common indication for oxygen therapy.
  - Left untreated, hypoxemia leads to hypoxia (low tissue oxygen) and possibly anoxia (absent tissue oxygen; Goldsmith, 2020; Heideric & Leone, 2020; Katheria & Finer, 2018; Niermeyer & Clarke, 2021; Owen et al., 2022; Ringer, 2017; Walsh, 2019).

Oxygen Delivery Methods

BLOWBY OXYGEN

- Begin oxygen blowby at a flow rate of 10 L/min and adjust the fraction of inspired oxygen (FiO$_2$) to meet the preductal saturations per minute-of-life target range. Deliver oxygen by mask, cupped hand holding the tubing over the neonate's face, flow-inflating bag and mask, or T-piece resuscitator. The closer the oxygen source to the face, the higher the oxygen concentration delivered.
- A flow-inflating bag (but not a self-inflating bag) can deliver high concentrations of blowby oxygen.
- If free-flow oxygen is to be continued for any period, it should be heated and humidified and given through wide-bore tubing.
- Begin blowby as needed when the HR is above 100 bpm and respiratory rate is adequate, but saturations remain below the NRP guidelines. Slowly withdraw oxygen as the infant's saturations reach the target range (Goldsmith, 2020; Niermeyer & Clarke, 2021; Pappas & Robey, 2021; Ringer, 2017).

POSITIVE PRESSURE VENTILATION (BAG AND MASK)

- Effective assisted ventilation is the single most important intervention in newborn resuscitation. The importance of effective PPV cannot be overstated. Delaying effective ventilation greatly impacts an infant's own respiratory efforts.
  - Adequacy of ventilation can be assessed by observing chest wall motion at the cephalad portions of the thorax and listening for equal breath sounds laterally over the right and left hemithoraces at the midaxillary lines.
- The aim of PPV is to provide effective ventilation and gas exchange, without causing lung injury, which can occur within a few large-volume positive pressure inflations (volutrauma).
- With adequate lung inflation, FRC is created and oxygenation maintained.

- The ideal target volumes for PPV of term and preterm infants after birth have not been established; animal studies demonstrate that initial high tidal volumes are detrimental.
- Begin PPV, after initial steps, if the infant is without respiratory effort (apnea) or has gasping respirations despite tactile stimulation. The lack of respiratory effort increases the partial pressure of carbon dioxide (PaCO$_2$), lowering blood pH and causing metabolic acidosis.
- Begin PPV If the HR is below 100 bpm even if the infant is breathing.
- Begin PPV if saturations are out of target range with 100% blowby or free-flowing oxygen (Heideric & Leone, 2020; Katheria & Finer, 2018; Niermeyer & Clarke, 2021; Pappas & Robey, 2021; Ringer, 2017).

STEPS IN GIVING POSITIVE PRESSURE VENTILATION

- Turn on the air low (10 L) and oxygen blend to the bag and mask.
- Begin at 21% for full-term infants and at 21% to 30% for infants under 35 weeks.
- Start with an initial positive end-expiratory pressure (PEEP) setting of 5 cm H$_2$O and a peak inspiratory pressure (PIP) setting of 20 cm H$_2$O.
- Prepare appropriate mask size. Masks should cover the chin, mouth, and nose, but not the eyes.
- Position the infant with their neck slightly extended to open airway.
- Make sure the airway is clear.
- Apply a mask and use proper seal with the fingers in "C" shape around the mask. Apply gentle pressure to the neonate's face. There should be no leaks between the mask and the face.
- If the provider is unable to obtain a good seal or there is no chest risk (indicating no air flowing into the lungs), implement MRSOPA (Box 11.1).
- Provide PPV at a rate of 40 to 60 breaths per minute.
- Use an initial PIP of 20 cm H$_2$O and increase to 30 cm H$_2$O or more as needed for chest movement. PIP should be limited to the lowest pressure required to create adequate chest rise and aeration of the lungs.
- Continue to frequently observe for good chest expansion, improved HR, and targeted saturations.
- Spontaneous breathing is a sign of effective ventilation and overall improvement.
- Delivering PEEP with PPV will improve FRC, inflate alveoli, and reduce work of breathing.
- Place orogastric tube through the mouth (to maximize ventilation through the nose) after several minutes of ventilation to prevent abdominal distention elevating the diaphragm and reducing lung volume (Ali & Sawyer, 2020; Goldsmith, 2020; Heideric & Leone, 2020; Katheria & Finer, 2018; Niermeyer & Clarke, 2021; Owen et al., 2022; Pappas & Robey, 2021; Ringer, 2017).

Box 11.1 MRSOPA Mnemonic

If unable to obtain a seal or there is no chest risk when giving positive pressure ventilation:

■ **M**ask repositioned on the face and check seal
■ **R**eposition the airway, avoiding hyperextension or flexion of the neck
■ **S**uction the mouth and nose
■ **O**pen the mouth slightly, with the jaw lifted forward
■ **P**ressure increased gradually as needed
■ **A**irway alternative with intubation or laryngeal mask airway

CONTINUOUS POSITIVE AIRWAY PRESSURE

■ Consider continuous positive airway pressure (CPAP) for infants who have labored breathing and are unable to maintain oxygenation within the target range despite increasing oxygen concentration.

■ Self-inflating bags cannot be used reliably to deliver free-flow oxygen and they require a special adapter to deliver CPAP. Flow-inflating bags require a complete seal between the mask and the face to deliver a tidal volume. They offer the capability to achieve high peak pressures and deliver PEEP and CPAP.

■ Once respirations and HR are established, CPAP will:
  ● Minimize lung injury caused by pressure ventilation
  ● Improve gas exchange
  ● Inflate the lungs
  ● Increase lung compliance by stabilizing the chest wall FRC

■ It is preferable to use a T-piece resuscitator with an appropriately sized mask (the mask must have a secure seal to deliver PEEP and oxygen).

■ PEEP may need to be increased for effective ventilation.

■ CPAP carries the risk of developing pneumothorax (Niermeyer & Clark, 2021; Owen et al., 2022; Pappas & Robey, 2021).

ENDOTRACHEAL INTUBATION

■ Endotracheal intubation is indicated in the following situations:
  ● Need for suction of the trachea
  ● Prolonged PPV use or failure to respond to initial resuscitation measures
  ● Presence of a diaphragmatic hernia or other congenital anomalies
  ● Need for surfactant administration

■ Placement is confirmed when the chest rises, breath sounds are audible, condensation is visible in the tube, HR increases, and a color change is noted on the colorimetric carbon dioxide detector.

■ The longer it takes to achieve effective PPV, the longer it takes for the infant's respiratory effort to become effective.

■ Intubation can cause trauma to the trachea, mouth, pharynx, and vocal cords. Hypoxia and bradycardia may occur if the procedure takes more than 30 seconds per attempt (Katheria & Finer, 2018; Niermeyer & Clarke, 2021; Pappas & Robey, 2021).

■ See Chapter 7 for more detailed information on an endotracheal intubation procedure.

LARYNGEAL MASK AIRWAY

■ Laryngeal mask airway (LMA) is useful if unable to intubate, or if intubation is inhibited by physical anomalies such as those found in infants with trisomy 21, Pierre Robin sequence, or other airway anomalies of the mouth, lips, pharynx, or neck.

■ LMAs are limited in that medications cannot be given through them, nor can the infant be suctioned through the LMA. Generally, it is not used for infants under 1.5 kg or under 31 weeks' gestation (Owen et al., 2021; Pappas & Robey, 2021).

CHEST COMPRESSIONS

■ Chest compressions squeeze the heart and pushes it against the spine, increasing intrathoracic pressure, creating blood circulation.

■ Beginning chest compression too early may interfere with proper ventilation.

■ Begin chest compressions per the NRP guidelines.
  ● If HR is less than 60 bpm despite 30 seconds of effective bag and mask (with time given for MRSOPA) in tandem with PPV, plan to intubate.

■ Increase FiO_2 to 100% once chest compressions begin.

■ The method of using two thumbs is preferred as it improves the depth of compressions, is more effective in increasing blood pressure during asphyxia asystole, is more accurate than the hand around the chest method, and is less fatiguing for the provider.
  ● Placement of thumbs should be on the lower one-third of the sternum between the nipples. A compression is straight down (to minimize lung or rib damage) to one-third of the anterior–posterior chest diameter while the hands encircle the chest.
  ● Compressions deeper than one-third of the chest diameter do not improve hemodynamics and increase the risk of injury.

■ Use a 3:1 ratio, with 90 compressions to 30 breaths.

■ The fingers or thumbs should remain on the chest to prevent complications from incorrect placement and unproductive time reestablishing correct placement (Katheria & Finer, 2018; Niermeyer & Clarke, 2021; Pappas & Robey, 2021; Ringer, 2017).

■ Complications may include:
  ● Liver laceration due to dislocation of the xiphoid process may occur if compressions are performed too low on the sternum.
  ● Rib fractures, flail chest when the rib breaks and becomes detached, and pneumothorax may occur if compressions are performed off to the side of the sternum (Niermeyer & Clarke, 2021).

▶ MEDICATIONS USED IN RESUSCITATION

See Chapter 14 for more information.

▶ APGAR SCORING

- The Apgar score guides the evaluation and decisions regarding resuscitation measures. It was designed to monitor neonatal transition and the effectiveness of resuscitation, and their utility remains essentially limited to the role. The scores are somewhat subjective, especially in the assessment of premature infants.
- The Apgar score consists of the total points assigned to five objective signs in the newborn, each sign is evaluated and given a score of 0, 1, or 2. The components of the score are the result of the assessments of infant's HR, respiratory effort, color, grimace elicited, and overall muscle tone. The total scores at 1 and 5 minutes are noted.
- To minimize the chance of adverse sequelae, resuscitation should begin as soon as there is evidence that the infant is unable to establish ventilation sufficient to maintain an adequate HR. Waiting until a 1-minute Apgar score is assigned before initiating resuscitation only delays potential therapies.
  - The 1-minute Apgar score generally correlated with umbilical cord blood pH and is an index of intrapartum depression. It does not correlate with outcome.
  - Apgar scores beyond 1 minute are reflective of the infant's changing condition and the adequacy of resuscitative efforts (Ringer, 2017).
    - ❏ If the 5-minute score is 6 or less (less than 7), then the infant is scored again at 5-minute intervals until it is greater than 6 (equal to or greater than 7; Ali & Sawyer, 2020; Cheffer & Rannalli, 2016; Goldsmith, 2020; Katheria & Finer, 2018; Owen et al., 2022; Pappas & Robey, 2021; Ringer, 2017).

▶ POSTRESUSCITATION CARE

- Infants who required resuscitation after birth have an increased risk of multiple organ injury. These complications may be anticipated and promptly addressed by careful assessment and appropriate monitoring. Even newborns who required only brief (<1 minute) PPV after birth have a higher risk of short-term respiratory and neurologic complications and should have postresuscitation monitoring.
- The goals of postresuscitation care are to evaluate the neonate's condition for complications, avoid intensifying conditions that may impair outcome

(e.g., hypothermia, hypoglycemia), and help diagnose and treat underlying disease.

SURFACTANT IN THE DELIVERY ROOM

- Prophylactic surfactant is still recommended for extremely premature neonate (less than 26 weeks' gestational age) due to the high risk of failing CPAP.
- Administration of surfactant is shown to be beneficial in neonates less than 30 weeks' gestation, even without immediate signs of respiratory distress.
- In cases of infants who fail CPAP, administration of surfactant and removal of the endotracheal tube back to CPAP may be successful (**IN**tubate-**SUR**factant-**E**xtubate or "INSURE"). Surfactant may also be administered using an LMA to avoid intubation.
- Surfactant may be given early (within 30–60 minutes after birth) or late (between 7 and 14 days of age). Early surfactant administration is associated with less time on mechanical ventilation but is not significantly protective against BPD.
- When surfactant is given after birth, rapid compliance changes may equal the need for reduction in pressures delivered.
- The neonatal nurse practitioner (NNP) should refrain from suctioning the infant for at least 4 hours following surfactant administration.

POSTRESUSCITATION ASSESSMENT AND OUTCOME

- After significant resuscitation, close assessment of the infant is crucial. Any or all the following may need to be assessed:
  - Vital signs, including temperature
  - Neurologic status
  - Breath sounds, work of breathing (look for grunting, nasal flaring, retractions, and symmetry of chest movement)
  - Ventilation and oxygenation through arterial (preferable) or capillary blood gases
  - Blood glucose and electrolytes
  - Anemia, hypovolemia, or polycythemia, and hyperviscosity
- Assess capillary refill time as an indication of overall perfusion.
- Infants who do survive a significant resuscitation may require special attention in the hours to days that follow. Frequent complications immediately following resuscitation include hypoglycemia, hypotension, and persistent metabolic acidosis (Ali & Sawyer, 2020; Gardner, Enzman-Hines, & Nyp, 2021; Heideric & Leone, 2020; Katheria & Finer, 2018; Niermeyer & Clarke, 2021; Owen et al., 2022; Pappas & Robey, 2021).

▶ COMPLICATED RESUSCITATION SITUATIONS

AIR LEAK SYNDROME

■ If the infant fails to respond to resuscitation despite apparently effective ventilation, chest compressions, and medication, consider the possibility of air leak syndrome. Pneumothoraces should be assessed for through transillumination and treated if present.

■ An unrecognized pneumothorax could prevent adequate pulmonary inflation and, if under tension, could impair cardiac function. If the pneumothorax is recognized and drained, both gas exchange and circulation can be improved (Ali & Sawyer, 2020; Heideric & Leone, 2020; Katheria & Finer, 2018; Ringer, 2017).

CHOANAL ATRESIA

■ Choanal atresia is a bony or soft tissue obstruction of the posterior nares. It may be unilateral or bilateral. Respiratory distress may be present immediately after birth due to blockage of the primary airway, the nose. Signs include noisy respirations, and cyanosis when not crying and pink when crying. Inability to pass small-gauge suction catheter or nasogastric tube through each nare may indicate choanal atresia (Pappas & Robey, 2021).

CONGENITAL DIAPHRAGMATIC HERNIA

■ Congenital diaphragmatic hernia is one such anomaly that is difficult to recognize on initial inspection of the infant but can cause significant problems with resuscitation. The abdominal organs are displaced into one hemithorax, and the lungs are unable to develop normally, causing ventilation to be quite difficult.

■ Delivery room management should focus on achieving an acceptable preductal oxygen saturation without causing lung injury from high ventilating pressure, excessive tidal volume, and oxygen toxicity. PPV with a face mask should be avoided to prevent gaseous distention of the herniated abdominal contents and increased lung compression.
  ● Cardinal signs include scaphoid abdomen, bowel sounds in the chest, or one-sided decreased breath sounds.
  ● 85% of the defects are found on the left side, as the right side is blocked by the liver (Heideric & Leone, 2020; Katheria & Finer, 2018; Owen et al., 2022; Pappas & Robey, 2021).

■ Maternal anesthesia or narcotic use affecting the infant may present as persistent respiratory depression.

● Reversal of narcotic depression is rarely necessary during the primary steps of resuscitation and is not recommenced.

■ One of the possible complications of intrapartum medication exposure is perinatal respiratory depression after maternal opiate administration. Because opiates can cross the placenta, the fetus may develop respiratory depression from the direct effect of the drug.

■ Naloxone has been used in the past during neonatal resuscitation as an opiate receptor antagonist to reverse the effects of fetal opiate exposure. However, due to a lack of evidence of beneficial effects and possible adverse effects, naloxone hydrochloride is no longer recommended for use in neonatal resuscitation. The infant may require respiratory support until the drug effect wears off (Heideric & Leone, 2020; Katheria & Finer, 2018; Ringer, 2017).

▶ CORD BLOOD GAS

■ In utero, the umbilical cord vein transports oxygenated blood from the placenta to the fetus, and the umbilical arteries transport blood back to the placenta.

■ The umbilical cord arterial blood gas is more valuable than the umbilical cord venous blood gas in determining neonatal acid–base status because it represents both the fetal and uteroplacental states.

■ Umbilical venous blood reflects the uteroplacental state only.

■ Metabolic acidosis occurs when decreased oxygenation leads to increased lactic acid, decreased bicarbonate, and increased base deficit (BD).

■ Cord blood gases provide information on how the fetus' condition is immediately prior to delivery (Table 11.3). The arterial cord gas can be a valuable representation of the fetal acid–base state prior to delivery.

■ If only one cord blood gas is reported, it may be from the umbilical vein, as this vessel is larger and more easily sampled. One clue that a single gas sample is of venous origin is the PaO_2 value. If the reported PaO_2

Table 11.3 Cord Blood Gas Ranges

Measure	Venous	Arterial
pH	7.25–7.45	7.18–7.38
$PaCO_2$ (mmHg)	26.8–49.2	32.2–65.8
PaO_2 (mmHg)	17.2–40.8	5.6–30.8
HCO_3 (mmol/L)	15.8–24.2	17–27
Base deficit (mmol/L)	0–8	0–8

HCO_3, serum bicarbonate level; $PaCO_2$, partial pressure of carbon dioxide in arterial blood; PaO_2, partial pressure of oxygen in arterial blood.
Source: Data from Goldsmith, J. P. (2020). Overview and initial management of delivery room resuscitation. In R. J. Martin, A. A. Fanaroff, & M. C. Walsh (Eds.), *Fanaroff & Martin's neonatal perinatal medicine: Diseases of the fetus and infant* (11th ed., pp. 516–529). Elsevier.

is >31 mmHg, it is highly likely to be a venous sample (Goldsmith, 2020).

- Cord blood samples are performed when events of pregnancy or labor are connected to adverse outcomes in the neonate. These may include:
  - Severe intrauterine growth restriction (IUGR)
  - Abnormal fetal HR tracings
  - Cesarean section for fetal compromise
  - A low 5-minute Apgar score
  - Preterm and postterm infants
  - Multiparous gestations
  - Thick meconium-stained amniotic fluid
- The cord can be saved for sample collection, but blood must be drawn by 1 hour after birth if at room temperature and by 6 hours if refrigerated.
- Adverse neurologic sequelae have been associated with a low arterial cord pH. An arterial cord pH less than 7.0 and a base excess greater than −16 have been used as criteria for therapeutic hypothermia in the treatment of intrapartum asphyxia.
  - The pH as a solo indicator is a poor predictor of long-term outcomes.
  - A pH less than 7.0 with abnormal neurologic assessment is associated with poor outcomes. Encephalopathy is seen in 10% of infants with BD of 12 to 16 mmol/L and in 40% of infants with BD over 16 mmol/L (Goldsmith, 2020; Niermeyer & Clarke, 2021).

▶ NEONATAL TRANSPORT AND REGIONALIZATION

- Regionalization of medical care enhances the ability to centralize resources and has improved patient outcomes. Most experts agree that whenever possible, it is preferable to transfer the mother safely and expeditiously to a center with the necessary resources prior to the delivery of a high-risk newborn.
- In situations in which the risk to the mother outweighs the benefit of their transfer during active labor, the timely dispatch of the neonatal transport team from the regional perinatal center for resuscitation and stabilization of the high-risk neonate may be considered the optimal approach to delivery of care when it occurs.
- When considering transport of neonatal patients, several situations can occur: *intrafacility* for specialty services within a particular institution; and *interfacility*, often between lower and higher levels of service capability, as well as between relatively equivalent levels of service because of capacity or other issues.
- The regionalization of neonatal care has led to the development of specialized teams to transfer infants from outlying hospitals to a higher level of care.
- The composition of the team is less significant than the experience and skill level of the team members. Transport teams often bring a level of care that may not

be available at the referral center and requires a high level of competency.

- The decision regarding the mode of transport is influenced by distance from the referring and receiving facilities and several additional considerations, such as availability of mode of transport, staffing and expertise, patient's current status, capabilities of the referring facility, and weather.
- Currently, there are guidelines but no national absolute criteria or standards to direct the choice of ground versus air transport. Each modality has its own risks and benefits.
- Safety of the transport system and its providers is paramount and must be assessed and ensured before any patient is transported.
- Modes of transport:
  - Ground transport is used most often. Advantages include a larger workspace, ability to accommodate multiple team members, and the option to stop the vehicle to assess the patient. Ground transport is not as weather-dependent and has no need for helipad, but has slower transportation speed.
  - Rotor-wing transport has the advantage of rapid response within a distance of 100 to 150 miles. There is no need for a runway and helicopters are able to avoid common traffic delays and ground obstacles and fly into areas that are otherwise inaccessible to other modes of transport. Disadvantages include the operation expenses, weather, and weight limitations. Helicopter (rotor wing) has no need for a runway but needs a helipad and is faster than ground, but is weather-dependent and has a small work area.
  - Fixed-wing transport is available for distances of approximately 150 miles. This modality has a larger patient cabin than that of a helicopter and the ability to fly above or around inclement weather. It requires an airport for landing and an ambulance to shuttle the medical team and patient to and from the hospital (Gonzalez, 2019; Kleinman, 2017; O'Mahony & Woodward, 2018; Rojas et al., 2021).

LEVELS OF CARE

The AAP and the American College of Obstetricians and Gynecologists in their Guidelines for Perinatal Care established the classifications of perinatal resources according to different levels of care. The levels of care are described as follows:

- *Level I:* well newborn nursery
  - Provide NRP and S.T.A.B.L.E (**S**ugar, **T**emperature, **A**irway, **B**lood pressure, **L**ab work, and **E**motional support), resuscitation at delivery, and postnatal care for stable full-term infants; stabilize and care for infants 35 to 37 weeks if stable; and stabilize ill infants and those less than 35 weeks to prepare for transfer

- *Level II:* special care nursery
  - Care for infants 32 weeks and above, infants after intensive care, and some assisted ventilation; stabilize infants less than 32 weeks for transport
- *Level III:* neonatal intensive care
  - Care for infants less than 32 weeks; provide full respiratory support, including high-frequency ventilation (HFV) and inhaled nitric oxide (iNO), and appropriate support services and subspecialties; and perform MRI and echocardiogram
- *Level IV:* regional NICU
  - Provide level III care, plus provide surgery and facilitate outreach (Kleinman, 2017; O'Mahony & Woodward, 2018; Rojas et al., 2021)

▶ CONCLUSION

The transition from intrauterine to extrauterine existence is a critical time with multiple, important, and necessary physiologic changes occurring simultaneously. Any disruption in these processes can threaten the life of the infant and/or create lifelong morbidities. Although the steps in neonatal resuscitation are clearly outlined by the AAP NRP, the NNP must have a thorough understanding of underlying physiologic principles to not only comprehend the "how to," but perhaps more importantly the "why." A basic tenet of neonatology is providing care appropriate for gestational age, and resuscitation measures must be correctly tailored and adjusted to each delivery to achieve the desired outcomes.

1. The neonatal nurse practitioner (NNP) assesses an infant's response to resuscitative efforts best by assessing the infant's:

    A. Cardiac rhythm
    B. Metabolic status
    C. Pulse oximetry

2. An appropriate situation in which to consider obtaining cord blood gases is when an infant is:

    A. Assigned a 5-minute Apgar of less than 3
    B. Classified as large for gestational age
    C. Noted to have a tight nuchal cord

3. The recommendations for the length of time to delay umbilical cord clamping after delivery of a well newborn is:

    A. 0 to 20 seconds
    B. 30 to 60 seconds
    C. 90 to 120 seconds

4. The MRSOPA mnemonic stands for:

    A. Mask adjustment, reposition airway, stimulation, open mouth, pressure increase gradually, and airway alternative
    B. Mask adjustment, reposition airway, suction, open mouth, pressure increase gradually, and airway alternative
    C. Mask adjustment, reposition airway, suction, oxygen delivery, pressure increase gradually, and airway alternative

5. The neonatal nurse practitioner (NNP) recognizes that, following delivery, infant oxygen saturation (SpO_2) levels should reach 85% to 95% by:

    A. 1 minute of age
    B. 5 minutes of age
    C. 10 minutes of age

6. The most important step in neonatal resuscitation is to:

    A. Assign the Apgar score
    B. Circulate blood volume
    C. Ventilate the lungs

7. The correct point in a neonatal resuscitation when blowby oxygen should be initiated is when the infant's respirations are:

    A. Absent and saturations remain below the target range
    B. Compromised by the infant grunting and retracting
    C. Present but saturations remain below the target range

1. A) Cardiac rhythm

Cardiac monitoring is more accurate than pulse oximetry in determining the infant's response to resuscitation. Pulse oximetry relies on circulation, which may be poor, while the cardiac monitor measures the heart's electrical activity. Assessing metabolic status could potentially delay care (Goldsmith, 2020; Katheria & Finer, 2018; Niermeyer & Clarke, 2021; Owen et al., 2022).

2. A) Assigned a 5-minute Apgar of less than 3

Cord blood samples are performed when events of pregnancy or labor are connected to adverse outcomes in the neonate. These may include severe intrauterine growth restriction (IUGR), abnormal fetal heart rate (HR) tracings, Cesarean section for fetal compromise, a low 5-minute Apgar score, preterm and postterm infants, multiparous gestations, and thick meconium-stained amniotic fluid. The presence of a nuchal cord and the classification as large for gestational age (LGA) alone are not indicators of cord blood gases (Goldsmith, 2020; Niermeyer & Clarke, 2021).

3. B) 30 to 60 seconds

Delayed umbilical cord clamping is defined as a 30- to 60-second pause before clamping the cord to allow for the placental transfusion of blood to the infant. A delay of 0 to 20 seconds is too short, while more than 90 seconds may delay necessary care (Katheria & Finer, 2018).

4. B) Mask adjustment, reposition airway, suction, open mouth, pressure increase gradually, and airway alternative

The MRSOPA acronym is a mnemonic to direct proper resuscitation steps if the neonatal nurse practitioner (NNP) is unable to obtain a seal or there is no chest risk when giving positive pressure ventilation. The MRSOPA mnemonic stands for **M**ask repositioned on the face and checking the seal; **R**epositioning the airway, avoiding hyperextension or flexion of the neck; **S**uctioning the mouth and nose; **O**pening the mouth slightly with the jaw lifted forward; **P**ressure increase gradually; and **A**irway alternative with intubation or laryngeal mask airway. The substitutions of oxygen delivery and stimulation are incorrect procedures (Pappas & Robey, 2021).

5. C) 10 minutes of age

Preductal oxygen levels generally should be above 85% to 95% after 10 minutes. Avoid hyperoxia by using the targeted SpO_2 ranges (Heideric & Leone, 2020; Katheria & Finer, 2018; Niermeyer & Clarke, 2021; Owen et al., 2022; Pappas & Robey, 2021; Ringer, 2017).

6. C) Ventilate the lungs

The goal of resuscitation is to prevent morbidity and mortality. The most important task is to provide effective ventilation. Circulating unoxygenated blood will not promote resuscitation and may prolong neonatal responses. Assignment of an Apgar score is done at the completion of resuscitation (Heideric & Leone, 2020; Katheria & Finer, 2018; Niermeyer & Clarke, 2021; Ringer, 2017).

7. C) Present but saturations remain below the target range

Begin blowby as needed when the heart rate is above 100 beats per minute (bpm) and respiratory rate is adequate but saturations remain below the Neonatal Resuscitation Program (NRP) guidelines. Slowly withdraw oxygen as the infant's saturations reach the target range. Initiating blowby oxygen when respirations are absent is ineffective, and the presence of grunting and retracting indicates the need for positive pressure rather than blowby (Goldsmith, 2020; Niermeyer & Clarke, 2021; Pappas & Robey, 2021; Ringer, 2017).

Growth and Nutrition

Karen Stadd, Hope McKendree, and Emmeline M. Tate

▶ INTRODUCTION

Proper nutrition is imperative to ensure optimal neonatal growth and development. Term infants often successfully accrue the appropriate amount of nutrients in utero. Contrarily, preterm infants present with lower reserves due to limited nutrient accretion rates in utero. The success of the preterm infant's postnatal growth and development is dependent on the management of the infant's medical conditions and nutritional demands. As medical technology continues to improve preterm survival rates, it is crucial to maximize nutritional requirements for optimal growth and development.

▶ PHYSIOLOGY OF DIGESTION AND ABSORPTION

PRINCIPLES OF GASTROINTESTINAL DEVELOPMENT AND FUNCTION

- Morphogenesis and cellular differentiation affect the embryologic formation of the gastrointestinal (GI) tract. However, functional digestive development continues following birth.
- Postnatal GI function and development are influenced by genetic endowment, gut trophic factors, and hormonal regulatory mechanisms involved with enteral feeding initiation and feeding type.
- Maintenance of GI development and function requires interaction with the intrauterine environment, followed with postnatal exogenous environmental exposures (Blackburn, 2018a; Dimmitt et al., 2018; McElroy et al., 2018; Parker, 2021).

EMBRYOLOGY OF THE GASTROINTESTINAL TRACT

- During the fourth week of gestation, a series of folding, lengthening, and luminal dilation results in the formation of the following:

  - Foregut (esophagus, stomach, duodenum, liver, and pancreas)
  - Midgut (jejunum, ileum, ascending colon, and transverse colon)
  - Hindgut (descending colon, sigmoid colon, and rectum)
- Due to rapid growth of the liver during the sixth week of gestation, the small intestines and colon herniate into the umbilical cord, permitting direct communication between the fetal GI tract and the in utero environment. Therefore, the fetal intestinal tract is bathed in amniotic fluid during the early second trimester. Intestinal villi appear during 8 to 11 weeks' gestation, acquiring finger-like shape by 14 weeks' gestation.
- By 20 weeks' gestation, the abdominal contents migrate into the abdominal cavity by rotating counterclockwise around the superior mesenteric artery, resulting in the anterior placement of the colon with the cecum located in the right lower quadrant. During this 270-degree rotation, the duodenum becomes fixed in the retroperitoneal position from the pylorus to the ligament of Treitz. Any failure of rotation and fixation can cause twisting of the bowel, with subsequent interruption of blood flow to the intestines.
- The basic morphogenesis of the fetal GI tract is completed by the second trimester, but additional in utero and postnatal functional maturation is still necessary (Dimmitt et al., 2018; Dingeldein, 2020a; McElroy et al., 2018).

ROLE OF AMNIOTIC FLUID

- Amniotic fluid is considered the first environmental exposure required for GI development, and this fluid may vary in volume and composition over the gestational period. This dynamic fluid initially consists of water and solute from maternal plasma. By the second half of pregnancy, the fetus actively contributes to the volume and composition of amniotic fluid via swallowing and urination.
- Amniotic fluid is enriched with hormones, cytokines, growth factors, nutrients, and other plasma proteins to

facilitate GI development and the associated immune system.

■ Fetal swallowing of amniotic fluid occurs by 8 to 11 weeks' gestation. By the end of the third trimester, amniotic fluid provides approximately 25% of the enteral protein intake of a term breastfed infant (McElroy et al., 2018; Poindexter & Martin, 2020).

MECONIUM PRODUCTION

■ Meconium consists of ingested amniotic fluid, lanugo, intestinal cells, bile salts, and pancreatic enzymes that are created by or swallowed by the fetus in utero. Meconium is first found at 10 to 12 weeks and moves into the colon by 16 weeks. Small amounts may enter the amniotic fluid in the second trimester before the development of anal sphincter function at 20 to 22 weeks' gestation (Blackburn, 2018a).

▶ GASTROINTESTINAL DEVELOPMENT

■ Phases of GI development span from early embryogenesis to the introduction of solid foods in late infancy to early childhood.
  ● *Phase 1:* This phase involves embryonic organogenesis and primitive gut formation (0–5 weeks' gestation).
  ● *Phase 2:* The GI tract becomes a tubular structure with the formation of villi, initiating the functional role of the intestinal epithelium (6–20 weeks' gestation).
  ● *Phase 3:* At this phase, there is rapid linear intestinal growth and cellular differentiation for specific physiologic functions (20–40 weeks' gestation).
  ● *Phase 4:* The intestinal microbiome is established immediately after birth from environmental exposures, including response to dietary factors present in human milk or formula (birth to 5 months).
  ● *Phase 5:* Refinement and maturation of structural intestinal development and mucosal immunity occur after weaning from breast milk or formula while introducing solid food (>5–6 months, after weaning; McElroy et al., 2018).

FUNCTIONAL DEVELOPMENT

■ GI organs develop and acquire different digestive capacities during embryogenesis.
■ Intestinal transport of amino acids (AAs) is seen by 14 weeks of gestation, followed by intestinal transport of glucose by 18 weeks' gestation and fatty acid by 24 weeks' gestation.
■ Major gut-regulating polypeptides (gastrin, motilin, cholecystokinin, pancreatic polypeptide, and somatostatin) act locally to regulate gut growth and development. They are present in limited amounts by the end of the first trimester and reach adult distribution by term.

■ Gastric gland secretion activity is seen by 20 weeks of gestation.
■ Lingual and gastric lipase are present by 26 weeks' gestation in limited volume and function (Blackburn, 2018a; Dimmitt et al., 2018; Parker, 2021).

Functions of the Gastrointestinal Tract

■ The primary function of the GI tract is digestion and absorption of ingested nutrients from food. The small intestine is responsible for digestion and absorption of nutrients, whereas the colon absorbs more than 80% of water left after passage through the small intestine.
■ The GI tract serves as the largest defense barrier and immune organ in the body by protecting against dietary and environmental antigens (Dingeldein, 2020a; McElroy et al., 2018).

IMMUNITY

■ Colonization of bacteria within the GI tract is acquired after birth with the introduction of environmental influences and food. Development of the gut microbiome is also influenced by the mode of delivery, maternal health conditions, early exposure to antibiotics, and the composition of nutrition (breast milk vs. formula).
■ Physical and chemical barriers within the GI tract prevent epithelial adherence and translocation of pathogens between paracellular spaces. The first layer of immune defenses includes the acidic stomach environment, compounded with numerous digestive enzymes and bile salts along the entire GI tract. Gastric acid, bile salts, and pancreatic secretions inhibit potential pathogenic bacterial growth.
■ Healthy intestinal microbiomes are necessary to compete with pathogenic organisms for cell surface binding sites. Consequently, protective gut flora regulates intestinal inflammation by increasing the production of anti-inflammatory cytokines and decreasing proinflammatory cytokines.
■ Preterm infants are at increased risk of altered mucosal immunity and intestinal bacterial colonization due to an underdeveloped immune system, hospital environmental exposures, and medical interventions.
■ Delayed or absent enteral nutrition leads to a lack of luminal nutrients, resulting in decreased intestinal mass, mucosal enzyme activity, and gut permeability (Brown et al., 2021; Dimmitt et al., 2018; McElroy et al., 2018; Parker, 2021; Poindexter & Martin, 2020).

DIGESTION

■ Digestion consists of the breakdown of carbohydrates, proteins, and fats into smaller molecules (monosaccharides, oligopeptides, AAs, free fatty acids, and monoglycerides), which are transported into absorptive intestinal epithelial cells, followed by the portal circulation.

- Biochemical and physiologic capacities for limited digestion and absorption are present by 28 weeks' gestation.
- Enteroglucagon promotes intestinal mucosal growth. Gastrin stimulates gastric mucosa and exocrine pancreas growth. Motilin and neurotensin stimulate the development of gut motility.
  - Preterm infants are born with an underdeveloped GI tract. There is limited production of gut digestive enzymes and growth factor. Decreased gut absorption of lipids occurs from low levels of pancreatic lipase, bile acids, and lingual lipase.
- Enteral feeding is a major stimulus for hormonal regulatory mechanisms needed to mediate gut development after birth in both preterm and term infants (Blackburn, 2018a; Dimmitt et al., 2018; Parker, 2021).

Gastrointestinal Motility

- *GI motility* refers to the coordinated movement of food from ingestion to elimination, including suck–swallow, esophageal, stomach, and intestinal peristalsis.
- Immature gut motility and gastric emptying are a major limitation to enteral digestion, which progressively improves after 30 to 32 weeks' gestation until term.
- Passage of meconium is an essential step in the initiation of intestinal function. Most full-term infants pass meconium within 48 hours of birth.
- Preterm infants are more likely to have a delay in the passage of meconium secondary to the immaturity of gut motility patterns; however, almost 70% of preterm infants will pass meconium by 48 hours of age (Blackburn, 2018a; Parker, 2021; Taylor et al., 2018).

▶ ASSESSMENT OF NEONATAL GROWTH

- Accretion of most nutrients occurs during the later portion of the second trimester and throughout the third trimester in preparation for a term delivery.
- Term infants have adequate minerals, glycogen, and fat stores to meet the demands of the first few days of relative starvation experienced immediately after birth.
- Nutrient stores of fat, glycogen, iron, calcium, and phosphorus are established during the last trimester. Consequently, preterm infants have minimal nutrient stores and higher nutrient requirements compared with full term infants. Links between neurodevelopmental impairment and early nutrition are well established (Anderson et al., 2017).

GROWTH AND NUTRITIONAL ASSESSMENT

- Postnatal growth begins with a period of weight loss, primarily due to extracellular water loss. Consequently, it is recommended to use the birth weight for nutritional calculations until birth weight is regained.

- Expected postnatal weight loss in the term infant can range from 5% to 10% of birth weight and usually reaches the lowest point by the third day of life. Early and optimal nutrition is essential for the attenuation of weight loss and a faster return to birth weight. Unless appropriate nutritional therapy is provided, infants rapidly expend their limited nutrient reserve of glycogen and nitrogen, resulting in hypoglycemia and catabolism. Early nutritional deficits can take weeks to months to replenish.
- Preterm infants are at higher risk for postnatal growth failure for many reasons, mainly the deficit between the nutritional needs and the nutrition provided.
  - These infants often receive less protein and calories than necessary for protein accretion and body growth immediately following birth.
  - In addition, these infants have increased energy expenditure due to environmental factors, including losses from low humidity and radiant and convective heat losses.
  - There are also the physiologic demands of maintaining normothermia, breathing, resistance to gravity, the process of digestion, absorption, and the synthesis of nutrients into body structure.
  - Stress-induced hormones, such as corticosteroids and catecholamines, are catabolic and limit the production and action of anabolic growth factors, particularly insulin and insulin-like growth factors (IGFs). This further prevents normal rates of growth and weight gain.
- The principal factor causing postnatal growth failure and unfavorable neurodevelopmental outcomes is delayed and inadequate intake of protein and energy.
- The accepted goal of postnatal nutrition in preterm infants is to achieve and maintain the comparable rate of intrauterine growth.
- See Table 12.1 for the goals of postnatal anthropometric growth in the preterm infant.
- At a minimum, infant growth monitoring should consist of a daily weight. The extremely low birthweight (ELBW) infant may require more frequent checks with the rapidly changing extracellular fluid status in the first few days of life. Monitoring weight gain on a weekly basis in grams per kilogram of weight gained daily (g/kg/d) may help in reducing postnatal growth restriction and positively affect long-term neurodevelopmental outcomes.
  - Linear growth and head circumference (HC) represent lean mass growth and may be beneficial in predicting neurodevelopmental outcomes. Measure length and HC weekly and plot on a growth chart.
- Utilization of a length board should be encouraged and can increase the validity of the measurements. The accuracy of the measurement can be improved by utilizing the tonic–neck reflex to straighten the hip and the knee (Adamkin & Radmacher, 2020; Anderson et al., 2017; Bell, 2021; Brown et al., 2021; Olsen et al., 2021).

Table 12.1 Goals for Postnatal Anthropometric Growth in the Preterm Infant

Gestational Age	Weight Gain
24–32 wk	15–20 g/kg/d
33–36 wk	14–15 g/kg/d
37–40 wk	7–9 g/kg/d
Corrected/adjusted age	
40 wk–3 mo	30 g/d
3–6 mo	12 g/d
6–9 mo	15 g/d
9–12 mo	10 g/d
Other anthropometric measures	
Length	1 cm/wk
Head circumference	1 cm/wk

Sources: Data from Adamkin, D., & Radmacher, P. (2020). Nutrition and selected disorders of the gastrointestinal tract. In A. Fanaroff & J. Fanaroff (Eds.), *Klaus and Fanaroff's care of the high-risk neonate* (7th ed., pp. 80–120). Elsevier; Anderson, D., Poindexter, B., & Martin, C. (2017). Nutrition. In E. Eichenwald, A. Hansen, C. Martin, & A. Stark (Eds.), *Cloherty and Stark's manual of neonatal care* (8th ed., pp. 248–284). Wolters Kluwer; Blackburn, S. (2018a). Gastrointestinal and hepatic systems and perinatal nutrition. In S. Blackburn (Ed.), *Maternal, fetal, & neonatal physiology: A clinical perspective* (pp. 420–434). Elsevier/Saunders.

POSTNATAL GROWTH VELOCITY

- Extremely preterm infants with a suboptimal growth trajectory while hospitalized are more likely to have weight, length, and HC below the 10th percentile at 18 months' corrected age.
- Optimal nutrition is essential for the attainment of appropriate growth and development. Therefore, it is important for the clinician to continuously assess the infant's nutritional status.
  - The nutritional assessment should include the infant's gestational age, intrauterine growth, and nutrition, as well as an assessment of the current nutritional status and an evaluation over time.
  - Nonnutritional status, including illness, medications, and stress (surgery and infection), should also be assessed.
  - It may be difficult to assess growth measurements in preterm infants during the first week of life due to calorie and fluid restrictions as a result of illness (Adamkin & Radmacher; Colaizy et al., 2018).

Weight

- It is important to obtain weights on the same scale and at the same time daily. The addition or subtraction of equipment should be noted, and an assessment of whether weight gain is reflective of true growth (new tissue deposition), excess fat deposition, or water retention should be completed.
- Weight gain should be expressed as g/kg/d in preterm infants.

- To calculate:

  (Change in weight in kg ÷ Current weight in kg)
  ÷ Number of days = g/kg/d

  - *Example:* A preterm infant weighs 1,500 g today. Seven days ago, the infant weighed 1,300 g. What is the daily weight gain in g/kg/d over the last 7 days?

  $$1{,}500 \text{ g} - 1{,}300 \text{ g} = 200 \text{ g in weight gain over 7 days}$$
  $$200 \text{ g} \div 1.5 \text{ kg} = 133.33 \text{ g/kg}$$
  $$133.33 \text{ g/kg} \div 7 \text{ days} = 19 \text{ g/kg/d}$$

- The average goal for a preterm infant's weight gain is 15 to 20 g/kg/d.
- Weight loss or inadequate weight gain is the initial effect of inadequate caloric intake (Adamkin & Radmacher, 2020; Brown et al., 2021; Olsen et al., 2021).

Length

- Lean mass growth is represented by an increase in length. Prolonged periods of inadequate nutrition can affect linear growth (Brown et al., 2021).

Head Circumference

- In normal infants, HC growth correlates with brain development.
- The rate of head growth for the sick preterm infant, during a period of acute illness, is less than that of the normal fetus. Head growth is comparable with that of the normal fetus during recovery, and therefore rapid "catch-up" growth in HC may occur. Despite high energy intake, normal head growth does not occur until the acute illness has recovered. The longer the infant has a suboptimal head size, the greater the neurodevelopmental risk.
- As a result of "brain sparing, HC growth is the least affected with inadequate nutrition" (Adamkin & Radmacher, 2020; Olsen et al., 2021).
- See Table 12.2 for the growth velocity of preterm infants from term to 24 months.

Ponderal Index

- Also known as the weight–length index, ponderal index is used to assess the quality of an infant's growth. Credible tissue accretion and organ growth are appreciated with an increase in both weight and length, which can be assessed using this index (Brown et al., 2021).

Growth Charts

- Growth charts provide a method of tracking serial weights, length, and HC measurements. Several charts are available; however, Fenton and Olsen charts are used for preterm infants. The Fenton chart allows the infant to be monitored from 22 to 50 weeks' postmenstrual age (Figures 12.1 and 12.2).

Table 12.2 Growth Velocity of Preterm Infants From Term to 24 Months

Age From Term (months)	Weight (g/d)	Length (cm/month)	Head Circumference (cm/month)
1	26–40	3–4.5	1.6–2.5
4	15–25	2.3–3.6	0.8–1.4
8	12–17	1–2	0.3–0.8
12	9–12	0.8–1.5	0.2–0.4
18	4–10	0.7–1.3	0.1–0.4

Source: Reproduced with permission from Adamkin, D., & Radmacher, P. (2020). Nutrition and selected disorders of the gastrointestinal tract. In A. Fanaroff & J. Fanaroff (Eds.), *Klaus and Fanaroff's care of the high-risk neonate* (6th ed., pp. 80–120). Elsevier.

- Term-infant growth charts also include incremental growth curves for weight, length, and HC, and are developed by the National Center for Health Statistics and the National Center for Chronic Disease Prevention and Health Promotion (Anderson et al., 2017; Parker, 2021).

Laboratory Assessment

- Electrolytes:
  - Sodium, potassium, chloride, and bicarbonate are used to assess renal function and fluid status.
- Blood urea nitrogen (BUN) and creatinine (Cr):
  - In the first weeks of life, BUN is not an accurate marker of protein intake or tolerance in the preterm infant. During this period, it should not be utilized as a biochemical marker as it reflects the fluid status. Cr and Cr clearance are appropriate biochemical markers for renal function assessment in the preterm infant.
  - The BUN level does not usually correlate with AA intake during the first postnatal weeks, even with changes in renal function. Studies have demonstrated safety with early protein administration without abnormal elevations of ammonia or BUN levels.
- Plasma triglyceride levels:
  - Monitor plasma triglycerides prior to initiating lipids, after each increase in the dose, and weekly thereafter. Aim to maintain a serum triglyceride level less than 200 mg/dL.
- Calcium, magnesium, phosphorus, and alkaline phosphatase:
  - Calcium, phosphorus, and alkaline phosphatase are used to assess metabolic bone disease and bone mineralization status.
  - Decreased calcium and phosphorus levels or increased alkaline phosphatase levels (levels greater than 500 mg/dL) are indicators of bone demineralization.
  - Magnesium is important for plasma membrane excitability, energy storage, transfer, and production. Additionally, it is significant in calcium and bone homeostasis.
- Elevated alkaline phosphatase levels generally precede radiographic changes by approximately 2 to 4 weeks.

- Serum phosphorus levels of <4 mg/dL may be early signs of decreased bone mineralization.
- Calcium levels may remain normal despite depletion of calcium bone stores.
- Vitamin D:
  - Vitamin D levels are important to assess when evaluating for metabolic bone disease of prematurity, also called *rickets of prematurity*. 25-hydroxycholecalciferol (25-OH vitamin D) levels are usually normal, while 1,25 dihydroxycholecalciferol (1,25-OH vitamin D) levels may be elevated due to increased parathyroid hormone levels and low serum phosphorus levels.
- Serum total protein, albumin, transferrin, retinol-binding protein, and transthyretin (prealbumin):
  - These biochemical markers can be used to assess protein malnutrition. The latter two are mainly indicative for premature infants. This monitoring is necessary to avoid total parenteral nutrition (TPN) complications (Adamkin & Radmacher, 2020; Denne, 2018; Olsen et al., 2021; Parker, 2021).

▶ NUTRITIONAL REQUIREMENTS FOR TERM INFANTS

- The goal of parenteral nutrition (PN) therapy is to provide adequate nutrients to prevent energy deficiency and negative nitrogen balance. In addition to prevention of negative balances, the goal is to promote appropriate weight gain and growth in the newborn until adequate enteral calories can be achieved.
- Indications for PN in newborns include very low birth weight (VLBW) and ELBW infants, infants with congenital and/or surgical disorders (e.g., gastroschisis, tracheal esophageal fistula, malrotation, obstruction, necrotizing enterocolitis [NEC], intestinal perforation, short bowel syndrome), and infants with renal failure. The sick term infant may also require PN. PN should be initiated on the first day of life for these infants (Anderson et al., 2017; Olsen et al., 2021; Parker, 2020).

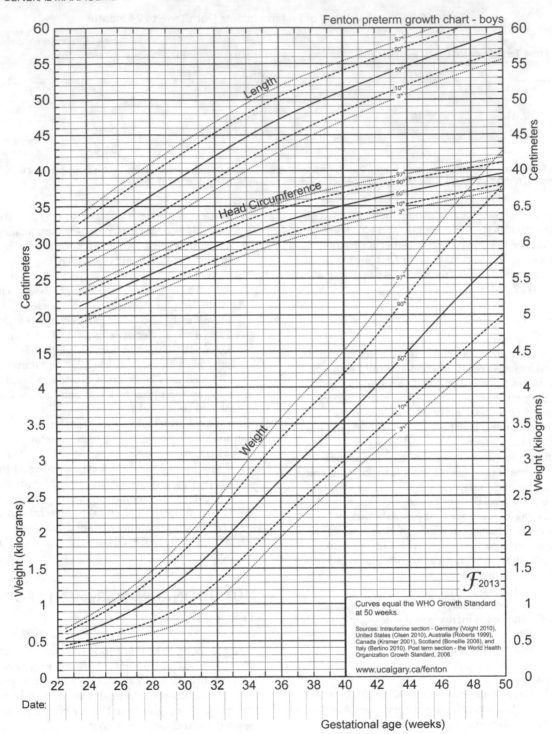

Figure 12.1 Fenton preterm growth chart for boys.

WHO, World Health Organization.
Source: Reproduced with permission from Fenton, T. (2013). *Fenton preterm growth chart site*. University of Calgary.

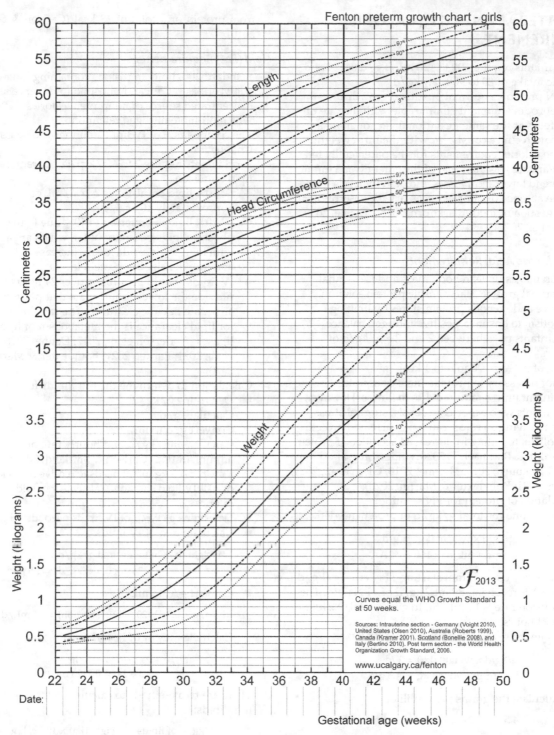

Figure 12.2 Fenton preterm growth chart for girls.

WHO, World Health Organization.

Source: Reproduced with permission from Fenton, T. (2013). *Fenton preterm growth chart site*. University of Calgary.

PARENTERAL ENERGY (CALORIE) REQUIREMENTS

- Term infants require 100 to 120 mL/kg/d of PN and a caloric intake of 80 to 90 kcal/kg/d.
  - PN promotes optimal postnatal growth and neurodevelopment comparable with the rate of a fetus at the same gestational age, or along a growth curve consistent with the birth weight.
  - The caloric requirements for the parenterally fed infant are less than that of the enterally fed infant due to lower fecal losses and activity levels (and the absence of calories necessary for absorption and digestion of food; Blackburn, 2018a; Denne, 2018 Parker, 2021).

Protein (Amino Acid) Requirements

- Protein makes up lean body mass and is essential for optimal growth. Early ample protein solutions preserve endogenous protein stores by limiting catabolism to ensure a positive nitrogen balance.
- Term infants need between 2 and 2.5 g/kg/d of protein.
  - 1 g of protein is equal to 4 kcal/g.
- It is not necessary to provide increased protein for the term infant unless required due to illness. However, term infants who experience sepsis, surgical stress, or are receiving steroids can have increased protein catabolism, resulting in decreased accretion of protein (Adamkin & Radmacher, 2020; Anderson et al., 2017; Blackburn, 2018a; Denne, 2018; Olsen et al., 2021; Parker, 2021; Poindexter & Martin, 2020).
- Calculation of protein for PN solution:
  - Determine the total g/kg/d of protein needed.

$$\text{g/kg/d} \times \text{weight (kg)} = \text{g/d}$$
$$(\text{g/d} \div \text{mL/d}) \times 100 = \% \text{ AA}$$

  - *Example:* A 3-kg infant starting TPN at 1.5 g/kg/d of AA is receiving 80 mL/kg/d of TPN fluid. The infusion rate is 10 mL/hr, to give a total of 240 mL in 24 hours.
- Calculate the grams of AA to add to TPN:

$$\text{g/kg/d} \times \text{weight (kg)} = \text{g/d}$$
$$1.5 \text{ g/kg/d} \times 3 \text{ kg} = 4.5 \text{ g/d}$$

  - Calculate the grams per milliliter:

$$4.5 \text{ g/d} \div 240 \text{ mL} = 0.1875 \text{ g/mL}$$

- Calculate the grams of AA per 100 mL of base solution or the % AA:
  Example: 0.1875 g/mL × 100 mL = 1.875 g of AA added to every 100 mL of base solution or 1.875% AA in the solution
- Calculate kilocalorie per kilogram delivered from protein:

$$1 \text{ g of protein} = 4 \text{ kcal}$$
$$4.5 \text{ g/d} \times 4 \text{ kcal/g} = 18 \text{ kcal}$$
$$OR$$
$$1.5 \text{ g/kg/d of AA} \times 4 \text{ kcal/g} = 6 \text{ kcal/kg/d}$$

from protein or a total of 18 kcal (Carlson & Shirland, 2010).

Lipid (Fat) Requirements

- Standard 20% lipid emulsions containing long-chain triglycerides (LCTs) and phospholipids serve as a concentrated source of nonprotein calories (NPC), which promote nitrogen retention.
- The composition of IV lipid solutions is discussed in Chapter 13.
- Term infants require 2 to 4 g/kg/d of parenteral, IV lipid emulsion.
  - IV 20% lipid emulsion is 2 kcal/mL or approximately 10 kcal/g.
  - IV 20% lipid is preferred to 10% due to fewer phospholipids per gram of fat, which are associated with high triglyceride levels, increased cholesterol, and low-density lipoprotein levels.
  - IV lipids should be infused over 24 hours to provide the lowest hourly rate that permits adequate hepatic clearance. The rate-limiting step for lipid clearance is the metabolism of lipoprotein lipases (Anderson et al., 2017; Denne, 2018; Olsen et al., 2021; Parker, 2021; Poindexter & Martin, 2020).
- Calculation to determine the intralipids for PN:
  - Determine g/kg/d.
  - Calculate g/d.
  - Convert g/d to mL/d.
  - Calculate mL/kg/d and hourly rate of administration (Carlson & Shirland, 2010).
  - *Example:* A 3-kg infant needs to receive 0.5 g/kg/d of 20% IV lipid solution. Calculate the fluid rate and calories.
  - Determine g/kg/d of IV lipids needed: 0.5 g/kg/d.
  - Calculate g/d of IV lipids.

$$\text{Weight of infant} \times \text{desired g/kg/d} = \text{g/d}$$
$$3 \text{ kg} \times 0.5 \text{ g/kg/d} = 1.5 \text{ g/d}$$

  - Convert g/d to mL/d.

$$1.5 \text{ d/g} \div 0.2 \text{ (IV 20\% lipid solution)} = 7.5 \text{ mL/d}$$

  - Calculate mL/hr of IV lipids.

$$\text{mL/d} \div 24 \text{ hr/d} = \text{mL/hr}$$
$$7.5 \div 24 = 0.3125 \text{ mL/hr}$$

- There are two methods to calculate calories from intralipids:

$$\text{g/kg/d of lipids} \times \text{weight (kg)} \times 10 \text{ kcal/g}$$

Example: A 3-kg term infant receives 0.5 g/kg of IV 20% lipid emulsion. How many kcal/kg is delivered?

$$0.5 \text{ g/kg of IV 20 \% lipid emulsion}$$
$$\times 10 \text{ kcal/g} = 5 \text{ kcal/kg mL/d}$$
$$\times 2 \text{ kcal/mL of lipid}$$

Example: A 3-kg term infant receives 7.5 mL of IV 20% lipid emulsion per day. How many kcal/kg/d is delivered?

$$7.5 \text{ mL/d} \times 2 \text{ kcal/mL} \div 3 \text{ kg} = 5 \text{ kcal/kg}$$

Carbohydrate (Glucose) Requirements

- Glucose is considered the IV source of carbohydrate and the key energy substrate for the infant receiving PN. Glucose is the primary energy substrate for the brain.
- With long-term PN, at least 50% of total calories should be provided as carbohydrates (Adamkin & Radmacher, 2020; Olsen et al., 2021; Poindexter & Martin, 2020).

GLUCOSE INFUSION RATE

- The glucose infusion rate (GIR) maintains normal plasma glucose concentrations to meet energy requirement demands. Endogenous glucose production is estimated at 4 mg/kg/min.
- An appropriate GIR for a full-term infant is approximately 3 to 5 mg/kg/min. Preterm infants require a higher GIR of 6 to 9 mg/kg/min.
  - 1 g of dextrose is equal to 3.4 kcal.
  - Maximize nutrition delivery by advancing the GIR by 1 to 2 mg/kg/min as able by increasing dextrose concentration and/or infusion rate to maximize caloric delivery without causing iatrogenic hyperglycemia (Anderson et al., 2017; Denne, 2018; Olsen et al., 2021; Poindexter & Martin, 2020).
- Glucose calculations for PN:
- Calculate the percentage of dextrose from the desired GIR.

$$mg/kg/min\,(desired) \times kg = mg/min\ of\ glucose$$
$$mg/min \div 1{,}000\ mg/g = g/min$$
$$g/min \times 1{,}440\ min/d = g/d$$
$$g/d \div total\ mL/d \times 100 = \%\ dextrose$$

  - *Example:* A 3-kg term infant is going to receive 80 mL/kg/d. The nurse practitioner would like to administer a GIR of 6 mg/kg/min. What percent dextrose should the practitioner order?
- Calculate mL/kg/d.

$$80\ mL/kg/d \times 3\ kg = 240\ mL/d\ of\ IV\ fluids$$

- Calculate the percentage of dextrose needed from the desired mg/kg/min (6 mg/kg/min).

$$mg/kg/min\ (desired) \times kg = mg/min\ of\ glucose$$
$$6\ mg/kg/min \times 3\ kg = 18\ mg/min\ of\ glucose$$
$$18\ mg/min \div 1{,}000\ mg/g = 0.018\ g/min\ of\ glucose$$
$$mg\ 1{,}000\ mg/g = g/min\ of\ glucose$$
$$g/min\ of\ glucose = g/d\ of\ glucose$$
$$\times 1{,}440\ min/d$$
$$0.018\ g/min\ of\ glucose = 25.92\ g/d$$
$$\times 1{,}440\ min/d$$
$$g/d \div mL/d\ (80\ mL/kg/d) \times 100 = \%\ dextrose\ needed$$
$$25.92\ g/d \div 240\ mL/d \times 100 = 10.8\%\ dextrose\ needed$$

- Calculate GIR from known dextrose concentration (%).

$$\%\ dextrose \div 100 \times mL/d = g/d$$
$$g/d \div 1{,}440\ min/d = g/min$$
$$g/min \times 1{,}000\ mg/g = mg/min$$
$$mg/min \div kg = mg/kg/min$$

Example: A term infant weighs 3 kg and is receiving 100 mL/kg/d of dextrose 15% solution.

$$mL/kg/d \times weight\ in\ kilogram = mL/d$$
$$100 \times 3 = 300\ mL/d\ of\ dextrose\ 15\%\ IV\ fluids$$
$$\%\ dextrose \div 100 \times mL/d = g/d$$
$$15 \div 100 \times 300\ mL/d = 45\ g/d$$
$$g/d \div 1{,}440\ min/d = g/min$$
$$45\ g/d \div 1{,}440\ min/d = 0.03125\ g/min$$
$$g/min \times 1{,}000\ mg/g = mg/min$$
$$mg/min \div kg = mg/kg/min$$
$$31.3\ mg/min \div 3\ kg = 10.4\ mg/kg/min$$

ENTERAL ENERGY (CALORIE) REQUIREMENTS

- The enteral caloric intake requirement for term and near-term infants is 100 to 120 kcal/kg/d.
- Breastfed term newborns require slightly less caloric intake than formula-fed term newborns for maintenance and growth due to the amount of energy required to metabolize the formula (Blackburn, 2018a; Parker, 2021).

Protein (Amino Acid) Requirements

- Enteral protein requirements range from 2 to 2.5 g/kg/d.
- Protein intake can be calculated based on the feeding regimen of the infant due to varying protein content of the formula versus breast milk (Parker, 2021).
- Calculation of enteral protein:
  - Calculate the total volume of feeds per day.
  - Determine how many grams of protein per 100 mL are in the current food.

$$Total\ mL\ of\ feed \times Protein\ content\ of\ feed = Total\ protein\ per\ day$$

  - *Example:* A 3.5-kg term infant is receiving 50 mL of unfortified human milk every 3 hours. How many grams of protein is the infant receiving?
  - Calculate the total volume of feeds per day.

$$50\ mL \times 8\ feeds\ (infant\ feeds\ every\ 3\ hours) = 400\ mL$$

  - Determine how many grams of protein per 100 mL are in breast milk.
  - Mature human milk has 0.9 g of protein per 100 mL.

$$Total\ mL\ of\ feed \times Protein\ content\ of\ feed = Total\ protein\ per\ day$$
$$400\ mL \times 0.9\ g/100\ mL = 3.6\ g\ of\ protein\ per\ day$$
$$Total\ g\ of\ protein\ per\ day = g/kg\ of\ protein \div Weight\ in\ kg$$
$$3.6\ g \div 3.5\ kg = 1.03\ g/kg\ of\ protein$$

Lipid (Fat) Requirements

- Enteral fat requirements for term infants range from 3 to 4 g/kg/d (Parker, 2021).
- Calculation of enteral fat:
- Calculate the total volume of feeds per day.
- Determine how many grams of fat per 100 mL are in the current feed.

Total mL of feed × Fat content of feed = Total fat per day

Total g of fat per day ÷ Weight in kg = g/kg of fat

- *Example:* A 3.5-kg term infant receives 50 mL of unfortified human milk every 3 hours. How many grams of fat does the infant receive?
- Calculate the total volume of feeds per day.

50 mL × 8 feeds (infant feeds every 3 hours) = 400 mL/d

- Determine how many grams of fat per 100 mL are in the current feed.
- Mature human milk has 3.5 g of fat per 100 mL.

Total mL of feed × Fat content of feed = Total fat per day

400 mL × 3.5 g fat/100 mL = 14 g of fat per day

Total g of fat per day ÷ Weight in kg = g/kg of fat

14 g ÷ 3.5 kg = 4 g/kg of fat

Carbohydrate (Lactose/Oligosaccharides) Requirements

- Term infants require approximately 40% of daily carbohydrate intake, or 8 to 12 g/kg/d enterally (Parker, 2021).
- To calculate enteral in kcal/kg/d:

Multiply g/kg/d × 3.4 kcal/g of carbohydrates = kcal/kg/d

Multiply kcal × Weight in kg = total kcal/d

OR

- Determine total enteral intake per day.

(Total volume of feeds in mL × [kcal of feed ÷ 30]) ÷ Weight in kg

- *Example:* A term 3.5-kg infant is receiving 8 g/kg/d of carbohydrates from enteral nutrition. How many kcal/kg/d does the infant receive?

g/kg/d × 3.4 kcal/g = kcal/kg/d of carbohydrates

8 g/kg/d × 3.4 kcal/g = 27.2 kcal/kg/d of carbohydrates

kcal × weight = Total kcal/d in kg

27.2 kcal × 3.5 kg = 95.2 total kcal from carbohydrates

- *Example:* A term 3.5-kg infant is receiving human milk fortified to 22 kcal/oz. The infant eats 60 mL every 3 hours. How many kcal/kg/d does the infant receive?

- Determine total enteral intake per day.

60 mL × 8 meals a day = 480 mL/d

$$\left(\frac{\text{Total volume of feeds}}{\text{Weight in kg/mL}}\right) \times [\text{kcal of feed} \div 30]$$

(480 mL × [22 kcal/oz ÷ 30]) ÷ 3.5 kg = 100 kcal/kg/d

- For the term infant, human milk can be fortified with powdered infant formula, medium-chain triglycerides (MCT) or corn oil, and/or SolCarb, also known as maltodextrin. Fortification should occur in 2 to 3 kcal/oz increments, with a maximum of 30 kcal/oz (Anderson et al., 2017).

▶ NUTRITIONAL REQUIREMENTS OF PRETERM INFANTS

GENERAL CONSIDERATIONS

- The goal of nutritional support for the high-risk infant is to provide postnatal support that will mimic in utero growth. Nutritional intake should account for tissue losses while permitting tissue accretion.
- Maximal nutritional support for the preterm infant is limited by the functional immaturity of the renal, GI, and metabolic systems, as well as any acute illnesses.
- Preterm infants are deprived of the fat, glycogen, iron, calcium, and phosphorus stores that accrue during the third trimester of pregnancy. The nutrient that is always limiting growth is protein. Sodium is considered a possible growth hormone in preterm infants, which may be deficient when having failure to thrive.
- Preterm infants require 120 to 150 mL/kg/d of fluid parenterally and 150 to 200 mL/kg/d enterally. See the calculation examples provided to equate this delivery into calories.
- The use of larger volumes of fluid (160–180 mL/kg/d) to prevent weight loss can increase the risk of developing patent ductus arteriosus (PDA), cerebral intraventricular hemorrhage (IVH), bronchopulmonary dysplasia (BPD), and NEC.
  - Mild fluid restriction that does not lead to dehydrations may decrease the incidence and/or severity of PDA, NEC, and BPD.
  - Preterm infants who develop postnatal growth failure may be at increased risk of neurodevelopmental delays (Adamkin & Radmacher, 2020; Brown et al., 2021; Parker, 2021; Wright et al., 2018).

Energy (Calorie) Requirements

- Preterm infant energy requirements are determined by total energy expenditure, energy excretion, and energy stored in new tissue for growth. Total energy expenditure comprises basal metabolic rate, thermoregulation, activity, digestion, and metabolism. Energy excretion encompasses heat loss by radiation and evaporation, as well as fecal and urinary losses.

- Extremely preterm infants require approximately 50 to 70 kcal/kg/d for weight maintenance and an additional 45 to 70 kcal/kg/d above maintenance for growth.
  - The European Society for Paediatric Gastroenterology, Hepatology and Nutrition (ESPGHAN) recommends an energy intake of 110 to 135 kcal/kg/d for preterm infants.
  - Small-for-gestational-age (SGA) infants and infants with increased metabolic needs, such as infants with intrauterine growth restriction (IUGR) who have a higher basal metabolic rate per kilogram body weight, may require higher energy intake to attain adequate growth (Adamkin & Radmacher, 2020; Poindexter & Martin, 2020).

Parenteral Energy (Calorie) Requirements

- Caloric needs of infants receiving PN are lower than infants enterally fed due to lower activity levels and fecal losses (Denne, 2018).
- Goal calories for full PN in the extremely preterm infants are 90 to 100 kcal/kg/d (Table 12.3).
  - An increase in caloric intake above 120 kcal/kg/d through the addition of calories does not result in proportionate increases in weight gain. The higher the caloric intake, the higher the energy consumed through excretion, tissue synthesis, and diet-induced thermogenesis.
  - An increase in the enteral protein-to-energy ratio is necessary to increase lean body mass and decrease fat deposition.
- In the parenterally fed preterm infant, NPCs are derived from glucose and lipids.
  - Providing a balanced carbohydrate and lipid approach (60:40) to NPCs improves protein accretion and minimizes overall energy expenditure.
  - Excess energy expenditure occurs if a disproportionate amount of NPCs is given as glucose. Even at a higher protein intake, a parenterally fed extremely preterm infant may require 80 to 90 kcal/kg of nonprotein energy supplies for growth (Adamkin & Radmacher, 2020; Blackburn, 2018a; Denne, 2018; Poindexter & Martin, 2020).

Protein Amino Acid Requirements

- The fetus receives a continuous supply of AAs via active transport from the placenta.
- Fetal protein accretion is 3 to 4 g/kg/d. The goal of providing AAs is to mimic in utero protein accretion.
- Infants receiving no AAs after birth lose more than 1.5% of their daily body protein when they should be

Table 12.3 Estimated Daily Energy Requirements for Preterm Infants

Factor	Enterally Fed (kcal/kg/d)	Parenterally Fed (kcal/kg/d)
Energy expenditure		
Basal metabolic rate	40–50	40–50
Activity	0–5	Less
Thermoregulation	0–5	0–5
Synthesis (energy cost of growth)	15	15
Energy stored	20–30	20—30
Energy excreted	15	Less
Total requirements	90–120	80–110

Sources: Data from Blackburn, S. (2018a). Gastrointestinal and hepatic systems and perinatal nutrition. In S. Blackburn (Ed.), *Maternal, fetal, & neonatal physiology: A clinical perspective* (pp. 387–434). Elsevier/Saunders; Brown, L., Hendrickson, K., Evans, R., Davis, J., & Hay, W. W., Jr. (2021). Enteral nutrition. In S. Gardner, B. Carter, M. Enzman-Hines, & J. Hernandez (Eds.), *Merestein & Gardner's handbook of neonatal intensive care: An interprofessional approach* (8th ed., pp. 377–418). Elsevier.

accumulating 2% per day. By 3 days, a 10% protein deficiency occurs.

- Protein loss in extremely preterm infants is approximately twofold higher than in term infants.
  - Starter or stock PN (premade AA solution with dextrose) is recommended for preterm infants within the first 24 hours of postnatal life to compensate for high protein losses, even if providing a lower caloric intake.
  - Administering 1 g/kg/d of AA can eliminate negative nitrogen balance, whereas providing 3 g/kg/d leads to protein accretion.
- In addition to preventing catabolism of body protein, early AAs may stimulate insulin secretion and improve glucose tolerance.
  - Inadequate protein intake can increase the risk of postnatal growth restrictions in preterm infants through alteration of growth factors, including serum IGF.
- Protein requirements are inversely related to body weight.
  - Protein requirement for infants weighing up to 1,000 g is 4.0 to 4.5 g/kg/d.
  - Protein requirement for infants weighing 1,000 to 1,800 g is 3.5 to 4.0 g/kg/d.
- See Table 12.4 for estimated daily nutrition for the term and preterm infant.
- The quality of protein or AA composition in PN is important for nitrogen utilization.
  - There are certain AAs that neonates are unable to produce (essential) or produce in limited quantities (semi-essential). Therefore, it is recommended to provide these AAs exogenously.
  - Essential AAs include cysteine, tyrosine, and taurine.

- Neonatal/pediatric crystalline AA solutions have a larger quantity of nonessential AAs, more branched-chain AAs, less methionine and phenylalanine, and more tyrosine, cysteine, and taurine than adult AA solutions. Neonatal/pediatric AA solutions also have a lower pH, allowing for greater concentrations of calcium and phosphorus.
- Preterm infants who are fed diets fortified with protein and energy have shown improved neurodevelopment test scores into adolescent years.
- Metabolic overload can occur with protein intake greater than 5 g/kg/d. Infants can experience irritability, late metabolic acidosis, azotemia, edema, fever, lethargy, diarrhea, and poor developmental outcomes (Adamkin & Radmacher, 2020; Blackburn, 2018a; Brown et al., 2021; Denne, 2018; Poindexter & Martin, 2020).

Lipid (Fat) Requirements

- Preterm birth leads to the early termination of fatty acid in utero accretion, which is essential for the developing brain and retina. Fat provides the major source of nonprotein energy for growing preterm infants, which should include approximately 50% of the postnatal caloric intake.
- Lipids provide energy in the form of essential fatty acids (EFAs), which are essential in preventing EFA deficiency. EFA deficiency may be noted in preterm neonates within 72 hours of birth.
  - Linoleic and linolenic acids are considered EFAs because they are not endogenously synthesized.
- Long-chain polyunsaturated fatty acids (LCPUFAs), like arachidonic acid and docosahexaenoic acid (DHA), are sources of omega-6 fatty acids and are essential to neurologic and vision development.
- Start lipid emulsions early with LCPUFA to prevent omega-3 deficiencies.
  - Providing 0.5 g to 1.0 g/kg/d of IV lipid can prevent the development of fatty acid deficiency.
  - Initiate IV lipids starting with 0.5 to 1 g/kg/d and advance by 0.5 to 1 g/kg/d as tolerated, to a maximum of 3 g/kg/d (Adamkin & Radmacher, 2020; Bell, 2021; Blackburn, 2018a; Denne, 2018; Poindexter & Martin, 2020).

Table 12.4 Estimated Daily Nutrition for Term and Preterm Infants

Nutritional Content	Term Infant	Preterm Infant
Fluid requirements (mL/kg/d)		
Parenteral	100–120	120–150
Enteral	120–150	150–200
Calories/energy (kcal/kg/d)		
Parenteral	80–90	80–110
Enteral	100–120	110–135
Protein (g/kg/d)		
Parenteral	1.5–2.5	3.5–4.5
Enteral	1.5–2.5	3.5–4.5
Fats/Lipid (g/kg/d)		
Parenteral	2–4	2–3.5
Enteral	3–4	3–4
Carbohydrates (g/kg/d)		
Parenteral	10–15	10–15
Enteral	8–12	8–12

Sources: Data from Blackburn, S. (2018a). Gastrointestinal and hepatic systems and perinatal nutrition. In S. Blackburn (Ed.), *Maternal, fetal, & neonatal physiology: A clinical perspective* (pp. 387–434). Elsevier/Saunders; Parker, L. (2021). Nutritional management. In M. T. Verklan, M. Walden, & S. Forest (Eds.), *Core curriculum for neonatal intensive care nursing* (6th ed., pp. 152–171). Elsevier; Poindexter, B., & Martin C. A. (2020). Nutrient requirements and provision of nutritional support in the premature neonate. In R. Martin, A. Fanaroff, & M. Walsh (Eds.), *Fanaroff & Martin's neonatal-perinatal medicine: Diseases of the fetus and infant* (10th ed., pp. 592–612). Elsevier.

CARNITINE

- Carnitine is an essential cofactor required for transport of long-chain fatty acids. Preterm infants have low plasma carnitine levels and limited carnitine reserves.
- Supplementing PN with L-carnitine results in increased tolerance to IV lipids.
  - It is recommended for low birth weight infants requiring PN for over 2 to 3 weeks.
  - Dosages of 8 to 10 mg/kg/d have been used without side effects (Adamkin & Radmachar, 2020).

Carbohydrate (Glucose) Requirements

- Serving as the main carbohydrate used for fuel, glucose is the principal energy substrate in PN for the preterm. Carbohydrates should provide 40% of postnatal caloric intake.
  - Preterm infants require parenteral carbohydrate administration at 13 to 15 g/kg/d of glucose.
  - Infants weighing above 1,000 g initially tolerate 10% glucose solution.
  - Extremely preterm infants have a predisposition toward hyperglycemia but may initially require a 5% glucose solution due to higher fluid needs from increased insensible losses.
  - Extremely preterm infants should start with a GIR of at least 4 to 6 mg/kg/min. Many small infants will initially be unable to tolerate a certain glucose load but will eventually develop tolerance.
- Excessive glucose infusion may result in increased energy expenditure, oxygen consumption, serum osmolality, osmotic diuresis, and fat deposition (Adamkin & Radmacher, 2020; Anderson et al., 2017; Burris, 2017; Denne, 2018; Parker, 2021; Poindexter & Martin, 2020).

Anions

- Anions are provided as either acetate or chloride.
  - The immature kidneys contribute to acidosis by failing to reabsorb HCO_3 and to excrete hydrogen. The addition of acetate aids with the correction of hyperchloremic metabolic acidosis.
  - The addition of chloride aids with the correction of metabolic alkalosis due to increased renal losses from diuretic therapy (Bell, 2021; Denne, 2018; Poindexter & Martin, 2020; Wright et al., 2018).

Vitamins, Mineral, and Trace Elements

- Preterm infants are born with low stores of trace elements because in utero accumulation occurs during the last trimester of pregnancy.
  - Dosing of trace elements in PN contributes less than 0.01% of total body weight. Requirements for preterm infants are not well defined.
- Peak fetal accretion of minerals occurs during the third trimester, placing preterm infants at increased risk for osteopenia.
  - The limited solubility of current PN solutions does not supply enough calcium and phosphorus to support optimal bone mineralization. However, adding cysteine to PN improves calcium and phosphorus solubility by lowering the pH (Adamkin & Radmacher, 2020; Denne, 2018; Poindexter & Martin, 2020).
- Preterm infants need:
  - 60 to 90 mg/kg/d of parenteral calcium
  - A ratio of calcium to phosphorus of 1.7 to 2.0:1, which should be the goal
  - 45 to 60 mg/kg/d of phosphorus
  - 4 to 7 mg/kg/d of magnesium
  - 120 to 160 IU/d of vitamin D
- Recommendations include adding zinc and selenium early in PN administration, whereas other trace elements are probably not needed until the first 2 weeks of life. Supplementing very preterm infants with selenium has been associated with reduced sepsis.
  - Iron is not recommended unless an infant is receiving PN for longer than 2 months.
  - It is recommended to reduce or omit copper and manganese from PN in patients with impaired biliary excretion and/or liver disease because they are excreted in the bile (Adamkin & Radmacher, 2020; Anderson et al., 2017; Denne, 2018; Olsen et al., 2021; Poindexter & Martin, 2020).
- The recommended intake of vitamins for term and preterm infants on PN is shown in Table 12.5.
- The recommended intake of trace elements in PN for term and preterm infants is shown in Table 12.6.

Complications of Parenteral Nutrition Delivery

- *Electrolyte imbalance/glucose instability:* This common, preventable complication can be corrected by manipulating the constituents of the infusate.
- *Hepatic dysfunction:* Infants who receive PN for greater than 2 weeks are at risk of cholestatic jaundice, with a noted direct bilirubin level greater than 2 mg/dL. The risk further increases with prematurity and duration of PN without enteral feedings.
- *Bacteremia/fungemia:* Sepsis is a potentially lethal complication of PN delivery from central line-associated bloodstream infections which increases with prematurity and prolonged duration of PN.
  - IV lipids provide a rich growth medium for skin flora that has colonized indwelling catheters.
  - There have been numerous reports of *Malassezia furfur* fungemia in infants receiving IV lipids.
- *Negative oxidant effects:* Exposure of PN to light may generate peroxides with negative oxidant effects. Increased oxidant stress induces vasoconstriction and is associated with higher occurrences of BPD. Photoprotection of bags, syringes, and tubing is recommended for PN delivery.
- *Adverse effects from IV lipids:* Lipid infusion rates in excess of 0.25 g/kg/hr can be associated with decreased oxygenation.
  - There is still hesitation to initiate early IV lipids for concern of exacerbating lung disease, displacing bilirubin from albumin, and aggravating sepsis (Adamkin & Radmacher, 2020; Olsen et al., 2021; Poindexter & Martin, 2020).

Table 12.5 Parenteral Vitamin Intake for Term and Preterm Infants

Vitamin	Term (Daily Dose)	Preterm (dose/kg/d)
Fat-soluble		
Vitamin A (IU)	2,300	700–1,500
Vitamin D (IU)	400	40–260
Vitamin E (IU)	7	2.8–3.5
Vitamin K (mcg)	200	10–80
Water-soluble		
Vitamin B_6 (mcg)	1,000	150–200
Vitamin B_{12} (mcg)	1	0.3–0.7
Vitamin C (mg)	80	15–32
Biotin (mcg)	20	5–8
Folic acid (mcg)	140	40–90
Niacin (mg)	17	4.0–6.8
Pantothenate (mg)	5	1–2
Riboflavin (mcg)	1,400	150–200
Thiamin (mcg)	1,200	200–350

Sources: Data from Anderson, D., Poindexter, B., & Martin, C. (2017). Nutrition. In E. Eichenwald, A. Hansen, C. Martin, & A. Stark (Eds.), *Cloherty and Stark's manual of neonatal care* (8th ed., pp. 248–284). Wolters Kluwer; Denne, S. (2018). Parenteral nutrition for the high-risk neonate. In C. Gleason & S. Juul (Eds.), *Avery's diseases of the newborn* (10th ed., pp. 1023–1031e2). Elsevier; Parker, L. (2021). Nutritional management. In M. T. Verklan, M. Walden, & S. Forest (Eds.), *Core curriculum for neonatal intensive care nursing* (6th ed., pp. 152–171). Elsevier.

Table 12.6 Parenteral Intake of Trace Elements for Term and Preterm Infants

Trace Element	Term (mcg/kg/d)	Preterm (mcg/kg/d)
Chromium	0.20	0.05–0.30
Copper	20	20–29
Iodide	1	1
Manganese	1	1
Molybdenum	0.25	0.25
Selenium	2	1.5–4.5
Zinc	250	400

Sources: Data from Denne, S. (2018). Parenteral nutrition for the high-risk neonate. In C. Gleason & S. Juul (Eds.), *Avery's diseases of the newborn* (10th ed., pp. 1023–1031e2). Elsevier; Parker, L. (2021). Nutritional management. In M. T. Verklan, M. Walden, & S. Forest (Eds.), *Core curriculum for neonatal intensive care nursing* (6th ed., pp. 152–171). Elsevier.

ENTERAL ENERGY (CALORIE) REQUIREMENTS

- The stable preterm infant will attain reasonable growth when 120 kcal/kg/d has been achieved (Blackburn, 2018a).

Protein (Amino Acid) Requirements

- Preterm infants have a higher protein fractional protein accretion rate than term infants. Therefore, they require 3.5 to 4 g/kg/d of enteral protein.
- Enteral protein sources include whey and casein. Preterm formulas contain a whey-to-casein ratio of 60:40 and have higher protein content compared with term formulas (Brown et al., 2021).

Lipid (Fat) Requirements

- Preterm infants require 3 to 4 g/kg/d of fat enterally.
- Preterm infants have a limited ability enterally to absorb and digest certain fats due to low levels of pancreatic lipase, bile acids, and lingual lipase.
- MCTs do not require bile for emulsification and are absorbed by passive diffusion. MCTs are better absorbed than LCTs; however, long-chain fatty acids are essential for brain development (Adamkin & Radmacher, 2020; Parker, 2021; Poindexter and Martin, 2020).

Carbohydrate (Glucose/Lactose/Oligosaccharides) Requirements

- The preterm infant's enteral carbohydrate requirement is 8 to 12 g/kg/d. Most preterm infant formulas include glucose polymers as a major source of carbohydrates. Glucose polymers provide increased caloric density without increasing osmolality (Poindexter & Martin, 2020).

Vitamins, Minerals, and Trace Elements

- Preterm infants can sustain normal vitamin D levels with 400 IU of vitamin D.
- In addition, they should receive:
  - 185 to 210 mg/kg/d of calcium
  - 123 to 140 mg/kg/d of phosphorus
  - 8.5 to 10 mg/kg/d of magnesium (Adamkin & Radmacher, 2020)

▶ ENTERAL FEEDINGS

FEEDING METHODS

- Enteral feeding is the preferred method of nutrient provision for nourishing all infants. However, high-risk neonates require gradual introduction of enteral feedings in conjunction with supplemental PN.
- Most high-risk infants begin feeding via nasogastric/orogastric (NG/OG) tubes; these feedings are commonly used for bolus/continuous feeding methods in the preterm or sick infant until determined safe to introduce oral feedings.
  - Neonatal feeding tubes consist of radiopaque material for radiographic visualization. Polyurethane or silicone-based feeding tubes are recommended for indwelling use up to 30 days. Polyvinylchloride-based feeding tubes are intended for nonindwelling intermittent use.
  - Optimal feeding tube size is determined by weight. Infants weighing ≤1,000 g require a 5-Fr gastric tube. Infants weighing ≥1,000 g require a 6- to 8-Fr gastric tube.
- Transpyloric (nasoduodenal and nasojejunal) feedings should be considered for lung protection secondary to the risk of aspiration in infants with severe chronic lung disease (CLD) and/or gastroesophageal reflux (GER). Transpyloric feedings are routinely placed under guided fluoroscopy and should always be infused continuously due to the intestine's limited capacity for expansion.
  - Lingual and gastric lipase secretions are bypassed when infants are receiving transpyloric feeding, resulting in increased risk of fat malabsorption.
- Gastrostomy tubes may be considered in infants who are unable to take sufficient oral feeding volumes for adequate growth/hydration (Anderson et al., 2017; Parker, 2021).

STANDARDIZED FEEDING GUIDELINES

- Enteral feeding practices vary from center to center, despite recommended evidence-based feeding guidelines for preterm infants. Standardized feeding guidelines have shown improved nutritional outcomes with optimized growth, reduced duration of PN, and decreased incidence of NEC (Poindexter & Martin, 2020).

Minimal Enteral Feedings

- Trophic/minimal enteral feedings are low-volume and hypocaloric to promote intestinal maturation, with a volume of <24 mL/kg/d. Trophic feedings improve feeding tolerance and maturation of the preterm intestine (both structurally and functionally) and reduce liver dysfunction. They do not contain sufficient calories to sustain somatic growth.
- Use full-strength colostrum/preterm human milk or pasteurized donor human milk (PDHM) to start gut priming. Full-strength 20 kcal/oz preterm formula is preferred over not feeding when human milk supply is insufficient or donor breast milk has been declined.
  - Contraindications for trophic feedings include, but are not limited to, severe hemodynamic instability, medical treatment for PDA, indications of ileus or clinical signs of intestinal pathology, or suspected or confirmed NEC (although evidence regarding this disease and the benefits of trophic feeds is constantly evolving; Anderson et al., 2017; Poindexter & Martin, 2020).

Rate of Advancement of Enteral Feeds

- Feeding practices vary among institutions due to limited data regarding the most appropriate way to advance feeding volume and caloric density in preterm infants.
- Use 20 kcal/oz human milk or preterm formula (full strength) and advance feeding volume in the following suggested manner:
  - Enteral feedings should cautiously be advanced by 20 to 30 mL/kg/d in preterm infants.
  - Extremely preterm infants may need slower advancement at 15 to 25 mL/kg/d.
  - As enteral volumes are increased, the PN or IV fluid volume should be decreased to balance the total fluid volume.
- Human milk fortification may be provided when the enteral intake is greater than 50 mL/kg/d, in an effort to optimize growth (Poindexter & Martin, 2020).

Gastric Residuals

- Although some institutions measure gastric residuals, there is no supportive evidence to discontinue enteral feedings solely based on gastric residuals. There are few data supporting the utility of gastric residuals in the diagnosis of feeding intolerance or NEC (Poindexter & Martin, 2020).

HUMAN MILK COMPOSITION AND USES

- Human milk remains the gold standard for healthy term infants and preterm infants. Human milk has a low renal solute load, has the ideal AA composition for newborns, is an easily digestible and absorbable form of lipid, and contains human milk bile salts.
- Colostrum has less carbohydrates, fats, and calories than mature milk. However, it contains more sodium, chloride, potassium, and protein than mature milk due to increased concentrations of globulins and lactoferrin. Colostrum has protective and anti-infective properties.
- Milk obtained from mothers of preterm infants differs from that of mothers of term infants. The initial milk composition of the preterm mother reflects the nutritional needs of the preterm infant. The mother's breast milk composition will resemble term milk by 1 month after delivery.
  - Preterm human milk is higher in cholesterol, phospholipids, and very-long-chain polyunsaturated fatty acids (PUFAs) than term milk. Preterm milk also has higher sodium and chloride levels than that of term milk. As lactation progresses, the total fat content increases and cholesterol and phospholipid content decreases.
  - The concentration of immunoglobulins, protein, lactoferrin, sodium, chloride, and carotenoids decreases. For example, the protein content and composition decrease from 2 g/dL at birth to 1 g/dL in mature milk. The whey-to-casein ratio changes from 80:20 at the start of lactation to 55:45 in mature milk.
- Freezing human milk can change its composition by reducing the antioxidant properties, rupturing the fat globules, altering the casein component of the protein, and decreasing the fat and caloric content.
- Human milk fat and MCT additives adhere to the feeding tube, altering the nutritional content of the milk (Anderson et al., 2017; Blackburn, 2018b; Hurst & Puopolo, 2017; Parker, 2021 ; Poindexter & Martin, 2020; Snell & Gardner, 2017).

Nutrient Components of Human Milk

PROTEIN

- The leading whey protein in human milk is alpha-lactalbumin, which is high in AAs. Other human milk proteins include lactoferrin, serum albumin, lysozyme, secretory immunoglobulin A (IgA), immunoglobulin G (IgG), immunoglobulin M (IgM), and casein.
- Human milk contains less protein than cow's milk. The higher levels of nonprotein nitrogen and the AA composition of human milk are easier for digestion.
- Human milk provides more than 45 enzymes, growth factors, and bioactive substances to promote growth and development, enhance gut maturation, and protect the infant from infection. It is ideal nutrition for the term and most preterm infants (Blackburn, 2018b).

FAT

- Serving as the primary source of energy in both human milk and most formulas, fats provide higher calories without increasing the osmotic load.
- Triglycerides are the primary component of human milk fat. Infants require both saturated and unsaturated fatty acids for neurologic and vision development.
- Fats make up about 40% to 52% of the total caloric density of human milk and formulas.
- At 3 days' lactation, the total fat content of human milk is about 2 g/dL. Mature milk has a fat content of 4 to 5 g/dL.
- The fat content of human milk varies with circumstance: Mothers of preterm infants have higher PUFA; phospholipids and cholesterol are higher in early lactation; higher volumes of human milk production are associated with lower fat content; mothers on low-fat diets are associated with milk production with a lower fat content; and milk fat content increases the longer a breastfeeding session continues (Blackburn, 2018b; Brown et al., 2021; Poindexter & Martin, 2020).

CARBOHYDRATES

- Carbohydrates comprise 40% to 50% of the caloric content of human milk and most formulas. Inadequate carbohydrates result in hypoglycemia. Excessive carbohydrates result in diarrhea.
- The primary carbohydrate in human milk is lactose. Lactose is an essential source of energy for the developing brain. Other carbohydrates include glucose, nucleotides, sugars, glycolipids, glycoproteins, and oligosaccharides.
- Lactose has been partially replaced in preterm infant formula to decrease the lactose load in the diet. Feedings containing lactose, specifically human milk, stimulate lactase activity and lactose utilization.
- Alternative carbohydrates can be used for infants who are unable to tolerate lactose or when greater carbohydrate absorption is needed. It is important to note that infants require some lactose for calcium and magnesium absorption.
  - Oligosaccharides are glucose polymers that function as prebiotics by promoting the development of intestinal bacterial flora and inhibiting bacterial adhesion, which minimize the risk of GI infections. Oligosaccharides are a major element in human milk (Adamkin & Radmacher, 2020; Blackburn, 2018b).

VITAMINS AND MINERALS

- The concentration of calcium and phosphorus in human milk is appropriate for the full-term infant. Supplementation with additional calcium, phosphorus, and vitamin D for preterm infants receiving human milk is recommended. This may be done simply with human milk fortifier. Insufficient consumption of calcium, phosphorus, and vitamin D can result in metabolic bone disease of prematurity, also known as *rickets of prematurity* (Adamkin & Radmacher, 2020).

Human Milk Fortification

- Preterm human milk, when compared with the preterm infant's nutritional requirement, is lower in protein, calcium, phosphorus, iron, vitamins, and sodium. Fortification of human milk can help minimize nutrient deficiencies for the preterm infant.
  - The preterm infant will not grow at the comparative rate of its fetal counterpart on human milk alone. To achieve similar intrauterine growth rates in the larger preterm infants, large volumes (180–200 mL/kg/d) of unfortified human milk would need to be consumed.
- Human milk fortifiers contain protein, carbohydrates, calcium, phosphate, vitamins, sodium, and other substances. Fortification can lead to increases in weight gain, length, and HC in the short term. However, some preterm infants may experience slower weight gain when compared with formula due to the variable protein content of human milk.
- Fortification allows for better mineral accretion compared with breast milk alone, resembling that of preterm formula-fed infants. The osmolarity of formulas and human milk mixtures increases by roughly the same percentage as the caloric density increases. The renal solute load and osmolarity must be considered when concentrating formulas/human milk beyond 24 cal/oz.
- Preterm infants less than 1,500 g should receive fortified human milk or fortified PDHM when available.
  - Human milk-fed infants weighing <1,500 g may be fortified with bovine milk-based human milk fortifier (HMF) when receiving approximately 100 mL/kg of feeding volume.
  - Larger infants may be considered for the addition of HMF once they reach full volume (Adamkin & Radmacher, 2020; Anderson et al., 2017; Blackburn, 2018a; Brown et al., 2021; Parker, 2021.

Pasteurized Donor Human Milk

- Donor human milk is pasteurized human milk obtained from an accredited milk bank and utilized in the preterm infant when maternal human milk supply is unavailable. The composition of donor milk may vary based on the gestational age at the time of donation. Additionally, donor milk changes throughout lactation.
  - VLBW infants and those born <32 weeks qualify for PDHM in most institutions due to the increased risk factors previously described. PDHM is used as supplementation until the mother can provide 100% human milk or as a replacement for formula if the mother chooses not to provide human milk (Anderson et al., 2017; Brown et al., 2021).

Human Milk Handling and Storage

■ It is important to collect, handle, and store breast milk appropriately to ensure nutritional quality and most importantly microbiological safety. Appropriate hand hygiene is required before beginning the human milk collection process. Human milk collection kits should be rinsed, cleaned with hot soapy water, and air-dried. Milk storage containers should be hard plastic or glass and each storage container should contain milk from one expression. The container should be labeled with a name, date, and time of pumping. Human milk should not be stored in plastic bags for preterm infants.

■ Human milk must be frozen if not used within 24 hours after collection. Freezing human milk preserves many of the immunologic and nutritional benefits. Human milk can be stored safely from 3 to 6 months in the rear of the freezer compartment or in a deep freezer for 6 to 12 months. It may be safe to freeze human milk for longer than recommended under appropriate conditions; however, the nutritional quality may decrease secondary to lipid degradation. Do not refreeze human milk after it has been thawed.

■ Human milk must be thawed completely, using tepid running water or a commercial human milk thawing machine. Never use hot water or warm in the microwave oven. Thawed human milk must be stored in a refrigerator at 4°C and used within 24 hours (Furman & Schanler, 2018; Hurst & Puopolo, 2017; Parker, 2021).

Lactation Support for Mothers

■ The benefits of providing human milk to preterm infants begin with early encouragement and education to mothers about expressing and storing human milk. Early discussions about the importance of human milk increase the incidence of lactation initiation without causing maternal stress and/or anxiety.

■ Pumping should begin soon after delivery to establish a generous milk supply. The first 24 to 48 hours postpartum may only yield a small amount of colostrum before sizable milk production begins. Mothers require encouragement to pump a minimum of eight times per day to establish an adequate milk supply. A break in frequency can cause a significant decrease in production.

■ Once milk production is established, the milk supply may be maintained by pumping a minimum of six times per day. Continue monitoring for ongoing success.

■ Providing a supportive environment to mothers in addition to regular breast massage with proper technique can facilitate optimal milk expression. Additionally, it is essential to have a properly fitted milk expression shield and to simultaneously pump both breasts with a high-quality breast pump (Hurst & Puopolo, 2017; Parker, 2017).

Contraindications for Human Milk

■ Illicit drugs concentrated in the mother's human milk can cause neonatal intoxication and death. See Chapter 5 for a discussion of breastfeeding in the presence of specific drugs. Some prescription or over-the-counter medications, including cytotoxic drugs, are contraindications to breastfeeding.

■ Mothers with active type 1 and 2 human T-lymphotropic virus infection should not breastfeed.

■ Varicella lesions must be crusted over before direct breastfeeding. Although pumped milk may be provided, the infant should be separated from the mother during an active varicella infection.

■ In developed countries, breastfeeding is contraindicated in mothers with HIV because of safer available alternative.

■ Infants with galactosemia are unable to digest lactose-containing milk and therefore unable to receive maternal human milk, donated human milk, or commercial bovine milk-based formulas (Furman & Schanler, 2018; Hurst & Puopolo, 2017; Parker, 2021; Snell & Gardner, 2017).

INFANT FORMULAS

Preparation of Formulas

■ Most standard formulas have a ready-to-feed, powder, and liquid concentrate form allowing the option of fortification. Unless there is no other option, the use of powder infant formulas or fortification should be avoided in hospitalized newborns due to the risk of *Cronobacter sakazakii* infection.

■ Caloric density of formula can be increased through addition of liquid concentrate, glucose polymers, or fat (e.g., vegetable or MCT oil). Formulas should not be concentrated to more than 30 kcal/oz due to the resulting high renal solute load.

■ When increasing the caloric density of a feeding, calculation of intake nutrients should be compared with recommended guidelines for appropriate distribution of carbohydrates, proteins, and fats. Total calories should be distributed as 35% to 65% from carbohydrates, 30% to 55% from fat, and 8% to 16% from protein (Adamkin & Radmacher, 2020; Brown et al., 2021).

Standard Infant Formulas

■ Most standard formulas are whey-predominant, with a whey-to-casein protein ratio of 60% to 40%. Casein-predominant cow's milk formulas have a whey-to-casein ratio of 18:82. Casein protein requires more energy to digest and is more likely to be incompletely digested due to its tougher curds. The curds of whey are softer.

- The fat content of standard formulas includes all LCTs from vegetable oils, including soy and coconut.
- Standard formulas are available as iron-fortified or nonfortified/low-iron forms. Iron-fortified formulas contain 12 mg/L of elemental iron, or 2 mg/kg/d for infants receiving 108 kcal/kg/d. Low-iron formulas contain 1.5 mg/L of elemental iron, or 0.2 mg/kg/d (Adamkin & Radmacher, 2020; Blackburn, 2018a; Poindexter & Martin, 2020).

Preterm Infant Formulas

- Preterm infant formulas have a lower lactose concentration and are whey-predominant, with a whey-to-casein ratio of 60:40. These formulas have a higher protein concentration of 3.6 to 4.2 g/kg/d of protein. Compared with human milk, whey-predominant formulas have higher levels of methionine, threonine, lysine, and branched AAs.
- High-protein infant formulas containing 2.7 to 2.9 g/100 mL are indicated:
  - For infants experiencing a cumulative deficit of protein; who are volume-restricted; for promotion of wound healing; for infants with inadequate growth in length and/or HC; and for infants with poor overall growth.
- Preterm formulas are available with low iron content of 3 mg/L of elemental iron and with an iron fortification content of 15 mg/L of elemental iron. The two options are available since infants may receive this type of formula for greater than 2 months postdischarge (Adamkin & Radmacher, 2020; Brown et al., 2021; Poindexter & Martin, 2020).

Soy Formulas

- Soy formulas are lactose-free and recommended for infants with galactosemia, with primary lactase deficiency, or for infants recovering from secondary lactose intolerance, vegan families, or infants with immunoglobulin E (IgE)-mediated cow's milk protein allergy. LCTs in the form of vegetable oils, usually coconut and soy oil, make up the fat content in soy formulas.
- Soy protein formulas are not recommended for preterm infants due to their low calcium and phosphorus content, poorer quality of protein, and lower digestibility and bioavailability. Preterm infants fed soy protein formulas are at increased risk of developing metabolic bone disease (osteopenia) and experience slower weight gain and have lower protein and albumin concentrations despite supplementation (Adamkin & Radmacher, 2020; Brown et al., 2021).

Protein Hydrolysate Formulas

- Protein hydrolysate formulas are designed for infants with allergies to cow's milk or soy protein and are sometimes used in the management of infants with bowel resections or intractable diarrhea. Elemental formulas have also been used in infants with severe liver disease and fat malabsorption, infants with short bowel syndrome, and those with dysmotility syndromes.
- The protein source in these elemental formulas are derived from free AAs, and many are lactose-free.
- Fat content comprises both medium-chain and long-chain triglycerides.
- Some of these formulas are elemental, with easily absorbable carbohydrates (e.g., monosaccharides or glucose polymers; Adamkin & Radmacher, 2020; Brown et al., 2021).

Postdischarge Transitional Formulas

- Postdischarge formulas have increased concentrations of calcium, phosphorus, zinc, vitamins, and trace elements to promote and support linear growth.
- Postdischarge transitional formula or fortified human milk should be provided to preterm infants who remain below normal weight at discharge.
- Preterm infants with normal weight for postmenstrual age at the time of discharge may be fed similar to term infants of the same gestational age (Adamkin & Radmacher, 2020; Brown et al., 2021).
- See Table 12.7 for the indications for use of different formulas.

ENTERAL SUPPLEMENTS

Oral Dietary Supplements

PROTEIN
- Extensively hydrolyzed casein protein offers 3.6 kcal/g or 4 kcal/6 mL (Parker, 2021).

FATS
- MCTs offer 8.3 kcal/g or 7.7 kcal/mL.
- LCTs offer 4.5 kcal/mL (Parker, 2021).

CARBOHYDRATES
- Maltodextrin (for use with term infants only) offers 3.8 kcal/g or 8 kcal/tsp (powder; Parker, 2021).

Enteral Electrolytes

- Sodium, potassium, and chloride are required for optimal growth and play a key role in water and acid–base balance. Many preterm infants, especially VLBW infants, may require sodium supplements until renal tubular function matures.
- Preterm human milk has higher sodium and chloride levels than that of mothers of term infants; however, these infants may still need additional supplementation until the renal tubular function matures.

Table 12.7 Indications for Use of Infant Formulas

Clinical Condition	Suggested Type of Infant Formula	Rationale
Allergy to cow's milk protein or soy protein	Extensively hydrolyzed protein or free amino acids	Impaired digestion/utilization of intact protein
Bronchopulmonary dysplasia	High-energy, nutrient-dense	Increased energy requirement, fluid restriction
Biliary atresia	Semi-elemental, containing reduced LCT (~45%), with supplemented MCT (~55%)	Impaired intraluminal digestion and absorption of long-chain fats
Chylothorax (persistent)	High-energy formula	Lower fluid and sodium intake, increased energy requirement
Cystic fibrosis	Semi-elemental formula, containing reduced LCT (~45%), with supplemented MCT (~55%) or standard formula with pancreatic enzyme supplementation	Impaired intraluminal digestion and absorption of long-chain fats
Galactosemia	Soy protein-based formula	Lactose-free
Gastroesophageal reflux	Standard formula, Enfamil A.R.	Consider small, frequent feedings
Hepatic insufficiency	Semi-elemental formula, containing reduced LCT (~45%), with supplemented MCT (~55%)	Impaired intraluminal digestion and absorption of long-chain fats
Lactose intolerance	Low-lactose formula	Impaired digestion or utilization of lactose
Lymphatic anomalies	Significantly reduced LCT (~15%), with supplemented MCT (~84%)	Impaired absorption of long-chain fats
Necrotizing enterocolitis	Preterm formula or semi-elemental formula, if indicated	Impaired digestion
Renal insufficiency	Similac PM 60/40	Low phosphate content, low renal solute load

LCT, long-chain triglyceride; MCT, medium-chain triglyceride.
Source: Reproduced with permission from Anderson, D., Poindexter, B., & Martin, C. (2017). Nutrition. In E. Eichenwald, A. Hansen, C. Martin, & A. Stark (Eds.), *Cloherty and Stark's manual of neonatal care* (8th ed., pp. 248–284). Wolters Kluwer.

- Preterm infant formulas contain higher amounts of sodium, potassium, and chloride than term infant formulas (Anderson et al., 2017; Parker, 2021).

Enteral Vitamins and Minerals

- Vitamins are organic substances that are essential to normal metabolism; however, they are not synthesized by the body.
- Infants of undernourished mothers as well as preterm infants have lower blood levels of water-soluble vitamins at birth.
- Vitamins are categorized by their solubility: Fat-soluble vitamins include vitamins A, D, E, and K. Water-soluble vitamins include vitamin B complex and vitamin C. Folic acid is not included in liquid multivitamins because there is a lack of stability; they can be given separately as indicated (Poindexter & Martin, 2020).

VITAMIN A

- Colostrum contains the highest amounts of vitamin A. Vitamin A content in preterm and term human milk are comparable, then decline as the human milk matures.
- Improving vitamin A levels in the preterm infant are associated with decreased incidence of BPD.
- Vitamin A supplementation in extremely preterm infants during the first month after birth positively affects survival without neurodevelopmental impairment (Colaizy et al., 2018; Picciano et al., 2021).

VITAMIN K (PHYTONADIONE)

- Human milk does not provide adequate amounts of vitamin K. There is also an association with human milk and the development of an intestinal microflora that makes less vitamin K. Therefore, it is a standard of care to administer vitamin K after birth to protect infants from hemorrhage.

- The recommended vitamin K dosing at the time of birth is 1 mg intramuscular (IM) injection in both term and preterm neonates of more than 1,000 g birth weight.
- Dosing for preterm infants less than 1,000 g is 0.3 mg (Furman & Schanler, 2018; Picciano et al., 2021; Poindexter & Martin, 2020).

VITAMIN D

- Vitamin D supplementation is recommended for exclusively breastfed infants or formula-fed infants taking less than 1,000 mL/d of vitamin D-fortified formula. Vitamin D plays a vital role in skeletal growth and maturation. Vitamin D in human milk is dependent on maternal vitamin D levels.
- Vitamin D supplementation is recommended in the exclusively breastfed infant secondary to the inadequate amounts of vitamin D in human milk. See current literature for up-to-date dosing amount recommendations (Abrams, 2017; Anderson et al., 2017; Beriln, 2020; Furman & Schanler, 2018; Picciano et al., 2021; Poindexter & Martin, 2020).

VITAMIN E

- Vitamin E supplementation in preterm infants has been debated by many experts. The American Academy of Pediatrics (AAP) does not recommend pharmacologic doses of vitamin E. Term and preterm human milk provides adequate amounts of vitamin E (Picciano et al., 2021).

IRON

- Preterm infants are more likely to develop iron deficiency, which can have a negative impact on brain development.
- Preterm infants who receive human milk are more likely to have iron deficiency secondary to the decrease in iron concentration during the progression of lactation.
- Given the iron content in many preterm formulas and human milk fortifiers, an additional source of iron may not be necessary.
- Infants receiving an erythrocyte-stimulating agent, such as erythropoietin, may need a higher dose of iron.
- Preterm infants require iron supplementation to be started between 2 and 4 weeks of age, with a recommended dose of 2 to 4 mg/kg/d (Anderson et al., 2017; Colaizy et al., 2018; Poindexter & Martin, 2020).

CALCIUM/PHOSPHOROUS

- The nutritional goal for preterm infants is to obtain a bone mineralization pattern similar to that of the fetus in an effort to prevent osteopenia and fractures. Calcium and phosphorus exist in ionized and complex

forms that are easily absorbed in human milk. Preterm human milk contains approximately 250 mg of calcium in addition to 140 mg of phosphorus per liter. Significant increases in calcium and phosphorus content may positively affect magnesium retention.
- The recommended daily requirement for enteral calcium is 120 to 200 mg/kg.
- The recommended daily requirement for phosphorus is 60 to 140 mg/kg.
- The calcium-to-phosphorus (Ca:P) ratio should be approximately 2:1, which is similar to the ratio in human milk (Colaizy et al., 2018; Poindexter & Martin, 2020).

OMEGA-3 FATTY ACIDS

- Omega-3 fatty acids play a vital role in visual and neurologic development, in addition to protecting the body from inflammation and decreasing the risk of many chronic degenerative diseases. Supplementing infants with LCPUFA has been shown to improve neural development, especially when infants are fed formula.
- Omega-3 fatty acids supplementation includes alpha-linolenic acid (ALA), LCPUFA metabolites, eicosapentaenoic acid (EPA), and DHA. Human milk contains a variety of omega-3 fatty acids and is dependent on the mother's diet.
- Infant formulas are made with corn, coconut, safflower, and soy oil unless they are fortified with LCPUFAs (Picciano et al., 2021).

ZINC

- Zinc is highly bioavailable in human milk; however, the quantity declines over the course of lactation.
- Preterm recommendations for zinc intake are 1 to 3 mg/kg/d and can be achieved through the use of term or preterm formulas as well as HMFs. Most formulas are supplemented with zinc to contain 5 to 7 mg/L, with preterm formulas containing roughly 5 to 10 mg/L (Picciano et al., 2021).

FLUORIDE

- Fluoride concentration in human milk is 4 to 15 mg/L, which results in intake of 3 to 12 mg/kg/d.
- Fluoride supplements are not recommended in infants under 6 months of age. Fluoride intake by infants can vary widely depending on whether the infant is fed human milk or formula. There is a difference in fluoride content in ready-to-feed formulas versus powder formulas that require reconstitution with water. Fluoride intake by formula-fed infants can be as high as 1.0 mg/d. However, there is variability based on the water source (Picciano et al., 2021).

IODINE

- Iodine is found in the developing brain, muscle, heart, pituitary, and kidney; however, it is concentrated in the thyroid gland.

- Iodine is the most common nutrient deficiency worldwide, causing transient hypothyroidism. However, iodine deficiency is not as common in the United States. Iodine content in human milk is contingent on maternal intake. Human milk and bovine milk-based infant formulas are typically a reliable source of this mineral.
  - Iodine deficiency disorders include learning disabilities, hypothyroidism, goiter, cretinism, and growth and developmental abnormalities (Picciano et al., 2021; Wassner & Belfort, 2017).

INFANTS WITH SPECIAL NUTRITIONAL REQUIREMENTS

Bronchopulmonary Dysplasia

- Infants with BPD often require a balance between proper nutrition and required fluid restriction. BPD can cause an increase in metabolic demand and energy requirements by 20% to 40%. It is essential to monitor growth parameters to ensure continued growth is not compromised.
- When fluids are restricted to minimize pulmonary edema, higher caloric concentrations are required to promote tissue healing and growth.
  - Infants with BPD often require a caloric density of 30 kcal/oz to achieve desired growth targets. Transitioning from gavage to oral feeding may require different approaches in the duration of feeding volume based on the infant's energy status and respiratory demands (Anderson et al., 2017; Parker, 2021).

Inborn Errors of Metabolism

- An individualized diet must be established based on metabolic defect. Modified formula preparation containing all except the aberrant AAs should be used.
  - An infant with galactosemia should be fed a lactose-free formula.
- It is important to withhold enteral feedings for infants with inborn errors of metabolism (IEM) until the infant is neurologically stable. Conversely, any infant who experiences acute decompensation following the initiation of enteral feeds should be evaluated for an IEM (Anderson et al., 2017).

Congenital Heart Disease

- Infants with cardiac defects have increased metabolic demand and tend to have poor growth. Higher metabolic rate and oxygen consumption secondary to increased cardiac and respiratory workload may cause fatigue, resulting in tachypnea and poor feeding.
  - Fortification of human milk/formula at an increased caloric density is imperative to ensure higher caloric needs are met in efforts to restrict total fluid intake (Parker, 2021).

Short Bowel Syndrome

- Infants with short bowel syndrome have reduced intestinal length and absorptive surface areas.
- Enteral feedings may potentially be achieved with a minimum of 25 cm (about 9.84 in.) of small bowel with an intact ileocecal valve, or with 40 cm of small bowel without an ileocecal valve. Regardless of the remaining intestinal length, failure occurs anytime the patient's energy, fluid, and electrolyte requirements are not met.
- Long-term PN may be required to promote linear growth, depending on the length of the remaining bowel and nutritional status. The goal of intestinal rehabilitation is to slowly advance enteral feeds and wean PN as the remaining bowel undergoes the process of intestinal adaptation (Javid et al., 2018; Parker, 2021).

Gastroesophageal Reflux

- Intestinal dysmotility and relaxation of the lower esophageal sphincter are common causes of emesis during the initiation and advancement of enteral feeds in the preterm infant. If these episodes do not compromise the infant's respiratory status or growth, only continued close monitoring is required.
- There is unambiguous evidence linking GER and apnea.
- Modifications of the feeding regimen can improve emesis in the preterm infant, including:
  - Lengthening the duration of the feeding (sometimes to the point of using continuous feeding)
  - Reduction in feeding volume
  - Removal of nutritional additives
  - Use of specialized formulas
- Therapeutic maneuvers to help decrease emesis include repositioning the infant to elevate the head and upper body, or positioning either prone or right side down.
- Infants may require an evaluation of their anatomy if the achievement of full-volume feeds is prevented by recurrent episodes of symptomatic emesis (Anderson et al., 2017; Richards & Goldin, 2018).

Intrauterine Growth Restriction

- IUGR infants have increased energy requirements secondary to low stores of energy, nutrients, and minerals. An individualized management plan is essential because these infants may not tolerate enteral feeding advancements or respond to the increased nutrient intake.
- Severe cases of IUGR (those with absent or reversed end-diastolic flow on prenatal ultrasound) are more susceptible to NEC. This population is also at increased risk for PN-associated liver disease for reasons not completely understood (Brown et al., 2021; Chu & Devaskar, 2020).

Necrotizing Enterocolitis

- NEC is the most acquired GI emergency in the NICU which predominantly affects preterm infants. Hypoxic–ischemic events and/or asphyxia episodes may place term infants at a higher risk of developing NEC.
- There are multiple bioactive factors in human milk that influence host immunity, inflammation, and mucosal protection. Preterm infants exclusively fed with expressed human milk are at decreased risk of developing NEC.
- Infants who are acutely ill with NEC are at risk of malnutrition secondary to increased nutrient losses and malabsorption. It is imperative to support the infants' nutritional needs with PN, specifically through the acute phase.
- In the case of surgical NEC, neonates are at increased risk for nutritional deficiencies caused by the stress of illness and surgery. Human milk feedings are preferred because they can preserve the integrity of the intestinal mucosa. Additionally, enteral feedings promote the continued development of the GI tract (Adamkin & Radmacher, 2020; Brown et al., 2021; Kudin & Neu, 2020; Weitkamp et al., 2017).

▶ CONCLUSION

The development and function of the GI system are vital to human growth and long-term survival. A thorough understanding of fluid, electrolytes, GI development, physiology, and disease process is crucial to ensure adequate growth and nutrition in the critically ill neonate. This chapter highlights GI embryology, physiology, and parenteral and enteral nutrition. The effects of nutrition on the neonate with multisystem disease processes are further discussed.

1. A 36-week infant born 1 month ago currently weighs 3.62 kg. The previous weight 7 days ago was 3.5 kg. What is the 7-day weight gain in grams per kilogram per day?

   A. 1.2 g/kg/d
   B. 3.3 g/kg/d
   C. 4.7 g/kg/d

2. An infant is eating 75 mL every 3 hours of human milk at 20 kcal/oz. The current weight is 3.62 kg. What is the intake in kilocalories per kilogram per day?

   A. 106 kcal/kg/d
   B. 111 kcal/kg/d
   C. 115 kcal/kg/d

3. Infants with necrotizing enterocolitis (NEC) are at high risk for malnutrition; therefore, it is imperative to support the infants' nutritional needs with:

   A. Intravenous iron
   B. Oral omega acids
   C. Parenteral nutrition

4. The neonatal nurse practitioner (NNP) recognizes a contraindication to breastfeeding includes an infant diagnosis of:

   A. Cytomegalovirus
   B. Galactosemia
   C. Microcephaly

5. The purpose of adding carnitine to parenteral nutrition (PN) is to facilitate the:

   A. Digestion of lactose
   B. Synthesis of bile acids
   C. Transport of fatty acids

6. Compared with infants being enterally fed, the caloric needs of infants receiving only parenteral nutrition (PN) are:

   A. Equal
   B. Higher
   C. Lower

7. The primary goal of delivering parenteral and enteral nutrition to a neonate in the ICU, regardless of disease state, is to:

   A. Achieve rate and composition of weight gain at the same postmenstrual age
   B. Enhance postnatal growth failure and suboptimal neurodevelopmental outcomes
   C. Increase protein and energy deficits during the early neonatal period

(See answers next page.) **187**

1. C) 4.7 g/kg/d

3,620 g − 3,500 g = 120 g/wk
then
120 g/wk ÷ 7 days = 17.14 g/d
then
17.14 g/d ÷ 3.62 kg = 4.73 g/kg/d

2. B) 111 kcal/kg/d

20 kcal/oz + 30 mL/oz = 0.67 kcal/mL
then
75 mL × 8 feeds/d = 600 mL/d
then
600 mL/d × 0.67 kcal/mL = 402 kcal/d
then
402 kcal/d ÷ 3.620 kg = 111 kcal/kg/d
OR
75 mL/feed × 8 feeds/d = 600 mL/d
then
600 mL/d + 3.62 kg = 166 mL/kg/d
then
166 mL/kg/d × 0.67 kcal/mL = 111 kcal/kg/d

3. C) Parenteral nutrition

Infants with NEC are at higher risk for malnutrition secondary to increased nutrient losses and malabsorption; therefore, it is imperative to support the infants' nutritional needs with parenteral nutrition (PN) specifically through the acute phase. Supporting with intravenous iron or oral omega acids alone is not sufficient to meet the infant's needs (Brown et al., 2021).

4. B) Galactosemia

Infants with galactosemia are unable to receive maternal human milk or donated human milk. Cytomegalovirus (CMV) and microcephaly are not contraindications to providing human milk (Furman & Schanler, 2018; Hurst & Puopolo, 2017).

5. C) Transport of fatty acids

Carnitine is an essential cofactor required for the transport of long-chain fatty acids. The digestion of lactose or synthesis of bile acids is not dependent on the presence of carnitine (Adamkin & Radmachar, 2020).

6. C) Lower

The caloric needs of infants receiving PN are lower than infants enterally fed due to lower activity levels and decreased fecal losses (Blackburn, 2018; Denne, 2018).

7. A) Achieve rate and composition of weight gain at the same postmenstrual age

The current goal of parenteral and enteral nutrition is to attain approximately the same rate and composition of weight gain as a normal fetus at the same postmenstrual age. Goals should never be to "enhance failure" or to "increase deficits" of neonatal nutrition (Poindexter & Martin, 2020).

Fluids and Electrolytes

Carolyn J. Herrington and Leanne M. Nantais-Smith

INTRODUCTION

Fluid and electrolyte management, acid–base homeostasis, and parenteral and enteral nutritional therapies are central in the management of the sick newborn. Management approaches have changed significantly over time, moving from restrictive fluid management approaches in the 1950s to the current, more liberalized approach. Those early restrictive approaches resulted in hyperosmolarity, exaggerated hyperbilirubinemia, and hypoglycemia, all of which further complicated the management and outcomes of these infants. The current approach recommends a more liberal approach to initial fluid management, but ideal approaches continue to remain somewhat uncertain. The principles of fluid and electrolyte management also vary based on the gestational age (GA) and the disease process.

PRINCIPLES OF FLUID AND ELECTROLYTE MANAGEMENT

- Physiologically, infants are different from children and adults in several ways. Basic metabolic rates are significantly higher in newborns, which creates a need for increased delivery per kilogram of body weight.
- Sodium excretion is only 10% of that of older children and adults because the glomerular filtration rate (GFR) is 5 to 10 times lower and sodium reabsorption in the proximal and distal renal tubules is decreased. This makes them more vulnerable to sodium overload.
- Total body water (TBW) distributions are also significantly different from those of older children and adults and vary significantly across GAs as well (Doherty, 2017; Nyp et al., 2021).

TOTAL BODY WATER

- TBW varies from 85% to 90% in the extremely low birth weight (ELBW) infant to 75% in the term newborn infant.
  - Prior to birth, the major factor controlling TBW is maternal status.

- After birth, the infant assumes the homeostatic control of TBW content, as well as fluid and electrolyte balance.
- TBW is composed of both the intracellular and extracellular fluid compartments (ICF and ECF, respectively). The ECF is further broken down into the intravascular space (IVS) and the interstitial space (IS; Bell, 2021; Doherty, 2017; Gomella et al., 2020b; Nyp et al., 2021).

Intracellular Fluid

- Water and biomolecules are contained within the cells surrounded by a cell membrane. The cell membrane allows movement of water and electrolytes inside and outside the cell via transport mechanisms, such as diffusion and sodium or potassium transport carriers.
  - Protein transporters in the cell membrane require energy to transport ions back and forth between the ICF and the ECF (e.g., sodium, potassium, and chloride movement).
  - The major intracellular solutes are proteins, which support cell function; organic phosphates, which participate in energy production and storage; and charged ions.
  - Potassium is the major cation of the ICF.
  - Any disorder or disease that disrupts maintenance of normal pH can affect fluid and electrolyte balance by interfering with normal cell function, such as limiting the production of protein cell membrane transport carriers or disabling oxygen-requiring active ion transport mechanisms (Bell, 2021; Nyp et al., 2021; Wright et al., 2018).

Extracellular Fluid

- The extracellular compartment comprises water and biomolecules contained outside the cell. The major cation of the ECF is sodium and the major anion is chloride. The ECF is divided into two compartments:
  - The IVS contains the fluid component of the blood, which circulates in the blood vessels.
  - The IS comprises fluid within the tissues that surround all cells that are not contained in the IVS.
- A capillary membrane divides the intravascular and interstitial compartments. The major differences in

the composition between the IVS and the IS are the proteins. Proteins in the IVS exert osmotic pressure.

- Movement of fluid between the IVS and the IS is determined by filtration and reabsorption.
- When capillary hydrostatic pressure (blood pressure) exceeds blood oncotic pressure, fluid moves from the IVS into the tissue (filtration).
- When capillary oncotic pressure (from circulating albumin) exceeds capillary hydrostatic pressure, fluid moves into the IVS (reabsorption).
  - ❑ Excess fluid not reabsorbed is drained by the lymphatic system and returns to the IVS via the subclavian veins.

■ The composition of the ICF and ECF differs in the concentration of each solute—for example, higher potassium concentration in the ICF, higher sodium concentration in the ECF—but the osmolality of the spaces must remain equal. This homeostasis is maintained by selective permeability of the cell membrane to solutes and energy-dependent protein transport carriers.

- Derailment in maintenance of normal fluid and electrolyte balance, caused by critical illness, asphyxia, cardiovascular compromise, and loss of capillary wall integrity, can lead to hypovolemia, cell damage from fluid overload shifts via osmosis, loss of oncotic pressure in the IVS from protein leakage and edema, or failure of electrolyte transport pumps due to hypoxia.
- The kidneys play a key role in maintaining normal fluid and electrolyte balance in the ECF via sodium and water reabsorption. This control is compromised in the preterm infant, leading to sodium and bicarbonate losses in the urine and the inability to manage large fluid volumes or sodium boluses.
- Management of fluid and electrolytes in the sick newborn and preterm infant is a careful balance between excesses or deficits in fluid or electrolytes, anticipated losses, growth needs, and challenges to normal function resulting from developmental compromise or critical illness (Bell, 2021; Doherty, 2017; Nyp et al., 2021; Wright et al., 2018).

MATERNAL, FETAL, AND PERINATAL INFLUENCES

■ Several factors must be evaluated in the assessment of fluid and electrolyte balance. An initial review of maternal history is critical since the newborn's status reflects the maternal status at birth, gradually reflecting the extrauterine transition over the first 24 hours of life. Oxytocin, maternal diuretic use, and infusion of hypotonic IV fluid may result in maternal and fetal hyponatremia.

■ Use of antenatal steroids can enhance lung maturation in the preterm infant and may also enhance skin maturation, which will decrease insensible water loss (IWL) and in turn reduce the risk of hyperkalemia. Fetal and perinatal factors, such as oligohydramnios, may be associated with congenital renal abnormalities such as renal agenesis, polycystic kidney disease, or posterior urethral valves. Severe hypoxia or asphyxia at birth can lead to renal tubular necrosis, which will require a decrease in total fluid goals for these infants (Doherty, 2017; Gomella et al., 2020b; Nyp et al., 2021).

TRANSITIONAL CHANGES AT BIRTH

■ Both GA and chronologic age affect the relationships between ICF and ECF compartments. These changes are primarily the result of maturation in the heart, kidney, and endocrine systems.

■ After birth, the infant enters a physiologic transitional phase as the body shifts from the intrauterine to extrauterine life. The degree of TBW loss and intercompartmental shifts is related primarily to GA.

■ These shifts are also influenced by the fat content of the infant (less fat content in the small-for-gestational-age [SGA] infant, for instance, and greater fat content in the infant of a diabetic mother [IDM]), as well as any disease processes in the infant (asphyxia, respiratory distress syndrome, and pneumonia). After birth, the first shift in fluid balance occurs as the ECF compartment contracts and the infant loses interstitial fluid through diuresis. This shift ideally occurs over the first 3 to 5 days of life.

- The preterm infant may lose 10% to 15% of the TBW, while the healthy term infant loses 5% to 10% of the TBW. Weight loss is generally regained over the first 7 to 10 days of life as muscle growth occurs and fat stores increase.

■ Diuresis is secondary to change in the glomerular filtration, which begins to increase after birth due to the increase in cardiac output, renal blood flow, and increasing glomerular permeability following clamping of the cord.

■ Diuresis is accompanied by natriuresis, which results in increased loss of sodium in the urine. This increased sodium loss produces an initial negative sodium balance but is not generally associated with a need for sodium supplementation in the first 24 to 48 hours of life. The goal of fluid and electrolyte management during this period is to provide sufficient fluid intake to allow the physiologic ECF losses to occur gradually over the first 3 to 5 days of life, while maintaining normal electrolyte balances and circulating IVS volumes to support cardiovascular function.

■ Subsequently, the goal of fluid and electrolyte balance is to provide the appropriate supplementation to maintain homeostasis and support growth (Doherty, 2017; Nyp et al., 2021; Wright et al., 2018).

INSENSIBLE LOSS/GAIN

- Another crucial factor that must be taken into consideration is the expected IWLs that occur in the newborn period through the pulmonary and cutaneous systems. Insensible losses cannot be directly measured, but are calculated as the provider assesses intake, output, and weight change in the infant. The external environment also influences the degree of insensible loss. Table 13.1 shows factors that affect IWL; the presence or absence of these conditions should guide the practitioner in planning fluid goals.
- IWL can be calculated using the following formula:
  - IWL = fluid intake − urine output + weight change
- The average IWLs for infants in incubators during the first 7 days of life are estimated at:
  - Birth weight (BW) 750 to 1,000 g = ~80 mL/kg/d
  - BW 1,001 to 1,250 g = ~50 mL/kg/d
  - BW 1,251 to 1,500 g = ~45 mL/kg/d
  - BW >1,501 g = ~25 mL/kg/d (Bell, 2021; Doherty, 2017; Gomella et al., 2020b; Nyp et al., 2021; Wright et al., 2018)

▶ ASSESSING FLUID AND ELECTROLYTE BALANCE

PHYSICAL ASSESSMENT

- A thorough assessment of the infant's status is critical to the management of fluid and electrolyte balance. All fluids administered must be accurately measured, including flushes for medications, especially in the most critically ill infants. Strict and accurate measurement of intake and output is critical.

Table 13.1 Factors That Affect Insensible Water Loss

Decrease IWL	Increase IWL
Clothes	Activity
Emollient use	Ambient temperature above thermoneutral
Heat shield or double-walled incubators	Fever
High relative humidity (ambient ventilator gas)	Inversely related to gestational age and weight
Plastic blankets	Phototherapy
	Radiant warmer
	Respiratory distress

IWL, insensible water loss.
Source: Reproduced with permission from Nyp, M., Brunkhorst, J. L., Reavy, D., & Pallotto, E. K. (2021). Fluid and electrolyte management. In S. L. Gardner, B. S. Carter, M. Enzman-Hines, & S. Niermeyer (Eds.), *Merenstein & Gardner's handbook of neonatal intensive care nursing: An interprofessional approach* (9th ed., p. 415). Elsevier.

Diapers must be weighed. Any source of measurable fluid loss must be measured and included in fluid evaluation. Daily weights are essential in helping to determine fluid losses and planning fluid goals. Acute changes in weight are reflective of TBW. Weight is the most sensitive indicator of IWL.
- Increases in weight may be indicative of fluid compartment shifts from IVS into the interstitial compartment, as seen in the infant with acute sepsis or peritonitis, or with long-term use of paralytic.
- Tachycardia can be seen in ECF excess (e.g., heart failure) as well as in hypovolemia (e.g., acute blood loss, intravascular fluid shifts).
  - Capillary refill should be less than 3 seconds and is best assessed over the forehead or sternum. Delayed capillary refill indicates decreased perfusion but is not a specific indicator of hydration.
  - Decreases in blood pressure are a late sign of hypovolemia.
- Normal urine output after the first 24 hours should be 1 to 3 mL/kg/hr; however, the ELBW infant may not have decreased urine output in response to ECF depletion early on due to marked renal immaturity.
- Although stool output is not calculated separately, normal fluid loss in the stool is estimated at 5 to 10 mL/kg/d.
- The skin and mucosal membranes are less helpful in evaluating overall hydration status unless dehydration is significant. Decreased skin turgor, sunken anterior fontanel, and dry mucous membranes are very late signs (Bell, 2021; Doherty, 2017; Nyp et al., 2021; Wright et al., 2018).

LABORATORY ASSESSMENT

- Serum electrolytes, blood urea nitrogen (BUN), creatinine (Cr), glucose, and acid–base status are central in managing fluids and electrolytes and should be measured in the ELBW infant every 4 to 6 hours in the first few days of life due to their increased rates of IWL.
- Urine electrolytes and specific gravity (SG) reflect renal concentration/dilutional capabilities and the quantity of sodium (Na^+) reabsorbed or excreted, but are altered when the infant is on diuretics.
- Fractional excretion of Na^+ (FENa) reflects the balance between GFR and tubular reabsorption of Na^+ and can be calculated as:

  FENa = (urine Na^+ × plasma Cr) / (plasma Na^+ × urine Cr) × 100
- Levels of <1% are indicative of prerenal failure secondary to decreased renal blood flow; levels of 2.5% are associated with acute kidney injury (AKI). However, levels of >2.5% are often noted in infants <32 weeks' GA due to renal immaturity, which results in increased Na^+ excretion.

■ Acid–base balance measured as arterial pH, partial pressure of carbon dioxide in arterial blood (PaCO²) and concentration of bicarbonate in arterial blood (HCO3-) provides indirect evidence of intravascular volume depletion related to the effect of decreased tissue perfusion and the development of lactic acidosis (Doherty, 2017; Nyp et al., 2021).

▶ FLUID

FLUID REQUIREMENTS IN THE FIRST 48 HOURS

■ The goal of fluid and electrolyte management is to allow appropriate initial losses during the first 5 to 6 days of life, while maintaining normal serum osmolality and intravascular volume.

■ Initial fluid goals will vary depending on the GA of the infant, considering the IWL, weight change, serum electrolytes, urine output, and cardiovascular stability.

■ Recommended initial fluid goal volumes vary significantly. Ongoing fluid adjustments must be guided by weight change, intake, measurable output, IWL, and electrolyte balance to maintain the gradual decrease in ECF to 5% to 10% for the term infant and 10% to 15% for the preterm infant in the first 5 to 6 days of life.

  ● At less than 24 hours of age:
    ❏ BW <1,000 g requires ~100 to 150 mL/kg/d.
    ❏ BW 1,000 to 1,500 g requires ~80 to 100 mL/kg/d.
    ❏ BW >1,500 g requires ~60 to 80 mL/kg/d.
  ● At 24 to 48 hours of life:
    ❏ BW <1,000 g requires ~120 to 150 mL/kg/d.
    ❏ BW 1,000 to 1,500 g requires ~100 to 120 mL/kg/d.
    ❏ BW >1,500 g requires ~80 to 120 mL/kg/d (Bell, 2021; Doherty, 2017; Gomella et al., 2020b; Nyp et al., 2021; Wright et al., 2018).

MAINTENANCE FLUID REQUIREMENTS AT MORE THAN 48 HOURS

■ Maintenance fluid volumes are calculated using anticipated IWL, urine and stool output, and any other measurable losses (e.g., gastrointestinal [GI] output, chest tubes). Table 13.2 shows the ranges of water loss expected in the first 7 days of age.

■ Maintenance fluid generally increases 20 to 40 mL/kg/d over the first few days of life. The actual fluid goal (mL/kg/d) must be guided by the latest evidence: Fluid maintenance must provide adequate hydration without increasing the risk of patent ductus arteriosus (PDA), necrotizing enterocolitis (NEC), and intraventricular hemorrhage (IVH).

■ Additional intake for phototherapy is at 20 to 30 mL/kg/d if the patient is in open warmer and has radiant phototherapy. No adjustment is needed if the baby is

Table 13.2 Ranges of Estimated Water Loss in the First 7 Days of Age

Weight (g)	Ranges of Water Loss (mL/kg/d)		Day 1[a]	Days 2–3[a]	Days 4–7[a]
<1,250	IWL[b]	40–170			
	Urine	50–100			
	Stool	5–10			
	Total	95–280	120	140	150–175
1,250–1,750	IWL[b]	20–50			
	Urine	50–100			
	Stool	5–10			
	Total	75–160	90	110	130–140
>1,750	IWL[b]	15–40			
	Urine	50–100			
	Stool	5–10			
	TOTAL	70–150	80	90	100–200

IWL, insensible water loss.
[a] Adjustment based on a urine flow rate of 2 to 5 mg/kg/hr and stable weight.
[b] May be reduced by 30% if the infant is on a ventilator.
Source: Reproduced with permission from Nyp, M., Brunkhorst, J. L., Reavy, D., & Pallotto, E. K. (2021). Fluid and electrolyte management. In S. L. Gardner, B. S. Carter, M. E. Hines, & J. A. Hernandez (Eds.), *Merenstein & Gardner's handbook of neonatal intensive care nursing: An interprofessional approach* (9th ed., p. 417). Elsevier.

in a humidified environment and/or has fiberoptic phototherapy source.

■ Additional intake for radiant warmer is at 20 to 30 mL/kg/d.

■ At more than 48 hours of life:
  ● BW <1,000 g requires ~140 to 190 mL/kg/d.
  ● BW 1,000 to 1,500 g requires ~120 to 160 mL/kg/d.
  ● BW >1,500 g requires ~120 to 160 mL/kg/d (Bell, 2021; Doherty, 2017; Gomella et al., 2020b; Nyp et al., 2021; Wright et al., 2018).

ELECTROLYTE REQUIREMENTS

■ Na+ and K+ supplementation is not required in the first 24 hours in newborn infants, but may be required after 24 to 48 hours of life based on fluid balance and electrolyte levels (Box 13.1).

■ Sodium is supplemented as chloride, acetate, or phosphate in the amount of 2 to 3 mEq/kg/d. Infants with mild metabolic acidosis may benefit from sodium acetate supplementation rather than chloride.

■ Potassium is not provided until adequate urine output has been established. Once urine output has been established, K+ supplementation is added in 1 to 2 mEq/kg/d, but requirements may increase to 3 to 4 mEq/kg/d.

Box 13.1 Maintenance Electrolyte Needs at >48 Hours of Age

- *Na:* 1–4 mEq/kg/d (2–8 mEq/kg/d in VLBW infants)
- *K:* 1–4 mEq/kg/d
- *Cl:* 1–4 mEq/kg/d
- *Ca:* 1 mEq/kg/d

VLBW, very low birth weight.

- Elemental calcium (Ca^{2+}) should be provided in the first days after birth for most newborns (20–60 mg/kg/d or 1.5–2.0 mmol/kg per day), increasing over the course of the first few days to 60 to 80 mg/kg/d (Denne, 2018; Doherty, 2017; Gomella et al., 2020b; Nyp et al., 2021; Olsen et al., 2021).

▶ GLUCOSE HOMEOSTASIS

FETAL PHYSIOLOGY

- Throughout pregnancy, the mother supplies most of the glucose for the fetus via facilitated diffusion across the placenta. Fetal glucose levels are approximately 70% of maternal values.
- During the fetal period, the fetus produces very little glucose, although the enzymes to facilitate gluconeogenesis are present in the third month of gestation. In periods of extreme stress, where maternal glucose levels fall, the fetus can utilize ketone bodies for energy.
- The fetus begins to produce glycogen as early as the ninth week of gestation and continues to increase production throughout gestation, with the majority of glycogen production and storage occurring in the last trimester.
- The fetus also stores energy as fat, with most of the fat storage occurring in the last trimester (Rozance et al., 2021).

NEONATAL PHYSIOLOGY

- At birth, the maternal glucose supply abruptly ceases with the separation from the placenta, and the infant assumes responsibility for glucose homeostasis. Several processes are required for successful adaptation.
  - Initially, catecholamine levels rise sharply as a result of delivery into a cooler, extrauterine environment and the physical separation of the placenta.
  - Glucagon levels rise, receptor sensitivity increases, and fetal glucagon-to-insulin ratios shift as catecholamine levels rise.
  - Rising glucagon and norepinephrine levels activate hepatic glycogen phosphorylase, and the rapidly decreasing glucose levels stimulate cortisol secretion, which stimulates hepatic glucose-6-phosphatase activity.

- The newborn's ability to achieve glucose homeostasis is dependent on the balance between hepatic glucose output and glucose utilization in the brain and peripheral tissues.
- Increased metabolic demands (e.g., prematurity, respiratory distress, and cold stress) will increase demand for glucose that may exceed hepatic rates of glycogenolysis and gluconeogenesis (Rozance et al., 2021).
- Box 13.2 lists the indications for routine blood glucose monitoring in the neonate.

Box 13.2 Indications for Routine Blood Glucose in the Neonate

Maternal Conditions
- Presence of diabetes or abnormal result of glucose tolerance test
- Preeclampsia and pregnancy-induced or essential hypertension
- Previous macrosomic infants
- Substance abuse
- Treatment with beta-agonist tocolytics
- Treatment with oral hypoglycemic agents
- Late antepartum to intrapartum administration of intravenous glucose

Neonatal Conditions
- Prematurity
- Intrauterine growth restriction
- Perinatal hypoxia–ischemia
- Sepsis
- Hypothermia
- Polycythemia–hyperviscosity
- Erythroblastosis fetalis
- Iatrogenic administration of insulin
- Congenital cardiac malformations
- Persistent hyperinsulinemia
- Endocrine disorders
- Inborn errors of metabolism

Source: Reproduced with permission from Rozance, P. J., McGowan, J. E., Price-Douglas, W., & Hay, W. W., Jr. (2021). Glucose homeostasis. In S. L. Gardner, B. S. Carter, M. E. Hines, & J. A. Hernandez (Eds.), *Merenstein & Gardner's handbook of neonatal intensive care: An interprofessional approach* (9th ed., pp. 433–434). Elsevier.

ASSESSING GLUCOSE HOMEOSTASIS IN THE NEWBORN

- Glucose concentrations in the newborn can be measured at the bedside (point of care [POC]) or in the laboratory. POC measurements rely on reagent strips and measure whole blood glucose.
- Reagent strips are subject to false positives and false negatives, and thus laboratory analysis must be performed to accurately determine hypoglycemia.
- POC glucose levels generally run 15% below plasma blood glucose samples run in the laboratory. Glucose concentrations calculated in the laboratory are completed on plasma and must be run quickly after

the sample is drawn to limit the uptake of glucose by the red blood cells in the sample (Burris, 2017).

HYPOGLYCEMIA

■ Agreement on absolute blood or plasma glucose concentrations that define hypoglycemia continues to vary, ranging from 20 mg/dL in premature infants (30 mg/dL in term infants) to plasma concentrations less than 45 mg/dL in the first day of life regardless of gestation. Beyond the first 48 hours of life, any infant with plasma glucose levels less than 60 mg/dL should be evaluated for hypoglycemia.

■ Signs of hypoglycemia may include tremors, jitteriness, exaggerated Moro, high-pitched or weak cry, apnea, tachypnea, irregular respirations, cyanosis, lethargy, hypotonia, poor feeding, hypothermia, or seizures (Armentrout, 2021; Burris, 2017; Rozance et al., 2021).

Management of the Asymptomatic Newborn at Risk

■ Initial screens for infants at risk for hypoglycemia (e.g., SGA infants, IDMs, large-for-gestational-age [LGA] infants, and late preterm infants) should be completed in the first hour of life.
  ● If the infant is otherwise stable and asymptomatic, the infant may be fed and the glucose rechecked 1 hour later. If the repeat glucose remains <25 mg/dL, the infant should be treated with IV glucose.

■ If the second blood glucose is 25 to 40 mg/dL, feeding may be considered rather than treating with IV glucose in the otherwise healthy infant. An alternative therapy that may be helpful for healthy breastfed infants is 40% dextrose gel placed in the buccal mucosa, in addition to putting the infant to breast. Studies have shown that the use of 40% dextrose gel may reduce the need for NICU admissions due to hypoglycemia and decrease the use of formula supplementation for these infants in the first 2 weeks of life (Burris, 2017; Garg & Devaskar, 2020; Rozance et al., 2021).

Management of the Symptomatic Infant

■ When the newborn is symptomatic, IV therapy should be initiated with a bolus of IV 10% dextrose solution (D10W). The bolus should be followed with maintenance intravenous fluids (IVFs) of D10W to provide a glucose infusion rate (GIR) of 6 to 8 mg/kg/min.

■ Refractive hypoglycemia, or hypoglycemia with onset beyond the first day of life, requires an endocrinology consult for further evaluation. Adjunct therapies for persistent hypoglycemia include:
  ● Corticosteroids may be used to decrease peripheral glucose utilization and enhance gluconeogenesis.
  ● Glucagon may be used in the term infant to stimulate glycogenolysis and release glycogen stores from hepatic stores when insulin concentrations are normal. If hyperinsulinism is present, the dose must be adjusted significantly.
  ● Diazoxide may be used to inhibit insulin secretion.

  ● Somatostatin may be used to inhibit insulin and growth hormone release.
  ● Pancreatectomy may be necessary to decrease insulin production and secretion (Armentrout, 2020; Burris, 2017; Garg & Devaskar, 2020; Rozance et al., 2021).

HYPERGLYCEMIA

■ Hyperglycemia is defined as capillary glucose level analyzed by point of care (POC) sampling of >120 to 125 mg/dL or plasma glucose level >150 mg/dL. Onset of hyperglycemia may be seen within the first day of life and usually begins within the first 3 days of life.

■ Signs of hyperglycemia may include glycosuria, dehydration, weight loss, fever, ketosis, metabolic acidosis, and failure to thrive.

■ The primary concern with hyperglycemia is related to hyperosmolarity and osmotic diuresis. An osmolarity of >300 mOsm/L is associated with osmotic diuresis, and each 18 mg/dL increase in blood glucose concentration will increase serum osmolarity by 1 mOsm/L.

■ When blood glucose reaches 450 to 720 mg/dL (hyperosmolar), the ICF can shift to the extracellular compartment. It is postulated that the resultant decrease in the ICF may result in IVH.

■ The primary goal of therapy is prevention and early detection of hyperglycemia.
  ● The initial GIR for all infants is 4 to 6 mg/kg/min. (Blood glucose should be checked regularly and adjustments to GIR made appropriately.)
  ● Care should be taken to calculate GIR with changes in total fluid goals to prevent significant increases in GIR.

■ If the newborn develops hyperglycemia significant enough to warrant treatment (>250 mg/dL), despite efforts to decrease GIR and subsequently decrease blood glucose, insulin therapy may be required. However, studies have reported that routine prophylactic use of insulin to prevent the development of hyperglycemia in the very low birth weight (VLBW) infant is associated with a significant increase in morbidity, including increases in hypoglycemic episodes, and that there was no improvement in long-term outcomes of infants treated with insulin (Armentrout, 2021; Burris, 2017; Rozance et al., 2021).

▶ DISORDERS OF FLUID AND ELECTROLYTE IMBALANCE

DEHYDRATION

■ Dehydration may occur when appropriate fluid management is not achieved. This may be the result of losses through uncommon routes (chest tubes, gastric tubes, ventriculostomy drainage) that were neglected in the intake and output. Fluid shifts due to NEC or sepsis and fluid loss due to gastroschisis or omphalocele can be difficult to measure.

- Signs of dehydration include weight loss greater than the anticipated physiologic losses, decreased urine output, and increased urine SG.
  - Other signs of dehydration include tachycardia and hypotension, metabolic acidosis, and increases in BUN.
  - The infant at less than 32 weeks' GA may not present with decreased urine output despite having a fluid deficit due to the inability of their immature renal tubules to concentrate urine.
- Fluids must be administered to correct the fluid deficit, and maintenance fluid requirements will need to be adjusted to reflect the intake and output.
  - Acute symptomatic dehydration with normal serum sodium can be treated with bolus(es) of normal saline (NS) at 10 mL/kg to improve cardiac function (Doherty, 2017; Nyp et al., 2021).

EDEMA

- Edema results when there is an abnormal accumulation of fluid in the IS. The etiology of edema can include decreased capillary oncotic pressure from inadequate protein intake or kidney glomerular disease, increased capillary hydrostatic pressure, increased capillary wall permeability from infection affecting the integrity of the capillary wall, or hypertension from venous obstruction.
- Excessive intake of isotonic fluids will precipitate edema and signs of fluid overload. Development of edema can also occur under conditions such as heart failure, sepsis, and long term use of paralytics
- Signs of edema often include exaggerated weight gain but may also include periorbital edema, edema of the extremities, and hepatomegaly.
- The goal of therapy in edema is Na^+ restriction (to decrease total body Na^+) and/or fluid restriction (in the case of low serum Na^+). Again, the overall fluid balance must be carefully assessed to ensure that the IVS is adequate (Bell, 2021; Doherty, 2017; Wright, 2018).

SODIUM

- Sodium is the primary extracellular cation and is intricately involved in water balance. Na^+ is the major electrolyte controlling tonicity of the fluid compartments. Sodium is also critical for normal growth.
  - Normal serum levels range from 135 to 145 mEq/L. Normal body Na^+ requirements are generally 2 to 4 mEq/kg/d, although in the case of the preterm infant higher Na^+ intake may be required due to greater renal Na^+ losses related to renal immaturity.
  - Elevated serum Na^+ creates a hyperosmolar situation where water shifts from intracellular to extracellular spaces, resulting in cellular dehydration.
  - Low serum Na^+ creates a hypoosmolar situation where water shifts from the extracellular space to the intracellular spaces, resulting in cellular edema (Bell, 2021; Gomella et al., 2020b; Wright et al., 2018).

Hyponatremia

- Evaluation of hyponatremia begins with determining whether the etiology is due to factitious hyponatremia related to hyperlipidemia, hypoosmolar hyponatremia due to osmotic changes, excess free water, or increased sodium losses.
  - *Hyponatremia* is defined as serum Na^+ less than 130 mEq/L. Severe hyponatremia (serum Na^+ <120 mEq/L) may cause seizures or coma.
- Hyponatremia can be classified as early-onset hyponatremia or late-onset hyponatremia. Hyponatremia with onset in the first week of life is termed *early-onset hyponatremia* and is most often related to acute fluid and electrolyte management. Hyponatremia with onset after the first week of life is termed *late-onset hyponatremia*. Late onset may be related to prematurity with subsequent increased renal sodium loss, or acute disease such as congenital adrenal hyperplasia and renal failure.
- Hyperlipidemia can create a factitiously low serum Na^+ because the elevated lipids remain in a solid phase in the serum after sample preparation and displace the water content in the serum, creating a lower Na^+ concentration per liter in the plasma (Bell, 2021; Doherty, 2017; Gomella et al., 2020b; Nyp et al., 2021; Wright et al., 2018).

EARLY-ONSET HYPONATREMIA

- *Hyponatremia due to ECF volume depletion* results from diuretic therapy, osmotic diuresis (secondary to significant hyperglycemia), renal losses related to immaturity of the preterm kidney, adrenal salt-losing disorders (e.g., congenital adrenal hyperplasia), excessive losses in GI secretions/diarrhea, and conditions that cause third spacing (e.g., NEC, tissue sloughing). Signs of volume depletion include decreased weight, poor skin turgor, tachycardia, rising BUN, and metabolic acidosis. Decreased urine output may be seen in infants with relatively mature kidneys (>32 weeks' GA) as well as increased SG (due to renal urinary concentration) and low FENa.
  - The goal of therapy is to decrease ongoing Na^+ loss, provide Na^+ supplementation, replace

fluid deficit, and adjust maintenance Na^+ and fluid supplementation. Serum Na^+ deficit can be calculated with the following formula: Sodium deficit = (sodium desired − actual serum sodium) × 0.6 × weight (kg)

- For example, a 1.5-kg infant has a serum Na^+ of 130 mEq/L. The target goal is 140 mEq/L. Substitute these values in the above equation:
  - ❑ Sodium deficit = (140 − 130) × 0.6 × 1.5 kg
        OR
  - ❑ Sodium deficit = 10 × 0.6 × 1.5
- The sodium deficit for this infant is 9 mEq. Generally, only one-half of this deficit is replaced, slowly over several hours, and the serum Na^+ level is checked again to avoid overcorrection and/or too rapid a change in serum osmolarity.

■ *Hyponatremia with normal ECF volume* can result from excess fluid administration and in syndrome of inappropriate antidiuretic hormone (SIADH). The etiologies for SIADH include pain, opiate administration, IVH, asphyxia, meningitis, pneumothorax, and positive pressure ventilation.

- Signs of SIADH include weight gain without apparent edema, decreased urine output, and increased SG. Signs of excessive fluid administration include high urine output and low SG.
- The goal of therapy is to restrict fluids unless the serum Na^+ is <120 mEq/L or there are neurologic symptoms such as seizure or coma. In mild hyponatremia, the goal of therapy is reduction of total fluids. When the serum Na^+ is <120 mEq/L, furosemide therapy may be initiated while decreasing fluid goals and replacing the urinary output with hypertonic NaCl (3%).

■ *Hyponatremia due to ECF volume excess* can result from conditions associated with fluid shifts from the IVS to the interstitial compartment (third spacing), such as overwhelming sepsis, heart failure, abnormal lymphatic drainage, and use of neuromuscular paralytics. Signs of third spacing include increase in weight with edema, low urine output, rising BUN, rising SG, and low FENa in infants with mature renal function (e.g., infants >32 weeks' GA).

- The goal of therapy is to treat the underlying etiology and restrict free water to normalize serum osmolality. Restricting Na^+ and improving cardiac output may be beneficial.

LATE-ONSET HYPONATREMIA

■ *Late-onset hyponatremia* in the otherwise healthy preterm neonate is most likely due to sodium depletion due to low or inadequate sodium intake resulting from higher sodium requirements and increased renal losses of the preterm neonate. Late-onset hyponatremia can also be caused by excess sodium loss due to diuretic therapy. Late-onset hyponatremia can also be seen in neonates with congenital adrenal hypoplasia (CAH) or renal failure, but these are less common, and the neonate will not present as otherwise "well."

■ Late-onset hyponatremia due to sodium depletion can be treated with oral sodium supplementation; management of late-onset hyponatremia in the neonate with CAH or renal failure will require acute management, as described under "Early-Onset Hyponatremia" (Bell, 2021; Doherty, 2017; Gomella et al., 2020b; Nyp et al., 2021; Wright et al., 2018).

Hypernatremia

■ Evaluation of hypernatremia begins with determining whether the condition results from increased Na^+ supplementation, decreased ECF volume, excessive urine output, or excessive administration of isotonic or hypertonic fluids. Hypernatremia is defined as a serum Na^+ >150 mEq/L.

■ *Hypernatremia with normal or deficient ECF volume* can result from increased renal losses (urine) and IWL in the VLBW infant. IWL may be increased due to skin sloughing, antidiuretic hormone (ADH) deficiency subsequent to IVH, and increased renal (urine) losses.

- Signs include weight loss, tachycardia, hypotension, metabolic acidosis, decreasing urine output, and increasing SG. SG may also be low in the infant with diabetes insipidus (DI), whether central or nephrogenic.
- The goal of therapy is to increase free water administration to reduce serum Na^+ while avoiding ECF excess. Serum Na^+ reduction should be achieved slowly, no greater than 1 mEq/kg/hr to avoid too rapid a change in the serum osmolality. Hypernatremia is not always indicative of excess body Na^+. The VLBW infant may present with hypernatremia in the first 24 hours of life due to free water deficits related to ECF contraction and IWL.

■ *Hypernatremia with ECF volume excess* can result from excessive administration of isotonic or hypertonic fluids, particularly in conditions resulting in decreased cardiac output.

Signs of hypernatremia with ECF include weight gain accompanied by edema. Vital signs such as heart rate, blood pressure, urine output, and SG are often normal, but the FENa will be elevated.

- The goal of therapy is to restrict Na^+ administration (Bell, 2021; Doherty, 2017; Gomella et al., 2020b; Nyp et al., 2021; Wright et al., 2018).

POTASSIUM

■ Potassium is the primary intracellular cation and is measured indirectly in the serum. K^+ shifts between the ICF and ECF based on pH of the serum. An increase of 0.1 pH units in the serum will result in a decrease of 0.6 mEq/L in serum K^+ concentration.

Normal total body K+ is a product of normal intake (1–2 mEq/kg/d) and excretion through the GI tract and renal system. Normal serum K+ levels range from 3.5 to 5.0 mEq/L (Bell, 2021; Doherty, 2017; Wright et al., 2018).

Hypokalemia

■ Evaluation of hypokalemia requires a determination of whether the primary etiology is increased loss of K+ or inadequate intake. Hypokalemia can result in arrhythmias, ileus, renal concentrating defects, and coma in the infant.

- Signs of hypokalemia include generalized muscle weakness, decreased T-waves, and ST depression measured on EKG.
- The goal of therapy is to decrease losses and gradually increase K+ supplementation. Hypokalemia related to the use of loop diuretics (e.g., furosemide) can be treated with K+ supplementation. Changing to K+-sparing diuretics (e.g., spironolactone) as early as possible when long-term diuretic therapy is indicated will reduce renal losses (Bell, 2021; Doherty, 2017; Eyal, 2020d; Nyp et al., 2021; Wright et al., 2018).

Hyperkalemia

■ Evaluation of hyperkalemia begins with determining the underlying etiology. The blood sample must be drawn centrally to confirm diagnosis, since capillary samples may be elevated due to squeezing causing cell lysis and release of intracellular K+.

- Initial therapy for hyperkalemia is often initiated emergently, but all therapies provide only temporary reduction in serum K+.
- Conditions commonly associated with hyperkalemia include acidosis (with or without tissue damage), cephalohematoma, hemolysis, hypothermia, asphyxia, ischemia, AKI, adrenal insufficiency, and IVH, or can be iatrogenic due to excess K+ administration.
- Nonoliguric hyperkalemia often occurs in the ELBW infant in the first few days of life even without K+ administration due to relatively low GFR and intra- to extracellular K+ shifts due to decreased activity of the Na–K ATPase system.
- Symptomatic hyperkalemia may be seen at levels >6 mEq/L.

■ Signs of hyperkalemia may include cardiovascular instability as bradyarrhythmias or tachyarrhythmias, or cardiovascular collapse, but the infant may also be asymptomatic in the early stages.

- EKG changes are often the first sign of hyperkalemia. Electrocardiographic findings are altered as the serum K+ rises, presenting with varying levels of peaked T-waves (secondary to increased repolarization of the cardiac tissue), flattened P-waves, and increased PR intervals (secondary to suppression of atrial conductivity).

These changes are followed by widening and slurring of the QRS complex (secondary to delay in ventricular conduction as well as delays in myocardial conduction), with eventual development of supraventricular tachycardia, ventricular tachycardia, bradycardia, or ventricular fibrillation.

■ The goal of therapy is to remove all sources of exogenous K+ (IV solutions, medications, enteral feedings if they contain K+), rehydrate if indicated, and evaluate serum and total ionized calcium (iCa) levels.

- There are three stages in pharmacologic therapy: stabilization of the conductive tissue, dilution, intracellular shifting of K+, and facilitating K+ excretion.
- If calcium levels are low, calcium supplementation is indicated to protect cardiac function.

■ Stabilization of the conductive tissue can be accomplished by Na+ or Ca2+ administration. Ca2+ is generally the first step, infusing 1 to 2 mL/kg IV of calcium gluconate over 15 to 30 minutes. In cases where the infant is also hyponatremic, NS bolus may be beneficial in adjusting the Na+ level and adding a dilutional factor.

■ Antiarrhythmic agents (lidocaine or bretylium) may be added to treat refractory ventricular tachycardia.

■ Dilution is accomplished by evaluating overall hydration and correcting fluid administration to promote adequate circulating volumes. Fluid administration must always be evaluated in the face of renal functionality; the infant with AKI will often not be able to accommodate additional fluid loads.

■ Sodium bicarbonate (NaHCO3) may be used to shift the pH slowly.

■ Insulin will enhance intracellular K+ uptake by stimulating the membrane-bound Na–K ATPase.

- Glucose infusion must always accompany insulin to maintain normal serum glucose. Insulin therapy may start with a bolus dose of insulin and glucose, followed by continuous infusion of D10W with human regular insulin. Many institutions have their own glucose/insulin cocktails that can be ordered from the pharmacy.
- Insulin binds to the plastic IV tubing, so the tubing must be flushed well in an attempt to saturate the binding sites prior to administration. Significant hypoglycemia and seizures may occur, which mandates frequent evaluation of blood glucose.

■ The use of beta-2-adrenergic agents (such as albuterol) will enhance K+ uptake as well, although they are not commonly used in the neonatal population; the mechanism for this is thought to be stimulation of the Na–K ATPase activity.

■ K+ excretion can be facilitated with diuretic therapy by increasing renal blood flow and improving Na+ delivery in the distal tubules.

■ In the infant with oliguria and reversible AKI, peritoneal dialysis and double-volume exchange transfusions may be considered as potentially lifesaving measures.

- Peritoneal dialysis can be successful in infants <1 kg and should be considered in situations where the newborn's overall clinical status is appropriate and there is a reasonable chance for recovery with good long-term outcome. Other sources suggest that peritoneal dialysis in the VLBW infant may be technically difficult to impossible, particularly in infants with accompanying NEC.
- Double-volume exchange transfusions should be conducted with fresh blood <24 hours old, or deglycerized red blood cells that have been reconstituted with fresh frozen plasma.
- Cation exchange resin solutions may also enhance K^+ excretion by exchanging Na^+ or Ca^{2+} ions for K^+ (Na^+ or Ca^{2+} polystyrene sulfonate). These resins may be given orally or rectally, although the literature remains inconclusive relative to their risk-to-benefit ratios in neonates (Bell, 2021; Bohannon et al., 2020; Doherty, 2017; Gomella et al., 2021; Nyp et al., 2021; Wright et al., 2018).

CALCIUM

- Calcium is essential for several biochemical processes, including coagulation, neuromuscular excitability, cell membrane integrity and function, and cellular enzymatic and secretory activity. Serum calcium levels are regulated by parathyroid levels and 1,25-dihydroxyvitamin D (calcitriol) and pH.
- Calcium can be measured as total serum calcium or as iCa. Normal ranges for calcium are 8.5 to 10.2 mg/dL for total serum calcium and 4.4 to 5.3 mg/dL for iCa. Calcium levels and distribution are also closely correlated with pH. In alkalosis, albumin affinity for calcium increases, which decreases ionized Ca^{2+} levels. Conversely, acidosis decreases albumin binding of calcium, thereby increasing iCa levels (Abrams, 2017; Abrams & Tiosano, 2020; Bell, 2021; Koves et al., 2018).

Hypocalcemia

- Hypocalcemia is a common finding in critically ill infants and is due to the interrelationship between calcium levels, parathyroid hormone, and calcitriol.
- At birth, the infant's calcium supply across the placenta ceases abruptly and parathyroid hormone responds by rising, which causes release of Ca^{2+} from the bone, increasing Ca^{2+} resorption in the renal tubule, and stimulating the renal production of calcitonin, resulting in a rise in serum Ca^{2+}. This response is gradual over the first 48 hours of life and is more diminished in the preterm and sick newborn. Normal Ca^{2+} nadir occurs at approximately 48 hours of life and is well tolerated in the healthy term newborn. Early Ca^{2+} supplementation may be required in the preterm

infant, the critically ill newborn, and the ill infant of the diabetic mother.

- The best approach is to prevent hypocalcemia by providing IV Ca^{2+} supplementation on the first day of life for infants at greatest risk for hypocalcemia.
- Conditions that are associated with low calcium due to hypoparathyroidism are DiGeorge sequence (hypoplasia or absence of the parathyroid) and Kenny–Caffey syndrome (pseudohypoparathyroidism, secondary to maternal hyperparathyroidism), hypomagnesemia, vitamin D deficiency, alkalosis and bicarbonate use, shock, sepsis, and phototherapy. The mechanism for phototherapy-induced hypocalcemia is thought to be secondary to decreased melatonin secretion, which increases bone absorption of Ca^{2+}. Late-onset hypocalcemia may be related to high phosphate intake, which decreases serum Ca^{2+}.
  - Signs of hypocalcemia may include jitteriness, irritability, or twitching; increased extensor tone; clonus; hyperreflexia; and stridor secondary to laryngospasm. Hypocalcemia is defined as total serum Ca^{2+} less than 7 mg/dL or iCa^{2+} less than 4 mg/dL (0.8–1 mmol/L). Calcium is present as total serum Ca^{2+} (free serum Ca^{2+} plus albumin-bound Ca^{2+}) and iCa. It is critical to measure ionized iCa when assessing for hypocalcemia since hypoalbuminemia will decrease the level of total circulating serum Ca^{2+}.
  - The goal of therapy is to provide calcium supplementation. Serum magnesium levels should be obtained prior to calcium supplementation to make certain that the serum magnesium is normal, since calcium and magnesium absorptions are interrelated. In circumstances where hypocalcemia occurs in the infant who is taking enteral nutrition, calcium glubionate syrup may be used orally; however, this will increase osmolarity and may cause GI irritation or diarrhea (Abrams, 2017; Abrams & Tiosano, 2020; Bell, 2021; Inayat, 2020; Koves et al., 2018; Nyp et al., 2021; Polin & Adamkin, 2020).

SPECIAL CONCERNS WITH INTRAVENOUS CALCIUM SUPPLEMENTATION

- Rapid infusion of Ca^{2+} may cause bradyarrhythmias.
- Calcium can cause hepatic necrosis if given through an umbilical venous catheter (UVC) that is improperly positioned in the hepatic portal veins.
- Rapid infusion of calcium into an umbilical arterial catheter (UAC) can cause arterial spasm, which may result in intestinal necrosis.
- Calcium and bicarbonate are incompatible and cannot be infused together.
- Extravasation of Ca^{2+} into the subcutaneous tissue can cause severe necrosis and calcifications (Abrams & Tiosano, 2020; Bell, 2021; Inayat, 2020; Koves et al., 2018; Nyp et al., 2021; Polin & Adamkin, 2020).

Hypercalcemia

- Hypercalcemia is defined as total serum Ca^{2+} >11 mg/dL or iCa >1.45 mmol/L. Infants with calcium levels in this range are often asymptomatic; however, infants presenting with total serum Ca^{2+} >16 mg/dL (iCa >1.8 mmol/L) may require immediate treatment. Conditions associated with hypercalcemia may be iatrogenic due to excessive vitamin D intake, excessive Ca^{2+} supplementation, or inadequate phosphorus supplementation in infants receiving parenteral nutrition (PN). Other conditions that may be associated with hypercalcemia include hyperparathyroidism, hyperthyroidism, Williams syndrome, and hypophosphatasia, or use of thiazide diuretics.
- If hypercalcemia is iatrogenic secondary to inadequately balanced Calcium (Ca^2+)/ phosphorus (Phos) supplementation in PN, adjusting the supplementation will correct serum Ca^{2+}.
- Iatrogenic hypercalcemia related to PN is often associated with the removal of phosphorous in an effort to decrease the Na or K supplementation.
- Hypercalcemia may also be seen in the ELBW infant as a result of an inability to utilize the amount of Ca^{2+} being provided by PN.
- Signs of hypercalcemia may include history of poor feeding, emesis, lethargy, irritability, constipation, and polyuria. Infants with hypercalcemia secondary to hyperthyroidism may present with hypotonia, encephalopathy, hepatosplenomegaly, anemia, and extraskeletal calcifications.
- The goal of therapy for infants with significant hypercalcemia depends on the etiology.
  - Emergent medical treatment for symptomatic infants or infants with total serum Ca^{2+} >16 mg/dL (iCa >1.8 mmol/L) is volume expansion (to provide dilution) with 0.9% NaCl to promote renal excretion of calcium.
    - Furosemide can be given to promote renal excretion of calcium. Inorganic phosphate may lower serum Ca^{2+} if the infant is hypophosphatemic, by inhibiting Ca^{2+} mobilization from the bone and promoting mineral accretion in the bone.
  - Glucocorticoids are effective in treating hypervitaminosis A and D and can also facilitate reduction of serum Ca^{2+} secondary to fat necrosis by inhibiting bone mobilization and intestinal absorption (Abrams, 2017; Abrams & Tiosano, 2020; Bell, 2021; Inayat, 2020; Koves et al., 2018; Nyp et al., 2021; Polin & Adamkin, 2020).

MAGNESIUM

- Magnesium is the second most abundant intracellular cation in the body. It is actively transported from the mother to the fetus using a transport mechanism different from calcium.
- Magnesium is required for optimal function of intracellular enzyme systems, including muscle contraction and carbohydrate metabolism. Additionally, it is critical for normal parathyroid function and bone–serum calcium homeostasis (Bell, 2021; Polin & Adamkin, 2020).

Hypomagnesemia

- Hypomagnesemia is defined as serum levels <1.6 mg/dL. Hypomagnesemia is uncommon in infants, but when present is most often seen in conjunction with hypocalcemia (Doherty, 2017).
- Signs of hypomagnesemia may include apnea and poor motor tone (Doherty, 2017).
- The goal of therapy for symptomatic hypomagnesemia is to provide magnesium supplementation with magnesium sulfate (Doherty, 2017). Serum calcium levels must also be measured, and if hypocalcemia is present it must be treated concurrently (Abrams, 2017; Abrams & Tiosano, 2020; Bell, 2021; Polin & Adamkin, 2020).

Hypermagnesemia

- Hypermagnesemia is defined as serum magnesium >3 mg/dL. The most common etiology for newborn hypermagnesemia is secondary to maternal therapy for preterm labor or preeclampsia.
- Signs of symptomatic hypermagnesemia include apnea, respiratory depression, lethargy, hypotonia, hyporeflexia, poor suck, decreased peristalsis, and delayed passage of meconium. Neonates are often asymptomatic until levels exceed 6 mg/dL.
- The goal of therapy for hypermagnesemia is the removal of exogenous magnesium. Enteral feedings are delayed until the infant demonstrates good suck and has adequate intestinal motility (Abrams, 2017; Abrams & Tiosano, 2020; Bell, 2021; Koves et al., 2018; Polin & Adamkin, 2020).
- Table 13.3 summarizes the ranges for serum electrolytes at the low (hypo-) normal, and high (hyper-) values.

COMMON PROBLEMS ASSOCIATED WITH FLUID AND ELECTROLYTE IMBALANCE

- SIADH occurs when the body is unable to excrete water due to an excessive amount of ADH. SIADH often develops after perinatal depression, exacerbating fluid and electrolyte imbalance by increasing fluid retention and risk of hyponatremia.
  - The resulting water retention leads to dilutional hyponatremia. Serum and urine chemistry and osmolality can assist in determining if SIADH is the etiology of hyponatremia. Oliguria, water retention, serum hyponatremia, low serum osmolality, increased urine osmolality, and no acid–base disturbance are suggestive of SIADH.

Table 13.3 Normally Accepted Ranges for Serum Electrolytes

	Hypo-	Normal	Hyper-
Na⁺ (mEq/L)	<130	135–145	>150
K⁺ (mEq/L)	<3.5	3.5–5.5	>6.5
Ca²⁺ (mg/dL)	<7	8.5–10.2	>11
iCa, mmol/L (mg/dL)	<1.1 (<4.4)	1–1.4 (4.4–5.3)	>1.45 (>5.8)
Mg²⁺ (mg/dL)	<1.5	1.5–2.5	>3

Ca²⁺, calcium; iCa, ionized calcium; K⁺, potassium; Mg²⁺, magnesium; Na⁺, sodium.
Sources: Data from Abrams, S.A., & Tiosano, D. (2020). Disorders of calcium, phosphorous, and magnesium metabolism in the neonate. In R. J. Martin, A. A. Fanaroff, & M. C. Walsh (Eds.), *Fanaroff & Martin's neonatal-perinatal medicine: Diseases of the fetus and infant* (11th ed., pp. 1611–1642). Elsevier; Bell, S. G. (2021). Fluid and electrolyte management. In M. T. Verklan, M. Walden, & S. Forest (Eds.), *Core curriculum for neonatal intensive care nursing* (6th ed., pp. 131–143). Elsevier.

- DI is an uncommon disorder in the newborn and is characterized by a decrease in ADH (vasopressin) secretion from the posterior pituitary (central DI) or lack of response to ADH by the renal tubules (nephrogenic DI), resulting in polyuria and hypernatremia. Serum and urine chemistry and osmolality show elevated serum sodium and osmolality, low urine osmolality, and low serum ADH levels.
- Oliguria is defined as urine output less than 1 mL/kg/hr. Investigation into the etiology of oliguria (prerenal, parenchymal, and postrenal) will determine the management. AKI has a significant effect on fluid, electrolyte, and acid–base balance. AKI can occur with or without oliguria (Dell, 2020; Nyp et al., 2021; Wright et al., 2018).
- PDA can be affected by fluid and acid–base imbalance (overhydration and metabolic acidosis) and may also affect fluid and electrolyte status.
  - Choice of pharmacologic management for closure of PDA (indomethacin vs. ibuprofen) will impact the severity of the fluid and electrolyte imbalance. Acetaminophen for closure of PDA may have less impact on fluid and electrolyte balance, but there is potential for hepatic dysfunction in the very preterm infant.
- Asphyxia secondary to insufficient oxygen delivery to the cells often results from decreased perfusion (ischemia) or inadequate ventilation (hypoxia/hypercarbia) and can damage renal tubules, resulting in decreased urine output. Management focuses on restriction of fluid delivery to basal needs plus insensible losses, strict output measurement of urine volume and sodium, and diligent fluid and electrolyte replacement during the oliguric and ensuing polyuric (tubule recovery) phases (Alpan, 2020; Dell, 2020; Nyp et al., 2021; Wright et al., 2018).
- Bronchopulmonary dysplasia (BPD) may result from the fluid and electrolyte management of the neonate, especially the necessary high fluid requirements

and the high sodium levels of the neonate in the first days after birth, accompanied by sluggish contraction of the ECF and expected loss of fluid on the first week of life.
- Infants with BPD, who require increased caloric support in the presence of high metabolic needs, are at increased risk for fluid and electrolyte imbalances.
- High nutrition and caloric needs often require higher daily fluid goals, which lead to volume overload and fluid retention, resulting in exacerbation of pulmonary disease.
- Diuretics are often used to manage fluid retention; however, this results in electrolyte abnormalities due to urine electrolyte losses. Diuretics have significant impact on both fluid and electrolyte and acid–base balance. The extent of the imbalances depends on the type of diuretic used in treatment (Dell, 2020; Doherty, 2017; Nyp et al., 2021; Wright, 2018). For specific information regarding diuretic medications, please see Chapter 14.

DELIVERY OF INTRAVENOUS FLUIDS

- The type of IV access that is available is a key factor to be considered when delivering IV fluids. For infants with relatively short-term requirements (<7 days), where nutritional requirements can be met with dextrose solutions no greater than 12.5%, peripheral access may be sufficient.
  - Maximum osmolarity for solutions to be delivered through peripheral catheters must not exceed 900 mOsm/L.
  - Osmolality limitations can result in limited nutrition delivery.
- For infants who are anticipated to require longer term PN (greater than 1 week) or whose nutritional needs will require dextrose >12.5%, central access will be required. Central access can be obtained with UVCs or peripherally inserted central catheters.
  - Central access must be obtained if the osmolarity of the PN will exceed 900 mOsm/L (Olsen et al., 2021).
  - Central venous delivery allows for more concentrated formulations and caloric density (Poindexter & Martin, 2020).
- Intralipid (IL) special circumstances:
  - Lipid oxidation also occurs with exposure to light. Covering PN and IL solutions, including tubing, may reduce these oxidant effects, enhance IL metabolism, and lower circulating triglyceride levels (Olsen et al., 2021).

▶ INTRAVENOUS LIPID INFUSIONS

- Recommended fat requirements vary depending on the source, but the most recent recommendation is to initiate 2 g/kg of lipid on the first day of life for infants <1,500 g, advancing to 3 g/kg on the second day of life.

- Preterm infants are at risk of essential fatty acid deficiency within 72 hours after birth. Essential fatty acid deficiency can be eliminated by providing 0.5 to 1 mL/kg/d of IL.
- The ELBW infant often has lower tolerance for IL, which may require initiating IL at a lower rate and/or advancing the dose more gradually.
- Lipids are infused over 24 hours to promote optimal clearance.

LIPID EMULSIONS

- Twenty percent lipid emulsion is the most commonly supplied formulation, and the most common lipid solutions used in the United States are soy-based or a combination of soy/safflower. Twenty percent solutions of IL provide 2.2 kcal/mL (or approximately 10 kcal/g).

SMOF

- SMOF lipid is a mixture of **S**oybean oil, **M**edium-chain triglyceride, **O**live oil, and **F**ish oil. It has been approved for use by the Food and Drug Administration (FDA) since 2016.
  - SMOF lipids are also higher in anti-inflammatory omega-3 fatty acids and have been introduced for management of parenteral nutrition-associated liver disease (PNALD).

OMEGAVEN

- Omegaven is 100% fish oil rich in n-3 fatty acids. It is a fish oil-based 10% fat emulsion and is high in anti-inflammatory omega-3 fatty acids. The use of fish oil emulsion is recommended in the management of parenteral nutrition-associated cholestasis (PNAC) or PNALD, but has not been demonstrated to prevent PNALD in infants. Omegaven was approved by the FDA in the United States in 2018 and is available by prescription.
- Although it provides alpha-linoleic acids, it lacks vital long-chain polyunsaturated fatty acids (LCPUFA), including docosahexaenoic acid (DHA), eicosapentaenoic acid (EPA), and arachidonic acid.
  - Concern exists that the high LCPUFA content of lipid emulsions (with excess mega-6 linoleic acid) leads to synthesis of prostaglandins and leukotrienes, which can increase vasomotor tone and result in hypoxemia.
- Fish-based emulsions help reverse cholestasis that develops in infants with short bowel syndrome after receiving prolonged soybean-based emulsion (Adamkin & Radmacher, 2020; Anderson et al., 2017; Denne, 2018; Parker, 2020; Poindexter & Martin, 2020).

▶ ACID–BASE BALANCE

- Cells function at their maximal metabolic function in a stable, homeostatic environment. The normal pH range is approximately 7.35 to 7.45. The Henderson–Hasselbalch equation calculates plasma pH. The pH is a negative logarithm that measures the level of hydrogen ions (H^+), which means that there is an inverse relationship between pH and H^+. The pH decreases with a rise in H^+ and increases with a fall in H^+. The pH remains normal when there is a balance in changes of carbon dioxide (CO_2) and bicarbonate (HCO_3).
- Regulation of pH is determined by chemical buffers in body fluids, elimination of PCO_2 (H^+ and water) by the lungs, and reabsorption or elimination of H^+ or HCO_3 by the kidneys. The classification of acidosis and alkalosis is determined by the system causing the pH derangement (Barry et al., 2021; Bell, 2021; Wright et al., 2018).
  - *Respiratory acidosis* results from inadequate alveolar ventilation, leading to an excess of CO_2 and a decrease in pH. Inadequate alveolar ventilation can result from prematurity, neurologic compromise, or medications.
    - In red blood cells, the enzyme *carbonic anhydrase* promotes the combination of a fraction of dissolved CO_2 with water to form carbonic acid (H_2CO_3), which then dissociates into a hydrogen ion (H^+) and a bicarbonate ion (HCO_3^-). This is demonstrated by the following equation: $CO_2 + H_2O = H_2CO_3 = [H^+] + [HCO_3^-]$.
  - *Respiratory alkalosis* results from alveolar hyperventilation, leading to a decrease in CO_2 and an increase in pH. Excessive alveolar ventilation can result from mechanical overventilation, tachypnea, or anxiety.
  - *Metabolic acidosis* results either from an excess of acid in the ECF or a loss of buffer, leading to a decrease in pH. Conditions such as hypoxia, immature renal tubular function, or diarrhea can result in metabolic acidosis, as well as hypovolemia, sepsis, hemorrhage, compromised cardiac function, or severe chronic anemia. Management of metabolic acidosis must focus on identification of the underlying cause of the disturbance and appropriately matched treatment (e.g., blood administration in the case of hemorrhage, improving cardiac contractility). The use of sodium bicarbonate is no longer recommended as the primary approach for treatment of metabolic acidosis due to the significant side effects that can be seen with use.
    - The anion gap helps distinguish metabolic acidosis from a pathologic condition, such as asphyxia, or a physiologic condition, such as an increased threshold for bicarbonate excretion in the neonate. The gap is calculated by subtracting

the chloride (Cl⁻) levels and bicarbonate (HCO3⁺) level from the sodium (Na⁺) amount measured in blood electrolytes. For example, Na⁺ of 135, K⁺ of 3.4, Cl⁻ of 110, and bicarbonate of 12 yield a gap of 13: Na⁺ 135 − (Cl⁻ 110 + HCO₃⁻ 12) = anion gap 13.

  ○ Decreases in anion gap (<5 mEq/L) indicate a loss of buffering agents.
  ○ Increases in anion gap (>15 mEq/L) indicate an excess accumulation of acid and may be caused by acute renal failure, inborn error of metabolism, lactic acidosis, or toxins (e.g., benzyl alcohol).

- *Metabolic alkalosis* results from a loss of acids or an increase in bases. Vomiting or diuretics can induce metabolic alkalosis. Treatment depends on the underlying cause and can be guided by urine chloride levels. For example, a low urinary chloride is suggestive of vomiting or continuous nasogastric suction, whereas high urinary chloride may be associated with hypokalemia or early diuretic therapy.
  ○ *Metabolic alkalosis in the presence of low urinary chloride* (<10 mEq/L) may be caused by GI losses (e.g., vomiting, gastric suction, diarrhea, or use of diuretic therapies).
  ○ *Metabolic alkalosis in the presence of high urinary chloride* (>20 mEq/L) may be caused by alkali administration, massive transfusion of blood products, diuretic therapy, or Bartter syndrome associated with mineralocorticoid excess.

■ *Management of respiratory and metabolic acidosis and alkalosis* is centered around the treatment of the underlying cause. Management of metabolic acidosis usually involves corrective action by treating the underlying circulatory problem and providing volume if indicated. In critically ill infants with metabolic acidosis, K⁺ levels must be closely monitored due to the intricate shifts of K⁺ and H⁺ ions during metabolic acidosis treated with sodium bicarbonate.

■ Normalization of respiratory acidosis or alkalosis may involve manipulation of ventilator rate (correction) acutely or involve kidney response by increasing bicarbonate reabsorption (compensation) in chronic permissive hypercapnia accompanying BPD.
  - *Correction* of a pH imbalance results from manipulation of the body system causing the problem, for example, correction of respiratory acidosis via manipulation of ventilator rate to control the level of CO_2 acid.
  - *Compensation* of a pH imbalance results from a response from the system not directly causing the pH imbalance, for example, kidney reabsorption of HCO_3 (buffer) as compensation for chronic respiratory acidosis (Barry et al., 2021; Bell, 2021; Dell, 2020; Doherty, 2017; Gomella, 2020; Wright et al., 2018).

■ Using the normal blood gas ranges identified in Table 13.4, blood gases can be assessed for acid–base

status; however, GA, disease, and clinical status must be considered when evaluating blood gases and acid–base status.

■ Table 13.5 demonstrates four examples of blood gases reflective of acid–base imbalances, possible causes, and possible corrective interventions to normalize acid–base balance.

FACTORS AFFECTING ACID–BASE BALANCE

■ Renal tubular acidosis (RTA) is most commonly associated with tubular damage in the kidney and should be considered in infants with metabolic acidosis with a normal anion gap and a urine pH less than 6.5. There are three types of RTA, and treatment varies depending on the type.

■ Dehydration has an impact on fluid and electrolyte and acid–base balance. The severity of the imbalance depends on the precipitating factors for dehydration, the etiology of the associated sodium balance (depleted, normal, or excess ECF water content), and the response to treatment.

■ *GI losses/surgery:* Intestinal decompression and postoperative metabolic response impact both fluid and electrolyte balance and acid–base homeostasis.

■ NEC is characterized by tissue edema and increased IS fluid, alteration in electrolytes due to GI decompression, and circulatory compromise affecting fluid/electrolyte and acid–base balance.

■ Diarrhea is a precipitating factor in metabolic acidosis with a normal anion gap. Treatment of the underlying cause and supportive treatment with fluid and electrolyte replacement are often necessary in severe diarrhea.

■ Vomiting places the infant at risk of metabolic alkalosis with low urinary chloride. Severe vomiting in the infant may require fluid and electrolyte replacement (Dell, 2020; Doherty, 2017; Nyp et al., 2021; Wright et al., 2018).

Table 13.4 Normal (Arterial) Blood Gas Values

pH	7.35–7.45
PaCO₂ (mmHg)	35–45
HCO₃⁻ (mEq/L)	18–26
Base excess	(−5 to +5)
PaO₂ (mmHg)	60–80
O₂ saturation (%)	92–94

HCO₃, concentration of bicarbonate in arterial blood; PaCO₂, partial pressure of carbon dioxide in arterial blood; PaO₂, partial pressure of oxygen in arterial blood.

Source: Data from Barry, J. S., Deacon, J., Hernandez, C., & Jones, M. D. (2021). Acid-base homeostasis and oxygenation. In S. L. Gardner, M. Carter, M. F. Hines, & J. A. Hernandez (Eds.), *Merenstein & Gardner's handbook of neonatal intensive care nursing: An interprofessional approach* (9th ed., pp 186–187). Elsevier.

Table 13.5 Acid–Base Imbalances: Causes and Interventions

Arterial Blood Gas: pH/PaCO$_2$ (mmHg)/PaO$_2$ (mmHg)/HCO$_3$ (mEq/L)	Acid–Base Imbalance	Cause/Mechanism (One Possible Cause)	Possible Intervention (Correction)	Expected Outcome (Repeat ABG)
7.25/60/50/22	Respiratory acidosis pH <7.35, PaCO$_2$ >45	CNS depression with hypoventilation	Mechanical ventilation with IMV	7.30/45/65/24
7.50/28/70/24	Respiratory alkalosis	RDS with mechanical hyperventilation	Decrease IMV	7.43/38/70/24
7.25/40/55/15	Metabolic acidosis pH <7.35, HCO$_3$ <22	Decreased tissue perfusion with lactic acid production	Reestablish perfusion Consider bicarbonate administration	7.30/45/62/20
7.49/38/72/28	Metabolic alkalosis pH >7.45, HCO$_3$ >26	Excessive base (acetate) in TPN	Change TPN additives (acetate to chloride)	7.43/40/70/24

ABG, arterial blood gas; CNS, central nervous system; HCO$_3$, concentration of bicarbonate in arterial blood; IMV, intermittent mandatory ventilation; PaCO$_2$, partial pressure of carbon dioxide in arterial blood; PaO$_2$, partial pressure of oxygen in arterial blood; RDS, respiratory distress syndrome; TPN, total parenteral nutrition.

Source: Data from Fraser, D., & Diehl-Jones, W. (2021). Assisted ventilation. In M. T. Verklan, M. Walden, & S. Forest (Eds.), *Core curriculum for neonatal intensive care nursing* (6th ed., pp. 440–441). Elsevier.

▶ CONCLUSION

Best practices in diagnosis and management of fluid and electrolyte abnormalities in the sick newborn require more than knowledge of physiologic principles. Astute clinical knowledge of disease processes and impact on the newborn, careful attention to changes in fluid and electrolyte levels, and timely adjustments in fluid and electrolyte supplementation to maintain homeostasis are equally critical in the safe and appropriate management of the sick newborn with fluid and electrolyte imbalances.

1. Calculate the insensible water loss (IWL) for a 2-kg infant with a total fluid intake of 150 mL/kg/d, a urine output of 3 mL/kg/hr, and a weight loss of 200 g.

   A. −124 mL

   B. −88 mL

   C. −44 mL

2. The neonatal nurse practitioner (NNP) is evaluating a 4-week-old, former 28-week neonate who is stable and on full enteral feedings. The serum electrolytes are: Na+ 121, K+ 3.8, and Cl− 97. Nutritional intake supplies 120 kcal/kg/d. Current weight is 1.5 kg, with a weight gain of 10 g/d over the past 7 days. This data reflects:

   A. Adequate weight gain; no nutritional changes required

   B. Insufficient weight gain most likely due to hyponatremia

   C. Poor weight gain most likely due to inadequate caloric intake

3. The neonatal nurse practitioner (NNP) is evaluating a 4-week-old, former 30-week infant who is currently on full enteral feedings of expressed mother's milk, fortified to 22 cal/oz with human milk fortifier. The neonate weighs 1.7 kg. The serum electrolytes this morning are: Na+ 130, K+ 4.0, Cl− 99, and HCO_3 18. Calculate the sodium deficit and choose the appropriate supplementation.

   A. NaCl 1.8 mEq

   B. NaCl 2.2 mEq

   C. NaCl 3.3 mEq

4. The neonatal nurse practitioner (NNP) recognizes the following as signs of syndrome of inappropriate antidiuretic hormone (SIADH) weight gain:

   A. Edema and low urine specific gravity

   B. Increased urine specific gravity and low urine output

   C. Urine specific gravity changes and high urine output

5. A term neonate now 72 hours of age continues to require total parenteral nutrition (TPN) due to persistent pulmonary hypertension and use of vasopressors. Birth weight (BW) was 4 kg and the total fluid goal is 100 mL/kg/d. The infant receives 60 mL of lipid concurrently with the TPN. Using BW, what percentage of dextrose does the neonatal nurse practitioner (NNP) need to order in the TPN to provide a glucose infusion rate (GIR) of 10 mg/kg/min?

   A. 12.5% dextrose

   B. 15% dextrose

   C. 17% dextrose

6. The kidney plays a key role in extracellular fluid (ECF) and electrolyte balance. The preterm neonate is less efficient with fluid and electrolyte regulation than the term infant, which predisposes the preterm infant to:

   A. Increased sodium losses

   B. Retention of sodium

   C. Retention of sodium bicarbonate

7. In the case of a neonate with hypoalbuminemia, the neonatal nurse practitioner (NNP) knows that serum calcium levels may be low due to the fact that lower serum albumin:

   A. Increases the number of Ca^{2+} binding sites

   B. Increases the amount of free Ca^{2+} in circulation

   C. Reduces the number of Ca^{2+} binding sites

1. C) −44 mL

IWL can be calculated using the following formula: IWL = fluid intake − urine output + weight change. Urine output = 3 mL/kg/hr × 2 kg × 24 hr/d = 144 mL/d; intake = 150 mL/kg/d × 2 kg = 300 mL/d. IWL = 300 −144 = 156 and 156 − 200 = −44 mL (Doherty, 2017).

2. B) Insufficient weight gain most likely due to hyponatremia

Weight gain for this infant should be 15 to 20 g/kg/d (22.5–30 g/d; Anderson et al., 2017). Caloric intake is appropriate and human milk is appropriately fortified (Anderson et al., 2017; Brown et al., 2021). Serum sodium is low (the normal serum sodium is 130–150 mEq/L; Doherty, 2017). There is no indication that the infant is on a diuretic; thus, the most likely etiology of the hyponatremia is late-onset hyponatremia of prematurity.

3. B) NaCl 2.2 mEq

First, the sodium deficit must be calculated. The target goal for serum Na^+ is typically 140 mEq/L (Nyp et al., 2021). The formula for calculating sodium deficit is: (goal sodium − current serum sodium) × 0.6 × weight (kg), so (140 − 130) × 0.6 × 1.7 = 10.2 mEq/L. This neonate is on oral feedings, so an oral sodium supplement is most appropriate. A deficit of 10.2 mEq/L would be required to restore the serum sodium to the desired level of 140 mEq/L, plus the daily sodium requirement. The usual approach is to replace half of the calculated deficit and recheck the electrolytes, so in this case the sodium deficit is 10.2 mEq. The goal for serum sodium adjustment is gradual to avoid too rapid a change in osmolarity, with half the calculated deficit as goal. 4.3 mEq PO 4× daily would provide 10.1/kg of sodium (the full calculated deficit, which is too rapid a correction). 2 mEq NaCl PO 2× daily would only provide 2.3 mEq of sodium supplement and waiting 48 hours after this insufficient supplementation is likely to result in little to no improvement, and if the infant is losing larger than normal urine sodium, the serum sodium will actually be lower in 48 hours.

4. B) Increased urine specific gravity and low urine output

With SIADH, too much antidiuretic hormone is secreted and thus the body retains fluid, resulting in weight gain, which is generally equally distributed in the interstitium and so edema is not observed. With low urine output, urine electrolytes are increased (due to reduction in renal water excretion), resulting in elevated specific gravity, not low urine specific gravity (Doherty, 2017).

5. C) 17% dextrose

The first step is to determine what rate the TPN will run at: 100 mL/kg/d × 4 kg = 400 mL of fluid. Next, subtract the lipid volume, which is 60 mL: 400 mL − 60 mL = 340 mL/d. Next, solve for rate per hour: 340 mL divided by 24 (hours) = 14.1 mL/hr. Then the NNP substitutes varying dextrose percentages to determine the percentage needed to provide 10 mg/kg/d. The formula for calculating GIR is: (D5 × rate) / (6 × weight in kg; Burris, 2017). Since we know that 80 mL/kg/d of 10% dextrose will provide a GIR of 5 mg/kg/min, we can estimate that we will need more than 10% dextrose to achieve the goal. Substituting 15% dextrose yields a GIR of 8.8 mg/kg/min, which is less than the desired goal. 17% dextrose will provide 9.9 mg/kg/min of glucose.

6. A) Increased sodium losses

The immature kidney is susceptible to both increased sodium and sodium bicarbonate wasting, as well as decreased ability to respond to fluid overload (Wright et al., 2018).

7. C) Reduces the number of Ca^{2+} binding sites

Low serum albumin levels decrease serum Ca^{2+} levels due to the decrease in available sites for the free Ca^{2+} to bind. Serum calcium levels do not rise with hypoalbuminemia, but may increase in hyperalbuminemia as a result of additional Ca^{2+} binding sites available on the albumin (Abrams & Tiosano, 2020; Doherty, 2017; Nyp et al., 2021).

Part IV: Pharmacology

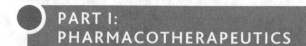

Principles of Neonatal Pharmacology and Common Drug Therapies

Tosha Harris and Amy R. Koehn

PART I: PHARMACOTHERAPEUTICS

Pharmacotherapeutics, or the use of medications to treat disease, is one of the most common responsibilities of the neonatal nurse practitioner (NNP) and requires knowledge of pharmacokinetics (PK) and pharmacodynamics (PD) during the perinatal period. There is great variability in PK and PD in the neonate and infant due to rapid changes in the physiology and the effect of various disease states on the neonate (Allegaert et al., 2018; Blackburn, 2018). Aspects of neonatal PK and PD are presented to assist the NNP in understanding various drug therapies. Specific drug treatments are presented in subsequent chapters.

▶ PRINCIPLES OF PHARMACOKINETICS

- PK is the mathematical relationship between drug dose and blood levels over time. PK processes include absorption, distribution, metabolism (biotransformation), and excretion (Allegaert et al., 2018; Blackburn, 2018; Wade, 2020).

ABSORPTION

- *Absorption* is the process of drug movement from the administration site (gastrointestinal [GI], intravenous [IV], intramuscular [IM], intrapulmonary/inhaled, and subcutaneous [SC]) across membranes and into the systemic circulation.
- *Bioavailability* is defined as the amount of drug administered that reaches the circulation or as the amount of drug delivered to the site of action.
- Intravenously administered drugs are considered 100% bioavailable and are the standard by which the bioavailability of orally and intramuscularly administered drugs is determined.
- Bioavailability of orally administered drugs may be limited by drug formulation, solubility, dissolution, or stability in an acidic environment, or be reabsorbed by enterocytes back into the gut lumen (Allegaert et al., 2018; Domonoske, 2021; Wade, 2020).

DISTRIBUTION

- *Drug distribution* is the movement of drugs from the circulatory system to the tissues, to the site of action, or to the extravascular space.
  - Drug properties that affect distribution include lipid solubility, size (molecular weight), and degree of ionization. Only free, unbound drug crosses membranes and can exert a pharmacologic action and be metabolized and excreted.
    - ❑ Drugs diffuse across membranes passively along a concentration gradient by facilitated carrier mediated transport, endocytosis, and exocytosis.
  - Physiologic differences among preterm infants, term infants, children, and adults that affect distribution include (a) total body water (TBW) content, (b) body fat content, (c) protein (primarily albumin) content, (d) protein binding affinity, and (e) competition for protein binding with other substances, primarily bilirubin.
    - ❑ TBW is higher in preterm infants (~85%) compared with term infants (~75%) and adults (~50%–65%), thus affecting the distribution of water-soluble drugs. Body fat content is lower in the newborn and increases during the first 5 months of infancy as TBW decreases, thereby affecting the distribution of lipophilic drugs. Protein binding is lower in the infant due to lower circulating proteins, and the circulating protein available has a lower binding affinity in the infant, thus more free drug is available for distribution

207

to tissues. Bilirubin freely binds with protein and competes with drugs for protein binding sites; thus, the amount of unbound drug varies with bilirubin levels.

- Measurements of serum drug concentrations include free and protein-bound drug; in the infant, the amount of free drug may be higher than in the adult due to the protein binding differences between infants and adults.
- Volume of distribution (Vd), also called the apparent volume of distribution, is the hypothetical amount of volume (L or L/kg) needed to dissolve a given amount of drug (mg or mcg/kg) in order to produce a measurable drug concentration (mg/L or mcg/L).
  - ❑ Drugs with high Vd are found extensively in the tissues rather than plasma and are not homogeneously distributed, whereas drugs found mostly in plasma have a smaller Vd.
  - ❑ Vd is influenced by gestational age due to the rapid changes in TBW and fluid shifts.
  - ❑ Infants with large extracellular fluid volumes have increased Vd for water-soluble drugs and may reduce peak drug values and affect drug excretion.
  - ❑ Decreased body fat in preterm and intrauterine growth-restricted infants decreases the Vd of lipophilic drugs (Allegaert et al., 2018; Blackburn, 2018; Domonoske, 2021; Holford, 2018; Katzung, 2018; McClary, 2020; Wade, 2020).

METABOLISM

- *Drug metabolism* is the biotransformation of drug into inactive and active metabolites. It occurs in the liver, kidney, intestinal mucosa, and lungs, and is generally classified as phase I or phase II metabolism.
  - *Phase I metabolism:* enzymatic drug conversion to metabolites via oxidation, reduction, and hydrolysis
    - ❑ Cytochrome P450 (CYP450) enzymes mediate phase I metabolism and are present in many tissues, but they are most highly concentrated in hepatic tissues.
      - ○ CYP450 enzymes have variable expression and maturation across the life span; thus, the enzyme responsible for metabolism of a given drug may be active in the infant depending on gestational and postnatal age.
      - ○ Examples of drugs metabolized via phase I reactions include phenytoin, phenobarbital, ibuprofen, diazepam, and indomethacin.
  - *Phase II metabolism:* enzymatic drug biotransformation via the addition (conjugation) of a substance to the drug metabolite
    - ❑ Phase II reactions are glucuronidation (glucuronide conjugation), acetylation,

methylation, glycine conjugation, glutathione conjugation, and sulfate conjugation.
  - ○ Primary enzymes in phase II metabolism include uridine 5'-diphosphoglucuronosyltransferases (UGTs), glutathione S-transferase, and sulfotransferase.
  - ○ Phase II enzyme activity is variable in infants, with glucuronidation activity typically low at birth and sulfate conjugation activity more active at birth.
  - ○ Examples of drugs metabolized via phase II reactions include morphine and acetaminophen via glucuronidation and dopamine and epinephrine via methylation.
- Factors affecting metabolism that may result in prolonged or unpredictable drug half-life and decreased drug clearance include age-related enzyme maturation, nutrition, illness, drug interactions, hepatic blood flow, drug transport, protein synthesis, protein binding, biliary secretion, and genetic variation (pharmacogenomics).
  - The rate of drug metabolism is low at birth in term infants and even lower in premature infants regardless of the route of metabolism. The development of individual drug-metabolizing enzymes varies widely among neonates and may be delayed in premature neonates.
  - Many enzymes responsible for metabolism of drugs have significant development during the first month of life; therefore, dosing regimens at birth may not be appropriate at 3 to 4 weeks of life, necessitating dose and dose interval adjustments.
  - Predicting clearance is difficult and dosing regimens must be individualized based on patient response, tolerance, and drug levels. Decreased clearance and prolonged half-life often require drug administration with longer dosing intervals (Allegaert et al., 2018; Blackburn, 2018; Domonoske, 2021; McClary, 2020b; Wade, 2020).

EXCRETION

- The excretion or elimination of unchanged drug or drug metabolites from the body occurs via the renal, biliary, cutaneous, and pulmonary systems. Renal excretion is an important excretory pathway for unchanged drugs or drug metabolites in neonates and infants.
  - Renal mechanisms of drug elimination include glomerular filtration, active secretion at the proximal tubule, and reabsorption at the distal tubule.
    - ❑ Altered renal elimination occurs in the neonate due to reduced renal function, glomerular filtration rate, and creatinine clearance. Pathologic processes such hypoxemia, poor perfusion, hypothermia, concurrent renal disease, and exposure to nephrotoxic drug can also alter renal excretion rates.

- Hepatic mechanisms of drug elimination include metabolism, bile excretion, fecal elimination, and enterohepatic recirculation.
  - Hepatic excretion can be affected by poor hepatic blood flow, alterations in hepatic enzyme activity, decreased albumin levels, and altered protein binding activity, and affect hepatic excretion (Allegaert et al., 2018; Blackburn, 2018; Domonoske, 2021; McClary, 2020b; Wade, 2020).

▶ MODELS OF PHARMACOKINETICS

- PK models describe the changes in drug concentration over time. These models involve mathematical equations that describe the relationship between the dose selected (mg/kg) and the desired serum concentrations (peak and trough). Factors that can influence these relationships include the body's ability to clear the drug, Vd, half-life ($T_{1/2}$), and elimination rate constant (K_{el}).
- The simplest way to identify and adjust for interindividual variability in drug response is to objectively measure the degree of effect and then adjust the dosing regimen accordingly. Rational pharmacotherapy requires a basic understanding of the way patients handle drugs (PK) and their response (effect) to specific drug concentrations (PD). PK may be simply defined as what the body does to the drug, as opposed to PD, which may be defined as what the drug does to the body (Allegaert et al., 2018; Mizuno et al., 2021; Wade, 2020).

ZERO-ORDER OR SATURATION PHARMACOKINETICS

- Constant *amount* of drug is eliminated over time regardless of serum concentration. Enzymes or transport system receptors are saturated with drug, thereby preventing proportional drug elimination. The K_{el} is variable, resulting in a smaller amount of the drug being eliminated first, followed by a larger amount closer to the end. Small dose increases result in large serum concentration changes until receptors are free from drug and large doses result in a longer half-life.
- Examples of drugs with zero-order kinetics include caffeine, diazepam, furosemide, indomethacin, and phenytoin (Allegaert et al., 2018; Wade, 2020).

FIRST-ORDER OR SINGLE-COMPARTMENT FIRST-ORDER KINETICS

- Constant percentage of drug is eliminated over time; it is a proportional rate of elimination.
- The compartment is the fluid and tissue where drugs penetrate. These spaces include vascular, interstitial, spinal fluid, and tissues.

- *Central compartment:* the vascular space where hydrophilic drugs accumulate, typically the blood volume
- *Peripheral compartment:* tissues and other fluid spaces where lipophilic drugs accumulate
- Diffusion between the central compartment and peripheral compartments is influenced by the molecular size of the drug, polarity of the drug, and protein binding of the drug.
- Circulating/plasma drug concentration is the mathematical relationship between drug dose and Vd and is expressed as: plasma drug concentration (mg/L) = dose (mg/kg)/Vd (L/kg).
- *Half-life* refers to the time needed for the concentration of drug in plasma to decrease by 50% due to elimination (Figure 14.1; Allegaert et al., 2018; Domonoske, 2021; Wade, 2020).

MULTICOMPARTMENT FIRST-ORDER PHARMACOKINETICS

- The biphasic elimination of drugs from the circulation is divided into the alpha phase and beta phase (Figure 14.2).
  - *Alpha phase:* This is the distribution and elimination phase of a drug in serum. This phase is typically rapid; however, the length of time varies as the alpha phase is drug-dependent. For example, the alpha phase for gentamicin is 60 minutes: 30 minutes to infuse and 30 minutes to complete the alpha phase.
  - *Beta phase:* This is the elimination phase, which is slower and longer than the alpha phase due to the elimination rate constant, clearance, and the Vd unique to each infant (Allegaert et al., 2018; Wade, 2020).

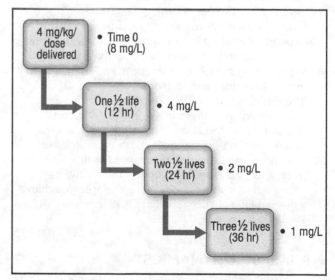

Figure 14.1 Example of a drug with a half-life of 12 hours. The drug plasma concentration decreases by one-half every 12 hours; thus, the half-life is equal to 12 hours.

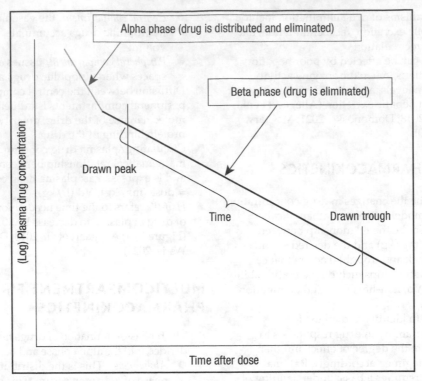

Figure 14.2 Multicompartment first-order pharmacokinetics is the basis for pharmacokinetics calculations. The length of the alpha phase is drug-dependent. Peak and trough drug levels are drawn during the beta phase of elimination when calculating drug kinetics. The drug peak is drawn at the beginning of the beta phase of elimination. The drug trough is ideally drawn at the time the next dose is due to be administered.

Source: Data from Allegaert, K., Ward, R. M., & Van Den Anker, J. N. (2018). Neonatal pharmacology. In C. A. Gleason & S. E. Juul (Eds.), *Avery's diseases of the newborn* (10th ed., pp. 419–431). Elsevier.

STEADY-STATE CONCENTRATION

- This occurs with repetitive drug dosing due to drug accumulation. The amount of drug administered equals the amount of drug eliminated and occurs after the fourth dose of drug given; however, the time it takes to reach steady-state concentration is mostly dependent on drug half-life and can be reached sooner if the dosing interval is shorter than the drug half-life.
- When steady state is reached, peak and trough levels will be the same after each dose.
- The clinician can use PK data when adjusting drug doses based on changes in Vd, elimination, and clearance. A sound knowledge of PK can assist the practitioner in predicting drug concentrations but does not provide information related to drug effects. In contrast, PD is a drug property the practitioner uses when selecting specific drug therapies to achieve a desired effect (Allegaert et al., 2018; Holford, 2018; Wade, 2020).

▶ PHARMACODYNAMICS

- PD is the relationship between drug concentrations in the serum and the effects of the drug on the body. These effects include therapeutic and toxic effects.

- PD properties are drug-specific and reflect the (a) mechanism of action, (b) potency, (c) toxicity characteristics, (d) efficacy, and (e) desired outcome.
- Many drugs bind to receptors and the PD of these receptor-binding drugs is altered in the neonate due to changes in receptor binding, receptor density (number of receptors available), downstream signal transduction, disease states, maturity, and concomitant use of other drugs.

PHARMACOKINETICS AND PHARMACODYNAMICS SPECIFIC TO ANTIBIOTIC THERAPY

- Selecting the optimal antimicrobial therapy is dependent on the consideration of both the PK drug exposure profile and the PD of the interaction between the drug and the microorganism or the minimal inhibitory concentration (MIC) of the organism.
- Antibiotics are grouped into three categories:
  - *Concentration-dependent:* Bacteria eradication is dependent on drug concentration; higher doses result in higher drug concentration and this increases the drug's bactericidal properties.

- *Time-dependent killing:* Bacteria eradication is dependent on the percent of time the drug concentration is above the MIC of the organism being treated.
- *Time-dependent killing with postantibiotic effect:* Bacteria eradication is not dependent on concentration. Instead, higher drug concentrations excrete sustained killing power even after drug concentration decreases (Domonoske, 2021; Holford, 2018; Wade, 2020).

▶ PRINCIPLES OF ADMINISTRATION

- The process of prescribing medications should be a multifactorial and multistep process. The clinician should choose an appropriate medication (route, dosage, and interval between doses) to achieve the desired effect in the patient while simultaneously considering the PK and PD principles previously described, as well as the likelihood of the neonate developing tolerance to the medication and/or experiencing withdrawal symptoms following discontinuation of the medication.

INTRAVENOUS ADMINISTRATION

- IV administration of medications is the most common and most effective route used in the neonatal population because it bypasses absorption barriers and an almost immediate medication response is achieved.
- Neonatal physiologic processes (such as dehydration, edema, prematurity) as well as extraneous factors such as slow IV infusion rates, small volumes of drugs, IV tubing dead space (IV-infused drugs need to be infused as close to the neonate as possible), and limits to volumes used to flush IV lines all play a role in achieving optimal therapy results (Allegaert et al., 2018; Domonoske, 2021).

ORAL ADMINISTRATION

- If feasible, medications administered intravenously and medications used to manage chronic conditions should be transitioned to oral administration as soon as possible.
- Oral drug absorption is dependent on gastric emptying time, gastric pH, intestinal enzyme activity, intestinal bacteria colonization, hepatic metabolism, and enterohepatic recirculation, which are altered in the preterm and ill neonate.
- Oral drug absorption is altered in the neonate due to decreased bile salts and pancreatic enzymes, slower gut transit time, delayed gastric emptying and motility, mucus in the stomach, gastric and duodenal pH differences, high levels of beta-glucuronidase, gut metabolic enzymes and drug transporters, intestinal flora, and intestinal surface area.

- Oral drug absorption matures by 4 to 5 months of life. The diseases that likely have the greatest impact on oral drug absorption are those affecting the total intestinal surface area, such as short bowel syndrome. This syndrome results from massive bowel resection complicating necrotizing enterocolitis (NEC), from volvulus, or from congenital anomalies like gastroschisis or multiple intestinal atresia (Allegaert et al., 2018, 2021; Blackburn, 2018; Domonoske, 2021).

INHALATION ADMINISTRATION

- This is the preferred route for medications whose site of action is the tracheobronchial tree (Domonoske, 2021).
- It may require endotracheal intubation to be properly administered (e.g., surfactant, epinephrine).

INTRAMUSCULAR AND SUBCUTANEOUS ADMINISTRATION

- IM administration is useful when the slow release of medication is desired; it should not be used as a substitute for IV administration for immediate effect or when multiple doses will be needed.
- Poor perfusion to the muscle limits absorption with these routes; drug may deposit and remain at the injection site for a prolonged period, and neonates are at risk of sclerosis at the injection site or abscess development.
  - Muscle and subcutaneous tissues are limited in the preterm and low birthweight infant, limiting the use of these sites for drug therapy.
  - Gestational age and health status of the neonate may result in delayed or erratic absorption from the muscle (Allegaert et al., 2018; Blackburn, 2018; Domonoske, 2021).

OTHER ADMINISTRATION ROUTES

- Buccal, lingual, rectal, and topical routes of administration are associated with variable rates of absorption.
  - Rectal absorption may be greater in neonates due to the well-vascularized rectum.
  - Topical absorption rate is inversely related to skin thickness and directly related to the neonate's hydration status. Increased skin permeability and surface area to body weight proportion puts the neonate at risk of toxic reactions from topically applied medications (Allegaert et al., 2018; Blackburn, 2018; Domonoske, 2021).

DOSAGE/INTERVAL

- Dosing and interval regimens are determined based on individual drug PK and PD properties. Therapeutic drug monitoring (TDM) assumes that total plasma drug concentrations correlate with drug dose and with circulating unbound drug concentrations and unbound drug concentrations at the site of action.

- *TDM:* TDM is a laboratory measurement of a drug's serum level that may directly influence the prescriber's dosing choice. It is useful (a) when there is a high correlation between therapeutic effect and serum level rather than dose; (b) the drug has a narrow therapeutic range; and (c) when maintaining the drug level within the range reduces toxicity and improves efficacy, thereby improving outcomes.
  - ❑ Therapeutic range is the drug concentration range that is highly efficacious with a low risk of toxicity in most patients.
  - ❑ Patient response is the goal of therapy, not whether the drug level is in a specified range.
  - ❑ Dose and interval determinations and changes in the neonate must take into consideration that drug metabolism is reduced in the neonate and improves over time as enzyme systems mature.
  - ❑ Drug clearance is reduced in neonates and improves as renal function improves. Vd is higher in neonates due to fluid shifts that change over the first week of life. The half-life of drugs is prolonged in the neonate and increases as drug metabolic processes mature during the first month to year of life. Dosages and intervals must be individualized in the neonate based on therapeutic response and monitoring of selected plasma drug concentrations (Allegaert et al., 2018; Domonoske, 2021; McClary, 2020b; Wade, 2020).

TOLERANCE AND WEANING

- Tolerance is the diminished response to a drug during a course of drug therapy, usually occurring over a long-term course; therefore, higher drug doses may be needed to achieve the same therapeutic effect.
- Tolerance develops due to receptor–drug interactions and the characteristic of the drug as either an agonist or antagonist when bound to receptor sites.
  - Receptors interact with a drug, initiating events leading to drug effects, with drug–receptor complexes determined by the number of receptors available, the affinity of the receptor for the drug, and the agonist or antagonist action of the drug–receptor complex.
  - Agonists are drugs that activate when bound with the receptor. Antagonists are drugs that interfere with the receptor–agonist interaction.
- The full action of some drugs may occur even if some receptors are not complexed with drug.
- The persistence of drug effects postdiscontinuation, while not tolerance per se, may occur due to the slow metabolism of the drug or the slow dissolution of protein–drug complexes, or when the drug has a high Vd due to lipophilic attributes and is slowly released to the central compartment after discontinuation.

- Downregulation of receptors at a rate faster than the genesis of new receptors may limit the strength and duration of drug effects, another type of tolerance.
- Opioids are a class of drugs where infants may develop tolerance when the drug is used long term, and dose adjustments should be made for the desired effect (Allegaert et al., 2018; Domonoske, 2021; McClary, 2020b; Schumacher et al., 2021; Trevor, 2018; Wallen & Gleason, 2018; von Zastrow, 2021).

Withdrawal

- Drug dependence is the physiologic condition whereby the neonate requires regular drug administration for physiologic well-being. Abrupt discontinuation of a drug on which a neonate or infant has developed dependence may result in withdrawal symptoms.
  - Drug withdrawal in the neonate is primarily related to antenatal fetal exposure to drugs or secondarily to long-term opioid treatment during the infant's hospitalization; however, other drugs may result in withdrawal-type signs and symptoms.
  - Among the maternal effects of opioid use that may affect the fetus are premature rupture of membranes and preterm birth, fetal death, and low birth weight.
    - ❑ Fetal effects of maternal opioid use may include exposure to infectious agents and fluctuating opioid concentrations resulting in intermittent withdrawal in utero.
    - ❑ Neonatal withdrawal occurs in 55% to 94% of neonates with antenatal exposure to opioids.
    - ❑ The onset of signs of withdrawal is variable depending on the opioid used by the mother, the type of opioid used, and the gestational age of the infant.
  - Infants who develop dependence may benefit from a tapered-dose regimen when discontinuing a drug to prevent withdrawal symptoms.
- Other drugs associated with signs of drug withdrawal that are not necessarily the same as opioid signs include nicotine, marijuana, benzodiazepines, cocaine, methamphetamine, and selective serotonin reuptake inhibitors (SSRIs); however, the neonatal signs seen in neonates whose mothers took SSRIs are believed to be due to the hyperserotonergic state resolving rather than drug withdrawal (Domonoske, 2021; Hudak, 2020; Wallen & Gleason, 2018).

▶ CONCLUSION

Drug therapy is one of the many responsibilities of the NNP. Safe drug prescribing depends on the NNP applying the basic principles of PK and PD to the neonate and infant (Allegaert et al., 2018). PK parameters (Vd, half-life, Cl) may be used in developing individualized dosing and drug dose intervals to achieve desired drug exposure levels; however, more PK studies in neonates are needed to ensure that effective dose and PD targets are achieved in the neonate and infant.

PART II: COMMON DRUG THERAPIES

This section of the chapter serves to review medications commonly used by neonatal clinicians. It is not intended to be an exhaustive list of all drug therapies and is not intended as an in-depth source on pharmacotherapeutics. Drug dosage and timing of onset and/or duration are not included as these will differ between neonates and among institutions. The reader is directed to medication reference resources for dosing and therapeutic monitoring guidelines. The focus of this chapter is on understanding the mechanisms of action of drugs, available routes, and things to consider when ordering and/or managing an infant receiving the therapy.

▶ ANALGESICS AND OPIOIDS (NARCOTICS)

ANALGESICS

24% Sucrose Solution (Sweet-Ease)
- *Use:* This is used to calm or soothe during times of stress and for short-term analgesia during minor procedures such as heel sticks, orogastric (OG)/nasogastric (NG) tube placement, and venipunctures. Sucrose is most effective when combined with other nonpharmacologic interventions such as nonnutritive sucking (NNS).
- *Mechanism of action:* Exact mechanism is unknown; it has been proposed that sucrose induces endogenous opioid release.
- *Route:* Oral (PO).
- *Considerations:* Give 2 minutes prior to a painful procedure; may be repeated. Place sucrose on the tongue or buccal surface. It is not effective if given NG. No long-term data are available. Some do not support use in extremely premature or critically ill infants (Eyal, 2020c; Gardner, Enzman-Hines, & Agarwal, 2021; Simons et al., 2021; Spruill & LaBrecque, 2017; Taketomo, 2021; Walden, 2021).

Acetaminophen (Tylenol)
- *Use:* Acetaminophen is used as analgesic and antipyretic.
- *Mechanism of action:* Analgesic effect is by inhibition of prostaglandin synthesis in the central nervous system (CNS) and peripherally, blocking pain impulse generation. Antipyretic effect is by inhibition of hypothalamic heat-regulating center.
- *Clearance:* Extensively metabolized by the liver primarily by sulfonation, and by glucuronidation to a much lesser extent; excretion by the kidney; prolonged elimination with liver dysfunction.
- *Route:* PO, per rectum (PR), IV.
- *Considerations:* Although acetaminophen may be effective in the short-term management of mild to moderate pain, it has not been demonstrated to be effective in acute procedure-related pain. A

synergistic effect is noted when IV acetaminophen is administered concurrently with opioid analgesia. Use with caution in hepatic failure; half-life may increase twofold or more. Do not use it in infants with glucose-6-phosphate dehydrogenase (G6PD) deficiency. Prophylactic administration prior to vaccination may decrease the immune response of some vaccines (Bohannon et al., 2020c; Domonoske, 2017; Gardner, Enzman-Hines, & Agarwal, 2021; Simons et al., 2021; Spruill & LaBrecque, 2017; Taketomo, 2021; Walden, 2021).

Ibuprofen (Motrin)
- *Use:* Ibuprofen is an antipyretic and mild analgesic used in the treatment of mild to moderate pain, fever, and inflammatory disease.
- *Mechanism of action:* It inhibits cyclooxegenase (COX)-1 and 2 enzymes, which results in decreased formation of prostaglandin precursors.
- *Clearance:* Hepatic metabolism, renal excretion.
- *Route:* PO.
- *Considerations:* It is not recommended for analgesia in infants <6 months of age. Side effects may include edema, hyperkalemia, and GI bleeding. Use with caution in infants with hepatic and renal failure (Bohannon et al., 2020c; Domonoske, 2017; Gardner, Enzman-Hines, & Agarwal, 2021; Taketomo, 2021).

OPIOIDS

Morphine Sulfate (Duramorph)
- *Use:* Morphine is administered to pediatric patients with prolonged pain, such as after surgery, and to uncomfortable ventilated premature newborns. It is also used in the management of moderate to severe acute and chronic pain, and palliative care management of dyspnea. Morphine is not a suitable drug for short painful procedures due to its pharmacologic properties, with a slow onset of action and a long half-life.
- *Mechanism of action:* The analgesic effect of morphine is mainly caused by an activation of μ receptors. It binds to opioid receptors in the CNS, causing inhibition of the ascending pain pathways, altering the perception of and response to pain. Morphine activates the descending inhibitory system within the basal ganglia and affects the limbic system by altering the emotional response to pain, making it more tolerable.
- *Clearance:* Hepatic metabolism (enterohepatic recirculation may result in higher plasma concentrations), renal and fecal excretion.
- *Route:* PO, IM, IV, and SC. When changing routes of administration in chronically treated patients, oral doses are approximately three to five times the parenteral dose.
- *Considerations:* Monitor for CNS and respiratory depression, hypotension, decreased gastric/intestinal motility, urinary retention, risk for NEC, and increased

intracranial pressure (ICP). It has a slower onset but longer duration than fentanyl. IV is the preferred route. Oral doses are half as effective as parenteral doses. Start with lower dosages in the opioid-naive infant; infants with previous or prolonged exposure may need higher dosing (Bohannon et al., 2020c; Domonoske, 2017; Gardner, Enzman-Hines, & Agarwal, 2021; Simons et al., 2021; Taketomo, 2021; Walden, 2021).

For discussion regarding morphine use in the treatment of neonatal abstinence syndrome (NAS), please see Chapter 5.

Fentanyl (Duragesic, Sublimaze)

- *Use:* Fentanyl may be the preferred analgesic agent for critically ill patients with hemodynamic instability, patients with symptoms related to histamine release during morphine infusion, or patients with morphine tolerance. Because of its relatively rapid onset of action and short duration of effect, fentanyl efficiently alleviates procedural pain.
- *Mechanism of action:* Fentanyl is a synthetic opiate which binds with stereospecific receptors at many sites within the CNS, increases pain threshold, alters pain perception, and inhibits the ascending pathways. It is highly lipophilic, redistributed into the muscle and fat. Its potency is about 100- to 300-fold that of morphine, with an effect on the μ receptor.
- *Clearance:* Hepatic metabolism, primarily excreted by kidneys as inactive metabolites.
- *Route:* IV or SC. Give intermittent IV doses slowly; rapid infusion may cause chest wall rigidity.
- *Considerations:* Fentanyl has a relatively rapid onset of 1.5 minutes and a short duration of action of approximately 60 to 120 minutes, with a peak effect of 20 to 30 minutes. Fentanyl has a wide margin of safety and beneficial effects on hemodynamic stability. Monitor for CNS and respiratory depression, hypotension, decreased gastric/intestinal motility, and urinary retention. Renal and/or hepatic dysfunction may alter PK properties (Bohannon et al., 2020c; Domonoske, 2017; Gardner, Enzman-Hines, & Agarwal, 2021; Simons et al., 2021; Taketomo, 2021; Walden, 2021).

OPIOID AGONIST

Naloxone (Narcan)

- *Use:* Naloxone is used for complete or partial reversal of opioid drug effects in circumstances of significant side effects of excessive opioids, most commonly respiratory depression, although pruritus and emesis may occur.
- *Mechanism of action:* It is a pure opioid antagonist that competes and displaces opioids at opioid receptor sites. Onset of action is within 1 to 2 minutes after IV injection and 8 to 15 minutes after intranasal inhalation.
- *Clearance:* Hepatic metabolism, renal excretion.
- *Route:* IM, IV, endotracheal tube (ET), SC.

- *Considerations:* Because naloxone's duration is shorter than most opioids, repeat dosing may be necessary. It is no longer recommended as part of initial resuscitative measures in the delivery room for neonates with respiratory depression due to unknown maternal use history and risk of precipitating acute withdrawal syndrome. Support ventilation to improve oxygenation and heart rate (Bohannon et al., 2020b; Domonoske, 2017; Simons et al., 2021; Taketomo, 2021).

▶ ANTICOAGULANTS

ANTICOAGULANT THERAPY

Heparin Sodium (Heparin)

- *Use:* Heparin sodium is used for systemic prophylaxis and treatment of thromboembolic disorders and as anticoagulant for extracorporeal membrane oxygenation (ECMO) and dialysis procedures. Local heparin lock solution maintains patency of IV sites.
- *Mechanism of action:* It potentiates the action of antithrombin III and thereby inactivates thrombin and prevents conversion of fibrinogen to fibrin. It also stimulates the release of lipoprotein lipase (lipoprotein lipase hydrolyzes triglycerides to glycerol and free fatty acids).
- *Clearance:* Metabolism in the liver and spleen, renal excretion.
- *Route:* IV.
- *Considerations:* Prior to start of systemic therapy, ensure imaging has been completed. Obtain baseline complete blood count (CBC) with differential, prothrombin time (PT), and partial thromboplastin time (PTT), then monitor serially.
- Adjustment of dose is based on clinical response, serial evaluation of thrombus, and lab values. Monitor PTT 4 hours after the initial bolus, change in dose, and then every 24 hours once therapeutic dose is achieved. Occurrence of heparin-induced thrombocytopenia is rare (Bohannon et al., 2020b; Domonoske, 2017; Taketomo, 2021).

Enoxaparin (Lovenox)/Low-Molecular-Weight Heparin

- *Use:* These are used for inpatient treatment of prophylaxis thromboembolic disorders and as anticoagulant for extracorporeal and dialysis procedures.
- *Mechanism of action:* It has a small effect on the activated PTT and strongly inhibits anti-Xa.
- *Clearance:* Hepatic metabolism, renal excretion.
- *Route:* SubQ.
- *Considerations:* Measure antifactor Xa levels 4 to 6 hours after a dose. After target level is reached, dosage adjustments may be required once or twice a month. Do not rub the injection site as bruising may occur. Compared with standard heparin, enoxaparin has much less activity against thrombin. Low antithrombin plasma

concentration reduces efficacy in neonates (Bohannon et al., 2020b; Domonoske, 2017; Taketomo, 2021).

REVERSAL OF ANTICOAGULATION

Protamine Sulfate (Protamines)

- *Use:* Protamine sulfate is used for treatment of heparin overdose.
- *Mechanism of action:* When given in the presence of heparin (strongly acidic and negatively charged), a stable salt is formed, and the anticoagulant activity of both drugs is nullified. In the presence of low-molecular-weight heparin (LMWH), protamine completely reverses the antifactory Xa activity of LMWH.
- *Clearance:* Renal excretion.
- *Route:* IV.
- *Considerations:* Administer slow IV push not more than 5 mg/min; rapid IV infusion causes hypotension. Monitor coagulation tests and cardiac status during administration (Bohannon et al., 2020b; Taketomo, 2021).

▶ ANTICONVULSANTS

PHENOBARBITAL (LUMINAL)

- *Use:* Phenobarbital remains the first-line management for neonatal generalized tonic–clonic seizures, status epilepticus, and cortical focal seizures. It may also be used for prevention and treatment of neonatal hyperbilirubinemia and for lowering bilirubin in chronic cholestasis.
- *Mechanism of action:* It promotes anticonvulsant activity by increasing the threshold for electrical stimulation of the motor cortex and depresses CNS activity by binding to the barbiturate site at the gamma-aminobutyric acid (GABA) receptor complex, enhancing GABA activity.
- *Clearance:* Hepatic metabolism, renal excretion. Initial half-life in neonates is 40 to 200 hours or longer, gradually declining to about 20 to 100 hours at 3 to 4 weeks of age.
- *Route:* PO, IV.
- *Considerations:* Phenobarbital is the drug of choice for neonatal seizures. Therapeutic level is 20 to 40 mcg/mL. Neonates may need additional respiratory support at higher doses (Bohannon et al., 2020b; Domonoske, 2017; Hall & Reavey, 2021; Lehr & Williams, 2021; Taketomo, 2021).

FOSPHENYTOIN (CEREBYX)

- *Use:* Fosphenytoin is used for management of generalized tonic–clonic status epilepticus. It is added if seizures are not controlled by phenobarbital alone.
- *Mechanism of action:* It is a diphosphate ester salt that acts as a water-soluble prodrug of phenytoin. Phenytoin acts by stabilizing neuronal membranes and decreasing seizure activity by increasing efflux or decreasing influx of sodium ions across cell membranes in the motor cortex during generation of nerve impulses.
- *Clearance:* Converted by hydrolysis to phenytoin; phenytoin undergoes hepatic metabolism and renal excretion.
- *Route:* PO, IM, IV. It must be prescribed in terms of phenytoin equivalents (PEs), with 1 mg PE equal to 1.5 mg fosphenytoin.
- *Dose:* Use the neonatal IV phenytoin dosing guidelines to dose fosphenytoin using doses in PEs equal to the phenytoin dose. Phenytoin 1 mg = fosphenytoin 1 PE. Do not change doses when changing between fosphenytoin and phenytoin as they are not equivalent on an mg-to-mg basis.
- *Considerations:* Measure trough serum phenytoin, not fosphenytoin. Obtain trough 48 hours after IV loading dose. Monitor CBC with differential and platelet count, serum glucose, and therapeutic level of total phenytoin, which is 8 to 15 mcg/mL (Bohannon et al., 2020b; Ditzenberger, 2021; Domonoske, 2017; Hall & Reavey, 2021; Lehr & Williams, 2021; Taketomo, 2021).

PHENYTOIN (DILANTIN)

- *Use:* Phenytoin continues to be used in pediatrics for status epilepticus, generalized tonic–clonic seizures, and partial seizures with or without secondary generalization.
- *Mechanism of action:* It stabilizes neuronal membranes and decreases seizure activity by increasing efflux or decreasing influx of sodium ions across cell membranes in the motor cortex during generation of nerve impulses.
- *Clearance:* Hepatic metabolism, renal excretion.
- *Route:* PO, IV. It should be administered IV directly into a large vein through a large-gauge needle or IV catheter; IV injections should be followed by normal saline (NS) flushes through the same needle or IV catheter to avoid local irritation of the vein.
- *Considerations:* Administer slowly at a maximum of 0.5 to 1 mg/kg/min to avoid cardiac arrhythmia. Monitor CBC with differential, liver function, and serum trough level. High serum levels can precipitate seizures. There is local tissue damage if extravasation occurs. Phenytoin is a vesicant, and there is conflicting information regarding use of hyaluronidase with infiltration (Bohannon et al., 2020b; Ditzenberger, 2021; Domonoske, 2017; Hall & Reavey, 2021; Lehr & Williams, 2021; Taketomo, 2021).

LEVETIRACETAM (KEPPRA)

- *Use:* Levetiracetam is used as adjunctive therapy in the treatment of partialonset seizures, myoclonic seizures, and primary generalized tonic–clonic seizures. It is only approved for use in combination with other seizure medications.
- *Mechanism of action:* The precise mechanism by which it exerts its antiepileptic effect is unknown; however, studies suggest one or more of the following are involved: inhibition of voltage-dependent N-type calcium channels; blockade of GABAergic inhibitory transmission through displacement of negative modulators; reversal of the inhibition of glycine currents; reduction of delayed rectifier potassium current; and/or binding to synaptic proteins that modulate neurotransmitter release.
- *Clearance:* Metabolized by enzymatic hydrolysis, renal excretion.
- *Route:* PO, IV. When switching from PO to IV formulation, the total daily dose should be the same.
- *Considerations:* There are few prospective studies. Monitor seizure frequency, severity, and duration, as well as CNS depression, diastolic blood pressure, renal function, and CBC (Bohannon et al., 2020b; Hall & Reavey, 2021; Lehr & Williams, 2021; Taketomo, 2021).

▶ CARDIOVASCULAR DRUGS

ANTIHYPERTENSIVE DRUGS

Alpha- or Beta-Receptor Antagonist

LABETALOL (TRANDATE)

- *Use:* IV formulation is used for treatment of severe hypertension and as oral treatment for hypertension alone or in combination particularly with thiazide or loop diuretics.
- *Mechanism of action:* Decreases in blood pressure occur through alpha-, beta-1-, and beta-2-adrenergic receptor blockade without causing significant reflex tachycardia or decrease in heart rate. It also reduces elevated renin levels. Responses are dose-related (i.e., higher doses more rapidly decrease systolic pressures).
- *Clearance:* Metabolized by the liver.
- *Route:* PO, IV.
- *Considerations:* Do not discontinue chronic use abruptly; should taper over 10 to 2 weeks. It is contraindicated in heart failure and bronchopulmonary dysplasia (BPD). Monitor blood pressure, heart rate, and EKG. When monitoring IV dosing, monitor for length of infusion and for several hours after infusion has been stopped due to prolonged duration of action (Bohannon et al., 2020b; Taketomo, 2021).

PROPRANOLOL (INDERAL)

- *Use:* Propranolol is used for management of hypertension, supraventricular arrhythmias, tetralogy of Fallot cyanotic spells, hypertension, and supraventricular tachycardia, especially if associated with Wolff–Parkinson–White syndrome.
- *Mechanism of action:* It decreases hypertension primarily by decreasing cardiac output. It inhibits the stimulation of renin production by catecholamines.
- *Clearance:* Hepatic metabolism, metabolites excreted in urine.
- *Route:* PO, IV.
- *Considerations:* For the PO route, monitor heart rate/blood pressure; a resting bradycardia may indicate need or dose change. For IV route, monitor EKG, blood pressure, and heart rate (Bohannon et al., 2020b; Taketomo, 2021).

Angiotensin-Converting Enzyme Inhibitors

CAPTOPRIL (CAPOTEN)

- *Use:* Captopril is used for treatment of hypertension, congestive heart failure (CHF), and reduction of afterload.
- *Mechanism of action:* Angiotensin-converting enzyme (ACE) inhibitors block the production of angiotensin II, leading to a decrease in release of aldosterone and norepinephrine. ACE inhibitors also increase the production of bradykinin. The result is a decrease in peripheral vascular resistance.
- *Clearance:* Cleared >95% unchanged via the renal system.
- *Route:* PO.
- *Considerations:* Monitor for hypotension; some experience significant drop in blood pressure, start with lower dosing. It may cause oliguria, hyperkalemia, and renal failure. Monitor blood urea nitrogen (BUN), serum creatinine, serum potassium, and CBC with differential. Try to give on an empty stomach; food decreases absorption (Bohannon et al., 2020b; Domonoske, 2017; Taketomo, 2021).

ENALAPRIL (ORAL)/ENALAPRILAT (INTRAVENOUS; VASOTEC)

- *Use:* These are used for management of hypertension, symptomatic heart failure, and symptomatic left ventricular dysfunction
- *Mechanism of action:* ACE inhibitors block the production of angiotensin II, leading to a decrease in release of aldosterone and norepinephrine. ACE inhibitors also increase the production of bradykinin. The result is a decrease in peripheral vascular resistance.
- *Clearance:* Hepatic metabolism, renal excretion Renal dysfunction will increase peak and trough levels.
- *Route:* PO; IV form used primarily for hypertensive crisis
- *Considerations:* It may cause prolonged hypotension. Use lower initial dose in patients with hyponatremia, hypovolemia, severe CHF, decreased renal function, or those receiving diuretics. It may cause oliguria, hyperkalemia, and renal failure, as well as dry, hacking cough. Monitor blood pressure, renal function, white

blood cell (WBC), serum potassium, and serum glucose. Monitor for angioedema and anaphylactoid reaction (Bohannon et al., 2020b; Domonoske, 2017; Taketomo, 2021).

Calcium-Channel Blockers

AMLODIPINE (NORVASC)
■ *Use:* Amlodipine istreatment of hypertension and is also useful in the management of chronic hypertension due its slow onset.
■ *Mechanism of action:* It decreases peripheral resistance and blood pressure by inhibiting calcium influx into the arterial smooth muscle cells.
■ *Clearance:* Hepatic (dysfunction will slow metabolism), renal excretion.
■ *Route:* PO.
■ *Considerations:* It may cause an increase in heart rate within 10 hours of administration secondary to vasodilating activity. Monitor blood pressure, heart rate, and liver function (Bohannon et al., 2020a; Taketomo, 2021).

NICARDIPINE (CARDENE)
■ *Use:* Nicardipine is used for short-term treatment of hypertension when PO is not feasible.
■ *Mechanism of action:* It decreases peripheral resistance and blood pressure by inhibiting calcium influx into the arterial smooth muscle cells.
■ *Clearance:* Hepatic metabolism, renal excretion. It will be altered with hepatic and/or renal dysfunction.
■ *Route:* IV—continuous infusion.
■ *Considerations:* Monitor blood pressure, heart rate, and hepatic and renal function. Monitor blood pressure carefully with initiation of therapy and dose changes (Bohannon et al., 2020c; Bohannon et al., 2020b; Taketomo, 2021).

Vasodilators

HYDRALAZINE (APRESOLINE)
■ *Use:* Hydralazine is used for management of moderate to severe hypertension and as an afterload-reducing agent to treat congestive heart failure.
■ *Mechanism of action:* It is a vasodilator that relaxes the smooth muscles of the arterioles, decreasing systemic vascular resistance and increasing cardiac output. It also increases renal, coronary, cerebral, and splanchnic blood flow.
■ *Clearance:* Hepatic metabolism, renal excretion.
■ *Route:* PO, IV.
■ *Considerations:* It may cause tachycardia. Give PO with food. Monitor blood pressure and heart rate. Due to concern for reflex tachycardia, concurrent use of beta-blockers is recommended in heart failure patients (Bohannon et al., 2020b; Taketomo, 2021).

▶ ANTIMICROBIALS

ANTIBACTERIALS: AGENTS THAT TARGET BACTERIAL CELL WALL SYNTHESIS

Beta-Lactam Compounds: Penicillins
■ *Use:* These are used for treatment of infections caused by susceptible organisms. They are active against some gram-positive organisms, some gram-negative organisms such as *Neisseria gonorrhoeae*, and some anaerobes and spirochetes.
■ *Mechanism of action:* Beta-lactam antibiotics inhibit bacterial growth by interfering with the transpeptidation reaction of bacterial cell wall synthesis. The exact mechanism of cell death is not completely understood, but autolysins are involved in addition to the disruption of cross-linking of the cell wall.
■ *Clearance:* Biliary and kidney excretion.
■ *Route:* IV, PO.
■ *Considerations/Examples:*
  ● *Natural penicillins:* penicillin G (Pfizerpen)
    ❑ These have the greatest activity against gram-positive organisms, gram-negative cocci, and non–beta-lactamase producing anaerobes.
  ● *Penicillinase-resistant penicillins:* methicillin, nafcillin (Nallpen), and oxacillin (Bactocill)
    ❑ These penicillins are resistant to staphylococcal beta-lactamases. They are active against *Staphylococcus* and *Streptococcus* spp.
  ● *Aminopenicillins:* ampicillin (generic) and amoxicillin (Amoxil)
  ● *Beta-lactam–beta-lactamase inhibitor combinations:* amoxicillin–clavulanic acid (Augmentin), ampicillin–sulbactam (Unasyn), and piperacillin–tazobactam (Zosyn)
    ❑ These drugs retain the antibacterial spectrum of penicillin and have improved activity against gram-negative rods (Beauduy & Winston, 2021b; Bohannon et al., 2020b; Domonoske, 2017; Sharma & Hammerschlag, 2021b).

Beta-Lactam Compounds: Cephalosporins
■ *Use:* Cephalosporins are used parenterally for treatment of lower respiratory tract, skin and skin structure, urinary tract, and bone and joint infections caused by susceptible gram-positive or gram-negative bacteria. They are also used parenterally for treatment of meningitis and septicemia/bacteremia caused by susceptible gram-positive or gram-negative bacteria. Cephalosporins are like penicillin but are more stable to many bacterial beta-lactamases and therefore have a broader spectrum of activity.
■ *Mechanism of action:* Cephalosporins interfere with the synthesis of peptidoglycan in the bacterial cell wall. They bind to and inactivate enzymes responsible for the synthesis of the bacterial cell wall.

- *Clearance:* Excreted mostly unchanged by the kidneys.
- *Route:* IV, PO.
- *Considerations/Examples:* Cephalosporins are classified into generations on the basis of their spectrum of microbiologic activity. This classification reflects increasing stability of the higher generations to various bacterial beta-lactamases.
  - *First generation:* First-generation cephalosporins are very active against gram-positive cocci, such as streptococci and staphylococci. *Escherichia coli*, *Klebsiella pneumoniae*, and *Proteus mirabilis* are often sensitive to first-generation cephalosporins.
    - ❑ Cefazolin (Ancef)
    - ❑ Cephalexin (Keflex)
  - *Second generation:* Second-generation cephalosporins are relatively active against organisms inhibited by first-generation drugs, but in addition they have extended gram-negative coverage. *Klebsiella* spp. (including those resistant to first-generation cephalosporins) are usually sensitive. As with first-generation agents, no member of this group is active against enterococci or *Pseudomonas aeruginosa*.
    - ❑ Cefoxitin (generic)
    - ❑ Cefuroxime (Ceftin)
  - *Third generation:* Compared with second-generation agents, third-generation cephalosporins have expanded gram-negative coverage, and some are able to cross the blood–brain barrier. Third-generation drugs may be active against *Citrobacter*, *Serratia marcescens*, and *Providencia*, and against beta-lactamase-producing strains of *Haemophilus* and *Neisseria*.
    - ❑ Cefotaxime (Claforan)
    - ❑ Ceftazidime (Fortaz)
    - ❑ Ceftriaxone (Rocephin)
  - *Fourth generation:* Fourth-generation cephalosporins are more resistant to hydrolysis by chromosomal beta-lactamases (e.g., those produced by *Enterobacter*). However, like the third-generation compounds, they are hydrolyzed by extended-spectrum beta-lactamases. Cefepime has good activity against *P. aeruginosa*, Enterobacteriaceae, methicillin-susceptible *Staphylococcus aureus*, and *Streptococcus pneumoniae*. It is highly active against *Haemophilus* and *Neisseria* spp. It penetrates well into the cerebrospinal fluid.
    - ❑ Cefepime (Maxipime; Beauduy & Winston, 2021b; Bohannon et al., 2020b; Domonoske, 2017; Sharma & Hammerschlag, 2021a)

Beta-Lactam Compounds: Carbapenems

- *Use:* Carbapenems are structurally related to other beta-lactam antibiotics and have a wide spectrum with good activity against most gram-negative rods, including *P. aeruginosa*, gram-positive organisms, and anaerobes. Carbapenems penetrate body tissues and fluids well, including the cerebrospinal fluid.

They are useful in the treatment of infections due to cephalosporin-resistant Enterobacteriaceae.
- *Mechanism of action:* They inhibit cell wall biosynthesis. They are not hydrolyzed by most beta-lactamases.
- *Clearance:* Renal hydrolyzation and excretion.
- *Route:* IV.
- *Considerations/Examples:*
  - Imipenem (Primaxin)
  - Meropenem (Merrem; Beauduy & Winston, 2021b; Bohannon et al., 2020b; Domonoske, 2017; Sharma & Hammerschlag, 2021b)

Glycopeptides

- *Use:* Glycopeptides are primarily active against gram-positive bacteria, especially against infections caused by methicillin-resistant *Staphylococcus* spp.
- *Mechanism of action:* They inhibit cell wall synthesis by binding firmly to the end of a developing peptidoglycan cell wall matrix. This prevents further elongation of peptidoglycan and cross-linking. The peptidoglycan is thus weakened and the cell becomes susceptible to lysis. The cell membrane is also damaged, which contributes to the antibacterial effect.
- *Clearance:* No apparent metabolism; renal excretion primarily through glomerular filtration.
- *Route:* IV, PO only in cases of colitis caused by *Clostridioides difficile*.
- *Considerations/Examples:*
  - Vancomycin (Vancocin; Beauduy & Winston, 2021b; Bohannon et al., 2020b; Domonoske, 2017; Sharma & Hammerschlag, 2021a)

AGENTS THAT TARGET PROTEIN SYNTHESIS

Aminoglycosides

- *Use:* Aminoglycosides are mostly used against aerobic gram-negative bacteria, especially when there is concern for drug-resistant pathogens or in critically ill patients.
- *Mechanism of action:* Aminoglycosides are irreversible inhibitors of protein synthesis, but the precise mechanism for bactericidal activity is unclear. Protein synthesis is inhibited by aminoglycosides in at least three ways: (a) interference with the initiation complex of peptide formation; (b) misreading of mRNA, which causes incorporation of incorrect amino acids into the peptide and results in a nonfunctional protein; and (c) breakup of polysomes into nonfunctional monosomes.
  - Aminoglycosides exhibit concentration-dependent killing; that is, higher concentrations kill a larger proportion of bacteria and kill at a more rapid rate. They also have a significant postantibiotic effect, such that the antibacterial activity persists beyond the time during which the drug is measurable. When administered with a cell wall active antibiotic (a beta-lactam or vancomycin),

aminoglycosides may exhibit synergistic killing against certain bacteria.
- The aminoglycoside-induced rate of bacterial killing as well as induction of resistance is peak concentration-dependent.
- *Clearance:* Mostly unchanged renal excretion.
- *Route:* IV.
- *Considerations/Examples:*
  - Amikacin (Amikin)
    - ❏ It is slightly more active against *P. aeruginosa*; *Enterococcus faecalis* is susceptible to both gentamicin and tobramycin, but *E. faecium* is resistant to tobramycin. Gentamicin and tobramycin are otherwise interchangeable clinically.
  - Gentamicin (Garamycin)
    - ❏ It is effective against both gram-positive and gram-negative organisms, and many of its properties resemble those of other aminoglycosides.
  - Tobramycin (Tobradex)
    - ❏ Tobramycin has almost the same antibacterial spectrum as gentamicin with a few exceptions. Gentamicin is slightly more active against *S. marcescens* (Allegaert et al., 2021; Beauduy & Winston, 2021a; Bohannon et al., 2020b; Domonoske, 2017).

Macrolides

- *Use:* Macrolides are a group of closely related compounds characterized by a macrocyclic lactone ring to which deoxy sugars are attached.
- *Mechanism of action:* The antibacterial action of macrolides may be inhibitory or bactericidal. Inhibition of protein synthesis occurs via binding to ribosomal RNA, and peptide chain elongation is prevented. As a result, peptidyl tRNA is dissociated from the ribosome.
- *Clearance:* Hepatic metabolism, excretion through feces.
- *Route:* IV, PO.
- *Considerations/Examples:* Macrolide antibiotics prolong the electrocardiographic QT interval due to an effect on potassium channels. Prolongation of the QT interval can lead to torsades de pointes arrhythmia. Recent studies have suggested that azithromycin may be associated with a small increased risk of cardiac death.
  - Erythromycin (Erythrocin)
    - ❏ Erythromycin is the traditional drug of choice in corynebacterial infections (diphtheria, corynebacterial sepsis, erythrasma), and in respiratory, neonatal, ocular, or genital chlamydial infections.
  - Azithromycin (Zithromax)
    - ❏ It is resistant to many enzymes that inactivate gentamicin and tobramycin and therefore can be used against some microorganisms resistant to the latter drugs. Many gram-negative bacteria, including many strains of *Proteus*, *Pseudomonas*, *Enterobacter*, and *Serratia*, are

inhibited by amikacin (Beauduy & Winston, 2021d; Bohannon et al., 2020b; Domonoske, 2017; Le & Bradley, 2021).

ANTIFUNGAL AGENTS

Amphotericin B (Fungizone)

- *Use:* This is used for treatment of progressive, potentially life-threatening susceptible fungal infections. Owing to its broad spectrum of activity and fungicidal action, amphotericin B remains a useful agent for nearly all life-threatening mycotic infections.
- *Mechanism of action:* It exploits the difference in the lipid composition of fungal and mammalian cell membranes (ergosterol is found in the cell membrane of fungi, whereas the predominant sterol of bacteria and human cells is cholesterol). Amphotericin B alters the cell membrane permeability in susceptible fungi, causing leakage of cell components and resultant cell death. Some binding to human membrane sterols does occur, probably accounting for the drug's prominent toxicity.
- *Clearance:* Renal excretion, eliminated over 7 days, and may be detected in urine for up to 7 weeks after being discontinued.
- *Route:* IV.
- *Considerations:* Therapy with amphotericin B is often limited by toxicity, especially drug-induced renal impairment. Monitor renal function frequently during therapy. Monitor liver function tests; abnormalities are occasionally seen, as is a varying degree of anemia due to reduced erythropoietin production by damaged renal tubular cells (Bohannon et al., 2020b; Lampiris, & Maddix, 2021; Smith et al., 2021).

Amphotericin B (Liposomal Formulation; AmBisome)

- *Use:* This is used for treatment of systemic fungal infection.
- *Mechanism of action:* It alters cell membrane permeability in susceptible fungi, causing leakage of cell components, resulting in cell death.
- *Clearance:* Exhibits nonlinear kinetics, excreted through the kidneys over 24 hours.
- *Route:* IV.
- *Considerations:* It is not preferred in neonates due to poor penetration into the CNS, kidney, urinary tract, and eyes. Monitor BUN, serum creatinine liver function tests, serum electrolytes, especially potassium and magnesium, and intake and output (I/O). Monitor for signs or symptoms of hypokalemia (Bohannon et al., 2020b; Lampiris, & Maddix, 2021; Smith et al., 2021).

Fluconazole (Diflucan)

- *Use:* Fluconazole is used for treatment of suspected or proven candidiasis. It has a high degree of water solubility and good cerebral spinal fluid (CSF) penetration. It is the drug of choice in the treatment and secondary prophylaxis of cryptococcal meningitis, and is most commonly used for treatment of mucocutaneous candidiasis.

- *Mechanism of action:* It interferes with fungal CYP450 activity, decreasing ergosterol synthesis and inhibiting cell wall synthesis.
- *Clearance:* Excreted mostly unchanged in urine.
- *Route:* IV, PO.
- *Considerations:* Due to fewer hepatic enzyme interactions and better GI tolerance, fluconazole has the widest therapeutic index of the azoles. Monitor liver and renal function, serum potassium, CBC with differential, and platelet count (Bohannon et al., 2020b; Lampiris, & Maddix, 2021; Smith et al., 2021).

Nystatin (Bio-Statin [Oral]/Nyamyc [Topical])

- *Use:* Nystatin is used for treatment of cutaneous and mucocutaneous fungal infections caused by susceptible *Candida* species.
- *Mechanism of action:* It binds to sterols in fungal cell membrane, changing the cell wall permeability, allowing for leakage of cellular contents.
- *Route:* PO, topical, cream, ointment (too toxic for parenteral administration).
- *Considerations:* The oral suspension should be retained in the mouth for as long as possible. Paint nystatin into the recesses of the mouth and avoid feeding for 5 to 10 minutes (Bohannon et al., 2020b; Lampiris, & Maddix, 2021).

ANTIVIRAL AGENTS

Acyclovir (Zovirax)

- *Use:* Acyclovir is used for treatment and prophylaxis for herpes simplex virus (HSV-1, HSV-2) infections, herpes simplex encephalitis, herpes zoster infection, and varicella zoster infections. It has poor acyclovir activity against cytomegalovirus (CMV) due to absence of thymidine kinase (TK).
- *Mechanism of action:* It is a competitive inhibitor of HSV DNA polymerase and terminates DNA chain elongation. Because it requires certain conditions for activation, the active metabolite accumulates only in infected cells.
- *Clearance:* Glomerular filtration and tubular secretion.
- *Route:* PO, IV.
- *Considerations:* Adequate hydration and infusion rate of at least 1 hour reduce the risk of transient renal impairment and crystalluria. Monitor urinalysis, BUN, serum creatinine, CBC, liver function, neuro and nephrotoxicity, and neutrophil count (Bohannon et al., 2020b; Poole et al., 2021; Safrin, 2021).

Ganciclovir (Cytovene)

- *Use:* Ganciclovir is used for treatment of congenital cytomegalovirus. Activity is up to 100 times greater than that of acyclovir.
- *Mechanism of action:* The activated compound inhibits viral DNA polymerase and causes termination of viral DNA elongation.
- *Clearance:* Renal excretion linearly related to creatinine clearance.
- *Route:* IV. Bioavailability of the PO formula is poor and no longer available.
- *Considerations:* Neutropenia, anemia, thrombocytopenia, and pancytopenia may occur. It may be dose-limiting. Monitor CBC with differential, and platelet count, serum creatinine, and liver enzymes. Closely follow urine output (UOP) and consider serial urinalysis studies. Monitor vitals signs, particularly blood pressures, and perform an ophthalmologic exam to screen for disease (Bohannon et al., 2020b; Poole et al., 2021; Safrin, 2021).

Valganciclovir (Valcyte)

- *Use:* Valganciclovir is used for long-term treatment of CMV, with the goal of reduced hearing loss and developmental delay. Chronic suppression therapy has reduced transmission rates. It is also effective in preventing CMV infection following transplantation.
- *Mechanism of action:* It rapidly converts to ganciclovir in the body and inhibits viral DNA synthesis.
- *Clearance:* Metabolized by intestinal mucosal cells and excreted through the kidneys.
- *Route:* PO.
- *Considerations:* Monitor CBC with differential and platelet count, serum creatinine at baseline, and periodically during therapy. It is also used for prevention of CMV disease in high-risk patients undergoing heart transplant 1 month of age and greater (Bohannon et al., 2020b; Poole et al., 2021; Safrin, 2021).

Zidovudine (Retrovir; azidothymidine [AZT])

- *Use:* Zidovudine decreases the rate of clinical disease progression and prolongs survival in HIV-infected individuals. Use during pregnancy shows significant reductions in the rate of vertical transmission.
- *Mechanism of action:* It interferes with the HIV viral RNA-dependent DNA polymerase, resulting in inhibition of viral replication.
- *Clearance:* Hepatic metabolism, renal excretion.
- *Route:* PO, IV.
- *Considerations:* Routinely monitor CD cell counts for immune status. Concurrent use of phenytoin and methadone may result in elevated zidovudine levels. In contrast, use of zidovudine may decrease phenytoin levels. Hazardous drug—use appropriate precautions for receiving, handling, administration, and disposal. Gloves should be worn during any handling (Bohannon et al., 2020b; Safrin, 2021; Taketomo, 2021).

▶ BIOLOGICALS/IMMUNITIES

HEPATITIS B IMMUNE GLOBULIN (HUMAN)

- *Use:* Hepatitis B immune globulin (HBIG) provides prophylactic postexposure passive immunity to infants born to hepatitis B surface antigen (HBsAg)-positive mothers. HBIG provides short-term protection (3–6 months) and is indicated in specific postexposure circumstances. Transmission of perinatal hepatitis B virus (HBV) infection can be prevented in approximately 95% of infants born to HBsAg-positive mothers by early active and passive immunoprophylaxis of the infant.
- *Mechanism of action:* HBIG is a nonpyrogenic sterile solution containing immunoglobulin G (IgG) specific to HBsAg. Standard immune globulin is not effective in postexposure prophylaxis against HBV infection because concentrations of anti-HBs are too low.
- *Route:* IM injection.
- *Considerations:* It may be given at the same time as hepatitis B vaccine but a different site should be used. Do not mix in the same syringe; vaccine will be neutralized. Do not shake the vial and avoid causing foaming of the content (Bohannon et al., 2020b; Taketomo, 2021).

VACCINATIONS: PASSIVE IMMUNIZATION

Hepatitis B Vaccination (Engerix; Recombivax HB)
- *Use:* Hepatitis B vaccination is used to immunize against all known subspecies of HBV. HepB vaccine is used for pre-exposure and postexposure protection and provides long-term protection. Pre-exposure immunization with HepB vaccine is the most effective means to prevent HBV transmission. Accordingly, HepB immunization is recommended for all infants, children, and adolescents through 18 years of age. Infants should receive HepB vaccine as part of the routine childhood immunization schedule.
- *Mechanism of action:* HepB vaccines stimulate immunity through the production of specific antibodies. Vaccines licensed in the United States have a 90% to 95% efficacy in preventing HBV infection and clinical HBV disease among susceptible children and adults.
- *Route:* IM.
- *Considerations:* See current infectious references for recommendations on dosing and schedule intervals. Hepatitis B vaccine preparations differ by concentration; when dosed by volume, the equivalent dose is the same between products (Bohannon et al., 2020b; Taketomo, 2021).

Diphtheria, Tetanus, and Acellular Pertussis (Daptacel, Infanrix)
- *Use:* Diphtheria, tetanus toxoids, and pertussis vaccine (DTaP) consists of a mixture of the detoxified toxins (toxoids) of diphtheria and tetanus and inactivated *Bordetella pertussis* that have been adsorbed onto an aluminum salt. Diphtheria and tetanus toxoids and acellular pertussis vaccines contain PT.
- *Mechanism of action:* It promotes active immunity to diphtheria, tetanus, and pertussis by inducing production of specific antibodies.
- *Route:* IM.
- *Considerations:* Same product should be used for the entire series; shake vial well prior to withdrawing (Taketomo et al., 2021).

Haemophilus Influenzae Type B
- *Use: Haemophilus influenzae* type B (Hib) is used for protection against *Haemophilus influenzae*. The Hib conjugate vaccine consists of the Hib capsular polysaccharide (polyribosylribitol phosphate [PRP]) covalently linked to a carrier protein. Protective antibodies are directed against PRP.
- *Mechanism of action:* It stimulates the production of anticapsular antibodies and provides active immunity to Hib. Vaccination provides protective antibodies to 95% of infants who are vaccinated with a two- or three-dose series.
- *Route:* IM injection.
- *Considerations:* The minimum age for the first dose is 6 weeks. Do not restart if doses have been missed; refer to current immunization guidelines for schedule and timing of dose based on patient age and previous number of doses (Taketomo, 2021).

Influenza Virus Vaccine, Inactivated (Fluzone)
- *Use:* The influenza virus vaccine promotes immunity to seasonal influenza virus. Strains selected for inclusion in the seasonal vaccine may change yearly in anticipation of the predominant influenza strains expected to circulate in the United States. The American Academy of Pediatrics (AAP) recommends annual use of inactivated influenza vaccines (IIVs) in all people 6 months and older.
- *Mechanism of action:* It promotes immunity by inducing specific antibody production.
- *Route:* IM.
- *Considerations:* Flu seasons vary in their timing and duration from year to year; vaccination should occur as soon as vaccine is available and, if possible, by the end of October. The effectiveness of influenza vaccines depends primarily on the age and immune competence of vaccine recipients, the degree of similarity between the viruses in the vaccine and those in circulation, and the outcome being measured (Taketomo, 2021).

Pneumococcal Conjugate (Prevnar 13)

- *Use:* Pneumococcal conjugate is used for immunization against *S. pneumoniae* infections.
- *Mechanism of action:* pneumococcal conjugate vaccine (PCV13) is composed of purified capsular polysaccharide serotypes which are all individually conjugated to a nontoxic variant of the diphtheria toxin carrier protein.
- *Route:* IM.
- *Considerations:* Do not restart if doses have been missed; refer to current immunization guidelines for schedule and timing of dose based on patient age and previous number of doses (Taketomo, 2021).

Inactivated Polio Vaccine

- *Use:* Inactivated polio vaccine (IPV) provides active immunity against the poliovirus.
- *Mechanism of action:* As an inactivated virus vaccine, polio vaccine induces active immunity against the three serotypes, which are grown in Vero cells or human diploid cells and then inactivated. Administration of IPV results in seroconversion in 95% or more of vaccine recipients to each of the three serotypes after two doses and results in seroconversion in 99% to 100% of recipients after three doses.
- *Route:* IM.
- *Considerations:* Do not restart if doses have been missed; refer to current immunization guidelines for schedule and timing of dose based on patient age and previous number of doses (Taketomo, 2021).

VACCINATIONS: ACTIVE IMMUNIZATION

Rotavirus Vaccine (Rotarix, RotaTeq)

- *Use:* The rotavirus vaccine is used for routine immunization to prevent rotavirus gastroenteritis.
- *Mechanism of action:* It is a live vaccine. It replicates in the small intestine and promotes active immunity to rotavirus gastroenteritis. Virus from live vaccines may be transferred to nonvaccinated persons by physical contact. Viral shedding occurs within the first weeks of administration.
- *Route:* PO. Administer to the inner cheek if the infant spits out portion of the dose; do not administer replacement dose.
- *Considerations:* It is not routinely administered in the NICU. Immunocompromised patients should not receive live vaccines. Series should not be restarted if a dose is missed. If doses have been given, restart with the applicable dose number and separate doses by 4 weeks, for a total of three doses. It is contraindicated in infants with a history of intussusception or severe combined immunodeficiency syndromes (SCIDS). The series should not be started after 15 weeks 0 days of age and should be completed by 8 months of age (Taketomo, 2021).

▶ CARDIOVASCULAR DRUGS

VASODILATORS/VASOPRESSORS

Dobutamine (Dobutrex)

- *Use:* Dobutamine is used for short-term management of patients with cardiac decompensation.
- *Mechanism of action:* It stimulates beta-1 receptors, resulting in increased myocardial contractility and cardiac output. It also has mild beta-2 agonist activity, which makes it useful for mild vasodilatation.
- *Clearance:* Hepatic metabolism, renal excretion.
- *Route:* IV, intraosseous (IO).
- *Considerations:* Infuse in a large vein. Monitor blood pressure, EKG, heart rate, and UOP.
- *To calculate rate of infusion:* (mL/hr) = dose (mcg/kg/min) × weight × 60 minutes divided by the concentration (mcg/mL; Bohannon et al., 2020b; Domonoske, 2017; Taketomo, 2021).

Dopamine (Intropin)

- *Use:* Dopamine increases cardiac output, blood pressure, and urine flow as an adjunct in the treatment of shock and hypotension which persist after adequate fluid volume replacement. It is also used in low doses to increase renal perfusion.
- *Mechanism of action:* It stimulates both adrenergic and dopaminergic receptors. Lower doses are mainly dopaminergic-stimulating and produce renal mesenteric vasodilatation; higher doses are both dopaminergic- and beta-1-adrenergic-stimulating and produce cardiac stimulation and renal vasodilatation. Large doses stimulate alpha-adrenergic receptors.
- *Clearance:* Renal, hepatic metabolism, renal excretion.
- *Route:* Continuous IV.
- *Considerations:* Monitor blood pressure, EKG, heart rate, and UOP. Monitor skin for temperature and color changes. Ensure proper IV placement. If extravasation occurs, do not flush line; stop infusion and attempt to aspirate the extravasated solution, then remove the catheter (Bohannon et al., 2020b; Domonoske, 2017; Taketomo, 2021).

Epinephrine (Adrenalin)

- *Use:* Epinephrine is used for treatment of bradycardia, cardiac arrest, and cardiogenic shock.
- *Mechanism of action:* It stimulates alpha-, beta-, and beta-2-adrenergic receptors, resulting in relaxation of the smooth muscle of the bronchial tree, cardiac stimulation (increasing myocardial oxygen consumption), and dilatation of skeletal muscle vasculature. Small doses can cause vasodilatation via beta-2-vascular receptors; large doses may produce constriction of skeletal and vascular smooth muscle.
- *Clearance:* Taken up by the adrenergic neuron and metabolized by monoamine oxidase (MAO), renal excretion.

- *Route:* IV, IO, ET.
- *Considerations:* Titrate by 0.01 mcg/kg/min as needed to stabilize mean blood pressure. Monitor EKG, heart rate, blood pressure, and site of infusion for excessive blanching/extravasation; cardiac and blood pressure monitoring is required during infusion (Bohannon et al., 2020b; Domonoske, 2017; Taketomo, 2021).

ANTIDYSRHYTHMIA DRUGS

Adenosine (Adenocard)

- *Use:* Adenosine is used for acute treatment of sustained paroxysmal supraventricular tachycardia for conversion to normal sinus rhythm.
- *Mechanism of action:* It slows conduction time through the atrioventricular (AV) node, interrupting the reentry pathway through the AV node, restoring normal sinus rhythm. Effects are mediated by depression of calcium slow-channel conduction and an increase in potassium conductance.
- *Clearance:* Removed from circulation by vascular endothelial cells and erythrocytes, metabolized intracellularly, excreted by the kidneys.
- *Route:* Rapid IV; half-life is less than 10 seconds, duration of action is 20 to 30 seconds.
- *Considerations:* EKG monitoring is required during use. Equipment for resuscitation and trained personnel should be immediately available. It may cause bronchoconstriction; use with caution in patients with a history of bronchospasm (Bohannon et al., 2020b; Domonoske, 2017; Taketomo, 2021).

Digoxin (Lanoxin)

- *Use:* Digoxin is used for treatment of mild to moderate heart failure and to slow ventricular rate in supraventricular tachyarrhythmias.
- *Mechanism of action:* Inhibition of sodium/potassium pump in myocardial cells results in an increase in intracellular sodium, which promotes calcium influx via the sodium–calcium exchange pump, leading to increased contractility.
- *Clearance:* Metabolism via sugar hydrolysis in the stomach or by reduction by intestinal bacteria, renal excretion.
- *Route:* PO, IV.
- *Considerations:* It has narrow therapeutic window. Dosage must be individualized. Consider renal function. When transitioning from IV to oral, decrease dose by 20% to 25%. Monitor heart rate and rhythm, periodic EKG, electrolytes, and renal function; sinus bradycardia is a sign of toxicity. Trough concentrations should be followed 3 to 5 days after start of therapy and after dose changes (Bohannon et al., 2020b; Domonoske, 2017; Taketomo, 2021).

Flecainide (Tambocor)

- *Use:* Flecainide is used for prevention and treatment of ventricular arrhythmia, and prevention of supraventricular tachycardia.

- *Mechanism of action:* It slows conduction of electrical impulses within the heart.
- *Clearance:* Excreted primarily as unchanged drug in urine.
- *Route:* PO.
- *Considerations:* Monitor EKG, heart rate, blood pressure, and periodic serum concentrations after fifth dose and after dose changes (Bohannon et al., 2020b; Taketomo, 2021).

Lidocaine (Xylocaine)

- *Use:* Lidocaine is used for treatment of ventricular arrhythmias.
- *Mechanism of action:* It suppresses automaticity of conduction tissue by increasing the electrical stimulation threshold of the ventricle. It blocks both the initiation and conduction of nerve impulses by decreasing the neuronal membrane's permeability to sodium ions.
- *Clearance:* Hepatic metabolism, renal excretion.
- *Route:* IV, IO, ET.
- *Considerations:* Continuous EKG monitoring is recommended. Monitor serum concentrations with continuous infusions. Do not exceed 20 mcg/kg/min in patients with shock, hepatic disease cardiac arrest, or CHF (Bohannon et al., 2020b; Taketomo, 2021).

DRUGS AFFECTING DUCTUS ARTERIOSUS PATENCY

Alprostadil (Prostaglandin E1; Prostin VR)

- *Use:* Alprostadil is used in any clinical condition in which blood flow must be maintained through the ductus arteriosus to sustain either pulmonary or systemic circulation until corrective or palliative surgery can be performed.
- *Mechanism of action:* It causes vasodilation of all vascular smooth muscle, including the ductus arteriosus.
- *Clearance:* 70% to 80% by oxidation during a single pass through the lungs.
- *Route:* IV.
- *Considerations:* Apnea is experienced by about 10% to 12% of neonates with congenital heart defects treated with alprostadil injection USP (U.S. Pharmacopeia). Apnea is most often seen in neonates weighing <2 kg at birth and usually appears during the first hour of drug infusion. Therefore, respiratory status should be monitored throughout treatment, and alprostadil should be used where ventilatory assistance is immediately available (Bohannon et al., 2020b; Domonoske, 2017; Taketomo, 2021).

Acetaminophen (Paracetamol)

- *Use:* Acetaminophen is used for patent ductus arteriosus (PDA) closure.
- *Mechanism of action:* It acts by inhibiting prostaglandin synthetase at its peroxidase segment, thereby reducing the production of prostaglandin E2. It is unknown

whether this is the only mechanism whereby acetaminophen affects the PDA.

■ *Clearance:* Hepatic metabolism, excretion in urine.
■ *Route:* IV.
■ *Considerations:* Case series have suggested that acetaminophen may be useful in some cases where postnatal age may mitigate against the success rate of indomethacin or ibuprofen or in cases where there is contraindication to their use. The primary concern in using acetaminophen in premature neonates is the potential for hepatic dysfunction (Alpan, 2020a; Taketomo, 2021).

Ibuprofen Lysine (NeoProfen)

■ *Use:* Ibuprofen lysine is used for PDA closure.
■ *Mechanism of action:* It inhibits COX-1 and 2 enzymes, which results in decreased formation of prostaglandin precursors.
■ *Clearance:* Hepatic metabolism, renal excretion.
■ *Route:* PO, IV.
■ *Considerations:* Ibuprofen has an advantage in that it does not reduce mesenteric and renal blood flow as much as indomethacin and is associated with fewer renal side effects. Monitor vital signs, CBC, serum electrolytes, BUN, electrolytes, glucose, bilirubin, and calcium. Monitor for bleeding, heart murmur, and echocardiogram (Alpan, 2020a; Bohannon et al., 2020b; Taketomo, 2021).

Indomethacin (Indocin)

■ *Use:* Indomethacin is used for closure of hemodynamically significant PDA, prophylaxis of PDA, and prevention of intraventricular hemorrhage.
■ *Mechanism of action:* It inhibits COX-1 and 2 enzymes, which results in decreased formation of prostaglandin precursors.
■ *Clearance:* Hepatic metabolism, renal excretion.
■ *Route:* IV.
■ *Considerations:* In general, it may be given at 12-hour intervals if UOP is ≥1 mL/kg/hr after first dose; use 24-hour interval if <1 mL/kg/hr after first dose. Dose should be held if UOP <0.6 mL/kg/hr or anuria is noted. Monitor electrolytes, platelet count, UOP, heart murmur, and echocardiogram (Bohannon et al., 2020b; Domonoske, 2017; Taketomo, 2021).

ENDOTHELIN RECEPTOR ANTAGONIST

Bosentan (Tracleer)

■ *Use:* Bosentan is used for treatment of pulmonary arterial hypertension (PAH) in patients with idiopathic or congenital PAH to improve pulmonary vascular resistance (PVR). It should be used in context whereby attempts have been made to optimize ventilatory support and complicating factors.
■ *Mechanism of action:* It is an endothelin receptor antagonist that blocks endothelin receptors on the endothelium and vascular smooth muscle (stimulation of these receptors is associated with vasoconstriction).
■ *Clearance:* Hepatic metabolism, excreted through feces.
■ *Route:* PO, 3 to 5 hours to achieve peak effect.
■ *Considerations:* While case series have reported on the successful use of bosentan, controlled trials have shown conflicting results, and further studies are needed to identify patients who may benefit from this drug. There have been reported cases of hepatic failure. Serum transaminase levels (aspartate aminotransferase [AST] and alanine aminotransferase [ALT]) and bilirubin should be determined prior to start of therapy and monitored at monthly intervals thereafter. Discontinue therapy in patients who develop elevated liver levels, including increased bilirubin. Bosentan is a hazardous agent; providers should wear gloves when handling tablets/capsules (Alpan, 2020; Taketomo, 2021).

▶ DIURETICS

LOOP DIURETICS

Furosemide (Lasix)

■ *Use:* Furosemide is used in the management of edema associated with heart failure and hepatic or renal disease. It is used alone or in combination with antihypertensives to treat hypertension.
■ *Mechanism of action:* It inhibits reabsorption of sodium and chloride in the ascending loop of Henle and proximal and distal renal tubules, causing increased excretion of water, sodium, chloride magnesium, and calcium.
■ *Clearance:* Hepatic metabolism, excretion through urine and feces.
■ *Route:* PO, IM, IV. Oral and IM/IV doses are not interchangeable.
■ *Considerations:* Monitor electrolytes, renal function, blood pressure, I/O, and hearing; there is risk of hypokalemia and renal calcifications with chronic use. Risk of ototoxicity increases in the premature infant due to prolonged half-life and with concomitant use of an aminoglycoside (Bohannon et al., 2020b; Domonoske, 2017; Taketomo, 2021).

Bumetanide (Bumex)

■ *Use:* Bumetanide is used for management of edema associated with heart failure and hepatic or renal disease, including nephrotic syndrome. It has been used to reverse oliguria in preterm neonates and is used alone or in combination with antihypertensives to treat hypertension.
■ *Mechanism of action:* It inhibits chloride and sodium reabsorption in the ascending loop of Henle and proximal renal tubule, causing increased excretion of water and electrolytes. It does not appear to act in the distal tubule.

- *Clearance:* Hepatic metabolism, renal excretion.
- *Route:* PO, IM, IV.
- *Considerations:* Higher end of dosing may be needed for patients in heart failure. It has been used to reverse oliguria in preterm infants. Monitor electrolytes, renal function, blood pressure, and UOP. It may displace bilirubin (Bohannon et al., 2020b; Taketomo, 2021).

THIAZIDE DIURETICS

Chlorothiazide (Diuril)

- *Use:* Chlorothiazide is used for treatment of edema due to heart and renal failure, management of hypertension alone or in combination with antihypertensive, treatment of BPD, and treatment of central diabetes insipidus (DI).
- *Mechanism of action:* It inhibits sodium and chloride reabsorption in the distal tubules, causing increased excretion of sodium chloride and water, resulting in diuresis. Loss of potassium, hydrogen ions, magnesium phosphate, and bicarbonate also occurs. Thiazide diuretics decrease calcium excretion.
- *Clearance:* Not metabolized, renal excretion as unchanged drug.
- *Route:* PO, IV.
- *Considerations:* Monitor electrolytes, BUN, creatinine, hyperglycemia, blood pressure, I/O, and weight (Bohannon et al., 2020b; Domonoske, 2017; Taketomo, 2021).

Hydrochlorothiazide (Microzide)

- *Use:* Hydrochlorothiazide (HCTZ) is used for management of edema related to heart failure, hepatic cirrhosis, corticosteroid therapy, or renal dysfunction; and for management of hypertension alone or in combination with other antihypertensives. It has also been used for BPD, central DI, and idiopathic hypercalciuria.
- *Mechanism of action:* It inhibits sodium and chloride reabsorption in the distal tubules, causing increased excretion of sodium chloride and water, resulting in diuresis. Loss of potassium, hydrogen ions, magnesium phosphate, and bicarbonate also occurs. Thiazide diuretics decrease calcium excretion.
- *Clearance:* Not metabolized, renal excretion as unchanged drug.
- *Route:* PO.
- *Considerations:* Monitor electrolytes, BUN, creatinine, hyperglycemia, blood pressure, I/O, and weight (Bohannon et al., 2020b; Domonoske, 2017; Taketomo, 2021).

POTASSIUM-SPARING DIURETICS

Spironolactone (Aldactone)

- *Use:* Spironolactone is used for management of edema and sodium retention, and as prophylaxis against hypokalemia patients on digoxin.

- *Mechanism of action:* It competes with aldosterone for receptor sites in the distal renal tubule, increasing sodium chloride and water losses, while conserving potassium and hydrogen ions.
- *Clearance:* Hepatic metabolism, renal excretion.
- *Route:* PO.
- *Considerations:* It is generally used in combination with a thiazide diuretic. Use with caution in infants with renal impairment. Monitor electrolytes, primarily hyperkalemia, renal function, I/O, and weight (Bohannon et al., 2020b; Domonoske, 2017; Taketomo, 2021).

COMBINATION DIURETIC THERAPY

Hydrochlorothiazide and Spironolactone (Aldactazide)

- *Use:* This combination therapy is used for symptom management of BPD, hypertension, and edema complicating the clinical status.
- *Mechanism of action:* See individual medications for description of mechanisms of action. This product is a fixed combination of components in equal milligram proportions.
- *Route:* PO.
- *Considerations:* Monitor serum electrolytes, BUN, creatinine, blood pressure, fluid balance, body weight, and heart rate (Domonoske, 2017; Taketomo, 2021).

INHIBITORS OF CARBONIC ANHYDRASE DIURETICS

Acetazolamide (Diamox)

- *Use:* Acetazolamide is used as a mild diuretic and for correction of metabolic alkalosis through treatment of renal tubular acidosis (RTA).
- *Mechanism of action:* Reversible inhibition of the enzyme carbonic anhydrase results in reduction of hydrogen ion secretion at the renal tubule and increased renal excretion of sodium, bicarbonate, and water. It decreases the production of aqueous humor in the eye.
- *Clearance:* Renal excretion.
- *Route:* PO, IV.
- *Considerations:* Monitor serum electrolytes, CBC, and platelet count (Bohannon et al., 2020b; Taketomo, 2021).

▶ GASTROINTESTINAL DRUGS

HISTAMINE H2 ANTAGONIST

Ranitidine (Zantac)

- *Use:* Ranitidine is used as short-term and maintenance treatment for duodenal ulcers, gastric ulcers, gastroesophageal (GE) reflux, and erosive esophagitis.
- *Mechanism of action:* Competitive inhibition of histamine at the H2 receptors of the gastric parietal

cells, which inhibits gastric acid secretion; gastric volume and hydrogen ion concentrations are reduced.

- *Clearance:* Hepatic metabolism, renal excretion.
- *Route:* PO, IV.
- *Considerations:* There is a sixfold increased risk of NEC, infection, and mortality in very low birthweight (VLBW) infants. Monitor AST/ALT, serum creatinine, and occult blood with GI bleeding (Bohannon et al., 2020b; Domonoske, 2017).

Famotidine (Pepcid)

- *Use:* Famotidine is used as short-term treatment for GE reflux.
- *Mechanism of action:* Competitive inhibition of histamine at the H2 receptors of the gastric parietal cells, which inhibits gastric secretion.
- *Clearance:* Hepatic metabolism, renal excretion.
- *Route:* PO, IV.
- *Considerations:* Monitor CBC, gastric pH, occult blood with GI bleeding, and renal function (Bohannon et al., 2020b; Domonoske, 2017; Taketomo, 2021).

PROKINETICS

Metoclopramide (Reglan)

- *Use:* Metoclopramide is used for symptomatic treatment of GE reflux.
- *Mechanism of action:* It blocks dopamine receptors and, when given in higher doses, also blocks serotonin receptors in the chemoreceptor trigger zone of the CNS. It enhances response to acetylcholine of tissues in the upper GI tract, causing enhanced motility and increased gastric emptying without stimulating gastric, biliary, or pancreatic secretions; and increases lower esophageal sphincter tone.
- *Clearance:* Hepatic metabolism, renal excretion.
- *Route:* PO, IM, IV.
- *Considerations:* Monitor blood pressure and heart rate when rapid IV administration is used., Monitor for dystonic reactions (Bohannon et al., 2020b; Domonoske, 2017; Taketomo, 2021).

Erythromycin (erythromycin ethylsuccinate [EES])

- *Use:* Erythromycin is a prokinetic GI motility agent.
- *Mechanism of action:* It inhibits RNA-dependent protein synthesis during elongation and blocks the transpeptidation binding to the 50S ribosomal subunit.
- *Clearance:* Hepatic metabolism, excreted in feces.
- *Route:* PO.
- *Considerations:* Therapy is started after the start of enteral feedings. Efficacy has not been demonstrated in the majority of trials. Use in neonates less than 14 days of age has been associated with a 10-fold increase in pyloric stenosis (Bohannon et al., 2020b; Taketomo, 2021).

PROTON PUMP INHIBITORS

Omeprazole (Prilosec)

- *Use:* Omeprazole is used as short-term treatment for GE reflux and erosive esophagitis.
- *Mechanism of action:* It suppresses gastric basal and stimulated acid secretion by inhibiting the parietal cell H+/K+ adenosine triphosphate (ATP) pump.
- *Clearance:* Hepatic metabolism, renal excretion.
- *Route:* PO.
- *Considerations:* Use of proton pump inhibitors (PPIs) may increase the rate of GI infections. Titrate to the lowest effect dose to minimize risks of developing osteoporosis and subsequent fractures. Consider supplementation of vitamin D and calcium (Bohannon et al., 2020b; Domonoske, 2017; Taketomo, 2021).

Pantoprazole (Protonix)

- *Use:* Pantoprazole is used for treatment of GE reflux, erosive esophagitis, and gastritis.
- *Mechanism of action:* It suppresses gastric basal and stimulated acid secretion by inhibiting the parietal cell H+/K+ ATP pump.
- *Clearance:* Hepatic metabolism, excreted in urine and feces.
- *Route:* PO, IV.
- *Considerations:* Thrombocytopenia, ascites, pulmonary deterioration, and renal and hepatic failure have been reported. Use of PPIs may increase the rate of GI infections. There is increased frequency of osteoporosis and fractures. Use the lowest effective dose. Consider supplementation of vitamin D and calcium (Taketomo, 2021).

▶ INHALANTS

INHALED STEROIDS, CORTICOSTEROIDS

Budesonide (Oral Inhalation; Pulmicort)

- *Use:* Budesonide is used as maintenance therapy and prophylaxis for bronchial asthma. It is NOT indicated for acute bronchospasm.
- *Mechanism of action:* It controls the rate of protein synthesis, depresses the migration of polymorphonuclear leukocytes and fibroblasts, and reverses capillary permeability and lysosomal stabilization. It has potent glucocorticoid activity and weak mineralocorticoid activity.
- *Route:* Oral inhalation, nebulization.
- *Considerations:* Orally inhaled corticosteroids may cause a reduction in growth velocity; titrate to the lowest effective dose. Monitor mucous membranes for signs of fungal infection. Monitor for signs and symptoms of hypercorticism or adrenal suppression. Prolonged use may increase the risk of secondary

infection, may mask acute infection or prolong/exacerbate viral infections, and limit response to vaccines (Taketomo, 2021).

INHALED STEROIDS, MINERALOCORTICOID

Fluticasone (Oral Inhalation; Flovent)

- *Use:* Fluticasone is an anti-inflammatory and antiasthmatic agent, and is used for treatment of BPD.
- *Mechanism of action:* Fluticasone belongs to a group of corticosteroids which utilize a fluorocarbothioate ester linkage at the 17-carbon position. It has extremely potent vasoconstriction and anti-inflammatory activity. The effectiveness of inhaled fluticasone is due to its direct effect.
- *Route:* Oral inhalation.
- *Considerations:* Monitor growth, mucous membranes for signs of fungal infection, ocular effects such as cataracts, increased ocular pressure, glaucoma, bone mineral density, hepatic impairment, and possible eosinophilic conditions. Monitor for signs of asthma. Monitor for hypothalamic-pituitary-adrenal (HPA) axis suppression (i.e., adrenal insufficiency caused by abrupt discontinuation of chronic glucocorticoids; Li & White, 2019; Taketomo, 2021).

▶ NEUROLOGIC AGENTS

ANESTHETICS AGENTS: GENERAL

Ketamine (Ketalar)

- *Use:* Ketamine is a rapid-acting general anesthetic agent for short diagnostic and minor surgical procedures that do not require skeletal muscle relaxation.
- *Mechanism of action:* It produces dissociative anesthesia by direct action on the cortex and limbic system. It is a noncompetitive N-methyl-d-aspartate (NMDA) receptor antagonist that blocks glutamate.
- *Clearance:* Hepatic metabolism, renal excretion.
- *Route:* IV, IM, PO.
- *Considerations:* Avoid use of ketamine in patients with increased ICP. There is risk of respiratory depression and apnea after rapid IV administration of high doses, as well as risks of inducing laryngospasms. Doses may lead to increased airway resistance, and cough reflex may be depressed. Increased muscle tone that may resemble seizures may occur in infants receiving high, repeated doses. Severe reactions can be treated with a benzodiazepine (Bohannon et al., 2020b; Taketomo, 2021).

Propofol (Diprivan)

- *Use:* Propofol is a nonbarbiturate anesthetic used for short-term procedural sedation and anesthesia. It is also used for induction of anesthesia.
- *Mechanism of action:* It causes global CNS depression presumably through agonism of $GABA_A$ receptors

and perhaps reduced glutamatergic activity through NMDA receptor blockade.

- *Clearance:* Hepatic metabolism, renal excretion.
- *Route:* IV; quick loss of consciousness (within 30 seconds) and short duration of action after a single bolus dose (3–10 minutes).
- *Considerations:* Side effects in neonates include prolonged hypotension, bradycardia, desaturations, and significant variability in pharmacokinetics (Davidson et al., 2020; Taketomo, 2021).

SEDATIVES/HYPNOTICS

Dexmedetomidine (Precedex)

- *Use:* Dexmedetomidine offers the benefit of rapid achievement of targeted sedation levels. The use of dexmedetomidine to facilitate extubation in children intolerant of an awake, intubated state may abbreviate ventilator weaning.
- *Mechanism of action:* It is a selective alpha-2-adrenoceptor agonist that, unlike traditional sedative agents, produces its sedative effect at least in part through an endogenous sleep-promoting pathway that does not produce respiratory depression.
- *Clearance:* Hepatic metabolism, renal clearance.
- *Route:* IV, onset of action 5 to 10 minutes.
- *Considerations:* The most common side effects of dexmedetomidine are hypotension and bradycardia, which generally resolve by decreasing the dose (Eyal, 2020c; Taketomo, 2021).

Diazepam (Valium)

- *Use:* Diazepam is used for treatment of seizures refractory to other combined anticonvulsant agents. It reduces anxiety and can be used for preoperative or preprocedural sedation. It is an alternative choice to lorazepam for status epilepticus.
- *Mechanism of action:* It binds to stereospecific benzodiazepine receptors on the postsynaptic GABA neuron at several sites in the CNS.
- *Clearance:* Hepatic metabolism, renal excretion.
- *Route:* IV.
- *Consideration:* It is not recommended as a first-line agent. Use only after multiple agents have failed. Observe for and be prepared to manage respiratory arrest. Rapid IV push may cause sudden respiratory depression, apnea, or hypotension (Bohannon et al., 2020b; Taketomo, 2021).

Lorazepam (Ativan)

- *Use:* Lorazepam is used for treatment of status epilepticus resistant to conventional anticonvulsant therapy, and for management of anxiety (anxiolytic) and as amnestic often used for preprocedure sedation.
- *Mechanism of action:* It binds to stereospecific benzodiazepine receptors on the postsynaptic GABA neuron at several sites in the CNS.
- *Clearance:* Hepatic metabolism, renal excretion.
- *Route:* IV.

Considerations: It may cause respiratory depression and hypotension; use the lowest effective dose. Dependence develops with prolonged use. Monitor respiratory status, blood pressure, heart rate, CBC with differential, and liver function with long-term use. Use with caution; there is concern regarding neurotoxicity (Bohannon et al., 2020b; Taketomo, 2021).

Midazolam (Versed)

- *Use:* Midazolam is used for preprocedural sedation, anxiolysis, and as amnestic for diagnostic or radiographic procedures. Infusions may be used in sedation of intubated and mechanically ventilated patients.
- *Mechanism of action:* It binds to specific GABA receptor subunits at CNS neuronal synapses, facilitating GABA-mediated chloride ion channel opening frequency, also enhances membrane hyperpolarization.
- *Clearance:* Hepatic metabolism, renal excretion.
- *Route:* IM, IV, intranasal.
- *Considerations:* It may cause severe hypotension and/or seizures with rapid administration; give over 2 to 5 minutes. Use the lowest effective dose. Dependence develops with prolonged use (Bohannon et al., 2020b; Taketomo, 2021).

▶ RESPIRATORY DRUGS

BRONCHODILATORS

Albuterol (Ventolin)

- *Use:* Albuterol is used for prevention and treatment of bronchospasm, and as a bronchodilator in respiratory distress syndrome (RDS) and BPD. It is probably the most commonly used aerosolized bronchodilator.
- *Mechanism of action:* It promotes primarily beta-2-adrenergic stimulation (bronchodilation and vasodilation) with minor beta-1 stimulation (increased myocardial contractility and conduction).
- *Route:* Oral inhalation, nebulization, duration is 2 to 5 hours.
- *Considerations:* Monitor serum potassium, oxygen saturation, heart rate, pulmonary function respiratory rate, use of accessory muscles during respiration, suprasternal retractions, and blood gases. It may cause insomnia and excitability (Bohannon et al., 2020b; Eyal, 2020b; Li & White, 2019; Taketomo, 2021).

Ipratropium (Oral Inhalation; Atrovent)

- *Use:* Ipratropium is used for treatment of bronchospasm associated with asthma and as a bronchodilating agent in BPD and neonatal respiratory distress. It is not sufficiently effective for use as a single agent in the treatment of acute bronchospasms.
- *Mechanism of action:* It blocks the action of acetylcholine at parasympathetic sites in bronchial smooth muscle, causing bronchodilatation.
- *Route:* Oral inhalation, nebulization.

Considerations: Data are limited, and optimal dosing has not been established (Li & White, 2019; Taketomo, 2021).

Levalbuterol (Xopenex)

- *Use:* Levalbuterol is used for treatment or prevention of bronchospasms in children. It produces acute improvement in lung mechanics and gas exchange in infants with BPD exhibiting symptoms of increased airway tone. Effect is time-limited.
- *Mechanism of action:* It is an inhaled beta-2 agonist and relaxes the bronchial smooth muscle by action on beta-2 receptor.
- *Clearance:* Metabolism in the GI tract, >80% excretion in urine.
- *Route:* Oral inhalation, nebulization.
- *Considerations:* It is composed of both (R) and (S) isomers of albuterol. Levalbuterol is the active isomer of albuterol (R-albuterol). The difference between levalbuterol and albuterol is modest, but levalbuterol has fewer side effects (Li & White, 2019; Taketomo, 2021; Zayek, 2020).

RESPIRATORY STIMULANTS

Caffeine Citrate (Cafcit)

- *Use:* Caffeine citrate is used for treatment of apnea of prematurity.
- *Mechanism of action:* It is a CNS stimulant that increases medullary respiratory center sensitivity to carbon dioxide, stimulates central inspiratory drive, and improves diaphragmatic contractility.
- *Clearance:* Hepatic metabolism, renal excretion.
- *Route:* IV, PO.
- *Considerations:* Monitor for tachycardia, number and severity of apnea spells, and serum caffeine levels—therapeutic 8 to 20 mcg/mL, potentially toxic >20 mcg/mL, and toxic >50 mcg/mL. Administer with caution in patients with gastric esophageal reflux, impaired renal or hepatic function, seizure disorders, or cardiovascular disease. It may be associated with risk of NEC (Bohannon et al., 2020b; Domonoske, 2017; Taketomo, 2021).

▶ STEROIDS

SYSTEMIC STEROIDS, CORTICOSTEROIDS

Dexamethasone (Systemic; Decadron)

- *Use:* Dexamethasone is used for prevention of RDS and as an anti-inflammatory.
- *Mechanism of action:* It is a long-acting corticosteroid with minimal sodium-retaining potential. It decreases inflammation by suppression of neutrophil migration, decreased production of inflammatory mediators, and reversal of increased capillary permeability.

- *Clearance:* Hepatic metabolism, renal excretion.
- *Route:* PO, IM, IV.
- *Considerations:* In premature neonates, the use of high-dose dexamethasone approximately >0.5 mg/kg/d for prevention or treatment of BPD has been associated with adverse neurodevelopmental outcomes, including higher rates of cerebral palsy, without additional clinical benefits of lower doses. Dexamethasone may increase the effects/toxicity of loop and thiazide diuretics. Monitor hemoglobin, occult blood loss, blood pressure, serum glucose, and serum potassium. Monitor for osteopenia with long/multiple courses of therapy (Bohannon et al., 2020b; Domonoske, 2017; Taketomo, 2021).

Hydrocortisone (Solu-Cortef)

- *Use:* Hydrocortisone is an anti-inflammatory and is used for treatment of primary or secondary adrenocorticoid deficiency; management of septic shock, hypoglycemia, and hypotension; and treatment of BPD.
- *Mechanism of action:* It is a short-acting corticosteroid with minimal sodium-retaining potential. It decreases inflammation by suppression of neutrophil migration, decreased production of inflammatory mediators, and reversal of increased capillary permeability.
- *Clearance:* Hepatic metabolism, renal excretion.
- *Route:* PO, IV.
- *Considerations:* Monitor electrolytes, serum glucose, and blood pressure. Monitor growth/weight. Monitor for suppression of HPA. It is associated with GI perforation in low birthweight infants (Bohannon et al., 2020b; Domonoske, 2017; Taketomo, 2021).

Prednisolone (Pediapred)

- *Use:* Prednisolone is an anti-inflammatory used in the treatment of BPD.
- *Mechanism of action:* It decreases inflammation by suppression of migration of polymorphonuclear leukocytes and reversal of increased capillary permeability. It suppresses the immune system by reducing the activity and volume of the lymphatic system.
- *Clearance:* Hepatic metabolism, renal excretion.
- *Route:* PO.
- *Considerations:* Dose depends on the condition being treated and response of the patient. Dosage for infants should be based on disease severity and patient response rather than rigid adherence to dosing guidelines. Consider alternate-day therapy for long-term therapy. Monitor blood pressure, weight, electrolytes, serum glucose, and bone mineral density with long-term therapy. Risk of fractures increases with >4 courses of corticosteroids (Bohannon et al., 2020b; Taketomo, 2021).

▶ CONCLUSION

Making decisions surrounding medication therapy for a neonate is a complex task deserving careful thought and consideration. Benefits of treatment weighed against risks of exposure to drugs should be balanced and discussed within the healthcare team and a pharmacist specializing in neonatal medicines if available. Drug therapy decisions should also take into account the particular medications available within a healthcare system, rules governing their use, and individualized abilities to administer and monitor their usage.

1. The administration of hepatitis B immune globulin (HBIG) is an example of the use of:

   A. Active immunization
   B. Passive immunization
   C. Torpid immunization

2. The neonatal nurse practitioner (NNP) recognizes that an infant who has undergone a gastrointestinal surgery resulting in significant loss of small bowel may require individualized adjustments to medications which are given:

   A. Intravenously
   B. Orally
   C. Subcutaneously

3. The neonatal nurse practitioner (NNP) is treating an infant with *Escherichia coli* sepsis with an aminoglycoside, knowing that maximal effective therapy is dependent on the medication's:

   A. Distribution of water
   B. First pass metabolism
   C. Peak concentration

4. Rational pharmacotherapy depends on a basic understanding of the way a drug affects the body of the neonate, which is known as:

   A. Pharmacodynamics (PD)
   B. Pharmacokinetics (PK)
   C. Pharmacosynthesis (PS)

5. The neonatal nurse practitioner (NNP) orders digoxin (Lanoxin) when the desired result is:

   A. A decrease in cardiac afterload and correction of acidosis
   B. An increase in heart rate and reduction in peripheral edema
   C. A slowing of heart rate and improved peripheral tissue perfusion

6. The neonatal nurse practitioner (NNP) understands a medication's ability to reach the site at the desired time in an effective concentration is determined by the medication's:

   A. Method of administration
   B. Protein binding capacity
   C. Total body water volume

7. The neonatal nurse practitioner (NNP) chooses the antifungal therapy with the widest therapeutic index by selecting:

   A. Amphotericin B (AmBisome)
   B. Fluconazole (Diflucan)
   C. Ganciclovir (Cytovene)

1. B) Passive immunization

HBIG provides prophylactic postexposure passive immunity to infants born to hepatitis B surface antigen (HBsAg)-positive mothers. HBIG provides short-term protection (3–6 months) and is indicated in specific postexposure circumstances (Bohannon et al., 2020b; Taketomo, 2021). Active immunity is conferred through inducing production of specific antibodies. "Torpid" denotes slow or sluggish responses and is not pertinent to discussions of immunization.

2. B) Orally

The diseases that likely have the greatest impact on oral drug absorption are those affecting the total intestinal surface area, such as short bowel syndrome. This syndrome results from massive bowel resection complicating necrotizing enterocolitis, from volvulus, or from congenital anomalies like gastroschisis or multiple intestinal atresia (Allegaert et al., 2021). Intravenous or subcutaneous administration is not affected by gastrointestinal tract integrity.

3. C) Peak concentration

Aminoglycosides exhibit concentration-dependent killing; that is, higher concentrations kill a larger proportion of bacteria and kill at a more rapid rate. The aminoglycoside-induced rate of bacterial killing as well as induction of resistance is peak concentration dependent. Distribution of medication throughout the body water does not affect rate of bacterial killing. First-pass metabolism refers to metabolism of the medication not the rate of bacterial killing (Allegaert et al., 2021).

4. A) Pharmacodynamics (PD)

The simplest way to identify and adjust for interindividual variability in drug response is to objectively measure the degree of effect and then adjust the dosing regimen accordingly. Rational pharmacotherapy requires a basic understanding of the way patients handle drugs (PK) and their response (effect) to specific drug concentrations (PD). PK may be simply defined as what the body does to the drug, as opposed to PD, which may be defined as what the drug does to the body (Mizuno et al., 2021). PS is a concept not applied to neonatal pharmacology.

5. C) A slowing of heart rate and improved peripheral tissue perfusion

Digoxin (Lanoxin) is used for treatment of mild-to-moderate heart failure, to slow ventricular rate in supraventricular tachyarrhythmias. Its mechanism of action is inhibition of sodium/potassium pump in myocardial cells, resulting in increase in intracellular sodium, which promotes calcium influx via the sodium–calcium exchange pump, leading to increased contractility. Monitor heart rate and rhythm, periodic EKG, electrolytes, and renal function. Sinus bradycardia is a sign of toxicity (Bohannon et al., 2020b; Domonoske, 2017; Taketomo, 2021).

6. A) Method of administration

For optimal therapeutics to be realized, a method of drug administration must be used that will enable the drug to reach its site of action at the desired time and in an effective concentration. Pharmacodynamics (PD) is the relationship between drug concentrations in the serum and the effects of the drug on the body. These effects include therapeutic and toxic effects. PD properties are drug-specific and reflect the (a) mechanism of action, (b) potency, (c) toxicity characteristics, (d) efficacy, and (e) desired outcome (Domonoske, 2021; Holford, 2018; Wade, 2020).

7. B) Fluconazole (Diflucan)

Due to fewer hepatic enzyme interactions and better gastrointestinal tolerance, fluconazole has the widest therapeutic index of the azoles (Bohannon et al., 2020b; Lampiris & Maddix, 2021; Smith et al., 2021). Amphotericin B has a very limited therapeutic index, while ganciclovir is an antiviral therapy rather than an antifungal.

Part V: Embryology, Physiology, Pathophysiology, and Systems Management

Genetics

Amy R. Koehn

▶ INTRODUCTION

Neonates born with a congenital anomaly, chromosomal defect, or an inborn error of metabolism require assessment and management by a multidisciplinary team of neonatal experts. Advances in medical technology provide clinicians with the ability to diagnose genetic abnormalities and diseases antenatally, but many may still not be evident until after delivery. A genetic evaluation can be multifaceted and quite complex, and may include a physical examination to identify dysmorphic features, a family history to identify lineage etiology, and advanced skill in interpreting laboratory results. The evaluation of an infant with a suspected genetic anomaly must use a logical and disciplined methodologic process to ensure accurate diagnosis. Early evaluation may guide appropriate treatment, provide timely diagnosis, and optimize the prognosis for infants and their families. This chapter provides an overview of genetic processes, diagnostic options, and treatments that may be currently available.

▶ GENETIC BASICS

TERMINOLOGY

- ▪ *Chromosome:* This is a structure in a cell nucleus that has genes and transports genetic information. It is composed of complex, linear DNA molecules with structural proteins. Chromosomes are located in the nucleus of a cell.
  - ● A normal human karyotype has 46 chromosomes (diploid number), 22 sets of autosomes, and 1 set of sex chromosomes. Genetic material is stained, and chromosomes are arranged by size and banding patterns. Each chromosome has a long arm, referred to as the *q arm*; and a short arm, or the *p arm*; these are joined by a centromere.
    - ❏ The term *diploid* indicates the presence of the normal two copies (46) of all chromosomes.
    - ❏ *Haploid* indicates only one copy of all chromosomes, for a total of 23 present.
    - ❏ *Triploidy* indicates three copies of all chromosomes, for a total of 69 present.
    - ❏ *Tetraploidy* indicates four copies of all chromosomes, for a total of 96 present.
    - ❏ The term *aneuploidy* is used to describe any genotype in which the total chromosome number is not a multiple of 23. This indicates a net loss or gain of genetic material (Gross & Gheorghe, 2020; Haldeman Englert et al., 2018; Matthews & Robin, 2021; Schiefelbein, 2021).
- ▪ *Gene:* A gene is the functional unit of heredity. This small unit is responsible for inherited single characteristics, such as biochemical, physical, or physiologic traits, and is aligned in a linear sequence along with other genes along a chromosome.
  - ● A person's *genotype* is the actual genetic makeup of an individual. This cannot be known without in-depth genetic analysis.
  - ● *Phenotype* is a term used to describe the identifiable features and possible dysmorphisms of an individual. In clinical practice, *phenotype* refers to a collection of specific traits and physical findings, and the results of medical tests such as laboratory, pathologic, and radiologic studies (Bennett & Meier, 2019; Matthews & Robin, 2021; Mitchell, 2020; Powell-Hamilton, 2020).
- ▪ *Genetics* is the study of a single or limited number of genes and their role in heredity.
- ▪ *Genomics* is the study of an individual's complete DNA sequence (genome).
- ▪ *DNA: Deoxyribonucleic acid* is a molecule that stores, processes, and duplicates vital hereditary information. It has two long strands which form a double helix. Each DNA strand is composed of four nucleotides: guanine (G), adenine (A), thymine (T), and cytosine (C).
- ▪ *Exons* are parts of the DNA sequence that code for proteins.

■ It is important to distinguish the concepts of *congenital* and *genetic*, terms that are often confused. A *congenital anomaly* is an internal or external structural defect that is present at birth. It may or may not be immediately visible. Congenital features can have genetic or nongenetic causes (Matthews & Robin, 2021; Mitchell, 2020; Powell-Hamilton, 2020).

GENETIC TESTING

Karyotype

■ To analyze the size, shape, and number of chromosomes, a karyotype is produced (Figure 15.1). A karyotype is the standard pictorial arrangement of chromosome pairs. The pairs are organized according to size and then evaluated for overall structure and banding pattern. Standardized reporting is guided by the International System for Human Cytogenetic Nomenclature (Matthews & Robin, 2021; Powell-Hamilton, 2020).

- *Chromosome report format:* total chromosomal number, sex chromosomes, abnormalities
  - ❏ *Example:* The report may read 47,XX, +21; this should be interpreted as 47 total chromosomes, XX (girl), extra 21st chromosome (trisomy 21; Gross & Gheorghe, 2020).

Chromosomal Microarray

■ Chromosomal microarray (CMA) is considered the first-line genetic test in neonates with multiple anomalies. This analysis allows for the detection of chromosomal deletions and duplications too small to be seen in a high-resolution analysis and can identify an additional 5% to 10% of cases with genomic imbalance compared with routine karyotyping.

■ CMA can also identify deletions or duplications, known as *copy number variants*, which may or may not be associated with the phenotype of the neonate. Thus, care must be taken when interpreting CMA results (Bacino, 2017; Lubbers, 2021; McCandless & Kripps, 2020; Mitchell, 2020; Powell-Hamilton, 2020).

Fluorescence In Situ Hybridization

■ A DNA probe is labeled with a fluorochrome, and the fluorescent signal is visible with microscopy. The number of signals can be counted (one signal = a specific genetic sequence). It is relatively rapid, but some chromosomal structural abnormalities may be missed as the test detects genetic sequence, not its location.

■ Fluorescence in situ hybridization (FISH) studies can be useful in the rapid detection of aneuploidies, especially for trisomies 13 and 18 and for sex chromosome testing in infants with ambiguous genitalia.

■ FISH testing is ordered if there is a high level of suspicion for a known microdeletion syndrome

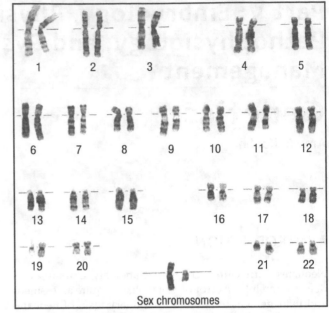

Figure 15.1 Karyotype of a normal male.

Source: Reproduced with permission from Bajaj, K., & Gross, S.J. (2015). Genetic aspects of perinatal disease and prenatal diagnosis. In R. Martin, A. Fanaroff, & M. Walsh (Eds.), *Fanaroff & Martin's neonatal-perinatal medicine: Diseases of the fetus and infant* (10th ed., pp. 130–146). Elsevier.

not detectable by routine cytogenetic analysis. An example is testing for 22q11 deletion/velocardiofacial/DiGeorge syndrome or Williams syndrome. A full karyotype should still be performed.

■ Testing with FISH has shown that a significant number of neonates with conotruncal heart defects have a 22q11 microdeletion; therefore, this testing is indicated in all patients with truncus arteriosus, interrupted aortic arch, and tetralogy of Fallot (TOF; Bacino, 2017; Gross & Gheorghe, 2020; Haldeman-Englert et al., 2018; Lubbers, 2021; McCandless & Kripps, 2020; Mitchell, 2020; Powell-Hamilton, 2020).

Comparative Genomic Hybridization Array

■ This technology blends molecular techniques with cytogenetics and allows the genome to be scanned at a higher resolution than conventional techniques. It is based on the comparison of a known genome from a normal individual against the test sample and is often done with a matched sex control.

■ It can measure the difference between two different DNA samples in copy number (dosage) of a particular segment of DNA. Thus, microscopic gains and losses from a patient sample can be quantified.

■ Chromosome microarrays can detect 14% to 16% more abnormalities than conventional cytogenetic studies. Disadvantages include inability to detect inversions, balanced chromosome translocations, and low-level mosaicisms (Bacino, 2017; Powell-Hamilton, 2020).

Exome Sequencing

- Exome sequencing studies are performed in infants with multiple anomalies but with a normal chromosome microarray study. This study allows sequencing of all the exomes of the genome (20,000 genes approximately) using next-generation sequencing (NGS). Exome sequencing detects the etiology in approximately 26% of patients whose etiology was not detected by previous studies (Bacino, 2017; Powell-Hamilton, 2020).
- Tests based on NGS technologies are rapidly replacing many single-gene sequencing tests. These tests use disease-targeted exon capture, whole-exome sequencing (WES), or whole-genome sequencing (WGS) strategies.
  - WES allows for all the exomes in the genome (the coding portion of DNA) to be examined and to identify disease-causing mutations.
  - WGS investigates an individual's entire genome (all components of genes, such as introns, regulatory elements, etc.) and is available clinically in some instances (Matthews & Robin, 2021).
- As technologies change and improve, it seems likely that whole-genome testing will become more standard, although our ability to interpret the full genome, including all the noncoding DNA, is likely to take many years to mature (McCandless & Kripps, 2020; Powell-Hamilton, 2020).

▶ CHROMOSOMAL STRUCTURE ABNORMALITIES

- A *deletion* denotes a loss of a chromosomal segment. This mechanism is responsible for partial monosomy in the affected chromosome.
  - Loss of material from the end of a chromosome is known as *terminal deletion*.
  - An *interstitial deletion* involves loss of chromosomal material that does not include the ends.
- *Duplication* of the DNA region that contains a gene results in a new mutation. It is considered partial trisomy of a chromosome.
- *Nondisjunction* occurs when paired chromosomes fail to separate during cell division. It is the most common mechanism for aneuploidy.
- *Translocation* occurs when a chromosomal agent attaches at an abnormal site, either in the wrong position on the same chromosome or attached to another chromosome.
- *Unbalanced translocation* results in partial trisomy or monosomy (Matthews & Robin, 2021; Schiefelbein, 2021).
- Figure 15.2 summarizes these structural anomalies.

ETIOLOGIES OF DYSMORPHOLOGY

- Anomalous external physical features are called *dysmorphisms* and can be clues to an underlying

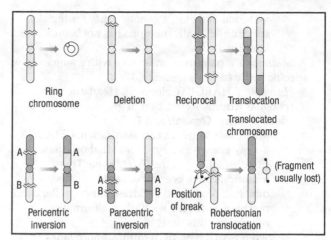

Figure 15.2 Schematic example of structural chromosomal abnormalities.

cause or developmental defect. A useful approach to determining the etiology of a congenital anomaly is to consider whether it represents a malformation, deformation, or disruption of normal development (Mitchell, 2020).

Malformation/Disruption/Deformation

- A *malformation* implies an abnormal morphogenesis of the underlying tissue owing to a genetic or teratogenic factor. Malformation is a primary structural defect that results from a localized error of morphogenesis and results in abnormal development. The effects are primary structural defects in tissue formation, such as a neural tube defect or a congenital heart defect.
- A *deformation* results from abnormal mechanical forces, such as intrauterine constraint, acting on otherwise normal tissues (e.g., dolichocephaly due to breech positioning). A variety of maternal factors can cause fetal constraint, and common examples include breech or other abnormal positioning in utero, oligohydramnios, and uterine anomalies.
- A *disruption* represents the destruction or interruption of intrinsically normal tissue. Disruptions usually affect a body part, not a specific organ (e.g., amniotic bands). Monozygotic twinning and prenatal cocaine exposure are common predisposing factors for disruptions based on vascular interruption (Bacino, 2017; Bennett & Meier, 2019; Lubbers, 2021; Matthews & Robin, 2021; Mitchell, 2020).

Association/Syndrome/Sequence

- An *association* refers to a nonrandom occurrence of multiple malformations for which no specific or common etiology has been identified.
  - *Example:* VATER/VACTERL **A**ssociation (**V**ertebral, **A**nal, **C**ardiac, **T**racheal, **E**sophageal, **R**enal, **L**imb [radial])
    - ❏ Although VACTERL association has been associated with certain conditions, such as

maternal diabetes, a genetic cause for the spectrum of malformations has not been identified.

- A *syndrome* is a pattern of anomalies with a single specific cause (usually genetic).
  - *Example:* CHARGE (**C**oloboma, **H**eart anomalies, choanal **A**tresia, **R**estriction of growth and development, **G**enital, and **E**ar)
    - ❏ Previously known as an association, CHARGE is now known as a syndrome that originates from mutations in the *CHD7* gene. These mutations have been discovered as causative in over half of affected children, although the exact mechanism for the multiple malformations is not clear at this time.
- *Sequence* refers to a pattern of multiple anomalies derived from a single known or presumed cause.
  - *Example:* Oligohydramnios sequence, often referred to as Potter syndrome; and Pierre Robin sequence
    - ❏ Potter syndrome demonstrates a constellation of features which are primarily due to a lack of amniotic fluid during gestation. Another example is Pierre Robin sequence, in which features are altered due to a malformed mandible, which causes the tongue to move backward and upward in the oral cavity (Bacino, 2017; Bennett & Meier, 2019; Lubbers, 2021; Mitchell, 2020).

▶ PRINCIPLES OF INHERITANCE

MENDELIAN INHERITANCE

Autosomal Disorders

- Single-gene traits for which mutations cause predictable diseases are described as exhibiting Mendelian inheritance because they follow the rules that Mendel originally described.
- Variants of a gene are called *alleles*. Some versions of the gene are *mutations*, not all of which cause disease. Mutations to genetic traits can either be inherited from the parents or develop de novo, meaning the mutation occurred as a random error.
- Autosomal dominant:
  - The phenotype of one (dominant) allele will express itself over a recessive allele.
  - Approximately half of Mendelian disorders are inherited in an autosomal dominant fashion. This indicates that the phenotype usually appears in every generation, with each affected person having an affected parent. For each offspring of an affected parent, the risk of inheriting the mutated allele is 50% if there is only one parent with the gene. If both parents carry the gene, it will be inherited in all offspring.
- Autosomal recessive:
  - An autosomal recessive condition occurs when an individual possesses two mutant alleles that were inherited from heterozygous parents.

- An individual with one normal allele does not manifest the disease because the normal gene copy is able to compensate. The phenotype of the recessive allele will not be expressed in the presence of a dominant allele. The phenotype of the recessive allele will be expressed only when two of the recessive alleles are present.
- If both parents are carriers of a mutated allele, there is a 25% chance of each offspring inheriting the condition.
  - ❏ Consanguineous parents (individuals who are second cousins or closer) present an increased risk of passing an autosomal recessive disorder to an offspring because there is a higher likelihood that both parents carry the same recessive mutation (Bennett & Meier, 2019; Gross & Gheorghe, 2020; Lubbers, 2021; Powell-Hamilton, 2020).

Sex-Linked

- Disorders may be caused by abnormalities on one of the sex chromosomes, and traits may be dominant or recessive. Disorders of genes located on the X chromosome have a characteristic pattern of inheritance that is affected by gender.
- X-linked recessive disorders are generally seen in males and rarely seen in females who are homozygous for the mutation.
  - Males with an X-linked mutant allele are described as being hemizygous for that allele. Males have a 50% chance of inheriting a mutant allele if the mother is a carrier.
  - Females can be homozygous dominant-type allele, homozygous mutant allele, or heterozygous (Gross & Gheorghe, 2020).

NON-MENDELIAN PATTERNS

- Multifactorial or *complex* inheritance disorders have a greater incidence than disorders secondary to chromosomal or single-gene mutations. These disorders affect certain families more than others, but do not follow Mendelian patterns of inheritance or fit into the non-Mendelian inheritance phenomenon. These occur when one or more genetic susceptibility factors combine with environmental factors and random developmental events.
- Mitochondrial DNA (mtDNA) is located only in the mitochondria of a cell and inherited entirely from the maternal side. More than 100 different mutations in mtDNA have been identified to cause disease in humans. Most of these involve the central nervous system or the musculoskeletal system.
  - Mitochondrial disease typically manifests as dysfunction in high energy-consuming organs, such as the brain, muscle, heart, and kidneys. Poor growth, muscle weakness, loss of coordination, or developmental delay are common.

- *Epigenetics* refers to modification of genes that determines whether a gene is expressed or not.
- *Imprinting* refers to a phenomenon in which genetic material is differentially expressed depending on whether it was inherited from the father or the mother. Classic examples of disorders related to genomic imprinting are Prader–Willi and Angelman syndromes. Both these syndromes involve the long arm of chromosome 15 (Gross & Gheorghe, 2020; Mitchell, 2020).

▶ GENETIC (CHROMOSOMAL) DISORDERS

TRISOMY

Trisomy 21 (Down Syndrome)

INCIDENCE AND ETIOLOGY

- Affected individuals have three copies of chromosome 21, for a total of 47 chromosomes.
  - More than 90% trisomy 21 syndromes occur secondary to meiotic nondisjunction, but 3% to 5% of cases are caused by a translocation that could be either de novo or inherited from a balanced translocation-carrier parent that subsequently becomes unbalanced and trisomic in the baby. Of these infants, 25% receive the extra chromosome from their father. Familial transmission is autosomal dominant. Mosaicism (combinations of diploid and triploid cells) may also occur. In mosaic Down, a certain percentage of the cells in the patient have three chromosome 21, while the rest of the cells have the expected chromosome complement containing two chromosome 21.
- The more common occurrence of Down syndrome in babies of mothers of advanced maternal age (AMA) led to the recommendation for prenatal karyotyping when the maternal age is >35 years at the time of conception.
  - The incidence is reported at 1 in 270 pregnancies in mothers aged 35 to 39 years and 1 in 100 in mothers aged 40 to 44 years. By the age of 45 to 50, mothers have 1 in 50 chance of conceiving an infant who will be affected with trisomy 21 (Haldeman-Englert et al., 2018; Lubbers, 2021; Schiefelbein, 2021).

CLINICAL FEATURES AND ASSOCIATED ANOMALIES

- If not diagnosed prenatally, most patients with Down syndrome are recognizable at birth due to the typical phenotypic features.
- Physical features may include brachycephaly, upslanted palpebral fissures, epicanthal folds, a flattened nasal bridge, small posteriorly rotated and/or low-set ears, a prominent tongue, and short neck with excessive nuchal folds. The hand may have single palmar creases and the fifth finger clinodactyly; the

foot may have an exaggerated gap between the first and second toes. Hypotonia is also often noted.
- Cardiac defects occur in 50% of infants with trisomy 21. The most frequent defects are atrioventricular canal defects, but also ventricular septal defect (VSD), autism spectrum disorder (ASD), TOF, and patent ductus arteriosus (PDA).
- Gastrointestinal anomalies may include duodenal atresia and Hirschsprung disease. Rarer findings are esophageal atresia, fistulas, and webs (Bacino, 2017; Bennett & Meier, 2019; Haldeman-Englert et al., 2018; McCandless & Kripps, 2020; Lubbers, 2021; Schiefelbein, 2021).

COMPLICATIONS AND OUTCOMES

- Patients with Down syndrome demonstrate a wide range of developmental abilities, with highly variable personalities. Central hypotonia with concomitant motor delay is most pronounced in the first 3 years of life, as are language delays. Early intervention and developmental therapy are necessary to maximize developmental outcomes.
- Significantly decreased postnatal growth velocity is encountered in these patients. Separate growth curves have been devised for patients with Down syndrome.
- A potential metabolic disorder that merits screening is hypothyroidism in approximately 5% of trisomy 21 patients, often with the presence of thyroid autoantibodies. Initial evaluation occurs with newborn screening programs, followed by additional measurement of thyroid-stimulating hormone and free thyroxine levels at 6 months, 12 months, and then yearly thereafter.
- An initial ophthalmologic evaluation is also indicated in the first few months of life, and then annually, because strabismus, cataracts, myopia, and glaucoma have been shown to be more common in children with Down syndrome.
- Bone marrow dyscrasias, such as neonatal thrombocytopenia, and transient self-resolving myeloproliferative disorders, such as leukemoid reaction, have been observed during the first year of life. An elevated rate of leukemia with a relative risk 10 to 18 times greater than normal up to age 16 years has been identified.
- The most common causes of death in patients with Down syndrome are related to congenital heart disease, infection (e.g., pneumonia) thought to be associated with defects in T-cell maturation and function, and malignancy. Once medical and surgical interventions for the correction of associated congenital malformations are complete and successful, the long-term survival rate is good. However, less than half of patients survive to 60 years and less than 15% survive past 68 years (Haldeman-Englert et al., 2018; Lubbers, 2021).

Trisomy 18 (Edwards Syndrome)

INCIDENCE AND ETIOLOGY

- Affected individuals have three copies of chromosome 18, for a total of 47 chromosomes.
- This occurs most frequently due to nondisjunction (80%), but may also be caused by partial trisomy, translocation, or mosaicism (5%).
- Trisomy 18 is associated with a high rate of intrauterine demise. It is estimated that only 5% of conceptuses with trisomy 18 survive to birth and that 30% of fetuses in whom trisomy 18 is diagnosed by second-trimester amniocentesis die before the end of the pregnancy (Haldeman-Englert et al., 2018; Lubbers, 2021; Schiefelbein, 2021).

CLINICAL FEATURES AND ASSOCIATED ANOMALIES

- Phenotypic features that are notable at birth include intrauterine growth restriction (IUGR) with a small narrow cranium with prominent occiput, open metopic suture, low-set and posteriorly rotated ears, and micrognathia. Characteristics are clenched hands with overlapping fingers, hypoplastic nails, and rocker bottom feet.
- Additional malformations include heart defects (ASD, VSD, PDA, pulmonic stenosis, aortic coarctation), cleft palate, clubfoot deformity, renal malformations (horseshoe, ectopic kidneys), brain anomalies, choanal atresia, eye malformations, vertebral anomalies, hypospadias, cryptorchidism, and limb defects (Bacino, 2017; Bennett & Meier, 2019; Haldeman-Englert et al., 2018; Lubbers, 2021; McCandless & Kripps, 2020; Schiefelbein, 2021).

COMPLICATIONS AND OUTCOMES

- There is a high rate of intrauterine demise. Death after delivery is usually from central apnea or congestive heart failure.
- Nondisjunction patterns can be associated with the outcomes:
  - *Severe pattern:* Handicaps are severe with short life expectancy.
  - *Mosaic pattern:* Some cells have the normal complement of genetic material; the remaining have the trisomy 18 pattern. Infants are less severely affected and have a longer life expectancy.
  - *Partial pattern:* Depending on the portion of the chromosome affected, effects range from minimal handicaps and few abnormalities to partial syndrome with less profound developmental delays and longer survival.
- The prognosis of this disorder is extremely poor, with more than 90% of babies succumbing in the first 6 months of life and only 5% alive at 1 year old. Causes of death include central apnea, infection, and congestive heart failure.

- Infants will full trisomy are usually fragile, and prognosis for survival is poor. Those who survive the first year deal with feeding, growth, and developmental issues. They are generally unable to walk unsupported and are capable of only limited verbal communication (Gross & Gheorghe, 2020; Haldeman-Englert et al., 2018; Lubbers, 2021; Schiefelbein, 2021).

Trisomy 13 (Patau Syndrome)

INCIDENCE AND ETIOLOGY

- Affected individuals have three copies of chromosome 13, for a total of 47 chromosomes. It is the fourth most common autosomal dominant disorder resulting from chromosomal nondisjunction.
- Approximately 2% to 3% of fetuses with trisomy 13 survive to birth, with a frequency of 1 in 12,500 to 1 in 21,000 live births.
- Abnormal noninvasive screening, such as ultrasound or maternal screens, identifies the risk and prompts genetic testing. There is a high rate of intrauterine demise. It is unusual for infants to survive out of the newborn period (Gross & Gheorghe, 2020; Haldeman-Englert et al., 2018; Lubbers, 2021).

CLINICAL FEATURES AND ASSOCIATED ANOMALIES

- Infants with trisomy 13 are known to have multiple midline malformations, which may include congenital heart disease, cleft palate, renal anomalies, and postaxial polydactyly. Eye anomalies and scalp defects can suggest the diagnosis. Brain malformations such as microcephaly and holoprosencephaly are found in more than half of patients with concomitant seizure disorders.
- Aplasia cutis congenita is a congenital absence of skin involving the scalp that is associated with but not limited to infants with trisomy 13. Lesions have sharp margins and may present as ulcers, bullae, or scars. Most defects are small and superficial.
- Congenital heart disease is present in approximately 80% of patients, usually VSD, ASD, PDA, or dextrocardia.
- Limb anomalies, such as postaxial polydactyly, single palmar creases, and hyperconvex narrow fingernails, are also seen (Bacino, 2017; Bennett & Meier, 2019; Haldeman-Englert et al., 2018; Lubbers, 2021; Schiefelbein, 2021).

COMPLICATIONS AND OUTCOMES

- The presence of holoprosencephaly is the single most important factor predicting survival.
- Prognosis is extremely poor, with 80% mortality in the neonatal period and less than 5% of patients surviving to 6 months old. Developmental delays

are profound, and many patients are blind and deaf. Feeding difficulties are typical (Haldeman-Englert et al., 2018; Lubbers, 2021; Schiefelbein, 2021).

MONOSOMY

Turner Syndrome (45,X)

INCIDENCE AND ETIOLOGY
- Turner syndrome describes a phenotype associated with loss of all or part of one copy of the X chromosome and occurs in approximately 1 in 2,500 female infants. Studies indicate that in approximately 80% of cases it is the paternally derived X chromosome that is lost.
  - The 45,X karyotype or loss of one entire X chromosome accounts for approximately half of the cases. A variety of X chromosome anomalies, including deletions and translocations, account for the remainder of the causes (Haldeman-Englert et al., 2018; Lubbers, 2021).

CLINICAL FEATURES AND ASSOCIATED ANOMALIES
- Turner syndrome exhibits a wide variety of presentations. At birth, notable findings are short stature, webbed neck, low posterior hairline, broad nasal bridge, low-set ears with anomalous auricles, ptosis of eyelids, shield chest, and lymphedema of the hands and feet. The syndrome is associated with congenital heart disease, which may include bicuspid aortic valve, coarctation of the aorta, valvular aortic stenosis, and mitral valve prolapse (Bennett & Meier, 2019; Haldeman-Englert et al., 2018; Lubbers, 2021).

COMPLICATIONS AND OUTCOMES
- Growth issues, especially short stature, are the predominant concern in childhood and adolescence; growth hormone therapy has been shown to increase final adult height, but the age of initiation of therapy has not yet been established.
- Primary ovarian failure caused by gonadal dysplasia (streak gonads) can result in delay of secondary sexual characteristics and primary amenorrhea (Haldeman-Englert et al., 2018; Lubbers, 2021).

DELETION SYNDROME

DiGeorge Syndrome—22q11.2 Deletion

INCIDENCE AND ETIOLOGY
- Patients with classically termed conditions DiGeorge, velocardiofacial, and conotruncal anomaly face syndromes all reflect features of the same genomic disorder, a deletion of 22q11.2, which is the most commonly occurring microdeletion syndrome in humans. Estimates indicate that 22q11.2 microdeletion syndrome occurs in approximately 1 in 1,000 fetuses.
- Most 22q11 deletions occur as de novo events, with less than 10% of them being inherited from an affected parent. Both parents must be tested to determine carrier status (Haldeman-Englert et al., 2018; Lubbers, 2021).

CLINICAL FEATURES AND ASSOCIATED ANOMALIES
- Most patients with a deletion receive the diagnosis following identification of significant cardiovascular malformations, conotruncal cardiac anomaly including interrupted aortic arch type B, truncus arteriosus, or TOF.
- Clinical features include facial dysmorphia, which may include hooded eyelids, hypertelorism, overfolded ears, bulbous nasal tip, a small mouth, and micrognathia.
- With further evaluation, often aplasia or hypoplasia of the thymus and parathyroid glands are noted, along with functional T-cell abnormalities and hypocalcemia.
  - Hypocalcemia occurs in 60% of neonates; severe cases will cause seizures (Bacino, 2017; Bennett & Meier, 2019; Haldeman-Englert et al., 2018; Lubbers, 2021; McCandless & Kripps, 2020).

COMPLICATIONS AND OUTCOMES
- Developmental delays or learning disabilities have been reported in most patients with 22q11.2 deletion syndrome, and a wide range of developmental and behavioral findings have been observed in young children.
  - In the preschool years, affected children were most commonly found to be hypotonic and developmentally delayed, with language and speech difficulties; however, one-third of patients functioned within the average range.
- Death is primarily related to severity of cardiac defects (Haldeman-Englert et al., 2018; Lubbers, 2021).

SINGLE-GENE DISORDER

Cystic Fibrosis

INCIDENCE AND ETIOLOGY
- Cystic fibrosis (CF), the most common autosomal recessive disease in live-born infants, is the result of mutations of a large gene on chromosome 7 that encodes the cystic fibrosis transmembrane conductance regulator (CFTR) protein.
- The carrier rate differs based on ethnic origin; individuals of Asian descent have the lowest carrier rates and Ashkenazi Jewish and

non-Hispanic White individuals have the highest (Gross & Gheorghe, 2020, 2020).

CLINICAL FEATURES AND ASSOCIATED ANOMALIES

- The screening program is less accurate in children with less common alleles; therefore, a normal newborn screen does not rule out the presence of CF. The diagnosis is confirmed by a sweat chloride test showing a chloride greater than 60 mEq/L, which is present in 99% of patients with CF. This study is generally not performed until >4 weeks of age.
- Multiorgan disorder impacts the pulmonary, pancreatic, and gastrointestinal systems, but does not affect intelligence.
- This disorder can present very early in life with meconium ileus, which is an obstruction of the ileum as a result of thick meconium plugs. On abdominal x-rays, the small bowel loops may have a ground-glass appearance (Neuhauser sign) resulting from dilated loops of the bowel with bubbles of gas and meconium without air–fluid levels.
  - Half of infants presenting with meconium ileus develop complications, including peritonitis, volvulus, atresia, and necrosis.
  - The presence of meconium plug syndrome, which is a temporary obstruction of the distal colon, should also raise concerns for the possibility of CF.
- Chronic diarrhea secondary to pancreatic fat malabsorption is a common presentation, leading to poor nutrient absorption and overall poor growth.
- Infants can present less commonly with extrahepatic biliary duct obstruction as a result of thick inspissated bile. Therefore, CF should be included in the differential diagnosis of any neonate with prolonged conjugated hyperbilirubinemia (Larson-Nath et al., 2020).

COMPLICATIONS AND OUTCOMES

- Early and presymptomatic diagnosis through screening leads to early nutritional therapy, pancreatic enzyme replacement, and antibiotic prophylaxis for pulmonary infection.
  - Median survival is approximately 37 years, with respiratory failure as the most common cause of death.
- It is important for providers to discuss with their patients that a negative screen decreases the risk of being a carrier but does not eliminate it completely because screening does not test for all possible mutations.
- Cell-based therapies, advances in bone marrow transplantation, direct treatment of metabolic disorders, and mutation-specific interventions for CF have all provided hope to families with a child diagnosed with CF, but not curative therapy. Now a new technology, clustered regularly interspaced short palindromic repeats (CRISPR)/CRISPR-associated

protein-9 nuclease (Cas9), holds out a new promise that targeted gene editing may be possible to apply on an individual basis (Cotton & Murray, 2018; Larson-Nath et al., 2020; Matthews & Robin, 2021; Sahai & Levy, 2018).

IMPRINTING DISORDER

Beckwith–Wiedemann Syndrome

INCIDENCE AND ETIOLOGY

- Beckwith–Wiedemann syndrome affects approximately 1 in 14,000 newborns and manifests itself as an overgrowth syndrome in the neonatal period.
- Genetic studies in patients with Beckwith–Wiedemann syndrome have identified three major subgroups of patients: familial, sporadic, and chromosomally abnormal. Sporadic causes 85% of cases, with the remaining being due to inherited autosomal dominant 11p15, methylation of H19/IGF2, and mutation of the *CDK1C* gene.
  - Mutations causing overexpression of the paternal allele or underexpression of the maternal allele can result in an imbalance of expression, leading to the overgrowth and tumor formation encountered in these patients.
  - It has been observed that pregnancies that are the result of assisted reproductive therapy (ART) are at an increased risk of rare imprinting disorders, such as Beckwith–Wiedemann syndrome, suggesting that epigenetic changes may occur as a result of ART (Garg & Devaskar, 2020; Gross & Gheorghe, 2020; Haldeman-Englert et al., 2018; McCandless & Kripps, 2020).

CLINICAL FEATURES AND ASSOCIATED ANOMALIES

- Often called *congenital overgrowth syndrome*, the characteristic findings are macrosomia, abdominal wall defect, and macroglossia. Hemihypertrophy caused by asymmetric growth is common, as is visceromegaly of various organs, including the spleen, kidneys, liver, pancreas, and adrenal gland.
  - Other common features are being large for gestational age (somatic overgrowth), macroglossia, transverse ear lobe crease, renal abnormalities, visceromegaly, hemihypertrophy, and abdominal wall defects (omphalocele in the majority).
- Hypoglycemia is present in at least half the cases and may be manifested soon after birth. Endocrine evaluation of the few reported cases has not been consistent. However, based on the clinical features of hypoglycemia with low free fatty acids (FFAs) and ketones and autopsy findings of islet cell hyperplasia, it is believed that hypoglycemia is caused by hyperinsulinism in this syndrome (Bennett & Meier, 2019; Garg & Devaskar, 2020; Haldeman-Englert et al., 2018).

COMPLICATIONS AND OUTCOMES

■ Treatment of hypoglycemia may require high caloric intake and therapy to inhibit insulin secretion. It may require a central line for increased glucose infusion rates. Medication therapy can include diazoxide and octreotide.

■ Infants with this disorder are predisposed to certain malignancies (adrenal carcinoma, nephroblastoma) and appear to have an increased risk for malignancies associated with hemihypertrophy.
  ● Routine ultrasonograms from the neonatal time through the school-age years (approximately 8 years old) are necessary due to the increased risk of malignant tumors, especially Wilms tumor. The estimated risk is as high as 8% in patients with hemihypertrophy (Garg & Devaskar, 2020; Haldeman-Englert et al., 2018).

▶ NONCHROMOSOMAL DISORDERS

MALFORMATION DISORDERS

Osteogenesis Imperfecta

INCIDENCE AND ETIOLOGY

■ This disorder is caused by mutations of the *COL1A1* and *COL1A2* genes on chromosomes 17q21 and 17q22.1. The result of the mutation is an abnormality of type I collagen. Overall incidence is 3 to 4 per 100,000. The more severe forms of osteogenesis imperfecta (OI) are the result of abnormal collagen synthesis rather than decreased production.

■ Types II and III are generally spontaneous, dominant-acting gene mutations with approximately 6% reoccurrence risk. Other types are mostly autosomal dominant and rare recessive forms (Haldeman-Englert et al., 2018; Lubbers, 2021; Tiller & Bellus, 2018).

CLINICAL FEATURES AND ASSOCIATED ANOMALIES

■ Six clinical types (in decreasing order of severity) have been identified; types I, II, and III are considered severe.

■ All clinical types share common findings of low birth weight, short stature, macrocephaly, triangular-appearing facies (with a bossed, broad forehead and a tapered, pointed chin), blue sclerae, and short-limbed extremities.
  ● Associated findings are hearing loss, platelet dysfunction, and scoliosis (Lubbers, 2021; Tiller & Bellus, 2018).

COMPLICATIONS AND OUTCOMES

■ Depending on the type of osteogenesis, treatment will vary extensively.

■ Of the affected babies, 60% are stillborn or die during the first day of life and 80% die by 1 month. Those severely affected with OI type II are not expected to survive the neonatal period (Lubbers, 2021; Tiller & Bellus, 2018).

INBORN ERRORS OF METABOLISM

INCIDENCE AND ETIOLOGY

■ The term *inborn errors of metabolism (IEM)* was coined in the early 20th century to describe diseases caused by errors and variations in chemical pathways.

■ IEMs are genetic biochemical disorders in which the function of a protein is compromised, resulting in alteration of the structure or amount of the protein synthesized. These gene mutations produce deficiencies in enzymes, cofactors, transport proteins, and cellular processes. Interruptions of any of the steps in the formation of the coenzyme can lead to disease.

■ IEM is most often due to an autosomal recessive inheritance. Other mechanisms of inheritance are autosomal dominant and sex-linked. The majority of mutations are of no consequence; however, others produce disease states ranging from mild to severe.

■ The March of Dimes and the American College of Medical Genetics and Genomics (www.ACGM.net) recommend 29 conditions for testing. Most of these conditions can be managed by medications and/or special diets, and treatment may be lifesaving.

■ IEM can be classified into three groups:
  ● Defects involving complex molecules result from the defective function of enzymes responsible for breaking down complex glycosaminoglycans and sphingolipids. Symptoms are not generally evident at birth as pathologic metabolites accumulate slowly.
  ● Disorders of fatty acid metabolism are defects concerning the intermediary metabolism of small molecules—glucose, lactate, amino acids, organic acids, and ammonia.
  ● Metabolic disorders in which there is insufficient generation of energy by the mitochondria are complex processes involving problems in either the manufacture, the failure of delivery, the inability to break down, or the deficient function of mitochondrial substrates and energy-generating systems (Bacino, 2017; Cotton & Murray, 2018; Lubbers, 2021).

CLINICAL PRESENTATION AND ASSOCIATED ANOMALIES

■ An infant may or may not present with IEM in the newborn period. Consider IEM as a differential diagnosis in any otherwise healthy infant with an acute decompensation of unknown etiology. Early recognition of the symptoms can lead to appropriate medical interventions, and a delay in treatment may have severe consequences, such as impaired neurodevelopmental outcomes or death.

■ Symptoms of possible IEMs include:

- Neurologic changes in activity and/or muscle tone, new onset of seizures
- Cataracts, glaucoma, dislocated lenses of the eyes
- Respiratory changes ranging from tachypnea to apnea
- Cardiomyopathies
- Onset of vomiting, long-term failure to gain weight
- Metabolic acidosis
- Jaundice, hepatomegaly, refractory hypoglycemia
- Unusual body or urinary odor

- An initial laboratory workup when IEM is suspected includes:
  - Blood gas analysis with lactate level, serum electrolytes, glucose, ammonia level, and urinalysis (urine pH, ketones)
- Second-line workup includes:
  - Serum and urine amino acids and urine organic acids
- Newborn screening:
  - Newborn screening is a practice to test all newborns for specific disorders that can cause serious health issues. The goal is to identify IEM that will lead to early treatment and prevention of major sequelae.
  - With the introduction of mass spectrometry, a single blood spot can detect greater than 50 disorders. Each state can choose which tests are collected; however, all states are required to screen for phenylketonuria (PKU), hypothyroidism, and galactosemia (Cederbaum, 2018; Lubbers, 2021; Matthews & Robin, 2021; Sahai & Levy, 2018).

COMPLICATIONS AND OUTCOMES

- Specific genetic biomarkers may be obtained later in the clinical course once a full family history is completed by the genetic or metabolic pediatric specialist, in addition to a full assessment of laboratory results and a full physical examination. Some IEMs may need to be supplemented with radiographic testing, such as an MRI of the brain.
- Genetic testing of the biological parents of the infant/child will be beneficial for future pregnancies (Matthews & Robin, 2021).

DISORDERS OF METABOLISM

- See Table 15.1 for a summary of IEMs by classification.

Carbohydrate Disorders

- The most common disorder is galactosemia, a defect in one of three enzymes in the galactose metabolic pathway.
- Most often presents in the newborn period.
- These disorders are identified on newborn screen (Table 15.2).

Urea Cycle Disorders

- *Defective process:* caused by an inhibited synthesis of urea from ammonia
- *Two common pathways:* proximal and distal urea cycle disorders
- Most often presents within the first 24 hours of life; poor feeding and lethargy most common clinical presentations
- Hyperammonemia present (Table 15.3).

Table 15.1 Summary of Classification of Inborn Errors of Metabolism

Amino Acid/Urea Cycle Disorders	Organic Acid Disorders	Fatty Acid Oxidation Disorders	Others
Phenylketonuria	Isovaleric acidemia	Medium chain acyl-CoA dehydrogenase deficiency	Congenital adrenal hyperplasia
Homocystinuria	Propionic acidemia	Short-chain acyl-CoA dehydrogenase deficiency	Galactosemia
Hypermethioninemia	Glutaric acidemia type I	Very long-chain acyl-CoA dehydrogenase deficiency	Sickle cell disease
Argininosuccinic acidemia	Isobutyryl-CoA dehydrogenase deficiency	Glutaric acidemia type II	Hemoglobinopathies
Citrullinemia	3-Hydroxy-3 methylglutaryl-CoA lyase deficiency	Carnitine palmityl transferase deficiency	Congenital hypothyroidism
Argininemia	2-Mehylbutyryl-CoA dehydrogenase deficiency	Carnitine/acylcarnitine translocase deficiency	
Tyrosinemia types I and II	3-Methylcrotonyl-CoA carboxylase deficiency	Multiple CoA carboxylase deficiency	
Maple syrup urine disease		Trifunctional protein deficiency	

Sources: Data from Matthews, A. L., & Robin, N. H. (2021) Genetic disorders, malformations, and inborn errors of metabolism. In S. L. Gardner, B. S. Carter, M. Enzman-Hines, & S. Niermeyer (Eds.), *Merenstein & Gardner's handbook of neonatal intensive care nursing: An interprofessional approach* (9th ed., pp. 969–995). Elsevier; Sahai, I., & Levy, H. (2018). Newborn screening. In C. Gleason & S. Juul (Eds.), *Avery's diseases of the newborn* (10th ed., pp. 332–346. e3). Elsevier.

Table 15.2 Carbohydrate Metabolism Disorder

Disorder	Defective Process	Characteristics
■ Galactosemia ■ GALT deficiency ■ GALK ■ Uridine diphosphate GALE	■ A defect in one of three enzymes in the galactose metabolic pathway	GALT ■ Clinical jaundice ■ Coagulopathy ■ Most common in the newborn period ■ Identified on NBS ■ Cataracts ■ *Escherichia coli* sepsis if untreated ■ Liver failure if untreated GALE ■ May be identified on NBS ■ Deficient enzyme activity in RBC ■ Liver failure if untreated GALK ■ Cataracts
■ GSDs ■ Hepatic glycogen storage diseases ■ Muscular glycogen storage diseases	■ Defective glycogen synthesis ■ Abnormal utilization for energy production ■ Categorized by how they affect liver	■ Hypoglycemia ■ Infantile cardiomyopathy ■ Muscular glycogen storage diseases—most common form of GSD in the neonatal period; also a lysosomal storage disease
■ Fructose metabolism ■ HFI	■ Abnormal enzyme activity in liver tissue and/or sequencing of *ALDOB*	■ Most often later infancy ■ Hypoglycemia, pallor, GI disturbances

GALE, galactose-4-epimerase; GALK, galactokinase; GALT, galactose-1-phosphate uridyltransferase deficiency; GI, gastrointestinal; GSDs, glycogen storage diseases; HFI, hereditary fructose intolerance; NBS, newborn screen; RBC, red blood cell.
Source: Data from Merritt, J. L., & Gallagher, R. (2018). Inborn errors of carbohydrate, ammonia, amino acid, and organic acid metabolism. In C. Gleason & S. Juul (Eds.), *Avery's diseases of the newborn* (10th ed., pp. 230–252.e4). Elsevier.

Amino Acid Metabolism Disorders

■ Most common disorder is PKU, which is caused by deficiency of phenylalanine hydroxylase, resulting in decreased levels of tyrosine
■ Severe phenotype if presents in the newborn period
■ Clinical presentation is developmental delays, intellectual delays, eczema, and hypopigmented skin and hair (Table 15.4)

Table 15.3 Urea Cycle Disorder

Disorder	Defective Process	Characteristics
■ Proximal UCD ■ NAGS deficiency ■ CPSI deficiency ■ OTCD ■ Distal UCD ■ Argininosuccinate synthetase deficiency ■ Argininosuccinate lyase deficiency ■ Arginase 1 deficiency	■ Inhibited synthesis of urea from ammonia	■ Onset ~24 hours of life ■ Poor feeding ■ Emesis ■ Hyperventilation ■ Altered level of consciousness; lethargy ■ Symptoms secondary to hyperammonemia ■ Encephalopathy ■ Seizures ■ Hallmark sign is hyperammonemia ■ Delayed treatment fatal

CPSI, carbamyl phosphate synthetase I; NAGS, *N*-acetylglutamate synthase deficiency; OTCD, ornithine transcarbamylase deficiency; UCD, urea cycle disorder.
Source: Data from Merritt, J. L., & Gallagher, R. (2018). Inborn errors of carbohydrate, ammonia, amino acid, and organic acid metabolism. In C. Gleason & S. Juul (Eds.), *Avery's diseases of the newborn* (10th ed., pp. 230–252.e4). Elsevier.

Organic Acidemias

■ Defects in pathways of catabolism of more than one of the following: leucine, isoleucine, and valine
■ Clinical presentation consistent with those of hyperammonemia
■ Most disorders in this category present within the newborn period, except for glutaric aciduria type 1 (Table 15.5)

Fatty Acid Oxidation Disorders

■ *Defective pathway:* failure of beta-oxidation within, or transport of fatty acids into, the mitochondria
■ Most common disorder is medium-chain acyl-CoA dehydrogenase (MCAD) deficiency
■ Presents in the newborn period (Table 15.6)

Ketone Metabolism Disorders

■ *Defective process:* inability to use ketone bodies, 3-hydroxybutyric acid, and acetoacetic acid for energy generation
■ Clinical presentation consistent with hyperammonemia

Primary Lactic Acidosis

■ *Defective process:* multifactorial abnormal energy metabolism; primary defect in the mitochondrial electron transport chain (ETC) or the tricarboxylic acid (TCA) cycle
■ Presents with profound metabolic acidosis
■ Moderate hyperammonemia (Table 15.7)

Table 15.4 Amino Acid Metabolism Disorder

Disorder	Defective Process	Characteristics
Maple syrup urine disease	■ BCKAD complex deficiency	■ Onset within 48 hours of life ■ Poor feeding ■ Irritability ■ Lethargy ■ Seizure-like activity ■ Apnea ■ High-pitched cry ■ Maple syrup odor
NKH	■ Defective synthesis of glycine	■ Onset approximately on the first week of life ■ Apnea ■ Seizures ■ Milder forms of NKH present later in infancy
Hyperhomocysteinemia and remethylation disorders	■ Deficiency of the cystathionine beta-synthase enzyme	■ Does not present in the newborn period
Phenylketonuria	■ Deficiency of phenylalanine hydroxylase resulting in decreased levels of tyrosine	■ Most common IEM ■ Severe phenotype if presents in the newborn period ■ Developmental delays ■ Intellectual delays ■ Eczema ■ Hypopigmented skin and hair

BCKAD, branched-chain alpha-ketoacid dehydrogenase; IEM, inborn errors of metabolism; NKH, nonketotic hyperglycinemia.
Source: Data from Merritt, J. L., & Gallagher, R. (2018). Inborn errors of carbohydrate, ammonia, amino acid, and organic acid metabolism. In C. Gleason & S. Juul (Eds.), *Avery's diseases of the newborn* (10th ed., pp. 230–252.e4). Elsevier.

Table 15.5 Organic Acidemias

Disorder	Defective Process	Characteristics
Methylmalonic acidemia	■ Elevation of methylmalonic acid	■ Onset days 2–3 of life ■ GI disturbances ■ Lethargy ■ Seizures ■ Identified with urine organic acids subsequent to an abnormal NBS
Propionic acidemia	■ Deficiency of propionyl-CoA carboxylase	■ Symptoms consistent with hyperammonemia ■ Identified with urine organic acids and DNA testing
Multiple carboxylase deficiency	■ Defects in holocarboxylase ■ Synthetase deficiency ■ Biotinidase deficiency	■ Metabolic acidosis ■ Lactic acidosis ■ Encephalopathy
Glutaric aciduria type 1	■ Deficiency of glutaryl-CoA dehydrogenase	■ Delayed onset ~6–18 months

GI, gastrointestinal; NBS, newborn screen.
Source: Data from Merritt, J. L., & Gallagher, R. (2018). Inborn errors of carbohydrate, ammonia, amino acid, and organic acid metabolism. In C. Gleason & S. Juul (Eds.), *Avery's diseases of the newborn* (10th ed., pp. 230–252.e4). Elsevier.

Table 15.6 Fatty Acid Oxidation Disorders

Disorder	Defective Process	Characteristics
	■ Failure of beta-oxidation within, or transport of fatty acids into, the mitochondria	■ Severe phenotypes present within 24–48 hours of life ■ Hypoglycemia ■ Liver disease/failure ■ Cardiomyopathy
MCADD		■ Most common FAOD ■ Most common etiology of SIDS ■ Severe phenotypes present in the newborn period

FAOD, fatty acid oxidation disorders; MCADD, medium-chain acyl-CoA dehydrogenase deficiency; SIDS, sudden infant death syndrome.
Sources: Data from Merritt, J. L., & Gallagher, R. (2018). Inborn errors of carbohydrate, ammonia, amino acid, and organic acid metabolism. In C. Gleason & S. Juul (Eds.), *Avery's diseases of the newborn* (10th ed., pp. 230–252.e4). Elsevier; McCandless, S. E., & Kripps, K. A. (2020). Genetics, inborn errors of metabolism, and newborn screening. In A. A. Fanaroff & J. M. Fanaroff (Eds.), *Klaus and Fanaroff's care of the high-risk neonate* (7th ed., pp. 121–147.e1). Elsevier.

Table 15.7 Primary Lactic Acidosis

Disorder	Characteristics
■ Pyruvate dehydrogenase complex deficiency	■ Profound lactic acidosis ■ Low to normal lactate-to-pyruvate ratio ■ Moderate hyperammonemia
■ Pyruvate carboxylase deficiency	■ Lactic acidosis in the newborn period ■ Developmental delays
■ Electron transport chain defects	■ Presents ~3 months of age
■ Benign infantile mitochondrial myopathy, cardiomyopathy, or both	■ Congenital hypotonia at birth
■ Barth syndrome	■ Anemia ■ Ringed sideroblasts ■ Exocrine pancreatic dysfunction
■ Early lethal lactic acidosis	■ Onset within the first 72 hours of life ■ Poor prognosis

Source: Data from Merritt, J. L., & Gallagher, R. (2018). Inborn errors of carbohydrate, ammonia, amino acid, and organic acid metabolism. In C. Gleason & S. Juul (Eds.), *Avery's diseases of the newborn* (10th ed., pp. 230–252.e4). Elsevier.

Lysosomal Storage Disorders
- *Defective process:* deficiency in a specific lysosomal enzyme/transport
- 20 lysosomal storage disorders (LSDs) will appear in the newborn period (Table 15.8)

Congenital Disorders of Glycosylation
- *Defective process:* defects in the process of modifying proteins, lipids, or sugar molecules/chains
- Onset variable based on phenotype (Table 15.9)

Peroxisomal Disorders
- *Defective process:* absence or dysfunction of a peroxisomal enzyme; may involve more than one enzyme
- Clinical presentation variable; may include dysmorphic craniofacial features, glaucoma, and cataracts
- Onset variable (Table 15.10)

Table 15.8 Lysosomal Storage Disorders

Disorder	Defective Process	Characteristics
Niemann–Pick C disease	■ Defective transport of lipoprotein	■ Variable onset ■ Conjugated hyperbilirubinemia in the newborn period
Gaucher disease type 2 (acute neuropathic)	■ Deficiency of lysosomal glucocerebrosidase	■ Infantile onset of severe CNS involvement
GM1 gangliosidosis	■ Deficiency in lysosomal beta-galactosidase	■ Coarse, thick skin ■ Hirsutism on forehead and neck ■ Dysmorphic facial features
Farber lipogranulomatosis	■ Deficiency of lysosomal acid ceramidase	■ Onset 2 weeks to 4 months of age ■ Aphonia ■ Poor weight gain ■ Intermittent fever
Galactosialidosis	■ Deficiency of two lysosomal enzymes, neuraminidase, and beta-galactosidase	■ Onset birth to 3 months of age ■ Ascites ■ Edema ■ Coarse facial features ■ Inguinal hernias ■ Hypotonia
Wolman disease	■ Deficiency of lysosomal acid lipase	■ Onset birth to first few weeks of life ■ GI disturbances ■ Failure to thrive ■ Abdominal distention

(continued)

Table 15.8 Lysosomal Storage Disorders (*Continued*)

Disorder	Defective Process	Characteristics
Infantile sialic acid storage disease	■ Defective lysosomal sialic acid transporter	■ Hepatosplenomegaly ■ Ascites ■ Hypopigmentation ■ Hypotonia
I-cell disease (mucolipidosis type II)		■ Corneal clouding ■ Organomegaly ■ Hypotonia ■ Gingival hyperplasia ■ Low BW

BW, birth weight; CNS, central nervous system; GI, gastrointestinal.
Source: Data from Thomas, J. A., Lam, C., & Berry, G. (2018). Lysosomal storage, peroxisomal, and glycosylation disorders and Smith–Lemli–Opitz syndrome presenting in the neonate. In C. Gleason & S. Juul (Eds.), *Avery's diseases of the newborn* (10th ed., pp. 253–272.e3). Elsevier.

Table 15.9 Congenital Disorders of Glycosylation

Disorder	Defective Process	Characteristics
Combined glycosylation defects	■ Defective glycosylation	■ Microcephaly ■ Seizures ■ Hypotonia ■ Cutis laxa ■ Hepatic involvement

Source: Data from Thomas, J. A., Lam, C., & Berry, G. (2018). Lysosomal storage, peroxisomal, and glycosylation disorders and Smith–Lemli–Opitz syndrome presenting in the neonate. In C. Gleason & S. Juul (Eds.), *Avery's diseases of the newborn* (10th ed., pp. 253–272.e3). Elsevier.

Table 15.10 Peroxisomal Disorders

Disorder	Defective Process	Characteristics
Zellweger syndrome	■ Fails to import newly synthesized peroxisomal proteins into the peroxisome	■ Cataracts ■ Glaucoma ■ Seizures ■ Dysmorphic facial features ■ Hepatomegaly ■ Generalized weakness ■ Hypotonia

Source: Data from Thomas, J. A., Lam, C., & Berry, G. (2018). Lysosomal storage, peroxisomal, and glycosylation disorders and Smith–Lemli–Opitz syndrome presenting in the neonate. In C. Gleason & S. Juul (Eds.), *Avery's diseases of the newborn* (10th ed., pp. 253–272.e3). Elsevier.

▶ CONCLUSION

Although individual conditions may be rare, the cumulative number of infants admitted to the NICU with a potentially genetic condition is significant. Recent advances in knowledge and technology have made the need for collaborative practice increasingly important. The neonatal provider requires multiple skills to be able to care for these infants and their families, including advanced physical assessment skills, the ability to identify dysmorphology, a working knowledge of how to start a basic genetic evaluation, and good communication skills to relay information to parents. These infants may require extensive multidisciplinary care and coordination, and the neonatal nurse practitioner (NNP) must act as an advocate for these infants and their families. The NNP's knowledge on infant physiology, testing, infant pain, and family stress as well as their role as coordinators of care make them uniquely qualified to act as advocates. The NNP must also possess skills not covered in this chapter, including the ability to compassionately deliver unexpected news and provide family support, and knowledge of local, regional, national, and online resources.

1. The term used to describe any genotype in which the total chromosome number is not a multiple of 23, noting a net loss or gain of genetic material, is:

   A. Aneuploidy
   B. Tetraploidy
   C. Triploidy

2. The neonatal nurse practitioner (NNP) chooses the correct genetic exam to assess for suspected DiGeorge syndrome by sending genetic material for analysis by:

   A. Exome sequencing (ES)
   B. Fluorescence in situ hybridization (FISH)
   C. Karyotype (KT)

3. The neonatal nurse practitioner (NNP) describes a neonate's physical features and possible dysmorphisms by noting the particulars of a/an:

   A. Exotype
   B. Genotype
   C. Phenotype

4. The neonatal nurse practitioner (NNP) correctly documents the finding of limb amputation secondary to amniotic bands syndrome as a:

   A. Deformation
   B. Disruption
   C. Malformation

5. The neonatal nurse practitioner (NNP) considers a neonate's complete clinical presentation and notes anomalies in the high energy-consuming organs of the brain, heart, and kidneys, and theorizes the origin of the diseases is a:

   A. Mendelian disorder
   B. Mitochondrial disease
   C. Multifactorial disorder

6. When managing an infant who is diagnosed with trisomy 21, the neonatal nurse practitioner (NNP) knows to evaluate for congenital cardiac disease, particularly:

   A. Ebstein anomaly (EA)
   B. Transposition of the great vessels (TOGV)
   C. Ventricular septal defect (VSD)

7. The neonatal nurse practitioner (NNP) recalls the finding of rocker bottom feet on physical exam is associated with a diagnosis of:

   A. Trisomy 13
   B. Trisomy 18
   C. Trisomy 21

1. A) Aneuploidy

The term *aneuploidy* is used to describe any genotype in which the total chromosome number is not a multiple of 23. This indicates a net loss or gain of genetic material. Triploidy indicates three copies of all chromosomes, for a total of 69 present. Tetraploidy indicates four copies of all chromosomes, for a total of 96 present (Gross & Gheorghe, 2020; Haldeman-Englert et al., 2018; Matthews & Robin, 2021; Schiefelbein, 2021).

2. B) Fluorescence in situ hybridization (FISH)

FISH testing is ordered if there is a high level of suspicion for a known microdeletion syndrome not detectable by routine cytogenetic analysis. An example is testing for 22q11 deletion/velocardiofacial/DiGeorge syndrome or Williams syndrome. A karyotype is the standard pictorial arrangement of chromosome pairs only, while exome sequencing studies are performed for infants with multiple anomalies but a normal chromosome microarray study.

3. C) Phenotype

Phenotype is a term used to describe the identifiable features and possible dysmorphisms of an individual. In clinical practice, *phenotype* refers to a collection of specific traits and physical findings. A person's genotype is the actual genetic makeup of an individual. *Exotype* is not a term used in genetic studies (Bennett & Meier, 2019; Matthews & Robin, 2021; Mitchell, 2020; Powell-Hamilton, 2020).

4. B) Disruption

A disruption represents the destruction or interruption of intrinsically normal tissue. Disruptions usually affect a body part, not a specific organ (e.g., amniotic bands). Deformation results from abnormal mechanical forces, such as intrauterine constraint, acting on otherwise normal tissues. A malformation implies an abnormal morphogenesis of the underlying tissue owing to a genetic or teratogenic factor (Bacino, 2017; Bennett & Meier, 2019; Lubbers, 2021; Matthews & Robin, 2021; Mitchell, 2020).

5. B) Mitochondrial disease

Mitochondrial DNA is located only in the mitochondria of a cell and has been identified to cause disease in humans. Most of these involve high energy-consuming organs such as the brain, muscles, heart, and kidneys. Mendelian disorders arise from single-gene traits for which mutations cause predictable disease because they follow the rules that he originally described. Multifactorial or complex inheritance disorders do not follow Mendelian patterns of inheritance or fit into the non-Mendelian inheritance phenomenon. These occur when one or more genetic susceptibility factors combine with environmental factors and random developmental events (Gross & Gheorghe, 2020; Mitchell, 2020).

6. C) Ventricular septal defect (VSD)

Cardiac defects occur in 50% of infants with trisomy 21. The most frequent defects are atrioventricular canal defects, but also VSD, autism spectrum disorder (ASD), tetralogy of Fallot (TOF), and patent ductus arteriosus (PDA). EA and TOGV are not routinely associated with trisomy 21 (Bacino, 2017; Bennett & Meier, 2019; Haldeman-Englert et al., 2018; Lubbers, 2021; McCandless & Kripps, 2020; Schiefelbein, 2021).

7. A) Trisomy 13

Phenotypic features of trisomy 18 that are notable at birth include intrauterine growth restriction (IUGR) with a small narrow cranium with prominent occiput, open metopic suture, low-set and posteriorly rotated ears, and micrognathia. Characteristics are clenched hands with overlapping fingers, hypoplastic nails, and rocker bottom feet. Rocker bottom feet are not associated with Trisomy 18 or 21 (Haldeman-Englert et al., 2018; Lubbers, 2021; Schiefelbein, 2021).

The Eyes, Ears, Nose, and Mouth/Throat Systems

Yvette Pugh

▶ INTRODUCTION

Complete understanding of the development and pathology of the structures of the eyes, ears, nose, and mouth/throat (EENM/T) is crucial to providing prompt and accurate evaluation and treatment of potentially life-threatening or debilitating disease processes. Craniofacial malformations affect multiple systems and can have an impact on breathing, vision, swallowing, and hearing. Issues concerning the physical examination and findings of EENM/T can be found in Chapter 6.

▶ THE EYES

EMBRYOLOGY

■ Optic evagination occurs during the first trimester at 24 days of embryonic development and the optic cups are formed at 30 days.
■ Lens development occurs between 34 and 44 days of embryonic development.
  ● Lens invagination occurs at 34 days, then at 38 days the lens is detached and pigmentation of the retina occurs.
  ● The eyelids are formed at 55 days. At 70 days, the iris and ciliary body form and the eyelids fuse.
  ● Pupillary light reaction is present at 28 to 30 weeks' gestation, and lid closure in response to bright light occurs at 30 weeks' gestation.
  ● Vestibular (doll's eye) rotations are well developed at 34 weeks' gestation.
  ● Visual fixation and conjugate horizontal gaze are well developed and present at birth (Blackburn, 2018; Graeber & Oatts, 2020; Órge, 2020).
  ● Visual milestones from 30 weeks' gestation to 6 months of age are summarized in Table 16.1.

POSTNATAL VISUAL PROGRESSION

■ Pupillary light reaction is well developed by 1 month. Color vision is present at 2 months and reaches adult level by 6 months. Infants can coordinate vision at 3 to 5 months.

Table 16.1 Visual Milestones Up to 6 Months' Corrected Gestational Age

Age	Visual Milestone Present
30 weeks' gestation	■ Pupillary response to light ■ Lid closure in response to bright light
34 weeks' gestation	■ Well-developed vestibular rotation (doll's eye reflex)
Full-term birth	■ Visual fixation ■ Well-developed conjugate horizontal gaze ■ Well-developed optokinetic nystagmus ■ Eyeball development 70% of adult diameter ■ Cornea development 80% of adult diameter
1 month	■ Well-developed pupillary response to light
2 months	■ Well-developed fixation ■ Color vision ■ Well-developed conjugate vertical gaze ■ Blink response to visual threat (present 2–5 months)
3 months	■ Well-developed visual following
4 months	■ Well-developed accommodation ■ Stable ocular alignment ■ Differentiation of fovea complete
6 months	■ Visual evoked potential acuity at adult level ■ Color vision at adult level ■ Stereopsis developed ■ Well-developed fusional convergence ■ Well-developed iris pigmentation

Sources: Data from Blackburn, S. (2018). The prenatal period and placental physiology. In S. Blackburn (Ed.), *Maternal, fetal, & neonatal physiology: A clinical perspective* (4th ed., pp. 61–114). Elsevier; Órge, F. (2020). Examination and common problems of the neonatal eye. In R. Martin, A. Fanaroff, & M. Walsh (Eds.), *Fanaroff & Martin's neonatal-perinatal medicine: Diseases of the fetus and infant* (11th ed., pp. 1934–1969). Elsevier.

■ The iris is immature at birth and the color tends to be gray or blue. The iris may become darker as the pigmented layer of the iris stroma becomes more fully developed. Pigmentation of the iris occurs by 6 months of age.

- The eyeball is 70% of adult diameter at birth and 95% of adult diameter at 3 years.
- Maximal vision is reached by 5 years (Blackburn, 2013; Campomanes & Binenbaum, 2018; Őrge, 2020).

CATARACTS

Definition

- *Cataract* is defined as any opacity or abnormality within the structure of the lens. Normally, the light from an object passes directly through the lens to a focal point on the retina, producing a sharp image. Cataracts result in a degraded image or no image at all (Fraser & Diehl-Jones, 2021; Graeber, 2020).

Incidence and Etiology

- The incidence of congenital cataracts is approximately 2 in 10,000 live births. Cataracts are responsible for 10% of blindness worldwide.
  - Congenital cataract is the most common form of preventable childhood blindness.
  - Infants with isolated unilateral cataracts often do not have a family history and rarely have associated systemic disorders.
- There are several causes of cataracts, including heredity, maternal infections, and congenital rubella. See Table 16.2 for a summation of possible etiologies of cataracts, including percentages of some of the etiologies (Campomanes & Binenbaum, 2018; Lissauer & Hansen, 2020; Őrge, 2020).

Presentation

- Normally, when light is directed at the pupils, they appear black to the naked eye of the examiner; cataracts, however, present as white pupils (leukocoria) that can be dense, milky white opacities in the lens. Dense central opacities greater than 3 mm are considered visually significant.
- The presence of nystagmus in conjunction with cataracts is a marker of poor visual prognosis.
  - Rapid, searching eye movements, or nystagmus, are elicited with rotational movements and are a normal variant until 3 to 4 months of age.
  - However, spontaneous horizontal, vertical, torsional, or persistent nystagmus (occurring greater than 4 months of age) is considered pathologic and warrants further intervention (Campomanes & Binenbaum, 2018; Fraser & Diehl-Jones, 2021).

Interventions and Outcomes

- Interventions should target the cause of cataracts; therefore, the following evaluations should be considered: TORCH (**T**oxoplasmosis, **O**ther, **R**ubella, **C**ytomegalovirus, **H**erpes virus) titers (including syphilis); urine tests for reducing substance (galactosemia), plasma urea, electrolyte, and urine amino acid levels (Lowe syndrome); quantitative amino acid levels and red blood cell

Table 16.2 Cataract Classification and Possible Etiologies

Classification of Cataracts	Possible Etiology
Hereditary (30%)	Most common mode of inheritance—autosomal dominant
Metabolic and endocrine disorders	Galactosemia, Fabry disease, hemolytic jaundice, neonatal hypoglycemia, diabetes mellitus, hypoparathyroidism
Traumatic/iatrogenic	Birth trauma, blunt trauma, perforating injuries, high-voltage electric shock, battered child syndrome
Idiopathic (30%)	Developmental variation; not associated with other abnormalities
Secondary	Maternal infection, inflammation, steroid use
Congenital rubella	Present in 30% of newborn infants with congenital rubella syndrome
Other congenital infections	Toxoplasmosis, CMV infection, herpes simplex, varicella
Chromosomal abnormalities	Down syndrome, trisomy 13, Turner syndrome
Renal disorders	Lowe, Alport, Hallermann–Streiff–François syndromes
Skeletal and connective tissue disorders	Smith–Lemli–Opitz, Marfan, Conradi, Weill–Marchesani syndromes
Clinical syndromes	Crouzon syndrome, Pierre Robin syndrome

CMV, cytomegalovirus.
Sources: Data from Campomanes, A. G., & Binenbaum, G. (2018). Eye and vision disorders. In C. Gleason & S. Juul (Eds.), *Avery's diseases of the newborn* (10th ed., pp. 1536–1557). Elsevier; Fraser, D., & Diehl-Jones, W. (2021). Ophthalmologic and auditory disorders. In M. T. Verklan, M. Walden, & S. Forest (Eds.), *Core curriculum for neonatal intensive care nursing* (pp. 691–704). Saunders, Elsevier; Őrge, F. (2020). Examination and common problems of the neonatal eye. In R. Martin, A. Fanaroff, & M. Walsh (Eds.), *Fanaroff & Martin's neonatal-perinatal medicine: Diseases of the fetus and infant* (11th ed., pp. 1934–1969). Elsevier.

enzyme levels (galactokinase, galactose-1-phosphate uridyltransferase); complete blood count and ferritin, blood glucose, calcium, and phosphate levels; genetic consultation; chromosome analysis and next-generation sequencing (focused on the 115 cataract-causing genes known to date); and ocular examination of the parents and siblings.
- Children with a family history of infantile or juvenile cataracts should be examined early by a pediatric ophthalmologist, and infants with cataracts may undergo selective diagnostic evaluation, especially if they have bilateral cataracts.
- Congenital cataracts are the main treatable cause of visual impairment in infancy and should be surgically removed within 6 to 8 weeks of birth. Aphakic (without a lens) glaucoma is one of the most common sight-threatening complications of cataract surgery in infants.

- Cataracts lead to varying degrees of visual impairment, from blurred vision to blindness, depending on the location and extent of the opacity. In neonates, cataracts may be transient, disappearing spontaneously within a few weeks.
  - Useful vision can be restored if the surgery is completed within the first 6 weeks after birth. Beyond this time, visual restoration becomes progressively more difficult due to irreversible deprivation amblyopia.
  - Visual prognosis depends not only on the extent of the cataract, age at removal, surgical outcome, and rapid optical correction, but also on the nature of other associated anomalies of the eye or syndromes.
- Intensive visual rehabilitation strategies must be implemented, and if the infant is left aphakic (without a lens) optical correction is achieved with special contact lenses or glasses.
  - Critical intervention involves adherence to the use of contact lenses and glasses; in the case of monocular cataracts, aggressive amblyopia treatment by penalizing (patching) the sound eye is critical and directly affects the child's ultimate visual outcome (Campomanes & Binenbaum, 2018; Fraser & Diehl-Jones, 2021; Graeber, 2020).

CONGENITAL GLAUCOMA

Definition

- *Glaucoma* is an optic neuropathy usually associated with raised intraocular pressure (IOP; Campomanes & Binenbaum, 2018; Graeber, 2020).

Incidence and Etiology

- Congenital glaucoma can occur as a primary disease or secondary to numerous other ocular conditions or systemic syndromes, such as aniridia, congenital rubella, Hallermann–Streiff syndrome, Lowe syndrome, Axenfeld–Rieger syndrome, Sturge–Weber syndrome, and neurofibromatosis.
  - One cause of congenital glaucoma is inadequate drainage of aqueous fluid that leads to increased pressure in the eye, resulting in damage of the optic nerve (Campomanes & Binenbaum, 2018; Graeber, 2020; Őrge, 2020).

Presentation

- Symptoms of congenital glaucoma can be apparent at birth or weeks to months later and include tearing, light sensitivity, blepharospasm (blinking), Haab striae (tears in the Descemet membrane, seen as lines in the red reflex), or lack of a red reflex.
- With acute glaucoma, high IOP is painful enough to manifest as crying, irritability, grimacing, poor feeding, or emesis in an infant. Tearing may be a sign of glaucoma, not just of a blocked tear duct. If the IOP is high enough for any prolonged period, irreversible optic nerve damage can ensue, with permanent vision loss.
- Cloudy corneas may be present in the premature or term baby during the first few days of life; however, a persistently hazy cornea beyond this period may be suggestive of birth trauma or glaucoma, and referral to an ophthalmologist is indicated.
  - Cloudy corneas represent glaucoma until proven otherwise and require prompt ophthalmologic evaluation even if buphthalmias is not present.
- As the disease progresses, increased IOP causes stretching of the eye, creating a cloudy cornea, corneal and eye enlargement (buphthalmias), progressive myopia (nearsightedness), and loss of vision.
  - Most newborn infants have a corneal diameter of about 9 to 10 mm. If this measurement exceeds 12 mm, congenital glaucoma must be considered, especially if corneal haze, tearing, and photophobia are present (Campomanes & Binenbaum, 2018; Graeber, 2020; Őrge, 2020; Walker, 2018).

Interventions and Outcomes

- Congenital glaucoma is a surgical disease that requires prompt intervention, frequently in the neonatal period. Medical management is used only for temporizing the condition or better visualization for various surgical procedures.
- The prognosis depends on the age of onset, time to diagnosis, and associated ocular and systemic conditions. Vision loss from glaucoma is typically irreversible. Genetic testing should be considered to rule out associated syndromes (Campomanes & Binenbaum, 2018; Őrge, 2020).

RETINOPATHY OF PREMATURITY

Definition

- *Retinopathy of prematurity (ROP)* is a disease of the developing retinal vasculature of premature infants. It first became a significant cause of blindness in children due to increased survival of premature infants mainly because of the use of supplemental oxygen (Campomanes & Binenbaum, 2018; Gaeber & Oatts, 2020; Leeman & VanderVeen, 2017; Sun et al., 2020).

Incidence and Etiology

- The incidence of ROP decreases with increasing gestational age. Over 80% of infants born at less than 26 weeks' gestation will develop some form of ROP compared with only 50% at 29 weeks.
  - In most cases, ROP develops at 31 to 33 weeks' postmenstrual age.
- The human retina is avascular until 16 weeks of gestation, after which a capillary network begins to grow, starting at the optic nerve and branching outward toward the ora serrata (edge of the retina).

The nasal periphery is vascularized by about 32 weeks of gestation, but the process is not complete in the more distant temporal periphery until 40 to 44 weeks.

- Lower gestational age and birth weight along with the loss of growth factors found in utero are the main risk factors for ROP, given that at lower gestational ages retinal development is less complete.

- Relative hyperoxia, aggravated by exogenous oxygen supplementation, damages existing retinal blood vessels and inhibits retinal secretion of vascular endothelial growth factor (VEGF), a hypoxia-induced vasoactive molecule responsible for normal and pathologic blood vessel development and growth in the body. ROP develops due to poor retinal vascularization, resulting in retinal hypoxia and pathologic neovascularization.

  - After the initial insult, vessel growth may proceed without ROP, or growth may remain arrested, and the vessels pile up within the retina, forming a ridge that might become very thick. If the new vasculature develops abnormally, these capillaries may extend into the vitreous body and/or over the surface of the retina (where they do not belong), and leakage of fluid from these weak, abnormally growing blood vessels may occur.

  - Blood and fluid leakage into various parts of the eye can result in scar formation and traction on the retina; visual acuity may be affected depending on the extent to which the macula is pulled out of position.

- Other risk factors for ROP are slow postnatal weight gain, low insulin-like growth factor-1 (IGF-1), hyperglycemia and insulin use, hyper/hypocapnia, sepsis, and other prematurity-related morbidities (Campomanes & Binenbaum, 2018; Fraser & Diehl-Jones, 2021; Gaeber & Oatts, 2020; Leeman & VanderVeen, 2017; Sun et al., 2020).

Classification

- The standardized approach to describing ROP, developed by the International Committee for the Classification of Retinopathy of Prematurity (2005), takes into account four components: anterior–posterior location of the retinopathy (zone), severity (stage), extent of the disease at the circumference of the vascularized retina (in clock hours), and the presence or absence of plus disease (Figure 16.1).
- The ROP status of an eye is determined by the highest stage and the lowest zone observed, along with presence or absence of plus disease.
  - *Plus disease* is defined as engorged and tortuous vessels of the posterior pole and is indicative of a more serious form of ROP (Campomanes & Binenbaum, 2018; Fraser & Diehl-Jones, 2021; Gaeber & Oatts, 2020; Leeman & VanderVeen, 2017; Sun et al., 2020).

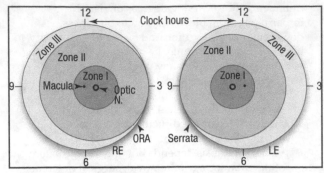

Figure 16.1 Clock hours and zones of retinopathy of prematurity.

LE, retina of the left eye; Optic N., optic nerve; RE, retina of the right eye. *Source:* Image used with permission from Campomanes, A. G., & Binenbaum, G. (2018). Eye and vision disorders. In C. Gleason & S. Juul (Eds.), *Avery's diseases of the newborn* (10th ed., p. 1551). Elsevier.

- See Table 16.3 for the classification of ROP.

Retinopathy of Prematurity Exam

- It is critical for clinicians to identify the at-risk baby so that timely examinations can be performed to reduce the likelihood of or prevent blindness. In the United States, the recommended guidelines for detection of serious ROP indicate that diagnostic examinations should be performed on:
  - Infants with birth weight less than 1,500 g or of 30 weeks' gestation, along with babies in the 1,501 to 2,000 g birth weight group thought to be at high risk, should undergo diagnostic examinations.
  - The first exam should occur 4 to 6 weeks after birth (approximately 31–33 weeks of postconceptional age).
- Infants who are found to have areas of retinal immaturity on initial examination should have repeated examinations every other week, then every 2 to 3 weeks until complete vascularization is achieved, when it has reached the ora serrata.
- If ROP is present during the initial examination, the infant should be examined weekly or every other week, depending on the severity of clinical findings (Campomanes & Binenbaum, 2018; Fraser & Diehl-Jones, 2021; Sun et al., 2020).

Interventions for Retinopathy of Prematurity

- Laser photoablation therapy for ROP is recommended for infants with the following classifications:
  - *Zone II:* plus disease with stage 2 or 3 ROP
  - *Zone I:* plus disease with stage 1 or 2 ROP
  - *Zone I:* stage 3 ROP
- Another treatment option that is in the experimental stages is anti-VEGF therapy. Anti-VEGF agents are being considered more frequently as a first-line treatment alternative, especially for eyes with zone I ROP because laser photoablation is relatively ineffective in decreasing retinal detachment in these cases.
- Bevacizumab (Avastin) is a monoclonal antibody that inhibits angiogenesis and is administered as an

Table 16.3 Classification of Retinopathy of Prematurity

Stage (Severity)	Stage Description	Zone (Anterior–Posterior Location of the Retinopathy)	Zone Description
Stage 0	■ Mildest form of ROP ■ Immature retinal vasculature	Zone I	■ Zone I is the most labile. ■ The center of zone I is the optic nerve. ■ Most severe retinopathy occurs in zone I or posterior zone II.
Stage 1	■ Mildly abnormal blood vessel growth ■ Presence of a fine, thin line of demarcation between the vascular and the avascular region	Zone II	■ Zone II is a circle surrounding the zone I circle, with the nasal ora serrata as its nasal border. ■ Most retinopathy occurs in zone II.
Stage 2	■ Moderately abnormal blood vessel growth ■ Ridge at the junction between vascularized and avascular retina	Zone III	■ Zone III is the crescent that the circle of zone II does not encompass temporally. ■ Aggressive disease is rarely seen in this zone. ■ ROP with an onset in zone III has good prognosis.
Stage 3	■ Severely abnormal blood vessel growth ■ Growth of vessels into the vitreous	x	x
Stage 4	■ Partial retinal detachment	x	x
Stage 5	■ Total retinal detachment	x	x
Plus disease	■ Blood vessels of the retina becoming enlarged and twisted, indicating a worsening of the disease	x	x

Note: See Figure 16.1 for the clock hours and zones of the retina ROP, retinopathy of prematurity.

Sources: Data from Campomanes, A. G., & Binenbaum, G. (2018). Eye and vision disorders. In C. Gleason & S. Juul (Eds.), *Avery's diseases of the newborn* (10th ed., pp. 1536–1557). Elsevier; Fraser, D., & Diehl-Jones, W. (2021). Ophthalmologic and auditory disorders. In M. T. Verklan, M. Walden, & S. Forest (Eds.), *Core curriculum for neonatal intensive care nursing* (6th ed., pp. 691–704). Saunders, Elsevier; Sun, Y., Hellstrom, A., & Smith, L. (2020). Retinopathy of prematurity. In R. Martin, A. Fanaroff, & M. Walsh (Eds.), *Fanaroff & Martin's neonatal-perinatal medicine: Diseases of the fetus and infant* (11th ed., pp. 1970–1978). Elsevier; Leeman, K. T., & VanderVeen, D. K., (2017). Retinopathy of prematurity. In E. Eichenwald, A. R. Hansen, C. Martin, & A. Stark (Eds), *Cloherty and Starks manual of neonatal care* (8th ed., pp. 986–992). Lippincott Williams & Wilkins.

intraocular injection and suppresses the development of blood vessels in the retina (Campomanes & Binenbaum, 2018; Fraser & Diehl-Jones, 2021; Gaeber & Oatts, 2020; Leeman & VanderVeen, 2017; Sun et al., 2020).

Outcomes From Retinopathy of Prematurity

■ Of cases of acute ROP, 90% (or more) resolve spontaneously with little or no loss of vision. Timely treatment has been shown to reduce the risk of blinding complications of ROP by 50%.

■ ROP located in the most immature zone, zone I, has the worst prognosis.

■ ROP with an onset in zone II, or a slower evolution of the disorder, more often leads to complete resolution. ROP with an onset in zone III has a good prognosis for full recovery.

■ Blindness or severe visual impairment commonly results from progression of the retinopathy to retinal detachment or severe distortion of the posterior retina (Campomanes & Binenbaum, 2018; Fraser & Diehl-Jones, 2021; Gaeber & Oatts, 2020; Leeman & VanderVeen, 2017; Sun et al., 2020).

STRABISMUS

Definition

■ *Strabismus* is the appearance of crossed eyes often seen in newborns due to weak eye musculature and lack of coordination (Tappero & Honeyfield, 2018).

Incidence and Etiology

■ Strabismus results from muscular incoordination and gives the appearance of crossed eyes. Transient deviations (neonatal ocular misalignments) occur very commonly in the first month of life in visually normal infants; at this age, it is not possible to distinguish infants who will progress to develop pathologic strabismus from those who will develop normal binocular vision.

■ Conjugate horizontal gaze (movement of both eyes with the visual axes parallel) should be evident in the newborn, while vertical conjugate gaze develops by 2 months of age (Campomanes & Binenbaum, 2018; Johnson, 2018; Őrge, 2020).

Presentation

- The most common form of strabismus is esotropia (crossed eyes), but exotropia (wall eye) and hypertropia (vertical misalignment of the eyes where one eye is higher than the other) also occur.
- Pseudostrabismus due to a flat nasal bridge usually resolves within a year and can be differentiated from strabismus by the presence of symmetrical corneal light reflexes.
- Strabismus may also produce abnormal or asymmetric red reflexes. An additional observation is the position of the light reflex on the corneal surface. Asymmetric positioning of this reflex can indicate misalignment of the eyes (strabismus; Campomanes & Binenbaum, 2018; Johnson, 2018; Stewart et al., 2017).

Interventions and Outcomes

- Premature and low birth weight infants are at increased risk of developing strabismus and other amblyogenic conditions throughout their childhood. Any constant strabismus beyond the age of 4 months requires further evaluation. This is especially important as, in some cases, strabismus can also be the first sign of serious ocular or systemic disorders.
- Strabismus may be treated with eye patching, atropine drops, and corrective lenses. Surgical intervention may be necessary depending on the cause.
- Premature infants have a higher incidence of myopia, amblyopia, and strabismus in childhood; therefore, careful follow-up of all children born prematurely is advisable to ensure early detection of these ocular conditions (Campomanes & Binenbaum, 2018; Örge, 2020; Stewart et al., 2017).

CONJUNCTIVITIS

Definition

- *Neonatal conjunctivitis* (*ophthalmia neonatorum*) is an inflammatory reaction resulting from invasion of the conjunctivae by pathologic organisms (Campomanes & Binenbaum, 2018; Fraser & Diehl-Jones, 2021; Örge, 2020).

Incidence and Etiology

- Conjunctivitis caused by bacterial and viral infections is typically acquired from the mother as the child passes through the birth canal, but can also occur after Cesarean section.
  - The incidence of neonatal conjunctivitis has decreased dramatically since the introduction of prophylaxis in 1881, but still blinds thousands of babies annually worldwide.
  - Chlamydial (*Chlamydia trachomatis*) conjunctivitis is the most common cause of neonatal conjunctivitis, and the rates are higher when there is absent prenatal care.

- About 20% to 50% of babies born vaginally to mothers with *C. trachomatis* infection of the cervix will develop conjunctivitis, and 10% to 20% develop pneumonia (Campomanes & Binenbaum, 2018; Fraser & Diehl-Jones, 2021; Örge, 2020).
- See Table 16.4 for the causes and treatment of conjunctivitis.

Presentation

- The infant with mucopurulent discharge must be distinguished from the infant who exhibits only excessive tearing and a relatively white eye, which is most likely nasolacrimal duct obstruction (NLDO); however, the possibility of congenital glaucoma must always be ruled out (Campomanes & Binenbaum, 2018).

Interventions and Outcomes

- Since the timing of the onset of conjunctivitis is not a reliable diagnostic clue, and because significant overlap exists among the different etiologic agents, diagnosis can be made more conveniently by Giemsa staining and polymerase chain reaction (PCR) tests.
- Infants with gonococcal conjunctivitis are at risk of having corneal ulceration, perforation, and subsequent visual impairment. Systemic complications involving the blood, joints, or central nervous system (CNS) may occur in a small number of infants.
- Chlamydial infections are spread through the nasolacrimal duct system and can lead to chlamydia-related pneumonia (Campomanes & Binenbaum, 2018; Fraser & Diehl-Jones, 2021; Örge, 2020).

▶ THE NOSE

EMBRYOLOGY

- Olfactory placodes, nasal swellings, choana, and primitive palate develop, and olfactory evagination occurs at 34 to 44 days of gestation.
- The lacrimal apparatus consists of structures that produce tears (lacrimal glands) and structures responsible for drainage of tears (upper and lower puncta, canaliculi, lacrimal sac, and nasolacrimal duct).
- Term and preterm newborn infants have the capacity to secrete tears as a reflex to irritants but usually do not secrete emotional tears until 2 to 3 months of age (Blackburn, 2018; Fraser & Diehl-Jones, 2021).

NASOLACRIMAL DUCT OBSTRUCTION

Definition

- NLDO is obstruction or stenosis of the nasolacrimal duct (dacryostenosis; Campomanes & Binenbaum, 2018; Graeber, 2020; Örge, 2020).

Table 16.4 Causes and Treatment of Conjunctivitis

Type	Causative Factor	Onset (Days)	Presentation	Treatment
Chemical	Instillation of silver nitrate or other antibiotic prophylaxis	1–2	■ Low amount of purulence ■ No organisms on Gram stain ■ Usually resolves in 1–2 days	None
Bacterial	*Neisseria gonorrhea*	3–4	■ Bilateral, hyperacute purulent conjunctivitis ■ Marked lid edema ■ Copious discharge	Ceftriaxone 25–50 mg/kg daily intravenously Topical irrigation Topical antibiotics useful only if corneal ulcer is present
	Chlamydia trachomatis ■ Most common cause of conjunctivitis in the neonatal period ■ Can lead to chlamydia-related pneumonia if left untreated	5–7	■ Mild mucopurulent, nonfollicular conjunctivitis ■ Lid edema ■ Pseudomembrane formation	Erythromycin, 12.5 mg/kg orally every 6 hours for 2 weeks or azithromycin suspension 20 mg/kg orally daily for 3 days
	Staphylococcus aureus, Streptococcus, and other bacteria	5–14	■ Nosocomial mucoid discharge ■ Conjunctival hyperemia and swelling	Broad-spectrum topical antibiotic (e.g., polymyxin B–trimethoprim, one drop every 4 hours for 7 days)
Viral	Herpes simplex virus	6–14	■ Unilateral or bilateral conjunctivitis ■ Serous discharge, associated lid vesicles	Acyclovir, 60 mg/kg/d in three divided doses for 2 weeks (3 weeks if there is CNS or disseminated disease), plus topical drops (1% trifluridine, 0.1% iododeoxyuridine, or 3% vidarabine)

CNS, central nervous system.

Sources: Data from Campomanes, A. G., & Binenbaum, G. (2018). Eye and vision disorders. In C. Gleason & S. Juul (Eds.), *Avery's diseases of the newborn* (10th ed., pp. 1536–1557). Elsevier; Fraser, D., & Diehl-Jones, W. (2021). Ophthalmologic and auditory disorders. In M. T. Verklan, M. Walden, & S. Forest (Eds.), *Core curriculum for neonatal intensive care nursing* (6th ed., pp. 691–704). Saunders, Elsevier; Örge, F. (2020). Examination and common problems of the neonatal eye. In R. Martin, A. Fanaroff, & M. Walsh (Eds.), *Fanaroff & Martin's neonatal-perinatal medicine: Diseases of the fetus and infant* (11th ed., pp. 1934–1969). Elsevier.

Incidence and Etiology

■ The duct is blocked at birth in 5% to 10% of newborns, resulting in epiphora (excessive tearing) and discharge in an otherwise white and quiet eye; 90% of such blockages clear by 1 year of age.
■ Congenital NLDO is usually caused by an imperforate membrane at the distal end of the nasolacrimal duct. NLDO is an ophthalmic manifestation of Goldenhar syndrome (Campomanes & Binenbaum, 2018; Fraser & Diehl-Jones, 2021).

Presentation

■ NLDO presents with epiphora (excess tearing) and usually does not occur until after the first 3 weeks of life, when the major portion of the lacrimal gland has become functional.
■ NLDO also presents with crusting or matting of the eyelashes, the spilling of tears over the lower lid and cheek, and absence of conjunctival infection.
  ● Chronic obstruction may lead to secondary infection in the lacrimal sac, a condition known as *dacryocystitis.*

● Dacryocystocele is formed when a proximal and a distal obstruction coexist in the lacrimal sac, and the lacrimal sac becomes distended.
  ❏ It is manifested as a bluish, nontender mass just inferior and medial to the canthus, causing bulging of the mucosa at the lower end of the nasolacrimal duct and can significantly compromise the airway (Campomanes & Binenbaum, 2018; Fraser & Diehl-Jones, 2021; Graeber, 2020; Örge, 2020).

Interventions and Outcomes

■ Simple NLDO usually requires conservative management. This consists of digital massage downward from the lacrimal sac over the nasolacrimal duct on the side of the nose. The massage empties the sac, reducing the opportunity for bacterial growth. Dacryocystocele should be ruled out by inspection of the nasal passage.
■ Once confirmed, treatment with topical or oral antibiotics is recommended to prevent infection of the dacryocystocele, and surgical treatment with a

- nasolacrimal probing may be performed between 6 and 12 months.
- Dacryocystitis, if not treated, can have potentially serious consequences in a neonate, including meningitis and septicemia (Campomanes & Binenbaum, 2018; Graeber, 2020; Őrge, 2020).

CHOANAL ATRESIA

Definition

- *Choanal atresia* is a membranous or bony obstruction in the nasal passage and may be bilateral or unilateral (Draus & Ruzic, 2020; Niermeyer & Clark, 2021; Otteson & Wang, 2020; Tappero, 2021).

Incidence and Etiology

- Choanal atresia occurs in approximately 1 in 5,000 to 7,000 live births, with up to two-thirds of cases being unilateral. Congenital anomalies are present in approximately 50% of cases, CHARGE syndrome being a main one. Other anomalies include polydactyly, hypertelorism, cleft palate, laryngomalacia, and Treacher Collins and Crouzon syndromes (Bennett & Meier, 2018; Otteson & Wang, 2020).

Presentation

- Choanal atresia presents with noisy breathing, cyanosis that resolves during crying, and apnea of the quiet infant. As infants are preferential nose breathers in the first 4 to 6 weeks of life, symptoms of bilateral choanal atresia can be severe and depends on the severity of the lesion. *Left untreated, the newborn with bilateral choanal atresia can asphyxiate and die.*
- Bilateral choanal atresia, as in other conditions with severe airway obstruction or swallowing dysfunction, commonly presents with polyhydramnios prenatally (Draus & Ruzic, 2020; Evans et al., 2018; Otteson & Wang, 2020; Walker, 2018).

Interventions and Outcomes

- Passage of a thin (6-Fr) catheter through both nostrils into the nasopharynx evaluates the newborn for potential choanal atresia.
  - An oral airway should be placed if bilateral choanal atresia is suspected. This can stabilize the airway by bypassing the choanal obstruction. Once the airway has been secured, a confirmatory CT scan of the nasal passages can be obtained.
- If the oral airway does not allow adequate air entry, endotracheal intubation may be required. In consultation with a pediatric otolaryngologist, transnasal stents may be placed to keep the nasal passages patent postoperatively after choanal atresia repair.
- Definitive therapy includes opening a hole through the bony plate with the use of a laser.

- Bottle feeding or breastfeeding is contraindicated in an infant with choanal atresia and the infant should be gavage-fed instead (Evans et al., 2018; Otteson & Wang, 2020; Ringer & Hansen, 2017; Walker, 2018)

▶ THE EARS

EMBRYOLOGY

- The structures of the ear begin to form at 9 weeks' gestation and continue until 32 weeks' gestation. The cartilage continues to mature until 40 weeks' gestation and is used as a criterion for gestational age assessment (Gross & Gheorghe, 2020; Trotter, 2018).

PREAURICULAR TAGS AND SINUSES

Definition

- *Preauricular tags* are minor malformations of the skin generally found on the anterior tragus.
- *Preauricular sinuses* are an indentation on the anterior tragus that may be blind or communicate with the inner ear or brain (Douma et al., 2017; Johnson, 2018).

Incidence and Etiology

- Preauricular and auricular skin tags are usually isolated and benign but warrant investigation as they are sometimes associated with other dysmorphic features or syndromes (e.g., CHARGE), a family history of deafness, renal anomalies, or a maternal history of gestational diabetes (Lissauer & Hansen, 2020).

Presentation

- Upon inspection, preauricular tags or sinuses are evident (Lissauer & Hansen, 2020; Tappero, 2021).

Interventions and Outcomes

- Preauricular sinuses are usually benign but carry an associated increased risk of deafness and renal anomalies. When single or bilateral preauricular tags are present with other abnormalities or risk factors, a renal ultrasound is indicated.
- Routine hearing screening should occur due to associations with congenital hearing loss (Douma et al., 2017; Lissauer & Hansen, 2020; Mitchell, 2020; Tappero, 2021).

MALFORMATION AND DEFORMITIES OF THE EAR

Definition

- Normal ear position occurs when the attachment of the ear is above the horizontal plane from the inner to the outer canthus. If the ear attachment falls below this plane, the ear is considered "low-set" (Johnson, 2018; Lissauer & Hansen, 2020).

Incidence and Etiology

■ Malformation of the ear occurs when the anatomic structures of the ear are not formed correctly due to a primary defect in tissue formation.
  ● Microtia is a disorganized, dysplastic, or dysmorphic external ear which may be unilateral or bilateral. Ears may also appear low-set. It is associated with atresia of the auditory meatus and conductive hearing loss and other malformations and abnormalities of the middle ear.
■ Congenital ear deformities in the setting of normal development but abnormal architecture may resolve spontaneously. To avoid surgery and improve cosmetic appearance, splinting of the ear has been recommended in the early neonatal period.
  ● The incidence of congenital malformations and deformations of the ear has not been identified (Lissauer & Hansen, 2020; Mitchell, 2020; Tappero, 2021; Walker, 2018).

Presentation

■ Normal ear placement is considered to be above the imaginary line drawn from the inner to the outer canthus of the eye toward the ear. If the insertion of the ear is lower than this point, the ear is considered low-set. Both ears should be examined for insertion and rotation, as one ear may be posteriorly rotated and appear low-set, while the other ear appears in normal position. Posterior rotation occurs when the ear deviates more than 10 degrees from the vertical axis.
■ Low-set, posteriorly rotated, or poorly formed ears may be associated with chromosomal abnormalities and syndromes. These abnormalities may also indicate additional anomalies of the middle and inner ear associated with hearing loss (Bennett & Meier, 2018; Johnson, 2018; Lissauer & Hansen, 2020; Mitchell, 2020).

Interventions and Outcomes

■ Microtia or posteriorly rotated or low-set ears should alert the provider to conduct further testing, such as hearing screening and possible genetic testing (Bennett & Meier, 2018; Johnson, 2018; Lissauer & Hansen, 2020; Mitchell, 2020).

CONGENITAL HEARING LOSS

Definition

■ Hearing loss is one of the most common major abnormalities present at birth. Neural hearing loss occurs with the pathology of the inner hair cells and eighth cranial nerve with intact outer hair cells. Failure of sound transmission within the cochlea, outer and inner hair cells, and eighth cranial nerve is a manifestation of sensorineural healing loss.
■ Hearing loss is classified as bilateral or unilateral, and as slight, mild, moderate, severe, or profound (Johnson, 2018; Vohr, 2020).

Incidence and Etiology

■ Approximately 50% of congenital hearing loss are hereditary. Genetic hearing loss is more likely to be nonsyndromic, autosomal recessive (30% syndromic and 70% nonsyndromic). Over 400 syndromes have an association with congenital hearing loss (Vohr, 2020).
■ See Box 16.1 for risk factors for hearing loss.

Presentation

■ Symptoms of hearing loss may be difficult to assess in the neonatal period; however, the infant should startle, cry, or respond to loud noises and should alert to voices (Johnson, 2018).

Interventions and Outcomes

■ Universal hearing screening is recommended for all infants in the United States. Two of the common physiologic tests performed prior to hospital discharge are the otoacoustic emissions (OAEs) and the auditory brainstem response (ABR).
  ● OAE and ABR do not require active responses; therefore, they can be performed while the infant

Box 16.1 Risk Factors for Congenital Hearing Loss

■ Caregiver concerns regarding hearing, speech, language, or developmental delay
■ Family history of permanent hearing loss
■ NICU admission for greater than 5 days,
■ Any of the following occurrences regardless of length of stay:
  ● Extracorporeal membrane oxygenation
  ● Assisted ventilation
  ● Exposure to ototoxic medications or loop diuretics
  ● Hyperbilirubinemia requiring exchange transfusion
  ● Intrauterine TORCH infection
  ● Craniofacial abnormalities involving the ear structures and temporal bone anomalies
  ● White forelock, associated with sensorineural or permanent conductive hearing loss
  ● Syndromes such as neurofibromatosis, osteopetrosis, and Usher syndrome, associated with progressive hearing loss
  ● Neurodegenerative disorders, that is, Hunter syndrome, or sensory motor neuropathies such as Friedreich ataxia or Charcot–Marie–Tooth disease
  ● Postnatal bacterial or viral infection confirmed with culture, including meningitis
  ● Head trauma requiring hospitalization
  ● Chemotherapy

TORCH, toxoplasmosis, other, rubella, cytomegalovirus, herpes virus.
Source: Data from Vohr, B. (2020). Hearing loss in the newborn. In R. Martin, A. Fanaroff, & M. Walsh (Eds.), *Fanaroff & Martin's neonatal–perinatal medicine: Diseases of the fetus and infant* (10th ed., pp. 1081–1089). Elsevier.

sleeps. Both OAE and ABR testing methods detect sensorineural and conductive hearing loss. However, false positive fail screenings can occur due to middle ear dysfunction, presence of fluid or debris (transient conductive hearing loss), or noise interference.

- Failed hearing screening should be referred to a pediatric audiologist for further diagnostic testing, including CT or MRI, genetic counseling, and pediatric ophthalmology.
- Providers should aim to identify infants with congenital hearing loss and enroll qualified infants into early intervention services by 3 months of age to optimize speech and language development.
- Outcomes depend greatly on the severity of hearing loss, time of diagnosis and treatment initiation, as well as presence of syndromes or comorbidities. Earlier identification and treatment leads to better achievement of age-appropriate speech and language milestones.
  - Fitting of hearing aids by 6 months of age has shown improved speech outcomes (Johnson, 2018; Stewart et al., 2017; Vohr, 2020).

▶ MOUTH AND THROAT

EMBRYOLOGY

- The mouth and throat structures develop between weeks 5 and 9 of gestation, with fusion of the lip and primary palate occurring at week 7 (Blackburn, 2018; Evans et al., 2018; Gross & Gheorghe, 2020).

CLEFT LIP AND/OR PALATE

Definition

- Cleft lip generally occurs at the lateral aspect, along one of the philtral ridges or along the midline. Cleft palate can occur on any area of the hard or soft palate (Evans et al., 2018; Gomella, 2020).

Incidence and Etiology

- The causes of orofacial clefting are usually nonsyndromic and unknown in 75% of infants with cleft lip with or without cleft palate and 50% of infants with isolated cleft palate. The prevalence of cleft lip and palate is approximately 0.8 per 1,000 births.
- See Table 16.4 for syndromes with potential oral anomalies.
- As an isolated anomaly, cleft palate is rarely associated with genetic anomalies. Midline cleft lip is associated with holoprosencephaly, whereas U-shaped clefts are associated with Pierre Robin sequence (Evans et al., 2018; Lissauer & Hansen, 2020; Mitchell, 2020).

Presentation

- Palpation of the hard and soft palate should be completed with exam visualizing the entire palate, possibly requiring a flashlight and depression of the tongue, in order to identify submucosal or posterior clefts.
- The location, shape, and degree of the cleft should be noted, as this information will guide the need for further genetic evaluation (Johnson, 2018; Lissauer & Hansen, 2020).

Interventions and Outcomes

- Presence of atypical cleft lip and/or palate, for example, midline cleft lip and U-shaped or V-shaped cleft palate, and any additional anomalies should lead the provider to complete genetic testing and genetic counseling referrals.
- Cleft lip/palate is not an automatic ICU admission. A multidisciplinary approach to management and early intervention follow-up is recommended. Nutritionist consultation should be considered as infants with cleft lip and palate may have higher caloric requirements and are at higher risk for failure to thrive.
  - Breastfeeding may pose a challenge due to inability to create adequate suction, especially in cases of cleft palate. Parents should be taught to feed the infant safely using a specialized bottle.
- Surgical intervention occurs around 6 months of age for cleft lip and 9 to 12 months of age for cleft lip and palate to optimize speech and language development.
- Outcomes vary depending on the type and location and any associated syndromes. Early diagnosis and repair will lead to optimized speech and language development (Evans et al., 2018).

LARYNGEAL CLEFTS

Definition

- *Laryngeal clefts* are clefts of the airway structures, which may include the larynx, trachea, and/or esophagus (Draus & Ruzic, 2020; Evans et al., 2018; Otteson & Wang, 2020).

Incidence and Etiology

- Laryngeal clefts are a result of failure of the trachea–esophageal septum fusion. Laryngeal clefts are not typically associated with cleft palate (Evans et al., 2018; Otteson & Wang, 2020).

Presentation

- Infants with laryngeal clefts may present with dysphagia, recurrent aspiration pneumonia, cyanosis, and respiratory distress (Draus & Ruzic, 2020; Evans et al., 2018; Otteson & Wang, 2020).

Interventions and Outcomes

- Definitive diagnostic testing for laryngeal cleft is microlaryngoscopy under general anesthesia. Early diagnosis is key to reduce lung inflammation and injury.
- A chest x-ray should be obtained to evaluate the airway and lung fields for aspiration. The primary concern is for aspiration of secretions and feeds.
  - Thickened feedings may be sufficient in mild cases; however, if aspiration or distress with feedings persists or the cleft is severe, gastrostomy tube placement may be necessary to prevent aspiration.
- Surgical treatment may initially require tracheostomy to allow growth and ensure airway patency (Evans et al., 2018; Ringer & Hansen, 2017).

MICROGNATHIA AND RETROGNATHIA

Definition

- *Micrognathia* is an excessively small jaw.
- *Retrognathia* refers to the position of the jaw being set further back.
- Infants may have a combination of micrognathia and retrognathia (Evans et al., 2018).

Incidence and Etiology

- Micrognathia is present in several syndromes, most commonly Pierre Robin sequence, Stickler syndrome, and Treacher Collins syndrome.
- Pierre Robin sequence occurs in 1 in 8,500 births and is one of the most common nonchromosomal deformation or disruption sequences in the neonatal period (Bennett & Meier, 2018; Evans et al., 2018; Mitchell, 2020).

Presentation

- Micrognathia and retrognathia are evident on exam of the infant's facies. Macroglossia (large, protruding tongue) may be exaggerated as the oral cavity is not large enough for the tongue.
  - Presence of respiratory distress with accompanying jaw deformity requires prompt intervention (Evans et al., 2018; Johnson, 2018; Mitchell, 2020).

Interventions and Outcomes

- Systematic examination of the oral cavity should be performed when micrognathia and retrognathia are present.
- Initial airway stabilization may include prone positioning, and nasopharyngeal or endotracheal airway placement. Nasopharyngeal airway is preferred as it is the least invasive treatment.
- Factors that determine treatment plan include presence of additional airway anomalies or presence of musculoskeletal or neurologic syndromes or skeletal dysplasias, which may contribute to the degree of airway obstruction.

- As the infant grows, subsequent growth of the mandible may occur and alleviate airway obstruction. A multidisciplinary approach should include consultations with otolaryngology and nutrition.
- Surgical treatments differ by facility and provider but may include mandibular distraction with osteogenesis, tongue–lip adhesion, or tracheostomy (Evans et al., 2018; Johnson, 2018; Pappas & Robey, 2021; Ringer & Hansen, 2017).

MACROGLOSSIA

Definition

- *Macroglossia* is the presence of a large tongue, which does not allow for complete closure of the mouth (Johnson, 2018).

Incidence and Etiology

- The incidence of macroglossia is unknown; however, it is commonly seen in genetic disorders such as Beckwith–Wiedemann syndrome and Down syndrome. It may also be associated with hypothyroidism and mucopolysaccharidosis (Bennett & Meier, 2018; Johnson, 2018).

Presentation

- Macroglossia is a large protruding tongue, which hinders the mouth from closing. Care should be taken when examining an infant with presumed macroglossia, as micrognathia may be the cause of the protruding tongue (Bennett & Meier, 2018; Johnson, 2018).

Interventions and Outcomes

- Interventions regarding airway obstruction and feeding difficulties are necessary if these issues arise and compromise the infant.
- Outcomes of macroglossia depend on the root cause and outpatient support. Infants with Beckwith–Wiedemann and Down syndrome may need outpatient services, such as physical, occupational, and speech therapies, to achieve optimum functioning.
- Table 16.5 describes the syndromes and potential associated oral anomalies.

▶ AIRWAY OBSTRUCTIONS

LARYNGEAL WEBS

Definition

- *Laryngeal webs* are a result of a failure to recanalize the laryngeal inlet at approximately 10 weeks' gestation (membranous tissue most commonly covering the glottis to the anterior vocal process; Otteson & Wang, 2020).

Table 16.5 Syndromes and Potential Associated Oral Anomalies

Syndromes	Associated Oral Obstructions
Pierre Robin sequence	Micrognathia, retrognathia, U-shaped bilateral cleft, glossoptosis
Treacher Collins syndrome	Micrognathia with glossoptosis
Crouzon syndrome	Retrognathia
Trisomy 21	Glossoptosis (downward placement or retraction of the tongue)
Trisomy 18	Microstomia (abnormally small mouth opening)
Cornelia de Lange syndrome, fetal alcohol syndrome	Thin upper lip, flattened philtrum
Beckwith–Wiedemann syndrome, hypothyroidism, mucopolysaccharidosis	Macroglossia, macrostomia (abnormally wide mouth)
Holoprosencephaly	Midline cleft lip or palate

Sources: Data from Evans, K. N., Hing, A. V., & Cunningham, M. L. (2018). Craniofacial malformations. In C. Gleason & S. Juul (Eds.), *Avery's diseases of the newborn* (10th ed., pp. 1417–1437). Elsevier; Johnson, P. (2018). Head, eyes, ears, nose, mouth, and neck assessment. In E. Tappero & M. E. Honeyfield (Eds.), *Physical assessment of the newborn* (6th ed., pp. 61–77). Springer Publishing Company; Mitchell, A. (2020). Congenital anomalies. In R. Martin, A. Fanaroff, & M. Walsh (Eds.), *Fanaroff & Martin's neonatal-perinatal medicine: Diseases of the fetus and infant* (10th ed., pp. 489–513). Elsevier.

Incidence and Etiology

- Laryngeal webs are classified into the following: type 1, where there is less than 35% glottic length involvement; type 2, with an incidence of 35% to 50%; type 3, with an incidence of 50% to 75%; and type 4 (thick web), with an incidence of up to 99% (Otteson & Wang, 2020).

Presentation

- Infants may not be symptomatic at birth, and depending on the thickness of the web they may present several weeks after birth with biphasic stridor. Cry may be soft or nonexistent.
  - Mild hoarseness with little airway obstruction (thin anterior laryngeal web)
  - Weaker voice, increased airway obstruction (thicker laryngeal web >75% glottic involvement)
  - Muffled or absent cry (laryngeal web or pharyngeal obstruction)
- When severe webbing is present at birth and causes severe respiratory distress, perforation with stiff endotracheal tube is necessary (Gomella, 2020; Otteson & Wang, 2020; Ringer & Hansen, 2017).

Interventions and Outcomes

- Biphasic stridor increases as age and activity level increase. Laryngeal webs should be evaluated endoscopically when presentation of such symptoms occur, usually at around 4 to 6 weeks of age.
- Interventions for thin webs are done endoscopically with web excision. Thicker webs may require tracheostomy and an open approach with laryngotracheal reconstruction and grafts (Otteson & Wang, 2020).

LARYNGOMALACIA

Definition

- Laryngomalacia is classified as congenital flaccid larynx or congenital laryngeal stridor (Otteson & Wang, 2020).

Incidence and Etiology

- Laryngomalacia comprises approximately 60% of all pediatric laryngeal problems and is the most common cause of stridor. The etiology is unknown, but is commonly thought to be caused by neurologic immaturity of the respiratory and digestive tracts (Gomella, 2020; Otteson & Wang, 2020).

Presentation

- Laryngomalacia is characterized as inspiratory stridor, generally presenting at 2 to 4 weeks of age, but stridor may be present at birth. Gastroesophageal reflex is commonly present with laryngomalacia (Otteson & Wang, 2020).

Interventions and Outcomes

- When not associated with cyanotic events, fiberoptic nasolaryngoscopy is performed to confirm diagnosis.
- Management includes prone positioning to decrease supraglottic collapse, and surgical intervention may be needed if the infant presents as *failure to thrive*. Agitation may worsen the degree of stridor. Direct laryngoscopy via rigid bronchoscopy may be warranted in atypical cases to evaluate for secondary obstructive lesion.
- Infants with laryngomalacia typically improve by 8 to 12 months of age and symptoms typically resolve with minimal intervention by 2 years of age (Otteson & Wang, 2020).

CONGENITAL SUBGLOTTIC STENOSIS

Definition

- *Congenital subglottic stenosis* is defined as a subglottic diameter <4 mm at birth in a term infant, generally a result of a malformed cricoid ring or excessive thickening of the subglottic tissue (Otteson & Wang, 2020).

Incidence and Etiology

- Congenital subglottic stenosis results from an abnormally shaped (elliptical) cricoid ring or thickened subglottic tissue. Many mild cases are undetected until 2 to 3 years of age (Otteson & Wang, 2020).

Presentation

- It presents as biphasic stridor and/or croup-like cough with absence of systemic signs of infection. Infants usually have normal cry, but tend to have respiratory distress with feeding, including tachypnea (Otteson & Wang, 2020).

Interventions and Outcome

- Endoscopic evaluation should be performed to diagnose subglottic narrowing.
- In most cases of congenital subglottic stenosis, treatment depends on the severity of the narrowing. Infants should be referred to otolaryngology for possible cricoid split or tracheostomy in severe cases (Otteson & Wang, 2020).

▶ CONCLUSION

Thorough assessment and understanding of the anatomy and pathology of EENM/T allows the practitioner to provide accurate diagnosis and implement appropriate interventions necessary to reduce the comorbidities associated with prematurity and genetic abnormalities.

1. The ophthalmologist reports an exam for retinopathy of prematurity (ROP) yielded findings as stage 1, zone III. The neonatal nurse practitioner (NNP) knows that ROP which originates in zone III has:

   A. Good prognosis for full recovery
   B. Slower progression of the disorder
   C. Worse prognosis than zone II

2. Upon examination of the eyes of a 7-day-old preterm infant, the neonatal nurse practitioner (NNP) notices cloudiness of the corneas of the eyes and recognizes the need to:

   A. Document this as a normal finding as preterm infants may have cloudy corneas for 2 weeks after birth
   B. Order genetic testing as this finding is consistent with osteogenesis imperfecta
   C. Request an ophthalmology consultation as any opacity is abnormal after the first few days of life

3. To treat conjunctivitis caused by *Chlamydia trachomatis*, the neonatal nurse practitioner (NNP) knows that the appropriate antibiotic therapy is:

   A. Intravenous acyclovir (Zovirax)
   B. Oral erythromycin ethylsuccinate (EES)
   C. Topical diphenhydramine (Benadryl)

4. In an infant who exhibits excessive eye tearing in the absence of other findings, the neonatal nurse practitioner (NNP) should evaluate for:

   A. Cataracts
   B. Glaucoma
   C. Strabismus

5. Eyelid colobomas are often diagnosed as part of which of the following syndrome?

   A. Beckwith–Wiedemann
   B. Goldenhar
   C. Trisomy 21

6. The neonatal nurse practitioner (NNP) is called emergently to a labor and delivery room for an infant in respiratory distress. Upon arrival, the NNP notes the infant has a small, recessed chin, a small jaw, an enlarged tongue, and has tachypnea and severe intercostal and subcostal retractions. The most appropriate first intervention is to:

   A. Immediately place the infant on their side or prone
   B. Position the infant in a sniffing position with a shoulder roll
   C. Provide continuous positive airway pressure mask

7. Upon doing an eye exam on a newborn, the neonatal nurse practitioner (NNP) does not see a red reflex. An appropriate next step is to:

   A. Dilate the eye, and if a red reflex is still not seen consult an ophthalmologist
   B. Reassess in 1 week as haziness in the first few days can interfere with eliciting a red reflex
   C. Suspend the exam for 48 to 96 hours so that the initial retained fluid from birth has evacuated

(See answers next page.)

1. A) Good prognosis for full recovery

ROP rates of progression are variable, and the worst prognosis is associated with onset of severe disease in zone I (most immature). Onset in zone II, or a slower evolution of the disorder, more often leads to complete resolution. ROP with an onset in zone III has a good prognosis for full recovery (Örge, 2020).

2. C) Request an ophthalmology consultation as any opacity is abnormal after the first few days of life

Cloudy corneas may be present in the premature or term baby during the first few days of life; however, a persistently hazy cornea beyond this period may be suggestive of birth trauma or glaucoma, and referral to an ophthalmologist is indicated (Örge, 2020). Cloudy corneas represent glaucoma until proven otherwise and require prompt ophthalmologic evaluation even if buphthalmos is not present (Walker, 2018). Osteogenesis imperfecta is associated with blue sclera, not cloudy corneas.

3. B) Oral erythromycin ethylsuccinate (EES)

The therapy of choice is oral EES (estolate preparation) for 14 days. Antiviral medications are not effective on bacterial infections, and topical antihistamines are equally ineffective (Fraser & Diehl-Jones, 2021).

4. B) Glaucoma

Infants presenting with persistent tearing (epiphora) need to be evaluated for congenital glaucoma. Tearing may be a sign of glaucoma, not just of a blocked tear duct (Fraser & Diehl-Jones, 2021). Cataracts and strabismus are notable as clinical findings on their own and are not associated with glaucoma.

5. B) Goldenhar

There are numerous ocular abnormalities and systemic findings associated with colobomas, including more than 200 syndromes such as CHARGE syndrome, 22q11 deletion, and Treacher Collins, Walker–Warburg, Aicardi, and Goldenhar (eyelid coloboma) syndromes. However, colobomas are *not* associated with trisomy 21 or Beckwith–Wiedemann syndromes (Campomanes & Binenbaum, 2018; Örge, 2020).

6. A) Immediately place the infant on their side or prone

The presence of respiratory distress with accompanying jaw deformity requires prompt intervention to relieve the airway obstruction (Evans et al., 2018). This is accomplished by positioning so that the structures are passively removed from the hypopharynx. If the infant remains supine, the obstruction will persist; therefore, continuous positive airway pressure (CPAP) mask will be ineffective and a sniffing position will increase the obstruction.

7. A) Dilate the eye, and if a red reflex is still not seen consult an ophthalmologist

The red reflex test is vital for early detection of vision-threatening conditions. If a red reflex cannot be seen, the pupils can be dilated with Cyclomydril eye drops. If a clear and equal red reflex is still not seen, the baby should be referred to an ophthalmologist (Örge, 2020). Delaying any consultation or intervention could result in lifelong visual impairment.

The Neurologic System

Kim Friddle

▶ INTRODUCTION

The nervous system is one of the first organ systems to begin development following conception. Fetal development and postnatal neurologic function may be influenced and/or altered by genetics and the environment, which include but not limited to maternal health, diet, pharmaceuticals, and pharmacologic therapies Sequelae associated with compromised neurodevelopment can range from treatable conditions to severe neurologic devastation. This chapter provides a review of fetal neurologic development and the most commonly encountered neurologic malformations and neuronal and neurologic disorders.

▶ EMBRYOLOGY AND GROWTH AND DEVELOPMENT OF THE NEUROLOGIC SYSTEM

- Neural crest/neural tube:
  - Normal development of the central nervous system (CNS) involves several steps. The steps of brain development and maturation are controlled by the interplay of individual genes and the environment in which these genes are exposed. *Neurulation* is the process by which neuroectodermal cells transform into the neural tube. The neural tube will then evolve into the brain and spinal cord. The following are the four steps of neurulation:
    - ❏ Neural plate formation begins on the third week of gestation.
    - ❏ Neural plate modeling continues during the third week of gestation.
    - ❏ Neural groove formation also develops in the third week of gestation.
    - ❏ Closure of the neural groove to form the neural tube starts on the fourth week of gestation beginning with formation of the neural crests. Closure begins in the lower medulla and moves both rostrally and caudally to form the neural tube. Closure of the neural tube is complete by approximately the 26th day of gestation (Gressens et al., 2020).

- Neuronal development and migration:
  - Neuronal proliferation primarily occurs during 8 to 16 weeks of gestation. However, some areas of the CNS continue neuron production throughout life.
  - Neuronal migration occurs primarily during the 12 to 24 weeks of gestation (Blackburn, 2018; Gressens et al., 2020).
- Porencephalic development:
  - The essential formation of the prosencephalon occurs through interaction between the notochord–prechordal mesoderm and the forebrain at the rostral end of the embryo.
  - Peak development occurs between the second and third months of gestation.
  - Key events:
    - ❏ *Prechordal mesoderm:* face and forebrain
    - ❏ *Prosencephalic cleavage:* optic and olfactory structures, cerebral hemispheres, as well as thalamus and hypothalamus
    - ❏ *Porencephalic midline development:* corpus callosum, septum pellucidum, optic nerve chiasm, and hypothalamus (du Plessis & Volpe, 2018b)
- Anatomy of the brain:
  - *Cerebellum:* complexity of neurons that influence voluntary muscle activity, coordination, muscle tone, posture, and equilibrium; contains the vermis and hemispheres and its development continues into the second year of life and hence the vulnerability of the preterm infant to cerebellar injury
  - Cerebrum–cerebral hemispheres:
    - ❏ *Cortical lobes:* consisting of frontal, parietal, temporal, and occipital
      - ○ *Frontal:* associated with executive function and decision-making
      - ○ *Parietal:* associated with hearing and understanding language, along with developing a sense of self
      - ○ *Temporal:* associated with memory, learning, and a sense of smell
      - ○ *Occipital:* associated with visual processing
    - ❏ *Corpus callosum:* largest bundle of nerve fibers connecting the hemispheres; completion of corpus callosum takes a minimum of 11

weeks with continued developing connections throughout adolescence
- ❑ Lateral ventricles and the fluid-filled space of the third ventricle
- ❑ Thalamus
- ❑ Hypothalamus
- *Brainstem:* Development of the following structures occurs after the neural tube is completed:
  - ❑ *Midbrain:* vision, hearing, sleep/wake, motor control, temperature regulation
  - ❑ *Pons:* carries sensory messages to the thalamus and conducts signals from the brain down to the cerebellum
  - ❑ *Medulla:* relays sensory information to other portions of the brainstem and is the control center for involuntary functions such as heart rate (HR), breathing, oxygen, and carbon dioxide levels (Darras & Volpe, 2018a; Ditzenberger, 2021; Huang & Doherty, 2018)

▶ CONGENITAL MALFORMATIONS OF THE CENTRAL NERVOUS SYSTEM

DISORDERS FROM THE PROSENCEPHALON

Agenesis of the Corpus Callosum

INCIDENCE AND ETIOLOGY
- The corpus callosum is the largest band of nerve fibers that connect the two hemispheres of the brain. When absent, the fiber bundles that would have run through the corpus callosum instead may run parallel to the ventricle in an anterior to posterior direction rather than connecting. These fibers are the Probst bundles and are a useful distinguishing feature on imaging, but not always present. When present, there is believed to be an improved prognosis. Agenesis of the corpus callosum (ACC) is a common malformation and represents ~50% of midline defects. It can be partial or complete and oftentimes involves loss of posterior segments. The prevalence in the general population is 0.5 in 10,000, whereas in children with neurodevelopmental disabilities the prevalence is 600 in 10,000.
- Formation of the corpus collosum is affected by genetic and environmental factors. Alcohol exposure has the highest incidence, where 7% of children with fetal alcohol syndrome are affected.
- Prenatal infection can cause ACC but it is rare. Infection more commonly results in a thinning of the corpus callosum.
- Multiple disorders have been shown to be associated with ACC with inheritance by all modalities of transference. Genetic syndromes associated with ACC will have additional malformations and are associated with significantly worse prognosis (du Plessis & Volpe, 2018b; Gressens et al., 2020; Hang & Doherty, 2018).

CLINICAL PRESENTATION AND ASSOCIATED FINDINGS
- ACC is often associated with other neuronal migration abnormalities, including craniofacial anomalies, midline ocular/nasal clefts or other defects, holoprosencephaly, and Dandy–Walker (DW) malformation. Metopic synostosis is also associated.
- Seventeen percent of the time, ACC is associated with chromosomal aneuploidy (chromosomes 13, 18, and 21).
- When isolated, ACC can go unnoticed (du Plessis & Volpe, 2018b; Huang & Doherty, 2018).

DIAGNOSIS
- *Prenatal:* Fetal ultrasound (US) may suggest ACC through indirect clues from change in brain structures due to ACC. A fetal MRI at 20 to 22 weeks' gestation may be helpful in identifying ACC and/or other cerebral findings; however, the diagnosis is challenging to make and should be confirmed with an MRI shortly after birth.
- *Postnatal:* Antenatal US can be helpful but has a false positive rate of up to 20%. MRI is the gold standard for diagnosis. Laboratory testing for genetic or chromosome anomalies in addition to metabolic testing will help determine the presence of any other associated abnormalities (du Plessis & Volpe, 2018b; Huang & Doherty, 2018).

TREATMENT AND OUTCOMES
- Long-term developmental follow-up is dependent on severity and may involve subspecialty consultations with neurology, ophthalmology, genetics, audiology, and developmental pediatrics.
- Patients with known ACC have been shown to have specific impairment in abstract reasoning, problem-solving, category fluency, and difficulty with higher level language comprehension. More severe cases associated with other anomalies of the nervous system have a high level of cognitive or neuromotor disturbances (du Plessis & Volpe, 2018b; Huang & Doherty, 2018).

Holoprosencephaly

INCIDENCE AND ETIOLOGY
- *Holoprosencephaly* refers to an entire spectrum of cleavage disorders sharing a common embryologic origin. The essential abnormality is the incomplete separation of the cerebral hemispheres along one or more of its three major planes–horizontal, transverse, and sagittal–occurring no later than the fifth and sixth weeks of gestation.
- Holoprosencephaly can be divided into three variants based principally on the severity of the cleavage abnormality in the cerebral hemispheres and deep nuclear structures. The DeMyer's classification scheme includes alobar, semilobar, and lobar divisions.

- Alobar holoprosencephaly is the most severe form where the brain fails to separate. It includes a single anterior ventricle contained within a holosphere with complete lack of separation of the prosencephalon. There may be a fusion of thalami and an absence of any or all of the interhemispheric fissure, corpus callosum, and third ventricle.
- Semilobar holoprosencephaly occurs when there is a failure of separation of the anterior hemispheres with presence of a posterior portion of the interhemispheric fissure and less severe fusion of deep nuclear structures. This somewhat milder form will still have distinct hemispheres and the presence of a portion of the posterior corpus callosum.
- Lobar holoprosencephaly is identified when the cerebral hemispheres are nearly fully separated, and the fissure is present along almost the entire midline and includes separation or near separation of the thalami. Deep nuclear structures are nearly or totally separated and the posterior callosum is well developed, although the anterior callosum may be somewhat underdeveloped. The third ventricle is present and frontal horns are partially formed and the corpus callosum is present; however, the frontal lobes may still be hypoplastic according to the severity of the malformation.

- Holoprosencephaly is the most common brain malformation, with its frequency estimated to be approximately 1 in 10,000 to 1 in 20,000 live births. This incidence is likely underestimated because many cases abort and mild variants may be unrecognized.
- Up to 45% of holoprosencephaly are caused by chromosomal abnormalities detectable by standard karyotyping, with 10% to 20% identifiable on chromosome microarrays. The most common chromosome abnormalities are trisomy 13 and 18. The most notable is trisomy 13, with 70% having this defect. Holoprosencephaly is also observed in several syndromes, including the Smith–Lemli–Opitz syndrome. Causes of holoprosencephaly are variable, with genetic, chromosomal, syndromic, and environmental etiologies. Some familial cases have been reported. Environmental factors include maternal diabetes, including gestational diabetes, and prenatal exposure to antiepileptic drugs (AED), alcohol, retinoic acid, and cytomegalovirus infection (du Plessis & Volpe, 2018b; Gressens et al., 2020; Huang & Doherty, 2018; Lazebnik et al., 2020).

CLINICAL PRESENTATION AND ASSOCIATED FINDINGS

- Disorders of prosencephalic development often have concurrent facial anomalies with ocular and olfactory malformations as well as forebrain alterations.
- Facial anomalies are present in up to 80% to 90% of holoprosencephaly cases. Findings may range from mild, with hypotelorism or a single central front tooth,

to more severe anomalies such as cyclopia (a single central eye) with a nose-like structure (proboscis) above the eye, or cebocephaly (a flattened single nostril situated centrally between the eyes). There may even be a complete absence of the eye or nasal structure. Severe facial malformations are often associated with more severe brain malformations.
- Neurologic features in the newborn period include low tone and microcephaly unless hydrocephalus is present. As severity increases, infants exhibit frequent apneic spells and stimulus-sensitive tonic spasms. Approximately 40% of children will have epilepsy, with one-third of these having intractable epilepsy. Seizures occur in a minority of patients.
- Endocrinologic abnormalities are very common. Various abnormalities of hypothalamic function may disturb temperature regulation, appetite, thirst, and sleep.
  - Diabetes insipidus occurs in up to 70% of patients, with hypothyroidism, hypoadrenocorticism, and growth hormone deficiency being less common (Blackburn, 2018; du Plessis & Volpe, 2018b; Huang & Doherty, 2018).

DIAGNOSIS

- Prenatal ultrasonography is adept at identifying a fetus with holoprosencephaly. A fetal MRI may then clarify the diagnosis and the severity of the malformation. Due to the high rate of chromosome abnormalities associated with holoprosencephaly, an amniocentesis for chromosome array and possibly DNA sequencing is indicated (Huang & Doherty, 2018).

TREATMENT AND OUTCOMES

- Treatment is supportive. Prognosis is related to the severity of the defect, involvement of other organ systems, and the genetic cause. The most severe forms of holoprosencephaly result in death in the first year. Subsequent neurologic deficits relate to the nature of the neuropathologic features (du Plessis & Volpe, 2018b; Huang & Doherty, 2018).

CORTICAL DEFECTS IN MIGRATION

Lissencephaly

INCIDENCE AND ETIOLOGY

- *Lissencephaly* is a neuronal migration disorder that results in a smooth appearance of the cortical surface of the brain caused by absent or reduced gyri.
  - The development of the normal fetal brain is smooth early in gestation, with convolutions forming throughout gestation. Neuronal migration is necessary to the cortical layers for gyri formation. Lissencephaly is a cortical migration disorder that impairs neuron development in all layers of the cortex, resulting in agyria (lack of gyration) or pachygyria (incomplete gyration).

- Clinically, lissencephaly is divided into two main types:
  - Classic or type I lissencephaly (LISI) is the type where the brain is smooth, similar to that of a 12-week-old fetus. Type I is estimated to occur in 1.2 per 100,000 births. Approximately 60% come from deletions and missense mutations of the *LIS1* gene, which gives way for absent or decreased gyri. Additional less common associated genes include *DCX*, *YWHAE*, and several tubulin genes, along with the *ARX* gene. Lissencephalies may be X-linked.
  - Cobblestone or type II lissencephaly (LISII) has reduced gyrations and a pebbly appearance to the cortex, and is associated with structural abnormalities of the cerebellum and brainstem. These are linked to Fukuyama congenital muscular dystrophy, Walker–Warburg syndrome and muscle–eye–brain disease.
    - ❏ Dominant and recessive mutations can be found and are related to different mutations of genes, creating sex-linked differences in the severity of of disorders.
    - ❏ Neuronal migration disorders can be linked to several environmental factors, such as prenatal exposure to cocaine, alcohol, or ionizing radiation, as well as infections with cytomegalovirus or toxoplasmosis (Blackburn, 2018; Gressens et al., 2020; Hall & Reavey, 2021; Huang & Doherty, 2018; Poduri & Volpe, 2018).

CLINICAL PRESENTATION

- Clinical features of lissencephaly include normal head size at birth, with developing microcephaly in the first year, hypotonia that will progress to hypertonia later in infancy, feeding problems, decreased movement, spastic quadriparesis, and seizures. Ambiguous genitalia may also be noted.
  - *Microcephaly* is defined as a head circumference measuring greater than 2 *SD* below the average for infants at that gestational age.
- Warburg syndrome with LISII generally presents with macrocephaly, cerebellar malformation, ventricular dilatation and/or hydrocephalus, retinal malformations, and muscular dystrophy.
- Miller–Dieker syndrome will demonstrate additional findings of dysmorphic facial features, such as depression or flattening on the sides of the skull known as *bitemporal hollowing*, micrognathia, malposition and/or malformed ears, short nose with upturned nares and low nasal bridge, long and thin upper lip, and late tooth eruption (Gressens et al., 2020; Hall & Reavey, 2021; Huang & Doherty, 2018; Poduri & Volpe, 2018).

DIAGNOSIS

- Prenatal US is adept at intrauterine diagnosis. In cases when the mother has no to limited prenatal care, individual clinical presentation and testing are key.

- Postnatally, EEG, CT cranial ultrasound (CUS), and MRI of the brain are all helpful in establishing a diagnosis (Ditzenberger, 2021; Huang & Doherty, 2018).

TREATMENT AND OUTCOME

- Microcephaly and myoclonic epilepsy are commonly noted to occur over the first year of life. Poor head growth resulting in microcephaly usually occurs within the first year in LIS1. Neonatal seizures may also occur, but seizures are more commonly present at 6 to 12 months of age.
- Like most disorders causing long-term neurodevelopmental delays, early interventions and identification of support are crucial. Prognosis of lissencephalies is very poor. Typically, seizures and spastic quadriparesis limit long-term achievements.
- Severe muscle disease with elevated serum creatine kinase (CK) often found in LISII can accentuate the weakness observed. Death in the first year is common (Huang & Doherty, 2018; Poduri & Volpe, 2018).

CONGENITAL CEREBELLAR ANOMALIES

Hydrocephalus

INCIDENCE AND ETIOLOGY

- *Hydrocephalus* is a category of ventriculomegaly that results in ventricular dilatation by an accumulation of cerebral spinal fluid (CSF) due to CSF production exceeding CSF absorption. It can result from abnormalities anywhere in the CSF pathway; however, majority of cases are caused by decreased absorption due to an obstruction.
  - Impaired CSF flow distal to the fourth ventricle foramina results in *communicating hydrocephalus*.
  - Enlargement of any or all ventricles due to an obstruction of CSF flow upstream or at the fourth ventricle foramina is called *noncommunicating hydrocephalus*.
- The etiology is typically heterogenous, but most cases result from developmental disorders of the brain and its CSF circulatory system. Major causes have been identified as DW malformation (7%), myelomeningocele (MMC) with Chiari type II malformation (28%), communicating hydrocephalus (22%), and aqueductal stenosis (33%), with the remaining 10% not defined.
  - DW malformation is the result of abnormal development of the rhombencephalon at weeks 7 to 10 in gestation. The exact etiology is unknown. The occurrence rate is approximately 1 per 25,000 to 30,000 births. The occurrence is usually sporadic, with few familial cases reported. DW consists of three major abnormalities: (a) enlargement of the posterior fossa (occipital cranial prominence) with upward displacement of the tentorium, (b) cystic dilatation of the fourth ventricle, and (c) partial or

complete ACC. By 3 months of age, 75% of infants with DW malformation will have hydrocephalus, with 90% or more ultimately developing hydrocephalus.

- Arnold–Chiari malformation (Chiari malformation type II) is a primary neurulation defect that occurs during weeks 3 to 4 in gestation and presents in the second trimester. There is displacement of the medulla, cerebellum, and fourth ventricle into the cervical canal, blocking adequate CSF drainage. It is almost always exclusively seen with open neural tube defects (NTD).
- Aqueductal stenosis is an obstructive noncommunicating hydrocephalus occurring when the CSF is unable to drain from the third ventricle into the fourth ventricle due to a congenital obstruction in the aqueduct of Sylvius connecting the third and fourth ventricle. CSF collects into the cranial cavity and leads to lateral and third ventricular dilatation, causing compression of blood flow and brain growth. This develops between 15 and 17 weeks' gestation, the time of rapid elongation of the mesencephalon and evolution of the normal constriction of the aqueduct (Blackburn, 2018; du Plessis, Robinson, & Volpe, 2018; Gressens et al., 2020; Huang & Doherty, 2018).

CLINICAL PRESENTATION AND ASSOCIATED FINDINGS

- Neonatal presentation is a markedly enlarging head, full anterior fontanel, separated cranial sutures, full (bulging) and tense fontanels, increased frontal-occipital circumference (FOC), "setting-sun" eyes, and visible scalp veins, as well as other nonspecific signs of increased intracranial pressure (ICP) such as vomiting, lethargy, and irritability.
- Sequelae of this hydrocephalus may include apnea, respiratory distress with inspiratory stridor, depressed gag, weak cry, quadriparesis, or dysphagia. These are typically the result of brainstem or cranial nerve dysfunction. Hindbrain dysfunction, like that found with Chiari type II malformation, can be the result of compression or ischemic factors. Brainstem dysfunction can be caused by the abnormal development of the cranial nerve nuclei in the brainstem. The highest mortality is seen when stridor, apnea, cyanotic spells, and dysphagia are all present.
- Ventricular dilatation occurs before rapid head growth or increased ICP is seen.
- Careful neonatal assessment should be made for signs of specific etiologic types of congenital hydrocephalus, such as the flexion deformity of the thumbs (which can often be detected by fetal US) characteristic of approximately 50% of cases of X-linked aqueductal stenosis, the occipital cranial prominence of the DW malformation, and the chorioretinitis of intrauterine infection by toxoplasmosis or cytomegalovirus

(Ditzenberger, 2021; du Plessis, Robinson, & Volpe, 2018; du Plessis & Volpe, 2018a; Huang & Doherty, 2018).

DIAGNOSIS

- Ventriculomegaly is usually readily recognized by experienced ultrasonographers on prenatal US, but may on occasion be mistaken for other fluid-filled supratentorial lesions, such as hydranencephaly or holoprosencephaly. These issues are resolved by fetal MRI (du Plessis, Robinson, & Volpe, 2018).

TREATMENT AND OUTCOMES

- The options for postnatal treatment of symptomatic hydrocephalus are individualized to the needs of each infant, and require consideration of comorbidities, overall prognosis, and parental preferences.
- Hydrocephalus that is symptomatic, regardless of etiology, can be managed with temporary procedures such as ventricular access device (VAD), ventriculosubgaleal shunt (VSGS), third ventriculostomy, or permanent ventriculoperitoneal (VP) shunt insertion.
  - The main complications of shunts include infections and malfunctions. The risk of early shunt infection has been reduced by implementation of specific protocols and typically averages 5% to 7.5%.
- The prognosis of congenital hydrocephalus is dependent on the underlying cause, the extent of secondary parenchymal brain injury, the treatment options, and the complications of the intervention. Overall, the incidence of serious associated brain anomalies in fetal hydrocephalus is approximately 60% to 70%.
  - Better neonatal intensive care and neurosurgical techniques are credited for the improving outcomes of these patients (du Plessis, Robinson, & Volpe, 2018).

ABNORMALITY OF THE CRANIUM

Craniosynostosis

INCIDENCE AND ETIOLOGY

- *Craniosynostosis* is the premature fusion of one or more of the sutures of the skull, which then prevents appropriate growth of the brain, and occasionally facial dysmorphisms. The overall incidence of all types is estimated to be 1 in 2,500 live births.
- Sagittal craniosynostosis is the most common nonsyndromic synostosis, occurring in 1.5 per 10,000 live births, and is commonly known as *scaphocephaly* (an elongated appearance of the skull). Known risk factors include male sex, intrauterine head restriction,

twin gestation, maternal smoking, and thyroid dysregulation.

- Unilateral coronal craniosynostosis is the second most common, with a prevalence of 0.7 per 10,000 live births. It is present when one of the coronal sutures is prematurely fused, creating some asymmetry in the eyes, forehead, and nose, and causing a flattening of the forehead on the same side of the fused suture. This is commonly known as *plagiocephaly*. Genetic syndromes are more common with coronal synostosis.
- Bilateral coronal craniosynostosis results when both coronal sutures are prematurely closed, causing flattening and widening of the skull structure.
- Metopic craniosynostosis has a prevalence of 0.8 per 10,000 live births and is identified by the triangular-shaped head with a point at the forehead (trigonocephaly), hypotelorism, and increased biparietal diameter.
- Lambdoid synostosis is the least common and is characterized by flattening of the ipsilateral occiput, displacement of the ear posterior–inferior, and a bulging of the mastoid process on the fused side. This type is occasionally confused with positional plagiocephaly; however, with positional plagiocephaly, the ears will be level on the same horizontal plane.
- Multiple suture synostosis is when there are two or more fused sutures. These are often associated with known syndromes such as Apert, Crouzon, Pfeiffer, Muenke, or Saethre–Chotzen syndrome (Evans et al., 2018; Hall & Reavey, 2021; Johnson, 2018; Temei & Smith, 2020; Volpe, 2018a).

CLINICAL PRESENTATION AND ASSOCIATED FINDINGS

- The primary findings are a misshapen head, facial asymmetry, bossing of the forehead, bony prominence at the cranial suture line, inability to move the suture, and hydrocephalus with signs of increased ICP. Viewing the head from above may facilitate assessment of skull shape.
- The most significant concerns for the newborn with craniosynostosis are airway compromise (specifically, upper airway obstruction) and intracranial hypertension. Obstructive sleep apnea is common in Apert, Pfeiffer, and Crouzon syndromes.
- Conductive and mixed hearing loss, most commonly due to middle ear disease, ossicular abnormalities, and external auditory canal stenosis or atresia, can be present in syndromic craniosynostosis.
- Syndromic associations most commonly related include:
  - Crouzon syndrome's common feature are brachycephaly, exophthalmos, and small maxillary bone.
  - Apert syndrome is a triad of dysmorphia noted at birth: craniosynostosis, small maxillary bone, and syndactyly of hands.

- Pfeiffer syndrome is similar to features of Crouzon syndrome, with addition of proptosis, broad and deviated thumbs and big toes, and partial syndactyly of the hands and feet. Three types of Pfeiffer syndrome exist, with type 2 presenting with cloverleaf scalp shape (Ditzenberger, 2021; Evans et al., 2018; Johnson, 2018; Temei & Smith, 2020).

DIAGNOSIS

- The diagnosis of craniosynostosis is usually made based on clinical criteria. A detailed physical exam should be done assessing head shape, suture mobility, and signs of increased ICP. Cases of single suture involvement may be identified by skull radiographs demonstrating sclerosis along all or part of the fused suture and compensatory changes. For complex cases, CT or three-dimensional CT scanning can help delineate the pathologic process (Ditzenberger, 2021; Evans et al., 2018; Tomei & Smith, 2020).

TREATMENT AND OUTCOMES

- A craniofacial team made up of appropriate specialties allows proper planning and coordination so that the patient may receive the best possible care. This includes members specializing in pediatrics, neurosurgery, ophthalmology, oral surgery, orthodontics, otolaryngology, nursing, nutrition, plastic surgery, and social work.
- Although the specific timing of the surgical treatment may differ between teams, it is generally accepted that individuals with synostosis should undergo cranial surgery in the first year of life. Cranioplasty involves release of fused sutures and repositioning and reconstruction of the calvaria so as to prevent increased ICP and progressive abnormal craniofacial development (Evans et al., 2018).

NEURAL TUBE DEFECTS

- NTDs occur when there is failure of the neural folds to fuse and form the neural tube. The neural tube forms the CNS, with the rostral portion developing into the brain and the caudal portion into the spinal cord. There is secondary malformation of the skeletal structure, muscle, and skin covering. These abnormalities cover a wide spectrum of defects, including anencephaly, encephalocele, meningocele, MMC, and spina bifida occulta. NTDs, as a group, are one of the most common congenital malformations in newborns, affecting 0.5 to 2 per 1,000 pregnancies (Blackburn, 2018; Hall & Reavey, 2021; Hansen & Warf, 2017; Huang & Doherty, 2018).

Anencephaly

INCIDENCE AND ETIOLOGY

- Anencephaly typically occurs within the first 4 weeks of gestation and is a complete failure of the rostral end of the neural tube. It is characterized by a lack of calvaria and intracranial contents, which are replaced by disorganized glial tissue and vascularization. It is the most devastating of all NTDs and represents nearly one-half of all open NTDs, with approximately 75% being stillborn. The incidence in live-born infants is about 0.28 per 1,000.
- The risk of anencephaly increases with decreasing social economic status and with a history of an affected sibling in the family. There have also been identified variations in prevalence based on geographic location, sex, ethnicity, race, season of the year, and maternal age (du Plessis & Volpe, 2018a; Hall & Reavey, 2021; Hansen & Warf, 2017; Huang & Dorty, 2018; Heaberlin, 2019).

CLINICAL PRESENTATION AND ASSOCIATED FINDINGS

- Three-fourths of anencephalic infants are stillborn. If born alive, most die within 24 hours of life. Some have been reported to survive up to 2 months of age.
- Due to the lack of normal cranial structures, the eyes appear to be large and protruding on US, giving distinct facies noted on US.
- It is seen in congruency with polyhydramnios and malposition as a later finding.
- At birth, the physical exam is notable for lack of brain and cranial vault (Gressens et al., 2020; Huang & Doherty, 2018; Lazebnik et al., 2020).

DIAGNOSIS

- Diagnosis often made by fetal US or MRI; anomalies may be evident as early as 10 weeks but are recognizable throughout gestation.
- Maternal serum alpha-fetoprotein (AFP) levels are very elevated.
- Physical exam can also help with diagnosis. Skull defects begin at the vertex and may extend to the foramen magnum. Hemorrhagic and fibrotic cerebral tissue may be exposed. The cranium is underdeveloped which results in shallow orbits and protruding eyes (Haeberlin, 2019; Hansen & Warf, 2017; Huang & Doherty, 2018; Lazebnik et al., 2020).

TREATMENT AND OUTCOMES

- Palliative care is provided to infants born alive. The majority of anencephalic infants die within the neonatal period.
- Prenatal detection rate is high; in turn, individuals often choose termination (du Plessis & Volpe, 2018a; Hall & Reavey, 2021).

Encephalocele

INCIDENCE AND ETIOLOGY

- Encephalocele arises from a failed closure of part of the rostral neural tube and most commonly occurs in the occipital region (70%–80%), with a sac protruding at the base of the skull or top of the neck. The remaining 20% to 30% are in the parietal, frontonasal, intranasal, or nasopharyngeal region.
- It occurs before 26 days post conception.
- These are cranial skull defects that contain brain tissue in the pocket that protrudes from the skull. Ten to twenty percent contain no neural elements.
- The severity depends on the location and the amount of brain tissue involved.
- Genetic factors also play a role in its development (Blackburn, 2018; Hall & Reavey, 2021; Hansen & Warf, 2017; Heaberlin, 2019; Huang & Doherty, 2018).

CLINICAL PRESENTATION AND ASSOCIATED FINDINGS

- Large mass is noted around the infant's skull or face.
- Wide-bridge nose and wide-spaced eyes can be a sign of internal encephaloceles.
- It may present with hydrocephalus due to the high relationship with other CNS defects, such as ACC, anomalous venous drainage, and Chiari malformations.
- The most common associated syndromes are Meckel syndrome and Walker–Warburg syndrome, both with autosomal recessive inheritance.
- Environmental factors such as maternal hyperthermia between 20 and 28 days of gestation have been associated with an increased incidence of NTDs including encephaloceles (du Plessis & Volpe, 2018a; Hall & Reavey, 2021; Huang & Doherty, 2018).

DIAGNOSIS

- It can be seen on fetal US.
- Postnatal transillumination can be used; x-rays, US, CT, MRI with angiography, and venography are preferred (Huang & Doherty, 2018).

TREATMENT AND OUTCOMES

- Surgery is indicated soon after birth in most cases.
- Palliative care should be provided to those without surgical options due to the severity of the lesion (Huang & Doherty, 2018).

Meningocele

INCIDENCE AND ETIOLOGY

- Meningocele is a skin-covered protruding sac that contains fluid and meninges herniated through the posterior vertebral column. The spinal cord is typically intact and unaffected; however, there are cases where there can be cord tethering, eventually causing symptoms.

- It occurs during gestational weeks 4 to 7, during secondary neurulation.
- It is located in the posterior lumbar, sacral, or thoracic spine (du Plessis & Volpe, 2018a; Hansen & Warf, 2017; Hills & Tomei, 2020; Huang & Doherty, 2018).

CLINICAL PRESENTATION AND ASSOCIATED FINDINGS

- In the neonatal period, infants do not tend to have neurologic deficits.
- Later deficits can include incontinence and disturbances in gait, all associated with tethered cord (du Plessis & Volpe., 2018a).

DIAGNOSIS

- It is often seen on prenatal US.
- Postnatal diagnosis consists of clinical assessment, spinal US, and MRI to assess for spine tethering (Huang & Doherty, 2018).

TREATMENT AND OUTCOMES

- Surgical correction is done shortly after birth.
- Folic acid supplementation has not been noted to decrease the incidence of closed spinal dysraphism. However, other studies have shown that 70% of NTDs can be prevented due to the practice of preconception supplementation (du Plessis & Volpe, 2018a; Hills & Tomei, 2020).

Myelomeningocele

INCIDENCE AND ETIOLOGY

- MMC is a result of failure of the posterior neural tube closure along with failed vertebral arc closure. MMC is characterized by herniation of a porous, cystic sac that contains meninges and neural tissues, or an open and exposed open spinal cord. It affects all layers of the spinal cord, vertebrae, nerves, and skin.
- Of these defects, 80% are located in the lumbar region.
- It occurs during gestational weeks 3 to 4, *during primary neurulation* (du Plessis & Volpe, 2018a; Hall & Reavey, 2021; Hansen & Warf, 2017; Heaberlin, 2019; Hills & Tomei, 2020).

CLINICAL PRESENTATION AND ASSOCIATED FINDINGS

- Defects that are open without a sac are known as *spina bifida aperta*, while those with a fluid-filled transparent sac intact are known as *spina bifida cystica*. Infants typically demonstrate neurologic deficits below the level of the defect, so the higher the defect the greater the neurologic impact.
- It is associated with Chiari type II malformation, with clinical signs of apnea, stridor, poor feeding, as well as signs of hydrocephalus with signs of increased ICP. Other conditions may include skeletal, renal, and gastrointestinal (GI) disorders (du Plessis & Volpe, 2018a; Hills & Tomei, 2020; Huang & Doherty, 2018).

DIAGNOSIS

- It is usually prenatally diagnosed through the use of ultrasonography. Increased AFP levels may also be indicative of MMC (Hansen & Warf, 2017).

TREATMENT AND OUTCOMES

- *Primary prevention:* Folate supplementation at the time of conception is estimated to prevent 50% to 72% of NTDs.
- *Intrauterine intervention:* Fetal MMC repair has been studied showing improved outcomes with decreased VP shunts, improved motor and mental composite scores, and less moderate to severe Chiari II malformations. This, however, comes with increased risk of prematurity and maternal complications.
- *Postnatal:* Surgical closure is the primary treatment, occurring approximately 48 to 72 hours after birth. Early intervention typically enhances cognitive outcomes and with decreased incontinence problems, but the infant remains at risk of chronic urinary tract infections.
- For significant hydrocephalus involvement, a VP shunt may be indicated.
- Long-term care of children with MMC includes a multiple disciplinary approach including urology, physical therapy, neurosurgery, occupational therapy (OT), physical therapy (PT), and developmental care (du Plessis & Volpe, 2018a; Hall & Reavey, 2021; Hansen & Warf, 2017; Huang & Dorty, 2018; Heaberlin, 2019).

Spina Bifida Occulta

INCIDENCE AND ETIOLOGY

- *Spina bifida occulta* is a closed defect of the lower part of the spinal cord with intact skin covering and is a result of defects in the caudal neural tube.
- It is the mildest form of spina bifida and is due to one or more vertebrae remaining open at the level of the spinous process; however, the spinal cord remains intact.
- It occurs during gestational weeks 4 to 7 or during secondary neurulation (du Plessis & Volpe, 2018a; Hills & Tomei, 2020; Huang & Doherty, 2018).

CLINICAL PRESENTATION AND ASSOCIATED FINDINGS

- Cutaneous alterations are frequently present. Examples include abnormal hair tufts, hemangiomas, pigmented spots, aplasia cutis congenita, cutaneous dimples or tracts, or subcutaneous mass.
- Neurologic impairments are rarely seen in the newborn period but can present with varying degrees of neurologic compromise later in life if associated with other closed spinal dysraphisms, such as syringomyelia, diastematomyelia, lipoma, fatty filum, dermal sinus, and/or a tethered cord (Hills & Tomei, 2020; Huang & Doherty, 2018).

DIAGNOSIS

- A spine x-ray with failed vertebral closure typically involving L5 and S1
- Spinal US to evaluate spinal cord mobility and MRI to define structural anomalies of the cord if needed (Huang & Doherty, 2018)

TREATMENT AND OUTCOMES

- Surgical management depends on the presence or progression of neurologic signs and symptoms (Huang & Doherty, 2018).

CONGENITAL NEUROMUSCULAR DISORDERS

Myotonic Dystrophy

INCIDENCE AND ETIOLOGY

- *Myotonic dystrophy* is an autosomal dominant disorder passed on by the mother that presents with hypotonia rather than myotonia associated with other myotonic disorders. This heredity pattern makes the disease more severe as generations pass it along to their kin due to the excessive amounts of cytosine–thymine–guanine (CTG) trinucleotides as DNA repeats. The greater the number of repeats, the more unstable the DNA and the worse disease expression (Darras & Volpe, 2018b; Walsh, 2019).

CLINICAL PRESENTATION AND ASSOCIATED FINDINGS

- Prenatally, there is frequently polyhydramnios due to poor fetal swallowing, decreased fetal movement, and premature birth.
- At birth, there is profound hypotonia, muscle atrophy, and generalized weakness, which may require resuscitation for respiratory insufficiency. The respiratory impairment may be so severe that the newborn infant fails to establish adequate ventilation and requires intubation and mechanical ventilation without lung disease. Additionally, they present with facial diplegia (paralysis), a characteristic tent-shaped triangular upper lip, feeding difficulties, arthrogryposis (especially of the lower extremities), and decreased or absent reflexes.
- A head circumference within the upper half of the normal range is more common than overt macrocephaly, although approximately 70% of infants will present with macrocephaly, with or without accompanying ventricular dilatation when examined on CT or MRI (Bass, 2020; Darras & Volpe, 2018b; Walsh, 2019).

DIAGNOSIS

- The diagnosis is suspected if the mother has clinical or electromyogram (EMG) features of myotonic dystrophy or has a confirmed genetic diagnosis; the diagnosis is made in the neonate by identifying the abnormally expanded CTG repeat in the *DMPK* gene.
  - The diagnosis is supported particularly by demonstrating myotonic discharges on the EMG elicited by direct muscular percussion of the neonate.
- Additional information can be obtained by evaluating the serum CK levels and CSF for protein levels. These levels will be normal and support the diagnosis of myotonic dystrophy.
- Nerve conduction studies are also generally normal. Slender ribs are commonly seen on chest radiography and support the diagnosis (Darras & Volpe, 2018b).

TREATMENT AND OUTCOMES

- The clinical course relates to the severity of the disease. Neonatal mortality can be as high as 40% in extreme cases, but typically ranges from 15% to 20%. For those who survive into young adulthood, GI problems occur in about 20%.
- For optimal development, adequate nutrition and ventilation must be ensured; respiratory support and tube feedings may be needed for extended periods of time.
- Significant learning difficulty or mental retardation is common. Most who survive the neonatal period will walk by 3 years of age (Bass, 2020; Darras & Volpe, 2018b; Walsh, 2019).

Spinal Muscular Atrophy

INCIDENCE AND ETIOLOGY

- *Spinal muscular atrophy* (*SMA*) is predominantly an autosomal recessive disorder characterized by degeneration of the anterior horn cells in the spinal cord and motor nuclei in the lower brainstem.
- Approximately 95% of individuals with SMA are homozygous for a deletion of exon 7 of the survival motor neuron (SMN) gene (*SMN1*) on chromosome 5q13. The incidence is approximately 1 in 10,000 live births. Onset and severity fall along a spectrum.
  - SMA type 0 or type 1A is the most severe form, with prenatal onset, multiple joint contractures, respiratory compromise, and death by 3 months age.
  - SMA type 1 is often referred to as Werdnig–Hoffmann disease. This severe form of SMA is the most common and is defined by onset before 6 months of age, failure to develop the ability to sit unsupported, and death usually by less than 2 years of age. Type 1 will be the focus of this section.
    - ❏ The respiratory effects of SMA type 1 include weakness of the bulbar, abdominal, and intercostal muscles, which makes a weak and ineffective cough. Poor airway clearance may result in recurrent pneumonias.

- SMA type 2 is defined as onset less than 18 months of age, ability to sit unsupported, failure to walk, and death after 2 years of age.
- SMA type 3 is defined by an onset after 18 months of age, the ability to stand and walk, and death in adulthood (Bass, 2020; Darras & Volpe, 2018c; Natarajan & Ionita, 2018; Walsh, 2019).

CLINICAL PRESENTATION AND ASSOCIATED FINDINGS

- Severe generalized hypotonia and symmetric flaccid paralysis generally greater in the legs than in the arms and greater in the proximal than in distal
- Severe muscle atrophy also generalized and more apparent as the infant ages
- Characteristic posture, demonstrated by a frog-leg posture with the upper extremities abducted and either externally rotated or internally rotated (jug handle) at the shoulders
- Respiratory distress with weak intercostal musculature; there is associated distention of the abdomen and intercostal recession during inspiration, known as *paradoxical breathing*, which gives rise to the characteristic bell-shaped chest deformity
- Poor suck/swallow reflex, weak cry, excess oral secretions with inability to self-clear due to weak bulbar muscles
- Particularly noteworthy differential diagnostic features in the neurologic examination include:
  - Presence of normal sphincter and sensory functions
  - An alert expression with a furrowed brow and normal eye movements due to the sparing of the upper cranial nerves (Bass et al., 2020; Darras & Volpe, 2018c; Walsh, 2019)

DIAGNOSIS

- Decreased or lost fetal movement is noted by the mother in the late stages of pregnancy.
- Once the clinical pattern is recognized and serum CK level is normal or only slightly elevated, genetic testing for the *SMN* gene is definitive (Bass, 2020; Darras & Volpe, 2018c).

TREATMENT AND OUTCOMES

- Decreased ability of sucking and swallowing early in infancy can lead to frequent aspiration; tube feeding is required for adequate nutrition.
- Tracheostomy and mechanical ventilation are often necessary, and surveillance for respiratory infection must be diligent.
- Quality of life discussions are important at various events throughout the infant's growth and development.
- In 2017, nusinersen became the first Food and Drug Administration (FDA)-approved drug treatment for SMA to address genetic changes in the *SMN* gene. This medication is given intrathecally and modifies the pre-mRNA splicing of the *SMN2* gene to promote increased SMN protein production. Clinical trials demonstrated a significant improvement in motor milestones and event-free survival (Bass, 2020; Darras & Volpe, 2018c).

CRANIAL HEMORRHAGES

Subdural Hemorrhage

INCIDENCE AND ETIOLOGY

- *Subdural hemorrhage* or *hematoma* is bleeding in the subdural space between the dura and the arachnoid layers.
- There are four major varieties based on the location of the blood vessel insult: tentorial laceration, occipital osteodiastasis, falx laceration, and superficial cerebral veins.
- It usually occurs in full-term infants and is most often related to trauma, especially when the lesion is large.
- It is most likely to occur under circumstances where the infant is subjected to unusual or rapid deforming stresses, such as compression, molding, or stresses on extraction during delivery.
- Additional risks include large head and/or small birth canal, an unusually compliant skull (premature infant), unusually rigid pelvic structures (primiparous or older multiparous mother), short duration of labor not allowing pelvis structures to dilate or an unusually long labor in which the head is subjected to prolonged compression and molding, atypical presentation (breech, face, or brow), difficult vacuum extraction, challenging forceps, or rotational maneuvers.
- It can result from coagulation disturbances or maternal injury with blunt force trauma to the abdomen.
- Incidence has been underestimated because these hemorrhages can be asymptomatic (Hall & Reavey, 2021; Heaberlin, 2019; Inder et al., 2018; Soul, 2017).

CLINICAL PRESENTATION AND ASSOCIATED FINDINGS

- Large infants above 4,000 g
- 1-minute Apgar score of 1
- Lethargy, stupor, or coma
- Bradycardia
- Ataxic respirations, respiratory arrest, facial paresis, and seizures
- Nuchal rigidity with retrocollis or opisthotonos
- Unequal pupils, skew deviation of eyes with lateral that is not altered by the "doll's eyes" maneuver, ocular bobbing
- *Signs of increased ICP:* irritability, full fontanel, and apnea (De Vries, 2020; Inder et al., 2018)

DIAGNOSIS

- MRI is the most effective; however, CT is useful for rapid diagnosis.
- Lateral skull x-rays and CUS are also used (Inder et al., 2018).

TREATMENT AND OUTCOMES

- Rapid surgical evacuation of blood with the more severe life-threatening lacerations that demonstrate neurologic deterioration
- Close surveillance in the absence of neurologic symptoms
- Subdural taps, which can be used to decrease signs of increased ICP
- Outcomes are based on the location and severity of the hemorrhage:
  - Major symptomatic lacerations of the tentorium and flax with large hemorrhage are nearly always fatal and the rare survivor will develop hydrocephalus.
  - Large occipital diastasis bleeds also have poor outcomes, but there is a possibility of improved interventional outcomes with early diagnosis.
  - Moderate or large superficial cerebral vein bleeds have a relatively good prognosis; 50% to 90% are well on follow-up.
  - Hydrocephalus can develop as a result of outflow obstruction and may require temporary external drainage. Some may need permanent shunt placement (De Vries, 2020; Inder et al., 2018).

Subarachnoid Hemorrhage

INCIDENCE AND ETIOLOGY

- *Primary subarachnoid hemorrhage* is blood within the subarachnoid space that is not a secondary extension from hemorrhage anywhere else within the skull (subdural, intraventricular, cerebellar, pia arachnoid). A primary subarachnoid hemorrhage should be suspected any time findings in the CSF demonstrate an elevated red blood cell count and an elevated protein count.
- Bleeding is believed to be from small vascular channels derived from involuting arteries present during brain development or bridging veins within the subarachnoid space.
- It is more commonly found in premature infants than term.
- The pathogenesis is not clear, but is believed to be related to trauma or circulatory events related to prematurity (Hall & Reavey, 2021; Heaberlin, 2019; Inder et al., 2018; Soul, 2017).

CLINICAL PRESENTATION AND ASSOCIATED FINDINGS

- There are minimal or no clinical signs with minor hemorrhage.
- Hydrocephalus can occur but less common than with subdural hemorrhage.
- Seizures can occur in term infants, with the onset most commonly at 2 days of age. Apnea may be a presenting sign in preterm infants.
- Massive hemorrhage with catastrophic deterioration is very rare but can occur. Usually, these infants have sustained a severe perinatal asphyxia or an element of trauma (Hall & Reavey, 2021; Inder et al., 2018).

DIAGNOSIS

- CT is the most accurate imaging method for detection of subarachnoid blood. Ultrasonography is insensitive in detecting subarachnoid hemorrhage but may be seen if large (Inder et al., 2018; Neil & Inder, 2018; Weinman et al., 2021).

TREATMENT AND OUTCOMES

- The management is essentially that of posthemorrhagic hydrocephalus (PHH) if CSF blockage occurs.
- The general prognosis for infants with subarachnoid hemorrhage without traumatic or hypoxic injury is good. The infant with minimal signs in the neonatal period does well.
- At least 90% of infants who present with seizures are normal on follow-up.
- The rare patient with a massive subarachnoid hemorrhage of unknown origin will develop hydrocephalus. Those with a catastrophic deterioration will die (Inder et al., 2018).

Cerebellar Hemorrhage

INCIDENCE AND ETIOLOGY

- Cerebellar hemorrhage occurs more commonly in preterm infants than in term, with the highest incidence in the very preterm infant weighing less than 750 g.
- Detection is difficult and dependent on the technique used. Rates for infants less than 32 weeks on mastoid-view CUS are 3% to 9% versus MRI rates of 15% to 37% (Limperopoulos et al., 2018; Soul, 2017).
- There are four major categories:
  - *Primary cerebellar hemorrhage:* This hemorrhage has a wide range of severity, from mild to near total destruction of cerebellum. It can occur unilaterally or bilaterally, and progress to cerebellar atrophy and reductions in cerebellar volumes.
  - *Venous infarction:* This hemorrhage is a complication of extremely preterm birth. It typically involves the bilateral inferior parts of the cerebellar hemispheres and often occurs in conjunction with supratentorial white matter injury, suggesting a hypoxic–ischemic (HI) insult.
  - *Extension of blood from intraventricular or subarachnoid spaces:* Intraventricular hemorrhage (IVH) accompanies 95% of cerebellar hemorrhages. It can result in injury to the underlying structures and impair the immature and rapidly developing cerebellum.

- *Traumatic injury:* This refers to laceration of the cerebellum or of cerebellar bridging veins. In preterm infants, the compliant skull is vulnerable to external forces that can affect the flow of venous blood and increase venous pressure to the cerebellum (Limperopoulos et al., 2018).

CLINICAL PRESENTATION AND ASSOCIATED FINDINGS

- In term infants, signs most commonly occur within the first 24 hours of life with larger hemorrhages. Signs are consistent with brainstem compression, such as apnea, respiratory irregularities, bradycardia, or CSF obstruction with full fontanel and separated sutures, and moderately dilated ventricles on MRI/CT scan or CUS. Other symptoms include skew deviation of the eyes, opisthotonos, and seizures. Seizures may occur by 36 hours of life.
- In preterm infants with smaller bleeds, clinical signs can be subtle or nonexistent. Clinical seizures and unexplained motor agitation have been seen.
- Thrombocytopenia
- Breech extraction or difficult forceps extraction (Limperopoulos et al., 2018)

DIAGNOSIS

- MRI is more likely than CT or US to establish the etiology of the hemorrhage and then anticipate long-term prognosis.
- US imaging is very sensitive to intracranial hemorrhage, and areas of increased echogenicity can be demonstrated (Soul, 2017; Weinman et al., 2021).

TREATMENT AND OUTCOMES

- Neurosurgical evaluation is recommended in infants who deteriorate quickly. These infants may need hematoma evacuation or a shunt for CSF obstruction.
- Neonatal mortality for term infants with major hemorrhage is as high as 10%. Survivors have an increased likelihood of neurologic deficits, language delays, behavioral difficulties, and cognitive and especially motor deficits. Approximately half develop hydrocephalus requiring VP shunt.
- Preterm mortality with major hemorrhage ranges from 14% to 50%. Survivors may exhibit cognitive deficits, language, behavioral problems, and autism spectrum disorders.
- In early studies, magnesium sulfate exposure in preterm infants <33 weeks was found to decrease MRI-detected cerebral hemorrhage, suggesting some degree of neuroprotection. More research is needed (Limperopoulos et al., 2018; Soul, 2017).

Intraventricular Hemorrhage of the Term Infant

INCIDENCE AND ETIOLOGY

- IVH is primarily a lesion in the premature infant but can also occur in term infants. Sources of hemorrhage include:
  - Choroid plexus, which is the most common (35%)
  - Thalamus associated with moderate to severe IVH and venous thrombosis (24%)
  - Subependymal germinal matrix, caudate (17%)
  - Periventricular cerebral parenchyma (14%)
  - Unclear source (10%)
- The pathogenesis is similar to the preterm infant with disturbances in cerebral blood flow, venous pressure, vascular integrity, as well as coagulation and trauma.
- Hypercoagulable states, disseminated intravascular coagulation (DIC), or extracorporeal membrane oxygenation (ECMO) were more common factors than in the preterm infant with thrombosis being more common.
- Mechanical trauma also seems to play a greater role in the term infant.
- Rates of IVH ranged from 2% to 3.5% in two large studies (Inder et al., 2018; Inder & Matthews, 2020).

CLINICAL PRESENTATION AND ASSOCIATED FINDINGS

- Infants with perinatal complications usually present early by 1 to 2 days of life with irritability, stupor, apnea, and predominantly with seizures.
- Seizures are usually multifocal or focal and occur in 50% to 65% of cases.
- Less common signs include fever, jitteriness, and signs of increased ICP.
- Infants without a clear cause present as late as 2 to 4 weeks of life (Inder et al., 2018).

DIAGNOSIS

- MRI is more sensitive than US or CT.

TREATMENT AND OUTCOMES

- Treatment includes supportive care and monitoring.
  - *Maintain cerebral perfusion:* Provide adequate arterial blood pressure, while avoiding abrupt increases in cerebral blood flow by avoiding hyper/hypocarbia, hypoxemia, acidosis, hyperosmolar solutions, rapid volume expansion, and pneumothorax.
  - Detect and treat seizures.
  - Treat coagulopathies.
- Follow with serial US to monitor for progressive ventricular dilatation.
- Outcomes are dependent on the size and location of the initial hemorrhage.
  - Fifty percent of infants will develop hydrocephalous requiring shunt placement, while 20% will develop hydrocephalous that will resolve without treatment.

- Forty percent will improve but have continued major neurologic deficits (e.g., cerebral palsy [CP]).
- Five percent of infants with hydrocephalus will die (Inder, 2020).

Intraventricular–Periventricular Hemorrhages of the Preterm Infant

INCIDENCE AND ETIOLOGY

- Germinal matrix/IVH is the most common neonatal intracranial hemorrhage and is characteristic of preterm infants.
- The hemorrhage originates in the subependymal germinal matrix. The germinal matrix is highly cellular, gelatinous in texture, active with cellular proliferation, and richly vascularized, especially in the premature infant, placing them at higher risk for hemorrhage.
- Venous drainage from the deep white matter flows into the germinal matrix and into the terminal vein, which is positioned just below the germinal matrix, eventually terminating in the great cerebral vein of Galen.
- The overall incidence of IVH in premature infants is 24% to 26%, with approximately 10,000 infants in the United States alone with IVH annually (Hall & Reavey, 2021; Heaberlin, 2019; Inder et al., 2018; Soul, 2017).
- IVH is graded into four classifications based on US examination. The grades of hemorrhage include:
  - *Grade I:* This is characterized by hemorrhage into the subependymal germinal matrix with minimal (<10%) or no IVH.
  - *Grade II:* This is characterized by blood in the lateral ventricle without ventricular dilatation. Blood fills less than 50% of the ventricles.
  - *Grade III:* This is characterized by hemorrhage with distention causing ventricle dilatation. Blood fills more than 50% of the ventricle. Clot formation may lead to an outflow tract obstruction most commonly at the level of the aqueduct of Sylvius, which leads to progressively worsening ventricle dilatation.
  - *Grade IV:* This is recognized as a hemorrhagic infarct or stroke in the periventricular white matter, not an extension of an IVH; however, it does relate to the severity of the IVH.
    - ❏ Changes in systemic and cerebral hemodynamics precede the bleeding and have revealed a pattern of hypoperfusion–reperfusion cycle. This is an important causative pathway (Back & Miller, 2018; De Vries, 2020; Hall & Reavey, 2021; Inder et al., 2018; Weinman et al., 2021).
- Autoregulation of cerebral blood flow:
  - A factor that puts premature infants at higher risk for hemorrhages is the lack of ability to autoregulate their cerebral blood flow. This concept refers to local control of blood flow in the brain.

Sustaining consistent blood flow to the brain is vital in regulating pressure in these fragile vessels. Without autoregulation, the cerebral blood flow is in a pressure-passive state, unprotected from wide swings or changes. The more premature the infant, the more time spent in a pressure-passive state.

- Other factors that increase the risk of IVH are related to common premature problems such as hypovolemia, hypoglycemia, hypercarbia, hypoxia, and acidosis. These states all affect cerebral autoregulation, thus increasing the risk of devastating hemorrhages (Inder et al., 2018; Neil & Volpe, 2018; Soul, 2017).

CLINICAL PRESENTATION AND ASSOCIATED FINDINGS

- Catastrophic syndrome evolves in minutes to hours: falling hematocrit, bulging anterior fontanel, hypotension, bradycardia, apnea, temperature instability, metabolic acidosis, inappropriate antidiuretic hormone (ADH) secretion, generalized tonic seizures, pupils fixed to light, flaccid quadriparesis, decerebrate posturing, and stupor leading to a coma.
- Saltatory syndrome evolves in hours to days: altered level of consciousness, decrease in the quantity and quality of spontaneous and elicited movements, hypotonia, subtle deviation from the normal eye position and movements, and tight popliteal angle.
- It is a clinically silent syndrome. Neurologic signs may be so subtle they can be easily overlooked. The most valuable sign can be an unexplained drop in hematocrit or failure of hematocrit to rise after transfusion. Of infants with IVH, 25% to 50% may fail to have any clinical signs indicative of a hemorrhage (Inder et al., 2018; Soul, 2017).

DIAGNOSIS

- US scan is effective in the identification of all levels of severity for IVH from isolated germinal matrix hemorrhage to major hemorrhage, with or without periventricular hemorrhagic infarction.
- A primary guideline for CUS screening in the United States is the Practice Parameter for Neuroimaging of the Neonate in 2002, which recommends screening with CUS of all infants with estimated gestational age (EGA) less than 30 weeks at 7 to 14 days and optimally again at 36 to 40 weeks.
  - Many hemorrhages develop within the first 48 hours of life and progress over 1 to 2 days, and only 10% of germinal matrix hemorrhage (GMH)-IVH occurs outside the first 7 days of age.
  - The more severe the hemorrhage, the higher the risk for posthemorrhagic ventricular dilatation to occur.
- Noncontrast CT is extremely sensitive and specific in the detection and localization of intracranial blood. Blood from acute hemorrhage has a density

on noncontrast CT higher than any normal structure, except the bone and calcium. Blood from acute hemorrhage is visualized as white as soon as a clot is formed, and this high density will slowly decrease over time.
- The radiation dose in CT, however, is significantly higher than that in routine radiography. CT now accounts for more than 60% of the radiation exposure from medical imaging in the United States (De Vries, 2020; Hall & Reavey, 2021; Inder et al., 2018; Soul, 2017; Weinman et al., 2021).

TREATMENT AND OUTCOMES
- Prevention is the best treatment.
  - *Prenatal:* Prevent premature birth. Antenatal betamethasone when delivery is not avoidable reduces the risk of IVH in single-born preterm infants, especially when a complete course is given.
  - *Optimal management of labor and delivery:* Transport in utero for delivery in a perinatal center specializing in high-risk deliveries. Avoid prolonged labor, breech delivery, perinatal asphyxia, and birth trauma. Delayed cord clamping by 30 to 120 seconds has been associated with decreased risk of IVH. Stabilize temperature.
- Acute management of IVH:
  - Maintain cerebral perfusion through the provision of adequate arterial blood pressure while preventing abrupt increases in cerebral blood flow by avoiding hyper/hypocarbia, hypoxemia, acidosis, hyperosmolar solutions, rapid volume expansion, and pneumothorax, and detecting and treating seizures.
  - Treat coagulopathies.
  - Follow with serial US to monitor for progressive ventricular dilatation (Back & Miller, 2018; Hall & Reavey, 2021; Inder et al., 2018; Soul, 2017).
- Outcomes of hemorrhages:
  - Grade I IVH has low mortality and rarely progresses to PHH.
  - Grade II IVH has increased mortality in only the less than 750-g population; 5% to 15% will progress to PHH.
  - Grade III IVH mortality rates increases to 30% in infants less than 750 g and 10% in infants greater than 750 g. Approximately 75% of the survivors will develop PHH.
  - Grade IV with periventricular infarction has 50% mortality in infants less than 750 g and approximately 20% rate in infants greater than 750 g. Nearly all survivors develop PHH (Inder et al., 2018).
  - PHH:
    - The likelihood and speed of the development of hydrocephalus due to CSF blockage after a ventricular bleed are directly related to the severity of the IVH. Hypothetically, with larger

IVHs, it may develop over days, and with smaller grade IVHs it may develop over weeks.
    - It usually develops within 1 to 3 weeks of hemorrhage.
    - Rapid head growth, signs of increased ICP, or both will follow ventricular dilatation by days to weeks.
    - It is diagnosed through serial US measuring ventricular dilatation, rate of head growth, and clinical signs of increased ICP.
    - Management and outcomes vary. Approximately 10% of infants with PHH will rapidly progress to VP shunt placement and 50% will progress or not progress. The remaining 40% will spontaneously stop increasing ventricular size (Hall & Reavey, 2021; Inder et al., 2018).

Encephalopathy of Prematurity
- *Encephalopathy of prematurity* is a term used to characterize nonhemorrhagic injury to the white and gray matter in the premature infant's brain from multiple potential causes. This damage reflects both destructions, also known as periventricular leukomalacia (PVL)/white matter injury and abnormal brain maturation with associated neuronal/axonal deficits.
- Neonatal encephalopathy results from an insult to the fetus or newborn causing a lack of oxygen and perfusion. It is associated with tissue hypoxia and acidosis.
  - Mild encephalopathy is associated with irritability, jitteriness, and hyperalertness.
  - Moderate encephalopathy is characterized by lethargy, hypotonia, a decrease in spontaneous movements, and seizures.
  - Severe encephalopathy is characterized by coma, flaccidity, disturbed brainstem function, and seizures (Heaberlin, 2019; Gressens et al., 2020; Neil & Volpe, 2018; Soul, 2017).

INCIDENCE AND ETIOLOGY
- *Periventricular* (around the ventricles), *Leuko* (white matter), *malacia* (softening or liquifying; PVL).
- These are areas of necrosis that form cysts in the deep white matter and often occur adjacent to the lateral ventricles.
- These are characterized as areas with scarcity of white matter, thinning of the corpus callosum, ventriculomegaly, and delayed myelination, in addition to decreased thalamic, striatal, hippocampus size, and cortical gray matter.
- Deep white matter is prone to necrosis due to presumed vascular end zones.
- Studies have shown that brain injury is initiated by two major mechanisms, hypoxic–ischemia and systemic infection/inflammation, which may interact and potentiate each other. These are especially

important during the vulnerable period of 23 to 32 weeks' gestation.

- Hypoxia–ischemia associated with fetal acidosis, severe respiratory distress syndrome (RDS), cardiac insufficiency, and hypotension
- Systemic inflammation due to maternal intrauterine infection, neonatal sepsis, or necrotizing enterocolitis (NEC)

- Preterm birth is a leading cause of long-term neurologic disabilities in children. This includes impairments in development, learning, behavior, and social interactions.
- A key hallmark in diffuse white matter damage is disrupted development, as seen with the blocked maturation or death of oligodendrocytes. Additionally, there is evidence of extensive involvement of axonal damage and white matter neuronal damage (Gressens et al., 2020; Neil & Volpe, 2018; Soul, 2017).

CLINICAL PRESENTATION AND ASSOCIATED FINDINGS

- The initial presentation is hypotonia and lethargy. All evaluations must be taken into consideration with the adjusted gestational age and may be difficult to interpret.
- It progresses in 6 to 10 weeks with irritability, hypertonia, increased flexion of arms with leg extension, frequent tremors and startles, and potentially abnormal Moro reflex.
- Infants may present with seizures (Neil & Volpe, 2018).

Cerebral Palsy

- CP refers to a group of nonprogressive, but often changing, motor impairment syndromes secondary to lesions of the developing brain.
  - Decreased gestational age ~100 out of every 1,000 births of infants <31 weeks are at higher risk, compared with 10 out of every 1,000 infants between 32 and 36 weeks and 1 out of every 1,000 term infants ≥37 weeks (Wilson-Costello & Payne, 2020a; Soul, 2017).
- Two common categories:
  - *Diplegia:* affects the symmetrical parts of the body
  - *Hemiplegia:* referring to spasticity isolated to one side of the body

DIAGNOSIS

- EEG may be helpful in detecting early seizures.
- CUS is good for detecting cystic PVL, although limited for detecting diffuse white matter injury.
- CT and MRI may also yield helpful diagnostic information (Gressens et al., 2020; Soul, 2017).

TREATMENT AND OUTCOMES

- Prevent preterm births.
- Provide antenatal magnesium, steroids, and antibiotics.

- Provide optimal management of labor and delivery with delayed cord clamping.
- Provide newborn management with adequate ventilation avoiding hypercarbia/hypocarbia, and adequate oxygenation avoiding hypoxia/hyperoxia; maintain adequate perfusion, recognizing pressure-passive cerebral circulation; and maintain normal arterial blood pressures for gestational age.
- Provide neurorestorative intervention: erythropoietin, optimal nutrition, individualized care, and early intervention programs.
- Periventricular white matter injury with motor deficits is frequently accompanied by reduced gray matter volume and intellectual delay.
- The major long-term morbidities seen with encephalopathy of prematurity, including PVL, are grouped together under the term *CP*.
- Long-term sequelae of PVL include spastic diplegia, and visual and cognitive deficits. Mainly there is greater spastic paresis on the lower extremities. In the more severe forms, the upper extremities are affected as well (Gressens et al., 2020; Neil & Volpe, 2018; Soul, 2017).

Hypoxic–Ischemic Encephalopathy

- *Perinatal asphyxia* refers to a condition during the first and second stage of labor in which impaired gas exchange leads to fetal acidosis, hypoxemia, and hypercarbia.
- *Perinatal hypoxia, ischemia,* and *asphyxia* are pathophysiologic terms to describe decreased oxygen, blood flow, and gas exchange, respectively.
- *Perinatal/neonatal depression* is a descriptive term pertaining to the condition of an infant upon physical examination within the first hour after birth.
- *Neonatal encephalopathy* is a clinical and not etiologic term to describe an abnormal neurobehavioral state. It does not imply an etiology.
- *Hypoxic–ischemic encephalopathy (HIE)* is used to describe clinical evidence of abnormal neurologic behavior in the term infant following perinatal asphyxia, with objective data to support the diagnosis.
- *HI brain injury* refers to the neuropathology evidenced by neuroimaging (Groenendaal & De Vries, 2020; Hall & Reavey, 2021; Hansen & Soul, 2017).

INCIDENCE AND ETIOLOGY

- HIE following severe perinatal asphyxia has an incidence of 1 to 2 per 1000 live births in the Western world. Worldwide, HIE is far more common and contributes to 20% to 40% of all neonatal deaths globally. HIE is a major cause of neonatal brain injury and mortality (Carlo, 2020; Groenendaal & De Vries, 2020; Hall & Reavey, 2021; Hansen & Soul, 2017; McAdams & Traudt, 2018).

- The etiology of HIE is multifactorial, but usually a result of a serious HI event which may be acute or prolonged.
  - Neonatal hypoxia–ischemia in most cases involves a combination of cerebral hypoxia and ischemia during bradycardia, followed by reperfusion and potential excessive oxygen distribution.
  - *Hypoxia* refers to a lack of oxygen within the circulation at the cellular level. *Ischemia* refers to deficient perfusion and, in the setting of HIE, insufficient cerebral blood flow.
  - Hypoxemia leads to brain injury principally by causing cardiovascular compromise and loss of cerebrovascular autoregulation and perfusion, which then leads to ischemia.
  - Animal experiments have shown that the immature brain is more resistant to hypoxia–ischemia than the brain of the term neonate (Groenendaal & De Vries, 2020; Hansen & Soul, 2017; Inder & Volpe, 2018a; McAdams & Traudt, 2018).
- Three features are considered to be important when considering the timing and nature of an HI event in the etiology of HIE:
  - Evidence of fetal distress and/or fetal risk of hypoxia–ischemia (e.g., fetal HR abnormalities, sentinel event, fetal acidosis)
  - The need for resuscitation and/or low Apgar scores
  - An overt neonatal neurologic syndrome in the first hours or day of life (Inder & Volpe, 2018b).
- HI injury may occur at any time shortly before birth, the birth process, or the neonatal period shortly after birth. The pattern of brain damage is reflected by the gestational age of the fetus at the time that the injury occurs (Groenendaal & De Vries, 2020; Hansen & Soul, 2017; Inder & Volpe, 2018b).
- The principal intrapartum events leading to HI fetal insults include maternal, uteroplacental, and fetal factors.
  - *Maternal:* cardiac arrest, asphyxiation, severe anaphylaxis, status epilepticus, hypovolemic shock, hypertension, and chronic vascular disease
  - *Uteroplacental:* abruptio placentae, cord prolapse, tight nuchal cord, and uterine rupture
  - *Fetal:* fetomaternal bleed, twin-to-twin transfusion syndrome, severe isoimmune hemolytic disease, fetal thrombosis, and cardiac arrest (Groenendaal & De Vries, 2020; Hansen & Soul, 2017; Inder & Volpe, 2018b; McAdams & Traudt, 2018)
- Selective neuronal necrosis is the most common variety of injury observed in neonatal HIE and refers to necrosis of the neurons in a characteristic and often widespread distribution.
- An acute HI insult leads to events that can be categorized as early (primary) and delayed (secondary) neuronal death.
  - Early or primary neuronal damage occurs as a result of cytotoxic changes caused by failure of the microcirculation, inhibition of molecular energy production, increasing extracellular acidosis, and failure of the Na+/K+-ATPase pump leading to excessive Na+ and Cl⁻ leakage into the cell with increased intracellular water (cytotoxic edema). Additional free radical production is triggered. Neuronal death occurs shortly after the time of insult if these processes are not reversed.
  - Late or secondary neuronal damage occurs as a result of recovery and reperfusion that occurs with resuscitation. This propagates a complex series of events that evolve rapidly to induce cell dysfunction and/or death (Groenendaal & De Vries, 2020; Hansen & Soul, 2017; McAdams & Traudt, 2018; Volpe, 2018b).

CLINICAL PRESENTATION AND ASSOCIATED FINDINGS

- At birth, neonates with HIE are depressed and display clinical signs consistent with neurologic injury within the first few hours after delivery. The clinical presentation may change over a period of 72 hours and is often categorized using the Sarnat staging scale.
  - *Sarnat stage 1 (mild encephalopathy):* Infants appear hyperalert with wide-open eyes, often with a "stunned look" or a blank stare, dilated pupils. Tone is normal with an increased Moro and a normal EEG.
  - *Sarnat stage 2 (moderate encephalopathy):* Infants present with decreased level of consciousness, low tone, weak suck, constricted pupils, decreased Moro reflex, and often have clinical seizures. EEG shows a low-voltage, periodic paroxysmal pattern.
  - *Sarnat stage 3 (severe encephalopathy):* Infants are difficult to arouse or are comatose with flaccid tone, intermittent decerebrate posturing (rare), absent reflexes (suck, gag, and Moro), and poorly reactive pupils. EEG has infrequent periodic discharges or is isoelectric (Groenendaal & De Vries, 2020; Hall & Reavey, 2021; Hansen & Soul, 2017; Inder & Volpe, 2018b; McAdams & Traudt, 2018).
- Clinical seizure-like activity often begins by 6 to 12 hours of age in approximately 50% to 60% of infants who ultimately have seizures.
  - Seizures occur in many infants who have sustained moderate and severe HI insult. In general, the more severe or prolonged the hypoxia–ischemia, the more seizure activity the infant will have. Seizures can be difficult to identify and may be subtle or clinically invisible. EEG is necessary for clear identification of seizure activity (Groenendaal & De Vries, 2020; Hansen & Soul, 2017; Inder & Volpe, 2018b; McAdams & Traudt, 2018).
- Multiorgan dysfunction may be evident following asphyxia.
  - The kidney is the most common organ to be affected, leading to acute tubular necrosis, oliguria, and a rise in serum creatinine.

- Cardiac dysfunction may present as ST depression and T-wave inversions. An echocardiogram may demonstrate decreased function and/or contractility.
- Pulmonary vascular resistance may remain high.
- DIC may result from liver dysfunction and depressed bone marrow production of platelets.
- GI effects include an increased risk of NEC (Hansen & Soul, 2017).

DIAGNOSIS

- The recognition of neonatal HIE depends primarily on information gathered from a careful history and a thorough neurologic examination, along with laboratory studies.
  - The history includes maternal risk factors (hypothyroidism, obesity, diabetes, fetal growth restriction, hypertension, chorioamnionitis), fetal distress (fetal HR, meconium passage, difficult labor and delivery, umbilical cord prolapse), and need for resuscitation at delivery.
  - The neurologic examination is critical in two ways. A systematic exam before 6 hours of age will allow recognition of any neonatal HIE that can lead to implementation of neuroprotective strategies, such as therapeutic hypothermia. Second, the regular and systematic neurologic examination of the infant over the first week of life carries important information for prognosis.
  - Laboratory studies are useful to evaluate multisystem organ failure common in babies with HIE. Some metabolic imbalances may significantly contribute to the severity and signs of the neurologic syndrome. A basic metabolic panel and arterial blood gas should be obtained to evaluate for hypoglycemia, hypocalcemia, hyponatremia (inappropriate secretion of ADH), hypoxemia, and acidosis that is frequently seen. Serum lactates are often elevated. Additionally, checking a complete blood count (CBC), coagulation studies, and hyperammonemia can help evaluate for metabolic complications and organ dysfunction that may occur to the liver, renal, and cardiac systems.
- Low Apgar scores (<5) at 5 and 10 minutes of age are consistent with an acute peripartum or intrapartum event resulting in HIE. Neonates with HIE who sustained an intrapartum hypoxic event typically have a fetal umbilical artery pH of less than 7.0 or base deficit greater than or equal to 12 to 15 mmol/L or both.
- Multisystem organ failure is common in babies with HIE, evidenced by metabolic and hematologic abnormalities, and hepatic, renal, GI, and cardiac dysfunction.
  - The diving reflex occurs during asphyxia to maintain blood flow to vital organs such as the brain at the expense of less vital organs. This is

believed to be the cause of systemic complications after a clinically significant HI insult. The heart, kidneys, and liver are the most vulnerable organs. Almost all babies with HIE show compromise in at least one organ system outside the brain.

- Monitoring for the presence of electrographic seizures is strongly recommended. Continuous video EEG (cEEG) is the gold standard for identifying neonatal seizures; however, amplitude-integrated EEG (aEEG) is a commonly used monitoring tool for assessing cortical electrical activity trends and detecting electrographic seizures.
- CUS is available for infants too clinically unstable to transport from the NICU; however, it has poor ability in the assessment of abnormalities of the brain or the full extent of the cerebral lesions in the full-term infant with HIE.
- CT is less sensitive than MRI in detecting changes in the central gray matter, which is the most common problem in full-term infants with HIE.
- MRI is the study of choice for neonates with HIE and is able to show different patterns of injury. MRI provides the highest sensitivity for both anatomic and functional detail and has an array of imaging options that can be tailored to the specific clinical question.
  - Conventional MRI shows the abnormalities in the first 3 to 4 days, but generally not on the first day. MRI done in the first week after birth (after rewarming, days 4–5) can assess for injury patterns consistent with HIE and rule out other potential causes.
  - MRI performed in the newborn period has a high predictive value, with and without therapeutic hypothermia treatment, for neurologic impairment at 18 months of age (Groenendaal & De Vries, 2020; Hansen & Soul, 2017; Inder & Volpe, 2018b; McAdams & Traudt, 2018).

TREATMENT AND OUTCOMES

- Ideally, prevention of HI insult is far more preferable to having to manage a newborn who has suffered an HI insult (Groenendaal & De Vries, 2020).
- Rapid recognition of peripartum HI insult is crucial and requires immediate interventions to stabilize systemic physiology, including respiratory, cardiovascular, and metabolic need, control of seizures, and commencement of neuroprotective therapy (therapeutic hypothermia), if indicated.
- Clinical and electrographic seizure activity should be assessed (e.g., with cEEG or aEEG) and controlled to limit further neurologic injury.
- Neonates with HIE often have renal injury manifesting with oliguria or anuria with elevated creatinine levels. Close monitoring of electrolytes and fluid restrictions to limit edema are recommended.
- Phenobarbital remains the preferred drug for treatment of seizures in neonatal HIE.

NEUROPROTECTIVE STRATEGIES

■ Available clinical and preclinical evidence confirms that moderate therapeutic hypothermia should be implemented as soon as possible as a standard-of-care for infants with moderate and severe HIE.

■ Timing of hypothermia for neuroprotection is based on this "therapeutic window" of 6 hours before the onset of secondary energy failure. Its effect is thought to be related to reduction of cerebral metabolism and adenosine triphosphate (ATP) consumption and downregulating many intracerebral metabolic processes associated with rapid expression of early gene activation (Chakkarapani & Thoresen, 2020; Groenendaal & De Vries, 2020; Hansen & Soul, 2017; Inder & Volpe, 2018b; McAdams & Traudt, 2018).

■ The selection of infants who may benefit from hypothermia therapy has been investigated. The American Academy of Pediatrics (AAP) endorses the following criteria for initiation of therapeutic hypothermia:
  ● Greater than 35 weeks' gestational age
  ● Less than 6 hours of age
  ● Evidence of asphyxia as defined by the presence of at least one to two of the following:
    ❑ Apgar score less than 6 at 10 minutes or continued need for resuscitation with positive pressure ventilation or chest compressions at 10 minutes
    ❑ Any acute perinatal sentinel events that may result in HIE (e.g., abruptio placentae, cord prolapse, severe fetal heart rate [FHR] abnormality)
    ❑ Cord pH <7.0 or base excess of −16 mmol/L or less; if cord pH is not available, arterial pH <7.0 or base excess less than −16 mmol/L within 60 minutes of birth
  ● Presence of moderate/severe neonatal encephalopathy on clinical examination (Chakkarapani & Thoresen, 2020; Hall & Reavey, 2021; Hansen & Soul, 2017; Inder & Volpe, 2018b)
  ● Following 72 hours of cooling, infants should be *slowly* rewarmed (0.5°C/hour). This rate is based on animal data demonstrating increased seizures and increased cortical apoptosis with rapid rewarming.

■ Long-term neurologic sequelae depend on the location of the neuronal injury. Unfortunately, despite treatment with therapeutic hypothermia, 44% of neonates with moderate to severe encephalopathy will still die or have major long-term neurodevelopmental disabilities such as CP with or without intellectual impairment (Chakkarapani & Thoresen, 2020; Groenendaal & De Vries, 2020; Hall & Reavey, 2021; Hansen & Soul, 2017; Inder & Volpe, 2018b; McAdams & Traudt, 2018).

NEONATAL SEIZURES

INCIDENCE AND ETIOLOGY

■ Neonatal seizures occur in 2 to 4 per 1,000 live births and are a cause of neonatal morbidity and mortality.

■ The incidence of seizures varies with gestational age and birth weight and is most common in the very low birth weight (VLBW) infant. The estimated incidence is 58 per 1,000 live births in the VLBW infant and 1 to 3.5 per 1,000 live births in the term infant.

■ Seizure in the neonate is the most distinctive and frequent expression of neurologic disease in the neonatal period. HIE is the most common cause of seizures in the neonatal period.

■ A *seizure* is defined clinically as a convulsive alteration in neurologic function (e.g., behavioral, motor, or autonomic function). Such a definition includes clinical activities that are associated with seizure activity identifiable on an EEG and therefore are clearly epileptic.
  ● Although the fundamental mechanisms of neonatal seizures are not entirely understood, current data suggest that excessive synchronous electrical discharge (depolarization) may occur due to the imbalance of neural excitation over neural inhibition.

■ Seizures in the newborn differ in their clinical appearances, electrographic characteristics, etiologies, management, and outcomes compared with seizures that occur later in life.

■ The majority of neonatal seizures occur in the context of acute neurologic disorders often within 1 week of the documented brain insult. Examples of the most common reasons include HIE, stroke, intracranial hemorrhage, intracranial infections, cerebral dysgenesis, hypoglycemia, and hypocalcemia. Less common but important etiologies include inborn errors of metabolism and neonatal epileptic syndromes, such as benign familial neonatal epilepsy, benign nonfamilial neonatal seizures, early myoclonic epilepsy, early infantile epileptic encephalopathy, and malignant migrating partial seizures of infancy.

■ The deleterious effects of seizures can be divided into prolonged seizures and recurrent seizures.
  ● Prolonged seizures are associated with hypoventilation and apnea, which result in hypoxemia and hypercapnia. A markedly increased cerebral metabolic rate may lead to a rapid fall in brain glucose, an increase in lactate, and a decrease in high-energy phosphate compounds. Moreover, the excessive synaptic release of certain excitotoxic amino acids (e.g., glutamate) may also lead to cellular injury.
  ● Recurrent seizures even if not prolonged are associated with long-term functional, morphologic, and physiologic deficits. The most consistent functional disorder involves deficits in cognition. Recurrent seizures also alter subsequent neuronal excitability and lead to previously normal brain tissue alteration to be more seizure-prone; in addition, ion channel changes also contribute to permanent changes in excitability (Abend et al., 2018; Hall & Reavey, 2021; Inder, 2020; Inder & Volpe, 2018b; McAdams & Traudt, 2018; Natarajan & Gospe, 2018; Sansevere & Bergin, 2017).

- Seizures are associated with a markedly accelerated cerebral metabolic rate, and this acceleration may lead to a rapid fall in brain glucose, an increase in lactate, and a decrease in high-energy phosphate compounds. Moreover, the excessive synaptic release of certain excitotoxic amino acids (e.g., glutamate) may also lead to cellular injury (Groenendaal & De Vries, 2020; Hansen & Soul, 2017; Inder & Volpe, 2018b; McAdams & Traudt, 2018).

CLINICAL PRESENTATION AND ASSOCIATED FINDINGS

- Recognition of seizures in the newborn period can be difficult due to subtle or absent clinical signs. EEG monitoring now plays a critical role in seizure recognition within the NICU.
- A consensus statement on neonatal EEG terminology by the American Clinical Neurophysiology Society defines three types of neonatal seizures: (a) clinical-only seizures, where there is a sudden paroxysm or abnormal clinical change that does not correlate with simultaneous EEG seizure; (b) electroclinical seizures, where there is a clinical seizure coupled with an associated EEG seizure; and (c) EEG-only seizures, where there is an EEG seizure that is not associated with any outward visible clinical signs, also known as subclinical, nonconvulsive, or occult seizures.
- Classifications of neonatal seizures:
  - A *clonic seizure* is defined as a seizure characterized by rhythmic movements of muscle groups which consist of a rapid phase followed by a slow return movement. Clonic seizures appear as repetitive and rhythmic jerking movements that can affect any part of the body, including the face, extremities, and even diaphragmatic or pharyngeal muscles. They are divided into focal and multifocal.
    - ❏ Focal seizures are rhythmic movements of muscle groups in a focal distribution that consist of a rapid phase followed by a slow return movement, to be distinguished from the symmetric movements of jitteriness. Gentle flexion of the affected body part does not suppress the tremor, whereas it will with jitteriness.
    - ❏ Multifocal or migratory clonic seizures spread over body parts either in a random or anatomic fashion. This seizure movement may alternate from side to side and appear asynchronously between the two halves of the body. The migration most often "marches" through the body (e.g., left arm jerking may be followed by right leg jerking).
  - *Tonic seizures* are defined as a sustained flexion or extension of muscle groups in the appendages. This can affect the limbs, but also the eye muscles, with sustained eye deviation or the head, resulting in head version. Tonic seizures may be epileptic

or nonepileptic, with bilateral tonic extension not having a correlate on EEG.

- *Myoclonic seizures* are demonstrated by movements which are rapid, lightning fast jerks. Myoclonus can occur at multiple levels of the nervous system: cortical regions, brainstem, and spinal cord. In some instances, myoclonus is benign, such as benign sleep myoclonus of the newborn. In preterm infants, myoclonus can occur without nervous system abnormalities.
  - ❏ There are three categories of myoclonic seizures: focal, multifocal, and generalized myoclonic seizures. Focal myoclonic seizures typically involve the flexor muscles of an upper extremity. Multifocal myoclonic seizures are characterized by asynchronous twitching of several parts of the body. Generalized myoclonic seizures are characterized by bilateral jerks and flexion of the upper and occasionally lower limbs.
- Subtle seizure activity is the most frequently observed category of neonatal seizures and includes repetitive buccolingual movements, orbital-ocular movements, unusual bicycling or pedaling, and autonomic findings such as tachycardia, elevated blood pressure, apnea, pupillary change, drooling, and cutaneous vasomotor phenomena. Subtle seizures are notoriously difficult to determine clinically, where often one must first be aware of the neonate's typical behaviors, movements, and autonomic findings and then identify unexplained alterations of these patterns.
- EEG-only (subclinical, nonconvulsive, occult) seizures have been identified to represent 80% to 90% of all seizures and can only be identified on EEG monitoring. There is no associated clinical activity to the electrographic seizure, which results in the inability to detect seizure without EEG monitoring and seriously underestimates true seizure frequency. Additionally, in infants with medically treated seizure activity, clinically evident seizure may terminate while electrographic seizure persists. This is known as electromechanical uncoupling on electromechanical dissociation (Abend et al., 2018; Hall & Reavey, 2021; Heaberlin, 2019; Inder, 2020; Natarajan & Gospe, 2018; Sansevere & Bergin, 2017).

DIAGNOSIS

- Sampling and examination of either blood and/or CSF may assist in identification of a possible etiology of the seizures.
- Neonatal seizures are often brief and subtle in appearance, thus raising diagnostic uncertainty when unusual movements are present. As newborns may have behaviors that mimic movements concerning for seizure, and those at high risk of seizures may develop movements that are nonepileptic in addition

to seizures, further testing is imperative to limit overtreatment as well as underrecognition of events.

- Conventional EEG is the gold standard for neonatal seizure detection. Continuous monitoring of neonates with EEG is recommended in certain populations, including instances where there is suspicion for neonatal seizures to occur, such as in acute brain injury secondary to perinatal asphyxia, neonates with clinically suspected seizures, or when neonatal epilepsy is suspected.
- Many institutions incorporate aEEG to aid in the detection of seizures. Two or four scalp leads are used to obtain a raw tracing of information. This signal is processed and time-compressed, creating a single channel tracing per hemisphere. Advantages of aEEG include bedside availability and interpretation, as well as reduced cost, as compared with cEEG monitoring. Disadvantages of aEEG include its inability to detect brief or low-amplitude seizures, or seizures that may occur in other parts of the brain not monitored by the two or four probes. Additional limitations include being prone to artifactual signals from movement, high-frequency oscillator ventilation, or ECMO.
- MRI can provide evidence of injury or malformation (Inder, 2020; Inder & Volpe, 2018b; Natarajan & Gospe, 2018; Sansevere & Bergin, 2017).

TREATMENT AND OUTCOMES

- Efforts should be geared toward detecting correctable causes of neonatal seizures. Hypoglycemia, hypocalcemia, or sodium disturbances should be corrected. Pyridoxine-dependent epilepsy is an important etiologic consideration requiring treatment with enteral vitamin B_6.
- AEDs are used once metabolic derangements are addressed. The initial first-line AED used is phenobarbital, administered intravenously in a loading dose of 20 mg/kg. This dosing is necessary to achieve a blood level of approximately 20 mcg/mL, which achieves a measurable anticonvulsant effect in the newborn. Maintenance dose is 4 mg/kg/d. Total loading doses of phenobarbital in excess of 40 to 50 mg/kg and levels above 40 mcg/mL generally do not provide extra benefit.
- Treatment choices beyond phenobarbital vary greatly between providers. The best evidence is for phenytoin or fosphenytoin. These drugs are often used as second-line medications for infants who continue to experience electrographic or clinical seizures after as much as 40 mg/kg of phenobarbital, or in the severely asphyxiated infant in whom less than the full phenobarbital loading dose is deemed appropriate due to cardiopulmonary concerns.
  - Fosphenytoin is dosed in *phenytoin equivalents* (1.5 mg of fosphenytoin yields approximately 1 mg of phenytoin), and the effective dose is essentially identical to that described for phenytoin. The 20 mg/kg loading dose of phenytoin results in a therapeutic blood level of approximately 15 to 20 mcg/kg.
- Approximately 20% or more of newborns with electrographic seizures do not respond to the

sequential administration of phenobarbital and phenytoin. Benzodiazepines, such as midazolam, diazepam, or lorazepam, may also be used to control refractory neonatal seizures.

- As a newer anticonvulsant medication, levetiracetam has become a medication used for treatment of refractory neonatal seizures. In some centers, it is used as a second-line agent before using phenytoin, benzodiazepines, or lidocaine. Although levetiracetam use is increasing, few data are available regarding its efficacy.
  - Other anticonvulsants used to treat seizures may include lidocaine, sodium valproate, carbamazepine, oxcarbazepine, felbamate, vigabatrin, and lamotrigine.
- The optimal duration of anticonvulsant therapy for newborns with seizures relates principally to the likelihood of seizure recurrence if the drugs are discontinued. Three key determinants are considered. First, an abnormal neonatal neurologic exam at the time of discharge increases the risk of seizure recurrence by 50%. Second, the initial cause of the seizure has different risks of recurrence. HIE has a risk of 30% to 60%, while the risk of cortical dysgenesis is 100%. Last is the background EEG pattern. Patterns with marked depression on the tracing developed subsequent epilepsy. The length of time to treat with AED therapy for neonatal seizures remains unknown. The length of treatment has been minimized due to additional concern of the effects of AEDs on the immature brain.
- The etiology of a newborn's seizure largely accounts for the overall outcome. Half of infants with seizures due to HIE will have normal development, while 10% of infants with seizures related to IVH will have normal development.
  - Newborns with seizures acutely in the neonatal period remain at an approximately 25% risk of developing epilepsy, defined as recurrent unprovoked seizures, later in life. Neonates with refractory seizures requiring multiple AEDs, those with severe brain injury, or those with persistent interictal epileptiform discharges on EEG have the highest risk.
  - The incidence of neurologic sequelae in infants with seizures is as much as 40-fold greater than the incidence in those without seizures (Abend et al., 2018; Hall & Reavey, 2021; Inder, 2020; Inder & Volpe, 2018b; Natarajan & Gospe, 2018; Sansevere & Bergin, 2017).

NONEPILEPTIC NEONATAL MOVEMENTS

INCIDENCE AND ETIOLOGY

- Infants are prone to a variety of movements that can raise concern for seizures but are actually nonneurologic in nature. Approximately 44% of healthy term infants have been noted to experience some such movements.

- These nonepileptic movements can be from maternal medications such as selective serotonin reuptake inhibitors (SSRIs) or illicit drug usage such as cocaine and marijuana. They can also be caused by metabolic derangements such as hypoglycemia or hypocalcemia, as well as intracranial hemorrhage and/or hypothermia (Natarajan & Gospe, 2018).

CLINICAL PRESENTATION AND ASSOCIATED FINDINGS

- Tremors can mimic subtle seizure activities like bicycling and chewing. The difference between tremors and seizures is that there are equal phases and amplitude of flexion and extension. Tremors can be asymmetric and spontaneous, and can occur with tactile and environmental stimulation.
- Jittery movements are rhythmic-like tremulous movement patterns that are characterized by trembling of the hands and feet. Five characteristics aid in distinguishing between jitteriness and seizure:
  - There are no eye movements involved with jitteriness.
  - Jitteriness is very sensitive to stimulus, while seizures are not.
  - Tremor (rhythmic, alternating movements with equal rate and amplitude) is the dominant movement in jitteriness, while the dominant movement in seizures is clonic jerking (movement with a fast and slow component).
  - Jitteriness can be stopped with passive flexion of the affected extremity, while seizures cannot.
  - Jitteriness is not accompanied by autonomic changes (tachycardia, elevated blood pressure, apnea, pupillary change, drooling, cutaneous vasomotor phenomena), while seizures often are.
- *Nonepileptic myoclonus* is defined as a sequence of repetitive nonrhythmic movement caused by sudden involuntary contraction or relaxation of the muscles. Preterm infants are most vulnerable to this nonepileptic movement. It is mostly noted while the infant is asleep or sleeping and resolves when awake. These movements can be exacerbated or provoked by

treatment with benzodiazepines and resolve within approximately 2 months.

- Pathologic myoclonus is attributed to a brainstem release from loss of cortical inhibition of the lower circuits. It is frequently seen in infants with severe global brain injury from HIE and severe IVH, as well as toxic-metabolic disturbances including drug withdrawal and glycine encephalopathy. These babies have abnormal neurologic exams and abnormal background EEG.
- Dyskinesias are involuntary movements that appear as abnormal posturing. In the neonate, it often represents intrapartum or antepartum injury particularly to the basal ganglia. This is commonly mistaken for seizures in the neonatal period. Dystonia is the involuntary sustained or intermittent co-contraction of agonist and antagonist muscles resulting in abnormal posture. EEG is necessary to correctly diagnose and treat (Abend et al., 2018; Inder, 2020; Natarajan & Gospe, 2018).

DIAGNOSIS
- cEEG (Natarajan & Gospe, 2018)

TREATMENT AND OUTCOMES
- When properly diagnosed, most infants do not need medical intervention and will outgrow these movements as the CNS matures.

▶ CONCLUSION

The developing neurologic system is fragile, yet resilient. Postnatal function depends heavily on uncompromised fetal development. Mitigating influences that can lead to neurologic dysfunction are often beyond our control. However, clinicians should maintain a high level of understanding regarding the physiologic and pathophysiologic processes of the neonatal neurologic system to aid in appropriately preventing, diagnosing, and managing the various types of neurologic insults. Health team members should also assess parents and caregivers for altered psychosocial integrity, knowledge deficits, and ineffective coping skills related to the uncertainty and/or finality of the short-term and long-term outcomes of neurologic dysfunction.

1. Seizures evidenced by repetitive rhythmic jerking of an extremity that starts in one arm and then moves to the other are known as:

   A. Clonic seizures

   B. Focal tonic seizures

   C. Multifocal clonic seizures

2. The neonatal nurse practitioner (NNP) distinguishes holoprosencephaly through the findings of:

   A. A hypoplastic nose, ocular hypotelorism, and abnormal dentition

   B. Midface hypoplasia and short limbs

   C. Overlapping suture and severe microcephaly

3. An intraventricular hemorrhage (IVH) with accompanying dilated ventricles best describes the hemorrhage at grade:

   A. II

   B. III

   C. IV

4. A 34-year-old primigravida came for antenatal checkup at 24 weeks of gestation. On examination, the size of the uterus is consistent with 32 weeks of gestation. Laboratory investigations show markedly increased serum alpha-fetoprotein, and ultrasonography shows an abnormally formed head with a defective skull. The neonatal nurse practitioner (NNP) recognizes this prenatal report indicates signs of possible failure of:

   A. Germ cell proliferation

   B. Migratory germ cells location

   C. Rostral neuropore tube closure

5. The neonatal nurse practitioner (NNP) knows that, based on pathologic processes, the presence and the maximum extent of an intraventricular hemorrhage (IVH) cannot be determined until:

   A. 3 days of age

   B. 5 days of age

   C. 7 days of age

6. The neonatal nurse practitioner (NNP) notes on physical exam asymmetry in the eyes, forehead, and nose, which results in a unilateral flattening of the forehead, and correctly documents the finding as:

   A. Cebocephaly

   B. Plagiocephaly

   C. Scaphocephaly

7. The neonatal nurse practitioner (NNP) educates neonatal nurses when providing care to the extremely premature neonate in the use of careful handling and positioning to avoid cerebral blood flow:

   A. Autoregulation

   B. Overflow

   C. Shunting

(See answers next page.)

1. C) Multifocal clonic seizures

Multifocal or migratory clonic seizures spread over body parts either in a random or anatomic fashion. This seizure movement may alternate from side to side and appear asynchronously between the two halves of the body. The migration most often "marches" through the body (e.g., left arm jerking may be followed by right leg jerking; Abend et al., 2018). Focal and clonic seizures are characterized by rhythmic movements of muscle groups which consist of a rapid phase followed by a slow return movement.

2. A) A hypoplastic nose, ocular hypotelorism, and abnormal dentition

Facial anomalies are present in up to 80% to 90% of holoprosencephaly cases. The findings may range from mild, with hypotelorism or a single central front tooth, to more severe anomalies, such as cyclopia (a single central eye) with a nose-like structure (proboscis) above the eye or cebocephaly (a flattened single nostril situated centrally between the eyes). There may even be a complete absence of the eye or nasal structure. Severe skull and facial malformations, such as overlapping sutures, severe microcephaly, and midface hypoplasia, are often associated with other types of malformations (du Plessis & Volpe, 2018b; Huang & Doherty, 2018).

3. B) III

Hemorrhage with distention causing ventricle dilatation. Blood fills more than 50% of the ventricle. Blood in the lateral ventricle without ventricular dilatation is consistent with grade II, and a grade IV hemorrhagic infarct or stroke in the periventricular white matter is not an extension of an IVH (De Vries, 2020).

4. C) Rostral neuropore tube closure

Encephalocele arise from a failed closure of part of the rostral neural tube and most commonly occurs in the occipital region (70%–80%) with a sac protruding at the base of the skull or top of the neck. The remaining 20% to 30% are in the parietal, frontonasal, intranasal, or nasopharyngeal region (Huang & Doherty, 2018). A neuronal migration that results in a smooth appearance of the cortical surface of the brain caused by absent or reduced gyri. Proliferation of germ cell layers is not visible on prenatal ultrasound.

5. C) 7 days of age

Studies have shown that the majority of all hemorrhages occur within the first week of life and a single scan at the end of that week shows 90% of all hemorrhages as well as their maximum extent. IVH identified at 3 or 5 days may still extend or increase by 7 days of age (De Vries, 2020).

6. B) Plagiocephaly

Premature fusing of a coronal suture creates asymmetry in the eyes, forehead, and nose, causing a flattening of the forehead on the same side of the fused suture. This is commonly known as plagiocephaly. Scaphocephaly denotes an elongated appearance of the skull, while cebocephaly denotes a flattened single nostril situated centrally between the eyes (Blackburn, 2018; du Plessis & Volpe, 2018b; Evans et al., 2018; Hall & Reavey, 2021; Huang & Doherty, 2018; Johnson, 2018; Temei & Smith, 2020; Volpe, 2018a).

7. B) Overflow

A factor that puts premature infants at higher risk for hemorrhage is the lack of ability to autoregulate their cerebral blood flow. Without autoregulation, the cerebral blood flow is in a pressure-passive state, unprotected from wide swings or changes and large volume shifts, possibly into overflows. The more premature the infant, the more time spent in a pressure-passive state. Shunting away from the brain by active physiologic means does not occur as the brain is sustained ahead of all other organs (Neil & Volpe, 2018).

The Metabolic/Endocrine System

Elena Bosque

▶ INTRODUCTION

Many neonatal nurse practitioners (NNP), as well as other care providers, are intimidated by neonatal metabolic or endocrine system problems due to the fear of making an incorrect diagnosis or treatment plan with, potentially, devastating consequences. The goal of this chapter is to alleviate those fears and to provide an overview of the problem in conceptual terms and a general approach to care which can be applied to cases that the NNP may encounter. The learner is encouraged to refer to the texts in the references for entire lists and explanations of all of the specific disorders.

The pathophysiology and treatment sections will be presented as metabolic and endocrine disorders. Metabolic disorders include those of carbohydrate, fat, and protein metabolism; problems of infants of diabetic mothers (IDM); and inborn errors of metabolism. Endocrine disorders include those of calcium, phosphorus, and magnesium metabolism; osteopenia; and thyroid, pituitary, and adrenal disorders, including disorders of sex development. There is some overlap among these categories because there is some overlap with these conditions. For example, problems of IDMs can be categorized as either or both a metabolic disorder, due to problems of carbohydrate metabolism, and an endocrine disorder, due to abnormal hormone production, with hyperinsulinism.

The NNP is expected to be able to identify typical clinical expressions of these disorders, to describe appropriate first line interventions in collaboration with a neonatologist, to refer to a subspecialist, and to talk to parents about these problems. These activities involve anticipatory guidance of all team members to establish rigorous systems for obtaining, reporting, and responding to newborn screening results. Expected competencies include familiarity with characteristic signs and symptoms, communication with and integration of family members related to diagnosis and plan of care, and communication with subspecialists regarding inpatient and follow-up services (Merritt & Gallagher, 2018).

▶ OVERVIEW OF DISORDERS

- Metabolic or endocrine disorders of the newborn include problems known as inborn errors of metabolism and encompass both metabolic and biochemical genetic diseases.
  - Some of the expressions of metabolic disorders overlap with endocrine disorders, such as hypothyroidism and congenital adrenal hyperplasia (CAH).
  - Most conditions involve gene mutation, which causes an absent or defective enzyme; or over- or underproduction of hormones, with life-threatening physiologic or biochemical system regulation dysfunction.
- Collectively, the incidence of metabolic or endocrine disorders is estimated to be approximately 1 per 1,000 to 2,000 live births. Newborn screening has identified disorders in 1 per 2,000 to 4,000 live births. The most common disorders, such as phenylketonuria (PKU), occur approximately 1 per 10,000 to 15,000 live births. Conversely, some disorders occur rarely, such as homocystinuria, which is diagnosed in approximately 1 per 1,800 to 1 per 900,000 live births.
- It is possible that the incidence of metabolic or endocrine disorders is underestimated if conditions are undetected. It is important to remember that multiple disorders of intermediary metabolism and energy metabolism are not detected through newborn screening. Intermediary metabolic disorders include aminoacidopathies, organic acidemias, and fatty acid oxidation disorders.
- Many of these disorders are present during the neonatal period and are revealed as the protective effect of the maternal placenta ceases. Disorders then develop as acute, chronic, or progressive diseases, with potential life-threatening harm.
  - The normal transition from the maternal–fetal transport of nutrients to extrauterine homeostasis of the neonate may be disrupted by metabolic problems or dysfunction of regulatory systems.

■ Most neonates with metabolic or endocrine disorders are healthy at birth and present with nonspecific signs in hours or days after birth, and most are inherited in an autosomal recessive manner.

■ If undiagnosed, many metabolic or endocrine disorders have profound negative consequences for the individual (El-Hattab & Sutton, 2017; Swartz & Chan, 2018; Wassner & Belfort, 2018). In modern neonatology, with the standard use of the expanded newborn screen, diagnosis and treatment usually occur early and before symptomatic presentation, and treatment can occur before the condition harms the individual.

■ Because some of the disorders present early, before the results of the newborn screen are known, or are not identified by the screen, it is important for health care providers to be able to identify clinical manifestations of these disorders, to provide initial care, and to recognize appropriate times to involve subspecialists.

■ Diagnosis of neonatal metabolic or endocrine problems is challenging for most clinicians. Nonspecific presentations and individual rarity of diseases mean limited exposure for clinicians. Inherited metabolic or endocrine disorders will not be diagnosed unless specific investigations for that disorder are undertaken. It becomes important to understand basic pathophysiology and to develop an approach to the investigation upon presentation of symptoms (Cederbaum, 2018; Divall & Merjaneh, 2018; El-Hattab & Sutton, 2017; Garg & Devaskar, 2020; Konczal & Zinn, 2020; Koves et al., 2018; Merritt & Gallagher, 2018; Thomas et al., 2018; Woo et al., 2021).

▶ PHYSIOLOGY AND PATHOPHYSIOLOGY

METABOLIC DISORDERS IN THE NEONATE

Disorders of Carbohydrate Metabolism

■ Although the fetus is entirely dependent on the mother for nutrients, it is hormonally independent. Maternal glucose is the major nutrient and the only source of fetal glucose. Fetal hormone responses are mediated by maternal supply of nutrients, even as maternal concentration fluctuates with pathology, as in the case of maternal diabetes.

■ At birth, when maternal supply of nutrients ceases, there is a surge of levels of epinephrine, norepinephrine, and glucagon in the neonate. This causes a fall in insulin level to mobilize glycogen and stimulate gluconeogenesis, resulting in an initial rise, then a steady glucose production.

■ In healthy full-term newborn infants, the plasma glucose concentration remains at a steady level of 40 to 80 mg/dL. Breastfed, small-for-gestational-age, and premature infants may have lower steady-state glucose levels.

● Most investigators have defined hypoglycemia as plasma glucose level lower than 45 mg/dL in the first 24 hours of life, and preprandial glucose less than 50 mg/dL up to 48 hours of age and less than 60 mg/dL after 48 hours of age as meeting the criteria for hypoglycemia (Garg & Devaskar, 2020; Mandy & Suresh, 2020).

HYPERINSULINEMIA

■ Transient hyperinsulinism may result in neonatal hypoglycemia secondary to being an IDM, being under perinatal stress, or being small for gestational age.

■ Hyperinsulinism, which results in incalcitrant hypoglycemia, is usually related to metabolic disorders associated with genetic mutations or tumors.

● Diagnostic criteria for the diagnosis of hyperinsulinism are based on a critical sample at the time of hypoglycemia and include:
  ❑ Insulin level >2 μIU/mL
  ❑ Beta-hydroxybutyrate level <1.8 mmol/L
  ❑ Free fatty acid level <1.7 mmol/L
  ❑ Glucose rise ≥30 mg/dL after glucagon administration
  ❑ Insulin-like growth factor-binding protein 1 level ≤110 ng/mL

● Normal insulin levels associated with transient hypoglycemia may be caused by immaturity, increased metabolic expenditure, or maternal conditions.

● If hypoglycemia persists in the presence of normal insulin levels, this may be caused by endocrine disorders such as hypopituitarism or primary adrenal insufficiency or inborn errors of metabolism (see later sections; Blackburn, 2021; Werny et al., 2018).

HYPOGLYCEMIA

■ Any alteration in either maternal metabolism or intrinsic metabolic problems of the neonate may cause hypoglycemia.

● Transient hypoglycemia, during the transition period after birth, may require brief surveillance and intervention, but resolves. It is usually the consequence of changes in the metabolic environment in utero, maternal drugs (e.g., tocolytics, diuretics, propranolol), or perinatally.

● Persistent or recurrent hypoglycemia is a problem which requires prolonged management, including high rates of glucose infusions for several hours, or potentially days, or pharmacologic intervention, such as use of diazoxide. Persistent hypoglycemia is the product of intrinsic metabolic problems of the infant, such as hyperinsulinism, congenital disorders, endocrine disorders, or inborn errors of metabolism.

■ Defects of any of the enzymes in the carbohydrate metabolic pathways will result in the pathogenesis of many organs, including the liver, kidney, brain, heart, intestine, ovaries, and skin.

- These disorders include galactosemia, glycogen storage diseases (GSD), and fructose-1-6-phosphatase deficiency.
- For example, infants with galactosemia often present with severe jaundice and coagulopathy, while infants with other disorders of carbohydrate metabolism may present with hypoglycemia, lactic acidosis, infection, or intestinal problems.

■ Many of the disorders of carbohydrate metabolism are confirmed through newborn screening and genetic testing. Hyperinsulinemia will be diagnosed with measurement of glucose, insulin, cortisol, beta-hydroxybutyrate, and free fatty acid levels. Treatment approaches vary by disorder, but may include dietary, medication, or vitamin management (Blackburn, 2018; Burris, 2017; Garg & Devaskar, 2020; Mandy & Suresh, 2020; Merritt & Gallagher, 2018; Werny et al., 2018).

INFANTS OF DIABETIC MOTHERS

■ The incidence of neonatal hypoglycemia in IDMs varies from 5% to 50%, with a lower incidence rate in infants of mothers with good glycemic control in pregnancy.

- The reported rates vary due to controversies and inconsistencies in the medical literature with the definitions of hypoglycemia.

■ IDMs, who experience intermittent fetal hyperglycemia in response to maternal hyperglycemia, develop hypertrophic pancreatic islets and beta cells with increased fetal insulin secretion.

- These fetuses and infants have high stores of glycogen and fat.
- These fetuses and infants are at risk of numerous morbidities, including congenital anomalies, heart failure, cardiac septal hypertrophy, surfactant deficiency, respiratory distress syndrome, persistent pulmonary hypertension, hyperbilirubinemia, hypoglycemia, hypocalcemia, hypomagnesemia, macrosomia, nerve injury related to birth trauma, renal vein thrombosis, small left colon, unexplained intrauterine demise, polycythemia, visceromegaly, neurosensory impairment, and predisposition to obesity and diabetes later in life.

■ Neonatal hypoglycemia in IDMs is most likely due to hyperinsulinism. The fetus was hyperglycemic in relation to maternal hyperglycemia and responded with production of insulin.

- Despite high energy stores, after birth, the amount of insulin production remains the same, with less neonatal glucose supply, so the neonate has hypoglycemia in the first few hours of life, which may persist for several days.

■ Symptoms may include sweating, pallor, tachycardia, tachypnea, tremor, "jittery," abnormal cry (weak or high-pitched), hypotonia, weak suck, lethargy, coma, and seizure. Polycythemia is an associated feature related to increased erythropoiesis.

- Not all infants with hypoglycemia, as defined in the medical literature, have symptoms or adverse effects.

■ Treatment of IDMs with hypoglycemia may include early feeding, frequent feeding, oral dextrose gel (40%), and intravenous dextrose administration. Central venous catheter placement is recommended for dextrose concentration greater than 12.5%, with careful calculation of fluids and glucose index rate (mg/kg/min), then judicious weaning over the first days or weeks of life (Burris, 2017; Dysart, 2020; Garg & Devaskar, 2020; Gorman, 2017; Werny et al., 2018).

Disorders of Fat Metabolism

■ Lipids are necessary for retinal and neuronal development, including myelin sheath synthesis.

- Essential fatty acids (EFAs) and linoleic acids are essential for brain, retinal, prostaglandin, thromboxane, and leukotriene development.
- Cholesterol is necessary for embryogenesis, cell membrane growth and function, bile acid synthesis, and steroid production.
- The fetus is somewhat dependent on placental transfer of lipids, with some lipogenesis occurring in the fetal liver and other tissue.

■ The transition of the fetus to extrauterine life includes lipid mobilization.

- As with carbohydrates, an increase in catecholamines and glucagon, with a decrease in insulin levels and a surge in thyroid hormones, promotes fatty acid mobilization and glucagon production.
- The newborn changes from glucose to fatty acid oxidative metabolism to conserve glucose for the brain.
- Free fatty acid production is used by the heart and brain in the absence of glucose and results in ketone bodies.

■ Lipogenesis is dependent on cholesterol metabolism and substrate availability. Lipogenic precursors include glucose, lactate, and ketone bodies. During anaerobic metabolism, for example, during asphyxia, inefficient anaerobic glycolysis cannot meet energy requirements, resulting in precursors of gluconeogenesis, including lactate, pyruvate, and glycerol.

■ Any disruption of enzyme activity in fatty acid metabolism will result in failure of oxidation within or transport of free fatty acids into the mitochondria. This transport activity depends on carnitine.

- These disorders lead to a deficit in energy production and can be life-threatening.
- Infants with these disorders present after a few days of life, in a catabolic state, with breakdown of fatty acids from adipose tissue. This may occur before newborn screening results are known.

- These infants may present with hypoglycemia, liver problems, cardiomyopathy, cardiac dysrhythmias, skeletal myopathy, and retinal degeneration.
- Diagnosis of many fatty acid oxidation disorders is made with plasma acylcarnitine levels, free carnitine levels, and genetic testing.
  - These disorders include long-chain acyl-coenzyme A (CoA) dehydrogenase deficiency (LCHADD), multiple acyl-CoA dehydrogenase deficiency (MADD), medium-chain acyl-CoA dehydrogenase deficiency (MCADD), short-chain acyl-CoA dehydrogenase deficiency (SCADD), and very-long-chain acyl-CoA dehydrogenase deficiency (VLCADD).
- Many of the devastating organ effects of these disorders may be avoided with early treatment. Some of these disorders require avoidance of dietary fat, so breastfeeding may be contraindicated.
- Treatment may include frequent feedings, avoidance of fasting, and diet, medication, or vitamin management (Blackburn, 2018; Garg & Devaskar, 2020; Merritt & Gallagher, 2018).

Disorders of Protein Metabolism

- Amino acids are necessary for protein synthesis and oxidative activities during organ development and tissue remodeling. Some amino acids are used for energy.
- After birth, the newborn is in a catabolic state relative to the anabolic state during fetal life. Serum amino acids are higher in newborns than later in life. The newborn infant has limited ability to synthesize amino acids, partly due to limited liver enzyme function.
- An infant with a disorder in protein metabolism may present with hypoglycemia, poor feeding, vomiting, odor, hypothermia, respiratory distress, hyperammonemia, azotemia, metabolic acidosis, ketosis, cholestasis, hepatosplenomegaly, lymphadenopathy, or hematologic problems.
  - These defects may lead to cirrhosis, renal dysfunction, cardiomyopathy, central nervous system abnormalities, developmental delay, or death.
- Some amino acid metabolic disorders are associated with dysmorphic features, while some are not. The most common inborn error of amino acid metabolism is PKU, which affects approximately 1 in 12,000 live births.
  - It is an autosomal recessive disorder from deficiency of phenylalanine hydroxylase required to convert phenylalanine to tyrosine.
  - PKU was the first disorder detected by the development of the newborn screen in the 1960s.
  - Since tyrosine is elemental to the production of dopamine and other essential neurotransmitters, infants with this disorder experience developmental and intellectual disabilities, skin problems, and epilepsy.
  - Treatment for PKU is lifelong dietary therapy.
- The diagnosis of amino acid metabolic disorders may be made, depending on the disorder, by newborn screening; plasma, urine, and cerebral spinal fluid amino acid analysis; plasma acyl-carnitine analysis; urine organic acid analysis; chromatography; tandem mass spectrometry; in vitro cell studies of cultured skin fibroblasts; enzyme assay; or genetic testing.
  - Treatment for some of these disorders may include diet, vitamin supplementation, or liver transplantation; however, with some of these disorders, there is no known effective treatment (Blackburn, 2018; El-Hattab & Sutton, 2017; Konczal & Zinn, 2020; Merritt & Gallagher, 2018; Sahai & Levy, 2018).

INBORN ERRORS OF METABOLISM

- Inborn errors of metabolism are also known as inherited metabolic disease.
  - Enzyme proteins normally catalyze metabolic processes, and thousands of enzymes are required to perform critical biochemical reactions for processing or transport of amino acids, carbohydrates, or fatty acids.
  - The substance upon which the enzyme acts is the substrate.
- With absence or deficiency of these enzymes, the substrate molecules accumulate and may be converted to products that are not usually present. These alternative end products also interfere with normal metabolic processes. Finally, there is an inability to degrade end products.
  - Symptoms result from increased levels of normal substrate that become toxic, or lack of normal end products necessary for cellular function.
  - The toxic levels of metabolites or deficient cellular function can lead to decreased muscle tone, seizures, organ failure, blindness, deafness, mental retardation, and death.
- Various strategies for conceptualization, classification, evaluation, and treatment of inborn errors of metabolism that present in the newborn period or later have been proposed.
  - Inborn errors of metabolism are presented in this chapter as small molecule disorders, lysosomal storage disorders, energy metabolism disorders, and heterogenous disorders.
  - In Table 18.1, classification groups, examples of metabolic problems, examples of some common specific disorders, and treatments are presented (Cederbaum, 2018; El-Hattab & Sutton, 2017; Konczal & Zinn, 2020).

Table 18.1 Example of a Classification System for Neonatal Inborn Errors of Metabolism

Group	Metabolic Problem	Disorder	Treatment
Small molecule disorders	▪ Amino acids ▪ Organic acids ▪ Sugars	▪ Include aminoacidemias, for example, phenylketonuria, organic acidurias, urea cycle disorders, sugar intolerances, for example, galactosemia	▪ Diet ▪ Extracorporeal procedures ▪ Renal replacement therapy ▪ Dialysis ▪ Drugs ▪ Vitamins
Lysosomal storage disorders	▪ Lipids ▪ Glycoproteins ▪ Glycolipids ▪ Mucopolysaccharides ▪ Sphingolipids	▪ Include diseases with lysosomal, defects, for example, glycogen storage disease type II (Pompe), Gaucher, Niemann–Pick type A or type B, Krabbe, Fabry disease, or mucopolysaccharidosis	▪ Mostly untreatable ▪ Some new or experimental enzyme, organ transplant, or gene therapy
Energy metabolism disorders	▪ Inborn errors of metabolism that affect the cytoplasmic and mitochondrial energetic processes ▪ Oxidation disorders ▪ Fatty acid mobilization and metabolism disorders ▪ Glycogen storage diseases	▪ Include cytoplasmic defects, encompass those affecting glycolysis, glycogenosis, gluconeogenesis, hyperinsulinism (most treatable) ▪ Creatine (partly treatable) and pentose phosphate pathways (untreatable) ▪ Mitochondrial defects including respiratory chain disorders, and Krebs cycle and pyruvate oxidation defects (mostly untreatable) ▪ Disorders of fatty acid oxidation and ketone bodies (treatable)	▪ For some, dextrose, diet, and supplements ▪ For others, no treatment
Heterogenous	▪ Carbohydrate-deficient glycoprotein disorders ▪ Peroxisomal biogenesis disorders ▪ Cholesterol biosynthetic disorders ▪ Disorders of biogenic amines, folate, and pyridoxine ▪ Transport disorders ▪ Purine and pyrimidine metabolism disorders ▪ Receptor disorders	▪ Include Smith–Lemli–Opitz syndrome, mevalonic aciduria, folate deficiencies, Fanconi syndrome, Menkes disease, Zellweger syndrome, X-linked adrenoleukodystrophy, and so on	▪ For some, nutritional, dietary, or vitamin supplements, medication, replacement therapy ▪ For others, no treatment

Sources: Data from Bacino, C. (2017). Genetic issues presenting in the nursery. In E. Eichenwald, A. Hansen, C. R. Martin, & A. Stark (Eds.), *Cloherty and Stark's manual of neonatal care* (8th ed., pp. 117–130). Lippincott Williams & Wilkins; Brown, Z., & Chang, J. (2018). Disorders of carbohydrate metabolism. In C. Gleason & S. Juul (Eds.), *Avery's disease of the newborn* (10th ed., pp. 1403–1416). Elsevier; Burris, H. (2017). Hypoglycemia and hyperglycemia. In E. Eichenwald, A. Hansen, C. R. Martin, & A. Stark (Eds.), *Cloherty and Stark's manual of neonatal care* (8th ed., pp. 312–334). Lippincott Williams & Wilkins; Cederbaum, S. (2018). Introduction to metabolic and biochemical genetic diseases. In C. Gleason & S. Juul (Eds.), *Avery's disease of the newborn* (10th ed., pp. 209–214). Elsevier; Cederbaum, S., & Berry, G. T. (2018). Inborn errors of carbohydrate, ammonia, amino acid, and organic acid metabolism. In C. Gleason & S. Juul (Eds.), *Avery's disease of the newborn* (10th ed., pp. 215–238). Elsevier; El-Hattab, A. W., & Sutton, V. R. (2017). Inborn errors of metabolism. In E. Eichenwald, A. Hansen, C. R. Martin, & A. Stark (Eds.), *Cloherty and Stark's manual of neonatal care* (8th ed., pp. 858–891). Lippincott Williams & Wilkins.

Small Molecule Disorders

▪ The small molecule disorders include aminoacidopathies, including PKU, organic acidurias, urea cycle defects, and sugar intolerances, including galactosemia. They result from the accumulation of toxic compounds before the blockage in the metabolic pathway or process.
  ● The infant may be symptom-free initially, then demonstrates acute or progressive intoxication. The infant presents with increased drowsiness and poor feeding after the metabolite accumulates, with stress, or when feeds are introduced.
  ● Without intervention, full decompensation will occur with acidosis, seizure, obtundation, coma, and death.

Lysosomal Storage Disorders

▪ Lysosomal storage disorders (LSDs) result from defective function of a catabolic hydrolase located in the lysosome, which is responsible for metabolism of glycosaminoglycans and sphingolipids (products of normal cellular turnover).
  ● Other disorders in this category include a group of metabolic disorders that share dysfunction and defects of glycosylation or cholesterol synthesis.

- With most of these disorders, pathologic metabolites accumulate slowly with time and may not present in the newborn period. However, there are a few disorders of mucopolysaccharides and glycolipids which do present in neonates, including Pompe disease and Krabbe disease. Pompe disease (acid alpha-glucosidase deficiency [abbreviated as GAA], also known as acid maltase deficiency or lysosomal alpha-1,4-glucosidase deficiency) is the only GSD that is also an LSD. The synonym for Krabbe disease, globoid cell leukodystrophy, is caused by a deficiency of lysosomal galactocerebroside beta-galactosidase. Deficiency of the enzyme results in storage of galactocerebroside.

Energy Metabolism Disorders

- Energy metabolism disorders are notable for insufficient generation of energy by the mitochondria. These include disorders such as fatty acid oxidation defects, disorders of ketogenesis, GSD type I, and disorders of gluconeogenesis. Infants may present at birth or later with hypoglycemia, lactic acidosis, or cardiac decompensation.
  - Mitochondrial disorders and long-chain fatty acid oxidation defects can present with many symptoms, especially neurologic or cardiac ones, but may also include disruptions of energy metabolism.

Heterogeneous Disorders

- Heterogenous disorders are very rare disorders resulting from absence or dysfunction of enzymes, which include carbohydrate-deficient glycoprotein disorders, LSD, peroxisomal disorders, disorders involving transport or receptor enzymes, or purine and pyrimidine disorders.
  - These complex molecules are key to embryogenesis, so infants with these disorders often present with dysmorphic features, which may be subtle at birth but become more pronounced as storage material accumulates.
  - These disorders usually present in the extended neonatal period and may be diagnosed with enzyme assay or genetic sequencing testing (Cederbaum, 2018; Merritt & Gallagher, 2018; Thomas et al., 2018).

ENDOCRINE DISORDERS IN THE NEONATE

Disorders of Calcium, Magnesium, and Phosphorus Metabolism

- The majority of calcium, phosphorus, and magnesium stores can be found in the human skeleton, but also in the intracellular and extracellular spaces. These minerals are necessary for many biochemical reactions and cell functions in the body, including cardiovascular, nervous system, muscular, and homeostatic processes.
  - Bone minerals are important for ion transport across cell membranes, enzyme activity, intracellular regulation of metabolic pathways, hormone activity, coagulation activity, muscle contractility, and nerve conduction.
- During fetal life, these nutrients are transferred across the placenta. After birth, the supply of calcium is dependent upon enteral absorption through active and passive transport in the intestine with adequate vitamin D levels. For this reason, serum calcium levels normally decline after birth.
  - Calcium is excreted by the kidney. Nutrient intake from unfortified human milk has been calculated to be inadequate compared with fetal levels.
- Serum calcium represents less than 1% of whole-body calcium. Of this, about 50% of total serum calcium is in the ionized form and is the only physiologically active fraction. About 40% of total serum calcium is bound to proteins.
- Serum calcium is regulated by parathyroid hormone and 1,25-dihydroxyvitamin D (calcitriol), which increases serum calcium, and by calcitonin, which decreases it. Total serum calcium can be decreased by hypoalbuminemia.
  - Ionized calcium levels may be decreased by alkalosis as this increases albumin affinity for calcium.
    - In the converse, acidosis decreases albumin binding and increases the ionized calcium.
- Phosphorus accounts for about 10% to 15% of stores and is present in soft tissues and in extracellular fluid. Phosphorus is absorbed in the intestine and reabsorbed and excreted by the kidney. Absorption depends on dietary phosphorus, as well as on relative concentrations of calcium and phosphorus. Deficiencies may result in muscle weakness, impaired leukocyte function, and abnormal bone metabolism.
- Magnesium is stored in the skeleton at about 60%, and the remainder can be found in the muscle, the nervous system, and organs with high metabolic rates. One-third of serum magnesium is bound to albumin.
  - Magnesium is absorbed in the intestine via both active and passive mechanisms. It is excreted and reabsorbed via the kidney to maintain homeostasis.
  - Magnesium is required for normal parathyroid secretory responses, protein synthesis, membrane integrity, nervous tissue, conduction, neuromuscular excitability, muscle contraction, hormone secretion, and intermediate metabolism.
- Homeostasis of all three elements—calcium, phosphorus, and magnesium—requires normal parathyroid hormone and calcitonin function, as well as sufficient vitamin D levels.
  - The parathyroid glands secrete parathyroid hormone, which mobilizes calcium and phosphorus from the bone and stimulates calcium reabsorption in the kidneys.
  - Calcitonin is synthesized by the thyroid in response to elevated serum calcium and lowers serum calcium and phosphorus secretions by inhibition of bone resorption and increased renal secretion.

- Vitamin D is synthesized through the skin after sunshine exposure or is absorbed from dietary sources in the intestine. It is transported to the liver, bound to protein, and metabolized in the kidney. Vitamin D maintains calcium and phosphorus balance through effects on the small intestine, through the synthesis of calcium-binding proteins, and on the kidney (Abrams & Tiosano, 2020; Blackburn, 2018; Koves et al., 2018).

Calcium, Phosphate, and Magnesium Imbalances

CALCIUM

- The definition of neonatal hypocalcemia varies with gestational age and birth weight, but has been defined as a serum calcium level of less than 7 mg/dL (1.8 mmol/L; total) or an ionized calcium less than 4 mg/dL (1 mmol/L). Definitions of normal values may also vary, slightly, depending on the reference source.
  - In sick infants, it may be useful to measure the ionized calcium, which is the physiologically active portion, transported across membranes and tightly regulated.
  - Early hypocalcemia in the first 3 days of life commonly occurs with prematurity, asphyxia, in IDMs, and with intrauterine growth restriction.
  - Late neonatal hypocalcemia, after 3 to 5 days of life, may be associated with high phosphate load, maternal vitamin D deficiency, congenital hypoparathyroidism including DiGeorge syndrome, maternal hyperparathyroidism, secondary to renal hypomagnesemia or renal tubular acidosis, abnormalities in vitamin D metabolism, and other rare causes.
- Signs of hypocalcemia are variable and may not correlate with calcium level, but may include jitteriness, poor feeding, vomiting, hematemesis, melena, hypotonia, apnea, tachycardia, prolonged cardiac QT interval, respiratory distress, high-pitched cry, hyperactivity, irritability, or seizures.
- Infants may not require treatment of hypocalcemia if stable and without symptoms.
  - Treatment during the acute stage may include a constant infusion of intravenous administration of calcium gluconate, if the calcium level is very low or if there are symptoms. Longer term treatment may include calcium supplementation, diet therapy, magnesium supplementation, or vitamin D treatment, depending on the cause.
  - Risks of calcium infusion include bradyarrhythmias with rapid boluses or subcutaneous tissue injury with infiltration.
- Neonatal hypercalcemia has been defined as total serum calcium greater than 11.0 mg/dL (2.75 mmol/L) or ionized calcium levels greater than 5.4 mg/dL (1.28 mmol/L).

- Hypercalcemia may occur when there is a disruption in the interactive activities of parathyroid hormone, calcium-sensing receptors, calcitonin, and vitamin D in the intestine and kidney.
- This may be caused by calcium-sensing receptor mutations with hyperparathyroidism, other forms of hyperparathyroidism, Williams syndrome, subcutaneous fat necrosis, iatrogenic excessive intake of calcium or vitamin D, iatrogenic decreased intake of phosphorus, or other rare causes.
- Hypercalcemia at low levels may be asymptomatic. Symptoms of hypercalcemia at high levels may include vomiting, respiratory distress, apnea, hypotonia, lethargy, polyuria, and seizures.
  - Treatment may include restriction of calcium and vitamin D, rehydration, or medication to treat acute effects, including calcitonin, loop diuretics, and steroids (Abrams, 2017; Blackburn, 2020; Koves et al., 2018; Polin & Adamkin, 2020).

MAGNESIUM

- Magnesium is actively transported from the mother to the fetus using a transport mechanism different from calcium. Furthermore, unlike calcium, this transfer is adversely affected both by placental insufficiency and by maternal magnesium deficiency caused by poor diet or disease.
- Neonatal hypomagnesemia has been defined as serum magnesium level less than 1.6 mg/dL. Neonatal hypomagnesemia is uncommon but may be associated with hypocalcemia or therapeutic cooling.
  - Symptoms may include apnea, poor tone, or seizures. Treatment of hypomagnesemia, with seizures, may include slow intravenous infusion of magnesium sulfate.
- Hypermagnesemia has been defined as serum magnesium level of greater than 3 mg/dL.
  - Hypermagnesemia is usually due to exogenous load that exceeds renal clearance, for example, magnesium that crosses the placenta after treatment for toxemia or preterm labor.
  - Common causes include maternal magnesium therapy, administration of neonatal antacids, excessive magnesium in total parenteral nutrition, or medication errors.
  - Signs of hypermagnesemia include apnea, respiratory depression, lethargy, hypotonia, hyporeflexia, poor suck, decreased intestinal motility, delayed passage of meconium, hypotension, arrhythmias, coma, complete heart block, and asystolic cardiac arrest.
  - Treatment is supportive until the magnesium is cleared by the kidney (Abrams, 2017; Koves et al., 2018; Polin & Adamkin, 2020).

PHOSPHATE

■ Normal term neonatal serum phosphate levels are 5.5 to 7.0 mg/dL and may be higher than adult levels due to released stores, decreased or immature renal function, increased energy demand, and delayed feeding. Phosphorus is absorbed in the small intestine. Absorption and metabolism of phosphorus are under the influence of vitamin D and parathyroid hormone.

● Phosphorus, along with calcium, is necessary for bone mineralization, skeletal and skin growth, glucose metabolism, cardiovascular function, neuromuscular depolarization, immune system function, and hormone regulation.

■ Hypophosphatemia is rare and usually related to parenteral or enteral nutritional causes, or rarely renal causes. Symptoms would be related to hypercalcemia, including feeding intolerance, lethargy, irritability, hypertension, or seizures.

■ Hyperphosphatemia is usually related to hypocalcemia, dietary excesses, or ordering error.

● Infants with hyperphosphatemia may be asymptomatic, or with symptoms related to hypocalcemia such as apnea, jitteriness, increased tone, hyperreflexia, abnormalities of cardiac function, or seizures.

● Treatment would include detection and correction of hypocalcemia, change in diet, or prevention of ordering errors (Abrams, 2017; Blackburn, 2018).

METABOLIC BONE DISEASE

■ *Metabolic bone disease* is defined as inadequate postnatal bone mineralization and is common among very low birth weight infants.

● It is often called *osteopenia* or *rickets of prematurity* and is caused by deficiency of calcium and phosphorus due to poor mineral intake and absorption.

● Less common causes include long-term fluid restriction, long-term total parenteral nutrition, furosemide therapy, or long-term steroid use.

● This condition can lead to osteoporosis, with fractures, due to decreased bone mineral density, or rickets, which involves the growth plate.

■ Rarely, metabolic bone disease may be associated with genetic disorders, including 1 alpha-hydroxylase deficiency or maternal vitamin D deficiency, Fanconi syndrome, or tumors.

● Diagnosis may be made by laboratory analysis of mineral and hormone levels, rapid increase in alkaline phosphatase value, fracture seen per radiograph, or rarely with genetic testing.

● Treatment includes diet management, diet fortification, mineral supplementation, vitamin therapy, passive physical activity, and surveillance

(Abrams, 2017; Koves et al., 2018; Rao, 2020; Wassner & Belfort, 2017).

Disorders of the Thyroid

■ Thyroid embryogenesis is complete by 10 to 12 weeks of gestation. At this time, the fetal thyroid gland starts to concentrate iodine and secrete triiodothyronine (T3) and thyroxine (T4).

● Thyrotropin/thyroid-stimulating hormone (TSH) secretion from the fetal pituitary gland increases, beginning midgestation. Maternal TSH does not cross the placenta, but maternal thyrotropin-releasing hormone (TRH) does cross.

● After birth, there is a dramatic surge of TSH, which peaks at 30 minutes and with continued hypersecretion for the next 6 to 24 hours of life. In the preterm, this surge is less marked.

■ Thyroid hormone is essential for fetal brain development and for growth and metabolism regulation throughout infancy and childhood.

● Thyrotropin/TSH is a pituitary hormone that stimulates the thyroid gland to secrete T3 and T4 into the circulation to regulate metabolism of thyroid-dependent tissues in the body.

■ Control of thyroid hormone secretion is centered in the hypothalamic–pituitary–thyroid axis (HPA).

● Thyroid hormones are iodinated amino acids.

● Iodine is required by the thyroid gland and made available, when ingested or absorbed, via an active transport process that requires oxidative phosphorylation.

● Thyrotropin is a glycoprotein that stimulates the thyroid to produce T4. T4 is converted to T3, which is the active hormone that stimulates metabolism in most body tissues.

● There are many intermediary hormones, antibodies, and other proteins that may affect normal thyroid function (Chuang & Gutmark-Little, 2020; Kim et al., 2018; Wassner & Belfort, 2017).

HYPOTHYROIDISM

■ Congenital hypothyroidism can be caused by primary hypothyroidism, including thyroid dysgenesis, inborn errors of thyroid hormone synthesis or secretion, mutations in the TSH receptor causing resistance, maternal ingestion of antithyroid drugs, or as a result of iodine deficiency (cretinism). Congenital hypothyroidism may also be due to central congenital hypothyroidism, a genetic disorder resulting from either inheritance or a mutation.

● This disorder has been attributed to difficult birth, birth injury, anoxia, and growth or pituitary hormone deficiencies, and may be associated with any midline congenital defect.

- Transient congenital hypothyroidism can be caused by antithyroid drugs, iodine excess or deficiency, transient hypothyroxinemia of prematurity, maternal TSH receptor-blocking antibodies, liver hemangiomas, and hypothyroxinemia associated with sick euthyroid syndrome. Most of these infants require treatment with thyroid hormone replacement, but will not require lifelong treatment.
- Diagnosis of congenital hypothyroidism is made, most often, through the newborn screen, which permits early diagnosis and treatment, with optimal outcome.
  - Clinical signs of hypothyroidism include constipation, hypothermia, poor tone, lethargy, inactivity, respiratory distress, mottled skin, prolonged jaundice, poor feeding, large tongue, periorbital edema, large anterior and posterior fontanels, pallor, perioral cyanosis, poor or hoarse cry, lingual thyroid, or goiter.
  - If clinical signs of hypothyroidism are present, thyroid function studies should be performed even if newborn screening results are negative.
  - Radiographic studies of bone maturation, radiograph or echocardiogram to evaluate for cardiomegaly, or ultrasound of the thyroid may be considered.
  - Other tests that should be considered may include cortisol and growth hormone levels and imaging of the hypothalamus and pituitary to rule out pituitary–hypothalamic defects.
- Treatment of hypothyroidism includes thyroid hormone replacement therapy and proper nutrition and vitamin support. Congenital hypothyroidism is one of the most preventable causes of intellectual disability (Blackburn, 2021; Chuang & Gutmark-Little, 2020; Kim et al., 2018; Srinivasan, 2020; Wassner & Belfort, 2017).

HYPERTHYROIDISM

- Neonatal hyperthyroidism is uncommon and usually transient.
  - Most infants with hyperthyroidism are born to mothers with Graves disease and results from transplacental transfer of stimulating TSH-receptor antibodies (TRAb) from the mother to the newborn. About 1% to 5% of infants born to mothers with Graves disease have neonatal hyperthyroidism.
  - Rarely, infants have permanent hyperthyroidism from an autosomal dominant trait resulting in activating mutation of the TSH receptor.
- Signs of hyperthyroidism and neonatal thyrotoxicosis include prematurity, intrauterine growth restriction, irritability, excessive movement, tremor, flushing of cheeks, hyperthermia, sweating, increased appetite, weight loss or poor growth, supraventricular tachycardia, arrhythmia, goiter, exophthalmos, lymphadenopathy, hepatosplenomegaly,

craniosynostosis, thrombocytopenia, hypoprothrombinemia, and coagulopathy.
  - Treatment includes antithyroid drugs. Supportive care may include beta-blockers such as propranolol to treat tachycardia or steroids.
  - Death may occur if the condition is not treated. If the condition is caused by genetic defect and is permanent, thyroid gland removal or ablation may be considered (Blackburn, 2021; Chuang & Gutmark-Little, 2020; Srinivasan, 2020; Wassner & Belfort, 2017).

Disorders of the Pituitary Gland

- Deficiencies of cortisol or growth hormone can cause neonatal hypoglycemia, in the context of hypopituitarism, with adrenocorticotropic hormone (ACTH) and growth hormone deficiency.
  - Hypopituitarism and altered functioning of the HPA are often associated with midline, facial, cranial, or intracranial defects.
  - Septo-optic dysplasia is often associated with pituitary hormone deficiencies.
  - Clinical signs of hypopituitarism include hypoglycemia related to growth and ACTH deficiencies, polyuria from antidiuretic hormone deficiency, microphallus in boys from gonadotropin hormone deficiency, nystagmus, and hypothyroidism.
  - Diagnosis is made with endocrine studies after other causes of symptoms are ruled out.
  - Treatment may include corticosteroids, as well as thyroid, sex, or growth hormone replacement (Blackburn, 2021; Garg & Devaskar, 2020; Werny et al., 2018).

Disorders of the Adrenal Gland

- Normal adrenal function is essential for fetal and extrauterine growth and homeostasis. Adrenal disorders can be life-threatening.
- The major adrenal hormones are cortisol and aldosterone, regulated in response to corticotropin-releasing hormone (CRH) from the hypothalamus and ACTH from the pituitary gland.
  - Glucocorticoids, primarily cortisol, are metabolized in the zona fasciculata and are responsible for the regulation of fluid and electrolyte balance, glucose stability, regulation of blood pressure, response to stress, and response to inflammation with immune suppression.
  - Mineralocorticoids are produced in the zona glomerulosa, which regulates fluid and electrolyte balance.
    - Epinephrine and norepinephrine, which have both glucocorticoid and mineralocorticoid properties, are produced in the adrenal medulla and are also involved in stress responses and cardiovascular function.

- Androgens are produced in the zona reticularis and in the gonads. Androgens are important for sexual differentiation.
- Disorders of the adrenal glands may include Cushing syndrome (too much cortisol secondary to tumor), Addison disease (primary adrenal insufficiency), hyperaldosteronism, pheochromocytoma or paraganglioma (primary tumors), or adrenal problems secondary to pituitary tumors, but these rarely present in the neonate (Blackburn, 2018; Blackburn, 2021).

CONGENITAL ADRENAL HYPERPLASIA

- CAH comprises a group of disorders in which there is an inherited defect in one of the enzymes required for the adrenocortical synthesis of cortisol from cholesterol. This leads to impaired cortisol production and elevated ACTH levels.
  - The clinical problems are caused by impaired synthesis of glucocorticoids, mineralocorticoids, or gonadal sex steroids, and overproduction of precursor steroids or their side products.
- CAH is a fairly common disorder, with a worldwide incidence of 1 per 16,000 births, and is included in newborn screening.
  - This disorder involves problems with both adrenal function and sex development.
- The most common cause of CAH is 21-hydroxylase enzyme deficiency, accounting for more than 95% of all cases. Other defects in the adrenal-steroid hormone synthesis pathway that can lead to disordered sex development include 11-beta-hydroxylase deficiency, 17-alpha-hydroxylase deficiency, and 3-beta-hydroxysteroid dehydrogenase deficiency.
  - The most common forms of CAH include the simple virilizing form, with increased secretion of androgens before the enzyme block.
  - In the female fetus, this leads to varying degrees of male differentiation of the external genitalia, but internal sex organs develop normally. In the male fetus, the effect of increased androgens is insignificant and penile enlargement is usually not recognizable as such. Both females and males may have increased pigmentation of the genitalia.
- Severe deficiency of the 21-hydroxylase enzyme with impairments of cortisol and aldosterone synthesis results in the salt-wasting form of CAH. Thus, the infant presents with adrenal insufficiency that can manifest with shock-like symptoms.
  - Hypoaldosteronism causes renal sodium wasting with depletion of total body sodium content and impaired ability to secrete potassium and hydrogen ions via the kidney. This may lead to hyponatremia, hyperkalemia, or metabolic acidosis.
  - Hypocortisolemia causes impairment of cardiovascular, metabolic, and other system functions, including the renin–angiotensin axis, which results in hypoglycemia and shock.

- Diagnosis of CAH is made via the newborn screen in most cases.
  - The most common disorder of sex development with presentation in the newborn period is a 46,XX female with CAH. Females with the salt-losing form of CAH may present with complete masculinization of the external genitalia, and some are incorrectly identified as male.
    - ❏ Infants born with ambiguous genitalia, non-palpable testes, or severe hyponatremia should be evaluated for adrenal disorders.
    - ❏ Although most disorders of sex development involve a virilized infant with 46,XX karyotypes and caused by CAH, it is important to understand the differential diagnoses, clinical assessment, appropriate referral, and parental support for all possible presentations. Males usually receive medical attention when they develop a salt-losing crisis caused by adrenal insufficiency.
- When CAH is suspected, diagnosis may be facilitated by readily available algorithms, as well as referral to pediatric subspecialists.
  - General concepts include performance of a complete physical exam with thorough documentation of symmetry, presence, and description of external genitalia; appropriate laboratory and genetic analyses; and imaging of the internal gonads.
- The goal of treatment of CAH is to normalize ACTH secretion and provide replacement or correction of cortisol, aldosterone, or gonadal sex steroid deficiencies.
  - Treatment of salt-wasting CAH may include glucocorticoid (cortisol) and mineralocorticoid replacement, sodium replacement, hydration, other supportive care, and surveillance.
  - These infants may require cortisol stress doses with any illness, surgery, or trauma (Blackburn, 2021; Fechner, 2018; McCandless & Kripps, 2020; Shnorhavorian & Fechner, 2018; Sorbara & Wherret, 2020; Swartz & Chan, 2017; Theda, 2020).

ADDITIONAL DISORDERS OF SEX DEVELOPMENT

- This heterogenous group of disorders is associated with developmental, genetic, or endocrine causes, and includes findings of ambiguous genitalia, cryptorchidism, hypospadias, microphallus, clitoromegaly, asymmetry of genitalia, and discordance of external genitalia with prenatal karyotype.
  - Because internal genital anatomy, karyotype, and sex assignment cannot be determined from external appearance, a rapid and thorough evaluation is required, including a suspicion of CAH, which would necessitate urgent treatment.

- The differential diagnosis for ambiguous genitalia includes categories of problems that include causes of 46,XX virilized female, 46,XY undervirilized male, gonadal differentiation and chromosomal disorders, and syndromes associated with ambiguous genitalia.
- General considerations in the approach to assessment and care of the newborn with ambiguous genitalia include initial history collection and physical exam, including notation of genitalia asymmetry; gonadal size, position, and descent; and description of associated anomalies.
    - Laboratory testing may include genetic testing and 17-hydroxyprogesterone before newborn screen results are available, pertinent adrenal precursors, hormones and chemistries, imaging of gonads and other pertinent structures, and possibly biopsies.
    - Referrals to appropriate subspecialists may include a neonatologist, pediatric surgeon, pediatric endocrinologist, pediatric urologist, geneticist, and child psychologist.
- Care of the family should include open and honest discussion of available assessment and test results, avoidance of premature sex assignment until a collaborative decision has been made by the multidisciplinary team and parents after thorough evaluation, and psychological support.
    - Until sex assignment is made, gender-specific names, pronouns, and other references should be avoided.
    - The main goal of sex assignment is to attempt to match the child's future gender identity (Blackburn, 2021; Shnorhavorian & Fechner, 2018; Swartz & Chan, 2017; Theda, 2020).

▶ ASSESSMENT AND TREATMENT OF METABOLIC AND ENDOCRINE DISORDERS

THE NEONATAL NURSE PRACTITIONER'S ROLE IN EVALUATION

- The NNP may not be able to identify the specific disorder, but they should be able to describe and document a complete history, physical, and first-line laboratory and radiographic evaluation. Any infant who presents with hypoglycemia, acidosis, lethargy, temperature instability, or neurologic abnormalities should be considered to possibly have a metabolic or endocrine disorder if there is concern that this infant's condition does not fit the pattern of sepsis or hypoxia.
- Because the care of the infant with suspected metabolic and endocrine disorders can be overwhelming, it is helpful to emphasize the priorities and interventions of the NNP, within the scope of practice granted by state licensure. All of these efforts will involve collaboration with the neonatologist.
    - These priorities include identification of abnormal symptoms, evaluation, stabilization, communication with parents, notification of colleagues and consultants, consideration of need for transport, and discharge planning (Blackburn, 2018; Cederbaum, 2018; El-Hattab & Sutton, 2017; Matthew & Robin, 2021; Wassner & Belfort, 2017).
    - A guide to the approach to care of infants with metabolic or endocrine disorders is presented in Table 18.2.

Table 18.2 Presenting Signs of Metabolic and Endocrine Disorders in Infants

Primary Organ System Involved	Presenting Signs	Metabolic/Endocrine Disorder
Neurologic	■ Encephalopathy ■ High-pitched cry ■ Jitteriness ■ Lethargy, hypotonia, or abnormal movements ■ Coma	■ Hypoglycemia, hypo/hypercalcemia, hypomagnesemia ■ Amino acid disorders ■ Organic acidemias ■ Respiratory chain defects ■ Urea cycle defects
	■ Seizures	■ Neurotransmitter disorders
	■ Seizures + microcephaly	■ 3-phosphoglycerate dehydrogenase ■ Glucose transporter type 1 deficiency
Eye	■ Cataracts	■ Galactosemia ■ Carbohydrate defects ■ Lysosomal storage disease ■ Peroxisomal disorders ■ Respiratory chain defects
	■ Retinopathies	■ Congenital disorders of glycosylation ■ Lysosomal storage disorders ■ Peroxisomal disorders
	■ Abnormal movements or gaze	■ Mitochondrial cytopathies or Gaucher disease

(continued)

Table 18.2 Presenting Signs of Metabolic and Endocrine Disorders in Infants (*continued*)

Primary Organ System Involved	Presenting Signs	Metabolic/Endocrine Disorder
Hepatic	■ Liver failure	■ Galactosemia ■ Hereditary fructose intolerance ■ Tyrosinemia type I ■ Phosphomannose isomerase (PMI)
	■ Jaundice, cholestasis	■ Galactosemia ■ Long-chain 3-hydroxy-acyl-CoA ■ dehydrogenase deficiency ■ Bile acid synthesis defects ■ Cerebrotendinous xanthomatosis
	■ Hepatosplenomegaly	■ Congenital erythropoietic porphyria
Cardiac	■ Cardiomyopathy ■ Arrhythmias	■ Fatty acid oxidation defects ■ Glycogen storage diseases ■ Lysosomal storage diseases ■ Respiratory chain defects
Endocrine	■ Hepatosplenomegaly ■ Metabolic acidosis ■ Hypoglycemia	■ Amino acid defects ■ Bile acid biosynthetic defects ■ Carbohydrate defects ■ Congenital disorders of glycosylation ■ Fatty acid oxidation defects ■ Peroxisomal disorders ■ Respiratory chain defects ■ Organic acidemias
	■ Severe hypoglycemia ■ Ambiguous genitalia	■ Congenital hyperinsulinism ■ Congenital adrenal hyperplasia
	■ Cardiac involvement	■ Fatty acid oxidation defects ■ Carnitine uptake defect
Gastrointestinal/ hepatic	■ Poor feeding ■ Jaundice, hepatomegaly, splenomegaly ■ Vomiting	■ Bile acid biosynthetic defects ■ Carbohydrate defects ■ Congenital glycosylation disorders ■ Fatty acid beta-oxidation disorders ■ Lysosomal storage disorders ■ Organic acidemias ■ Respiratory chain defects ■ Glycogen storage diseases
Hair/skin/skeletal anomalies	■ Increased skin pigmentation ■ Fair hair and skin ■ Brittle, coarse hair ■ Alopecia ■ Rash ■ Unusual odor ■ Fractures	■ Amino acid disorders ■ Organic acidemias ■ Menkes disease ■ Phenylketonuria ■ Osteopenia of prematurity
Hematologic anomalies	■ Neutropenia ■ Thrombocytopenia ■ Anemia ■ Pancytopenia	■ Organic acidemias ■ Respiratory chain defects

CoA, coenzyme A; PMI, phosphomannose isomerase.

Sources: Data from Bacino, C. (2017). Genetic issues presenting in the nursery. In E. Eichenwald, A. Hansen, C. R. Martin, & A. Stark (Eds.), *Cloherty and Stark's manual of neonatal care* (8th ed., pp. 117–130). Lippincott Williams & Wilkins; Brown, Z., & Chang, J. (2018). Disorders of carbohydrate metabolism. In C. Gleason & S. Juul (Eds.), *Avery's disease of the newborn* (10th ed., pp. 1403–1416). Elsevier; Burris, H. (2017). Hypoglycemia and hyperglycemia. In E. Eichenwald, A. Hansen, C. R. Martin, & A. Stark (Eds.), *Cloherty and Stark's manual of neonatal care* (8th ed., pp. 312–334). Lippincott Williams & Wilkins; Cederbaum, S., & Berry, G. T. (2018). Inborn errors of carbohydrate, ammonia, amino acid, and organic acid metabolism. In C. Gleason & S. Juul (Eds.), *Avery's disease of the newborn* (10th ed., pp. 215–238). Elsevier; El-Hattab, A. W., & Sutton, V. R. (2017). Inborn errors of metabolism. In E. Eichenwald, A. Hansen, C. R. Martin, & A. Stark (Eds.), *Cloherty and Stark's manual of neonatal care* (8th ed., pp. 858–891). Lippincott Williams & Wilkins.

CLINICAL PRESENTATION

- Generally, newborn infants with metabolic or endocrine disorders have relatively nonspecific types of presenting symptoms. The most common presenting symptoms include dysmorphic features (sometimes), hypoglycemia, poor feeding, vomiting, poor growth, jaundice, organomegaly, acidosis, cardiomyopathy, respiratory distress, lethargy, apnea, hypotonia, hypothermia, cyanosis, seizures, encephalopathy, obtundation, coma, and sudden death.
  - Since some of these symptoms may be caused by a common neonatal problem, such as breastfeeding difficulty, jaundice, benign cardiac murmur, or infection, it becomes clear why a consistent, thorough, differential, and systematic approach is necessary for the assessment of all infants (Blackburn, 2018; Cederbaum, 2018; El-Hattab & Sutton, 2017; Konczal & Zinn, 2020; Werny et al., 2018).

Perinatal History

- Parents and family members should be asked about a history of neonatal death or sudden, unexplained death of any infant or child within the family, as well as any incidence of mental retardation, developmental delay, or heart problems.
- It is helpful to remember that X-linked conditions have male predominance, but females may have milder forms, so it may be important to listen, carefully, to how mild abnormalities are described, especially of female relatives.
- Parents should be asked if they are related at all, as autosomal recessive disorders are more likely to occur with parental consanguinity.
- Although pregnancy history may be available in the medical record, parents should still be questioned since information may be lacking or prenatal care may have been received elsewhere without transfer of records.
  - Infants with metabolic or endocrine disorders are often born to mothers with normal pregnancies. However, in some cases, the pregnancies may have had associated severe hyperemesis, liver dysfunction, fatty liver of pregnancy, or HELLP (including hemolysis, elevated liver enzymes, and low platelet count) syndrome.
  - Fetal ultrasound results may have revealed congenital malformations associated with genetic metabolic disorders (Bacino, 2017; El-Hattab & Sutton, 2018).

Systematic Physical Examination

- In this chapter, only the organs or systems most commonly affected by metabolic or endocrine disorders, which may be identified during a physical exam, are presented.
- The physical exam should be performed with a consistent, thorough approach of all organs or systems

to identify all abnormalities to assist in the evaluation and care of the infant.

- It is important to start with a general assessment of the infant for evaluation of phenotype and activity, as there may or may not be phenotype abnormalities with specific metabolic or endocrine disorders; however, a thorough evaluation may reveal physical dysmorphology that is present with some disorders.
- It is also important to initiate a neurologic evaluation of the infant at rest in terms of position, tone, and activity before they are disturbed.
- It is possible to have confounding problems, as in the case, for example, of an infant with a metabolic disorder who also has respiratory distress due to meconium aspiration syndrome.
- A more complete description of the presenting signs of metabolic and endocrine disorders in infants is presented in Table 18.2 (Cederbaum, 2018; Garg & Devaskar, 2020; Konczal & Zinn, 2020; Thomas et al., 2018).
- An eye examination may reveal, or suggest, galactosemia, sphingolipids, mitochondrial cytopathies, Kearns–Sayre syndrome, and other metabolic or endocrine disorders.
  - Infants with these conditions may present with cataracts, cherry spots, retinopathies, or abnormal gaze.
  - It is possible to miss some of these anomalies during the initial eye exam, without dilation of the pupils, so if a metabolic or endocrine disorder is suspected, a referral to a pediatric ophthalmologist is appropriate (Cederbaum, 2018; Thomas et al., 2018).
- Infants may present with respiratory distress, including tachypnea (Cederbaum, 2018).
- A cardiac exam should be performed in any infant with suspected metabolic disorder. However, for some disorders, the cardiac problem, when accompanied by hemodynamic instability, is the presenting symptom.
  - The symptoms of metabolic or endocrine disorders with cardiac involvement may include cardiac murmur, arrhythmia, cardiomyopathy with signs of failure, or hemodynamic decompensation.
  - There may be significant cardiac problems and symptoms with mitochondrial disorders, for example, mitochondrial respiratory chain disorders, or GSD, for example, Pompe disease (Blackburn, 2018; Cederbaum, 2018; Thomas et al., 2018).
- The abdomen should be evaluated for distension, associated with vomiting or diarrhea, and may be assessed for many of the intoxication disorders.
  - Liver, or spleen, involvement is common to many metabolic or endocrine disorders.
  - Signs of liver failure may be seen with disorders such as galactosemia and tyrosinemia.
  - Hepatosplenomegaly may be seen with congenital erythropoietic porphyria or LSD, for example,

Gaucher disease (Cederbaum, 2018; Thomas et al., 2018).

■ Genitalia should be assessed for appropriateness for gestational age and for any abnormalities.
  ● Abnormalities such as ambiguous genitalia in a female may be associated with endocrine disorders such as CAH.
  ● Other abnormalities may be related to other sex development disorders (Blackburn, 2018; Thomas et al., 2018).

■ Extremities should be assessed for bone fracture by inspection or radiologic determination that may be associated with osteopenia of prematurity, also called *metabolic bone disease* or *rickets of prematurity* or *physiologic osteoporosis of infancy* in term infants.
  ● Subcutaneous fat necrosis, associated with birth trauma, may be associated with hypercalcemia later as calcification resolves (Abrams & Tiosano, 2020; Thomas et al., 2018).

■ Abnormal neurologic signs may present in many infants with metabolic or endocrine disorders.
  ● Sometimes, these are subtle and ubiquitous signs, such as "poor feeding." However, infants may present with progressive or significant neurologic symptoms.
  ● Infants with either metabolic or endocrine disorders, such as hypoglycemia, may present with irritability, high-pitched cry, apnea, jitteriness, tremors, feeding difficulty, lethargy, stupor, seizures, hypothermia, sweating, or hypotonia.

● With many of the acidemia disorders, and lysosomal storage, as well as heterogenous disorders, the infant will present with neurologic signs, including hypotonia, seizures, and obtundation, and may progress to coma. They may also have accompanying abnormal, distinctive odors of urine, breath, saliva, or sweat.
● Abnormal odor may be an important diagnostic feature of some disorders, such as PKU, which presents with a stale, mousy, barn-like smell, or tyrosinemia, which presents with a rancid smell, like sulfur (Abrams & Tiosano, 2020; El-Hattab & Sutton, 2017; Garg & Devaskar, 2020; Kim et al., 2018; Thomas et al., 2018).

FIRST-LINE INVESTIGATIONS

■ If metabolic or endocrine disorders are suspected, the goal is to promote cardiopulmonary and metabolic stability and to obtain some basic measures that are routinely available before more specialized investigation. Even if the NNP is uncertain about ordering some of these first-line studies before discussion with a neonatologist, much may be revealed by, at least, blood sugar levels and arterial blood gas tests, as well as some other commonly ordered metabolic tests (Table 18.3).

Table 18.3 Screening Tests for Metabolic or Endocrine Disorders That Should Be Considered

Test	Reason	Clinical Importance and Abnormalities That May Be Associated With the Disorders
Glucose—metabolic or endocrine disorders should be suspected in any infant with prolonged, persistent hypoglycemia	■ Normal, low, or high	■ *Small molecule disorders:* glucose with poor feeding, obtundation ■ *Energy metabolism disorders:* normal ■ *Lysosomal storage disorders:* may be normal ■ *Endocrine:* hypoglycemia, TSH, T3, T4
Arterial blood gas	■ To determine metabolic acidosis	■ *Small molecule disorders:* pH, CO_2 with coma and respiratory failure, or CO_2 with hyperventilation ■ *Energy metabolism disorders:* pH with lactic acidosis, base deficit, CO_2 with alkalosis ■ *Lysosomal storage disorders:* may be normal
Electrolytes/minerals	■ Especially serum bicarbonate, to determine metabolic acidosis ■ To determine anion gap with acidosis	■ *Small molecule disorders:* abnormal electrolytes with vomiting and acidosis ■ *Energy metabolism disorders:* bicarbonate, abnormal with acidosis ■ *Lysosomal storage disorders:* may be normal ■ *Endocrine:* sodium, potassium, calcium magnesemia, alkaline phosphatase
Liver function studies with bilirubin, coagulopathy studies	■ To determine liver involvement and jaundice	■ *Small molecule disorders:* liver function tests ■ *Energy metabolism disorders:* liver function tests ■ *Lysosomal storage disorders:* bilirubin or normal
Ammonia	■ May be elevated	■ *Small molecule disorders:* may be elevated ■ *Energy metabolism disorders:* may be elevated ■ *Lysosomal storage disorders:* may be elevated or normal

(continued)

Table 18.3 Presenting Signs of Metabolic and Endocrine Disorders in Infants (*continued*)

Test	Reason	Clinical Importance and Abnormalities That May Be Associated With the Disorders
Lactate	■ May be elevated	■ *Small molecule disorders:* lactate ■ *Energy metabolism disorders:* lactate ■ *Lysosomal storage disorders:* may be normal
Urinary ketones	■ To determine if present, which is abnormal	■ *Small molecule disorders:* ketones ■ *Energy metabolism disorders:* normal or ketones ■ *Lysosomal storage disorders:* may be normal

CO2, carbon dioxide; T3, triiodothyronine; T4, thyroxine; TSH, thyroid-stimulating hormone.
Sources: Data from Bacino, C. (2017). Genetic issues presenting in the nursery. In E. Eichenwald, A. Hansen, C. R. Martin, & A. Stark (Eds.), *Cloherty and Stark's manual of neonatal care* (8th ed., pp. 117–130). Lippincott Williams & Wilkins; Brown, Z., & Chang, J. (2018). Disorders of carbohydrate metabolism. In C. Gleason & S. Juul (Eds.), *Avery's disease of the newborn* (10th ed., pp. 1403–1416). Elsevier; Burris, H. (2017). Hypoglycemia and hyperglycemia. In E. Eichenwald, A. Hansen, C. R. Martin, & A. Stark (Eds.), *Cloherty and Stark's manual of neonatal care* (8th ed., pp. 312–334). Lippincott Williams & Wilkins; Cederbaum, S., & Berry, G. T. (2018). Inborn errors of carbohydrate, ammonia, amino acid, and organic acid metabolism. In C. Gleason & S. Juul (Eds.), *Avery's disease of the newborn* (10th ed., pp. 215–238). Elsevier; El-Hattab, A. W., & Sutton, V. R. (2017). Inborn errors of metabolism. In E. Eichenwald, A. Hansen, C. R. Martin, & A. Stark (Eds.), *Cloherty and Stark's manual of neonatal care* (8th ed., pp. 858–891). Lippincott Williams & Wilkins.

● First-line investigations of blood often include blood glucose levels; arterial pH, carbon dioxide, bicarbonate, and base deficit; complete blood count; serum lactate, ammonia, amino acids, and liver function studies; and clotting studies.

● First-line investigations of urine include ketones, organic acids (including orotic acid), reducing substances (if suspecting galactosemia), and amino acids.

■ If any of the physical examination findings or laboratory test results are abnormal, or if the clinician is concerned despite normal results, then this may be the appropriate time to ask for a consult from a pediatric subspecialist. Depending on the case and stability of the infant, it may be appropriate to request a consult from a pediatric endocrinologist, biochemical geneticist, neurologist, cardiologist, gastroenterologist, infectious disease specialist, dermatologist, and so on. Depending on the suspected disorder, further testing will be performed (Cederbaum, 2018; El-Hattab & Sutton, 2017; Matthew & Robin, 2021; Swartz & Chan, 2017; Wassner & Belfort, 2017).

Newborn Screening

■ Newborn screening is a successful public health program that began, in 1963, with drops of blood on filter paper and a process of bacterial inhibition assay to detect PKU, a preventable cause of mental retardation. In the following years, more screening tests were developed to detect a few more conditions. As conditions were identified, treatment and follow-up recommendations were established.

■ In the 1990s, with the application of tandem mass spectrometry, many metabolic and hematologic disorders could be detected, and the list of conditions was broadened.

  ● Examples of some of the disorders that can be detected include endocrine disorders, hemoglobinopathies, immunodeficiencies, and cystic fibrosis, as well as PKU and other inborn errors of metabolism (Blackburn, 2018; Sahai & Levy, 2018).

■ Presently in the United States, newborn screening programs are mandated, and more than 60 conditions are included, although specific tests done will vary state to state. In some states, parents are allowed to refuse screening.

■ All states require screening for PKU, hypothyroidism, CAH, sickle cell disease, S-beta thalassemia, and galactosemia. Additional disorders most often screened for include amino acid disorders (homocystinuria, maple syrup urine disease), organic acids (glutaric, methylmalonic, and propionic acidemias), disorders of fatty acid metabolism (medium-chain and very-long-chain acyl-CoA dehydrogenase deficiency), hemoglobinopathies including sickle cell anemia, and others such as biotinidase deficiency, CAH, and cystic fibrosis.

  ● The goal is to screen all infants and provide the necessary follow-up evaluation and intervention to prevent death or disability. However, some experts question if there exists clear scientific evidence of the long-term benefits of screening and treatment. Controversies exist among experts in different countries about the benefits and risks of certain therapies, especially with disparate availability of resources, and about which disorders should be included in the screen.

■ A positive screen result must be followed by a confirmatory diagnostic test. Moreover, if there is clinical suspicion of a particular disorder despite a negative screening result, further diagnostic testing is warranted.

■ The concept of "newborn screening" has been broadened to include other technologies such as hearing screening, with automated auditory brainstem response (ABR) to screen for hearing loss, and critical congenital heart disease (CHD) screening, with pulse oximetry.

- In the future, it may be possible to perform a genetic and mutational scan across the whole genome of the fetus, in a noninvasive manner, by analyzing cell-free fetal DNA in maternal blood as early as the fifth week of gestational age. This technology and approach remains controversial due to methodologic, ethical, and political issues (Matthew & Robin, 2021; Sahai & Levy, 2018).

SECOND-LINE INVESTIGATIONS

- Second-line investigations are usually performed as a result of consultants' recommendations, and may include urine, cerebral spinal fluid, or serum samples for metabolites or markers, such as urine succinylacetone, cerebral spinal fluid glycine, serum acylcarnitines, and other markers or metabolites. Chromosomes and other specific genetic studies may also be requested.
- Organ or organelle-specific investigations may include studies such as long-chain fatty acids, transferrin isoelectric focusing, and peroxisomal function tests. Skin, muscle, and liver biopsies may be performed at this time, if possible and appropriate, or during postmortem studies.
- Specific imaging may include tandem mass spectrometry, as well as other radiographic or ultrasound studies.
- Depending on the resources at the facility where the infant was born or evaluated, sometimes the infant must be transported to a regional pediatric medical center for some of these tests.
- For second-line investigations, it is important to determine, with the collaborative team, an appropriate medical order to prevent excessive exsanguination and handling.
  - It is also important to contact the laboratory personnel in the facility to determine if the tests are analyzed at that facility or must be sent out, to plan for optimum collection and processing of the samples.
  - To accomplish this goal, one must establish proper timing (e.g., not before a long weekend if the sample needs to be sent to another lab), confirm proper tubes, proper handling (e.g., if the sample needs to be placed on ice), and notice to the lab technologists when these tests are to be sent so that they are processed immediately (Cederbaum, 2018; El-Hattab & Sutton, 2017; Kim et al., 2018; Swartz & Chan, 2017; Wassner & Belfort, 2017).

TREATMENT GOALS

Acute Management

- The goals of acute management of metabolic or endocrine problems are to stop further decompensation and buildup of toxic metabolites and to support with appropriate nutrient, substrate, enzyme, or hormone. This may be accomplished through the following:
  - Reducing or eliminating any food or drug that cannot be metabolized properly
  - Replacing missing or inactive enzymes or other chemicals if possible
  - Removing toxic products of metabolism that accumulate due to the metabolic disorder
- If the infant's oral feedings are stopped at the time of evaluation, 10% dextrose with electrolytes should be administered, or high glucose rate of infusion if hypoglycemic.
  - The exception to this strategy would be if congenital lactic acidosis or mitochondrial disorders were suspected, since higher carbohydrates exacerbate acidosis. In this situation, 5% dextrose with electrolytes should be administered.
  - If the infant is hyperglycemic, insulin should be considered rather than decrease the dextrose infusion index.
  - If fat oxidation defects are excluded from the evaluation, provide lipids.
- For disorders of calcium, phosphorus, and magnesium, intravenous correction or adjustment should occur while laboratory investigation is pending. Treatment of rare conditions involving toxicities may include parenteral rehydration, diuretics, corticosteroids, antacids, and enemas.
- Electrolytes should be monitored due to intravenous fluid therapy and underlying conditions.
  - Potassium levels should be monitored if acidotic, since potassium falls as acidosis is corrected.
  - Both sodium and potassium should be ordered if certain endocrine disorders are suspected which alter electrolyte balance.
- With certain disorders, it may be necessary to remove or divert toxic metabolites. All of these interventions can be determined in collaboration with the neonatologist and appropriate subspecialist consultants (Abrams & Tiosano, 2020; Cederbaum, 2018; El-Hattab & Sutton, 2017; Konczal & Zinn, 2020; Koves et al., 2018; Swartz & Chan, 2017; Thomas et al., 2018; Wassner & Belfort, 2017).

Long-Term Management

- Lifelong treatment may include diet management, provision of a deficient substance, or vitamin therapy such as vitamin B_{12}, biotin, riboflavin, thiamine, pyridoxine, or folate.
- Supportive therapy includes early intervention, education, family, genetic counseling, and continued follow-up with the pediatrician and appropriate pediatric subspecialists, depending on the case.
- Some of the treatments for metabolic or endocrine disorders are listed in Table 18.4 (El-Hattab & Sutton, 2017; Koves et al., 2018; Merritt & Gallagher, 2018; Thomas et al., 2018).

Table 18.4 Neonatal Nurse Practitioners' Guide for Approach to Care of
Infant With Suspected Metabolic or Endocrine Disorder

Priority	Intervention
Proper identification of abnormal symptoms	■ Complete physical assessment and documentation of abnormalities. ■ Obtain family, maternal, pregnancy, and labor and delivery histories.
Initial evaluation	■ Obtain other tests as indicated (laboratory, radiologic, pulse oximetry, echocardiogram).
Initial stabilization	■ Provide basic stabilization per the Neonatal Resuscitation Program guidelines and systems approach to problems. ■ Treat acid–base imbalances. ■ If metabolic disorder is suspected, consider nothing per mouth and intravenous dextrose infusion. ■ Do not transfuse without consultation with at least the neonatologist since genetic studies may be required before transfusion.
Communicate with parents initially	■ Provide honest description of what is observed as abnormal findings. ■ Do not offer a diagnosis, unless it is confirmed. ■ Reassure parents that further tests will be performed, the infant will be supported, and specialists are available if needed.
Proper notification of colleagues	■ Notify the neonatologist per institutional and practice expectations.
Consider need for transport	■ Based on the stability of the infant and resources in the institution, consider need for transport to regional children's hospital with subspecialist support at this time.
Further evaluation	■ Consider the remainder of first-line investigation studies, if not already obtained.
Consideration of need for subspecialist consultation	■ If symptoms persist or worsen and diagnosis is unclear, consider subspecialist consultation request. The type of consultation depends on the case presentation and the systems involved.
Support recommendations of consultant	■ Based on discussion with team, as recommended by consultants, order further second-line diagnostic tests. ■ Provide supportive interventions per recommendations.
Plan family conference	■ Once a diagnosis or plan for diagnostic tests is made, conduct an interdisciplinary family conference to answer all questions, provide information regarding possible differential diagnoses, and identify goals of hospitalization, for example, cardiorespiratory stability, feeding (oral, nasogastric, etc.), and discharge to home or eventual transport. ■ If necessary, discuss the need for transport to regional children's hospital.
Plan for functional goals	■ Identify an appropriate plan for functional goals of the infant. ■ Communicate plan to the entire team (neonatology, nursing, support staff). ■ Refer to a social worker for support.
Discharge planning	■ Identify a pediatrician comfortable with following an infant with the disorder. ■ Plan for support, if appropriate; for example, home oxygen and home support for tube feedings. ■ Support nurses to write specific discharge teaching plan. ■ Plan for discharge medications, metabolites, vitamins, and diet, and allow time to obtain the necessary supplements before discharge. ■ Avoid discharge on weekend or holiday unless all necessary items are obtained.
Make appropriate referrals and follow-up appointments	■ If able to be discharged from the institution without transport to regional children's hospital, then: ● Make pediatrician follow-up appointment. ● Complete referral documentation for subspecialist outpatient clinic referrals. ● If appropriate, complete paperwork to obtain special formulas through government-funded programs. ● If necessary, make first appointments at subspecialist clinics. ● If diagnosis is known, refer parents to appropriate support groups.

Sources: Data from Bacino, C. (2017). Genetic issues presenting in the nursery. In E. Eichenwald, A. Hansen, C. R. Martin, & A. Stark (Eds.), *Cloherty and Stark's manual of neonatal care* (8th ed., pp. 117–130). Lippincott Williams & Wilkins; Brown, Z., & Chang, J. (2018). Disorders of carbohydrate metabolism. In C. Gleason & S. Juul (Eds.), *Avery's disease of the newborn* (10th ed., pp. 1403–1416). Elsevier; Burris, H. (2017). Hypoglycemia and hyperglycemia. In E. Eichenwald, A. Hansen, C. Marin, & A. Stark (Eds.), *Cloherty and Stark's manual of neonatal care* (8th ed., pp. 312–334). Lippincott Williams & Wilkins; Cederbaum, S., & Berry, G. T. (2018). Inborn errors of carbohydrate, ammonia, amino acid, and organic acid metabolism. In C. Gleason & S. Juul (Eds.), *Avery's disease of the newborn* (10th ed., pp. 215–238). Elsevier; El-Hattab, A. W., & Sutton, V. R. (2017). Inborn errors of metabolism. In E. Eichenwald, A. Hansen, C. R. Martin, & A. Stark (Eds.), *Cloherty and Stark's manual of neonatal care* (8th ed., pp. 858–891). Lippincott Williams & Wilkins.

▶ CONCLUSION

The evaluation and treatment of metabolic and endocrine disorders can be daunting for the NNP care provider due to the nonspecific, rare presentations, and complexities of the disorders. An overview of metabolic or endocrine disorders has been presented, including a strategy for evaluation and treatment, to guide the NNP. This approach includes a thorough assessment, first-line investigation, second-line investigation, short- and long-term management options,

referrals, discharge planning, and follow-up. The key concepts presented emphasize that an infant may have subtle symptoms of metabolic or endocrine problems that may be in common or coexist with other problems. If a thorough systems approach is applied and referrals to consultants are made at appropriate times, one does not need to feel intimidated by these problems. The goal is, as with all other neonatal problems, to support the infant and the family with the goal of discharge to home with the necessary support, follow-up care, and referrals.

1. The neonatal nurse practitioner (NNP) recognizes most metabolic or endocrine disorders are inherited in a/an:

   A. Autosomal recessive manner
   B. Dominant autosomal manner
   C. Outcome of a new mutation

2. Many metabolic or endocrine problems present in the neonatal period due to:

   A. Cessation of the protective effect of the maternal placenta
   B. Presentation of protein from breast milk or formula
   C. Stimulation of abnormal metabolic processes after birth

3. The neonatal nurse practitioner (NNP) identifies that the importance of health care providers' ability to identify clinical manifestations of metabolic or endocrine disorders in neonates is related to the fact that some disorders:

   A. Necessitate confirmative genetic or endocrine testing
   B. Present before the newborn screen results are known
   C. Require treatments that are not available everywhere

4. The neonatal nurse practitioner (NNP) identifies that the goal of treatment of neonatal metabolic or endocrine disorders is to:

   A. Identify the need for dialysis or renal replacement therapy
   B. Refer to appropriate subspecialists as soon as possible
   C. Stop further decompensation and buildup of toxic metabolites

5. A term infant had been transferred to the NICU due to poor feeding and lethargy. A bacterial and viral sepsis evaluation has been performed and antimicrobial therapy was initiated. The complete blood count was normal and blood culture was negative. The neonatal nurse practitioner (NNP) should consider next testing the infant's serum:

   A. Calcium level
   B. Lactate level
   C. Sodium level

6. A term infant was admitted to the NICU for transient tachypnea of the newborn, which has resolved. The nurses report that the infant is feeding poorly, still requires the radiant warmer due to low temperatures, and has poor tone. A sign on physical exam that would support the neonatal nurse practitioner's (NNP) suspicion of hypothyroidism would be a/an:

   A. Exaggerated Moro reflex
   B. Large anterior fontanel
   C. Small and shortened tongue

7. A 38-week gestational age infant with birth weight of 3.47 kg is admitted to the NICU with hypoglycemia and respiratory distress. A chest x-ray reveals an enlarged heart, and occasional abnormal cardiac rhythm is noted on the EKG. Physical exam reveals an enlarged liver, and laboratory results demonstrate an elevated direct bilirubin of 2.9 mg/dL. This presentation is most consistent with a problem of:

   A. Amino acid metabolism
   B. Fatty acid metabolism
   C. Hyperinsulinism

1. A) Autosomal recessive manner

Most neonates with metabolic or endocrine disorders are healthy at birth and present with nonspecific signs in hours or days after birth, and most are inherited in an autosomal recessive manner. Metabolic or endocrine disorders do not originate from new mutations and are not transmitted via a dominant autosomal manner (El-Hattab & Sutton, 2017; Konczl & Zinn, 2020).

2. A) Cessation of the protective effect of the maternal placenta

Many of these disorders are present during the neonatal period and are revealed as the protective effect of the maternal placenta ceases. Disorders then develop as acute, chronic, or progressive diseases, with potential life-threatening harm. Disorders can appear in infants who receive formula, not just breast milk, and metabolic processes are passive responses to conditions, not the result of a direct stimulation (Cederbaum, 2018; Merritt & Gallagher, 2018; Thomas et al., 2018).

3. B) Present before the newborn screen results are known

Because some metabolic or endocrine disorders present early—before the results of the newborn screen are known—or are not identified by the screen, it is important for health care providers to be able to identify clinical manifestations of these disorders, to provide initial care, and to recognize appropriate times to involve subspecialists. Disorders may require confirmatory testing or need specialty intervention; however, this occurs after the initial identification of metabolic or endocrine disorders and are more effective with prompt recognition (Cederbaum, 2018; Merritt & Gallagher, 2018; Konczal & Zinn, 2020).

4. C) Stop further decompensation and buildup of toxic metabolites

The goals of acute management of metabolic or endocrine problems are to stop further decompensation and buildup of toxic metabolites and to support with appropriate nutrient, substrate, enzyme, or hormone. This may be accomplished by reducing or eliminating any food or drug that cannot be metabolized properly, replacing missing or inactive enzymes or other chemicals if possible, and removing toxic products of metabolism that accumulate due to the metabolic disorder. Referral is necessary but not a primary goal of intervention. Dialysis and/or renal replacement are a singular action in response to some disorders, again not an overarching goal of intervention (El-Hattab & Sutton, 2017; Swartz & Chan, 2017; Wassner & Belfort, 2017).

5. B) Lactate level

First-line investigations of blood often include blood glucose levels; arterial pH, carbon dioxide, bicarbonate, and base deficit; complete blood count; serum lactate, ammonia, amino acids, and liver function studies; and clotting studies. First-line investigations of urine include ketones, organic acids (including orotic acid), reducing substances (if suspecting galactosemia), and amino acids. Serum electrolyte levels such as calcium and sodium alone will not provide appropriate information for management decisions (Cederbaum, 2018; El-Hattab & Sutton, 2017; Swartz & Chan, 2017; Wassner & Belfort, 2017).

6. B) Large anterior fontanel

Physical features of hypothyroidism include a large tongue, periorbital edema, large anterior and posterior fontanels, pallor, perioral cyanosis, poor or hoarse cry, lingual thyroid, or goiter. Clinical signs of hypothyroidism include constipation, hypothermia, poor tone, lethargy, inactivity, respiratory distress, mottled skin, prolonged jaundice, and poor feeding. An exaggerated Moro reflex and a small tongue are not associated with neonatal hypothyroidism (Chuang & Gutmark-Little, 2020; Wassner & Belfort, 2017).

7. B) Fatty acid metabolism

Any disruption of enzyme activity in fatty acid metabolism leads to a deficit in energy production and can be life-threatening. Infants with these disorders present in a catabolic state, with breakdown of fatty acids from adipose tissue, and may present with hypoglycemia, liver problems, cardiomyopathy, cardiac dysrhythmias, skeletal myopathy, and retinal degeneration. Disorders of amino metabolism present with the addition of a high-pitched cry, metabolic acidosis, and hair and nail anomalies. Hyperinsulinism results in incalcitrant hypoglycemia and does not involve the liver (Merritt & Gallagher, 2018).

The Cardiac System

Karen Wright and Jacqueline M. Hoffman

▶ INTRODUCTION

Congenital heart disease (CHD) is one of the more common birth defects, occurring in 6 to 13 per 1,000 births as a result of genetic or environmental factors. Of these infants, 25% have critical CHD requiring intervention. A delay in the diagnosis of critical CHD compromises neonatal outcomes. CHD is the most common genetic anomaly and the leading noninfectious cause of death during the first year of life. Cardiac development is a complex multifactorial process involving a convergence of risk factors resulting in CHD. Congenital disorders of the cardiac system, if left untreated, will compromise neonatal well-being and survival.

▶ CARDIAC SYSTEM DEVELOPMENT

- The cardiac tract arises as a complex process derived from embryogenic cells from multiple origins. The fetus is dependent. Disorders of cardiac development result in abnormal fetal "programming" of tissues and may result in long-term neurobehavioral consequences as well as later health concerns.
- Cardiac development is a complex process occurring early in gestation and in general prior to when pregnancy is known. The heart is one of the first organs to be functional in life and arises from the cardiogenic mesoderm.
- The following are the primary concepts of cardiac development:
  - Gastrulation, the arrangement of the three germ layers
  - Establishment of the first and second heart fields
  - Development of the heart tube
  - Cardiac looping, convergence, and wedging
  - Evolution of septa (common atrium, atrioventricular [AV] canal)
  - Development of the outflow tract
  - Formation of the cardiac valves
  - Design of the coronary arteries and aortic arches
  - Arrangement of the conduction system (Swanson & Erickson, 2021)
- Figure 19.1 depicts the cardiac tube formation during the first 8 weeks.

GESTATIONAL WEEKS 3 TO 12

- Between days 16 and 18 (around week 2), progenitor cells from the endoderm form the splanchnic mesoderm from which the cardiac tube is formed. Fetal development of the heart begins with the cardiac tube from which the cardiac structures arise.
  - The top (cephalic) part of the heart tube gives rise to the aortic arches, and from the bottom (caudal) portion the ventricles. By day 19 (weeks 2–3), angiogenic cells form the two endocardial tubes which develop synchronously. Near day 21 (week 3), the tubes migrate together in a cranial–caudal progression, then fuse and form in a single tube. The inside of the endocardial tube becomes the endocardium and the outside the myocardium (muscular wall) of the heart.
  - The heartbeat begins at days 22 to 23 (week 3) of life and begins pumping blood during week 4. The heart begins as a heart tube, which undergoes complex developmental tasks such as looping, shifting, and septation to result in a circulatory pattern. Venous–arterial communication evolves from a primitive to a complex state.
  - Complete cardiac development occurs at 6 weeks of embryologic age.
  - Disorders of this period include transposition of the great arteries and dextrocardia.
- Septation of the primordial atrium begins by the end of week 4. The atrial septum is derived from the septum primum and the septum secundum. The foramen ovale (FO) forms as a result of the septum secundum overlapping the foramen secundum.
- Ventricular septation from the endocardial cushions is coordinated with formation of the AV valves and semilunar valves. Spiraling of the truncus arteriosus and the bulbus cordis results in a single trunk separating into two vessels: the aorta and the pulmonary artery (PA). The aortic and aortic branches develop during this time.
- The major structures of the heart are completed by 8 weeks after fertilization (10 weeks' postmenstrual age). Most major defects arise during weeks 6

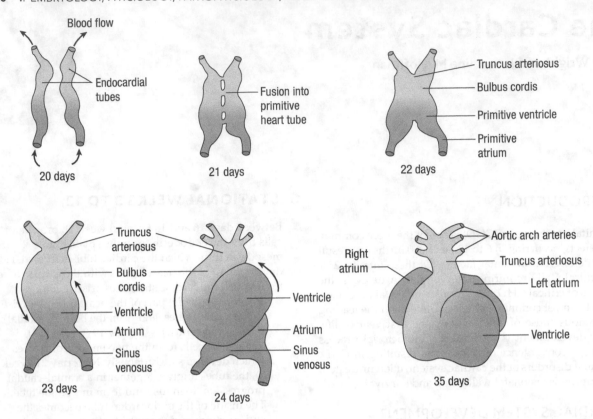

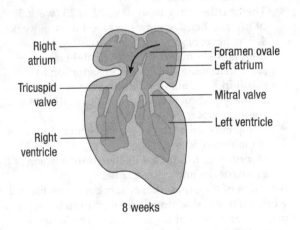

Figure 19.1 The developing heart tube.

to 7 of development. Disorders arising from this developmental period include the following:

- Failure of the AV valves to form *results* in tricuspid and mitral valve abnormalities.
- Failure of proper formation of the septum *results* in ventricular septal defect (VSD), atrial septal defects (ASD), AV septal defect, or endocardiac cushion defect.
- Failure of the vessels to form and separate *results* in coarctation of the aorta (COA) or an interrupted arch.

■ The etiology of most congenital heart defects is completely understood but is thought to include both genetic and environmental factors in most nonsyndromic congenital heart defects (Blackburn, 2018; Dees & Baldwin, 2018; Ford et al., 2020; Sadowski & Verlan, 2021; Swanson & Erickson, 2021).

■ Figure 19.1 depicts the cardiac tube formation during the first 8 weeks.

▶ **INCIDENCE AND RISK FACTORS FOR THE DEVELOPMENT OF CONGENITAL HEART DISEASE**

■ Prenatal diagnosis often occurs due to the widespread use of antenatal ultrasound, suggesting cardiac anomalies 39% of the time. Ultrasound leads to fetal echocardiography for diagnosis of CHD.
  ● The timing for fetal echocardiography should be between 18 and 20 weeks' gestational age.
  ● Only 39% of CHDs are diagnosed prenatally despite prenatal ultrasound. Prenatal diagnosis of congenital heart defects improves patient outcomes and decreases morbidity and mortality, allowing for interventions at delivery if needed.
■ The incidence of CHD in live-born infants is 3 to 9 per 1,000 live births, or approximately 1% of live births, and remains constant. In general, risk factors are not evident; however, certain maternal and fetal conditions are associated with risk of CHD (Cottrill & Hidestrand, 2020a; Sadowski & Verklan, 2021; Swanson & Erickson, 2021; Vernon & Lewin, 2018).

MATERNAL HEALTH

■ Maternal diabetes prior to conception adds two to four times the risk of CHD. Elevated insulin levels result in hypertrophic cardiac tissue.
  ● Maternal presence of anti-Ro or anti-La antibodies related to maternal systemic lupus erythematosus results in placental passage of immunoglobulin C antibody, which deposits *complement* near the AV node, resulting in fetal heart block or possible hydrops.
  ● Females with diabetes mellitus, especially those who are dependent on insulin, have a five times greater risk of delivering an infant with a CHD.
    ❑ The defects *most identified* in infants of diabetic mothers (IDMs) are transposition of the great vessels (TOGV), VSD, cardiomyopathy, and a variety of complex CHDs.
■ Maternal lupus disease is associated with fetal and neonatal complete congenital heart block and dilated cardiomyopathy.
■ Maternal infections with viral or bacterial illnesses can be associated with an increased risk of CHD.
  ● Rubella and cytomegalovirus (CMV) are strongly associated with persistent ductus arteriosus (PDA), pulmonary stenosis (PS) and *branch* PA stenosis, ASD, and VSD.
■ Cardiac teratogens include alcohol, tobacco, anticonvulsants, anticoagulants, lithium, amphetamines, and selective serotonin reuptake inhibitors (SSRIs; Cottrill & Hidestrand, 2020a; Sadowski & Verklan, 2021).

GENETIC FACTORS

■ The single greatest risk factor for CHD is genetic. The overall incidence of CHD in patients with a chromosome aberration is 30%.
  ● The incidence of CHD varies with each chromosomal aberration. Syndromes that should raise suspicion for CHD include trisomies 13, 18, and 21; Turner syndrome; microdeletion syndromes (e.g., DiGeorge and Noonan syndromes); and Beckwith–Wiedemann, VACTERL (**V**ertebral anomalies, **A**nal atresia, **C**ardiac defects, **T**racheo**E**sophageal fistula, **R**enal anomalies, and **L**imb abnormalities), and CHARGE (**C**oloboma, **H**eart defects, **A**tresia choanae, growth **R**etardation, **G**enital abnormalities, and **E**ar abnormalities) syndromes (Blackburn, 2018; Cottrill & Hidestrand, 2020a; Sadowski & Verklan, 2021; Swanson & Erickson, 2021).

FAMILY HISTORY

■ Familial history of CHD increases the incidence, with a higher incidence in closer relatives (parents and siblings). The risk of CHD in a newborn with a sibling with CHD is more than double (Sadowski & Verklan, 2021; Scholz & Reinking, 2018; Swanson & Erickson, 2021).

SEX

■ Male infants are more likely to experience coarctation of the aorta (COA), aortic stenosis (AS), TOGV, and hypoplastic left heart syndrome (HLHS).
■ Female infants are more likely to experience ASD and PDA (Sadowski & Verklan, 2021).

GESTATIONAL AGE

■ The majority of infants with CHD are born at term.
■ Infants born prematurely are more likely to experience PDA, VSD, and AV canal defects (Sadowski & Verklan, 2021).

▶ **CLINICAL PRESENTATION OF AN INFANT WITH CONGENITAL HEART DISEASE**

■ The time and presentation of CHD depend on the severity and physiology of the underlying disorder. CHD may present at delivery through the first few weeks of life. Birth transition and ductal closure, in conjunction with cardiopulmonary physiology, impact the presentation of the disorder.
■ The critical findings of CHD are cyanosis, respiratory distress, congestive heart failure (CHF), diminished cardiac output, abnormal cardiac rhythm, and cardiac murmurs (Breinholt, 2017; Swanson & Erickson, 2021).

DIFFERENTIAL DIAGNOSIS

■ Differential diagnosis of CHD is a clinical challenge in the NICU due to the similarity in presentation to intrapulmonary right-to-left shunting. Pulmonary etiologies that are similar to CHD in presentation include pulmonary hypertension (HTN), pneumonia, respiratory distress syndrome (RDS), congenital diaphragmatic hernia (CDH), pneumothorax, and airway obstruction. Overall considerations for differential diagnosis of CHD include:
  ● Persistent pulmonary hypertension of the newborn (PPHN)
  ● Respiratory etiologies (RDS, aspiration)
  ● Central nervous system disorders (lesions, neuromuscular disease)
  ● Chest compression (CDH, pneumothorax)
  ● Septicemia
  ● Airway obstruction (Pierre Robin, tracheal stenosis, thoracic dystrophies)
  ● Methemoglobinemia (Breinholt, 2017)

PHYSICAL EXAMINATION

■ A complete physical examination will provide clues to cardiac pathology. Physical examination of the newborn is holistic and not necessarily focused only on heart sounds.

NEUROLOGIC ASSESSMENT

■ The assessment of the neonate should begin with a general observation of the infant's overall appearance and behavior. A newborn with CHD may exhibit decreased activity and/or appear flaccid (Vargo, 2019).

CARDIAC/PERFUSION ASSESSMENT

Color

■ Cyanosis is a bluish color of the lips, tongue, mucous membranes, skin, earlobes, and nail beds due to deoxygenated venous blood. Cyanosis occurs when blood shunts "right to left," causing deoxygenated blood to enter the system and bypass the lungs for oxygenation. Cyanosis is visible after 3 g/dL of desaturated hemoglobin is present in the arterial system.
■ Central cyanosis must be differentiated from noncardiac etiologies, such as:
  ● Acrocyanosis, which refers to bluish hands and feet and is a normal finding
  ● Pulmonary HTN or respiratory disease, which may result in cyanosis secondary to cardiac right-to-left shunting
  ● Central nervous system disorders that result in hypoxemia
  ● Methemoglobinemia, which is not due to hypoxemia but rather a blood disorder

■ Pallor and mottling should also be considered, as infants with CHD may appear pale due to vasoconstriction and/or shunting.
■ Capillary refill should be less than 3 seconds to be considered normal (Sadowski & Verklan, 2021; Scholz & Reinking, 2018; Swanson & Erickson, 2021; Vargo, 2019).

Pulses

■ Peripheral pulses should be assessed for rate, rhythm, volume, and character. Pulses represent an approximate determination of cardiac output. The axillary, palmar, brachial, radial, femoral, popliteal, posterior tibial, and dorsalis pedis may be palpated using the index finger.
  ● Two methods to grade:
    ❑ From 0 (absent) to 4+ (bounding)
    ❑ From 0 (absent) to 3+ (full or bounding)
■ Abnormalities in peripheral pulses may be present. It is helpful to compare upper to lower and side to side for discrepancies.
  ● Weak pulses indicate shock, myocardial failure, or left outflow obstructions.
  ● Bounding pulses indicate cardiac runoff (surplus), such as PDA, aortic insufficiency, *and* systemic to pulmonary shunts (Phelps et al., 2020; Sadowski & Verklan, 2021; Vargo, 2019).

Cardiac Sounds

■ Murmurs are common and may be normal or abnormal. All neonates at one time have a murmur due to the closure of the PDA. Auscultation of a murmur requires consideration and evaluation. Most innocent murmurs are systolic.
■ Loudness or intensity of the murmur should be determined and recorded by the "grade":
  ● *Grade I:* barely audible; audible only after a period of careful auscultation
  ● *Grade II:* soft, but audible immediately
  ● *Grade III:* of moderate intensity (but not associated with a thrill)
  ● *Grade IV:* louder (may be associated with a thrill)
  ● *Grade V:* very loud; can be heard with the stethoscope rim barely on the chest (may be associated with a thrill)
  ● *Grade VI:* extremely loud; can be heard with the stethoscope just slightly removed from the chest (may be associated with a thrill)
■ If a murmur is not heard, the infant may still have severe heart disease.
■ Significant murmurs indicative of disease (pathologic) appear associated with the associated physiology. Diastolic murmurs are considered pathologic, and the severity of the murmur can be diagnostic.
  ● Valvular stenosis or insufficiency generally occurs shortly after birth. Systolic murmurs (occurring during systole) are heard in mitral, tricuspid insufficiency, VSD, tetralogy of Fallot (TOF), ASD,

and total anomalous pulmonary venous return (TAPVR).

- In the newborn with suspected CHD, listen with a stethoscope over the fontanel and liver for a continuous bruit murmur, indicating an arteriovenous malformation (AVM; Sadowski & Verklan, 2021; Scholz & Reinking, 2018; Swanson & Erickson, 2021; Vargo, 2019).

RESPIRATORY ASSESSMENT

- Respiratory distress, such as grunting, flaring, and retractions, is not normally found in infants with CHD. Cyanosis from CHD will not be impacted by inspired oxygen (if a right-to-left shunt is present).
  - If respiratory distress is present with CHD, it would most often occur with pulmonary overcirculation which is not draining due to pulmonary vein or left heart anomalies, as in pulmonary edema. In these cases, infants do exhibit respiratory distress (grunting, flaring, and retractions); a chest x-ray will be helpful in these cases, but not diagnostic of CHD.
- Diaphoresis may be evident if the infant is in CHF due to stimulation of the autonomic nervous system resulting in an increase in metabolic demands (Swanson & Erickson, 2021).

ABDOMINAL ASSESSMENT

- An abdominal examination should be done to assess for hepatomegaly due to systemic venous overload and hepatic venous congestion (Swanson & Erickson, 2021).

VITAL SIGNS

- For term infants, the normal heart rate is 120 to 160 for 0 to 7 days of life. Premature infants have a higher resting heart rate.
- Respiratory rate is 30 to 60 breaths per minute. The less mature the infant, the more likely the breathing pattern is to be irregular.
- Blood pressure (BP) varies by gestational age, wellness, temperature, postnatal age, behavior state, and cuff size. For accuracy, BP cuff should be 25% larger than the arm width.
  - BP differences between the upper and lower extremities (>10–15 mmHg) may be due to aortic arch abnormalities.
- Observe the color of the infant's skin and mucous membranes. Normally, the lips and mucous membranes should be pink and well perfused. Acrocyanosis (bluish coloration of the hands and feet) after birth is common and may persist during transition (up to 24 hours) following delivery (Blackburn, 2018; Breinholt, 2017; Cottrill & Mohan,

2020; Fraser, 2019; Sadowski & Verklan, 2021; Vargo, 2019).

DIAGNOSTIC TESTING

- Ability to oxygenate is determined by the hyperoxia test, which is conducted by obtaining an arterial partial pressure of oxygen in arterial blood (PaO_2) in room air and in 100% oxygen, allowing 10 minutes in each prior to the test and comparison of the values.
  - Evaluate pre- and postductal PaO_2s; preductal oxygenation is determined from blood sampling the right radial or temporal artery, postductal oxygenation is determined from blood sampling obtained from an umbilical artery catheter (UAC). Obtain simultaneously for most accurate comparison; results will be preductal <100 mmHg for cardiac disease and >100 mmHg for pulmonary disease.
  - Testing may include pre- and postductal pulse oximetry as additional information.
  - Testing assists in the differential diagnosis of congenital heart defect versus respiratory etiology.
- Obtaining a chest x-ray assists with the identification of pulmonary findings. A chest x-ray allows for evaluation of visible cardiac characteristics such as abnormal shape, size, and position.
- A cardiothoracic ratio greater than 60% suggests enlargement.
- Cardiac shapes may indicate an underlying disease. Classic findings include:
  - Transposition of the great vessels (TOGV) appears as an "egg on a string."
  - TOF appears "boot-shaped."
  - TAPVR appears like a "snowman."
- The following are types of malposition:
  - *Dextrocardia:* This is a mirror image of its normal position, with the apex pointed to the right.
  - *Mesocardia:* The apex of the heart is in the midline.
  - *Extrathoracic:* The heart develops outside the thoracic cavity, as in ectopia cordis.
- The position of other organs in relation to the heart is also incorporated into the definition of cardiac malposition. Positions of the abdominal organs are as follows:
  - *Situs solitus:* normal location of the atria and abdominal organs
  - *Situs inversus:* right atrium on the left, stomach and spleen on the right, liver on the left
  - *Situs ambiguous:* variable atrial position, but liver and stomach midline
- EKG is used to evaluate arrhythmias but is not as useful in detecting structural heart disease. EKG can add definition to the type of structural heart disease or may appear normal even if there are structural cardiac defects. EKG is helpful in evaluating cardiac defects with

abnormalities of the conduction system, such as sinus node dysfunction, heart block, or accessory pathways.
- Stand T-wave changes indicate myocardial ischemia.
- The normal complex is P-wave, then QRS wave.
- The normal P-wave is 0.04 to 0.08 seconds; the PR interval is 0.09 to 0.12 seconds.
- Echocardiography with Doppler is the gold standard for evaluating cardiovascular anatomy and function. Using two-dimensional (2D) echocardiography, the anatomy, physiologic pressure gradients, and cardiac function can be evaluated. Enhanced echocardiograph includes contrast (to evaluate flow), color flow (to evaluate patterns and direction of blood flow), 2D (evaluating anatomic relationships), and three-dimensional (3D; cross-sectional images; Breinholt, 2017; Cottrill & Hidestrand, 2020a; Phelps et al., 2020; Sadowski & Verklan, 2021; Swanson & Erickson, 2021; Trotter, 2021; Vernon & Lewin, 2018).

LABORATORY ASSESSMENT

- Lab work may be useful to determine a diagnosis of CHD versus other etiologies.
  - Arterial blood gases with a normal partial pressure of carbon dioxide in arterial blood ($PaCO_2$) may be present with CHD unless coinciding respiratory distress or CHF is present. A blood gas revealing a metabolic acidosis may indicate low cardiac output and decreased tissue perfusion.
  - An elevated lactate level indicates poor tissue perfusion and may reflect low cardiac output.
  - A metabolic panel is helpful in evaluating renal function by following blood urea nitrogen (BUN) and creatinine levels.
  - Hypoglycemia may be a secondary effect of CHD due to genetic abnormalities, medications treating CHD, and poor feeding. Diuretic therapy for CHF warrants monitoring of sodium, potassium, and chloride levels.
  - A complete blood count (CBC) is useful to detect significant anemia as well as assist with the differential or coinciding diagnosis of sepsis. Decreased hemoglobin worsens hypoxemia and increases the workload of the heart in infants with CHD (Swanson & Erickson, 2021).

▶ CYANOTIC HEART DEFECTS

- Right-to-left shunting due to CHD results in cyanosis due to the mixture of pulmonary and systemic venous return. These babies may present clinically with tachypnea, poor feeding, hepatomegaly, and pulmonary edema. Cyanotic defects decreasing pulmonary blood flow result in CHF-like symptoms (Scholz & Reinking, 2018).

EBSTEIN ANOMALY

Definition and Pathophysiology

- In fetal life, Ebstein anomaly results from a lack of formation of the tricuspid valve, resulting in a hypoplastic right ventricle. Ebstein anomaly is uncommon and involves a displaced tricuspid valve with a tethered leaflet with functional pulmonary atresia and right-to-left atrial shunting; the right ventricle pumps inefficiently. The valve is displaced into the right ventricle, resulting in a smaller right ventricle and a decrease in ventricular output. The displaced tricuspid valve allows the regurgitation of blood, resulting in a negative impact of blood allowed systemically through the PA.
- With severe tricuspid atresia (TA; regurgitation), only an insignificant amount of blood is passed into the PAs. This results in a ductal-dependent lesion, which may be severe with severe valvular displacement (Breinholt, 2017; Swanson & Erickson, 2021; Phelps et al., 2020).

Diagnosis

- Clinical presentation is cyanosis ranging from mild to severe based on the degree of right-to-left shunting at the FO and is able to be sent to the PA. Heart sounds are of a holosystolic murmur varying from grade I to VI based on the degree of tricuspid regurgitation. Diminished S2 and diastolic murmurs may be heard. Symptoms of CHF are due to volume overload.
- Diagnostic evaluation includes arterial blood gases, which will report low PaO_2 levels of 20 or above; and echocardiography to evaluate for valvular displacement, presence of pulmonary atresia, and shunting. Lactate levels are normal unless the cardiac output is diminished.
- Chest x-ray is markedly abnormal for massive cardiomegaly secondary to right atrial dilatation and decreased pulmonary vascularity depending on alternative sources of pulmonary blood flow. Cardiomegaly may be profoundly related to the severity of tricuspid insufficiency.
- EKG is positive for abnormal P-waves, supraventricular tachycardia (SVT), and right bundle branch block. It may be associated with Wolff–Parkinson–White syndrome, COA, ASD, and PA (Phelps et al., 2020; Swanson & Erickson, 2021; Trotter, 2021).

Management

- Medical management involves giving a large amount of oxygen to keep oxygen saturations greater than 75%, indicating adequate pulmonary blood flow. Prostaglandin E1 (PGE1) may be needed to increase pulmonary blood flow and help relieve hypoxemia.

- Advancements in catheter-based technology and techniques have allowed for some of these patients to be palliated by implantation of a stent in the ductus arteriosus (DA). This interventional palliation procedure can last many months until the patient can undergo complete surgical repair.
- Extracorporeal membranous oxygenation (ECMO) may be indicated. Surgical management is indicated for infants demonstrating severe illness.
- The surgical procedure is annuloplasty (repair of the leaking mitral valve) and repositioning of the valve to minimize mitral regurgitation and plication. A Blalock–Taussig (BT) shunt (creation of a pathway between the right subclavian and pulmonary arteries) may be needed in severe cases, followed by a Glenn surgery (connect the inferior vena cava [IVC] to the PA), then Fontan surgery (Bocks et al., 2020; Swanson & Erickson, 2021).

Outcomes

- Prognosis depends on the amount of tricuspid regurgitation; infants requiring surgery typically have less favorable outcomes. The most successful neonatal outcomes come from either subsequent single palliative care excluding the right ventricle and forming a single ventricle, or cardiac transplant. Replacement of the valve has not been useful in neonates (Swanson & Erickson, 2021).

TETRALOGY OF FALLOT

Definition and Pathophysiology

- TOF is the most common cyanotic congenital heart defect, occurring in about 1 in 5,000 live births, and causes 10% of all congenital cardiac malformations
- TOF presentation relates to the degree of PS. The cause of TOF is unknown but is considered to be genetic. TOF is characterized by four (Fallot) related disorders:
  - Pulmonary stenosis with right ventricular outflow tract (PS/RVOT) obstruction, with severity that directly impacts clinical presentation; a complete RVOT (pulmonary atresia) is a critical form of TOF, and PS varies greatly with TOF
  - VSD
  - An overriding aorta (OA)
  - Right ventricular hypertrophy (RVH; Cottrill & Hidestrand, 2020a; Sadowski & Verklan, 2021; Scholz & Reinking, 2018; Swanson & Erickson, 2021)
- Figure 19.2 demonstrates TOF with mild pulmonary atresia.

Diagnosis

- Diagnosis of TOF is by echocardiogram, which aids in determining the degree of PS, the size of the VSD, and the direction of blood flow across the septum.

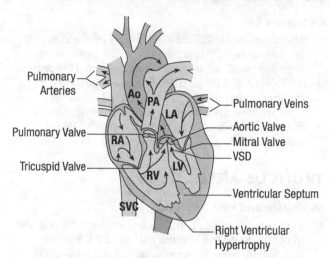

Figure 19.2 Tetralogy of Fallot with mild pulmonary stenosis.
Ao, aorta; LA, left atrium; LV, left vetricle; PA, pulmonary artery; RA, right atrium; RV, right ventricle; SVC, superior vena cava; VSD, ventricular septal defect.

- Blood gases will show normal pCO_2 and pH, and the pO_2 will be low based on the degree of right-to-left shunting.
- Chest x-ray shows a "boot-shaped" heart (due to a small, concave PA and a prominent cardiac apex as a result of RVH) without cardiomegaly. Pulmonary vascularity is more commonly diminished. EKG is nonspecific and shows RVH.
- CBC will provide information about possible coinciding anemia or sepsis.
- Hypercyanotic spells or "tet spells" are acute episodes that can develop in patients with TOF when there is dynamic subpulmonary obstruction of the RVOT. An increased gradient across the RVOT forces deoxygenated blood across the VSD into the aorta, resulting in cyanosis (Breinholt, 2017; Bocks et al., 2020; Cottrill & Hidestrand, 2020a; Swanson & Erickson, 2021; Trotter, 2021).

Management

- Medical management of TOF is generally nonemergent unless there is severe PS. TOF may be ductal-dependent, requiring continuous PGE1 infusion (vasodilator) to maintain ductal patency. Episodes of hypoxia may be managed with oxygen and morphine.
- The treatment for hypercyanotic episodes is to find ways to decrease the subpulmonary obstruction, encourage more pulmonary blood flow, and increase the relative degree of left-to-right shunting at the ventricular level. If these maneuvers are followed, hypercyanotic spells can often be treated quickly before the infant is hypoxic for an unsafe amount of time.
- Surgery to patch the pulmonary valve is completed during the first year of life. If there are periods of severe hypoxia, a BT shunt will be performed (Bocks et al., 2020; Cottrill & Hidestrand, 2020a; Bocks et al., 2020; Swanson & Ericson, 2021).

Outcomes

■ The outcome of TOF is based largely on the size of the PA. Repair of TOF is achievable in the presence of a normal-sized PA. Neonates with cyanotic TOF require a BT shunt and repair during the newborn period.

■ Prognosis after surgical repair is good; however, most will require future surgery or intervention for pulmonary valve replacement later in childhood (Swanson & Erickson, 2021).

TRUNCUS ARTERIOSUS

Definition and Pathophysiology

■ In truncus arteriosus, during embryology, the outflow tract fails to divide into the aorta and PA, both of which arise from the semilunar valve. The result is a single trunk responsible for pulmonary, systemic, and coronary circulation. One great artery overrides the VSD and either divides into right and left arteries (type 1 and type 2) or has separate origins (type 3) and results in pulmonary overcirculation, causing left ventricular (LV) hypertrophy. In utero, there is complete mixing of the systemic and pulmonary venous return above the truncal valve; therefore, because blood flow through the heart is normal, the rest of the heart develops normally.

■ Postnatally, the flow of the PAs and systemic arteries is a function of the relative resistances in the two circuits. As pulmonary venous return increases, CHF develops.

■ Truncus arteriosus is associated with extracardiac anomalies in 20% to 40% of cases, such as dysplastic valves, PS, and truncal valve stenosis. Of neonates with truncus arteriosus, 35% to 40% have 22q11 deletion syndrome (DiGeorge; Blackburn, 2018; Sadowski & Verklan, 2021).

Diagnosis

■ Clinical presentation varies from mild desaturation to cyanosis based on the amount of pulmonary blood flow. Classic physical examination findings include a hyperdynamic precordium, a left precordial bulge, a loud single S2 with an early systolic ejection click, and a systolic ejection murmur along the left sternal border. As pulmonary blood flow increases, the patient develops wide pulse pressure and bounding pulses due to continuous diastolic flow into the PAs and an apical rumble from increased flow across the mitral valve.

■ CHF symptoms may be present based on the amount of pulmonary blood flow. In basic truncus, the pulse oximetry is close to 85% until pulmonary vascular resistance falls and pulmonary blood flow increases. A desaturated infant may be due to increased pulmonary vascular resistance. Poor perfusion and bounding pulses may also be present (Cottrill & Hidestrand, 2020a; Phelps et al., 2020; Sadowski & Verklan, 2021; Scholz & Reinking, 2018; Swanson & Erickson, 2021).

■ Diagnosis is by echocardiography and Doppler flow, noting the number of truncal valve leaflets and valve stenosis.

■ Arterial blood gases may demonstrate normal pH and pCO_2, and pO_2 may or may not be normal based on pulmonary blood flow.

■ EKG will show combined ventricular hypertrophy and atrial enlargement.

■ Chest x-ray will demonstrate cardiomegaly with increased pulmonary vascularity secondary to pulmonary overcirculation. As CHF develops, pulmonary vessels become indistinct and obscured by pulmonary edema.

■ CBC will evaluate the hematocrit and possible origin for sepsis (Cottrill & Hidestrand, 2020a; Phelps et al., 2020; Swanson & Erickson, 2021; Trotter, 2021).

Management

■ Medical management involves treating CHF, such as with diuretics and digoxin, avoiding oxygen to decrease pulmonary overcirculation, and monitoring calcium levels. Calcium levels should be monitored due to the possibility of DiGeorge syndrome.

■ Surgical treatment involves separating the pulmonary arteries and patching the VSD with a homograph (skin from another human), then creating a conduit connected to the PA valve (Cottrill & Hidestrand, 2020a; Phelps et al., 2020; Swanson & Erickson, 2021).

Outcomes

■ The mortality rate for truncus arteriosus is 10% to 20% based on the severity of the disease and degree of truncal valve regurgitation or stenosis and associated genetic and extracardiac anomalies (Swanson & Erickson, 2021).

D-TRANSPOSITION OF THE GREAT VESSELS

Definition and Pathophysiology

■ The most common cyanotic cardiac defect in the newborn is TOGV, specifically d-transposition of the great vessels (d-TOGV), or complete transposition, in which the aorta is left of the PA. In TOGV, the deoxygenated blood returns to the right ventricle and is circulated by the aorta, and oxygenated blood returns to the left ventricle, then to the lungs, resulting in parallel circulation, hypoxia, and cyanosis if there is not a connection between systems. Opportunities for mixing blood include the ASD (best and needed for survival), PDA, and VSD if present.

■ TOGV is more common in males and accounts for 5% of all CHDs. The associated anomalies make a tremendous impact on the presentation of the disorder due to the opportunities for mixing blood. Associated defects include VSD (25%) and RVH. Genetic abnormalities are not normally associated.

- Presentation of d-TOGV depends on the degree of communication between the systems. TOGV presents as cyanosis and tachypnea with increased work of breathing (WOB), a holosystolic murmur (with VSD), or no murmur (Basu & Dobrolet, 2020; Blackburn, 2018; Phelps et al., 2020; Sadowski & Verklan, 2021; Scholz & Reinking, 2018; Swanson & Erickson, 2021).
- Figure 19.3 depicts the defects comprising TOGV.

Diagnosis

- Diagnosis of d-TOGV is by echocardiography, which also identifies associated defects (VSD, COA, interrupted aortic arch [IAA]) and determines the size of the ASD and PDA.
- Arterial blood gases reveal a low PAO$_2$ if there is an intact septum without a VSD. Lactic acid levels should be normal.
- Chest x-ray will demonstrate a cardiac silhouette in the shape of an "egg on a string" due to the narrowing of the mediastinum, but is not diagnostic. Pulmonary vascularity may be increased or decreased. EKG may be normal or show RVH (Basu & Dobrolet, 2020; Phelps et al., 2020; Scholz & Reinking, 2018; Swanson & Erickson, 2021).

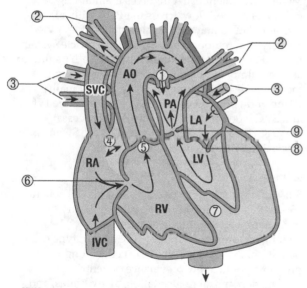

KEY:

① PDA	⑥ Tricuspid Valve
② Pulmonary Arteries	⑦ Ventricular Septum
③ Pulmonary Veins	⑧ Mitral Valve
④ ASD	⑨ Pulmonary Valve
⑤ Aortic Valve	

Figure 19.3 Transposition of the great vessels.

AO, aorta; ASD, atrial septal defect; IVC, inferior vena cava; LA, left atrium; LV, left ventricle; PA, pulmonary artery; PDA, persistent ductus arteriosus; RA, right atrium; RV, right ventricle; SVC, superior vena cava.

Management

- Medical management of d-TOGV is to infuse PGE1 continuously to maintain a PDA and treat metabolic acidosis as d-TOGV may be ductal-dependent to improve oxygenation and atrial shunting.
- Surgical treatment involves the arterial switch procedure, whereby the PA is anastomosed to the right ventricle and the pulmonary valve converted to become the functional aortic valve. Atrial balloon septostomy improves mixing by tearing the FO into an ASD for patients with a small patent foramen ovale (PFO), or with hypoxia and acidosis with a patent ductus. Surgical management is usually completed within 1 week of delivery and is the arterial switch procedure in which the aorta and the PA are switched (Basu & Dobrolet, 2020; Bocks et al., 2020; Phelps et al., 2020).

Outcomes

- Without surgery, 30% will die in the first week, 50% in the first month, and 90% within the first year.
- Infants who are not preterm or without RVH experience favorable outcomes with the arterial switch procedure. Complications after repair are myocardial ischemia and infarction, aortic and/or pulmonary supraventricular stenosis, and dysrhythmias (Basu & Dobrolet, 2020; Sadowski & Verklan, 2021)

TOTAL ANOMALOUS PULMONARY VENOUS RETURN

Definition and Pathophysiology

- TAPVR is a collection of congenital heart defects involving the anatomy of the pulmonary veins which return to the right heart circulation instead of normally returning to the left atrium. During fetal life, the pulmonary venous system development results in the absence of communication between the common pulmonary vein and the splanchnic plexus into the dorsal wall of the left atrium.
- There are four types of pulmonary venous return:
  - *Supracardiac:* 50% and is the most common; routes into the superior vena cava (SVC) and right atrium (RA)
  - *Infracardiac:* 15%; routes through the diaphragm and liver into the IVC to RA
  - *Cardiac:* 25%; routes pulmonary veins through the coronary sinus or RA
  - *Mixed type:* 10%; routes left pulmonary veins through the systemic veins and right pulmonary veins to the RA; ASD or PFO needed for survival; associated with left heart defects, TOGV, TOF, and heterotaxy (Basu & Dobrolet, 2020; Blackburn, 2018; Breinholt, 2017; Cottrill & Hidestrand, 2020a; Phelps et al., 2020; Swanson & Erickson, 2021)

Diagnosis

■ Clinical presentation varies because there are different variations, all present differently and at different times in the neonatal period. Cyanosis of a newborn varies with saturations less than 80%. If there is obstructive TAPVR, the result is venous congestion and decreased pulmonary blood flow. Murmurs are not usually present with TAPVR unless the infant is in CHF. Less severe types of TAPVR are usually asymptomatic in the neonatal period (if unobstructed); infracardiac presents in the neonatal period. Diagnosis of TAPVR is by echocardiogram with 2D imaging and color flow to map the blood flow.

■ Chest x-ray demonstrates a snowman sign (caused by widening of the superior mediastinum secondary to dilated mediastinal veins), although this is not diagnostic. Chest x-ray may also show pulmonary edema secondary to pulmonary venous obstruction. There may be cardiomegaly and increased pulmonary vascular markings. EKG may show RVH and right atrial enlargement (Basu & Dobrolet, 2020; Cottrill & Hidestrand, 2020a; Phelps et al., 2020; Trotter, 2021).

Management

■ Medical management of obstructive TAPVR is respiratory, metabolic support, and possibly ECMO until surgical anastomosis.

■ Obstructive TAPVR requires immediate surgery to increase blood flow and is based on the type of TAPVR. Surgery may involve reimplantation of the common vein or directing the anomalous veins to the left atrium (Basu & Dobrolet, 2020; Bocks et al., 2020; Cottrill & Hidestrand, 2020a; Phelps et al., 2020; Swanson & Erickson, 2021).

Outcomes

■ Prognosis of TAPVR is good unless the pulmonary veins are hypoplastic. Complications that may occur include dysrhythmias and pulmonary venous obstruction. The mortality rate of TAPVR varies from 10% to 25% (Phelps et al., 2020; Swanson & Erickson, 2021).

TRICUSPID ATRESIA

Definition and Pathophysiology

■ In TA, the right atrium and right ventricle are not connected due to agenesis of the tricuspid valve, resulting in right ventricular hypoplasia and PA hypoplasia with VSD and possible hypoplastic right ventricle. Blood shunts across the ASD and blood goes to the lungs via left-to-right shunting via the PDA or a VSD with relative hypoxia.

■ TA may be associated with transposition of the great arteries (30%–50%) and COA and relies on the presence of an ASD for neonatal survival at birth (Basu & Dobrolet, 2020; Blackburn, 2018; Breinholt, 2017; Phelps et al., 2020; Sadowski & Verklan, 2021; Swanson & Erickson, 2021).

Diagnosis

■ TA presents as varied cyanosis with ductal closure and based on pulmonary blood flow. Murmurs from an associated VSD or PDA may be audible. Symptoms of CHF may also be present (e.g., possible murmur, possible hepatomegaly).

■ Echocardiogram is the gold standard for diagnosis, demonstrating a large right atrium, an absent tricuspid valve, and the presence of right-to-left shunting across the atria, as well as a coexisting VSD or PDA.

■ Chest x-ray may be normal or show cardiomegaly. Pulmonary vascularity varies based on the amount of pulmonary blood flow.

■ EKG will have a left-axis deviation with a counterclockwise loop.

■ Arterial blood gases will show normal pH and pCO_2, with low to normal pO_2 based on the amount of shunting that is present. CBC will determine if anemia is present and aid in the screening of coinciding sepsis (Basu & Dobrolet, 2020; Swanson & Erickson, 2021; Trotter, 2021).

Management

■ Medical treatment of TA involves maintaining pulmonary blood flow across the PDA with a PGE1 infusion and so may be ductal-dependent.

■ Surgery is to remodel to a single left ventricle system for cardiac output. The infant may need a BT shunt to assure pulmonary blood flow, and PA banding if there is excessive pulmonary circulation. Finally, Glenn and Fontan procedures (diversion of the IVC and SVC blood to the PA) may also be necessary (Basu & Dobrolet, 2020; Bocks et al., 2020; Swanson & Erickson, 2021).

Outcomes

■ Survival through all three stages is variable; generally 85% with single left ventricle anatomy. Heart transplant may eventually be needed.

■ Among children who undergo the Fontan type of operation, those with TA have excellent long-term prognosis, with a low prevalence of ventricular dysfunction, mitral regurgitation, arrhythmias, and systemic venous congestion (Basu & Dobrolet, 2020; Swanson & Erickson, 2021).

PROSTAGLANDIN E1 (ALPROSTADIL) USE IN CYANOTIC HEART DISEASE

■ PGE1 (alprostadil) is a smooth muscle vasodilator, as is the ductus arteriosus (DA). During fetal life, the placenta is the source of PGE1. The action of PGE1 is to establish ductal patency and promote the shunting of blood from the PA (oxygenated) to the aorta (less oxygenated), establishing a flow that is right to left.

PGE1 increases blood flow through the PA, which promotes shunting across the atria.
- In infants with suspected CHD, begin PGE1 empirically until the diagnosis is confirmed and continue until corrective treatments are completed.
- PGE1 dose is peripheral intravenous (IV) or umbilical venous catheter (UVC) based on clinical situation. A larger ductus on echocardiogram indicates a lower continuous dose (0.01 mcg/kg/min) is needed, while a smaller ductus indicates a higher dose (0.05 mcg/kg/min), then titrate to the lowest possible dose needed to avoid side effects. The maximum dose is 0.10 mcg/kg/min.
- Apnea is the major side effect of PGE1 and should be prepared for respiratory assistance prior to beginning infusion. Other side effects include hypotension and tachycardia. Long-term use of PGE1 will result in periosteal thickening or gastric outlet thickening.
- Prior to transport, consider intubation of the infant receiving continuous PGE1 (Bocks et al., 2020; Breinholt, 2017; Cottrill & Hidestrand, 2020a; Phelps et al., 2020; Swanson & Erickson, 2021).

▶ ACYANOTIC DEFECTS

VENTRICULAR SEPTAL DEFECT

Definition and Pathophysiology
- A VSD may be isolated or part of a congenital cardiac disease and is the most common congenital heart defect. Openings in the septum divide the right and left ventricle.
- There are multiple types of VSD based on size and location. VSD may impact valve function and may result in complications if left patent. Shunting of the VSD is left to right. A small VSD is not clinically significant, while a large VSD may result in clinical symptoms by sending blood back to the lungs, resulting in pulmonary overcirculation, CHF, respiratory distress, and pulmonary edema. The severity is related to the severity of pulmonary vascular resistance. Infants may also experience poor growth. VSD is associated with COA.
- The four types of VSD are (a) inlet, (b) muscular (60%), (c) perimembranous (membranous, infracristal), and (d) outlet (Basu & Dobrolet, 2020; Blackburn, 2018; Cottrill & Hidestrand, 2020a; Phelps et al., 2020; Scholz & Reinking, 2018; Swanson & Erickson, 2021).

Diagnosis
- Clinical presentation is related to the size of the VSD. VSDs are acyanotic and present with a grade II, holosystolic, harsh murmur. The murmur may not be audible until pulmonary vascular resistance decreases. Larger VSDs result in symptoms of CHF.
- Postnatal diagnosis involves chest x-ray, which may show a normal heart size or cardiomegaly and increased pulmonary vascular markings.

- EKG is usually normal or may indicate biventricular hypertrophy. A VSD is diagnosed by 2D echocardiography and color flow for multiple VSDs (Basu & Dobrolet, 2020; Phelps et al., 2020; Swanson & Erickson, 2021; Trotter, 2021).

Management
- Management of VSD involves medical or surgical management. Medical management is pharmacologic to control CHF and includes digoxin, diuretics, afterload reducers (enalapril), and nutritional caloric supplementation for optimal nutrition. If the infant is not growing due to the VSD, surgical approach is indicated. Monitoring growth and nutrition is indicated.
- Larger VSDs of any type can result in considerable left-to-right shunting with pulmonary overcirculation and associated symptomatology, including tachypnea, increased WOB, poor feeding, and suboptimal weight gain.
- Surgical repair is through the right atrium and tricuspid valve. PA banding may be necessary for palliative reduction in pulmonary blood flow (Basu & Dobrolet, 2020; Scholz & Reinking, 2018; Swanson & Erickson, 2021).

Outcomes
- Spontaneous closure of VSD is common. However, a large VSD may instigate CHF and result in pulmonary vascular occlusive disease. Half of small VSDs close spontaneously (Phelps et al., 2020).

COARCTATION OF THE AORTA

Definition and Pathophysiology
- COA is obstruction or constriction of the aortic arch near the PDA, but can occur anywhere above the aortic valve and anywhere from the transverse arch to the bifurcation of the iliac arteries. Coarctation generally develops postnatally but may be detected prenatally. The incidence is 7% of cardiac lesions and is associated with Turner syndrome. More severe obstruction results in LV failure or poor cardiac output. There are three types of coarctation based on location (Figure 19.4):
  - Type A: before the subclavian
  - Type B: between the left carotid artery and the left subclavian
  - Type C: between the first and second head and neck vessels
- COA is a ductal-dependent lesion that affects blood supply to the descending aorta and is associated with a bicuspid aortic valve and a VSD. VSDs are invariably associated with an interrupted aortic arch. Other anomalies associated with COA include an aortopulmonary window, truncus arteriosus, and transposition of the great arteries. Associated genetic conditions include DiGeorge Syndrome and Turner syndrome (Basu & Dobrolet, 2020; Blackburn, 2018;

Bocks et al., 2020; Breinholt, 2017; Scholz & Reinking, 2018; Swanson & Erickson, 2021).

Diagnosis

- Clinical presentation is directly impacted by the degree of aortic narrowing. COA presents as critical illness after ductal closure due to obstructed LV blood flow and poor cardiac output past the obstruction. Signs and symptoms of newborns with coarctation are due to CHF and poor cardiac output.
- The hallmark of COA is diminished femoral pulses. Coarctation may or may not present with an audible grade I to IV soft systolic murmur audible in the left sternal border.
- Echocardiography is used to identify aortic narrowing and any additional left-sided obstructive lesions. EKG will be positive for RVH.
- Right-to-left shunting is found at the DA and indicates a larger left ventricle. Chest x-ray is usually normal. If cardiomegaly is present, this may be associated with other lesions or ventriculomegaly after ductal closure. Ductal closure will also result in increased pulmonary vascularity secondary to pulmonary venous congestion.

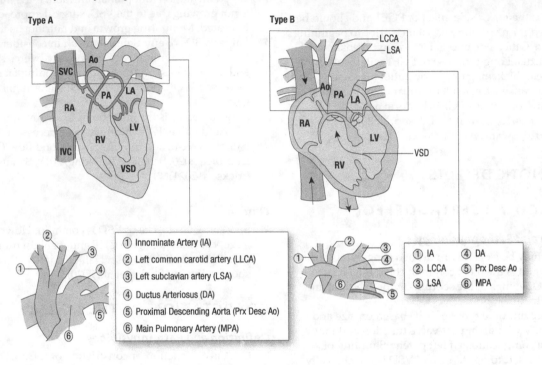

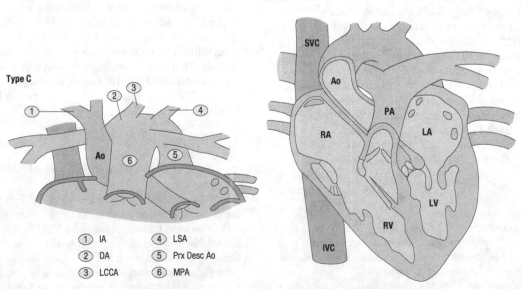

Figure 19.4 Three types of coarctation of the aorta.

IVC, inferior vena cava; PA, pulmonary artery; SVC, superior vena cava; VSD, ventricular septal defect.

- Pulse oximetry and arterial blood gas measurements document shunting (Basu & Dobrolet, 2020; Scholz & Reinking, 2018; Swanson & Erickson, 2021; Trotter, 2021).

Management

- Medical management involves continuous prostaglandin (PG) infusion for infants with poor perfusion or signs of CHF prior to surgery. Continuous inotropes such as dopamine and dobutamine are suggested for cardiovascular support, and metabolic acidosis should be corrected.
- Surgical repair determined by the severity of symptomatic infants by end-to-end anastomosis is completed, as well as closure of the VSD (Basu & Dobrolet, 2020; Bocks et al., 2020; Phelps et al., 2020; Scholz & Reinking, 2018; Swanson & Erickson, 2021).

Outcomes

- The mortality rate after surgical repair of COA is just above 5%. Of COAs, 10% to 15% recur and are managed with balloon angioplasty.
- Long-term growth of the repaired aortic segment might be an issue in up to 30% of infants, resulting in significant aortic narrowing or recurrent coarctation, particularly in premature infants. Balloon aortic angioplasty has become the preferred treatment for recurrent coarctation in infants and young children, with demonstrated safety and efficacy (Basu & Dobrolet, 2020; Scholz & Reinking, 2018).

ATRIAL SEPTAL DEFECT

Definition and Pathophysiology

- An ASD may be part of a complex cardiac disease or isolated. During fetal life, the atrial opening between the left and right atria is patent. The opening between the atria is patent in fetal life (PFO), or ASD may be ostium primum, secundum (most), or endocardial cushion. If the opening is less than 6 mm in a term infant, it will likely close spontaneously and is considered to be a PFO. The ASD is generally not diagnosed prenatally due to the presence of the PFO.
- The four most common types of ASD are:
  - *Secundum:* most common; associated with Holt–Oram
  - *Primum:* associated with the AV canal
  - *Sinus venosus:* a variation of anomalous venous return
  - Coronary sinus (Basu & Dobrolet, 2020; Cottrill & Hidestrand, 2020a; Sadowski & Verklan, 2021; Scholz & Reinking, 2018; Swanson & Erickson, 2021)

Diagnosis

- Clinical presentation of ASD is acyanotic because the shunting of blood is primarily from the left to the right atrium. Oxygen saturation is normal and a large

amount of left-to-right shunting results in a large ejection murmur, as in mild PS. A large ASD does not cause CHF.
- Diagnosis is by echocardiography. Arterial blood gas values are normal with an ASD. Electrolytes and renal function labs should be normal, as well as chest x-ray. An ASD may result in cardiomegaly later in life. EKG would be normal.
- Chest x-ray may be normal, with small defects. With large left-to-right shunts, there are moderate cardiac enlargement and increased pulmonary vascularity obscured by pulmonary edema (Basu & Dobrolet, 2020; Swanson & Erickson, 2021; Trotter, 2021).

Management

- Transcatheter devices are now commonly used for secundum ASD closure, especially for those defects that are very large or result in intractable CHF. Surgical repair is required for the ASD that cannot be closed by cardiac catheterization interventions (Basu & Dobrolet, 2020; Sadowski & Verklan, 2021).

Outcomes

- A balanced, complete ASD with no significant common AV valve abnormalities, ventricular dysfunction, or outflow tract anomalies is repaired on an elective basis in the first 4 to 6 months of life with a high degree of success.
- Most ASDs (80%) close spontaneously by 2 years of life. Surgical management is indicated for a primum ASD, sinus venosus, or secundum ASD that cannot be closed by cardiac catheterization later in life. Cardiac catheterization may be an option to insert a device to "plug the hole." Surgery by suture closure or patch of the defect is generally for older children (Basu & Dobrolet, 2020; Swanson & Erickson, 2021).

HYPOPLASTIC LEFT HEART SYNDROME

Definition and Pathophysiology

- A popular theory is that HLHS may result from in utero obstruction of blood flow to the left ventricle, thus preventing the growth of the ventricle and nearby vascular structures. HLHS is usually diagnosed prenatally whenever four chambers are not viewed.
- HLHS is characterized by coinciding spectrum disorders:
  - Aortic valve atresia
  - Mitral valve atresia
  - Severe LV hypoplasia
  - Aortic hypoplasia and COA
- An ASD is required to mix blood and decrease pulmonary edema. If the ASD is too small, it is life-threatening. The only available circulation is blood traveling from the PA through the DA to the aorta.
- HLHS is critically ductal-dependent to prevent systemic hypoperfusion, acidosis, and organ perfusion. Too much blood sent to the lungs will result in poor perfusion, and too little blood to the lungs results in hypoxia.

- HLHS is associated with multiple associations such as Turner syndrome, trisomy 9, trisomy 13, trisomy 18, Holt–Oram, Smith–Lemli–Opitz, and Jacobsen syndrome (Basu & Dobrolet, 2020; Breinholt, 2017; Cottrill & Hidestrand, 2020a; Phelps et al., 2020; Scholz & Reinking, 2018; Swanson & Erickson, 2021).
- Figure 19.5 depicts the defects associated with HLHS.

Diagnosis

- HLHS presents as tachypnea and cyanosis and may or may not have a murmur. Perfusion and palpable pulses diminish with ductal closure. Oxygen saturations may be low, with poor systemic perfusion. Listening to heart sounds may reveal a single S1 and S2. If too much blood is sent to the lungs, infants will show signs of CHF, and if too little hypoxia.
- Diagnosis is by echocardiography showing right ventricular dilatation, a small left ventricle, and a hypoplastic mitral and aortic valve. Echocardiogram will also be useful in determining the size of the ASD and PDA, as well as cardiac function.
- Chest x-ray may appear normal until significant cardiac decompensation occurs when the DA starts to close. This results in pulmonary edema, and the chest x-ray demonstrates cardiomegaly and increased pulmonary vascular markings followed by significant

pulmonary congestion. EKG will be abnormal with RVH and right-axis deviation.
- Arterial blood gases should indicate normal pH with low pO_2 and normal pCO_2 when pulmonary and systemic blood flow is balanced; an increased oxygen saturation with acidosis reflects increased pulmonary blood flow with decreased systemic perfusion. CBC should be done to evaluate for anemia, which can aggravate hypoxia (Basu & Dobrolet, 2020; Sadowski & Verklan, 2021; Swanson & Erickson, 2021; Trotter, 2021).

Management

- Medical management of HLHS includes preventing excessive pulmonary blood flow and a continuous infusion of PGE1 to maintain ductal patency. Because oxygen is a vasodilator, it should be avoided with HLHS. Volume expansion and inotropes help balance pulmonary and systemic circulation. Milrinone is an afterload reducer and pulmonary vasodilator if ventricular function is decreased and BP is stable. If this is not achieved, surgical management is indicated.
- The Norwood procedure increases systemic blood flow and decreases excessive pulmonary blood flow in three surgical steps:
  - *Norwood procedure:* enlarges ASD, ligates PDA, anastomoses the PA to the ascending aorta, reconstructs the aortic arch, and *creates a* BT shunt (aorta to PA)
  - *Glenn procedure:* connects the SVC to the PA (5–9 months of age)
  - *Fontan procedure:* connects the IVC to the PA (3–5 years of age; Basu & Dobrolet, 2020; Cottrill & Hidestrand, 2020a; Scholz & Reinking, 2018; Swanson & Erikcson, 2021)

Outcomes

- Cardiac transplantation is sometimes an option for HLHS babies as primary palliation. A Norwood procedure is performed during the wait for transplantation and the availability of a donor heart.
- Long-term morbidity and mortality may occur secondary to recurrent coarctation or arch obstruction, AV valve regurgitation, sinus node dysfunction, various arrhythmias, and ventricular dysfunction. Increasing data are demonstrating the association of HLHS and higher risk of neurodevelopmental issues (Basu & Dobrolet, 2020; Scholz & Reinking, 2018).

ENDOCARDIAL CUSHION DEFECT (ATRIOVENTRICULAR CANAL)

Definition and Pathophysiology

- AV canal defects are also known as endocardial cushion defects. The endocardial cushion fails to form the center

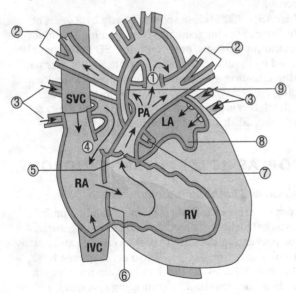

KEY:

1. Large PDA
2. Pulmonary Arteries
3. Pulmonary Veins
4. ASD
5. Pulmonary Valve
6. Tricuspid Valve
7. AV atresia
8. Hypoplastic LV with mitral valve atresia
9. Hypoplastic aortic arch and ascending aorta

Figure 19.5 Hypoplastic left heart syndrome.

ASD, atrial septal defect; AV, atrioventricular; IVC, inferior vena cava; LA, left atrium; LV, left ventricle; PA, pulmonary artery; PDA, persistent ductus arteriosus; RA, right atrium; RV, right ventricle; SVC, superior vena cava.

of the heart. It may be a severe large defect (complete AV canal), common AV canal and large VSD, transitional (less severe and small ASD and VSD), and small (common AV valves, cleft of the mitral valves, no VSD).
- There is a strong association between AV canal and trisomy 21 (Basu & Dobrolet, 2020; Breinholt, 2017; Cottrill & Hidestrand, 2020a; Phelps et al., 2020).

Diagnosis
- It presents as desaturation and cyanosis due to right-to-left shunting until PVR decreases and flow is reversed (left to right), as in CHF. Murmur may or may not be audible.
- Diagnosis of AV canal is by echocardiogram to determine the type of AV canal, ventricular size, valvular insufficiency, and identify associated anomalies. EKG will show a QRS axis deviation and RVH.
- Chest x-ray findings are based on the degree of RVOT/PS. Pulmonary vascular resistance usually remains high enough to delay the onset of CHF until after the first 1 to 2 weeks, after which marked cardiomegaly and vascular congestion are evident on x-ray (Basu & Dobrolet, 2020; Phelps et al., 2020; Scholz & Reinking, 2018; Trotter, 2021).

Management
- Medical management involves addressing cyanosis with supplemental oxygen to keep saturations >75%, or care of CHF, which may involve furosemide, digoxin, and an afterload reducer. However, oxygen should be avoided in the presence of CHF as it may increase pulmonary blood flow.
- Infants with concurrent pulmonary HTN or complicated CHF management will require surgical correction early, between 2 to 6 months of age. Otherwise, infants are repaired at 4 to 6 months of age (Basu & Dobrolet, 2020; Scholz & Reinking, 2018).

Outcomes
- Following complete repair, long-term issues primarily involve AV valve function (stenosis or regurgitation). Infants with a partial AVSD can often wait until almost 1 year of age for complete repair in the absence of any respiratory, feeding, or growth issues. Mortality for surgical repair is under 5%, up to 20% will develop mitral regurgitation, and 9% will require another surgical procedure (Basu & Dobrolet, 2020; Sadowski & Verklan, 2021).

AORTIC STENOSIS

Definition and Pathophysiology
- AS is a valvular disease resulting in left-sided outflow obstruction with subsequent shock and poor perfusion. The most common type is bicuspid aortic valve disease. Due to stenosis, the leaflets of the valve are thick and immobile, causing outflow obstruction. As the stenosis progresses, pumping blood becomes more difficult for the left ventricle. When AS becomes severe or critical, it results in decreased systemic output and cardiogenic shock.
- The incidence is 1% to 3%, and males are affected three times more often than females. This disorder is considered to be related to the NOTCH1 gene. AS is associated with Williams syndrome (Basu & Dobrolet, 2020; Phelps et al., 2020; Scholz & Reinking, 2018).

Diagnosis
- Clinical presentation of AS is based on severity and location. Shock with poor perfusion due to decreased blood flow in critical AS is similar to HLHS. Inadvertent closure of the DA results in worsening cardiogenic shock, acidosis, and multiorgan failure. Harsh midsystolic murmur is audible with systolic ejection click. A palpable thrill at the suprasternal notch should be evident. Pulse oximetry will demonstrate a gradient between the upper and lower extremities due to right-to-left shunting or show signs of CHF.
- Diagnosis is by echocardiogram to visualize the aorta and to determine the aortic valve anatomy and the size and degree of blood flow of the aorta.
- EKG would be normal. Chest x-ray may show pulmonary edema.
- Electrolytes and blood gases may show acidosis if AS decreases perfusion (Basu & Dobrolet, 2020; Scholz & Reinking, 2018).

Management
- If AS is mild or moderate and without illness, no treatment is needed other than follow-up. Medical management of AS requires continuous PGE1 to prevent cardiogenic shock. If the newborn demonstrates signs of CHF, a balloon or surgical valvotomy may be emergently indicated. The newborn may also need a Norwood procedure to provide alternative circulation to bypass the left ventricle (Basu & Dobrolet, 2020; Phelps et al., 2020; Scholz & Reinking, 2018).

Outcomes
- Mild AS requires no intervention, but moderate to severe AS requires monitoring for CHF. Surgical valvotomy remains an alternative as a primary intervention or secondary measure if balloon aortic valvuloplasty is unsuccessful (Basu & Dobrolet, 2020).

PATENT DUCTUS ARTERIOSUS

Definition and Pathophysiology
- During fetal life, the DA allows blood to flow from the right ventricle and PA to the descending aorta,

then the placenta, and is a normal finding. After birth, as PA pressures decrease and systemic BP increases (aortic pressure), blood flows from right to left across the PDA. Flow is reversed to this after birth due to decreased pulmonary vascular resistance and increases as pulmonary vascular resistance drops (i.e., lung disease improves), resulting in pulmonary edema. Functional closure occurs within the first 4 days of age in term, healthy newborns.

- DA patency is determined by the balance between dilating and constricting forces. The factors known to play a prominent role in DA regulation involve those that promote constriction (oxygen, endothelin, calcium channels, catecholamines, and Rho kinase) and those that oppose it (intraluminal pressure, PGs, nitric oxide [NO], carbon monoxide, potassium channels, and cyclic adenosine monophosphate [cAMP] and cyclic guanosine monophosphate [cGMP]).

- Functional closure of the ductus occurs in almost 50% of full-term infants by 24 hours, in 90% by 48 hours, and in nearly 100% by 72 hours after birth.
  - There are several events that promote ductus constriction in the full-term newborn following delivery: (a) an increase in arterial pO_2, (b) a decrease in BP within the ductus lumen, (c) a decrease in circulating prostaglandin E2 (PEG2), and (d) a decrease in the number of PGE2 receptors in the ductus wall.

- The incidence is 100% in the developing fetus as this is a normal finding in embryologic life. The incidence of PDA related to cardiac disease is 3.6%. Persistent PDA is more common in females and may be linked to chromosome 12.

- In contrast to the full-term ductus, the premature ductus is less likely to constrict after birth. The preterm ductus is thin-walled and less likely to constrict with birth due to the presence of immature myosin isoform, channels that are less responsive to oxygen inhibition. Systemically higher levels of PG secondary to decreased clearance by immature lungs also inhibit constriction.
  - The most important mechanism that prevents the preterm ductus from constricting after birth is its increased sensitivity to the vasodilating effects of PGE2.
  - Preterm infants of 30 weeks' gestation or more (including those with RDS) will close their ductus by the fourth day after birth. Infants born at less than 30 weeks' gestation have a 65% incidence of persistent ductus patency beyond day 4.

- In preterm infants, the ductus frequently remains open for many days after birth. Even when it does constrict, the premature ductus frequently fails to develop profound hypoxia and anatomic remodeling. The preterm infant requires a greater degree of ductal constriction than the term infant to develop a comparable degree of hypoxia. The preterm ductus requires complete cessation of luminal flow before it can develop the same degree of hypoxia as found at term.

- The pathophysiologic features of a PDA depend both on the magnitude of the left-to-right shunt and on the cardiac and pulmonary responses to the shunt (Alpan, 2020; Basu & Dobrolet, 2020; Benitz & Bhombal, 2020; Blackburn, 2018; Clyman, 2018; Phelps et al., 2020; Scholz & Reinking, 2018; Swanson & Erickson, 2021).

Diagnosis

- There are three general physiologic characteristics of a PDA in the preterm infant: (a) increased flow through the lungs with diastolic volume overload; (b) increased flow through the left atrium, LV, and aorta; and (c) left-to-right shunting to the pulmonary circulation.

- Clinical presentation stems from left-to-right shunting, which may also decrease cardiac output and increase the workload of the left side of the heart and result in decreased blood flow to vital organs, and presents as a left upper quadrant (LUQ) systolic "machinery" murmur, bounding pulses, visible precordium, worsening respiratory status due to pulmonary edema, and widened pulse pressure.

- Postnatal diagnosis is primarily by Doppler echocardiogram to determine the significance of a left-to-right shunt and rules out ductal dependence. EKG may be normal or show ventricular hypertrophy. Echocardiography determines the size and significance of the PDA and rules out ductal-dependent lesions.

- Chest x-ray may be normal or may have increased pulmonary vascularity if the PDA is large, with eventual cardiomegaly.

- Arterial blood gases are usually normal. A significantly large PDA may result in a mixed acidosis, electrolyte abnormalities (if managed by diuretics), and decreased renal function (Alpan, 2020; Basu & Dobrolet, 2020; Benitz & Bhombal, 2020; Clyman, 2018; Phelps et al., 2020; Swanson & Erickson, 2021).

Management

- Management of a PDA may be medical or surgical. Medical management is determined by symptomatology. If the newborn is asymptomatic, monitoring for CHF, oxygen need, and failure to thrive is indicated. Often, fluid restriction and observation are the approaches to the management of PDA.

- Inhibition of PG synthesis with indomethacin and ibuprofen appears effective; however, both have been associated with several potential adverse effects in the newborn. Indomethacin produces significant reductions in renal, mesenteric, and cerebral blood flow. Indomethacin also reduces cerebral oxygenation. Alterations in creatinine clearance and oliguria are common problems. The renal function returns to normal after the initial doses of indomethacin or after drug discontinuation.
  - While there may be a general consensus on the efficacy of indomethacin for treatment of a PDA, questions about proper dosage, treatment duration,

and optimal timing of treatment remain quite controversial.

- Ibuprofen has been further shown to be equally effective for ductal closure with fewer renal side effects.

■ Severe symptoms require ductal closure either pharmacologically (indomethacin, ibuprofen) or surgical ligation. Medications for ductal closure require monitoring of urine output and creatinine, which may indicate the need to discontinue the medication.

■ Surgical closure has been the gold standard for over 60 years and remains the standard approach when medical therapy fails. Surgical ligation is usually performed by an incision of the lateral thorax if the infant can tolerate the procedure and has failed medical management. Much of the morbidity and mortality of PDA surgical ligation are related to the preoperative clinical status of the neonate, and therefore the timing of when patients are referred for surgical ligation is crucial.

■ The Food and Drug Administration (FDA) recently approved the first device designed for occlusion of a PDA in a neonate. The most common complication is arterial vascular injury. When the venous access route is used, obstruction of the left branch PA or the descending thoracic aorta is the next most commonly observed issue. This is usually discovered before the device is released by angiography or transthoracic echocardiogram, at which time the device can be safely removed, or the patient is referred for surgical ligation (Alpan, 2020; Basu & Dobrolet, 2020; Benitz & Bhombal, 2020; Bocks et al., 2020; Clyman, 2018; Swanson & Erickson, 2021).

Outcomes

■ Prognosis is generally excellent with management; mortality from surgery is <1%.

■ Clear evidence is lacking for or against many of the approaches to PDA treatment. Although a prolonged, persistent moderate-to-large, left-to-right shunt through a PDA shortens the life span of animals and humans, there has been a growing debate in recent years about which is preferable: (a) to close the PDA (either surgically or pharmacologically) or (b) to deal with the pulmonary edema and hypotension through other means while awaiting spontaneous ductus closure; it needs to be closed during the neonatal period (Alpan, 2020; Benitz & Bhombal, 2020; Clyman, 2018; Swanson & Erickson, 2021).

CONGESTIVE HEART FAILURE

Definition and Pathophysiology

■ CHF may be caused by pressure overload (AS, COA), volume overload (left-to-right shunting such as PDA, truncus arteriosus, TOF, VSD, AV canal, single ventricle, AVM), a combination of pressure and volume overload (IAA, COA with VSD, AS), or myocardial dysfunction (inborn errors of metabolism genetic disorders, myocarditis, tachyarrhythmias, perinatal asphyxia, sepsis, premature closure of the PDA).

■ CHF may be subtle or obvious in the newborn and should be suspected in infants with a known VSD (Swanson & Erickson, 2021).

Diagnosis

■ Clinical presentation of CHF is hallmarked by decreased cardiac output and decreased tissue perfusion. Infants with CHF may have tachypnea, sinus tachycardia (to increase cardiac output), and hepatomegaly. Worsening CHF may involve retractions and grunting. Grunting respirations are a particularly concerning sign in a newborn and often accompany severe heart failure and decreased systemic perfusion.

■ Later symptoms of CHF include poor feeding and growth. As CHF progresses, the newborn may have decreased peripheral pulses, decreased urine output, and edema. Diagnosis is done by echocardiogram, chest x-ray, and metabolic acidosis. Discharge pulse oximetry is useful to find infants with subtle CHF (Scholz & Reinking, 2018; Swanson & Erickson, 2021).

Management

■ Medical management is multifocal, including the use of therapies to decrease oxygen consumption such as a neutral thermal environment, supplemental oxygen, and assisted ventilation; fluid restriction; increased calories without volume; and monitoring weight gain. The use of glucose polymers or medium-chain triglyceride (MCT) oil enhances caloric content without significant volume increase.

■ Correct acidosis and any metabolic derangements (e.g., hypoglycemia or hypocalcemia).

■ Pharmacologic management includes PGE1 if CHF is due to a ductal-dependent lesion, diuretic therapy, inotropes, digoxin, or afterload reducers (Sadowski & Verklan, 2021; Swanson & Erickson, 2021).

Outcomes

■ The outcome of CHF is based on the underlying cause (Breinholt, 2017; Sadowski & Verklan, 2021).

▶ NEONATAL SHOCK AND HYPOTENSION OR CARDIOVASCULAR COMPROMISE

DEFINITION AND PATHOPHYSIOLOGY

■ Shock may occur a result of hypovolemia, myocardial dysfunction, or abnormal peripheral vasoregulation. Hypovolemia is a decrease in circulating blood volume due to conditions resulting in a nonspecific inflammatory response (sepsis, asphyxia, major surgery) and afterload reducers (PGE1, milrinone). Dysfunction of systole or diastole may result in failed circulation.

- There are three phases of neonatal shock:
  (a) compensatory, involving perfusion of vital
  organs versus nonvital organs by vasodilatation
  and vasoconstriction; (b) uncompensated, with the
  development of hypotension, decreased cardiac
  output, and poor perfusion to vital organs; and
  (c) irreversible shock, resulting in permanent organ
  damage.
  - In the "compensated phase," complex
    compensatory mechanisms maintain perfusion and
    oxygen delivery in the normal range to the vital
    organs (brain, heart, and adrenal glands) at the
    expense of decreased perfusion to the remaining
    organs (nonvital organs).
  - If adequate treatment is not commenced,
    compensatory neuroendocrine and autonomic
    mechanisms begin to be exhausted, and
    hypotension develops as the shock enters its
    "uncompensated phase." Systemic perfusion
    (cardiac output) will decrease, perfusion of
    all organs including the vital organs becomes
    compromised, and lactic acidosis develops.
  - If treatment is ineffective in the uncompensated
    phase of shock, multiorgan failure develops, and
    shock may enter its "irreversible phase," where
    permanent damage to the various organ systems
    occurs (Khan, 2017; Noori et al., 2018; Scholz &
    Reinking, 2018).

DIAGNOSIS

- The is no standard method for diagnosing
  circulatory compromise, although BP is the standard
  parameter for diagnosis and treatment. Continuous
  BP measurement is crucial to managing neonatal
  shock and hypotension. A cautionary note: Available
  data suggest that sole reliance on BP can lead to
  inaccurate or, in other cases, significantly delayed
  diagnosis of circulatory compromise, especially
  in the very preterm infant during the immediate
  postnatal period.
- At the onset of shock, normal compensatory
  mechanisms may be able to maintain adequate BP
  by diverting blood away from nonessential organs.
  During this compensated shock, clinical findings may
  be subtle and include decreased peripheral perfusion.
  Once compensatory mechanisms are insufficient to
  maintain BP, systemic hypotension ensues.
  - Other observations for the diagnosis of circulatory
    compromise include heart rate, slow skin capillary
    refill time, increased core temperature gradient, low
    urine output, and acidosis with increased lactate
    production.
- Changes in serum lactate levels are informative
  of changes in the cardiovascular status; this
  indirect measure of cellular oxygen delivery
  and consumption has been used in clinical
  practice. Combining a capillary refill time of more
  than 4 seconds with an elevated serum lactate

concentration of more than 4 mmol/L has a
specificity of 97% in detecting a low SVC flow state
in very low birth weight (VLBW) neonates during
the first postnatal day.

- With the use of Doppler ultrasonography and more
  recently near-infrared spectroscopy (NIRS), blood
  flow to various organs can be assessed at the bedside.
  NIRS uses the difference in the absorption spectra
  of oxygenated and deoxygenated hemoglobin to
  indirectly assess flow. Advances in NIRS technology
  have allowed continuous assessment of brain, renal,
  mesenteric, and muscle oxygenation (i.e., blood flow)
  at the bedside.
- The mainstay of diagnosing neonatal circulatory
  compromise has been a combination of BP
  measurement and evaluation of the previously
  described clinical parameters. However, none of these
  parameters have a sufficient degree of accuracy to
  allow them to be relied on as the sole evaluator of
  systemic blood flow and tissue perfusion. Therefore,
  the addition of echocardiographic and NIRS
  hemodynamic assessment to BP monitoring and
  thorough continuous clinical evaluation of the patient
  are necessary to better understand changes in organ
  blood flow and tissue perfusion, especially in preterm
  neonates (Khan, 2017; Noori et al., 2018; Scholz &
  Reinking, 2018).

MANAGEMENT

- Selection of the most appropriate treatment strategy
  for neonatal shock requires identification of its
  pathogenesis. A large proportion of care is supportive.
- Supportive measures during cardiovascular
  compromise include maintaining intravascular
  volume, arterial pH, and serum calcium levels. Positive
  pressure ventilation may decrease ventricular afterload
  and decrease WOB.
- Hypovolemia treatment is based on volume
  administration. Volume administration with
  myocardial dysfunction may increase morbidity and
  mortality, indicating that volume administration
  is cautious. The exception to this is volume
  administration to infants with neonatal sepsis, and
  in that situation decreases mortality. Isotonic saline
  administration has been demonstrated to be effective.
  If the infant has a history of blood loss, packed
  red blood cells with a hematocrit of 55% or greater
  following administration of a crystalloid (normal
  saline) are indicated.
- Pharmacologic management includes:
  - Dopamine is an endogenous catecholamine that
    produces a cardiovascular response based on the
    dose administered intravenously; stimulating a
    response from dopaminergic, alpha-adrenergic,
    beta-adrenergic, and serotoninergic receptors
    impacts preload, myocardial contractility, and
    afterload (peripheral systemic vascular resistance
    [SVR]), resulting in increased BP.

- Dobutamine is a cardioselective sympathomimetic amine with significant alpha-adrenoreceptor-mediated and beta-adrenoreceptor and direct inotrope, which decreases total peripheral vascular resistance. Dobutamine works best in newborns with primary cardiac dysfunction and elevated pulmonary vascular resistance. Using dobutamine in addition to dopamine in infants with RDS also increases BP.
- Epinephrine is an alpha- and beta-adrenergic agonist and sympathomimetic agent that increases BP and cerebral vascular blood flow.
- Milrinone is a phosphodiesterase 3 inhibitor which reduces afterload in neonates with CHD or with low cardiac output. It has been shown to improve the oxygenation index of infants with PPHN.
- Vasopressin is a synthetic antidiuretic hormone that impacts the cardiovascular system by vasoconstriction. The benefits of vasopressin are similar to dopamine.
- Hydrocortisone is a glucocorticoid steroid that improves BP, but due to the potential for adverse effects is not a first-line treatment for neonatal hypotension but rather a rescue treatment. Hydrocortisone stabilizes cardiovascular status in the infant with vasopressor-resistant hypotension (Khan, 2017; Noori et al., 2018; Sadowski & Verklan, 2021; Scholz & Reinking, 2018).

OUTCOMES

- Outcome is based on the underlying cause of cardiovascular compromise. For example:
  - The physiology of the VLBW neonate in the immediate postnatal period includes poor vasomotor tone, immature myocardium, and dysregulated NO production.
  - The physiology of the septic infant involved hypovolemia, myocardial dysfunction, peripheral vasodilation, and increased pulmonary pressures secondary to acidosis.
  - The physiology of a term infant postperinatal depression involved the release of endogenous catecholamines, leading to normal or increased SVR, evidenced by mottling and myocardial dysfunction (Khan, 2017).

▶ NEONATAL DYSRHYTHMIAS

DEFINITION AND PATHOPHYSIOLOGY

- Arrhythmias in neonates may have normal and abnormal variations. The beginning of electrical activity in neonates is the sinus node, with input from the sympathetic and parasympathetic nervous system. Conduction between the atria and the ventricles is linked by the bundle of His.
- The normal pathway is sinus node → atrial myocardium → AV node → bundle of His → right and left bundle branches → ventricular myocardium → depolarization. Accessory pathways provide one direction (concealed pathway) or bidirectional (manifest pathway) conduction pathways. Newborns are sensitive to vagal stimulation, which fluctuates from bradycardia and tachycardia, based on newborn activity.
- The sinus node has inputs from both sympathetic and parasympathetic nervous systems. The balance of the two inputs determines the heart rate at any given moment. At rest and during sleep, vagal nerve stimulation is increased, causing slowing of the heart rate and potentially sinus bradycardia. During periods of stress, stimulation, or activity, sympathetic tone predominates, leading to an increase in heart rate and potentially sinus tachycardia.
- Tachyarrhythmias originate from areas other than the sinus node, such as conduction via the conduct through the AV node, bundle of His, and right and left bundle branches, and result in P-wave changes. Prolonged arrhythmias may result in cardiac failure or sudden death.
- Normal sinus rhythm or resting heart rate in newborns is 90 to 60 beats per minute (bpm).
- Sinus bradycardia is a heart rate below 60 bpm.
  - It is usually episodic and usually a physiologic response and not usually cardiac dysfunction. In neonates, it may be caused by increased vagal tone from intubation, gastroesophageal reflux, apnea, suctioning, seizures, and more uncommonly increased intracranial pressure, abdominal pressure, or medications. With sinus bradycardia, the need for ventilation must be ruled out first.
- Sinus tachycardia is a heart rate >160 to 180 bpm.
  - It may be a result of anemia, fever, agitation, infection, or pain. However, SVT must be considered and ruled out if the rate is >220 bpm, or if the P-wave is abnormal, the PR is prolonged, or an echocardiogram is normal.
- Premature atrial contractions (PACs) are early depolarization of the atria but are not from the sinus node. True PACs are followed by a QRS complex, and not just P-waves. *Bigeminy* refers to EKGs characteristic of a PAC every other beat. PACs are generally asymptomatic.
- Atrial flutter (AF) is a type of reentry tachycardia via the atrial myocardium at the tricuspid valve.
  - AF is characterized by sawtooth flutter waves. The rate of neonatal AF is 300 to 600 bpm with a lower ventricular rate (2:1, 3:1, or 4:1), protected by the AV node. Ventricular beats may exceed 200, resulting in the need for intervention.
- Atrial fibrillation (AFib) is a continuous dysrhythmia rarely seen in neonates and associated with CHD such as Ebstein anomaly and Wolff–Parkinson–White. It differs from atrial ectopic tachycardia (AET) in that AET is a chaotic rhythm.

- Supraventricular tachycardia is usually reentrant SVT, which uses nonconducting tissue pathways resulting in an electrical loop, which results in tachycardia resulting in narrow complexes.
  - This is usually caused by an accessory pathway but can be due to reentry at the AV node (rarely in neonates). Wolff–Parkinson–White is a manifest (atria to ventricle, one-way) accessory pathway and is generally sporadic.
- A premature ventricular contraction (PVC) is an early beat due to spontaneous ventricular depolarization of the ventricles.
  - If the heart is structurally normal, the baby is asymptomatic, family history is negative, and they disappear at higher bpm, PVCs can be considered benign.
- Ventricular tachycardia (VT) is an abnormal tachycardia arrhythmia, but idioventricular rhythm appears the same but is a benign rhythm.
  - VT originates below the bundle of His and may impact the baby's hemodynamic and cardiac function and requires intervention.
- Complete AV heart block (third-degree block) indicates a dysfunctional AV node, making the atria and ventricles independent of each other.
  - Complete heart block is associated with maternal lupus erythematosus. Other types of heart block are type I (prolonged PR interval >200 msec) and type 2 (prolonged P-wave conduction without a prolonged PR interval), which requires pacing (Breinholt, 2017; Cannon & Snyder, 2020; Cottrill & Mohan, 2020; Phelps et al., 2020; Swanson & Erickson, 2021).

DIAGNOSIS

- When evaluating any infant with an arrhythmia, it is essential to assess the electrophysiology and hemodynamic status. Emergency treatment should precede definitive diagnosis. Signs of pathologic arrhythmias include tachypnea, poor skin perfusion, lethargy, hepatomegaly, and rales on pulmonary examination.
- Three broad categories for arrhythmias in neonates are (a) tachyarrhythmias, (b) bradyarrhythmias, and (c) irregular rhythms.
- When analyzing the EKG for the mechanism of arrhythmia, a stepwise approach should be taken in three main areas: rate (variable, too fast, too slow), rhythm (regular, irregular, paroxysmal, or gradual), and QRS morphology. EKG ensures that there is no evidence of a pathologic arrhythmia, such as heart block (bradycardia) or SVT (tachycardia). Bedside monitoring may have artifact requiring a 12-lead EKG for confirmation.
- Laboratory studies should include electrolyte, calcium, and magnesium levels. Blood gas to evaluate for acidosis should also be done. If applicable, drug levels of digoxin or caffeine should be obtained to evaluate for toxicity

(Breinholt, 2017; Cottrill & Mohan, 2020; Phelps et al., 2020; Swanson & Erickson, 2021).

MANAGEMENT

- The majority of arrhythmias do not require urgent management. Urgent or chronic arrhythmias may be treated in a variety of ways. Treat the underlying cause such as infection or anemia, or no treatment. For bradycardias, evaluate the need for resuscitation. It is essential to have early accessible resuscitation equipment available before proceeding with antiarrhythmic interventions.
- Defibrillation and cardioversion are used for rapid termination of tachyarrhythmia from the atrium or ventricle that is unresponsive to basic treatment or is causing the patient to have cardiovascular compromise.
  - Cardioversion denotes synchronized delivery of energy (shock) during QRS complex. It uses lower energy (0.5–1 J/kg). This is indicated in an unstable patient with tachyarrhythmia who have a perfusing rhythm but evidence of poor perfusion.
  - Defibrillation denotes asynchronized, random delivery of energy (shock) during the cardiac cycle. It uses higher energy (2 J/kg). This is indicated in pulseless arrest with a shockable rhythm and in between CPR (Breinholt, 2017; Cottrill & Hidestrand, 2020b).
- For medication specifics used in the treatment of arrhythmias, please see Chapter 14.

OUTCOMES

- Neonatal arrhythmia outcomes are based on the type of arrhythmia and the underlying cause of arrhythmia (Breinholt, 2017).

▶ HYPERTENSION

DEFINITION AND PATHOPHYSIOLOGY

- The definition of neonatal HTN is sustained BP above the 95th percentile for infants of similar size, gestational age, and postnatal age.
- After birth, the BP is expected to decrease over the first few hours due to fluid shifts and then gradually rises by 6 days of age. HTN occurs in 1% to 2% of term and preterm infants and is most often seen in infants with a concurrent condition, such as chronic lung disease, renal disease, or a history of umbilical arterial catheterization. Differential diagnoses include renal/renovascular disorders (most common), cardiac disorders (arch abnormalities including COA and PDA), neurologic disorders (seizures, pain), adverse effects of meds, and bronchopulmonary dysplasia (BPD).
  - Renal arterial thromboembolism secondary to UAC is the most common cause of renovascular HTN;

IDM, sepsis, dehydration, and perinatal asphyxia place the infant with UAC at higher risk for thrombotic events.

■ Other causes of neonatal HTN include renal disorders such as acute kidney injury (AKI), autosomal recessive polycystic kidney disease, and obstructive uropathy. The most significant nonrenal cause of neonatal HTN is BPD. Medications such as corticosteroids, vasopressors, caffeine, theophylline, and bronchodilators have been associated with elevated BP in neonates (Vargo, 2019; Vogt & Springel, 2020).

DIAGNOSIS

■ The majority of neonates with HTN are asymptomatic, as elevated BPs are typically noted on routine monitoring.

■ Clinical presentation other than elevated BP during routine vital signs varies depending on etiology. Cardiorespiratory symptoms may include tachypnea, changes in perfusion, vasomotor instability, CHF, and/or hepatosplenomegaly. Clinical signs of hypertensive crisis may include cardiopulmonary failure, neurologic dysfunction, and concerns for AKI.

■ Diagnostic evaluation includes history and physical examination. The first step is to determine whether the elevated BP persists when the infant is quiet and relaxed. BPs are preferably measured in the upper arm, as leg BP measurements tend to overestimate the true BP.

● The infant should be examined carefully for signs of volume overload, including peripheral edema, cardiac gallop, or rales. The abdomen should be carefully inspected for presence of abdominal or flank masses or renal bruits. Ambiguous genitalia in a hypertensive infant should raise suspicion for congenital adrenal hyperplasia.

■ Laboratory evaluation should include a basic metabolic panel for evaluation of electrolytes and renal function and a urinalysis. Other laboratory evaluations may include evaluation of renin, aldosterone, cortisol, and thyroid function.

■ Ultrasound of the abdomen/kidneys with a Doppler flow study should be done to evaluate for renal or renovascular abnormalities. In more difficult cases, CT, MRI with angiography, or echocardiography may help with establishing diagnosis (Vogt & Springel, 2020).

MANAGEMENT

■ Management is aimed toward the underlying cause, including improper measurement technique,

vasopressor administration, volume overload, narcotic withdrawal, or inadequately controlled pain.

■ If BP remains elevated above the 99th percentile, experts advocate antihypertensive treatment with an IV or oral antihypertensive agent to prevent adverse effects on the kidneys, heart, and central nervous system.

■ The goal of antihypertensive agents is a gradual decrease in BP not dropping below the 95th percentile for the first 24 to 48 hours of treatment. IV therapy is preferred initially, with a switch to oral agents once BP is more stable. There are various antihypertensive agents that can be considered, including vasodilators, calcium channel blockers, and alpha-/beta-blockers.

■ If the HTN cannot be controlled medically or a massive aortic thrombosis results in major complications, thrombolysis with urokinase, streptokinase, or tissue plasminogen activator may be considered. If severe HTN persists, surgical thrombectomy or nephrectomy may be contemplated (Vogt & Springel, 2020).

OUTCOMES

■ Outcomes depend on the etiology. HTN related to BPD and complications from UAC typically resolves over time. Infants with renal abnormalities can have hypertensive issues that persist.

■ There is growing evidence that neonates born prior to completion of nephrogenesis at 34 to 36 weeks' gestation may be at increased risk of development of HTN and chronic kidney disease in adolescence or adulthood (Vogt & Springel, 2020).

▶ CONCLUSION

CHD is the most universal congenital disorder in neonates. Critical CHD requiring clinical intervention comprises 25% of CHDs and is a preeminent cause of infant mortality during the neonatal period. CHD can appear as shock, cyanosis, respiratory distress, or contrarily with subtle signs and symptoms. Delay in the recognition and management of CHD increases the risk of morbidity and mortality. Recognizing risk factors, clinical presentation, and inclusion of CHD as an in tandem differential diagnosis in the consideration of neonatal management decisions are key. Finally, consider that CHD may not be evident until days 3 to 5 of life or later due to corresponding physiologic changes. Pulse oximetry screening for hypoxemia is indicated for all newborns to detect imminent critical CHD lesions prior to hospital discharge.

1. The neonatal nurse practitioner (NNP) identifies a pathologic cardiac arrhythmia characterized by presence of a short PR interval and a delta wave as:

    A. Junctional atrial flutter (AF)

    B. Supraventricular tachycardia (SVT)

    C. Wolff–Parkinson–White (WPW)

2. Pharmacologic management of an infant with a large patent ductus arteriosus (PDA) using indomethacin (Indocin) is contraindicated in which of the following findings?

    A. Clinical presentation of congestive heart failure

    B. Previous treatment with inhaled corticosteroids

    C. Serum creatinine of greater than 1.7 mg/dL

3. A 10-day-old term infant with a clinical appearance of trisomy 21 presents with tachypnea and a systolic ejection murmur, leading the neonatal nurse practitioner (NNP) to suspect a diagnosis of:

    A. Atrioventricular canal or ventricular septal defect

    B. Coarctation of the aorta or aortic stenosis

    C. Tetralogy of Fallot or an anomalous aortic arch

4. A term infant presents at 6 hours of age with cyanosis but without respiratory distress. No murmur is audible and peripheral pulses are normal. The neonatal nurse practitioner (NNP) performs a hyperoxia test, and there is no change in the infant's oxygen saturation level. The most likely diagnosis for the NNP to consider is:

    A. Ebstein anomaly

    B. Tetralogy of Fallot (TOF)

    C. Transposition of the great arteries (TOGA)

5. A neurologic malformation which may present in part as congestive heart failure is:

    A. Agenesis of the corpus callosum

    B. Arteriovenous malformation

    C. Communicating hydrocephalus

6. The neonatal nurse practitioner (NNP) recognizes a finding associated with the diagnosis of complex congenital heart disease such as dextrocardia with situs solitus is:

    A. Asplenia

    B. Horseshoe kidney

    C. Pancreatic malformation

7. A neonate with congestive heart failure is being administered furosemide (Lasix). The neonatal nurse practitioner (NNP) uses a conservative management approach as a known complication of this medical therapy is:

    A. Hypercreatinemia

    B. Leukopenia

    C. Ototoxicity

1. C) Wolff–Parkinson–White (WPW)

WPW syndrome is characterized by a short PR interval and delta wave with a slow upstroke of the QRS complex. Atrial flutter is characterized by sawtooth flutter waves. SVT results in narrow complexes (Gomella, 2020).

2. C) Serum creatinine of greater than 1.7 mg/dL

An elevated serum creatinine of 1.7 mg/dL, frank renal and/or gastrointestinal (GI) bleeding, necrotizing enterocolitis (NEC), and sepsis are contraindications of indomethacin in premature infants. Indomethacin therapy may be repeated if needed for ductal closure. Symptoms of congestive heart failure (CHF) are an indication for indomethacin. Clinical presentation of CHF and previous treatment with inhaled corticosteroids are not contraindications (Gomella, 2020).

3. A) Atrioventricular canal or ventricular septal defect

Atrioventricular (AV) canal and ventricular septal defect (VSD) are associated with Down syndrome. Coarctation of the aorta and aortic stenosis are associated with Turner syndrome (XO). Tetralogy of Fallot and aortic are anomalies associated with DiGeorge syndrome (Gomella, 2020).

4. C) Transposition of the great arteries (TOGA)

Transposition of the great vessels presents with cyanosis, tachypnea, and normal pulses. Hypoplastic left heart syndrome presents variably, but most likely with cyanosis and poor perfusion. TOF presents based on the degree of pulmonary stenosis. In addition to tachypnea and profound cyanosis, Ebstein anomaly presents with cardiovascular collapse (Fanaroff, 2020).

5. B) Arteriovenous malformation

Arteriovenous malformations (AVMs) are malformations resulting in a direct connection between the cerebral arteries and veins. AVMs presenting during the neonatal period present as congestive heart failure. At birth, systemic vascular resistance increases, increasing blood flow from the AVM into the systemic circulation. A cranial bruit may also be audible. There are no overt clinically visible signs of agenesis of the corpus callosum. Communicating hydrocephalus may result in hypoperfusion rather than cardiac overload (Fanaroff, 2020).

6. A) Asplenia

Asplenia syndrome or bilateral right-sidedness should be suspected whenever complex cardiac defects are identified, such as dextrocardia with situs solitus. Horseshoe kidney and pancreatic malformations are not associated with dextrocardia or situs solitus (Fanaroff, 2020).

7. C) Ototoxicity

Ototoxicity is a complication of furosemide therapy. Other complications include hyponatremia, hypocalcemia, hypokalemia, and hypercalciuria, which can result in nephrocalcinosis. Leukopenia and thrombocytopenia are not associated with furosemide (Gomella, 2020).

The Respiratory System

Janice Wilson, Jennifer Fitzgerald, Dawn Mueller-Burke, and Mary Walters

▶ INTRODUCTION

The most common admission to the NICU is due to pathology of dysfunction of the respiratory system. Therefore, the understanding of lung development, physiology, function, and mechanics as well as the understanding of disorders that contribute to pulmonary dysfunction are critical to the care of all newborns (Fraser, 2021; Kallapur & Jobe, 2020; Keszler & Abubakar, 2022a).

▶ LUNG DEVELOPMENT

- Lung development is a complex interrelationship between genetic signaling and physical, biochemical, hormonal, and structural factors. Lung development and maturation are reflected in five overlapping anatomic phases.

PHASES OF LUNG DEVELOPMENT

- *Embryonic phase (weeks 3–6):* Denotes development of the proximal airways. The lung bud develops within the mesenchyme from the primitive embryonic foregut. The single lung bud divides into the right and left lung buds as well as the trachea. Rudimentary airway branching, pulmonary vein, and pulmonary artery formation occur during this stage. Abnormal development during the embryonic phase can result in tracheal agenesis, tracheal stenosis, tracheoesophageal fistula (TEF), and pulmonary sequestration.
- *Pseudoglandular phase (weeks 6–16):* During this phase, 20 generations of conducting airways are formed. Simultaneously, lymphatic vessels and bronchial capillaries also develop. The lung at this stage has the "gland-like" (pseudoglandular) appearance of an exocrine organ due to the surrounding loose mesenchyme tissue. Abnormal development during this phase can result in bronchogenic cysts, congenital lobar emphysema, and congenital diaphragmatic hernia (CDH).
- *Canalicular phase (weeks 16–26):* The acinar or respiratory units develop, which include airway

generations from 21 to 23. Pulmonary capillaries grow closer to the primitive acinus or respiratory unit. Cuboidal cells develop into type I cells (those responsible for gas exchange) and type II cells (those responsible for surfactant production and secretion). Gas exchange may occur near the end of this stage but is dependent on the approximation of the capillaries to the acinar units.
- *Terminal sac or saccular phase (weeks 26–36):* The primitive acini develop into saccules that continue to septate via the development of secondary crests. The saccules will develop into alveoli. The capillary network moves closer to the alveoli, facilitating rudimentary gas exchange. Type II cells increase the production and release of surfactant. As lung size increases, an increase in the surface area responsible for gas exchange occurs. Infants delivered during this phase may develop respiratory distress syndrome (RDS; surfactant deficiency), pulmonary insufficiency (reduced surface area, increased distance between alveoli and capillaries, immature lung mechanics), pulmonary interstitial emphysema (PIE), and bronchopulmonary dysplasia (BPD).
- *Alveolar phase (36 weeks–3 years):* Alveoli continue to increase in number and maturity and may continue to develop into early adulthood. Several factors can influence alveolarization, such as antenatal/postnatal administration of glucocorticoids, chorioamnionitis, hypoxia or hyperoxia, and poor nutrition. Continued alveolarization past the newborn period may assist in normalization of lung function of infants born prematurely (Joyner, 2019; Kallapur & Jobe, 2020; Keszler & Abubakar, 2022a).

▶ THE ROLE OF FETAL LUNG FLUID AND FETAL BREATHING

- Fetal lung fluid is produced at 4 to 5 mL/kg/hr and is facilitated by the active transport of chloride from the interstitium. Fetal lung fluid and its constituents, such as phospholipids, contribute to the amniotic fluid volume and as such can be evaluated as a test of fetal lung maturity.

- The lecithin-to-sphingomyelin (L:S) ratio and the phosphatidylglycerol (PG) levels can be used to assess lung maturity.
  - Lecithin (phosphatidylcholine) is produced by the fetal lung.
  - Sphingomyelin is a nonfetal membrane lipid found in amniotic fluid and begins to fall by 32 weeks.
  - An L:S ratio of 2:1 is indicative of fetal lung maturity. Its use is not accurate in infants of diabetic mothers. PG increases in production at around 35 weeks. The presence of PG indicates lung maturity. Fetal lung maturity can also be assessed by measuring the ratio of surfactant to albumin. A ratio of greater than 70 indicates lung maturity.
- Chronic stress (fetal, maternal, placental) can facilitate early lung maturation. Growth restriction and preeclampsia do not facilitate lung maturation.
- Fetal breathing movements (FBMs) can be seen as early as 11 weeks and are important for lung development. With fetal breathing, lung fluid moves up the trachea and is swallowed, and some makes its way out into the amniotic fluid. Fetal tracheal pressure is higher than amniotic fluid pressure maintaining a distending pressure, which promotes lung development. FBM increases cardiac output and blood flow to the heart and placenta. Decreased movement of the diaphragm has been associated with the development of pulmonary hypoplasia (Fraser, 2021; Hansen & Levin, 2019; Joyner, 2019; Kallapur & Jobe, 2020; Patrinos, 2020).

▶ THE ROLE OF SURFACTANT

- Surfactant is produced in type II alveolar cells. It is packaged and stored in the lamellar bodies. Lamellar bodies are extruded into the alveoli by exocytosis, forming tubular myelin. Tubular myelin is a lattice-like structure with the hydrophobic end of the phospholipid extending into the alveolar air and the hydrophilic end binding with water at the air–liquid interface. This process reduces surface tension. Surfactant components are also "recycled" by the lamellar bodies or broken down by lysosomes.
  - Surfactant is a combination of phospholipids (80%) and proteins (12%). The primary phospholipids in surfactant are dipalmitoyl phosphatidylcholine (DPPC; at 60%), unsaturated phosphatidylcholine (25%), phosphatidyl glycerol (15%), and phosphatidylinositol. Surfactant production begins at 25 to 30 weeks of gestation and production continues to term.
- Phospholipids (primarily DPPC) are responsible for the reduction of alveolar surface tension and stabilization of the alveolar membrane, preventing alveolar collapse at the end of expiration.
  - There are four surfactant proteins; two are hydrophilic (surfactant proteins A and D, or SP-A and SP-D) and two are hydrophobic (surfactant proteins B and C, or SP-B and SP-C). See Table 20.1.
  - Genetic mutations may result in SP-B deficiency and cause respiratory distress that is fatal in the newborn period. If SP-B is deficient, SP-C production is also reduced. Genetic mutations that result in SP-C deficiency can result in respiratory distress and/or interstitial lung disease in infancy and childhood.
    - ❏ The adenosine triphosphate (ATP)-binding cassette transporter gene (*ABCA3*) is responsible for lipid transport in the lamellar bodies. Genetic aberrancies in the *ABCA3* gene can result in severe RDS, similar to SP-B deficiency (Fraser, 2021; Gautham & Soll, 2022; Guttentag, 2017; Kallapur & Jobe, 2020; Zanelli & Kauffman, 2019).

Table 20.1 Surfactant Proteins

Surfactant Protein Type	Surfactant Protein Function(s)
SP-A, hydrophilic (water-soluble)	■ Active in lung host defense mechanisms and regulation of lung inflammation ■ Binds to pathogens and facilitates phagocytosis by macrophages
SP-B, hydrophobic (water-insoluble)	■ Cosecreted with phospholipids ■ Works in conjunction with phospholipids in stabilizing the alveolar membrane ■ Important in the formation of tubular myelin and in surfactant recycling ■ Only protein present in commercial surfactants
SP-C, hydrophobic (water-insoluble)	■ Assists with surfactant dispersal, spreading, and recycling of surfactant in conjunction with SP-B
SP-D, hydrophilic (water-soluble)	■ Performs lung host defense support similar to SP-A

SP-A, surfactant protein A; SP-B, surfactant protein B; SP-C, surfactant protein C; SP-D, surfactant protein D.
Sources: Data from Kallapur, S. G., & Jobe, A. H. (2020). Lung development and maturation. In R. J. Martin, A. A. Fanaroff, & M. C. Walsh (Eds.), *Fanaroff & Martin's neonatal-perinatal medicine: Diseases of the fetus and infant* (11th ed., pp. 1124–1142). Saunders; Gautham, S. K., & Soll, R. F. (2022). Exogenous surfactant therapy. In J. Goldsmith, M. Keszler, & S. K. Gautham (Eds.), *Assisted ventilation of the neonate* (7th ed., pp. 172–174). Elsevier; Fraser, D. (2021). Respiratory distress. In M. T. Verklan, M. Walden, & S. Forest (Eds.), *Core curriculum for neonatal intensive care nurses* (6th ed., p. 395). Elsevier.

▶ THE ROLE OF ANTENATAL STEROIDS

■ Treatment with maternal corticosteroids less than 24 hours before preterm delivery is associated with a decrease in mortality, RDS, and intraventricular hemorrhage (IVH), and is considered the standard of care for mothers at risk of preterm delivery.

■ Administration of steroids causes increased production of proteins that control the manufacture of surfactant by the type II cells in the fetal lung. Maximum benefit to the fetus is achieved following 48 hours after administration. Steroid administration should be considered when preterm delivery is anticipated within 7 days. A course of steroids is recommended for pregnant patients at 24 to 34 weeks of gestation at risk of preterm delivery within 7 days. Recommendations for steroid use have expanded to include pregnancies between 34 and 36 weeks. Use of antenatal steroids in infants less than 24 weeks has been less well studied but may be beneficial in infants who will be resuscitated. Betamethasone (Celestone) and dexamethasone (Dexasone) are the steroids of choice.

■ Multiple repeated courses of antenatal steroids are not recommended due to an associated increased risk of negative neurodevelopmental outcomes.
  ● A second dose of steroids may be considered if more than 7 days to 2 weeks have passed since the first dose and if preterm delivery is still a risk (Fraser, 2021; Hamar & Hansen, 2019; Kallapur & Jobe, 2020; Zanelli & Kaufman, 2019).

▶ CONGENITAL/DEVELOPMENTAL RESPIRATORY DISORDERS

PULMONARY HYPOPLASIA

Definition and Pathophysiology

■ Pulmonary hypoplasia is part of a subset of pulmonary underdevelopment diseases, which include pulmonary agenesis and pulmonary aplasia, and decreased numbers of alveoli, bronchioles, and arterioles. It can be either unilateral or bilateral. Both alveolar and pulmonary arteries are impacted.
  ● Primary hypoplasia is a result of an intrinsic failure of normal lung development.
  ● Secondary hypoplasia is a result of abnormal processes that interfere with lung development.
    ❑ Oligohydramnios resulting from renal anomalies (Potter sequence), early amniotic fluid leak/loss, and/or placental abnormalities
    ❑ Intrauterine growth retardation (IUGR)
    ❑ Space-occupying lesions that compress the lungs, inhibiting growth, such as CDH, cardiomegaly, and/or cystic lung diseases

    ❑ Abnormal diaphragmatic movement secondary to a central or peripheral nervous system disorder or musculoskeletal disease, with inhibition of FBM and lack of chest wall expansion restricting normal growth
    ❑ Infants at the highest risk for pulmonary hypoplasia are those with fetal growth restriction (FGR), altered FBM, prolonged polyhydramnios, decreased nutrient supply, nicotine exposure, and preterm birth (Blackburn, 2018; Crowley, 2020; Fraser, 2021; Jensen et al., 2022; Joyner, 2019; Pappas & Robey, 2021; Van Marter & McPherson, 2017).

Diagnosis

■ Antenatal assessments can be helpful in the identification of pulmonary hypoplasia. Antenatal ultrasound (US) evaluation of thoracic circumference (TC), TC to abdominal circumference, and thoracic to heart area can be evaluated. It is more useful with secondary versus primary hypoplasia. This is more reflective of chest wall measurement and not lung measurement. Antenatal three-dimensional MRI has been used to evaluate lung volume.

■ A high index of suspicion for pulmonary hypoplasia should be considered in infants with FGR, altered FBM, prolonged polyhydramnios, decreased nutrient supply, nicotine exposure, and preterm birth.

■ The most common presentation is severe respiratory distress.
  ● Infants with pulmonary hypoplasia may exhibit hypoxia and hypercapnia, and are at risk of pulmonary air leak syndrome (pneumothorax).
  ● Chest radiographs demonstrate decreased lung volumes.
  ● Abnormal pulmonary vasculature development may lead to persistent pulmonary hypertension of the newborn (PPHN) symptoms.
  ● Poor lung compliance requires higher pressures to ventilate (Blackburn, 2018; Crowley, 2020; Fraser, 2021; Pappas & Robey, 2021).

Management and Outcome

■ Intubation and assisted ventilation:
  ● Avoid hypoxia, hyperoxia, hypercarbia, hypocarbia, and acidosis.
  ● Minimize overexpansion and consider high-frequency oscillatory ventilation (HFOV) if peak inspiratory pressure (PIP) is greater than 25 cm H_2O.
  ● Administer surfactant.
  ● Consider the use of inhaled nitric oxide (iNO) if PPHN is present.
  ● Implement pain management and sedation protocols.
  ● Provide hemodynamic support (volume expansion, inotropes, and vasopressors).
  ● Use extracorporeal membrane oxygenation (ECMO).

■ The mortality rate is high and the degree of hypoplasia dictates the outcome. Infants who survive are at an elevated risk of development of chronic lung disease (CLD). While postnatal lung growth is rare, it is possible if treatment and supportive care are successful.

■ Survival of infants with pulmonary hypoplasia depends on the degree to which lung growth is restricted and the underlying cause of hypoplasia. Mortality rate is high. Management is difficult, but the infant can function adequately if treatment and support can be continued until lung growth occurs, although this outcome is rare (Crowley, 2020; Fraser, 2021; Keszler, 2022; Keszler et al., 2022; Pappas & Robey, 2021).

CONGENITAL DIAPHRAGMATIC HERNIA

Definition and Pathophysiology

■ CDH results from a developmental defect in the formation of the fetal diaphragm, allowing abdominal contents to herniate into the thoracic cavity, creating a mass effect that impedes lung development.
  ● Most defects occur on the left side. Posterolateral defects (Bochdalek) are the most common and account for 70% of CDH. Anterior defects (Morgagni) are less common, accounting for 25% to 30%. Central or bilateral defects are rare and usually fatal.

■ Overall incidence has been estimated at 1 per 2,000 to 3,000 live births, with the left side more commonly affected. Most are diagnosed antenatally.

■ CDH can be an isolated occurrence, but approximately 40% are associated with other anomalies (central nervous system [CNS], cardiovascular, skeletal, gastrointestinal [GI], and genitourinary [GU] defects), as well as chromosomal abnormalities like trisomies 13, 18, and 21, and 45,X.

■ Pulmonary hypoplasia is common, secondary to lung compression of the herniated contents.

■ Severity of respiratory distress is related to the severity of the defect and the degree of hypoplasia.

■ These infants are also at high risk for barotrauma and subsequent pneumothoraces (Bradshaw, 2021; Crowley, 2020; Draus & Ruzic, 2020; Hansen & Levin, 2019; Koo et al., 2022; Madenci et al., 2019).

Diagnosis

■ Measurement of lung-to-head ratio (LHR) on prenatal US can predict the severity of pulmonary hypoplasia. Infants with low observed to expected (O/E) LHRs are at the highest risk for significant pulmonary hypoplasia. Fetal MRI can help assess total fetal lung volume.

■ If undiagnosed antenatally, infants can present with severe respiratory distress, cyanosis, and scaphoid abdomen.

■ Breath sounds are diminished or absent on the affected side, and cardiac sounds may be shifted toward the opposite side. Bowel sounds may be heard over the chest on the affected side.

■ Chest radiographs are consistent with abdominal contents in the thorax, shift of mediastinal structures to the unaffected side, and the abdomen may be gasless (Bradshaw, 2021; Crowley, 2020; Draus & Ruzic, 2020; Lakshminrusimha et al., 2022; Madenci et al., 2019; Trotter, 2021).

Management and Outcome

■ Treatment is supportive and aimed at preventing respiratory failure. Delivery at a tertiary center and as close to term as possible optimizes management and patient outcomes.

■ Immediate intubation and positive pressure ventilation are required.
  ● Avoid bag mask ventilation. Swallowed air leads to gastric distention and further compression of the lung by the herniated portions of the GI system. Use of cuffed endotracheal tubes may further reduce gastric distention.
  ● Implement ventilation strategies that minimize barotrauma, such as HFOV, use of PIP less than 25 cm H_2O, permissive hypercapnia, preductal saturation levels greater than or equal to 85%, and pH greater than or equal to 7.25.

■ Perform gastric decompression via a nasogastric (NG) tube under continuous suction.
  ● It is advisable to perform decompression maneuvers prior to intubation to further minimize unintentional distention with air.
  ● It minimizes gastric distention and further elevation of the diaphragm and compression of the lung.

■ Provide hemodynamic support and treatment of PPHN.
  ● Inotropes, pulmonary vasodilators, and volume expanders maintain systemic blood pressure and decrease right-to-left shunting.
  ● iNO may be used in infants with severe hypoxemia. iNO dilates the pulmonary arteries, decreases pulmonary vascular resistance (PVR), and decreases right-to-left shunting across the ductus arteriosus.
    ❑ Additional vasodilator therapies include vasopressin, milrinone, and sildenafil.
  ● Pulmonary hypertension complicates most CDH cases, and ECMO may be necessary.

■ Pain management and sedation in conjunction with careful blood pressure monitoring is critical to the care of CDH infants.

■ Surgical repair can be done when physiologic stability has been achieved. CDH is no longer considered a surgical emergency and immediate surgical repair is thought to be detrimental.

- Overall prognosis is related to the size of the defect and the degree of pulmonary hypoplasia. Surgical repair does not reverse the complications of CDH.
  - Survival is highest in tertiary centers and with use of multidisciplinary standardized treatment guidelines. Mortality is high with larger defects, when the liver is involved in the defect, with presence of other defects, and with severe hypoplasia.
  - CDH infants are at a higher risk for long-term pulmonary, GI, neurologic, and skeletal system morbidities due to delayed lung maturation, altered pulmonary vasculature, and defects in surfactant maturation.
- With improvement in survival, there has been a focus on improving long-term morbidity of survivors. Coordinated long-term follow-up is required, as some survivors demonstrate neurologic issues: abnormal muscle tone and delayed neurocognitive and language skills.
  - Infants born with CDH have multiple long-term morbidities affecting the pulmonary, GI, neurologic, and skeletal systems. Respiratory complications include pulmonary vascular abnormalities, presumably causing pulmonary hypertension, a higher incidence of obstructive airway disease, and a restrictive lung function pattern that continues into adulthood. Gastroesophageal reflux disease (GERD), sometimes in combination with failure to thrive, is a well-recognized complication in patients with CDH, and several patients require antireflux surgery. It has been reported that infants with CDH are at a higher risk of having neuromotor delay, hypotonia, and delayed language skills. There is also a high percentage of these infants with sensorineural hearing loss (Bradshaw, 2021; Crowley, 2020; Draus & Ruzic, 2020; Fraser, 2021; Lakshminrusimha et al., 2022; Madenci et al., 2019).

▶ CONGENITAL CYSTIC LUNG LESIONS

BRONCHOGENIC CYST

Definition and Pathophysiology

- Bronchogenic cysts occur due to the abnormal budding of the embryonic foregut or maldevelopment of the tracheobronchial tree.
- Cysts are usually single in nature and commonly located near the carina, but may be found in the parenchyma, pleura, and diaphragm. They can enlarge over time and become infected (Crowley, 2020; Madenci et al., 2019).

Diagnosis

- Bronchogenic cyst may be diagnosed antenatally by US or fetal MRI.

- Postnatally, the chest x-ray may demonstrate fluid-filled cysts or air–fluid levels in cysts within the airway, and CT scan and bronchoscopy may confirm the diagnosis.
- Symptoms are related to airway compression/obstruction.
  - Symptoms of respiratory distress and stridor may occur later in the neonatal period or childhood (Crowley, 2020; Madenci et al., 2019).

Management and Outcome

- Respiratory support may include supplemental oxygen, intubation, and ventilation depending on whether airway obstruction is complete or partial, or if the airway is displaced anteriorly or posteriorly.
- Treatment for bronchogenic cyst consists of surgical resection and can be done thoracoscopically. Partial or total lobectomy yields uniformly good results. Early excision aims to prevent malignant changes over time.
- Outcomes are excellent after excision, with no long-term complications. Without excision, there is a risk of bleeding, rupture, infection, and malignancy (Crowley, 2020; Keller et al., 2018; Madenci et al., 2019).

CONGENITAL PULMONARY AIRWAY MALFORMATION

Definition and Pathophysiology

- Congenital pulmonary airway malformation (CPAM) was formerly known as cystic adenomatoid malformations (CCAMs). Revisions were made to the classification system to include less common proximal and distal malformations.
- While cystic lung diseases overall are rare, CPAM is the most common congenital cystic lung disease. It has an estimated incidence of 1 in 11,000 to 30,000 live births.
- The malformation is due to the abnormal branching of the fetal bronchial tree during the pseudoglandular period. The lesion is connected to the tracheobronchial tree and has a pulmonary blood supply. Cysts can be microcystic or macrocystic and can affect all lobes.
  - Up to 15% of these lesions appear to "disappear" in the prenatal period, usually after 28 weeks' gestation, when the growth of these lesions tends to plateau; however, in most cases, a postnatal CT scan or fetal MRI will show persistence of the anomaly.
- CPAMs have been classified into four types (Table 20.2; Crowley, 2020; Keller et al., 2018).

Diagnosis

- While CPAM can be diagnosed using prenatal imaging (fetal MRI), it can also be diagnosed in the postnatal period (CT scan). Prenatal US may identify a congenital lung lesion, but may not help differentiate

Table 20.2 Classification of Congenital Pulmonary Airway Malformations

Type	Disease Description
Type 0	■ Multiple small cysts, associated with other anomalies (cardiac, renal, dermal, and pulmonary hypoplasia) ■ Involves all lobes ■ The rarest and commonly lethal
Type 1	■ Large cysts surrounded by small cysts ■ Mass effect in utero can lead to hydrops and pulmonary hypoplasia ■ Cysts can collapse antenatal, with normal growth of unaffected lobes ■ Most common type
Type 2	■ Multiple small cysts, associated with other anomalies (renal, cardiac, CDH, extralobar sequestrations)
Type 3	■ Multiple small cysts that appear as a solid mass ■ Associated with hydrops, polyhydramnios, and pulmonary hypoplasia
Type 4	■ Large, thin-walled, air-filled cysts in the lung periphery ■ May be asymptomatic at birth

CDH, congenital diaphragmatic hernia.
Sources: Data from Crowley, M. A. (2020). Neonatal respiratory disorders. In R. J. Martin, A. A. Fanaroff, & M. C. Walsh (Eds.), *Fanaroff & Martin's neonatal-perinatal medicine: Diseases of the fetus and infant* (11th ed., pp. 1203–1230). Saunders; Fraser, D. (2021). Respiratory distress. In Verklan, M. T., Walden, M., & Forest, S. (Eds.), *Core curriculum for neonatal intensive care nursing* (6th ed., pp. 394–416). Elsevier.

CPAM from other cystic lung lesions. Microcystic lesions and the presence of hydrops are predictors of poor outcome. The degree of respiratory distress is influenced by the magnitude of mediastinal shift, cardiac compression, presence of lung hypoplasia, and association with other anomalies.

■ When diagnosed antenatally, fetal MRI is recommended throughout gestation to follow lesion growth, mediastinal shift, pulmonary hypoplasia, and impaired venous return that may result in the development of hydrops.

■ In nonemergent situations, a postnatal CT should be done to evaluate mass size, which facilitates surgical intervention if deemed necessary (Crowley, 2020; Fraser, 2021; Keller et al., 2018; Madenci et al., 2019; Ringer & Hansen, 2017).

Management and Outcome

■ Microcystic and large volume lesions may require fetal surgery (excision) if hydrops is present. If fetal surgery is not possible (see discussion in Chapter 3), antenatal steroids may reduce the size of microcystic lesions and resolve hydrops.

■ The degree of respiratory/ventilatory support will be indicated by the severity of the lesion. Severely affected infants may require iNO or ECMO support. The management of pulmonary hypertension, if present, is critical to the prevention of hypoxemia, maintenance of pulmonary and systemic perfusion, and preservation of end-organ function.

■ Postnatally, if respiratory distress is severe, immediate surgical excision is required.
  ● In asymptomatic infants, prophylactic early elective surgical removal may reduce the risk of infection and may improve lung growth and later malignancy.

■ Generally, children who have undergone resection for CPAMs are healthy. Pulmonary function data demonstrate normal vital capacity, residual volume, and expiratory flows between 1 and 2 years post lobectomy. However, the prognosis for infants with CPAM is related to the severity of other associated anomalies, and mortality is high when associated with pulmonary hypoplasia and hydrops. Long-term ventilatory assistance may be required when CPAM is more severe.

● There is an increased risk of bronchioloalveolar carcinoma (type 1) for lesions that are not removed. The intact lesion also remains a persistent reservoir for lower respiratory tract infection (Crowley, 2020; Keller et al., 2018; Madenci et al., 2019).

▶ ACQUIRED RESPIRATORY DISORDERS

RESPIRATORY DISTRESS SYNDROME

Definition and Pathophysiology

■ Insufficient or inactivated pulmonary surfactant leads to hypoxia, hypoventilation, and progressive atelectasis.

■ Pulmonary edema from serum proteins leaking into the alveoli contributes to the loss of functional residual capacity (FRC) and alterations in ventilation–perfusion ratio.
  ● Lung maturity or inadequate production of surfactant from type II alveolar cells is the most significant risk factor.
  ● Inflammation, as with infection, can negatively impact surfactant production and function.
  ● Increased fetal insulin in response to maternal diabetes inhibits proteins critical for surfactant production.
  ● Mutations in SP production or surfactant packaging can result in reduced production or functioning of surfactant.

- RDS incidence is inversely proportional to gestational age.
  - The incidence is higher in males (the male-to-female ratio is 2:1), as the presence of fetal androgens inhibits surfactant phospholipid production, and is higher in Caucasian infants.
  - Maternal administration of corticosteroids enhances lung maturity, antenatally inducing lung structural maturation by increasing the surface area for gas exchange and stimulation of surfactant production (Blackburn, 2018; Fraser, 2021; Guttentag, 2017; Hansen & Levin, 2019; Jensen et al., 2022; Kallapur & Jobe, 2020; Shepherd & Nelin, 2022; Tammela, 2020; Van Kaam, 2022; Yoder & Grubb, 2022).

Diagnosis

- Symptoms of RDS present soon after delivery, and respiratory difficulty increases within the first few hours of life, to include tachypnea, retractions, audible expiratory grunting, nasal flaring, cyanosis, and increased oxygen requirement.
  - Diagnostics include chest x-ray, arterial blood gas (ABG) measurements, blood cultures, and blood glucose monitoring.
  - Breath sounds may be diminished with poor air entry. Crackle, paradoxical seesaw respirations, and tachycardia may be present with disease progression, as well as pallor, central cyanosis, decreased capillary fill time, and progressive edema of the face, palms, and soles.
  - A chest x-ray will present with ground-glass or hazy appearance, low lung volumes, air bronchograms (more prominent as disease progresses), and microatelectasis. Complete atelectasis is characterized as "white-out" on chest x-ray.
  - Hypoxemia, hypercarbia, and acidosis can be seen on blood gas analysis.
  - Oliguria is a common presentation in the first 48 hours and lung improvement is seen at 2 to 4 days with diuresis.
- Symptoms gradually worsen and peak by 2 to 3 days, with improvement by 72 hours of life (Blackburn, 2018; Fraser, 2021; Guttentag, 2017; Hansen & Levin, 2019; Jensen et al., 2022; Lagoski et al., 2020; Shepherd & Nelin, 2022; Tammela, 2020).

Management and Outcome

- Exogenous surfactant administration augments endogenous surfactant production, improves lung compliance, and stabilizes the alveolar membrane, reducing alveolar collapse and atelectasis. Treatment is supportive to prevent further lung damage until the infant can produce adequate surfactant.
  - The brand or type of the surfactant used will vary with provider experience and preference and with commercial availability. Each has individual advantages and drawbacks.
- Mechanical ventilation strategies help establish and maintain FRC, recruit collapsed alveoli, and assist in improved oxygenation and ventilation.
- Caffeine therapy promotes respiratory drive.
- Evaluation for inflammatory/infectious processes and treatment with antibiotics may be necessary. Group B *Streptococcus* (GBS) pneumonia and RDS are often indistinguishable on chest x-ray.
- Resolution of RDS results in minimal to no complications in infants born at or over 32 weeks' gestation. Surfactant therapy reduces both the risk and severity of RDS and has been associated with a 30% reduction in mortality.
- Long-term sequelae are related to specific complications: CLD, IVH, retinopathy of prematurity (ROP), and respiratory syncytial virus (RSV) infection.
  - With severe RDS requiring prolonged ventilation, lung injury may be more severe and recovery delayed. The risk of development of CLD is highest in the lowest birth weight groups.
  - Readmissions for treatment of respiratory infections in the first year of life are not uncommon and lung disease may persist into adulthood (Blackburn, 2018; Bohannon et al., 2020b; DiBlasi, 2022; Fraser, 2021; Gautham & Soll, 2022; Guttentag, 2017; Hansen & Levin, 2019; Kallapur & Jobe, 2020; Tammela, 2020; Yoder & Grubb, 2022).

PNEUMONIA

Definition and Pathophysiology

- Multiple pathogens can be implicated with infection of the lung and can present early (within the first 3 days of life) or late (after 3 days of life). Organisms responsible for pneumonia vary by early and late onset (Table 20.3).
  - Congenital, or early-onset, pneumonia is acquired by vertical transmission in utero from aspiration of infected amniotic fluid, ascending infections from the birth canal, or via the transplacental route.
  - Late-onset pneumonia is common in infants requiring prolonged ventilation and is often hospital-acquired or nosocomial, caused by both bacterial and viral pathogens.
- Risk factors for pneumonia include prematurity, prolonged rupture of membranes, GBS colonization, chorioamnionitis, intrapartum maternal fever, sepsis, invasive procedures, presence of central lines, aspiration, and prolonged ventilation.
  - *Escherichia coli* is the most common bacterial isolate in the premature population (Crowley, 2020; Fraser, 2021; Hansen & Levin, 2019; Jensen et al., 2022; Rudd, 2021).

Diagnosis

- Symptoms of pneumonia are often indistinguishable from other respiratory diseases, RDS, and sepsis. Symptoms include grunting, nasal flaring, retractions,

Table 20.3 Organisms Responsible for Early- Versus Late-Onset Pneumonia

Early-Onset	Late-Onset
■ Group B *Streptococcus*	■ *Staphylococcus* spp.
■ *Escherichia coli*	■ *Streptococcus* pneumoniae
■ *Klebsiella* spp.	■ *Escherichia coli*
■ *Enterobacter* spp.	■ *Klebsiella* spp.
■ Group A *Streptococcus*	■ *Serratia* spp.
■ *Staphylococcus aureus*	■ *Enterobacter cloacae*
■ *Listeria monocytogenes*	■ *Pseudomonas* spp.
■ Herpes simplex virus (types 1 and 2)	■ *Candida* spp.
■ Adenovirus	■ *Citrobacter* spp.
■ Enterovirus	■ Respiratory syncytial virus
■ Rubella virus	■ Adenovirus
■ Cytomegalovirus	■ Enterovirus
■ *Treponema pallidum*	■ Parainfluenza
■ *Toxoplasma gondii*	■ Rhinovirus
■ *Candida* spp.	■ Influenza viruses
■ *Mycobacterium tuberculosis*	■ Cytomegalovirus
■ *Haemophilus influenzae*	■ *Chlamydia trachomatis*
■ *Chlamydia trachomatis*	
■ *Ureaplasma urealyticum*	

Source: Data from Fraser, D. (2021). Respiratory distress. In M. T. Verklan, M. Walden, & S. Forest (Eds.), *Core curriculum for neonatal intensive care nurses* (6th ed., pp. 394–416). Elsevier.

cyanosis, desaturations requiring supplemental oxygen, poor feeding, lethargy, irritability, temperature instability, and unwell appearance.
■ Chest x-ray findings may be nonspecific (unilateral or bilateral) and include alveolar infiltrates, areas of confluent opacities, diffuse interstitial pattern, and pleural effusions. Ground-glass appearance and air bronchograms may be present.
  ● Radiographic findings with postnatally acquired infections often change from normal to severely abnormal in a few days and may include pulmonary edema, pleural effusions, pneumatoceles, evidence of barotrauma, and cardiomegaly, depending on the severity of the disease process.
■ Infants should be evaluated for accompanying or concurrent septicemia: lethargy, temperature instability, apnea, poor feeding, and metabolic acidosis (Crowley, 2020; Fraser, 2021; Hansen & Levin, 2019; Rudd, 2021; Trotter, 2021).

Management and Outcome
■ Ventilation; circulatory support; management of hypoxia, acidosis, hypoglycemia, and electrolytes; and adequate nutrition help reduce mortality and morbidity.
■ Sepsis evaluation to rule out septicemia should be performed and should include a complete blood cell count with differential, blood culture, and polymerase chain reaction (PCR) to detect herpes viruses. Gram stain and culture of intubated infants, urine cultures,

and cerebrospinal fluid (CSF) cultures may also be helpful in determining the origin of infection.
  ● Positive tracheal aspirates after 8 hours of life may correlate with tracheal colonization and not infection.
■ Empiric antibiotics may be started before the identification of an organism. Antibiotic choice is based on the index of suspicion.
■ Suspected early-onset pneumonia is usually treated with ampicillin and gentamicin. Late-onset pneumonia is treated with vancomycin and gentamicin. Antivirals may be administered for herpes simplex or other pneumonias of viral origin.
■ Blood gas evaluation is important because metabolic acidosis may be severe. Tracheal aspirates may assist in the identification of a predominant infectious organism. CSF cultures should be obtained when the infant is stable since meningitis often accompanies pneumonia.
■ Length of antibiotic treatment is dictated by the organism responsible for the infection; treatment for 10 to 14 days is usually effective.
■ Outcome depends on the causative organism and response to antibiotic therapy. Complications include cardiopulmonary sequelae, systemic inflammatory response syndrome, disseminated intravascular coagulopathy, air leak, persistent pulmonary hypertension, and eventual development of CLD from prolonged ventilation.
■ Rapid identification of the infecting organism and timely treatment help minimize morbidity and mortality (Crowley, 2020; Fraser, 2021; Hansen & Levin, 2019; Rudd, 2021).

TRANSIENT TACHYPNEA OF THE NEWBORN

Definition and Pathophysiology

- Transient tachypnea of the newborn (TTN) is a delayed clearance of fetal lung fluid resulting in pulmonary edema. FRC may be reduced and thoracic gas volume may be increased secondary to air trapping.
  - The disease is characterized by tachypnea (up to 60–140 breaths per minute), mild to moderate retractions, grunting, cyanosis, decreased oxygen saturation (SO_2), hypercapnia, and respiratory acidosis, with a duration of 1 to 5 days.
- Risk factors include precipitous birth, preterm delivery, macrosomia, maternal diabetes, maternal asthma, multiple gestations, male gender, breech presentation, maternal sedation, and Cesarean delivery with or without labor.
  - TTN usually affects late preterm or term infants, occurring in 0.3% to 0.6% of term deliveries and 1% of preterm deliveries.
- Delayed clearance of fetal lung fluid is thought to be related to a delayed transition of the lungs from the in utero secretory fetal lung mode to the absorptive mode, and the absence of the hormonal changes that accompany spontaneous labor, including a surge in glucocorticoids and catecholamines. Impaired sodium channel clearance and active transport of chloride have also been implicated (Blackburn, 2018; Fraser, 2021; Gregory, 2017; Hansen & Levin, 2019; Jensen et al., 2022; Shepherd & Nelin, 2022; te Pas, 2020).

Diagnosis

- A diagnosis of TTN requires the exclusion of other potential etiologies for respiratory distress occurring in the first 6 hours of life, including RDS, sepsis, pneumonia, meconium aspiration syndrome (MAS), pulmonary hypertension, cyanotic congenital heart disease, central nervous system injury, pneumothorax, congenital malformations, metabolic acidosis, and polycythemia.
  - TTN is commonly seen in the first 6 hours of life and can persist for up to 72 hours. Air exchange is good and breath sounds may initially be moist, but clear quickly.
  - Chest x-rays exhibit increased pulmonary markings with perihilar streaking clearing at the periphery and fluid-filled interlobar fissures. Hyperaeration with widened intercostal spaces, mild cardiomegaly, mild hyperexpansion, mild pleural effusions, flattened diaphragm, and occasionally air bronchograms may also be present.
  - Decreased lung compliance results in tachypnea and increased work of breathing (WOB), cyanosis, grunting, retractions, and nasal flaring, all beginning within a few hours of birth.

- Infants may have a depressed diaphragm, an increased anteroposterior diameter, and a barrel-shaped chest secondary to hyperinflation.
- Laboratory screening evaluations may include serial complete blood count (CBC) and C-reactive protein (CRP) levels as well as appropriate cultures to rule out possible pneumonia or sepsis (Blackburn, 2018; Fraser, 2021; Gregory, 2017; Hansen & Levin, 2019; Jensen et al., 2022; Shepherd & Nelin, 2022; te Pas, 2020; Trotter, 2021).

Management and Outcome

- Treatment is mainly supportive and includes close observation, blood gas evaluation, and continuous positive airway pressure (CPAP) with or without supplemental oxygen therapy to prevent hypoxia. CPAP to improve lung recruitment may be indicated in more severe cases of TTN; however, CPAP is associated with an increased risk of air leak.
- If tachypnea and hypoxemia persist, evaluate for PPHN.
- Empiric broad-spectrum antibiotics may not be necessary if there are no risk factors for infection.
- Oral feedings should be deferred if respiratory rates are sustained consistently above 60 to 80 breaths per minute or high levels of positive pressure support (PS) are required (e.g., CPAP or high-flow nasal cannula [HFNC]). Restricting fluid intake may decrease the duration of support when TTN is severe.
- TTN is usually a self-limiting disease, generally improving within the first 48 to 72 hours of life, and in general there are no significant long-term negative outcomes.
  - There may be a link between TTN and the development of wheezing or reactive airway disease later in childhood (Crowley, 2020; Fraser, 2021; Gregory, 2017; Hansen & Levin, 2019; Jensen et al., 2022; Shepherd & Nelin, 2022; te Pas, 2020).

MECONIUM ASPIRATION SYNDROME

Definition and Pathophysiology

- MAS is the aspiration of meconium-stained amniotic fluid (MSAF) into the lungs in term or postterm infants, when the fetus gasps in the presence of fetal stress before, during, or immediately after delivery.
  - With intrauterine stress or asphyxia, peristalsis is stimulated and the anal sphincter relaxes, releasing meconium into the amniotic fluid. Fetuses at term (37+0 to 41+6 weeks gestational age [GA]) and postterm (beyond 42+0 weeks GA) pass meconium more readily than less mature fetuses.
  - The severity of MAS is related to the amount of fluid aspirated and the degree of asphyxial insult. It is frequently accompanied by air leak.
- Risk factors for MSAF are postterm (>41 weeks), small for gestational age, fetal distress, placental insufficiency, oligohydramnios, cord compression, and intrauterine hypoxia.

- Meconium can inactivate both endogenous and exogenous surfactants and inhibit surfactant production, causing airway obstruction, severe respiratory distress, impaired gas exchange, hypoxia, and increased PVR.
  - The obstructive phase is accompanied by acute airway obstruction, markedly increased airway resistance, scattered atelectasis with alveolar ventilation (V) / perfusion (Q) mismatching, and lung hyperexpansion secondary to air trapping and ball-valve effects.
  - The inflammatory phase, from the release of cytokines and vasoactive substances, occurs 12 to 24 hours later, leading to chemical pneumonitis and further alveolar involvement. Infants delivered with MSAF have an increased risk of pneumonia and PPHN (Blackburn, 2018; Crowley, 2020; Fraser, 2021; Hansen & Levin, 2019; Jenson et al., 2022; Plosa, 2017a; Yoder & Grubb, 2022).

Diagnosis

- MAS may present with birth depression requiring vigorous resuscitation.
- Symptoms of respiratory distress may range from mild and transient to severe and prolonged, and include grunting, flaring, retractions, tachypnea, and cyanosis.
  - Physical examination may reveal a barrel-shaped chest secondary to hyperinflation, with audible rales on auscultation.
    - Physical examination findings consistent with meconium aspiration related to postmaturity include peeling/cracking skin, loss of weight, long meconium-stained nails, and meconium-stained umbilical cord.
    - Diffuse, asymmetrical patchy infiltrates, areas of consolidation, hyperexpanded lucent areas mixed with areas of atelectasis, and a flattened diaphragm are classic findings on chest radiography (Blackburn, 2018; Crowley, 2020; Fraser, 2021; Hansen & Levin, 2019; Jensen et al., 2022; Trotter, 2021).

Management and Outcome

- Respiratory failure requiring mechanical ventilation is not uncommon, although most infants with mild cases do well with noninvasive support. Use of positive pressure may result in air leak due to the ball-valve effects of MAS. Low levels of positive end-expiratory pressure (PEEP; 4 to 5 cm H_2O) splint open partially obstructed airways and equalize V/Q matching. When airway resistance is high but lung compliance is normal, use of a slow rate and moderate pressure or volume is indicated.
  - Infants with severe MAS may require the use of high-frequency ventilation (HFV), nitric oxide, and/or ECMO, if PPHN develops.
- MAS management is primarily supportive and should include ventilatory/oxygen support (including close monitoring of blood gases) to maintain peripheral SO_2 between 95% and 99%, cardiovascular stabilization, blood PS, as well as avoidance of hypoxia and acidosis.
  - Antibiotic administration is required to treat pneumonia/sepsis.
  - Surfactant therapy may improve lung compliance and oxygenation. Surfactant administration is thought to reduce the severity of respiratory distress and may reduce disease progression and the need for ECMO, a last resort therapy.
  - Infants may need iNO if PPHN develops.
  - Sedation (morphine [Duramorph], fentanyl [Duragesic], lorazepam [Ativan], or midazolam [Versed]) and muscle relaxation (pancuronium bromide [Pavulon] and vecuronium [Norcuron]) may lower the risk of air leak in severe MAS.
  - Nonpharmacologic interventions may help decrease agitation and limit the need for sedation, and include limiting stimulation by lowering environmental light, noise, and any unnecessary tactile stimulation.
- Recovery and weaning of respiratory support are proportional to the resolution of airway obstruction, degree of inflammation, and extent of lung injury.
- Mild cases of MAS generally have excellent prognoses unless the MAS is accompanied by PPHN or severe asphyxia. MAS complicated by PPHN carries an increased risk of mortality.
  - A small number of infants who survive MAS will continue to require oxygen at 1 month and their pulmonary function may be abnormal.
  - Prolonged ventilatory support resulting from PPHN may result in CLD (Blackburn, 2018; Crowley, 2020; Eichenwald, 2017; Fraser, 2021; Gautham & Soll, 2022; Hansen & Levin, 2019; Jensen et al., 2022; Plosa, 2017a; Yoder & Grubb, 2022).

PULMONARY HEMORRHAGE

Definition and Pathophysiology

- Pulmonary hemorrhage is defined as the presence of erythrocytes in the alveoli and/or the lung interstitium and occurs in 3% to 5% of preterm infants ventilated for RDS. The highest incidence is in the very low birth weight and extremely low birth weight population. Of pulmonary hemorrhages in preterm infants, 80% occur within 72 hours of birth or between days 2 and 4 of life.
- Pulmonary hemorrhage is thought to result from hemorrhagic pulmonary edema rather than direct bleeding into the lung. It results in poor lung compliance, surfactant inactivation, and pulmonary edema. Other mechanisms contributing to pulmonary hemorrhage may include increased pulmonary capillary pressure and injury to the capillary endothelium from acute left ventricular failure; altered epithelial–endothelial barrier; and coagulation

disorders, which may worsen, but not initiate, the condition.

- It is rarely an isolated condition and is typically exhibited by the clinical presence of hemorrhagic fluid (pink or red frothy fluid) in the trachea, accompanied by respiratory decompensation requiring increased respiratory support or intubation within 60 minutes of the appearance of hemorrhagic fluid.
- Predisposing factors linked to pulmonary hemorrhage include patent ductus arteriosus (PDA), exogenous surfactant administration, sepsis, severe systemic illness, extreme prematurity, coagulopathy, IVH, heart disease, perinatal asphyxia, hypothermia, male gender, and multiple birth.
  - Other causes of blood in the airway not related to pulmonary hemorrhage include direct trauma to the airway and aspiration of blood (Crowley, 2020; Fraser, 2021; Hansen & Levin, 2019; Jensen et al., 2022; Plosa, 2017b).

Diagnosis

- Acute respiratory distress symptoms include cyanosis, bradycardia, apnea, gasping, hypotension, increased WOB, hypoxia, and hypercapnia.
  - Presence of pink frothy fluid is noted in the airway or endotracheal tube.
  - Chest x-ray findings may be nonspecific and include the presence of fluffy infiltrates or opacification of one or both lungs with air bronchograms.
  - A fall in hematocrit, metabolic, or mixed acidosis coagulopathy can also be seen.
- An echocardiogram should be done to assess and treat PDA and evaluate ventricular function (Crowley, 2020; Fraser, 2021; Gomella, 2020b; Hansen & Levin, 2019; Jensen et al., 2022; Plosa, 2017b).

Management and Outcome

- Provide ventilatory support, including high mean airway pressure and high PEEP of 6 to 8 cm H_2O, as well as ventilation strategy that maintains gas exchange and tamponades or minimizes further accumulation of interstitial and alveolar fluid. Aggressive airway suctioning should be avoided.
  - Consider surfactant administration to treat primary RDS or secondary surfactant deficiency from airway edema caused by the hemorrhage. However, the efficacy of surfactant therapy is not well established and its routine use is questionable.
  - Endotracheal administration of epinephrine will cause restriction of the pulmonary capillaries.
- Volume resuscitation, including packed red blood cell (PRBC) replacement, in addition to administration of vasoactive medications, may be required.
- Assess for and treat PDA and clotting abnormalities.

- If the hemorrhage is isolated or small, the outcome will depend on the underlying disease. If bleeding is massive, death will quickly occur in spite of aggressive management. Mortality is 30% to 40%.
- Pulmonary hemorrhage may be associated with a higher incidence of cerebral palsy, cognitive delay, periventricular leukomalacia, and seizures, with the highest mortality rates occurring in the extremely low birthweight population (Crowley, 2020; Fraser, 2021; Gautham & Soll, 2022; Gomella, 2020b; Hansen & Levin, 2019; Jensen et al., 2022; Plosa, 2017b).

PERSISTENT PULMONARY HYPERTENSION OF THE NEWBORN

Definition and Pathophysiology

- PPHN can be described as the failure of normal pulmonary adaptation resulting in sustained elevation in PVR and pulmonary artery pressure, leading to right-to-left shunting across persistent fetal channels (PDA, patent foramen ovale [PFO]), decreased pulmonary perfusion, severe systemic hypoxemic respiratory failure, acidemia, and lactic acidosis.
  - Adequate oxygenation after delivery depends on lung inflation, closure of the fetal shunts, decreased PVR, and increased pulmonary blood flow.
- Antenatal conditions linked to PPHN include asphyxia; pulmonary parenchymal disease (pneumonia, surfactant deficiency, aspiration syndromes); abnormal pulmonary development and structure (CDH, pulmonary hypoplasia, space-occupying lesions); congenital heart disease; myocardial dysfunction; prenatal pulmonary hypertension (systemic or secondary to premature closure of the ductus arteriosus associated with maternal aspirin or nonsteroidal anti-inflammatory drugs); pneumonia, bacterial, or viral sepsis; and genetic predisposition. Contributing mechanical pathology includes low cardiac output and hyperviscosity, associated with polycythemia, and abnormal pulmonary vasoreactivity and adaptation.
- Perinatal risk factors include MSAF, maternal fever, urinary tract infection (UTI), anemia, diabetes, or pulmonary disease, as well as selective serotonin reuptake inhibitor exposure, hypothermia, and Cesarean delivery.
  - PPHN is most common in full-term and postterm infants at a rate of 1 to 2 per 1,000 live births.
  - The most common precipitating factors for PPHN are intrauterine asphyxia and hypoxic respiratory failure (HRF). PPHN and HRF can be primary with no associated lung disease, or secondary to lung diseases such as MAS, RDS, TTN, and pneumonia (Blackburn, 2018; Fraser, 2021; Hansen & Levin, 2019; Keszler & Abubakar, 2022a;

Lakshminrusimha & Keszler, 2022; Steinhorn, 2020; Van Marter & McPherson, 2017).

Diagnosis

- PPHN is suspected based on history and clinical course.
- Respiratory distress and cyanosis with a gradient of 10% or more, between pre- and postductal SO_2, are helpful in making the diagnosis.
  - A hyperoxia test is one of the most helpful early screens to determine if cyanosis has cardiac or pulmonary origin. A right-to-left shunt is demonstrated if the partial pressure of oxygen (PaO_2) does not increase with 100% oxygen administration, indicating either PPHN or congenital heart disease.
- A single or narrowly split and accentuated second heart sound can be heard, as well as a systolic murmur.
- EKG findings include normal right ventricular predominance, evidence of myocardial ischemia, or infarction.
- Laboratory studies should be done to evaluate metabolic abnormalities such as hypoglycemia, hypocalcemia, and metabolic acidosis. Clotting studies may be abnormal secondary to end-organ damage from asphyxia.
- The chest x-ray usually appears normal but may reveal associated pulmonary disease.
- Echocardiogram findings include intracardiac or ductal shunting, tricuspid valve regurgitation, and flattened/bowing of ventricular septum. Echocardiogram assists in the diagnosis of congenital heart disease (Fraser, 2021; Hansen & Levin, 2019; Lakshminrusimha & Keszler, 2022; Van Marter & McPherson, 2017).

Management and Outcome

- Intubation and mechanical ventilatory support are required to improve oxygenation while minimizing hyperoxia and hyperventilation. The main goal is to correct hypoxia and acidosis, as well as to promote dilation of the pulmonary vascular bed.
  - HFV, HFOV, or high-frequency jet ventilation (HFJV) may be required if conventional mechanical ventilation fails.
- Maintaining postductal SO_2 between 93% and 98% may help promote adequate tissue oxygenation, avoid hypoxia-induced vasoconstriction, and minimize free radical release secondary to hyperoxia, which may also worsen the PPHN.
  - High oxygen (the most potent pulmonary vasodilator) concentrations may be required to reverse hypoxemia and pulmonary vasoconstriction.
- Arterial access assists in the monitoring of blood gases and blood pressure.

- Hemodynamic support to maintain systemic blood pressure and improve cardiac output may be required.
  - This may include the use of volume expanders: normal saline and packed red cells in the face of anemia.
  - Pharmacologic management includes the use of inotropic agents such as dobutamine and milrinone, or the administration of vasopressors such as dopamine, epinephrine, and/or vasopressin.
  - Correction of hypoglycemia and hypocalcemia promotes myocardial function and improves the response to inotropic drugs.
- Administration of iNO promotes smooth muscle relaxation and pulmonary vasodilation for term and near-term infants with minimal to no impact on systemic arterial pressure. Nitric oxide is also a naturally occurring substance that is produced by pulmonary endothelial cells. It is a selective pulmonary vasodilator that decreases PVR and can be administered via the ventilator at 1 to 20 parts per million (ppm).
  - Methemoglobin is a by-product of iNO therapy and should be monitored regularly.
  - Ventilatory support as well as iNO should be weaned gradually to avoid rebound hypoxemia and PPHN.
- Infants who fail ventilatory management and/or iNO therapy may require ECMO. The calculation of the oxygen index (OI) helps identify infants who might benefit from ECMO.
  - The OI index is a measure of the severity of respiratory failure and can be calculated as follows: OI = mean airway pressure (P_{aw}) × fraction of inspired oxygen (FiO_2)/PaO_2 × 100. Two OIs of greater than 40 within 1 hour, one OI of 60 on HFV, and one OI of 40 combined with cardiovascular instability are indicators of the need for ECMO.
- Reduction in noise and minimal stimulation and handling may facilitate shunt reduction. Administration of sedatives and analgesics (fentanyl citrate or morphine sulfate) is also useful in minimizing agitation and shunting, if there is no systemic hypotension.
- Infants with PPHN are at a higher risk for negative neurodevelopmental, cognitive, and audiologic (sensorineural hearing loss) impairments. Survival is dependent on the center where care is delivered, and the underlying disease process. The combined availability of iNO and ECMO has reduced PPHN mortality and the occurrence of CLD incidence in infants with hypoxemic respiratory failure (Arensman et al.; Barrington & Dempsey, 2022; Fraser, 2021; Hansen & Levin, 2019; Lakshminrusimha & Keszler, 2022; Steinhorn, 2020; Van Marter & McPherson, 2017; Wolf & Arnold, 2017).

PULMONARY AIR LEAK SYNDROMES

Definition and Pathophysiology

■ Pulmonary air leaks occur secondary to alveolar distention and rupture, with a common etiology of high transpulmonary pressures that damage terminal airways and alveoli and allow air to enter the interstitium, resulting in PIE. If transpulmonary pressures remain high, air may continue to dissect along the perivascular sheaths into the visceral pleura, the hilum, and the pericardium, resulting in pneumothorax, pneumomediastinum, and pneumopericardium.

■ The primary risk factors contributing to air leak syndromes are mechanical ventilation and underlying lung disorders, which result in decreased compliance or obstruction with air trapping. Air leaks can occur spontaneously if there is unequal air distribution at birth or iatrogenically from excessive use of airway pressure during resuscitation or with assisted ventilation (Eyal, 2020a; Fraser, 2021; Hansen & Levin, 2019; Jensen et al., 2022; Markham, 2017).

Diagnosis

■ Clinical findings can range from subtle changes in vital signs to cardiovascular collapse if the air leak is large. Symptoms include sudden respiratory deterioration (tachypnea, grunting, flaring, retractions), cyanosis, oxygen desaturation, increased oxygen requirement, hypotension, bradycardia, chest asymmetry or a barrel-shaped chest, a shifted point of maximum impulse (PMI), and distant heart sounds.

  ● Other symptoms may result from air continuing to dissect into subcutaneous tissues, producing subcutaneous emphysema, pulmonary emboli, as well as pneumoperitoneum.

  ● Chest radiography remains the gold standard but may not be timely. Transillumination may be helpful in emergent situations but can be prone to false negative or positive results (Eyal, 2020a; Fraser, 2021; Hansen & Levin, 2019; Markham, 2017; Shepherd & Nelin, 2022; Trotter, 2021).

Management and Outcome

■ See Table 20.4 for management overview of air leak syndromes.

■ Outcomes depend on the underlying pathology. There are high mortality rates with pneumoperitoneum, bilateral pneumothoraces, and bilateral PIE. The risk of CLD is high with bilateral PIE (Fraser, 2021; Hansen & Levin, 2019).

CHRONIC LUNG DISEASE

■ Respiratory management improved with the onset of more advantageous approaches to ventilation in the 1960s. More preterm infants survived, but with severe chronic lung damage, which was first described as BPD.

● The terms CLD and BPD are used interchangeably, and the current definition focuses on specific criteria which include the need for and duration of oxygen or ventilatory support at specific postmenstrual ages. CLD can be classified as mild, moderate, or severe, and the incidence is inversely proportional to gestational age and birth weight.

● Pathogenesis is multifactorial and includes gestational age, birth weight, lung immaturity, arrested lung development, and acute lung injury from maternal chorioamnionitis; barotrauma; volutrauma; and lung injury secondary to mechanical ventilation. Inflammation, oxygen toxicity (hyperoxia), excessive early IV fluid administration, PDA, intrauterine/perinatal infection, IUGR, decreased surfactant synthesis/function, nutritional deficits, and abnormal repair processes also play a role (Bancalari & Jain, 2020; Blackburn, 2018; Fraser, 2021; Goldsmith and Raju, 2022; Hansen & Levin, 2019; Parad & Benjamin, 2017; Van Kaam, 2022).

Diagnosis

■ CLD is a disease of exclusion. Clinical presentation typically reveals tachypnea, retractions, and rales on auscultation and inability to wean from respiratory support. ABG analysis often reflects hypoxemia, hypercarbia, and respiratory acidosis.

  ● Chest radiographs are consistent with abnormal lung parenchyma.
    ❑ Initial presentation includes diffuse haziness, increased density, and low to normal lung volumes.
    ❑ Chronic changes in more severe disease include regions of opacification and hyperlucency, as well as superimposed air bronchograms, and may also include hyperinflation, infiltrates, blebs, and cardiomegaly.

  ● Fluid intolerance often occurs despite no change in fluid intake, as evidenced by increased edema, weight, and decreased urine output.

  ● Complications of CLD include intermittent bronchospasm, recurrent respiratory tract infections, gastroesophageal reflux (GER), and developmental delays (Fraser, 2021; Hansen & Levin, 2019; Parad & Benjamin, 2017; Trotter, 2021).

  ● Table 20.5 shows a summary of the CLD/BPD diagnostic criteria.

Management and Outcome

■ Aggressive enteral and parenteral nutrition helps optimize growth and repair. Infants with CLD may require higher caloric intake (150–180 kcal/kg/d), as well as higher protein, vitamin, and mineral intake. Fortification of human milk is recommended.

■ Evaluation for cor pulmonale and right ventricle hypertrophy using serial electrocardiography and echocardiography is imperative.

Table 20.4 Management Overview of Air Leak Syndromes

Air Leak Syndrome	Signs and Symptoms	Diagnosis	Management
PIE	Respiratory distress, hypotension, bradycardia, hypercarbia, hypoxia, and acidosis	■ Common in the first 48 hours after birth ■ Linear cyst-like cysts lucencies on x-ray ■ Cysts can be large and bleb-like	■ Decrease P_{aw}, PEEP, and inspiratory time. ■ High-frequency ventilation may help reduce TV.
Pneumothorax	Respiratory distress may be severe, cyanosis, chest asymmetry, diminished/distant breath sounds, shift in point of maximum impulse, acute deterioration of vital signs, decreased cardiac output	■ Hypoxia, hypercarbia, acidosis ■ Transillumination positive for air on the affected side ■ Hyperlucent hemithorax on x-ray and may see shift of mediastinal structures	■ Manage with thoracentesis/needle aspiration, thoracotomy/chest tube insertion, and insertion of pigtail catheter. ■ Ventilatory management to reduce P_{aw}, PEEP, TV, and high-frequency ventilation may be the strategy of choice.
Pneumomediastinum	Heart sounds may be distant, cardiopulmonary decompensation is rare	■ Central air collections seen on x-ray and lifting of thymus from the heart (sail sign); may be more prominent in lateral view	■ Implement strategies to reduce P_{aw}.
Pneumopericardium	Acute hemodynamic instability, with hypotension, decreased pulse pressure, bradycardia, and cyanosis with distant heart sounds	■ Muffled heart sounds, with air surrounding heart on x-ray ■ May be identified by transillumination	■ Perform needle aspiration if cardiac tamponade is present.

P_{aw}, mean airway pressure; PEEP, positive end-expiratory pressure; PIE, pulmonary interstitial emphysema; TV, tidal volume.
Sources: Data from Fraser, D. (2021). Respiratory distress. In M. T. Verklan, M. Walden, & S. Forest (Eds.), *Core curriculum for neonatal intensive care nurses* (6th ed., pp. 394–416). Elsevier; Hansen, A., & Levin, J. (2019). Neonatal pulmonary disorders. In B. K. Walsh (Ed.), *Neonatal and pediatric respiratory care* (5th ed., pp. 407–452). Elsevier; Jensen, E. A., Fraga, M. N., Biko, D. M., Raimondi, F., & Kirpalani, H. (2022). Imaging: Radiography, lung ultrasound, and other imaging modalities. In M. Keszler & K. S. Gautham (Eds.), *Assisted ventilation of the neonate* (7th ed., pp. 76–93). Elsevier; Markham, M. (2017). Pulmonary air leak. In E. Eichenwald, A. Hansen, C. Martin, & A. Stark (Eds.), *Cloherty & Stark's manual of neonatal care* (8th ed., pp. 482–490). Wolters Kluwer; Sheppherd, E. G., & Nelin, L. D. (2022). Physical examination. In M. Keszler & K. S. Gautham (Eds.), *Assisted ventilation of the neonate* (7th ed., pp. 70–75). Elsevier; Trotter, C. W. (2021). Radiologic evaluation. In M. T. Verklan, M. Walden, & S. Forest (Eds.), *Core curriculum for neonatal intensive care nursing* (6th ed., pp. 219–243). Elsevier.

Table 20.5 Summary of Chronic Lung Disease/Bronchopulmonary Dysplasia Diagnostic Criteria

Gestational Age	<32 weeks	≥32 weeks
Timing of assessment	36 weeks PMA or discharge to home (whichever comes first)	>28 postnatal days, but less than 56 postnatal days, or discharge to home (whichever comes first)
	Treatment with >21% oxygen for at least 28 days PLUS the following:	
Mild BPD	Breathing 21% oxygen at 36 weeks' PMA or at discharge (whichever comes first)	Breathing 21% oxygen at 56 postnatal days or discharge to home (whichever comes first)
Moderate BPD	Need for <30% oxygen at 36 weeks' PMA or at discharge (whichever comes first)	Need for <30% oxygen at 56 postnatal days or at discharge to home (whichever comes first)
Severe BPD	Need for ≥30% oxygen or PPV or NCPAP at 36 weeks' PMA or at discharge (whichever comes first)	Need for ≥30% oxygen or PPV or NCPAP at 56 postnatal days or at discharge to home (whichever comes first)

BPD, bronchopulmonary dysplasia; NCPAP, nasal continuous positive airway pressure; PMA, postmenstrual age; PPV, positive pressure ventilation.
Source: Reproduced with permission from Bancalari, E. H., & Jain, D. (2020). Bronchopulmonary dysplasia. In R. Martin, A. A. Fanaroff, & M. C. Walsh (Eds.), *Fanaroff & Martin's neonatal-perinatal medicine: Diseases of the fetus and infant* (11th ed., pp. 1256–1269). Elsevier.

- Fluid restriction (130–140 mL/k/d) with reduction in salt intake can help reduce pulmonary edema and right-sided heart failure.
- Diuretics can be used to treat pulmonary edema. These include furosemide, spironolactone, chlorothiazide, hydrochlorothiazide, and hydrochlorothiazide with spironolactone.
  - If diuretics are used, serum electrolytes should be monitored for hyponatremia, hypokalemia, resultant hypochloremia, and metabolic alkalosis, which may impair growth. Supplementation of electrolytes may be needed.
  - Long-term use of furosemide is associated with hypercalciuria, bone demineralization, nephrolithiasis, and ototoxicity.
- Administration of bronchodilators assists in the reduction of bronchospasm and resistance to airflow related to smooth muscle hypertrophy commonly seen in CLD.
- Caffeine citrate promotes airway bronchodilation and has a mild diuretic effect and has both a lung protective and a brain-protective effect.
- Postnatal corticosteroid therapy reduces inflammation, improves lung function, and facilitates weaning from the ventilator.
  - Administration of corticosteroids postnatally has not been found to have a substantial impact on long-term respiratory outcomes and is controversial due to the potential for adverse neurologic outcomes with prolonged therapy.
- Blood transfusion of PRBCs to maintain a hematocrit of 30% to 35% while still on supplemental oxygen or ventilator support is helpful.
- RSV prophylaxis is recommended.
- Overall mortality is low. The highest mortality occurs in cases of severe CLD. Infants with CLD have a higher rate of readmission in the first year of life secondary to lower respiratory tract infections and reactive airway disease. CLD survivors have a higher incidence of wheezing episodes in the first 2 years of life, which may require hospitalization.
  - Pulmonary function may be reduced and may remain abnormal into adulthood.
  - Cor pulmonale and pulmonary hypertension can develop secondary to severe hypoxemia and can result in respiratory failure and death.
- Higher rates of neurologic delays or deficits are seen with severe CLD. Cerebral palsy is more common, as well as sensorineural hearing loss and visual difficulties (Bancalari & Jain, 2020; Blackburn, 2018; Fraser, 2021; Fraser & Diehl-Jones, 2021; Hansen & Levin, 2019; Parad & Benjamin, 2017).

▶ APNEA

DEFINITION AND PATHOPHYSIOLOGY

- *Apnea* is defined as the cessation of breathing for 15 to 20 seconds or less, if there is evidence of corresponding desaturations with pallor or cyanosis, bradycardia, and hypotonia.
- Apnea is pathologic (an apneic spell) when absent airflow is prolonged (usually 20 seconds or more) or accompanied by bradycardia (heart rate <100 beats per minute) or hypoxemia that is detected clinically (cyanosis) or by SO_2 monitoring. Bradycardia and desaturation are usually present after 20 seconds of apnea, although they typically occur more rapidly in the small premature infant.
  - Periodic breathing (recurrent sequences of pauses lasting 5 to 10 seconds followed by 10 to 15 seconds of rapid respiration) is considered normal in preterm and early term infants. Periodic breathing is not accompanied by cyanosis or heart rate changes.
  - Respiratory pauses may be caused by immature peripheral chemoreceptors unable to respond to changes in $PaCO_2$ via increased respirations. The resulting acidosis may be responsible for apnea episodes. Central chemoreceptors are found throughout the brainstem.
- Apnea of prematurity (AOP) is a developmental disorder resulting from immaturity and disorganization of neurotransmitters gamma-aminobutyric acid (GABA) and adenosine. Brainstem immaturity contributes to the lack of respiratory drive and generally resolves by 36 to 37 weeks in infants born beyond 27 weeks' gestation. Among more immature infants, apnea can often persist past term gestation. It reflects a "physiologic" rather than "pathologic" immature state of respiratory control.
- Apnea can be categorized as central, obstructive, mixed, primary, secondary, and idiopathic.
  - *Central apnea:* Respiratory efforts cease without evidence of obstruction.
  - *Obstructive apnea:* Breathing motions have no effect due to a blocked airway.
  - *Mixed apnea:* This is characterized by combined upper airway obstruction and central cessation of respiratory efforts. 50% to 60% of apnea episodes are obstructive in origin.
  - Mixed is the most common type of apnea (50%), followed by central (40%) and then obstructive (10%).
- Most apneas occur during active sleep. Preterm infants are asleep 80% of time, and 50% of sleep is active. This relationship lasts until 6 months of age. The ventilatory response to hypoxia and ventilatory sensitivity to carbon dioxide (CO_2) are more depressed during active sleep. Activation of serotonin-containing neurons, which are part of the arousal system of the brainstem, decreases by nearly half during slow-wave sleep and becomes nearly silent during rapid eye movement sleep via activation of GABAergic inputs (Churchman, 2020; Gomella, 2020a; Gomella & Palla, 2020; Patrinos, 2020; Stark, 2017).

DIAGNOSIS

- AOP is a diagnosis of exclusion; therefore, it is important to diagnose and treat any secondary cause.

Causes of apnea and bradycardia events (colloquially called *As & Bs*) can be classified according to diseases and disorders of various organ systems, gestational age, or postnatal age.

- Full-term infants rarely have apnea; the incidence is low and it is usually not due to physiologic causes, as in premature infants. The onset of apnea in a term infant at any time is a critical event that requires immediate investigation.

- History and physical examination must include a review of maternal risk factors, medications, birth history, and feeding intolerance. Physical examination should include a search for abnormal neurologic signs and signs of sepsis.

- Laboratory studies may include a complete septic workup, screening for metabolic disorders, radiography to evaluate for abdominal or cranial abnormalities, or EEG to rule out seizures as apnea may be the sole presentation of seizures.

- Polysomnography is the collective process of monitoring and recording physiologic data during sleep. It includes respiration, perioral electromyography, SO_2, heart rate, electroencephalography, electrocardiography, and electrooculography. The addition of a thermistor to detect change in the mouth and airflow results in a thermistor pneumocardiogram examination.

  - An impedance pneumography measures chest wall movement, heart rate, SO_2, and nasal airflow by thermistor or CO_2 probe (four-channel). Esophageal pH may also be measured through the use of a probe (five-channel testing; Churchman, 2020; Gomella, 2020a; Gomella & Palla, 2020; Patrinos, 2020; Stark, 2017).

MANAGEMENT AND OUTCOME

- All infants less than 35 weeks should be monitored for apnea, which should include the use of cardiorespiratory monitors and pulse oximetry. Apnea monitors alone may not differentiate breathing efforts through an obstructed airway from normal breathing patterns; therefore, heart rate should be monitored in addition to respiration.

- *Positioning:* Maintain the neck in a neutral position; use a neck roll for support as needed. Prone positioning may help reduce frequent obstructive apnea events related to impaired airway protective mechanisms (e.g., micrognathia).

- Provide respiratory support as required.

  - Adaptive backup ventilation for apnea is available using invasive or noninvasive means. If the infant is apneic or becomes hypoxic, the modality provides a preset mandatory breathing rate. Early studies show these modalities can better match the varying ventilatory needs of preterm or ill infants than conventional mandatory ventilation.

- CPAP increases end-expiratory lung volume, splints the upper airway and compliant chest wall, and prevents obstruction.

- Methylxanthines stimulate the central respiratory chemoreceptors and increase ventilatory response to CO_2 through the antagonism of the neurotransmitter adenosine. Methylxanthine therapy also increases the respiratory drive and thereby reduces the number of periodic breathing events.

- Apnea generally resolves by 36 to 40 weeks' postconceptional age (PCA); however, for extremely preterm infants, events may extend until 43 to 44 weeks.

  - Home cardiorespiratory monitoring may be an option for infants with a history of apnea events who are discharged prior to 44 weeks' PCA to avoid prolonged hospital stays.

  - Indications for home monitoring include premature infants with idiopathic apnea who are otherwise ready for discharge, a history of a sibling death from sudden infant death syndrome (SIDS), a sleep apnea syndrome secondary to a neurologic condition, or other conditions attributable to a high-risk infant.

    - Home monitoring is not intended as SIDS prevention in symptom-free, healthy infants.

  - In 80% of infants, home monitoring may be discontinued at 45 weeks' PCA.

- Infants discharged from a NICU often experience multiple comorbidities, which complicates an analysis to determine a relationship between apnea. However, evolving evidence suggests a link between delayed apnea resolution and the severity of the apnea course with impaired neurodevelopmental outcome (Churchman, 2020; Claure & Bancalari, 2022; Gauda & Martin, 2018; Kandasamy & Carlo, 2022; Patrinos, 2020; Stark, 2017).

▶ ADDITIONAL CAUSES OF RESPIRATORY DISTRESS

- See Table 20.6 for a summary of other disorders that contribute to respiratory distress in the neonate.

▶ NEONATAL RESPIRATORY MECHANICS AND RESPIRATORY SUPPORT

OXYGEN PHYSIOLOGY

- At sea level, maternal hemoglobin is 96% oxygenated at 100 mmHg. Fetal tissues are ~80% oxygenated with a PaO_2 of 30 to 40 mmHg and fully oxygenated at 50 to 60 mmHg. This illustrates why oxygen supplementation can be detrimental to the tissues of preterm infants.

- The gradient of higher maternal oxygen level diffuses through the placenta to the hypoxic fetus. In utero, fetal hemoglobin (HgF) has a greater binding capacity to attract oxygen molecules.

- Increasing the maternal oxygen level does not significantly increase the fetal PaO_2. The fetus responds to variability in oxygen levels by changes in cardiac output.
- Placental insufficiency decreases oxygen availability to the fetus, diminishing growth and resulting in intrauterine growth restriction.

- The neonate transitions over the first 3 to 6 months of life to the production of adult hemoglobin (HgA) with increased 2,3-diphosphoglycerate (DPG) production. The transition from HgF to HgA is associated with reduced oxygen affinity and rightward shift of the oxyhemoglobin dissociation curve.

Table 20.6 Summary of Other Disorders That Contribute to Respiratory Distress in the Neonate

Disorder	Etiology	Diagnosis	Management
CHD	■ 25% of congenital defects may be critical CHD lesions ■ The most common lesions appear in the first weeks of life and may be associated with other disorders or syndromes	■ Cyanosis, respiratory distress, tachypnea, murmur, CHF, difference in upper and lower extremities ■ Hyperoxia test, ■ echocardiogram ■ EKG	■ Respiratory support as needed ■ Stabilization and transport if intervention is required ■ Administration of prostaglandins may be required to support patency of fetal channels
Choanal atresia	■ Bony abnormality causing obstruction to flow ■ Bilateral is the most common cause of complete nasal obstruction ■ Can be associated with other anomalies (CHARGE)	■ Obligate nose breathers, so minimal to no oral air intake causing cyanosis, respiratory distress Symptoms may worsen with sucking ■ If bilateral, symptom improvement seen with crying ■ Failure to pass small-caliber tube may be diagnostic	■ Bilateral and severe will require immediate repair ■ Intubation may be required ■ Respiratory support as needed
Laryngomalacia	■ Obstructive disorder in which the supraglottic structures collapse into the laryngeal inlet during inspiration	■ Wheezing and/or stridor with or without respiratory distress Presence of cough or weak cry ■ Diagnosed via laryngoscopy or bronchoscopy	■ Surgical repair only in most severe cases ■ Prone positioning supports airway
Tracheomalacia	■ Airway obstruction caused by the collapse of the trachea during expiration ■ May develop from compression of the adjacent structures, connective tissue disorders, or prolonged mechanical ventilation	■ Expiratory stridor associated with respiratory distress ■ Diagnosed by bronchoscopy	■ Respiratory support as required ■ If severe may require tracheostomy ■ Humidification of airway to thin secretions
Micrognathia	■ Mandibular hypoplasia and can be associated with Pierre Robin sequence	■ Severe respiratory distress, airway obstruction, and feeding difficulties	■ Prone positioning, use of oral airway and if severe immediate surgical intervention ■ Tracheostomy may be required
Anemia	■ Accelerated loss/destruction of RBCs, defects in production ■ Decreased oxygenation and tissue perfusion	■ Cyanosis, pallor, tachycardia, tachypnea, apnea, respiratory distress, jaundice	■ Follow CBC and Hct and reticulocyte counts of those at risk ■ Transfuse with PRBCs if symptomatic (oxygen/respiratory support)
Polycythemia	■ Venous hematocrit ■ >65% leading to hyperviscosity ■ Risk factors include IUGR, SGA, LGA, IDM, and postdates, delayed cord clamping, cord stripping, maternal–fetal transfusion, twin–twin transfusion, sepsis, dehydration	■ If capillary hematocrit >65, draw central sample ■ Infants are ruddy/plethoric Prominent vascular markings on x-ray ■ Respiratory distress, heart murmur, jaundice, hypoglycemia, hypocalcemia, thrombosis, lethargy, poor feeding, apnea, seizures	■ Exclude other causes of symptoms ■ Partial exchange transfusion ■ If asymptomatic, increase fluid intake and follow hematocrit

(continued)

Table 20.6 Summary of Other Disorders That Contribute to Respiratory Distress in the Neonate (*continued*)

Disorder	Etiology	Diagnosis	Management
Cystic hygroma	■ Most commonly seen neck mass due to development of cyst secondary to sequestrated lymph channels	■ Supraclavicular mass of varying size that transilluminates ■ Diagnosis confirmed by US, MRI/CT	■ Respiratory support as required ■ Needle aspiration for rapid decompression ■ Surgical excision is treatment of choice

CBC, complete blood count; CHD, congenital heart disease; CHF, congestive heart failure; Hct, hematocrit; IDM, infant of diabetic mother; IUGR, intrauterine growth restriction; LGA, large for gestational age; PRBC, packed red blood cell; RBC, red blood cell; SGA, small for gestational age; US, ultrasound.
Sources: Data from Bennett, M., & Meier, S. R. (2019). Assessment of the dysmorphic infant. In E. P. Tappero & M. Honeyfield (Eds.), *Physical assessment of the newborn* (6th ed., pp. 219–237). Springer Publishing Company; Breinholt, J. P. G. (2017). Cardiac disorders. In E. C. Eichenwald, A. R. Hansen, C. R. Martin, & A. R. Stark (Eds.), *Cloherty and Stark's manual of neonatal care* (8th ed., pp. 510–575). Wolters Kluwer; Letterio, J., Poteva, I., Petrosiute, A., & Ahuja, S. (2020). Hematologic and oncologic problems in the fetus and neonate. In R. J. Martin, A. A. Fanaroff, & M. C. Walsh (Eds.), *Fanaroff & Martin's neonatal-perinatal medicine: Diseases of the fetus and infant* (11th ed., pp. 1416–1475). Elsevier; Lissauer, T., & Hansen, A. (2020). Physical examination of the newborn. In R. J. Martin, A. A. Fanaroff, & M. C. Walsh (Eds.), *Fanaroff & Martin's neonatal-perinatal medicine: Diseases of the fetus and infant* (11th ed., pp. 440–457). Elsevier; Madenci, A. L., Rice-Townsend, S. E., & Weldon, C. B. (2019). Surgical disorders in childhood that affect respiratory care. In B. K. Walsh (Ed.), *Neonatal and pediatric respiratory care* (5th ed., pp. 453–468). Elsevier; O'Reilly, D. (2017). Polycythemia. In E. C. Eichenwald, A. R. Hansen, C. R. Martin, & A. R. Stark (Eds.), *Cloherty and Stark's manual of neonatal care* (8th ed., pp. 624–629). Wolters Kluwer; Otteson, T. D., & Wang, T. (2020). Upper airway lesions in the neonate. In R. J. Martin, A. A. Fanaroff, & M. C. Walsh (Eds.), *Fanaroff & Martin's neonatal-perinatal medicine: Diseases of the fetus and infant* (11th ed., pp. 1244–1153). Elsevier; Mitchell, A. L. (2020). Congenital anomalies. In R. J. Martin, A. A. Fanaroff, & M. C. Walsh (Eds.), *Fanaroff & Martin's neonatal-perinatal medicine: Diseases of the fetus and infant* (11th ed., pp. 489–513). Elsevier; Patrinos, M. E. (2020). Neonatal apnea and the foundation of respiratory control. In R. J. Martin, A. A. Fanaroff, & M. C. Walsh (Eds.), *Fanaroff & Martin's neonatal-perinatal medicine: Diseases of the fetus and infant* (11th ed., pp. 1231–1243). Elsevier.

- The oxyhemoglobin dissociation curve demonstrates SO_2 and PaO_2. Never static, the curve shifts to the left with well-saturated hemoglobin or to the right with less saturated hemoglobin.
- The Bohr effect describes the changes in oxygenation and blood pH depending on the acidity, shifting the curve to the right with lower pH and/or hypercarbia (Greenberg et al., 2019; Meschia, 2019; Travers & Ambalavanan, 2022).

Oxygen Toxicity

■ Oxygen is probably the most widely used drug in neonatology. Oxidative processes provide most of the ATP needed by the body, especially for aerobic-dependent tissues known as *oxyregulators*, such as the brain, which cannot adapt to the absence of oxygen.

■ Reactive oxygen species (ROS) are a series of molecules derived from incomplete reduction of molecular oxygen. A small percentage of electrons "leak," leaving the oxygen molecule only partly reduced. ROS can be extremely aggressive free radicals and can cause direct structural and/or functional damage to the body.

- The term *free radical* refers to the molecule that has escaped from the partial reduction of oxygen. Free radicals easily decompose and lead to the formation of toxic products. These products may cause damage to DNA, proteins, and lipids. Under very stressful conditions (ischemia–reperfusion, inflammation, or hyperoxia), damage caused by free radicals can lead to marked cellular dysfunction and/or cell death by necrosis or apoptosis.

■ Several examples of oxygen overuse are present in the history neonatology.

- *ROP:* In early neonatology, oxygen was used liberally in the treatment of preterm infants with respiratory distress. This unrestricted use of oxygen resulted in a devastating eye disease, retrolental fibroplasia (RLF) or ROP. ROP occurs when the eye vessels thicken and become tortuous to the point the retina detaches with a corresponding loss of sight. Based on this discovery, oxygen use was then curtailed; however, subsequent restriction of oxygen use resulted in hypoxic states and increased respiratory failure.

- *CLD:* High oxygen levels result in the formation of ROS and free radicals, which in turn causes tissue injury and changes in lung function and distribution of gas. These changes are a primary contributor to the development of CLD (Vento, 2022; Walsh & Chatburn, 2019).

Algorithms for Oxygen Use

■ Oxygen (O_2) binds reversibly to up to four molecules of oxygen. The hemoglobin-bound portion of the O_2 content is nonlinear with respect to PaO_2. This relationship is illustrated by the oxyhemoglobin dissociation curve, which is sigmoid in shape (Figure 20.1). Conditions which increase the O_2 affinity of hemoglobin will shift the oxyhemoglobin dissociation curve to the left. This means that the same level of hemoglobin saturation can be achieved at lower PaO_2 values. Conditions which reduce O_2 affinity shift the oxyhemoglobin dissociation curve to the right. These shifts in the oxyhemoglobin dissociation curve promote O_2 uptake in the lungs, O_2 release at the tissue level, or both (Keszler & Abubakar, 2022a).

■ Judicious oxygen delivery maximizes the benefits of oxygen while minimizing potential morbidities. Evidence-based oxygen uses algorithms to help minimize the toxic effects of oxygen administration,

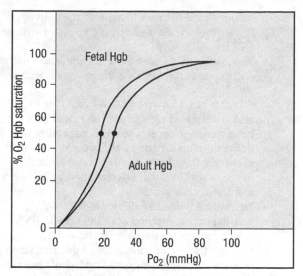

Figure 20.1 Oxygen dissociation curve.

Hgb, hemoglobin; PaO₂, partial pressure of oxygen in arterial blood.
Source: Reproduced with permission from Bradshaw, W., & Tanaka, D. T. (2016). Physiologic monitoring. In S. Gardner, B. Carter, M. Hines, & J. Hernandez (Eds.), *Merenstein & Gardner's handbook of neonatal intensive care* (8th ed., pp. 126–144.e1). Elsevier.

particularly in the very low birth weight group of infants or infants <1,500 g (Walsh, 2019).

FETAL AND NEONATAL PULMONARY MECHANICS

- Cord clamping initiates air breathing and lung filling for the establishment of FRC. In the newborn, the FRC is only slightly above closing volume.
- With lung expansion, surfactant is released, which helps maintain FRC by homogeneously decreasing surface tension and creating a pressure gradient for lung fluid removal through the alveoli.
- In premature infants, lack of surfactant results in alveolar collapse and atelectasis, causing a diminished FRC. The FRC can also be affected by disease states such as MAS, which plugs the airways, resulting in air trapping and a high FRC.
- Diaphragmatic activity controls breathing, while accessory muscles stabilize the chest wall. A premature infant has a more compliant chest wall and decreased intercostal muscle tone, and is therefore more prone to a concave rib cage during breathing.
  - Exhaustion of these muscles can lead to respiratory failure in a compromised infant.
- The neonatal chest is more cylindrical compared with the elliptical shape in the adult. Neonatal ribs have a more horizontal orientation, resulting in a relative shortening of the intercostal muscles. The compliant neonatal chest wall, in combination with noncompliant lungs, fewer interalveolar communications, less alveoli, and minimal surfactant production, can lead to chest wall collapse on expiration and atelectasis. This results

in an increase in WOB (intercostal/subcostal retractions) and exaggerated abdominal breathing (Keszler 2022; Keszler & Abubakar, 2022a).

RESPIRATORY SUPPORT IN THE NEONATE

Definitions

- *Oxygenation:* The PaO₂ within the arterial blood reflects the exchange of oxygen. Factors that impact oxygenation include percentage of oxygen delivered and mechanical mean airway pressure.
- *Ventilation: Ventilation* refers to the removal of CO₂. Infant-generated breaths contribute to CO₂ removal. Pulmonary blood flow can also impact CO₂ removal.
  - In conventional ventilation strategies, CO₂ removal is most affected by tidal volume (amplitude of the breath defined by PIP minus PEEP) and frequency.
  - In HFV strategies, CO₂ removal is a product of the frequency and the square of the tidal volume (amplitude).
- *PIP:* This refers to the peak pressure at which each breath is delivered and is measured in cm H₂O.
- *PEEP:* This is the amount of airway pressure in the lung at the end of expiration and is measured in cm H₂O. It promotes and improves FRC. Lack of PEEP results in alveolar collapse, and high PEEP can result in barotrauma.
- Mean airway pressure (P$_{aw}$) is the average pressure applied to the lungs during the respiratory cycle. P$_{aw}$ is affected by PEEP, PIP, inspiratory time, frequency, and gas flow. Excessive P$_{aw}$ can contribute to barotrauma and lung damage.
- The rate or frequency of the ventilator, in combination with tidal volume, influences the exchange of CO₂ during ventilation. Tidal volume has a higher impact on minute ventilation than the rate delivered.
- *Inspiratory time* (T$_i$) refers to the length of time of the inspiratory phase of the breath. As inspiratory time increases, mean airway pressure also increases.
- *Expiratory time* (T$_e$) is the length of time of the expiratory phase of the breath. If expiratory time is shortened, it can also contribute to an increase in mean airway pressure. Increases in expiratory time may facilitate CO₂ removal. Very prolonged expiratory times can result in gas/air trapping.
- *Tidal volume* (TV or V$_T$) is the amplitude of a mechanical breath and is determined by the difference between the PIP and the PEEP. Normal neonatal tidal volumes vary, but the normal can be considered to be between 4 and 6 mL/kg (Donn & Attar, 2020; Eyal, 2020b).

Assisted Ventilation

- An infant's gestational age, overall history, and clinical condition dictate the mode of ventilation to be used. There are many types of ventilators and respiratory support devices available. Selection of the device will be practitioner- and institution-dependent (Bancalari et al., 2018).

NONINVASIVE RESPIRATORY SUPPORT: PURPOSE

■ Noninvasive respiratory support provides continuous distending pressure and causes less injury to the lungs than mechanical ventilation. It is the preferred mode of ventilation for patients with a sustainable respiratory drive and is considered an appropriate therapy in preterm infants <29 weeks' gestation. Indications for initiation of noninvasive respiratory support include postdelivery respiratory support, management of infants with disorders of impaired gas exchange, postextubation management of airway obstruction secondary to airway collapse, and management of AOP.

■ Noninvasive ventilation modes increase or maintain FRC and stabilize the chest wall, supporting better lung inflation, improving compliance, decreasing WOB, and promoting improved oxygenation. Close monitoring is necessary as it can cause abdominal distention and would be contraindicated in patients with acute abdominal disease processes (Donn & Attar, 2020; Manley et al., 2022; Walsh, 2019c).

Noninvasive Respiratory Support: Devices

■ Nasal continuous positive airway pressure (NCPAP):
  ● Heated humidified gas is delivered as either continuous or variable flow via nasal prongs or nasal masks to the infant's airway at varying pressures measured in cm H_2O pressure.
  ● It can be delivered through a ventilator (continuous flow), a stand-alone NCPAP device (variable flow), or a "bubble" CPAP system (continuous flow).
■ HFNC:
  ● HFNC is a variable flow system which delivers blended, heated, and humidified oxygen generally at flows >1 L/min.
  ● There is a general lack of control over the pressure generated by HFNC, leading to variability in the pressure experienced by the infant. The distending pressure is dependent on cannula size, gas flow rates, and air entrainment secondary to the leak around the cannula, resulting in both low and high distending pressures.
  ● It may be delivered by standardized nasal cannulae. Commercial devices are also available (Bancalari et al., 2018; Donn & Attar, 2020; Eyal, 2020b; Manley et al., 2022; Walsh, 2019c).
■ Noninvasive nasal ventilation:
  ● Modes of noninvasive nasal ventilation include nasal intermittent positive pressure ventilation (NIPPV), synchronized bilevel CPAP (SiPAP), and synchronized NIPPV (SNIPPV).
    ❏ In all three modes, ventilator "breaths" augment CPAP, while PEEP, PIP, set respiratory rate, and inspiratory time can all be manipulated in order to achieve the delivery of higher mean pressures when compared with CPAP.
    ❏ The goal is to improve lung volume and FRC, at end expiration, with a visible improvement in WOB.
    ❏ SiPAP is also known as bilevel CPAP or BiPAP and is delivered by a flow driver device. A baseline CPAP level is set with the ability to deliver mandatory or "sigh" breaths set slightly above the baseline pressure level. The frequency of the "sigh" breaths is determined by setting a respiratory rate.
    ❏ Neurally adjusted ventilator assist (NAVA) ventilation is a method of delivering SNIPPV which recognizes diaphragmatic activity through the use of a naso- (oro-) gastric catheter. Inflation is patient-triggered by signals from the diaphragm (Bancalari et al., 2018; Donn & Attar, 2020; Manley et al., 2022; Walsh, 2019c).

INVASIVE MECHANICAL VENTILATION

■ Indications for use of invasive respiratory support include apnea, increased WOB (retractions, nasal flaring, tachypnea, and grunting), hypercapnia, hypoxia, inadequate respiratory effort, unresponsiveness to noninvasive interventions, and overall worsening of clinical condition (falling blood pressure, respiratory failure, and bradycardia). Efforts should be done to provide ventilation with minimal adverse effects while striving to extubate at the earliest opportunity (Kezler, 2022; Walsh & Chatburn, 2019).

Conventional Methods of Ventilation

■ *Intermittent mandatory ventilation (IMV):* Scheduled ventilator breaths are not influenced by the patient's intrinsic breathing rate. Scheduled breaths may interfere with an infant's own spontaneous breathing, which can be detrimental to the infant.
■ *Synchronized intermittent mandatory ventilation (SIMV):* Ventilator breaths are scheduled and are triggered by the infant's respiratory efforts. Ventilator breaths are triggered in the presence of apnea, and breaths beyond the preset number of scheduled breaths are only supported by PEEP.
■ *Assist control (AC):* Every breath that the infant initiates triggers a ventilator breath (pressure- or volume-assisted), with a preset number of assisted breaths.
■ *PS ventilation:* Spontaneous breaths above the set rate are controlled by a preset peak pressure, although lower than the set ventilator-delivered breaths. Inflation time, with a variable V_T, is dependent on lung compliance and resistance.
■ *Volume-controlled (VC) ventilation:* Preset V_T is delivered with each breath. To reach the set V_T requires ventilator adjustments to the inspiratory pressure depending on lung compliance and resistance.

- *Volume guarantee (VG):* A preset V_T is determined for each breath. The acceptable peak pressure limit is predetermined and automatically adjusted according to lung compliance as measured by the exhaled tidal volume.
- *NAVA ventilation:* This is a newer modality (and can be used invasively) that recognizes diaphragmatic activity through the use of a nasogastric catheter containing electrodes. Ventilator pressure changes in response to the activity of the diaphragm, which may improve tidal volume with less respiratory effort. While useful as a method of delivering noninvasive support as with SNIPPV, NAVA is not recommended for routine use as an invasive mode of ventilation since research has demonstrated inconsistent outcomes across preterm populations (Claure & Bancalari, 2022; Donn & Attar, 2020; Eyal, 2020b; Keszler & Abubakar, 2022b; Keszler & Mammel, 2022; Manley et al., 2022).

High-Frequency Ventilation

- There are three main types of HFV: high-frequency oscillator ventilation, HFJV, and high-frequency flow interruption (HFFI). All use very high breathing rates and small tidal volumes (less than or equal to the anatomic dead space volume) to enhance gas exchange. HFV, of all types, employs multiple mechanisms of gas delivery to the alveoli, enabling small changes in V_T to have a larger impact on CO_2 removal. HFV enables near-independent management strategies for CO_2 removal and oxygenation challenges.
  - *HFOV:* A defining difference of HFOV from other methods of HFV is the mechanism of action during inspiration and expiration. Inspiration and expiration occur as an active process through the actions of an electromagnetically operated piston which generates the oscillations. The amplitude of the oscillations within the airway determines the V_T delivered to the lungs (ventilation) around a constant mean airway pressure (oxygenation). It is often used when conventional modes of ventilation fail or for use with specific diseases, such as MAS or PPHN.
  - *HFJV:* The mechanism of action for exhalation during HFJV occurs as a result of passive lung recoil. Gas delivery is a result of direct pulses of pressurized gas into the endotracheal tube and the upper airway through a narrow-bore cannula or jet injector. It requires concurrent use of a conventional ventilator for the provision of PEEP and "sigh" breaths to facilitate improved aeration. It is most commonly used for air leak and air trapping disorders, although it is gaining more widespread use for RDS depending on user experience. With HFJV, CO_2 removal can be achieved at lower peak and mean airway pressures than with either HFV or HFOV.
  - *HFFI:* This form of HFV does not fit the definition criteria of an oscillator or jet ventilator and has had limited use until the release of the Bronchotron, a popular transport ventilator. High-frequency pressurized gas pulses enter a piston mechanism and create pulses of gas flow by the rapid movement of a spring mechanism that balances inspiratory and expiratory pressures (Donn & Attar, 2020; Keszler et al., 2022).

Inhaled Nitric Oxide

- iNO is a potent vasodilator derived from the amino acid L-arginine and works selectively on the pulmonary vasculature adjacent to an inflated, operating alveolus. Once absorbed by the pulmonary vasculature, iNO binds to hemoglobin, leading to smooth muscle relaxation and increased pulmonary blood flow. The result is increased oxygenation, improved pulmonary perfusion, and reduced lung inflammation.
- It is used in the treatment of HRF and pulmonary hypertension and may reduce the need for ECMO (Bohannon et al., 2020b; Eyal, 2020b; Parad & Banjamin, 2017; Plosa, 2017a; Walsh, 2019a).

Extracorporeal Membrane Oxygenation

- ECMO is the use of a modified cardiopulmonary bypass facilitating oxygenation and CO_2 elimination for infants in respiratory or cardiac failure that have not responded to conventional management strategies.
- Respiratory indications for use of ECMO include respiratory failure deemed to be reversible, such as in MAS, PPHN, CDH, sepsis, pneumonia, and RDS or severe air leak syndromes.
  - Venoarterial (VA) ECMO is indicated in instances of primary cardiac failure or respiratory collapse, combined with secondary cardiac dysfunction. Blood is drained from a vein, most often the internal jugular vein, and returned to the arterial system usually via the right common carotid artery.
  - Venovenous (VV) ECMO is indicated in instances of severe respiratory failure with sufficient cardiovascular function. Deoxygenated blood is drained, and oxygenated blood is returned to the patient through a catheter within a single vein, but does not provide the same amount of oxygenation as VA ECMO (Arensman et al., 2022; Wheeler, & Le, 2019; Wolf & Arnold, 2017).

RESPIRATORY SUPPORT MONITORING

- Refer to Chapter 7 for discussion on the techniques and equipment for cardiorespiratory monitoring in the NICU.

RESPIRATORY SUPPORT AT DISCHARGE

- Infants may meet the basic criteria for discharge home (adequate weight gain, competent caretakers, appropriate outpatient follow-up, free of apneic and bradycardic events, and overall stable condition) but still require some form of respiratory support.

- Oxygen support:
  - It is not uncommon for infants delivered at less than or equal to 28 weeks' gestation to require oxygen therapy at the time of discharge. The most frequent indicator of home oxygen use is CLD and/or hypoxia.
  - Other risk factors related to the need for home oxygen therapy include small-for-gestational age infants, congenital anomalies requiring ventilatory support in the first 72 hours of birth, and PDA.
  - The goal of home oxygen therapy is to minimize the effects of chronic hypoxemia, which include pulmonary vasoconstriction and pulmonary vascular remodeling, which both can lead to pulmonary hypertension, bronchial constriction, and airway obstruction.
- Ventilatory support:
  - Infants requiring long-term ventilatory support can be discharged home on mechanical ventilation.
  - Airway stabilization is critical to patient safety when mechanical ventilation is provided in the home setting. Tracheostomy may assist in consistent and stable airway management in these infants.
- Patient care management at discharge must be a well-coordinated effort involving primary care

providers, pulmonology specialists (as well as other specialists as required), discharge coordinators, home care staff, family caregivers, and medical equipment suppliers. Plans of care need to be clearly delineated for all providers.

- Both family and professional caretakers must be sufficiently educated and able to safely care for the infant. Emergency planning must be clearly mapped out and should include common scenarios that require urgent intervention, notification of community rescue and ambulance services for emergency treatment or transport might be required, and notification of local utilities that interruption of power will impact ventilator function (Rhein, 2022; Vento, 2022)

▶ CONCLUSION

Many of the pathology and management challenges faced by neonatal providers are directly related to the respiratory system and the sequelae of respiratory dysfunction. A thorough understanding of fetal and neonatal lung development as well as an understanding of basic respiratory physiology and respiratory pathology are crucial to their ability to implement successful evidence-based management strategies while caring for this very vulnerable population.

1. A full-term infant delivered by repeat Cesarean section is now 2 hours of age and is demonstrating mild nasal flaring, intermittent retractions, and episodes of coughing with cyanosis during breastfeeding. The bedside nurse reports an inability to pass an orogastric (OG) tube. What is the most likely diagnosis?

   A. Choanal atresia (CA)

   B. Esophageal atresia (EA)/tracheoesophageal fistula (TEF)

   C. Transient tachypnea of the newborn (TTN)

2. What stage of lung development can be expected in a 42-week postmenstrual age infant with moderate bronchopulmonary dysplasia?

   A. Alveolar

   B. Pseudoglandular

   C. Saccular

3. Initial management of an infant with severe respiratory distress secondary to meconium aspiration syndrome (MAS) includes:

   A. Intubation and antibiotic administration

   B. Intubation and direct suctioning at delivery

   C. Intubation and surfactant administration

4. Neonatal transition from fetal hemoglobin (HgF) to the production of adult hemoglobin (HgA) is associated with:

   A. Increased 2,3-disphophoglycerate (DPG) production and increased oxygen affinity

   B. Increased DPG production and reduced oxygen affinity

   C. Unchanged DPG production and reduced oxygen affinity

5. A common finding that can be seen in infants with congenital diaphragmatic hernia (CDH) and congenital pulmonary adenomatoid malformations (CPAM) is:

   A. Congenital pneumonia

   B. Pulmonary hypoplasia

   C. Renal agenesis

6. The neonatal nurse practitioner (NNP) is caring for a 2-day-old, 28-week gestation female infant who was extubated to nasal continuous positive airway pressure (NCPAP) +6 at 24 hours of age. In the past 12 hours, the infant has had seven apnea and bradycardia events and an increasing oxygen requirement from 21% to 55% oxygen. The following blood gas was obtained: pH 7.24, partial pressure of carbon dioxide in arterial blood ($PaCO_2$) of 69, partial pressure of oxygen in arterial blood (PaO_2) of 65 mmHg, concentrated bicarbonate level in arterial blood (HCO_3) of 19 meq/L, and base deficit (BD) of −8. On what mode of ventilation would the NNP place this infant?

   A. Nasal intermittent positive pressure ventilation (NIPPV)

   B. Pressure control (PC)/volume guarantee (VG) ventilation

   C. Synchronized intermittent mandatory ventilation (SIMV)

7. The neonatal nurse practitioner (NNP) is caring for an intubated full-term neonate with pulmonary hypertension and hypoxemia who is on high-frequency oscillatory ventilation (HFOV). The chest x-ray demonstrates inflation to 9.5 ribs with an endotracheal tube (ETT) at the level of T2. What management strategy should the NNP employ to improve oxygenation?

   A. Increase the mean airway pressure

   B. Initiate inhaled nitric oxide (iNO)

   C. Initiate referral for extracorporeal membrane oxygenation (ECMO)

1. B) Esophageal atresia (EA)/tracheoesophageal fistula (TEF)

EA is an anatomic interruption of the esophagus. The inability to successfully pass an OG tube is a common symptom. Chest x-rays of infants with this type are consistent with an OG/nasogastric tube visibly coiled in a blind pouch (Bradshaw, 2021; Madenci et al., 2019; Ringer & Hansen, 2017). TEF is a subset of combined anomalies of the esophagus and trachea, while TTN describes pulmonary fluid accumulation and is not related to esophageal patency.

2. A) Alveolar

The alveolar phase of lung development occurs between 36 weeks and up to 3 years of age and may continue to develop into adulthood. Continued alveolarization past the newborn period may assist in the normalization of lung function of infants born prematurely. The pseudoglandular phase occurs between weeks 6 and 16. The saccular phase can be seen between weeks 26 and 36. Infants born in this stage develop respiratory distress secondary to surfactant deficiency/insufficiency and pulmonary insufficiency, and commonly develop chronic lung disease (CLD) or bronchopulmonary dysplasia (Joyner, 2019; Kallapur & Jobe, 2020; Keszler & Abubakar, 2022a).

3. A) Intubation and antibiotic administration

Respiratory failure requiring intubation and ventilatory support is common in infants with severe MAS. High-frequency ventilation may be required. Antibiotic administration is required to treat pneumonia/sepsis. Surfactant is not an initial management strategy; however, surfactant therapy may improve lung compliance and oxygenation. Surfactant administration is thought to reduce the severity of respiratory distress and may reduce disease progression and the need for extracorporeal membrane oxygenation (ECMO), a last resort therapy. In initial delivery room management, routine suctioning at delivery of vigorous or depressed infants born through meconium-stained amniotic fluid (MSAF) is not beneficial and is no longer recommended (Blackburn, 2018; Crowley, 2020; Fraser, 2021; Gautham & Soll, 2022; Hansen & Levin, 2019; Plosa, 2017a; Yoder & Grubb, 2022).

4. B) Increased DPG production and reduced oxygen affinity

The neonate transitions over the first 3 to 6 months of life to the production of HgA with increased DPG production. The transition from HgF to HgA is associated with reduced oxygen affinity and rightward shift of the oxyhemoglobin dissociation curve (Travers & Ambalavanan, 2022)

5. B) Pulmonary hypoplasia

Secondary (as opposed to primary) hypoplasia can occur as a result of processes that interfere with lung development. Space-occupying lesions, like CDH and CPAM, compress the lungs, which inhibits normal lung growth. Congenital pneumonia can be acquired in utero, from exposure/aspiration of infected amniotic fluid, from ascending infections from the birth canal, and transplacentally. Pneumonia is not commonly associated with pulmonary hypoplasia (Blackburn, 2018; Crowley, 2020; Fraser, 2021; Hansen & Levin, 2019; Jensen et al., 2022; Pappas & Robey, 2021; Rudd, 2021; Van Marter & McPherson, 2017).

6. A) Nasal intermittent positive pressure ventilation (NIPPV)

The NNP should choose the level of respiratory support that provides continuous distending pressure while causing the least amount of injury to the lungs. NIPPV is a form of noninvasive respiratory support that is indicated for infants who have impaired gas exchange and apnea of prematurity, as is demonstrated in this example. The ventilator "breaths" provided through NIPPV allow for achievement of a higher mean airway pressure, when compared with continuous positive airway pressure (CPAP), as the positive end-expiratory pressure (PEEP), peak inspiratory pressure (PIP), and inspiratory time can all be manipulated. This would lead to improved lung function, functional residual capacity (FRC), and a decrease in the work of breathing. Both PC/VG and SIMV modes are invasive methods of ventilation. The NNP should consider invasive modes only when the patient is unresponsive to noninvasive interventions (Bancalari et al., 2018; Donn & Attar, 2020; Kezler, 2022; Manley et al., 2022; Walsh, 2019; Walsh et al., 2019).

7. B) Initiate inhaled nitric oxide (iNO)

iNO works selectively on the pulmonary vasculature to facilitate smooth muscle relaxation and pulmonary vasodilation through delivery of the gas to adjacent, inflated, and operating alveoli. This neonate demonstrates adequate inflation as noted on chest x-ray; therefore, initiation of iNO would be warranted. Although mean airway pressure changes would be necessary if poor lung inflation or atelectasis was noted, increases in the mean airway pressure (Paw) may cause overdistension of the lungs, impairing venous return and cardiac output. An ECMO referral would be warranted in the case of pulmonary hypertension that is refractory to conventional management strategies such as initiation of iNO (Walsh, 2019; Wolf & Arnold, 2017).

The Gastrointestinal System

Jacqueline M. Hoffman and Karen Wright

▶ INTRODUCTION

This chapter highlights gastrointestinal (GI) disorders in the neonate and is to be used in conjunction with all recommended resources from the National Certification Corporation for a more in-depth review. Disruption of normal developmental processes can result in an array of congenital GI disorders located anywhere from the esophagus to the anus, such as atresia/stenosis, abdominal wall defects, nonfixation of the intestines, and anorectal malformations. Functional obstruction may also occur due to abnormal intestinal mucous gland production or lack of neuronal migration of ganglion cells. It is crucial for the neonatal nurse practitioner (NNP) to be aware of the timing of clinical presentation and the physical examination findings to determine the best diagnostic workup, which may end up being therapeutic, as well as to assist in determining the final diagnosis.

▶ GASTROINTESTINAL SYSTEM DEVELOPMENT

■ The GI tract extends from the oral cavity to the anus and includes all the associated organs and glands that secrete hormones necessary for function. The fetus is dependent on placental transfer of maternal nutrients for normal fetal growth and development. Disorders of maternal nutrition result in abnormal fetal "programming" of tissues and may result in long-term neurobehavioral consequences, as well as later health concerns such as hypertension, cardiovascular disease, and obesity.

■ During the embryonic stage, from the third through the eighth week of gestation, anatomic development is prevalent.
  ● The primordial gut forms by the fourth week and can be divided into three parts: foregut (some resources separate this into pharyngeal and foregut), midgut, and hindgut (Table 21.1).
  ● Failure of the tracheobronchial diverticulum to divide into the ventral respiratory primordium and the dorsal esophagus at 4 to 5 weeks results in tracheoesophageal fistula (TEF).
  ● The lumen of many of the GI structures becomes temporarily obliterated due to rapidly growing epithelium. Recanalization of these structures must occur; otherwise, stenosis or atresia occurs.
    ❑ Failure of the duodenum to recanalize during the sixth to seventh week results in duodenal atresia; partial recanalization results in duodenal stenosis.

Table 21.1 The Primordial Gut

Primitive Component	Neonatal Structure	Blood Supply	Defects That May Occur
Foregut	Primordial pharynx and its derivatives, lower respiratory tract, esophagus, stomach, liver, upper portion of the duodenum distal to the entry of the bile duct, liver, biliary tree, and pancreas	Celiac artery	TEF with or without EA, isolated EA, esophageal stenosis, pyloric stenosis, duodenal atresia/stenosis, biliary atresia, and annular pancreas
Midgut	Small intestine (except for the upper duodenum), cecum, appendix, ascending colon, and proximal portion (one-half to two-thirds) of the transverse colon	Superior mesenteric artery	Abdominal wall defects, intestinal stenosis/atresia, and malrotation
Hindgut	Distal (one-third to one-half) transverse colon, descending and sigmoid colons, rectum, superior part of (upper) anal canal, epithelium of the bladder, and urethra	Inferior mesenteric artery	Hirschsprung disease, anorectal malformations such as persistent cloaca, imperforate anus, and anal stenosis/atresia

EA, esophageal atresia; TEF, tracheoesophageal fistula.

357

❏ Failure of the esophagus to recanalize during the eighth week results in esophageal atresia (EA); partial recanalization results in esophageal stenosis.

❏ Failure of the hepatic bile ducts to recanalize results in biliary atresia.

■ Due to rapid growth and elongation of the intestinal loops and growth of the liver during the sixth week of gestation, there is not enough room in the abdomen, leading to the intestinal loops herniating into the umbilical stalk, termed *physiologic herniation*. The midgut loop rotates 90 degrees counterclockwise around the axis of the superior mesenteric artery while it is in the umbilical cord, with the caudal end being on the left and the cranial limb on the right.

■ During the fetal stage, from the ninth week to birth, development of the functional components (hormones, enzymes, reflexes) is evident (Exhibit 21.1).

■ During the 10th week of gestation, retraction occurs, with the small intestine returning to the abdominal cavity, first occupying the central region of the abdomen, followed by the large intestines which rotate an additional 180-degree counterclockwise rotation, occupying the right side of the abdomen. At this time, the duodenojejunal junction is in the left upper quadrant of the abdomen, with fixation in the location of the ligament of Treitz (this becomes important to note when evaluating for malrotation/ volvulus).

■ By the end of the 11th week of gestation, rotation of the midgut is complete, with the cecum fixed in the right lower quadrant and the hindgut (splenic flexure of the colon to the rectum) fixed in the left hemiabdomen.

● The hindgut ends at the cloacal membrane. Development of the hindgut and the urogenital system is interrelated.

■ The intestinal length increases 100-fold during gestation, with a doubling in length during the last trimester.

■ Many of the GI disorders result from abnormalities during embryogenesis and can be associated with other conditions or anomalies related to systems/organs that are also developing at the same time (Table 21.2).

■ After birth, there is coordinated function of the hormone and enzymes needed for digestion, in addition to maturation of the suck–swallow mechanism (Bradshaw, 2021; Dingeldein, 2020a; Ditzenberger, 2018; Gallagher et al., 2021).

▶ GENERALIZATION ABOUT GASTROINTESTINAL TRACT DISORDERS

DEFINITIONS AND PATHOPHYSIOLOGY

■ A *mechanical obstruction* refers to a specific point of obstruction either by abnormal tissue growth or malpositioning of the organs.

■ A *functional obstruction* is not associated with an anatomic malformation; it is most commonly related to a problem with bowel motility.

■ An *atresia* occurs when there is complete congenital defect obstructing the intestinal lumen, ranging from a short web segment to complete loss of a segment of the intestine and the mesentery, or to multiple areas of discontinuity resulting in multiple atresias.

■ A *stenosis* occurs when there is a narrowing of the intestinal lumen; it remains continuous and ranges from involving a partial web to involving the entire thickness of the intestinal lumen (Dingeldein, 2020b; Flynn-O'Brien et al., 2018).

DIAGNOSIS

■ Polyhydramnios and large gastric aspirates at birth suggest a more proximal obstruction.

■ Of term infants, 95% pass meconium by 24 hours; almost 100% will pass meconium by 48 hours unless there is a mechanical or functional obstruction. Meconium passage is delayed in preterm infants. Passage of meconium does not exclude an obstruction as it may initially be passed from the bowel distal to the site of obstruction.

■ There is a direct relationship between the amount of abdominal distention and the level of the obstruction; the more distal the obstruction, the greater the amount of distention.

■ When the obstruction is distal to the ampulla of Vater, bilious emesis will be present. Bilious emesis in an otherwise healthy neonate is considered a midgut volvulus until proven otherwise and is therefore a medical emergency as prompt diagnosis is necessary to minimize the amount of necrotic bowel.

■ Abdominal x-ray is the initial study to evaluate an infant with a concern for obstruction; it is possible to miss an obstruction if x-ray is obtained too early as enough gaseous distention may not be present. The "thumb sign" refers to the dilated diameter of the bowel loop as large as the surgeon's thumb. The Neuhauser sign describes the mixture of air with meconium (Bradshaw, 2021; Dingeldein, 2020b; Gallagher et al., 2021; Gomella, 2020b; Odackal & Swanson, 2020; Ringer & Hansen, 2017).

MANAGEMENT

■ Generalized preoperative management includes nothing by mouth (NPO), gastric decompression such as Replogle to suction (decreases the risk of emesis and aspiration, improves bowel wall perfusion), parenteral fluid support, correction of electrolytes if emesis has been ongoing, surgical consult, and antibiotic therapy to provide coverage for enteric organisms.

■ Pain management of bowel obstruction and any surgical intervention are vital parts of neonatal management and should be attended to through best evidence and interdisciplinary collaboration (Bradshaw, 2021; Gallagher et al., 2021).

Exhibit 21.1 Highlights of Anatomic and Hormone Development

Week 3	Week 4	Week 5	Week 6	Week 7	Week 8	Weeks 9–10	Week 12	Second Trimester	Third Trimester
■ Tubular intestine, yolk sac, and mesentery form.	■ Primordial gut forms. Primordium of the stomach is evident. Esophagus and trachea separate. ■ TEF, EA (4–5 wk)	■ Intestine elongates into a loop and rotation begins. Pancreas is present. Cloaca is divided into two parts by the urorectal septum. ■ Anorectal malformation (5–8 wk)	■ Midgut herniates into the umbilical cord; 90-degree counterclockwise rotation. Temporary duodenal occlusion occurs. ■ Stomach dilates, enlarges, and rotates 90 degrees around an anteroposterior axis.	■ Esophagus reaches final length. There is lengthening and 90-degree counterclockwise rotation of intestinal loops in the umbilical cord. ■ Urorectal septum fuses with the cloacal membrane. Perineum is formed when urorectal and cloacal membranes fuse.	■ Esophagus, duodenum, and small intestine recanalize. Intestinal villi develop. Diaphragm is complete. ■ Duodenal atresia (8–10 wk), jejunoileal atresia, primary defect (8–10 wk), omphalocele (8–11 wk)	■ Rupture of pit in anal membrane; there is now open communication between the rectum and the exterior body. Intestines reenter the abdominal cavity with 180-degree counterclockwise rotation around the superior mesenteric artery. ■ Gastroschisis (9–11 wk)	■ Intestinal muscular layer is present. Ganglion cell migration is complete. Pancreatic islet cells appear. Lactase appears. ■ Hirschsprung disease	■ Meconium is present and swallowing is observed at week 16. Rectal ganglion cells are present by week 24. Jejunoileal atresia, secondary defect (after 12 weeks)	■ Coordination of sucking and swallowing occurs during weeks 34–36. ■ Maturation of GI system is complete by week 38.

EA, esophageal atresia; GI, gastrointestinal; TEF, tracheoesophageal fistula.

Table 21.2 Conditions Associated With Gastrointestinal Defects

GI Disorder	Associated Conditions
Duodenal atresia	Fetal hydantoin syndrome, trisomy 21
Esophageal atresia/tracheoesophageal fistula	Apert syndrome, CHARGE syndrome, trisomy 18, VACTERL association
Hirschsprung disease	DiGeorge syndrome, Smith–Lemli–Opitz syndrome, trisomy 21
Intestinal malrotation	Trisomy 13, trisomy 18
Imperforate anus	VACTERL association
Pyloric stenosis	Apert syndrome, trisomy 18, trisomy 21
Umbilical wall defects	Beckwith–Wiedemann syndrome (chromosome 11), fetal hydantoin syndrome (umbilical hernia), trisomy 13, trisomy 18, trisomy 21

CHARGE, Coloboma of the eye, Heart defects, Atresia of the choanae, Restriction of Growth, and Ear abnormalities; GI, gastrointestinal; VACTERL, Vertebral anomalies, Anal atresia, Cardiac defects, TracheoEsophageal fistula, Renal anomalies, and Limb abnormalities.

OUTCOMES

- Prognosis will depend on the presence of additional anomalies, amount of bowel loss (if any), and other long-term complications (Bradshaw, 2021; Gallagher et al., 2021).

▶ ABNORMALITIES IN THE DEVELOPMENT OF THE FOREGUT

ESOPHAGEAL ATRESIA/ TRACHEOESOPHAGEAL FISTULA

Definition and Pathophysiology

- The spectrum of EA/tracheoesophageal fistula (TEF) defects occurs during the fourth to seventh week of gestation when there is failure in normal development of the esophagus and/or incomplete separation of the trachea from the esophagus in the primitive foregut. This may occur due to hedgehog signaling abnormalities, other genetic alterations, or environmental insults.
- EA is an interruption in the esophagus resulting in a blind pouch. There are five variations seen in the neonate with an EA: 85% to 90% of neonates with an EA will have an associated distal TEF, 8% will only have an isolated EA, and less commonly neonates will have an EA with a proximal TEF or with a double (proximal and distal) TEF (Figure 21.1).
- TEF is an abnormal connection between the esophagus and the trachea; 5% of infants with TEF will have an isolated fistula between the esophagus and the trachea, or the "H-type" (see Figure 21.1; Bradshaw, 2021; Dingeldein, 2020b, 2020c; Gallagher et al., 2021; Ringer & Hansen, 2017).

Diagnosis

- Prenatal findings suggesting EA may include small or absent stomach on fetal ultrasound (US; especially after 14 weeks of gestation), along with polyhydramnios (related to the inability of swallowed amniotic fluid to flow through the digestive system).
- EA is postnatally diagnosed by the inability to pass a gastric tube—often coming back out of the mouth; x-ray will show the catheter coiled in the proximal esophageal pouch, typically at the second or third thoracic vertebrae, above the carina. Excessive oral secretions may also be noted. Air in the GI tract on x-ray indicates the presence of an EA with distal TEF, an EA with double TEF, or an isolated TEF. A gasless abdomen on an x-ray with a scaphoid-appearing abdomen indicates the presence of an EA with proximal TEF or an isolated EA.
- Clinical presentation depends on the type of defect and may include excessive oral secretions, drooling, coughing/choking, regurgitation of undigested formula/breast milk, and a scaphoid abdomen.
  - Respiratory distress is due to airway obstruction from excess oral secretions, from aspiration of saliva/feeds, or from reflux of gastric contents up the distal esophagus into the lungs through the abnormal connection. If an infant with a patent esophagus (i.e., a catheter can pass to the stomach), but the infant experiences coughing/choking during feedings and recurrent pneumonia—think "H-type" TEF (Bradshaw, 2021; Dingeldein, 2020b, 2020c; Draus & Ruzic, 2020b; Flynn-O'Brien et al., 2018; Gallagher et al., 2021; Ringer & Hansen, 2017; Trotter, 2021).

Management

PREOPERATIVE

- Placement of a Replogle catheter into the proximal esophageal pouch to low continuous suction will prevent aspiration of oral secretions.
- Elevation of the head will minimize aspiration of oral secretions that accumulate in the proximal esophageal pouch, as well as minimize gastric reflux through the fistula into the lungs.
- Provide comfort measures to minimize crying; crying increases air in the stomach and abdominal distention, and may be associated with increased risk of aspiration of gastric contents into the trachea. To minimize and prevent complications such as pneumonitis, consider administration of gastric reflux medications.
- Avoid continuous positive airway pressure (CPAP) or positive pressure ventilation (PPV) if possible; use low

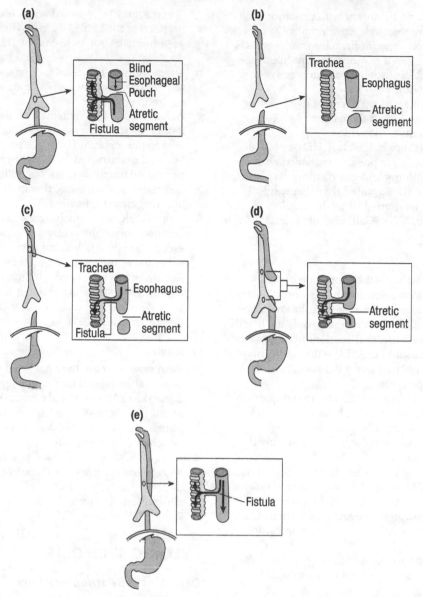

Figure 21.1 Five types of esophageal atresia/tracheoesophageal fistula: **(a)** esophageal atresia with distal tracheoesophageal fistula (85%), **(b)** isolated esophageal atresia (8%), **(c)** esophageal atresia with proximal tracheoesophageal fistula (1%), **(d)** esophageal atresia with double tracheoesophageal fistula (1%), and **(e)** isolated tracheoesophageal fistula (5%).

mean airway pressure if on conventional ventilation or use high-frequency oscillatory ventilation (HFOV) to minimize shunting of tidal volume from the trachea to the stomach. If respiratory support is required, these infants require surgery sooner for ligation of the TEF. Placement of gastrostomy is needed if there is increased abdominal distention compromising effective ventilation.

■ Evaluate for other anomalies. Operative repair is not an emergency except in the case of a preterm infant with respiratory distress syndrome (RDS) when TEF is distal and results in severe gastric distention.
  ● Echocardiogram should be done prior to surgery as presence of cardiac defect may influence the surgical approach. Abdominal US of the kidneys/

genitourinary tract and plain radiographs of the spine and limbs can be done after surgery (Bradshaw, 2021; Dingeldein, 2020b, 2020c; Gallagher et al., 2021; Flynn-O'Brien et al., 2018; Odackal & Swanson, 2020; Ringer & Hansen, 2017).

SURGICAL INTERVENTIONS

■ Surgical interventions vary depending on the defect(s) present. If possible, complete repair is preferred (division and ligation of the fistula with primary anastomosis of the esophageal segments).
■ Staged repair with early placement of a gastrostomy tube for decompression and feeding and division of fistula when the gap is too large between two esophageal segments are recommended in the very

premature infant and the infant with pneumonia or other coexisting morbidities. An alternative approach when the gap is too large for primary anastomosis is the use of high-powered magnets, the magnamosis technique, to create a sutureless anastomosis of the esophagus often within 4 to 7 days.

■ In rare cases, esophageal replacement using gastric or colon segment is done if the gap between two esophageal segments is too wide.

■ If severe congenital heart defects (CHDs) or lethal chromosomal defects are present, palliation with cervical esophagostomy and gastrostomy may be done; later it can be determined if further surgical interventions are warranted (Bradshaw, 2021; Dingeldein, 2020b, 2020c; Gallagher et al., 2021; Ringer & Hansen, 2017).

POSTOPERATIVE

■ Of primary importance is the protection of the anastomosis site to prevent suture disruption leading to anastomosis leak or a recurrent fistula. Protection is afforded particularly by suctioning only the length of the endotracheal tube; or if suctioning the posterior pharynx, a premeasured catheter is used. The infant should also be ventilated using the lowest mean airway pressure possible.

  ● Do not extubate until it is certain that respiratory status is stable with minimal risk of requiring reintubation. Only skilled personnel should attempt reintubation if the infant self-extubates or fails elective extubation.

  ● Also, the orogastric/nasogastric tube placed during surgery should not be replaced at the bedside if accidental dislodgment occurs, as doing so could inadvertently rupture the anastomosis site. Only replace with surgical and radiologic speciality involvement.

■ Monitor chest tube and gastric drainage; chest tube drainage suggests leakage from the esophageal anastomosis.

■ The head of the bed should be elevated to prevent aspiration. Consider gastric acid blockers, such as histamine antagonists or proton pump inhibitors (PPIs), to minimize reflux sequelae.

■ Brief course of systemic antibiotics is often dictated by surgeon preference.

■ Enteral nutrition is typically started after esophagram confirms the anastomosis site has healed with no leaking (usually at least 5–10 days postoperatively).

■ Pain management is indicated (Bradshaw, 2021; Gallagher et al., 2021; Flynn-O'Brien et al., 2018; Ringer & Hansen, 2017).

POSTOPERATIVE COMPLICATIONS

■ Anastomotic strictures requiring periodic esophageal dilation are the most common postoperative complication; may be exacerbated by gastroesophageal reflux (GER).

  ● GER may be lessened with elevation of the head of the bed, slow low-volume feeds, and administration of histamine (H2) antagonists or PPIs.

■ Dysmotility in the distal esophageal segment may require gastrostomy feeds to minimize vomiting and aspiration.

■ Anastomosis site problems include leak or recurrent fistula (usually as a result of a leak). Aspiration may lead to pneumonia. These site problems may be avoided or corrected by delaying feeds and providing parenteral nutrition (PN), maintaining chest tube, determining if antibiotic therapy is needed, and allowing time for healing.

■ Complications also include tracheomalacia due to compression of the posterior trachea by the proximal esophageal pouch, leading to deformation and softening of the tracheal cartilages.

■ Recurrent laryngeal nerve injury, vocal cord dysfunction, and unilateral diaphragmatic paralysis may also occur (Bradshaw, 2021; Dingeldein, 2020c; Gallagher et al., 2021).

Outcomes

■ With staged repair, the final stage of anastomosis of the proximal and distal esophagus segments is typically done at 6 to 12 months of age; until that time, the infant will require a mechanism to keep the esophageal pouch emptied (continuous suction of the proximal pouch or esophagostomy).

■ Long-term survival (22%–97%) depends on birth weight and the presence/type of comorbidities, such as prematurity with RDS, CHD, or presence of lethal chromosomal defects (Bradshaw, 2021; Dingeldein, 2020c; Gallagher et al., 2021).

PYLORIC STENOSIS

Definition and Pathophysiology

■ Pyloric stenosis is a stricture of the outlet from the stomach to the small intestine due to hypertrophy, mainly of the circular muscles of the pylorus; this results in obstruction of the passage of liquids (human milk or formula).

■ The exact etiology is unknown. There is an increased association between infants whose mothers had increased gastrin secretion during the third trimester and infants who received prostaglandin E. There have been some suggested associations in infants who receive erythromycin in the first 6 weeks of life. There is also a proposed genetic component as 10% to 20% of affected infants are born to mothers who had the same disorder and a higher rate of occurrence in monozygotic twins. It is more common in firstborn, male, full-term, and White infants.

■ It is commonly associated with trisomies 18 and 21 and Apert syndrome; otherwise, associated anomalies are uncommon (Bradshaw, 2021; Dingeldein, 2020c; Flynn-O'Brien et al., 2018).

Diagnosis

- Clinical presentation does not typically occur until after 2 to 3 weeks of life (can present as early as 1 week and as late as 5 months of age), with nonbilious emesis that over time, due to progressive gastric outlet obstruction, becomes projectile.
  - On palpation, a small, firm, mobile, oval-shaped pyloric mass, "olive," in the right upper quadrant can be felt.
- Diagnosis is by abdominal radiography showing distended stomach with little or no abdominal gas pattern below the duodenum. US confirms the diagnosis in majority of cases.
  - If diagnosis is still unclear, a contrast upper GI can be done which will show delayed or no gastric emptying, with an elongated pyloric channel referred to as a "string sign" (Bradshaw, 2021; Dingeldein, 2020c; Flynn-O'Brien et al., 2018; Ringer & Hansen, 2017; Trotter, 2021).

Management and Outcome

- Preoperative management includes gastric decompression, correcting any electrolyte or acid–base abnormalities, and fluid resuscitation as a result of persistent vomiting.
- Surgical repair is most often a pyloromyotomy, where an incision is made into the circular and longitudinal muscles of the pylorus, releasing the stricture.
- Postoperative management includes:
  - Never place or replace an orogastric or nasogastric feeding tube postoperatively as perforation of the surgical repair site may occur.
  - NPO until awake and then feedings are progressed over 24 hours. Persistent emesis in the first couple of days postoperatively may occur until normal gastric emptying times resume; this may alarm parents as the infant does not seem improved after surgery.
- Prognosis is excellent with no residual effects. Strictures are uncommon (Bradshaw, 2021; Dingeldein, 2020c; Flynn-O'Brien et al., 2018).

DUODENAL ATRESIA

Definition and Pathophysiology

- Duodenal atresia occurs when there is failure of vacuolization (during weeks 5–6 of gestation) and recanalization of the intestinal lumen (weeks 8–10 of gestation). A genetic component may also contribute to the occurrence.
  - Prenatal findings include dilated stomach and duodenum on fetal US, the classic "double bubble" echogenicity, more commonly noted in the third trimester when the duodenum becomes more dilated. There may also be polyhydramnios.

- Congenital obstruction of the duodenum is the most common portion of the bowel involved when considering the group of intestinal atresias. Partial or complete obstruction of the duodenum can be caused by extrinsic lesions, such as malrotation and annular pancreas, or by intrinsic lesions, such as duodenal stenosis or atresia.
- There are three common types (see Figure 21.2):
  - *Type 1:* membranous web, often associated with common bile duct abnormalities
  - *Type 2:* fibrous atretic cord connecting the two segments of the duodenum
  - *Type 3:* complete separation of the two atretic ends of the duodenum; may be associated with annular pancreas
- Commonly associated anomalies include trisomy 21 (up to 30%), CHDs (up to 30%), and other GI anomalies including annular pancreas, malrotation of the small intestine, small bowel atresia, and imperforate anus (Bradshaw, 2021; Dingeldein, 2020b, 2020c; Ditzenberger, 2018; Draus & Ruzic, 2020c; Flynn-O'Brien et al., 2018; Gallagher et al., 2021; Ringer & Hansen, 2017).

Diagnosis

- Clinical presentation includes bilious emesis (obstruction usually distal to the ampulla of Vater) within a few hours to 24 hours after birth (exclusively breastfed infants may not present in the first days of life), minimal abdominal distention limited to the upper abdomen, and failure to pass meconium.
  - Radiography that demonstrates the classic "double bubble" air in the stomach and upper duodenum but no air distally in the small or large intestine is diagnostic.
  - "Double bubble" with air present distally suggests duodenal stenosis (Bradshaw, 2021; Dingeldein, 2020b, 2020c; Gallagher et al., 2021; Odackal & Swanson, 2020; Ringer & Hansen, 2017; Trotter, 2021).

Management and Outcome

- Preoperative management includes generalized preoperative management and evaluation for other anomalies (e.g., send chromosomes if dysmorphic features are consistent with trisomy 21 or echocardiogram to rule out CHD). Antibiotics to cover enteric organisms are based on surgeon preference.
- Surgical management for intrinsic lesions includes excision of the atretic portion with primary end-to-end anastomoses via laparotomy or laparoscopically (duodenoduodenostomy). If the duodenal obstruction is related to annular pancreas or other causes compressing the duodenum, the goal of surgery is to remove or redirect the tissue causing the duodenal obstruction.
- Postoperative management includes using a Replogle to suction until return of bowel function (typically 3–10

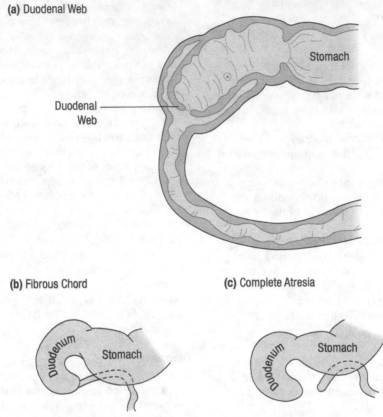

Figure 21.2 Three types of duodenal atresia: A) Type 1–membraneous web; B) Type 2–fibrous atretic cord; C) Type 3–complete atresia with separation of segments.

days), then initiation of enteral nutrition slowly due to delayed gastric emptying and microcolon distal to the repair site resulting in feeding intolerance. Fluid and electrolyte replacement may be required initially based on gastric output.

■ A survival rate of 95% is reported in those who are deemed satisfactory surgical candidates.

■ Prognosis is generally good, with long-term outcomes determined by associated anomalies. Early complications may include anastomotic leak and stricture; potential long-term problems may include dysmotility of the stomach and duodenum. A significant number of infants with corrected duodenal atresia also experience GER, which may be exacerbated by an impairment in gastric emptying (Bradshaw, 2021; Dingeldein, 2020c; Flynn-O'Brien et al., 2018; Gallagher et al., 2021).

▶ ABNORMALITIES IN THE DEVELOPMENT OF THE MIDGUT

MALROTATION/VOLVULUS

Definition and Pathophysiology

■ Malrotation describes failure of normal rotation and retroperitoneal fixation of the intestines which

normally occur during weeks 6 to 11 of gestation during the return from the extracoelomic position of the embryonic intestine to the fetal abdominal cavity. The hedgehog signaling pathway is responsible for transmitting information to the embryonic cells required for proper cell differentiation. Therefore, it is felt that abnormal hedgehog signaling can result in rotation and fixation abnormalities.

■ Normal rotation of the intestines occurs during physiologic midgut herniation and upon return to the abdominal cavity during weeks 10 to 12 of gestation, at which time there is fixation to the retroperitoneum in a precise pattern. The normal position of the intestines is the distal duodenum crossing to the left of the vertebral column, joining the jejunum to a normally positioned ligament of Treitz; the cecum and the ascending colon attaching to the right-lateral posterior body wall; and the descending colon attaching to the left-lateral body wall. The blood supply to the entire midgut is attached to the retroperitoneum from the ligament of Treitz in the upper left quadrant of the abdomen to the cecum in the right lower quadrant.

● Partial malrotation involves only one segment being improperly fixed.

● Mixed rotation results when the midgut only rotates 180 degrees, leading to the terminal ileum reentering first, resulting in the cecum being subpyloric and fixed to the abdominal wall; this results in compression of the duodenum. If the initial rotation is clockwise, the transverse colon ends up behind the duodenum.

- With complete nonrotation, the midgut only rotates 90 degrees and the entire intestines return en masse to the abdomen, resulting in the entire small bowel lying on the right side of the abdomen and the colon lying on the left, commonly coined *left-sided colon*. The intestines are loosely suspended by the superior mesenteric artery and vein but are not fixed to the retroperitoneal surface; in this case, the intestines are basically free-floating, resulting in high risk of volvulus.

■ Volvulus is twisting of the unfixed intestine, most commonly around the superior mesenteric artery, leading to compromise of the blood supply, with rapidly evolving ischemia, bowel infarction, and necrosis, and potential loss of the entire midgut (Figure 21.3).

■ It is associated with other GI abnormalities including intestinal atresia, Ladd's bands causing duodenal obstruction, and abdominal wall defects including congenital diaphragmatic hernia, omphalocele, and gastroschisis. It is seen more commonly in males compared with females (Bradshaw, 2021; Dingeldein, 2020b, 2020c; Ditzenberger, 2018; Flynn-O'Brien et al., 2018; Gallagher et al., 2021; Ringer & Hansen, 2017).

Diagnosis

■ Clinical presentation of malrotation *with volvulus* is sudden onset of bilious emesis in an otherwise healthy infant who has been stooling and feeding normally. Majority of infants will become symptomatic within the first week of life, the remaining present within the first month of life; presentation after 1 month of life is less common. In cases where there is intermittent kinking of the bowel, these infants will have intermittent bilious emesis, abdominal tenderness, and poor growth. As bowel ischemia increases, the infant becomes more symptomatic with abdominal distention, lethargy, pain, bloody emesis and/or stool, and signs of hypovolemia and sepsis.

■ Clinical presentation of malrotation *without volvulus* is similar to infants with proximal intestinal obstruction, including symptoms of feeding intolerance followed by bilious emesis; in some cases, the abdomen may be scaphoid on exam.

■ A barium enema may show obstruction with failure of barium to pass beyond the transverse colon; it may show the cecum in the abnormal position, confirming malrotation, but provides no information about the presence or absence of a volvulus.

■ Abdominal radiograph may show a pattern of obstruction with a dilated stomach and proximal duodenum, but it does not confirm or rule out malrotation; if the malrotation is intermittent, the abdominal x-ray may be normal.

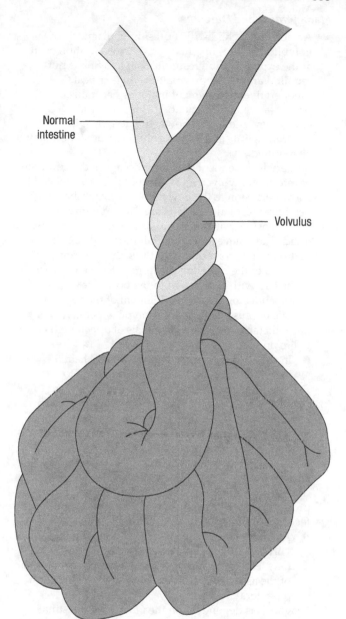

Figure 21.3 Anatomic illustration depicting a volvulus.

■ Abdominal US can be helpful if there is malrotation with volvulus which shows the "whirlpool sign," a twisting of the mesentery, and the abnormal relationship of the mesenteric vessels; however, it is user-dependent.

■ The gold standard for diagnosis is an upper GI that shows absent or abnormal position of the ligament of Treitz (confirms malrotation); presence of what appears as a bird's beak suggests complete midgut obstruction.

■ If there is any doubt after doing diagnostic workup for malrotation with volvulus, an exploratory laparotomy is mandatory, as a missed diagnosis may lead to significant loss of bowel (Bradshaw, 2021; Dingeldein, 2020b, 2020c; Gallagher et al., 2021; Odackal & Swanson, 2020; Ringer & Hansen, 2017; Trotter, 2021).

Management and Outcome

- An acutely ill child with a presumed diagnosis of volvulus requires urgent operative intervention even at the expense of full resuscitation. Imaging is not required and not appropriate. Time is critical.
- Preoperative management includes generalized preoperative management. This is a surgical emergency, and loss of bowel due to ischemia can occur in as little as 4 hours. Volume resuscitation may be required.
- Surgery is dependent on the pathology and the amount of intestinal involvement. The volvulus is untwisted to allow perfusion to the bowel to be reestablished; any necrotic intestinal segments are excised with creation of an ileostomy; if Ladd's bands are present, they are divided to relieve any potential duodenal obstruction; malrotation is corrected with the small intestine returned to the right and the large intestine returned to the left, with attachment to the posterior wall; and an appendectomy is done. Removal of the appendix is done because the final location postoperatively is unpredictable, making a diagnosis of appendicitis later in life problematic.
  - In the event of significant intestinal ischemia, marginal areas are not excised, and in 24 to 36 hours the marginal area is reevaluated for additional need for resection; this approach allows time to see if recovery is possible for the marginally viable intestinal portion and hopefully result in less total bowel resection.
- Postoperative management includes Replogle to suction until return of bowel function (typically 4–6 days on average in the infant undergoing a Ladd procedure); parenteral support is continued until full feedings are tolerated.
  - A major postoperative complication with midgut volvulus is short bowel syndrome (SBS), which may lead to the infant being PN-dependent and all of the associated morbidities related to long-term parenteral needs.
- Prognosis is dependent on the amount of intestinal resection and presence of other anomalies. Mortality is increased in the presence of intestinal necrosis and prematurity. Midgut volvulus accounts for nearly 20% of cases of short gut syndrome in the pediatric population (Bradshaw, 2021; Dingeldein, 2020c; Flynn-O'Brien et al., 2018; Gallagher et al., 2021).

GASTROSCHISIS

Definition and Pathophysiology

- Gastroschisis results from a herniation of abdominal contents (most commonly the stomach and bowel) through a full-thickness anterior abdominal wall defect usually to the right of an intact umbilical ring and cord. Due to lack of covering, the abdominal contents are exposed to the amniotic fluid.
- There are several theories as to the cause of the defect:
  - Occurs due to a vascular accident involving the right omphalomesenteric artery, which weakens the anterior abdominal wall during the seventh week of gestation
  - Failure of differentiation of the lateral fold somatopleure after return of the bowel to the peritoneal cavity and before the umbilical ring has formed
  - Failure in the formation of the umbilical coelom at the base of the umbilical cord due to rupture of the amniotic membrane
  - Intrauterine rupture of the incarcerated hernia into the umbilical cord
  - Alterations in the normal involution of the second umbilical vein or ischemic damage leading to weakness in the abdominal wall
- It occurs three to four times more frequently than an omphalocele; this defect is associated with preterm birth and small for gestational age.
- It is not commonly associated with major congenital anomalies or syndromes; however, association with anomalies of the GI tract is common. Malrotation is usually seen in *all* of these infants; up to 25% may have an associated intestinal atresia/stenosis as a result of the initial vascular accident or from constriction of the fascial defect compromising the affected bowel segment (Bradshaw, 2021; Dingeldein, 2020b, 2020c; Ditzenberger, 2018; Gallagher et al., 2021; Ledbetter et al., 2018; Ringer & Hansen, 2017; Wolf, 2019).

Diagnosis

- Prenatal findings may include elevated serum alpha-fetoprotein. Fetal US can confirm diagnosis early in the second trimester, with multiple loops of bowel seen freely floating in the amniotic fluid, with a typical "cauliflower" appearance. Early delivery may be warranted if there is progressive bowel distention or thickening suggesting intestinal obstruction or severe inflammation. There is minimal risk of bowel injury during vaginal delivery; therefore, vaginal delivery is not contraindicated.
- Delivery should occur at a tertiary center where surgery and complex medical problems can be managed.
- Clinical presentation includes eviscerated intestinal viscera, typically small and large intestines, which may be matted, thickened, and edematous, with no membranous sac; the defect is generally to the right of the umbilical cord, therefore the cord will be intact (Bradshaw, 2021; Dingeldein, 2020b, 2020c; Gallagher et al., 2021; Ledbetter et al., 2018; Wolf, 2019).

Management

PREOPERATIVE

- The preferred method is to place the infant's torso in a bowel bag to maintain sterile environment and allow

visualization of the exposed viscera; covering the defect also minimizes heat and fluid losses.
- Increased insensible water loss due to the exposed bowel may require up to three times maintenance volume.
- An alternative option is wrapping in warm saline-soaked gauze and covering with plastic wrap, taking caution to prevent kinking of the mesenteric blood supply; gauze dressing will adhere to the viscera and cause tissue trauma when removed if not kept moistened. There is increased risk of hypothermia as saline cools over time.
- Minimize handling of viscera to prevent damage; handle with sterile gloves.
- Place the infant with the right side slightly angled down to prevent kinking of the viscera resulting in vascular compromise.
- Maintain NPO with gastric decompression to prevent restriction of intestinal blood flow due to intestinal distention.
- Provision of PN is important to provide protein.
- Latex-free products should be used in all infants with congenital conditions that may require multiple procedures to minimize excessive exposure to latex and potential for development of allergies.
- Administer broad-spectrum antibiotics (Bradshaw, 2021; Dingeldein, 2020c; Gallagher et al., 2021; Ledbetter et al., 2018; Ringer & Hansen, 2017).

SURGICAL INTERVENTION

- The preferred method is primary repair with return of all contents back into the peritoneal cavity with closure of the fascia and skin. If atresia is present, the surgeon may or may not repair during initial surgery, depending on the presence of inflammation and matting of the intestine. If the defect is too large or if during primary repair there is impediment of intestinal blood supply from increased intra-abdominal pressure or impaired venous return, a staged repair should be done.
- There are three options for staged repair:
  - One intervention involves placement of a prosthetic sac or "silo" that is sutured to the edge of the defect or secured underneath the fascia. Support of the silo at a 90-degree angle promotes reduction of defect by gravity and decreases the risk of vascular compromise.
  - A second intervention is to apply a spring-loaded silo over the exposed viscera under the fascia; this approach is associated with fewer complications, fewer ventilator days, and shortened length of stay.
  - The third intervention for staged repair involves placement of an umbilical turban with coiling of the umbilical cord over the defect; this allows epithelization to take place but may result in an umbilical hernia.
  - Regardless of the approach, reduction occurs by gravity with the application of gentle pressure during daily or twice daily reduction; this gentle

reduction allows the respiratory and vascular systems to slowly adjust to the increased pressure of the organs. Once the intestines are at the level of the fascia, the silo is removed and the fascia is closed. Final closure of the defect and abdominal wall is attempted by 10 days; after this time, risk of infection and dehiscence of silo become major concerns (Bradshaw, 2021; Dingeldein, 2020c; Gallagher et al., 2021; Ledbetter et al., 2018).

POSTOPERATIVE

- In the immediate postoperative period, there is risk of intestinal obstruction, abdominal compartment syndrome, sepsis, skin necrosis over the repaired defect, and complications if there is diminished venous return distal to the repair. Monitoring of oxygen saturations, urine output, and blood pressure continuously is imperative to detect compromise, especially after primary repair.
- Maintain NPO with gastric decompression until gastric output is minimal and bowel sounds indicate readiness to begin feeds.
  - Infants with gastroschisis may have a prolonged ileus, making feeding advancement a challenge. Low-osmolality feeds are preferred; soy or elemental formulas may be needed for continued feeding intolerance or absorption.
- Provide PN through central lines such as peripherally inserted central catheter (PICC) or Broviac until able to tolerate full enteral feeds.
- Pain management is indicated.
- Aseptic dressing changes and antibiotics postoperatively prevent sepsis (Bradshaw, 2021; Dingeldein, 2020c).

Outcomes

- Prognosis is dependent on the size of the defect (large defects have higher mortality risk) and associated GI anomalies.
  - The amount of intestinal dysfunction impacts morbidity (impaired absorption, reduced enzymes, and significant dysmotility may result in SBS). Long-term complications include intestinal stricture, incisional hernia, and adhesive bowel obstruction (Bradshaw, 2021; Dingeldein, 2020c; Gallagher et al., 2021; Ledbetter et al., 2018).

OMPHALOCELE (EXOMPHALOS)

Definition and Pathophysiology

- Omphalocele is a developmental defect that is felt to occur as a result of a primary folding abnormality of the germ disc during weeks 4 to 7 of gestation. There is a concomitant failure of the intestines to return during midgut herniation during weeks 8 to 11 of gestation (bowel-containing omphalocele) and an associated failure of the ventral abdominal musculature at the junction of the umbilical cord to close.

■ It is characterized by a midline ventral wall defect with herniation of the abdominal viscera through the umbilical ring into the umbilical cord with a thin, avascular membranous sac; this covering consists of the peritoneum on the inside, amnion on the outside, and Wharton's jelly between these two layers. The umbilical cord passes through the mass and inserts into the membrane as opposed to the abdominal wall. The umbilical arteries and vein are inserted into the apex of the defect.

■ This defect has high association (up to 80%) with other congenital anomalies. Chromosomal defects (including trisomies 13, 18, and 21) and CHD are seen in approximately 50% of infants with this defect. It may also be associated with other midline defects such as genitourinary, craniofacial, musculoskeletal (including limb), or vertebral defects. Omphalocele can be present in several recognizable syndromes, including Beckwith–Wiedemann syndrome (which includes macrosomia, macroglossia, and hypoglycemia, in addition to the omphalocele), cloacal exstrophy, OEIS complex (omphalocele, exstrophy, imperforate anus, and spinal anomalies), and pentalogy of Cantrell (including defects in the diaphragm, sternum, heart, and pericardium, in addition to the omphalocele; Bradshaw, 2021; Dingeldein, 2020b, 2020c; Ditzenberger, 2018; Gallagher et al., 2021; Ledbetter et al., 2018; Ringer & Hansen, 2017; Wolf, 2019).

Diagnosis

■ Prenatal findings include serum alpha-fetoprotein which may not be uniformly elevated as seen with gastroschisis defect. Fetal US provides definitive diagnosis after the first trimester. If detected on fetal US, other potential anomalies should be evaluated, especially if there is absence of the liver within the omphalocele, as this is associated with aneuploidy. Fetal echo should be done. Liver herniation or herniation of other abdominal contents may warrant a Cesarean section to minimize potential trauma; otherwise, as with gastroschisis, vaginal delivery can be considered.

■ Clinical presentation of defect ranges from small to large mass at the base of the umbilical cord. The defect may be covered by an intact, thin, avascular membrane, or the membrane may have ruptured, leaving the herniated contents exposed to the amniotic fluid, as in a gastroschisis. Herniated contents can range from a few loops of intestines to potentially any abdominal organ being present, including the liver, spleen, stomach, bladder, and reproductive organs. There is a larger fascia defect with an omphalocele compared with a gastroschisis.

● Care should be taken always to examine any thickened umbilical cord closely prior to placing a cord clamp, as it may be a small omphalocele (Bradshaw, 2021; Dingeldein, 2020c; Ditzenberger, 2018; Gallagher et al., 2021; Ledbetter et al., 2018; Ringer & Hansen, 2017; Wolf, 2019).

Management

PREOPERATIVE

■ As with gastroschisis, place in a bowel bag to maintain sterile environment. Handle carefully to prevent tearing of the membrane.

■ Alternative options include covering with a nonadherent dressing to protect the sac, or wrapping in warm saline-soaked gauze and covering with plastic wrap. A gauze dressing will adhere to the viscera and cause tissue trauma when removed if not kept moistened; however, there is an increased risk of hypothermia as saline cools over time. Do not attempt to reduce the sac as it may rupture, interfere with venous return, or cause respiratory compromise.

■ Minimize handling of viscera to prevent damage; handle with sterile gloves.

■ Evaluate for other potential anomalies:
  ● Echocardiogram to rule out CHD
  ● Chest and abdomen radiograph to assess bony structures and for other anomalies
    ❏ Abdominal US to assess structures and the integrity of the urinary tract
    ❏ If uncorrectable due to congenital anomalies, provide palliative care

■ Maintain NPO with gastric decompression to prevent restriction of intestinal blood flow due to intestinal distention.

■ Provide PN and circulating volume support as needed. If the sac is intact, there is less evaporative loss; therefore the infant may not need as much volume support as compared with an infant who has a ruptured sac at birth.

■ Use latex-free products.

■ Administer broad-spectrum antibiotics (Bradshaw, 2021; Dingeldein, 2020c; Gallagher et al., 2021; Ledbetter et al., 2018; Ringer & Hansen, 2017).

SURGICAL INTERVENTION

■ Surgery is more emergent if sac is ruptured. Primary repair, the preferred surgical intervention, involves removal of sac or remnants, return of all contents back into the peritoneal cavity, and closure of the fascia and skin.

■ If the defect is too large or if during primary repair there is impediment of intestinal blood supply from increased intra-abdominal pressure or impaired venous return, *OR* if the infant has uncorrectable congenital anomalies, the defect is painted with an escharotic agent such as silver nitrate, with eschar formation and epithelization occurring within 10 to 20 weeks. After epithelization is complete, an elastic wrap or specially made brace is used for gentle compression to assist in reducing the contents back into the abdomen; the infant will require later surgical repair of the resultant ventral hernia.

- If painting with escharotic agent, assess for potential adverse systemic effects from the agent used (Bradshaw, 2021; Dingeldein, 2020c; Draus & Ruzic, 2020b; Gallagher et al., 2021; Ringer & Hansen, 2017).

POSTOPERATIVE

- If primary repair done, in the immediate postoperative period there is risk of intestinal obstruction, abdominal compartment syndrome, sepsis, and complications if there is diminished venous return distal to the repair. Monitoring of oxygen saturations, urine output, and blood pressure continuously is imperative to detect compromise.
- Maintain NPO with gastric decompression until gastric output is minimal and bowel sounds indicate readiness to begin feeds.
  - Feeding advancement is typically not a problem unless the sac was not intact and then, like infants with gastroschisis, there may be a prolonged ileus, making feeding advancement a challenge.
- Provide PN through central lines such as PICC or Broviac until able to tolerate full enteral feeds.
- Pain management is indicated.
- Aseptic dressing changes and antibiotics postoperatively minimize risk of sepsis (Bradshaw, 2021; Dingeldein, 2020c; Gallagher et al., 2021).

Outcomes

- Prognosis is related to the size of the defect, the severity of associated congenital anomalies, and if there are any challenges to closing the defect.
  - Possible short- and long-term complications include intestinal stricture, incisional hernia, and adhesive bowel obstruction (Bradshaw, 2021; Dingeldein, 2020c; Gallagher et al., 2021; Ledbetter et al., 2018).

▶ ABNORMALITIES IN THE DEVELOPMENT OF THE HINDGUT

HIRSCHSPRUNG DISEASE (CONGENITAL MEGACOLON, AGANGLIONIC MEGACOLON)

Definition and Pathophysiology

- Hirschsprung disease is congenital absence of the ganglion cells of a segment of the colon resulting in a functional obstruction. It more commonly affects the

rectum or the rectosigmoid portion of the colon, and less commonly may extend to the proximal colon. It is the most common cause of large bowel obstruction in the newborn.

- It is caused by failure of the ganglion cells prior to 12 weeks of gestation to migrate cephalocaudally, resulting in partial or complete aganglionosis of the submucosal and mesenteric plexuses of the colon. Absence of ganglion cells prevents the inhibitory relaxation normally regulated by parasympathetic nerves, leading to functional obstruction because the affected segment is unable to relax and becomes dysfunctional, resulting in an inability to effectively pass stool through the aganglionic area and beyond.
- There is increased hypertrophy of the normally innervated proximal portion of the colon as it attempts to overcome the functional obstruction. The presence of ganglion cells to the area of no ganglion cells is referred to as the *transition zone*. The time at which migration of the ganglion cells stopped determines the length of bowel involved.
- There are at least eight genomes associated with Hirschsprung disease, explaining family history in up to one-third of cases. Almost 20% of patients with Hirschsprung disease may have chromosomal abnormalities, most commonly trisomy 21.
- The oral, facial, and cranial ganglia arise from the same neural crest as the ganglionic plexus of the bowel, so other associated anomalies may also be present, such as sensorineural deafness with central alveolar hypoventilation, ocular neuropathies, systemic anomalies associated with Smith–Lemli–Opitz syndrome, and cardiovascular with skeletal and limb anomalies seen in DiGeorge syndrome. Colonic atresia and imperforate anus may also be present. Males are affected four times more often than females (Bradshaw, 2021; Dingeldein, 2020b, 2020c; Flynn-O'Brien et al., 2018; Gallagher et al., 2021; Gomella, 2020b).

Diagnosis

- Clinical presentation in the newborn includes failure to pass meconium spontaneously by 48 hours of age, increased abdominal distention, and bilious emesis. Rectal stimulation often results in passage of stool. If the obstruction continues, risk of enterocolitis increases—evidenced by diarrhea, obstipation (inability to pass stool or gas), progressive abdominal distention, vomiting, poor feeding with failure to thrive, lethargy, and fever. Hirschsprung disease in some cases does not present until in older infancy or childhood with chronic constipation problems.
- A contrast barium enema suggests diagnosis showing the contracted rectosigmoid colon with contrast material entering the proximal dilated bowel. In newborns, the conical tapering demonstrating the

transition zone is not always evident. Barium retained for greater than 24 hours after a contrast enema is suggestive of Hirschsprung disease.

■ Abdominal x-ray demonstrates proximal bowel distention, with absence of air at the point of the obstruction to the rectum demonstrating a bowel obstruction; air–fluid levels in the colon may be present.

■ Rectal biopsy is the gold standard to confirm diagnosis, demonstrating absence of ganglion cells and hypertrophic nonmyelinated axons in the nerve plexus. Histochemical tests of the biopsy samples show an increase in acetylcholine. A newer monoclonal antibody, anti-MAP2 antibody neuronal marker, detects ganglionic cells on rectal biopsy specimens with exceptional specificity and sensitivity. Suction or punch biopsy can be done at the bedside; however, full-thickness biopsy needs to be done under general anesthesia.

■ In the infant with very short segment aganglionosis, contrast studies may be normal; anal manometry in this case may be useful in establishing diagnosis (Bradshaw, 2021; Dingeldein, 2020b, 2020c; Flynn-O'Brien et al., 2018; Gallagher et al., 2021; Odackal & Swanson, 2020; Ringer & Hansen, 2017; Trotter, 2021).

Management and Outcome

■ Medical management includes fluid resuscitation and gentle rectal irrigations (not enemas) with warm saline solution twice a day to empty the colon and minimize the risk of enterocolitis until surgery.
  ● If the rectal irrigations evacuate stool, feedings can continue.
  ● If unable to evacuate stool and there is increased abdominal distention with emesis, feedings are stopped and preoperative management includes generalized preoperative management for bowel obstruction.

■ The goal of surgery is to bring the normal ganglionated bowel down to the anus using an endorectal or transanal pull-through procedure. During surgery, multiple seromuscular biopsies are done to identify where the normally innervated bowel occurs; if this area is not correctly identified, the infant will remain symptomatic due to an area of aganglionosis remaining. If the infant develops enterocolitis, is preterm, is less than 2 kg, or has significant proximal bowel distention, the abnormally innervated area of the colon is removed and a colostomy is done, with a pull-through procedure done later, typically between 3 and 6 months of age.

■ Postoperative management is similar to other GI obstruction disorders. In addition, these infants receive routine rectal irrigations with normal saline postoperatively to decrease the risk of recurrent enterocolitis.
  ● Postoperatively, if colostomy is required, there is a need to monitor for prolapse, skin dehiscence with excoriation, and stomal ulceration and bleeding. Parents need to be taught stoma care.
  ● Approximately 2 weeks postoperatively following primary pull-through, a series of anal dilations occur in infants who had a primary pull-through procedure.

■ Feedings are resumed when the infant has passed stool with endorectal procedure or when anastomosis site has healed. Diet adjustments may need to be made to improve stool consistency. In some cases, loperamide (Imodium) may be required to reduce stool frequency (commonly seen in the immediate postoperative period but typically normalizes over time) or kaolin–pectin suspensions to solidify stools.

■ Genetic counseling should be offered to the family.

■ Prognosis is based on the time of diagnosis, development of enterocolitis, and amount of bowel affected. Postoperative complications may include anastomotic leak or stricture. Morbidity associated with continued elimination problems despite removal of the aganglionic segment can be seen. Surgical intervention is not curative as, despite surgical resection, there is still an abnormally innervated anal sphincter. These infants remain at risk of persistent constipation, fecal incontinence, and life-threatening enterocolitis, with functional outcomes not known until the child reaches the age of toilet-training.

■ Long-term results indicate that approximately 90% of these patients ultimately achieve normal or near-normal bowel function (Bradshaw, 2021; Dingeldein, 2020c; Flynn-O'Brien et al., 2018; Gallagher et al., 2021; Ringer & Hansen, 2017).

ANORECTAL MALFORMATIONS

Definition and Pathophysiology

■ Anorectal malformations are a broad spectrum of anomalies characterized by an absent or abnormally located anus outside the normal sphincter muscles. This can be a stenotic or atretic anal canal that may be isolated, include a fistulous communication between the urogenital tract or vagina and the rectum, or in females a complex persistent cloaca.

■ These are caused by failure of differentiation of the urogenital sinus and cloaca during early embryonic development. Persistent cloaca in females is the result of arrest of development during weeks 4 to 6 of gestation of the gut and the complete separation from the urogenital tract. If the disruption of the cloacal membrane occurs before the urorectal septum has separated the urinary bladder from the hindgut, cloacal exstrophy occurs, whereas if the disruption of the cloacal membrane occurs after septation, exstrophy of the bladder occurs.

■ Imperforate anus is classified based on the level of the defect:
  ● High lesions are above the levator muscle component of the anal sphincter muscle complex

(can be estimated by drawing an imaginary pubococcygeal line); a low defect occurs below this area. High defects are more common in contrast to low lesions, are more common in males, generally more complex with rectourinary or rectovaginal fistulas, more likely to be associated with other malformations, and more likely to have incontinence if sacral anomaly is present due to lack of innervation to the bowel and/or bladder.
- Low lesions occur in both sexes equally and commonly may have a perineal fistula.
- There is a common association between **V**ertebral anomalies, **A**nal atresia, **C**ardiac defects, **T**racheo**E**sophageal fistula, **R**enal anomalies, and **L**imb abnormalities (VACTERL) anomalies and trisomy 21 and anorectal malformations. There is also a high incidence of cryptorchidism in males, as well as spinal dysraphism. Imaging of the spine should be done, as well as other evaluations based on physical exam (Bradshaw, 2021; Dingeldein, 2020b, 2020c; Flynn-O'Brien et al., 2018; Gallagher et al., 2021; Gomella, 2020b; Ringer & Hansen, 2017).

Diagnosis

- Clinical presentation may include absence of an anal opening with imperforate anus. In the case of anal stenosis or an anal membrane, there is visually a normal-appearing rectum but failure to pass meconium, with increasing abdominal distention prompting further evaluation.
- Diagnosis of imperforate anus is based on physical examination reflecting absence of an anal opening. Presence of a fistula needs to be determined. A fistula may not be evident until up to 24 hours of life. Presence of meconium in the urine is diagnostic of a rectourinary fistula, and presence of meconium in the vaginal vault is diagnostic of a rectovaginal fistula.
- Abdominal radiograph shows increased bowel gas pattern with lack of air in the rectum. An inverted lateral radiograph is sometimes done in an attempt to determine the level of the air-filled rectal pouch.
- A perineal US may be helpful in determining the termination of the rectum and its distance from the skin.
- A perineal fistula visible on physical exam does not usually require any imaging. A contrast study of the urethra in males will determine if fistula is present or not, and a contrast genitogram in females will determine the anatomic relationships of a persistent cloaca (Bradshaw, 2021; Dingeldein, 2020c; Gallagher et al., 2021; Ringer & Hansen, 2017).

Management and Outcome

- Preoperative management includes generalized preoperative management while evaluation is underway. Echocardiogram, spine radiographs, and renal/spinal US should be done to rule out other anomalies that are commonly seen. Infants with a fistula are at high risk of developing a hyperchloremic acidosis due to colonic absorption of urine.
- Surgery is always necessary, but the procedure is dependent on the level of the defect.
  - Intermediate and high defects require a colostomy, with a pull-through procedure done later (ranges from 3 to 8 months). Colostomy closure is done about 6 to 8 weeks after anorectoplasty if no stricture is present.
  - Low defects have good outcome, with anorectoplasty that may be done in the newborn period or by first month of life. With low defects, if there is no associated fistula, a colostomy will be required temporarily.
  - If there is a perineal fistula and early repair is not possible, dilation twice daily is done to promote elimination of stool until able to have a surgical procedure performed.
- Postoperative management includes stoma care and parent teaching if colostomy has been done with later definitive repair. Anal dilation is started 2 weeks postoperatively to prevent anal stenosis and may be continued for 4 to 6 months. If the fistula has not been divided, antibiotic prophylaxis for urinary tract infections should be administered and bicarbonate supplementation may be necessary.
- Long-term outcomes are affected by the type of malformation, sacral development, and presence of spinal abnormalities. Prognosis is generally excellent with low defects. There is an increased risk of constipation, which may require anal dilation if related to a stricture, and in rare cases revision of the anoplasty may be required. Prognosis of infants with high defects is determined by the amount of sphincter muscle development and innervation, with bowel incontinence strongly associated long term. Long-term complications may also include urinary and stool incontinence, ejaculatory dysfunction, and erectile dysfunction.
  - These patients need lifelong follow-up. Constipation is the most common sequela in patients with anorectal malformations, and it can be most severe in the benign group of malformations. The more complex malformations have poorer prognosis in terms of bowel control but less chance of constipation. Constipation must be treated aggressively. Prolonged use of laxatives in this population is indicated (Bradshaw, 2021; Dingeldein, 2020b, 2020c; Gallagher et al., 2021; Flynn-O'Brien et al., 2018).

▶ DISORDERS INVOLVING THE SMALL AND LARGE INTESTINES

MECONIUM ILEUS/MECONIUM PLUG

Definition and Pathophysiology

- A meconium ileus is a mechanical obstruction of the distal lumen of the *ileum* due to thick, tenacious meconium; the proximal segment of the bowel is dilated. More complex forms may be associated with volvulus, intestinal atresia, or perforation with meconium peritonitis.

■ A meconium plug results in a mechanical obstruction of the distal lumen of the *colon* due to thick, tenacious meconium in the absence of enzymatic deficiency or abnormalities of the ganglion cells.

■ Of infants with meconium ileus, 90% have cystic fibrosis (CF) due to an autosomal recessive gene defect on chromosome 7, resulting in alteration of the chloride channel transporter and transport of fluid across the epithelial cells.

■ Two implicating factors are hyposecretion of pancreatic enzymes or abnormal viscid secretions from the mucous glands of the small intestine. Pancreatic enzymes are necessary for digestion of intestinal contents; when lacking, there are abnormal amounts of proteins and glycoproteins, causing the meconium/stool to be thick and viscid. In patients with CF, there are gene mutations in the *cystic fibrosis transmembrane regulator (CFTR)* that affect transport of bicarbonate and chloride, resulting in the characteristic meconium that adheres to the intralumen of the bowel wall, resulting in obstruction (Bradshaw, 2021; Dingeldein, 2020b, 2020c; Flynn-O'Brien et al., 2018; Gallagher et al., 2021; Ringer & Hansen, 2017).

Diagnosis

■ Prenatal findings of a meconium ileus may include polyhydramnios, ascites, hyperechoic appearance, or dilation of the bowel; pathognomonic for meconium ileus is in utero meconium peritonitis, with perforation noted as intra-abdominal calcifications. Meconium ileus may also be suspected prenatally when there is a family history of CF or when parents are carriers of the *CFTR* mutations; in these cases, diagnosis can be confirmed by fetal DNA analysis.

■ An infant with an uncomplicated meconium ileus presents between 24 to 48 hours of age with bilious emesis, progressive abdominal distention, failure to pass meconium despite digital stimulation, and a dough-like sensation on palpation due to the thickened meconium in the distal bowel. These may manifest more abruptly and progress more quickly in complex forms with abdominal distention within the first 24 hours of life, an erythematous edematous abdomen, and respiratory distress.

■ Clinical presentation of meconium plug includes failure to pass meconium by 48 hours of life, hyperactive bowel sounds, and increasing abdominal distention; bilious emesis is a late sign. Seventy-five percent of newborns expel the plug spontaneously.

■ The gold standard for diagnosis of either disease, which may also be therapeutic, is a water-soluble contrast enema showing a microcolon and pellets of meconium at the site of the distal obstruction. In up to 60% of the cases, fluid is drawn into the intestine during the contrast study, dislodging the meconium and allowing normal intestinal activity. A contrast enema is contraindicated in the infant with a pneumoperitoneum or if there are concerns for peritonitis.

■ On abdominal x-ray, there are distended loops of bowel with few air–fluid levels due to the viscous nature of the meconium. In addition, Neuhauser sign can be seen and the distal intestine may have a "soap bubble" appearance as tiny air bubbles are mixed within the meconium.

● In complex cases, there may be scattered calcification if an intrauterine perforation occurred (Bradshaw, 2021; Dingeldein, 2020b, 2020c; Flynn-O'Brien et al., 2018; Gallagher et al., 2021; Gomella, 2020f; Ringer & Hansen, 2017).

Management and Outcome

■ Surgery may be required to relieve the intestinal obstruction if the contrast enema(s) fails to relieve the meconium obstruction or if there are calcifications on abdominal x-ray suggestive of in utero perforation.

■ Medical management of a plug includes rectal stimulation, which may expel the plug in some circumstances, and enemas of warm saline, meglumine diatrizoate, or acetylcysteine.

■ Medical management of the ileus includes Replogle to low suction, parenteral fluid support, and water-contrast enema (Gastrografin or Cysto-Conray are common agents used).

● Maintenance fluids up to 1.5 normal needs are required due to rapid fluid shifts from the contrast agents that can lead to hypovolemic shock; this is seen more commonly with use of hyperosmolar agents. Additional enemas may be required if meconium is not completely evacuated.

● It is important to monitor for the first 48 hours after the enema for potential intestinal perforation; the risk of perforation increases with each successive enema.

● In some cases, *N-acetylcysteine* (Mucomyst) enemas are used to break up the abnormal meconium and relieve the obstruction.

■ Due to high association with CF, chest physiotherapy (CPT), supplemental humidity, and aerosolized mucolytic agents such as Mucomyst are provided to prevent atelectasis and pneumonia. These infants also require supplementation of feedings with pancreatic enzymes.

■ Parental education on pulmonary hygiene, infection prevention, nutritional supplements, and genetic counseling is important.

■ One-year survival is excellent. Long-term survival is dependent on the presence of associated anomalies and the number and degree of organs involved as a result of CF (Bradshaw, 2021; Dingeldein, 2020b, 2020c; Flynn-O'Brien et al., 2018; Gallagher et al., 2021; Gomella, 2020b; Ringer & Hansen, 2017).

SMALL LEFT COLON SYNDROME

Definition and Pathophysiology

- Small left colon syndrome is a form of meconium plug syndrome. A functional distal bowel obstruction caused by transient dysmotility in the descending colon results in normal meconium becoming impacted in the distal portion of the colon. In meconium plug syndrome, the obstruction is generally in the sigmoid colon. In small left colon, the site of obstruction is the splenic flexure, which is small in caliber.
- Up to 50% of cases of small left colon syndrome are seen in infants of diabetic mothers (Dingeldein, 2020b; Gorman, 2017).

Diagnosis

- Clinical presentation includes failure to pass meconium within the first 24 to 36 hours of life and generalized abdominal distention with bilious emesis.
- The gold standard for diagnosis is water-contrast enema; this procedure may also be therapeutic, resulting in evacuation of stool.
- Abdominal radiography may show dilation of the proximal colon with abrupt narrowing of the distal colon usually at the splenic flexure (Dingeldein, 2020b; Gorman, 2017; Trotter, 2021).

Management and Outcome

- Medical management is conservative treatment with enemas.
- Prognosis is excellent, with resolution of stooling difficulties occurring in the first month of life (Dingeldein, 2020b; Gorman, 2017).

▶ ACQUIRED DISORDERS OF THE GASTROINTESTINAL TRACT

NECROTIZING ENTEROCOLITIS

Definition and Pathophysiology

- Necrotizing enterocolitis (NEC) is the most common acquired disease, mainly of preterm infants, characterized by inflammation of the bowel wall and necrosis. The terminal ileum and proximal ascending colon are the most frequently involved sites.
- NEC is a multifactorial disease resulting from complex interactions between intestinal immaturity, abnormal microbial colonization with poor host response to injury, and feedings. The interplay of these results in mucosal injury, intestinal inflammation, and ischemia progressing to necrosis, and bacterial translocation across the compromised intestinal barrier with a proinflammatory response.
  - The innermost intestinal mucosa is affected first, but as the disease progresses the muscular and subserosal layers of the intestine become involved. Proliferation of colonizing bacteria leads to the

release of endotoxins and cytokines. Bacterial fermentation leads to gaseous distention, further compromising intestinal blood flow.

- Although enteral feedings appear to be a key trigger, keeping a preterm infant NPO actually increases the incidence of NEC and is not protective.
- Risk factors in preterm infants include:
  - Prematurity is the single greatest risk factor, with increasing risk with decreasing gestational age.
  - Immaturity of the intestinal tract related to decreased immunologic factors, increased gastric pH, immature intestinal epithelial barrier allowing translocation to occur, and dysmotility of the intestine are also risk factors.
  - Up to 90% of infants who develop NEC have been fed. It is hypothesized that feeds and oral medication increase intestinal oxygen demand during absorption, resulting in tissue hypoxia. In addition, fluid shifts into the intestine occur, resulting in decreased intestinal blood flow and intestinal ischemia.
- Risk factors in term infants include:
  - Presence of cyanotic CHD (Figure 21.4), polycythemia, sepsis, hypotension, asphyxia, intrauterine growth restriction, cocaine exposure in utero, and history of gastroschisis
- Transfusion-related NEC is a distinct entity that can also lead to NEC. This phenomenon requires separate discussion and will not be covered in this chapter.
- Preventive measures include prevention of preterm birth and antenatal steroids with threatened preterm delivery.
- Measures associated with lowering risk of NEC include exclusive human milk diet, standardized feeding protocol especially in the very low birth weight (VLBW) population, and avoiding use of H2 blockers (this allows the acidic environment to remain). There is some potential benefit with the use of *Bifidobacterium* probiotics (Ahmad, 2020a; Bradshaw, 2021; Caplan, 2020; Ditzenberger, 2018; Gallagher et al., 2021; Javid et al., 2018; Kudin & Neu, 2020; Weitkamp, et al., 2017).

Diagnosis

- Postnatal onset is inversely related to birth weight and gestational age, with a mean gestational age for presentation of NEC typically between 28 and 32 weeks.
- Clinical presentation varies from a subtle course to an overwhelming fulminant course associated with high rate of mortality and morbidity.
  - A subtle presentation may include general systemic signs mistaken for sepsis including lethargy, temperature instability, increased apnea and bradycardia events, and poor feeding, in addition to GI symptoms including feeding intolerance (emesis, increased gastric aspirates), abdominal

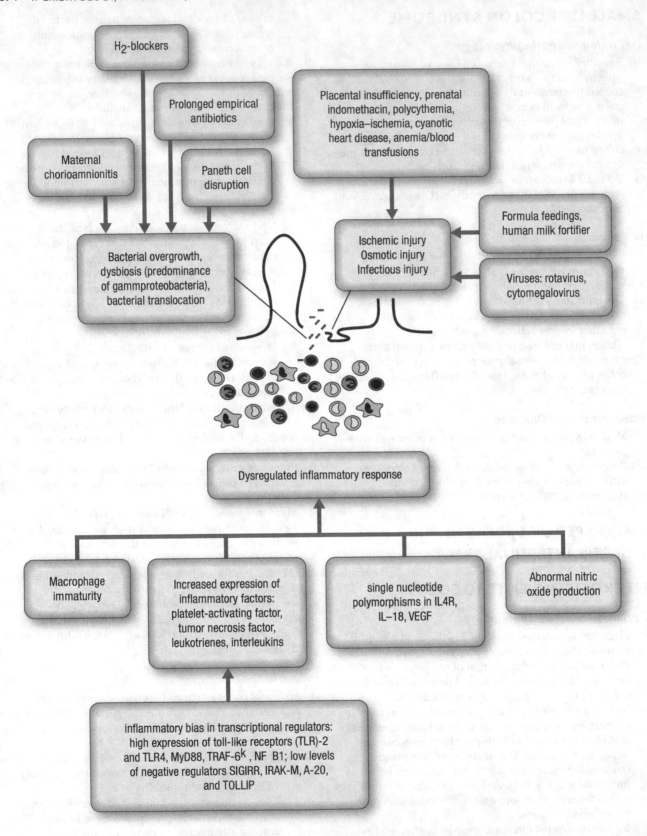

Figure 21.4 Multifactorial causes of necrotizing enterocolitis.

IL, Interleukin; MyD88, myeloid differentiation primary-response gene 88; NF-κB1, nuclear factor kappa B1; VEGF, vascular endothelial growth factor.
Source: Reproduced with permission from McElroy, S., Frey, M., Torres, B., & Maheshwari, A. (2018). Innate and mucosal immunity in the developing gastrointestinal tract. In C. Gleason & S. Juul (Eds.), *Avery's diseases of the newborn* (10th ed., pp. 1054–1067.e5). Elsevier.

distention with or without tenderness, abdominal wall erythema, and bloody stools.
- If undetected, the clinical course will progress, displaying increased systemic signs such as respiratory distress, decreased perfusion, hypotension, metabolic acidosis, oliguria, and coagulopathies.
- Laboratory findings are nonspecific; however, a common triad is thrombocytopenia, persistent metabolic acidosis, and refractory hyponatremia.
- Radiologic findings are diagnostic with presence of pneumatosis intestinalis (hallmark finding of hydrogen gas in the bowel wall), portal venous gas (air that has escaped from the bowel into the portal venous system), and/or pneumoperitoneum (free air in the peritoneal cavity).
  - Plain radiograph (anterior–posterior view) is used to evaluate for pneumatosis intestinalis and portal venous gas. To monitor for free air, a left lateral decubitus (left side down) view should be obtained; this view demonstrates peritoneal air that rises and layers out over the liver.
  - A fixed bowel loop on serial studies and stacking of intestinal loops support the concern for NEC. Presence of periumbilical air collection noted on an anterior–posterior x-ray is referred to as the "football sign."
  - US can also be used to evaluate for presence of portal venous gas and pneumatosis.
- Bell staging is an important tool that allows comparison of infants across clinical sites but can also be helpful in guiding management.
  - *Stage 1 (suspected):* clinical signs and symptoms as discussed above and inconclusive radiologic findings
  - *Stage 2 (definite):* clinical signs and symptoms with presence of *pneumatosis or portal venous gas* on x-ray; further divided into *2A* for mildly ill infant and *2B* for moderately ill infant with systemic clinical signs
  - *Stage 3 (advanced):* also divided into two stages—*3A* is the same as stage *2B* but now a critically ill infant with concern for impending perforation, while *3B* has proven intestinal perforation with *pneumoperitoneum* on x-ray (Ahmad, 2020a; Bradshaw, 2021; Caplan, 2020; Gallagher et al., 2021; Gomella, 2020a; Javid et al., 2018; Kudin & Neu, 2020; Trotter, 2021; Weitkamp et al., 2017)

Management

MEDICAL MANAGEMENT
- Medical management is geared toward supportive care.
  - Stage 1 NEC management includes bowel rest (NPO), fluid resuscitation, Replogle to suction to decompress and allow better intestinal bowel wall perfusion, monitoring labs (complete blood count [CBC], electrolytes), blood culture with

broad-spectrum antibiotics to cover enteric flora, abdominal x-rays every 4 to 8 hours (for progression of disease), and discussion with pediatric surgery specialists.
- Management for stage 2 NEC includes the same medical management as stage 1, but in addition lateral decubitus x-rays should be done due to increased risk of pneumoperitoneum now that there is pneumatosis intestinalis and/or portal venous air. Addition of anaerobic agent should also be considered, as well as placement of central line when blood cultures remain negative at 48 hours, supportive care, and official pediatric surgery consultation.
- Management for stage 3 NEC includes supportive care (treatment of coagulopathies and hypotension, may need intubation and mechanical ventilation) and pediatric surgery consultation with intervention.
- Medical management is successful in more than 50% of infants, but there is a risk of later stricture formation requiring surgical intervention (Ahmad, 2020a; Bradshaw, 2021; Gallagher et al., 2021; Javid et al. 2018; Kudin & Neu, 2020; Trotter, 2021; Weitkamp et al., 2017).

SURGICAL INTERVENTION
- Surgery is indicated if abdominal free air is present. It may also be indicated if the clinical picture is worsening despite maximal medical management, presence of portal venous gas, or if there is a persistent fixed intestinal loop on serial x-rays in the symptomatic infant.
  - Traditionally, the goal of surgery has been to excise necrotic bowel while preserving as much viable intestine as possible and creation of an ostomy. If there is extensive involvement, no or minimal intestinal resection is done, with a second operation in 24 to 48 hours to determine if some of the questionable areas are viable.
  - If the infant is extremely unstable or in extremely low birth weight (ELBW) infants, a peritoneal drain may be placed as a temporizing measure. In some cases, additional surgery may be initially everted, but there is a suggested increased incidence of strictures (as the inflamed intestine heals, there is scarring of the intestinal wall; Ahmad, 2020a; Bradshaw, 2021; Caplan, 2020; Gallagher et al., 2018; Javid et al., 2018; Kudin & Neu, 2020; Weitkamp et al., 2017).

POSTOPERATIVE
- Bowel rest for 10 to 14 days.
- Provide PN through central lines such as PICC or Broviac until able to tolerate full enteral feeds; once intestinal motility is present, slow introduction of low osmolar elemental feeds or breast milk can be started.

■ Antibiotics should be continued.

■ Pain management is indicated.

■ Stoma closure with reanastomosis is typically done 6 to 8 weeks after the initial surgery; a preoperative contrast enema is done prior to this to evaluate for presence of strictures (Bradshaw, 2021; Gallagher et al., 2021; Weitkamp et al., 2017)

Outcomes

■ Prognosis is dependent on numerous factors. There are decreased mortality rates in agencies that have standardized therapeutic protocols defining medical and surgical management and with early diagnosis. Mortality depends on the gestational age, birth weight, extent of bowel involvement, and need for surgical intervention. The overall mortality due to NEC ranges from 20% to 30%.

■ Infants with stage 2B and higher have an overall higher incidence of mortality, growth delay, and poor neurodevelopmental outcomes. Infants who require surgical intervention also have increased mortality secondary to sepsis, respiratory failure, and parenteral nutrition-associated liver disease (PNALD).

  ● Up to one-third of infants treated medically develop an intestinal stricture in the large bowel as a result of cicatricial scarring of the previous inflamed bowel; these infants present with bloody stools, feeding difficulties, diarrhea, and failure to thrive. Additional morbidity in the immediate postoperative period includes stoma prolapse or retraction, wound dehiscence, sepsis, and recurrent NEC.

■ Long-term morbidity can include SBS (if less than 40 cm of bowel remains with no ileocecal value, or if <20 cm with presence of ileocecal valve, which will be discussed later in this chapter), malabsorption and chronic diarrhea, cholestasis secondary to long-term PN, failure to thrive, metabolic bone disease, and increased risk of impaired neurodevelopmental outcome. There is a risk of recurrent NEC in up to 6% of infants; however, in these cases, medical management is usually successful (Ahmad, 2020a; Bradshaw, 2021; Caplan, 2020; Gallagher et al., 2021; Gomella, 2020a; Javid et al., 2018; Kudin & Neu, 2020; Weitkamp et al., 2017).

SPONTANEOUS INTESTINAL PERFORATION

Definition and Pathophysiology

■ Spontaneous intestinal perforation (SIP) is an isolated perforation not associated with intestinal ischemia or necrosis. This is a distinctly different disease process compared with NEC. It typically involves the antimesenteric border of the distal ileum; there is a well-defined margin of focal hemorrhagic necrosis, with the adjacent bowel appearing normal.

■ Prematurity is the only well-established risk factor. Other associated risk factors include the presence of an umbilical artery catheter (UAC), early administration of indomethacin or ibuprofen, early administration of postnatal steroids, or having a patent ductus arteriosus (PDA) or intraventricular hemorrhage (IVH) in the extremely preterm infant. There is also an association with a history of maternal chorioamnionitis in some of the cases (Bradshaw, 2021; Dingeldein, 2020b; Javid et al., 2018; Weitkamp et al., 2017).

Diagnosis

■ Clinical presentation is usually in the first 1 to 2 weeks of life with acute abdominal distention, often with a blue discoloration of the abdominal wall as a result of meconium butting up against the thin, abdominal wall. There is less hemodynamic instability and less metabolic acidosis compared with NEC. The onset of presentation is much earlier than seen with NEC.

■ The gold standard for diagnosis is clinical presentation, with abdominal radiography (anterior–posterior, left lateral decubitus, or cross-table lateral imaging) showing a pneumoperitoneum with absence of pneumatosis, portal venous gas, or other radiographic findings that can be seen in infants with NEC (Ahmad, 2020b; Bradshaw, 2021; Dingeldein, 2020b; Javid et al., 2018; Odackal & Swanson, 2020; Weitkamp et al., 2017).

Management and Outcome

■ Preoperative management includes NPO with Replogle to low suction, supportive care for respiratory or cardiac instability, and antibiotic therapy including an anaerobic agent.

■ Surgical options include placement of a peritoneal drain (if the infant is unstable) or laparotomy with resection of the segment of the bowel with the perforation, followed by an end-to-end anastomosis or an ostomy created with reconnection, typically after 8 to 12 weeks from the procedure.

■ Prognosis is similar in regard to mortality and neurodevelopmental impairment in infants with SIP compared with infants with intestinal perforation from NEC, but higher than those without SIP or NEC. Infants with SIP are at risk of developing bronchopulmonary dysplasia (BPD), late-onset sepsis, severe IVH, cystic periventricular leukomalacia, and growth failure (Ahmad, 2020b; Dingeldein, 2020b; Javid et al., 2018; Weitkamp et al., 2017).

SHORT BOWEL SYNDROME

Definition and Pathophysiology

■ Normal GI function consists of digestion and absorption of nutrients. Carbohydrates, proteins, and fats must be broken down into smaller molecules of monosaccharides, oligopeptides, amino acids and free fatty acids, and monoglycerides so that absorption into the intestinal epithelial cells and into the portal circulation can occur. Understanding this process makes the understanding of alterations in digestion or absorption with loss of bowel clearer.

- Following surgical resection, malabsorption and malnutrition as a result of loss of intestine absorptive surface area may result in SBS. The amount of malabsorption and malnutrition is dependent on the following:
  - How much and what segments of the intestine remain as this will determine the amount of surface area for absorption and which functions of the resected segment were lost
  - Whether or not the ileocecal valve was able to be preserved; the ileocecal valve slows down transit time to increase absorption and prevent bacterial colonic overgrowth in the small intestine (Bradshaw, 2021; Dimmitt et al., 2018)

Diagnosis

- Diagnosis of SBS varies and may be based on the length of the remaining bowel or on the presence of intestinal failure. Intestinal failure due to inadequate length or function occurs with any length of the remaining bowel that is unable to meet fluid, electrolyte, and energy requirements of the infant. Intestinal adaptation involves significant structural and functional alterations, the progress of which is often unpredictable and individualized (Javid et al., 2018).

Management and Outcome

- Medical management is complex and requires multidisciplinary care. Management includes PN and providing as much enteral nutrition as possible, even if only in small amounts. Cycling of PN may be necessary if the infant develops cholestasis. Skin care is important at the ostomy site and after reanastomosis in the perianal area due to diarrhea. Speech involvement is important to provide appropriate oral stimulation. Vitamin replacement and other medications may be required if steatorrhea, persistent diarrhea, or bacterial overgrowth is present.
- When medical management fails, surgical bowel-lengthening procedures to increase intestinal surface area or to decrease motility may be attempted. Small bowel transplant is considered when other surgical procedures fail and the patient cannot attain enteral autonomy.
- Following surgery, the remaining bowel will over 1 to 2 years make adaptive changes that lead to increased digestion and absorption of nutrients. Initially, the proximal bowel dilates to increase the mucosal surface area for absorption. In addition, there is increased crypt depth, increased villous height, and an increase in the number of enterocytes to allow for mucosal hyperplasia. This period of adaptation may continue over several years.

Table 21.3 Implications of Intestinal Loss

Area of Intestine	Function	Complications Associated With Loss
Jejunum	Digestion and absorption	Nutritional deficiencies, steatorrhea, cholestasis
Ileum	Absorption of fat-soluble vitamins, vitamin B_{12}, and bile salts	Metabolic and nutritional consequences

Adaptation occurs less in the jejunum compared with the ileum. However, other areas of the intestine can perform the functions lost by the jejunum; therefore, these infants tend to do better than infants with loss of the ileum (Table 21.3).

- The past decade has demonstrated significant improvements in long-term survival of children with SBS. These improvements are multifactorial and include improved delivery of PN, prevention of infection, and innovative bowel-lengthening techniques.
  - Survival is possible with as little as 15-cm small bowel with an intact ileocecal valve or with 30- to 45-cm small bowel with absence of the ileocecal valve. Eventual tolerance of full feeds is possible with as little as 25-cm small bowel with an intact ileocecal valve or with more than 40 cm bowel and no ileocecal valve (Bradshaw, 2021; Ditzenberger, 2018; Javid et al., 2018).

▶ OTHER CONCERNS INVOLVING THE GASTROINTESTINAL TRACT

INGUINAL HERNIA

Definition and Pathophysiology

- Inguinal hernia is bulging of the intra-abdominal contents through the normal internal and external ring openings of the abdominal wall muscles in the groin.
  - If only fluid protrudes through the opening, it is a hydrocele.
- Inguinal hernia occurs when the tunica vaginalis and the peritoneal cavity fail to close, resulting in a persistent processus vaginalis.
- Inguinal hernias occur more commonly in preterm, small-for-gestational age, and male infants. It occurs more frequently on the right side compared with the left; however, it can also be bilateral (Dingeldein, 2020b; Ledbetter et al., 2018; Ringer & Hansen, 2017).

Diagnosis

- Clinical presentation of inguinal hernias includes a bulge in the groin that can extend into the scrotum in males or labia in females. Hydroceles can be differentiated by transillumination of the scrotal sac and inability to be reduced (Draus & Ruzic, 2020b; Ledbetter et al., 2018).

Management and Outcome

- Surgery is indicated if the hernia contents become strangulated or prior to discharge as these do not spontaneously heal but get larger over time.
  - With strangulation (incarceration), sedation to relax infant with steady firm pressure and elevation of feet may reduce the hernia back into the abdomen; once edema has resolved, surgery should be done promptly.
  - Hydroceles usually resolve by 1 year of age if they are present at birth; hydroceles that persist after this time should be surgically repaired.
- Prognosis is excellent if not incarcerated. The most common complication postoperatively is apnea (Dingeldein, 2020b; Draus & Ruzic, 2020b; Ledbetter et al., 2018; Ringer & Hansen, 2017).

GASTROESOPHAGEAL REFLUX

Definition and Pathophysiology

- GER is the physiologic movement of gastric contents up into the esophagus, with or without regurgitation. Gastroesophageal reflux disease (GERD) is the pathologic passage of those gastric contents into the esophagus that is associated with failure to grow, a variety of significant symptoms, and complications such as respiratory distress or esophagitis.
- There are several factors in the neonate and infant correlated with reflux, including a shorter and narrower esophagus, relaxation of the lower esophageal segment, delayed esophageal clearance, excessive air in the stomach, delayed gastric emptying, and/or decreased esophageal motility.
  - The lower esophageal segment forms a pressure barrier between the esophagus and the stomach, and in the neonate is positioned primarily above the diaphragm, allowing reflux to occur.
- It is more common in preterm than term infants, in infants with neurologic or GI disorders, in infants with BPD, or as adverse effect of some medications such as methylxanthines (Bradshaw, 2021; Ditzenberger, 2018; Hibbs, 2020; Richards & Goldin, 2018).

Diagnosis

- Clinical presentation includes feeding difficulties, fussiness or irritability, or back arching. It is important to rule out other underlying causes of these symptoms, such as cow's milk protein allergy, neurologic disorders, excessive gassiness, or constipation.
- Diagnosis is most often based on physical symptoms.
  - Upper GI series may miss reflux events since they can be transient (false negative).
  - Esophageal pH probe studies do not detect nonacid reflux, which is more common in neonates due to milk-based diet.

- Endoscopy is helpful in identifying esophageal erosion (Bradshaw, 2021; Hibbs, 2020; Richards et al., 2018).

Management and Outcome

- Medical management strategies include elevating the head of the bed at least 45 degrees and trying to keep upright for 30 minutes after feedings, positioning prone or in lateral position if there is severe reflux or administering gavage feedings over a longer time period, small frequent feeds if oral feeding, frequent burping, and thickening of feeds.
- There are currently no approved U.S. Food and Drug Administration (FDA) medications for pharmacologic management of GER in infants. None of the medications commonly used to treat GERD in the NICU have been demonstrated to be safe and effective, and many have the potential to cause harm.
  - Medications that have been trialed, such as metoclopramide, a prokinetic, have been associated with significant adverse reactions and should not be used. PPIs in the infant with documented esophagitis may be trialed and if no improvement in irritability should be discontinued.
- When conservative and pharmacologic management fails and the infant develops consequences from GERD, such as strictures, erosive esophagitis, failure to thrive, aspiration, recurrent pneumonia, wheezing, and asthma, the most common surgical procedure considered is Nissen fundoplication.
- Prognosis is good as it typically self-resolves in majority of infants by 1 to 1½ years of age. A small percentage of infants require prolonged medical management or even surgery.
  - In infants with GERD, morbidity includes worsening of BPD, aspiration, esophagitis, strictures, and failure to thrive (Anderson et al., 2017; Bradshaw, 2021; Ditzenberger, 2018; Hibbs, 2020; Parad & Benjamin, 2017; Richards & Goldin, 2018).

▶ CONCLUSION

GI obstructions are one GI disorder that may be seen in the neonate and can occur anywhere from the esophagus to the anus. Most GI obstructions are not considered surgical emergencies except for malrotation with volvulus. It is often difficult to differentiate between the different disorders; however, a thorough history and physical examination may help guide the diagnostic workup.

1. The classic x-ray finding in an infant with duodenal stenosis is a dilated stomach and dilated duodenum (double bubble) with:

   A. Air visible past the dilated duodenum
   B. Included dilation of the proximal jejunum
   C. No air visible past the dilated duodenum

2. The neonatal nurse practitioner (NNP) identifies the expected increase in intestinal length during gestation is:

   A. 25-fold
   B. 50-fold
   C. 100-fold

3. The neonatal nurse practitioner (NNP) assesses a 14-hour-old, 38.6-week estimated gestational age infant for increasing respiratory distress. During the exam, the NNP notices the infant has mucousy oral secretions with occasional cough, respiratory rate of 76 with no grunting or nasal flaring, and an abdomen with scaphoid appearance. On further discussion with the mother, it was reported that the baby seems to be drooling a lot because the mother's chest keeps getting wet during skin-to-skin. The NNP lists at the top of the differential diagnosis a/an:

   A. Congenital diaphragmatic hernia
   B. Esophageal atresia with tracheoesophageal fistula
   C. Malrotation with midgut volvulus

4. During physiologic herniation of the intestine during the sixth week of gestation and then the return of the intestines into the abdominal cavity during the 10th week, the normal total rotation of the intestines is:

   A. 90 degrees
   B. 180 degrees
   C. 270 degrees

5. The neonatal nurse practitioner (NNP) cares for a 37.6-week estimated gestational age (EGA) infant who had surgical repair of an esophageal atresia and ligation of a tracheoesophageal fistula done 7 days ago. The infant has a Replogle to continuous low suction with minimal clear mucous drainage for the past 24 hours and a chest tube that continues to have 5- to 10-mL drainage every day. The NNP realizes these findings suggest a/an:

   A. Leak of the anastomosis site
   B. Normal postoperative course
   C. Return of normal bowel function

6. The neonatal nurse practitioner (NNP) examines a 28-hour-old, 35.6-week late preterm infant who has not stooled since delivery. The maternal history reveals polyhydramnios noted at the time of delivery. The NNP knows the best diagnostic study for diagnosis of gastrointestinal (GI) disorder in this infant is a/an:

   A. Abdominal x-ray
   B. Contrast enema
   C. Upper GI scan

7. A term infant born to a mother with gestational diabetes that required insulin had no stool at 48 hours, with increased abdominal distention. A contrast enema was done with evacuation of a meconium plug. The neonatal nurse practitioner (NNP) updates the parents on the prognosis and focuses the conversation on the fact that:

   A. Further diagnostic studies are not needed as long as normal stooling patterns persist
   B. Meconium ileus is associated with cystic fibrosis and diagnostic workup is warranted
   C. Stooling issues will persist throughout infancy and the parents need to learn rectal irrigations

(See answers next page.)   **379**

1. A) Air visible past the dilated duodenum

The x-ray of an infant with duodenal atresia or double stenosis is similar to the classic "double bubble." The distinguishing difference is the absence or presence of air beyond the dilated duodenum; with an atresia, there is no air as the intestinal lumen is not continuous, whereas with a stenosis the intestinal lumen is narrowed, allowing air to continue to pass (Bradshaw, 2021; Gallagher et al., 2021; Ringer & Hansen, 2017; Trotter, 2021).

2. C) 100-fold

The intestinal length increases 100-fold during gestation, with doubling in length in the last trimester (Bradshaw, 2021). This is important to keep in mind as a 24-week gestational age preterm infant who loses 25 cm of intestinal length will have much less absorptive properties compared with a 40-week gestational age term infant who loses 25 cm of intestinal length.

3. B) Esophageal atresia with tracheoesophageal fistula

Based on clinical presentation and x-ray findings, this infant most likely has an esophageal atresia (EA) with a proximal tracheoesophageal fistula (TEF). Infants who are exclusively breastfed may not present as clearly due to limited volumes of human milk/colostrum on the first day of life. The finding of "drooling a lot" is concerning for the infant being unable to clear oral secretions related to immaturity, an obstruction, or neurologic disorder. The additional respiratory findings are concerning as the infant is aspirating the oral secretions. On x-ray, the gasless abdomen suggests that there is no air passing from the mouth to the stomach and intestines. All of these point to EA with proximal TEF (Bradshaw, 2021; Gallagher et al., 2021; Flynn-O'Brien et al., 2018).

4. C) 270 degrees

Complete intestinal rotation is 270 degrees; the midgut rotates 90 degrees counterclockwise during herniation into the umbilical cord, and as the intestines return to the abdominal cavity there is an additional 180-degree counterclockwise rotation (Ditzenberger, 2018; Gallagher et al., 2021).

5. A) Leak of the anastomosis site

The continued presence of chest tube drainage is concerning for leakage at the esophageal anastomosis site and needs to be further evaluated by surgery prior to starting feeds. Postoperatively after gastrointestinal (GI) surgery, the Replogle will have high drainage output that is often bilious, and as bowel function resumes the volume of drainage will become less and become more clear, supporting that feeds can be started with close observation as long as no other problems are present (Bradshaw, 2021; Flynn-O'Brien et al., 2018; Gallagher et al., 2021; Ringer & Hansen, 2017).

6. B) Contrast enema

A contrast enema is the gold standard for diagnosis of bowel obstructions as the contrast material will not reflect the area where the obstruction occurs. The other radiographic studies listed will not provide definitive evidence and an enema would need to be done regardless. In this case, the infant has jejunoileal atresia and the contrast study would reflect a microcolon with no reflux into the proximal bowel as a result of the atresia (Gallagher et al., 2021).

7. A) Further diagnostic studies are not needed as long as normal stooling patterns persist

Based on the history of maternal diabetes, which can be associated with decreased bowel motility and lead to a meconium plug, the clinical presentation, and the evacuation of this via contrast enema, it would be anticipated that this infant will have normal stooling patterns and that no further interventions or workup will be required. If this infant had abnormal stooling patterns after the contrast enema, further evaluation is warranted to rule out cystic fibrosis, which is associated with meconium ileus or Hirschsprung disease, which can be medically managed with rectal irrigations (Bradshaw, 2021; Dingeldein, 2020b; Gallagher et al., 2021; Ringer & Hansen, 2017).

The Renal and Genitourinary System

Cheryl A. Carlson and Lori Baas Rubarth

▶ INTRODUCTION

In the past 30 years, the field of neonatal nephrology has expanded in conjunction with that of neonatology, influenced by the development of therapies and interventions to promote survival among the smallest of infants. The use of prenatal ultrasounds has created new paradigms for prenatal management of renal tract anomalies. The improved survival of infants who develop significant chronic lung disease has led to new renal-focused complications (Bates & Schwaderer, 2018; Engen & Hingorani, 2018).

Acute kidney injury (AKI) has supplanted the term *acute renal failure* as the accepted terminology to describe acute changes in renal function across medicine, including neonatology. Currently, the Kidney Disease: Improving Global Outcomes (KDIGO) defines AKI, and a neonatal classification of AKI parallels the KDIGO adult definition (Askenazi et al., 2018; Cadnapaphornchai et al., 2021; Kogon & Truong, 2020; McEwen & Vogt, 2020; Samuels et al., 2017; Vogt & Springel, 2020). This chapter provides a brief review of the embryology, physiology, and pathophysiology of the renal system.

▶ ANATOMY AND PHYSIOLOGY

KIDNEY

- The kidney is located in the retroperitoneal space on both sides of the vertebral column. The kidney is approximately 4.0 to 5.0 cm in length in a full-term infant; the length is related to gestational age in millimeters.
- The kidney develops from the pronephros, mesonephros, and metanephros into the true kidney, which begins functioning at about 9 to 10 weeks of gestation. Nephrogenesis, the process of nephron formation, is complete by about 34 to 36 weeks of gestation, with the critical development time between 31 and 36 weeks. Once nephrogenesis is complete, the kidney contains 800,000 to 1.2 million nephrons and there is only growth of individual nephrons after completion of nephrogenesis.
  - The metanephros' origins are in the pelvis and then ascends to the abdomen between the fifth and ninth week of gestation.
- The nephron is the functional unit of the kidney, with each kidney containing a glomerulus, renal tubules, and the collecting system.
  - The glomerulus lies within the Bowman's capsule and filters plasma, allowing nonprotein components of the plasma to pass into the Bowman's capsule and then into the renal tubule system.
  - The renal tubular system is a plasma filtration system.
    - ❏ The proximal tubules lie in the cortex of the kidney and continue to become the loop of Henle, which descends into the renal medulla making a loop and ascending back into the cortex.
    - ❏ The distal convoluted tubule joins nephrons to form the collecting tubules and the collecting duct. The tubules and the loop continue to grow after birth.
- Renal blood flow (RBF) is dependent on cardiac output. Renal arteries come off the aorta at L1 to L2.
- Circulation of the nephrons is supported by two capillary beds: the afferent arterioles that supply oxygenated blood to the glomerulus and the efferent arterioles that drain blood unable to enter the Bowman's capsule, continuing to form the peritubular capillary system.
  - The peritubular capillary system follows along the renal tubular system, allowing for the specific functions of the tubular system. Venous blood leaves the kidneys through the renal veins, emptying into the inferior vena cava (IVC).
- Bladder formation begins between 4 and 6 weeks of gestation. The ureters go from the kidneys to the bladder and are functionally open at about 9 weeks of gestation. The urethra's development is complete by 12 to 13 weeks of gestation.
- The glomerular filtration rate (GFR) is the amount of filtrate formed within the glomerulus each minute.

- The GFR is calculated using serum and urinary creatinine levels. The GFR is low in utero and increases initially due to increases in glomerular perfusion pressure, after which the increase in GFR is related to the increase in RBF.
- The major determinant of GFR is blood pressure in the peritubular capillary system. Other factors that influence the GFR are (a) hydrostatic pressure in the glomerular capillaries and Bowman's capsule and (b) the colloid osmotic pressure within the capillaries (Blackburn, 2018; Cadnapaphornchai et al., 2021; Cavaliere, 2019; Engen & Hingorani, 2018; McAleer, 2018; McEwen & Vogt 2020; Merguerian & Rowe, 2018; Samuels et al., 2017; Vogt & Springel, 2020).

RENAL TUBULES

- *Filtration* is the process where the plasma filtrated from the vascular space in the afferent arterioles into the Bowman's capsule forms filtrate in the renal tubules in the glomerulus.
- *Reabsorption* is the movement of substances from the renal tubules across the tubular epithelium into the peritubular capillaries.
- *Secretion* is the movement of substances from the peritubular capillaries across the tubular epithelium into the renal tubules.
- *Excretion* is the loss of metabolic wastes and toxins, as well as the fluid that makes up urine. Substances such as urea, creatinine, uric acid, urates, and toxins are filtered in the glomerulus and not reabsorbed, allowing for their excretion in the urine (Blackburn, 2018; Maguire, 2021).

TUBULAR FUNCTION

- Proximal tubules are reabsorptive generally and will reabsorb water, sodium, potassium glucose, amino acids, bicarbonate, phosphorous, magnesium, chloride, and calcium. Substances such as organic acids and hydrogen (H^+) ions are secreted.
- Distal convoluted tubules secrete potassium and H^+ ions, with water reabsorption in the presence of arginine vasopressin. Reabsorption of sodium is variable and dependent on the presence of aldosterone.
- The loop of Henle and the collecting ducts dilute or concentrate urine. Preterm infants have a decreased ability to concentrate urine and respond to a fluid load (Maguire, 2021; Vogt & Springel, 2020).

URINE FORMATION

- Formed from filtrate in the Bowman's capsule
- Movement of substances between the tubular lumens and the plasma in the peritubular capillaries
- RBF and GFR affect function of the renal tubules (Cadnapaphornchai et al., 2021; Maguire, 2021)

HORMONAL REGULATION

- The kidney is responsible for maintaining both systemic blood pressure and RBF.
- Autoregulation of RBF is accomplished through the vasorelaxation and vasoconstriction of the afferent and efferent arterioles to maintain a constant blood supply to the kidneys, despite variations in systemic blood pressure (hypotension or hypertension).
  - It is regulated by the renin–angiotensin–aldosterone–antidiuretic hormone (ADH) system and atrial and B natriuretic factors.
  - Other vasoreactive factors affecting RBF include endothelin, nitric oxide, and prostaglandins.
- Renal perfusion is measured indirectly by monitoring the concentration of sodium chloride by the macula densa cells in the ascending loop of Henle.
  - A decrease in sodium chloride will cause a relaxation of the afferent arteriole, allowing for increased blood flow into the glomerulus.
  - The macula densa cells will stimulate the juxtaglomerular cells, located in the afferent and efferent arterioles.
  - This will release renin, activating the renin–angiotensin–aldosterone–ADH system.

THE RENIN–ANGIOTENSIN–ALDOSTERONE–ANTIDIURETIC HORMONE SYSTEM

- The goal is to maintain adequate renal perfusion and blood flow to vital organs by increasing sodium chloride and water reabsorption by the peritubular capillaries to increase intravascular volume, increasing cardiac output and blood pressure.
- *Renin* is released in response to decreased RBF and will convert angiotensinogen released from the liver to angiotensin I.
- *Angiotensin I* will undergo further conversion to angiotensin II in the lungs and renal endothelium under the actions of the angiotensin-converting enzyme (ACE).
- *Angiotensin II* is a potent vasoconstrictor of peripheral blood vessels and the efferent arteriole that increases tubular sodium, chloride, and water reabsorption in the renal tubules.
- *Aldosterone*, a mineral–corticoid hormone, is released by the adrenal cortex in response to angiotensin II, adrenocorticotrophic hormone, or hyperkalemia. Aldosterone increases intravascular volume through sodium, chloride, and water reabsorption and excretion of potassium and H^+ ion.
- *Arginine vasopressin* or *ADH* is produced in the hypothalamus, stored in the posterior pituitary, and released in response to decreased intravascular volume or an increase in plasma osmolality and angiotensin II.
  - Arginine vasopressin increases the permeability of the collecting ducts to water and allows increased

water reabsorption into the peritubular capillaries, increasing intravascular volume.

- *Atrial natriuretic protein (ANP)* and *B natriuretic protein (BNP)* reverse the renin–angiotensin–aldosterone–ADH system.
  - ANP is secreted by the cardiac atria myocytes in response to increased intravascular volume; BNP is released in response to left ventricular dilation. It acts by decreasing renin level, decreasing conversion of angiotensin I to angiotensin II, and decreasing release of aldosterone.
  - Overall effects are peripheral vasodilation, decreased blood pressure, decreased intravascular volume, and increase in diuresis (Maguire 2021; McAleer, 2018).

▶ MAJOR FUNCTIONS OF THE KIDNEY

- At birth, the kidneys become the major homeostatic organs, replacing the placenta in functions such as:
  - Removal of metabolic wastes
  - Regulation of fluid volume and electrolyte composition
  - Acid–base homeostasis
  - Kidneys will release the nonvolatile acids produced from the metabolism of proteins to maintain acid–base homeostasis. In the presence of acidosis, the kidneys will secrete H^+ ions and reabsorb filtered bicarbonate ions. In the presence of alkalosis, the tubules will reabsorb H^+ ions.
  - Regulation of blood pressure
  - Regulation of red blood cell production through release of erythropoietin, a hormone that stimulates the production of erythrocytes by the bone marrow
  - Regulation of calcium, phosphorous, and magnesium homeostasis through metabolism of vitamin D into active metabolite (Maguire, 2021; Samuels et al., 2017)

NEWBORN RENAL FUNCTION

- There are gestational age differences in renal function due to tubular developmental and functional maturity at birth. Premature infants will have decreased renal function until nephrogenesis is complete. Renal function will improve with an increase in RBF, GFR, and tubular function due to postnatal transition in all infants, in spite of gestational age at birth.
- Asphyxia or ischemic damage may occur prenatally, during birth, or after birth, further affecting renal function.
- The following are overall differences in newborn and adult kidney function:
  - Decreased RBF in the neonate
  - Reduced GFR, especially in preterm infants <34 weeks' gestation due to immature renal development and function, and incomplete nephrogenesis

- Reduced ability to excrete fluid and solute
- Altered tubular function in term infants after birth
- Decreased response of renal tubules to aldosterone, especially in preterm infants (Blackburn, 2018; McAleer, 2018)

▶ ASSESSMENT OF INFANTS WITH ABNORMAL KIDNEY FUNCTION

FAMILY AND PRENATAL HISTORY

- Family history of renal disorders includes urinary tract abnormalities, polycystic kidney disease (PKD), or familial diseases such as autosomal recessive polycystic kidney disease (ARPKD) or congenital nephrotic syndrome. Prenatal ultrasound can be used to evaluate fetal kidney and urinary tract.
- Prenatal history includes maternal disease state, medications during pregnancy and labor, amniotic fluid volume, and prenatal ultrasound.
  - Elevated maternal serum or amniotic alpha-fetoprotein levels may indicate obstructive uropathy, renal agenesis, or congenital nephrotic syndrome.
  - Oligohydramnios can be associated with decreased fetal urine output (UOP), renal agenesis, dysplasia, PKD, or urinary tract obstruction.
  - Polyhydramnios may be due to renal tubular dysfunction and decreased ability to concentrate urine.
  - Maternal use of ACE inhibitors, indomethacin (nonsteroidal anti-inflammatory drugs [NSAIDs]), or angiotensin receptor blockers will affect renal capillary pressure, leading to a decrease in GFR.
  - Perinatal asphyxia/depression during or after delivery is associated with hypoxic or ischemic damage to the kidneys (Askenazi et al., 2018; Cadnapaphornchai et al., 2021; Gomella, 2020; Vogt & Springel, 2020).

PHYSICAL ASSESSMENT

- Although lower urinary tract and renal anomalies are seldom the presenting features of chromosomal disorders, they frequently form part of a multisystem malformation syndrome.
- Renal disorders seen with chromosomal disturbance can include fused kidneys, duplication defects, renal agenesis or hypoplasia, hydronephrosis and hydroureter, renal dysplasia or cystic disease, hypospadias, micropenis, and cryptorchidism.
- Other findings include:
  - Presence of abdominal mass on examination
  - Abdominal wall defects
  - Abnormal facies, ear malformations
  - Abnormal genitalia

- Hypospadias/epispadias
- Single umbilical artery
- Palpation of bladder
- Vital signs to note are:
  - Signs of volume depletion or volume overload
  - Heart rate and blood pressure
  - UOP
  - Voiding in the first 24 hours in approximately 90% of newborns and 99% by 48 hours of age
  - Range of urine formation 0.5 to 5 mL/kg/hr
  - Presence of edema
  - Total fluid intake, including medications and flush volume (Cadnapaphornchai et al., 2021; Cavaliere, 2019; Gomella, 2020)

LABORATORY ASSESSMENT

- Serum electrolytes:
  - Blood urea nitrogen (BUN) may be elevated in AKI or in hypercatabolic states or with increased protein intake (BUN >29 mg/dL or increase of 1 mg/dL/d).
  - Creatinine is initially reflective of maternal renal function and depending on gestational age will either remain the same and then decrease as kidneys mature. An increase in serum creatinine is suggestive of renal dysfunction (creatinine >1.5 mg/dL or increase of >0.2 mg/dL/d).
    - Preterm infants will often have increased creatinine levels over the first week of life due to decreased GFR.
  - BUN-to-creatinine ratio:
    - *Prerenal azotemia:* disproportionate rise
    - *Intrinsic AKI:* proportionate rise
  - Sodium may be decreased due to fluid overload from decreased UOP or loss of sodium in the urine.
  - Potassium is often elevated in AKI due to decreased renal excretion.
  - Calcium and phosphorous levels may be abnormal due to renal tubular dysfunction.
- Complete blood count and differential to evaluate for sepsis
- Urinalysis and culture
- Urine electrolytes if significant serum electrolyte abnormalities
- Serum albumin
- Renal and bladder ultrasound
- Urinalysis
  - Specific gravity should be about 1.021 to 1.025 in full-term infants due to limited concentrating ability.
  - Protein excretion will vary with gestational age and is higher in preterm infants <34 weeks' gestation. In term infants, protein excretion after 2 weeks of life is minimal. If present, it is associated with damage to the glomerulus.
  - Glycosuria is common in preterm infants <34 weeks due to decreased tubular resorption of glucose in infants that is increased with lower gestational ages.
  - Hematuria is an abnormal presentation and may indicate intrinsic kidney injury due to acute tubular necrosis (ATN).
- Calculation of fractional excretion of sodium (FENa; %):
  - The amount of urinary sodium excretion is the percentage of the filtered sodium, reflecting the balance between glomerular filtration and tubular reabsorption of sodium.
  - FENa (%) = (urine Na × plasma creatinine)/plasma Na × urine creatinine) × 100%
    - FENa >3.0% is indicative of intrinsic renal injury.
    - FENa <2.5% is indicative of prerenal injury.
    - FENa values are not helpful in preterm infants less than 32 weeks' gestation due to normal baseline values being as high as 6%, and may be as high as 15% in very low birthweight (VLBW) infants during the first week of life and decreases by 1 month of age (Askenazi et al., 2018; Cadnapaphornchai et al., 2021; Doherty, 2017; Gomella, 2020; McEwen & Vogt, 2020; Samuels et al., 2017; Vogt & Springel, 2020).

NEPHROTOXICITY

- Nephrotoxic drugs can damage the kidney of the fetus or the newborn infant. Drugs that cross the placenta and may damage the kidney are heavy metals (e.g., lead and mercury), organic solvents (such as toluene), and phthalates. Alcohol intake by the mother can cause fetal alcohol syndrome (FAS), which involves the kidney.
- Drugs given to the neonate may also damage the kidney. A recent study found 87% of the cohort were exposed to at least one nephrotoxic medication, and on average these neonates were exposed to over 14 days of nephrotoxic medications. The following are drugs used to treat the infant in the NICU that may affect renal functions:
  - Aminoglycosides, amphotericin B (Fungizone), cephalosporins, radiocontrast agents, rifampin (Rifadin), and vancomycin (Vancocin), all of which cause direct tubular damage
  - ACE inhibitors, diuretics, and indomethacin (Indocin), which result in decreased renal perfusion and direct tubular damage
  - Acyclovir (Zovirax), which can result in tubular obstruction and decreased GFR
- Nephrotoxicity may manifest clinically as nonoliguric renal failure, with a slow rise in serum creatinine and hypo-osmolar urine. Other alterations may include proteinuria and increase in BUN (Askenazi et al., 2018; Bennett & Meier, 2019; LaBronte, 2019).

▶ ACUTE KIDNEY INJURY

DEFINITION AND PATHOPHYSIOLOGY

- AKI is characterized by an abrupt decline in renal function, which manifests as a decrease in GFR, increase in serum creatinine, accumulation of nitrogenous waste products, and deranged fluid and electrolyte homeostasis.
- The most common cause of AKI in neonates is related to hypoperfusion or decreased blood flow to the kidney. This may be a result of neonatal asphyxia, causing both anoxic and ischemic damage to the kidney, blood loss, fluid loss from intravascular compartment due to sepsis or third space losses, dehydration, or shock. Tubular function and reabsorption are intact in most cases of prerenal azotemia.
- Incidence ranges from 8% to 24%; however, known risk factors include:
  - VLBW and extremely low birth weight (ELBW)
  - Low 5-minute Apgar score
  - Maternal medications, especially antibiotics and NSAIDs
  - Intubation at birth
  - Respiratory distress syndrome (RDS)
  - Patent ductus arteriosus (PDA)
  - Phototherapy
  - Neonatal drug administration (NSAIDs, antibiotics, and diuretics)
  - Congenital diaphragmatic hernia
  - Extracorporeal membrane oxygenation
- There are many causes of AKI in the newborn. It is helpful to classify these etiologies as prerenal, intrinsic renal, and postrenal (obstructive).

Prerenal

- Prerenal azotemia occurs in response to decreased RBF and accounts for up to 85% of AKI. The kidney remains intrinsically normal. Potential causes of renal hypoperfusion include:
  - Hypotension/hypoperfusion
  - Congestive heart failure
  - Respiratory distress/hypoxia
  - Dehydration
  - Hypoalbuminemia
  - Nephrotoxic medications such as ACE inhibitors, intrauterine exposure to NSAIDs, Cyclooxygenase-2 (COX-2) inhibitors, angiotensin receptor antagonists, aminoglycosides
- When low RBF occurs, renal autoregulation preserves GFR by increasing renal sympathetic tone, activation of the renin–angiotensin–aldosterone system, and increased activation of hormones such as vasopressin and endothelin. Renal hemodynamic changes lead to a decrease in water and sodium losses, to maintain systemic volume expansion and blood pressure.
- Once parenchymal damage occurs, renal tubular cell damage (ATN) occurs even if renal perfusion is restored.

Intrinsic

- Intrinsic renal injury is often considered synonymous with ATN and includes both tubular and vascular lesions. This may result as a prolongation of prerenal causes of renal injury, ischemic injury, or injury as a result of obstructive causes of renal injury. Causes would include:
  - Perinatal asphyxia (associated with intrinsic renal failure in approximately 40% of affected term neonates)
  - Congenital abnormalities
  - Inflammation/infection due to congenital viral or yeast infections
  - Vascular/ischemia hypoperfusion such as aortic or artery thrombosis
  - Nephrotoxic medications either in utero or postnatal administration
  - ATN, which may be due to perinatal asphyxia or secondary to nephrotoxic medications and is the most common cause of intrinsic kidney injury
- Intrinsic damage can be divided into several phases, which is helpful in the diagnosis, management, and prognosis of the disorder. These are early, initiation, maintenance, and recovery phases.
  - *Early (prerenal) phase:* This phase may be associated with hypoperfusion of the kidney due to prerenal causes.
  - *Initiation phase:* This phase includes the initial insult and the effect on the GFR.
  - *Maintenance phase:* Tubular dysfunction and low GFR are seen in the maintenance phase and the duration will depend on the extent and duration of the initial insult.
  - *Recovery phase:* This phase can take months, during which there is a gradual improvement in GFR and tubular function.

Postrenal

- Postrenal AKI is primarily due to obstructive kidney dysfunction occurring in utero secondary to congenital malformations, although postnatal causes include renal calculi or fungal balls. Depending on the cause and associated damage to the kidneys, relief of the obstruction will markedly improve renal function. Other causes include:
  - Posterior urethral valves (PUVs)
  - Bilateral ureteropelvic junction obstruction (UPJO)
  - Bilateral ureterovesical junction obstruction
  - Neurogenic bladder
  - Obstructive nephrolithiasis

DIAGNOSIS

■ Diagnosing AKI in the neonate is difficult due to the physiologic differences in neonatal renal function which complicate the interpretation of serum creatinine and UOP. Serum creatinine reflects maternal creatinine for the first 48 to 72 hours of life (longer in preterm infants), and thereafter its concentration is dependent on lean body mass, which is low in the neonate.

- A neonatal classification of AKI used to define AKI in critically ill neonates uses the lowest serum creatinine (SCr) as a baseline for subsequent SCr values. National guidelines define AKI when there is a rise in SCr of 0.3 mg/dL over 48 hours or a decrease in UOP. These criteria define neonatal AKI in infants under 120 days of age as an increase in serum creatinine of 0.3 mg/dL (or higher) or 50% or more from the previous lowest value and/or UOP less than 0.5 mL/kg/hr. Three stages of neonatal AKI are defined by relative changes in serum creatinine from baseline.
- The modified neonatal KDIGO criteria provide the current and most accepted definition of AKI in neonates.

■ A careful history should focus on prenatal ultrasound abnormalities, history of perinatal asphyxia, pre- or postnatal administration of nephrotoxic medications, and a family history of kidney disease.

■ The physical examination should focus on signs of volume depletion or volume overload, the abdomen, and the genitalia, and a search for other congenital anomalies or signs of oligohydramnios (Potter) syndrome.

- Decrease in body weight, tachycardia, dry mucous membranes, poor skin turgor, flattened anterior fontanel, and elevation in serum sodium can be seen in those with low intravascular volumes.

■ Laboratory evaluation may include electrolytes, BUN, creatinine, calcium, phosphorus, albumin, and uric acid. Urine should be sent for urinalysis, culture (when the etiology is unclear), and sodium and creatinine levels. Laboratory markers of prerenal azotemia include low urinary sodium excretion, low FENa, low renal failure index, and high BUN-to-SCr ratio.

- Elevated serum creatinine
- Hyperkalemia, defined as a serum level obtained by a central sample that is >6 to 6.5 mEq/L
- Metabolic acidosis, which may develop acutely in severe AKI due to decreased tubular reabsorption of bicarbonate and decreased excretion of H^+ ion
- Hypocalcemia, which may be a result of increased calcium deposition in injured tissues, resistance to parathyroid hormone (PTH) and skeletal release of calcium, due to decrease in vitamin D metabolism in injured kidney; also seen in nephrotoxic AKI especially due to aminoglycoside toxicity; associated with hyperphosphatemia

- Hypomagnesemia, which may be a result of tubular loss; can also cause abnormal parathyroid activity
- Hyperphosphatemia
- Prolonged half-life for renally excreted medications

■ Newer diagnostic techniques will lead to quicker identification of kidney injury and differentiate between functional and/or structural damage. Renal ultrasound should be completed to assess the presence of urine in the bladder, RBF, and presence of obstruction to UOP (Askenazi et al., 2018; Cadnapaphornchai et al., 2021; Gomella, 2020; Kogon & Truong, 2020; McEwen & Vogt, 2020; Samuels et al., 2017; Vogt & Springel, 2020).

MANAGEMENT AND OUTCOME

■ Initial management for prerenal kidney injury is a fluid challenge with an isotonic solution such as normal saline of 10 to 20 mL/kg over 30 minutes to replace intravascular volume and determine intravascular fluid loss.

■ Fluid management should be based on individual infants' fluid and electrolyte status: fluid restriction with low-output renal injury and fluid replacement with high-output renal injury.

■ Electrolyte supplementation is based on individual needs.

- Supplementation of electrolytes is dependent on serum and urine electrolytes during high-output phase. No additional potassium, magnesium, or phosphate should be added during oliguric phase due to tubular dysfunction.

■ Use of low-dose dopamine may increase RBF but has not been shown to improve overall survival.

■ Avoid nephrotoxic drugs and follow serum drug levels in those with kidney injury if these drugs are used (e.g., gentamicin, vancomycin).

■ Furosemide for fluid overload may be helpful, but it has not been shown to prevent or change the course of AKI.

■ Dialysis is indicated if tubular damage results in an inability to appropriately balance potassium and other electrolytes.

- Peritoneal dialysis requires placement of peritoneal catheter and is most commonly used in neonates due to the large area for dialysate insertion and no need for vascular access or use of anticoagulation.
- Hemodialysis or continuous renal replacement therapy (CRRT) requires vascular access using large-diameter catheters placed in the internal jugular or femoral vein. The extracorporeal circuit requires reliable vascular access and frequent monitoring of anticoagulants and temperature, and carries the risk of rapid fluid shifts. It has limited use in infants weighing less than 2.5 kg. Management includes access, frequent monitoring

of anticoagulants and temperature, and risk of rapid fluid shift.

■ Prompt recognition and treatment will improve prognosis. Risk of progressive renal disease and chronic kidney disease, hypertension, and renal tubular acidosis (RTA) with impairment of renal tubular growth has been recognized in long-term survivors of AKI (Askenazi et al., 2018; Cadnapaphornchai et al., 2021; Gomella, 2020; Kogon & Truong, 2020; Vogt & Springel, 2020).

PREVENTION OF ACUTE KIDNEY INJURY

■ Maintenance of circulatory volume; monitor blood pressure, heart rate, and UOP to prevent hypoperfusion of the kidney

■ Fluid and electrolyte management to follow serum electrolytes, urine electrolytes as indicated, and accurate volume intake and output

■ Prompt diagnosis and treatment of respiratory, infectious, or hemodynamic conditions

■ Monitoring of nephrotoxic medications through serum levels and avoiding use in infants at risk if possible (e.g., aminoglycoside antibiotics, indomethacin, IV contrast, diuretics; Askenazi et al., 2018; Cadnapaphornchai et al., 2021; Gomella, 2020l; Kogon & Truong, 2020; McEwen & Vogt, 2020; Samuels et al., 2017; Vogt & Springel, 2020)

▶ RENAL TUBULAR ACIDOSIS

DEFINITION AND PATHOPHYSIOLOGY

■ The kidneys excrete H^+ ion and reabsorb bicarbonate (HCO^-) ion to compensate for acidosis in the bloodstream. This disorder is the failure of the kidneys to respond and/or attempt to compensate for metabolic acidosis.

■ There are four types of RTA:
  ● *Type 1:* Distal RTA is a defect in the ability to secrete the H^+ ion.
  ● *Type 2:* Proximal RTA is a defect in the ability to reabsorb bicarbonate.
  ● *Type 3:* This is a combination of types 1 and 2.
  ● *Type 4:* Hyperkalemic tubular type is due to a problem with aldosterone, either aldosterone deficiency or aldosterone resistance, which then results in high serum potassium levels (Cadnapaphornchai et al., 2021; Maguire, 2021; Richardson & Yonekawa, 2018; Samuels et al., 2017).

DIAGNOSIS

■ Infants with RTA will have signs of polyuria and weight loss despite adequate caloric intake.

■ Serum electrolytes with anion gap, blood gas for acidosis and bicarbonate level, and urine analysis for pH should be tested when the infant is acidotic. Infants with RTA will have a normal anion gap (Richardson & Yonekawa, 2018).

MANAGEMENT AND OUTCOME

■ Treatment of infants with RTA is with sodium bicarbonate or Bicitra to correct the acidosis. Type 4 may require sodium supplementation and potassium restriction.

■ Infants with type 2 RTA may also have Fanconi anemia, and this needs to be explored.

■ Treatment may result in resolution of the symptoms and resolve the problem in some infants, but it depends on the cause of the tubular acidosis (see sections on renal dysplasia, obstruction, and hydronephrosis; Cadnapaphornchai et al., 2021; Richardson & Yonekawa, 2018; Samuels et al., 2017).

▶ BILATERAL RENAL AGENESIS (ALSO CALLED "POTTER SEQUENCE")

DEFINITION AND PATHOPHYSIOLOGY

■ Bilateral renal agenesis is the failure of renal development or the complete absence of the kidneys.

■ There is an incidence of about 1 in 3,000 or up to 10,000 births, with a slight male predominance (Cadnapaphornchai et al., 2021; Engen & Hingorani, 2018; Maguire, 2021; Samuels et al., 2017; Vogt & Springel, 2020).

DIAGNOSIS

■ Potter facies (or "squished face") is a unique appearance of the face and body of the fetus/infant due to fetal compression in utero. The infant has a flat face and a "pushed-in" or blunted nose with a depressed nasal bridge. These infants may have micrognathia or receded chin, with wide-spaced eyes, epicanthal folds, low-set or malformed ears, and wrinkled skin.

■ The diagnosis of bilateral renal agenesis can be accomplished by renal ultrasound either prenatally or after birth. The kidneys can also be evaluated using radionuclide scintigraphy (radioisotope renal scan) after birth (Bates & Schwaderer, 2018; Engen & Hingorani, 2018; Samuels et al., 2017; Vogt & Springel, 2020).

■ Table 22.1 lists the signs and symptoms of Potter sequence.

MANAGEMENT AND OUTCOME

■ Options for treatment include (a) providing comfort measures due to pulmonary hypoplasia and poor outcome; (b) peritoneal dialysis if pulmonary hypoplasia is not severe; and/or (c) renal transplant, which can be considered if death does not occur within the first few days of life.

Table 22.1 Clinical Presentation of Potter Sequence

Prenatal	Newborn
■ Oligohydramnios ■ Breech position (more common) ■ Intrauterine growth restriction ■ Fetal compression	■ Anuria or oliguria ■ Potter facies or "squished face" ■ Abnormal genital development ■ Leg deformities ■ GI defects ■ Broad, flat hands ■ Contractures ■ Respiratory distress due to pulmonary hypoplasia ■ No kidneys on palpation

GI, gastrointestinal.

- The mortality rate is almost always 100%, incompatible with life, due to lack of kidney function, resulting in pulmonary hypoplasia. Most infants die within 24 to 48 hours after birth and the stillborn rate is about 40%.

- Due to the compression of the fetus and oligohydramnios, the infant's lungs are hypoplastic, causing respiratory failure. With early ventilation and stiff lungs, the infant can develop pneumothorax. Acute renal failure occurs due to lack of kidney development or complete agenesis (Engen & Hingorani, 2018; Maguire, 2021; Samuels et al., 2017).

▶ POLYCYSTIC KIDNEY DISEASE

DEFINITION AND PATHOPHYSIOLOGY

- PKD is an autosomal recessive cystic kidney disorder which usually occurs in both kidneys soon after birth. The autosomal recessive type occurs in the neonatal period, but there can be delayed presentation until later childhood with the autosomal dominant version.
  - The disorder requires each parent to have the abnormal gene, with a 25% chance of passing it on to each child. The autosomal recessive type of PKD is linked to a specific gene, *PKHD1* gene on chromosome 6p21.
- The incidence of ARPKD is about 1 in 20,000 to 40,000 live births, with equal incidence in both males and females (Cadnapaphornchai et al., 2021; Engen & Hingorani, 2018; Samuels et al., 2017; Vogt & Springel, 2020).

DIAGNOSIS

- Prenatally, infants with autosomal recessive bilateral polycystic kidneys usually have a history of oligohydramnios depending on the extent of renal failure prior to birth. After birth, these infants will have palpable flank masses bilaterally, systemic hypertension, and oliguria. The large flank masses can result in abdominal distension and a palpable liver.

- With the oligohydramnios, there are hypoplastic lungs resulting in respiratory distress. Other signs of renal failure are elevated BUN and creatinine, elevated K^+ and phosphorus/phosphate (PO_4), low serum calcium (Ca^{++}), hematuria, and proteinuria. Congenital hepatic fibrosis usually also occurs with this disorder.

- A renal ultrasound can diagnose this disorder by noting enlarged, nodular, or cystic kidneys. Abdominal x-rays can also assist with diagnosis by seeing cystic areas on the kidneys.

- Genetic testing is necessary to distinguish between autosomal recessive and autosomal dominant forms (Bates & Schwaderer, 2018; Engen & Hingorani, 2018; Samuels et al., 2017; Vogt & Springel, 2020).

MANAGEMENT AND OUTCOME

- Management of renal failure includes dialysis, kidney transplant, or supportive care. Renal and respiratory monitoring is needed for infants with PKD to evaluate the degree of renal and respiratory involvement. Fluid overload and electrolyte abnormalities are treated with diuretics, antihypertensives, and supplementation with dialysis. Management also includes genetic counseling of the parents.

- Complications from PKD include renal failure, hypertension, frequent urination, urinary tract infections (UTI), esophageal varices, congestive heart failure from fluid overload, and portal hypertension leading to hepatic failure. Liver involvement occurs in most infants, but only about 40% of infants with the recessive type of PKD show signs of liver damage.

- Infants with severe renal or respiratory involvement may die in the neonatal period, but survival rates have improved with aggressive treatment to 70% to 75%. If infants survive the neonatal period, they may develop renal insufficiency in childhood or adolescence (Engen & Hingorani, 2018; Samuels et al., 2017; Vogt & Springel, 2020).

▶ MULTICYSTIC DYSPLASTIC KIDNEY DISEASE

DEFINITION AND PATHOPHYSIOLOGY

- Multicystic dysplastic kidney (MCDK) disease is a developmental renal disorder which usually occurs in only one kidney. The cysts are described as "grape-like" clusters. The parenchyma of the kidney is abnormal, with few normal nephrons. The proximal ureter is usually stenotic or nonpatent, which contributes to renal failure in that kidney. The disorder is usually nongenetic but can be associated with certain genes or genetic disorders.

- The incidence of MCDK disease is 1 in 2,400 to 4,300 infants, with a small male predominance (Engen & Hingorani, 2018; Maguire, 2021; Vogt & Springel, 2020).

DIAGNOSIS

- These infants may present with a history of oligohydramnios depending on the extent of renal involvement. After birth, the infant may present with an abdominal mass which is usually unilateral, of irregular shape, and usually on the left side. The other kidney is often larger than normal but usually non-cystic; however, there is a risk of UPJO. This disorder is one of the most common causes of abdominal mass in a newborn infant.
- MCDK disease is diagnosed mainly by renal ultrasound (or fetal ultrasound). Visualization of the multiple "grape-like" cysts is diagnostic. The ureter is usually atretic. There is no communication between the dysplastic tissue and the renal pelvis in the nonfunctioning kidney. A renal scan may not be needed for accurate visualization. A voiding cystourethrogram (VCUG) is controversial (Bates & Schwaderer, 2018; Engen & Hingorani, 2018; Samuels et al., 2017).

MANAGEMENT AND OUTCOME

- Management of MCDK disease has two possible plans: (a) nonoperative plan with close follow-up; or (b) operative plan with removal of the cystic, nonfunctional kidney (nephrectomy).
- Complications of MCDK disorders include hypertension, infection, hematuria with or without proteinuria, and pain.
- If multicystic kidneys occur in both kidneys (bilateral), the infant will die without dialysis or kidney transplant. If the multicystic kidney occurs in just one kidney (unilateral), the infant survives. A possible malignancy may occur later in life within the nonfunctional kidney, necessitating removal. Otherwise, the unilateral kidneys may regress by about 5 years of age (Engen & Hingorani, 2018; Maguire, 2021; Samuels et al., 2017; Vogt & Springel, 2020).

▶ ECTOPIC KIDNEY OR SUPERNUMERARY KIDNEY

DEFINITION AND PATHOPHYSIOLOGY

- An ectopic kidney results from disruption of the normal embryologic migration to usual positioning during fetal development. Ectopic kidneys are associated with other genital or cloacal anomalies, especially in females.
- Horseshoe kidney is a U-shaped kidney where there are two kidneys which are connected at the bottom in the midline of the abdomen. This type of kidney results in a higher incidence of Wilms tumor in childhood.
- Crossed renal ectopia refers to kidneys which have ureters entering the bladder from the wrong side.
- A supernumerary kidney is a rare phenomenon where the extra kidney and its collecting system is somewhere in the abdomen, but not related to the functioning kidneys.
- An ectopic kidney occurs in about 1 in 700 infants as seen on fetal ultrasound (Merguerian & Rowe, 2018). The incidence of a horseshoe kidney is about 1 in 400 infants and more common with Turner syndrome (Engen & Hingorani, 2018; Maguire, 2021; Merguerian & Rowe, 2018).

DIAGNOSIS

- It is typically asymptomatic; approximately 90% of patients are never diagnosed. It is usually only diagnosed if the ectopic/supernumerary kidney becomes infected or obstructed (Engen & Hingorani, 2018; Maguire, 2021; Merguerian & Rowe, 2018).

MANAGEMENT AND OUTCOME

- Surgical removal may be necessary if supernumerary kidney and/or malignancy occur.
- Prognosis for the ectopic kidney is good, with no evidence of adverse effects on blood pressure or renal function. It is not associated with hypertension, proteinuria, or chronic kidney disease. Patients are typically not followed unless there is evidence of reflux or obstruction (Engen & Hingorani, 2018; Merguerian & Rowe, 2018).

▶ HYDRONEPHROSIS

DEFINITION AND PATHOPHYSIOLOGY

- Hydronephrosis is damage to the kidney from a congenital obstruction in the urinary tract, resulting in backup of urine into the kidneys, which dilates the renal pelvis and calyces and may also dilate the ureters (hydroureters). The etiology of the obstruction is unknown.
- Common causes of obstruction to urine flow include:
  - *UPJO:* This is one of the most common causes of hydronephrosis and is more common in males. UPJO can occur from failure to recanalize a portion of ureter, abnormal development of ureter, or other reasons including genetic defects. About

1 in 1,000 fetuses have congenital UPJO, which results in hydronephrosis with hydroureter either unilaterally or bilaterally, although unilateral hydronephrosis is more common.

- *PUV:* This is the most common lower urinary tract/bladder obstruction in males. The obstruction is due to a membrane, not really a valve, which causes an obstruction or partial obstruction, with urine backing up into the kidneys and ureters causing hydroureters and hydronephrosis in utero and in neonatal life. PUVs occur only in males, with an incidence of 1 in 5,000 to 8,000 live births.

- Another potential cause of hydronephrosis is vesicoureteral reflux (VUR), a condition that results in urine flowing backwards from the bladder into the ureters, causing hydroureters and possibly hydronephrosis. Hydronephrosis can result in damage to the renal parenchyma due to the backup of urine into the kidney. Hypertension can also be a complication of kidney damage. UTI is common, with VUR from the urine refluxing from the bladder (Cadnapaphornchai et al., 2021; Engen & Hingorani, 2018; Maguire, 2021; McEwen & Vogt, 2020; Merguerian & Rowe, 2018; Samuels et al., 2017; Vogt & Springel, 2020; Wang et al., 2018).

DIAGNOSIS

- Hydronephrosis is frequently seen on prenatal ultrasounds. Most of these will resolve or improve prior to birth and are not due to an obstruction in the urinary tract. It may occur due to delayed maturation of the ureters during fetal development. Often the hydronephrosis can disappear after birth.

- After birth, infants with moderate to severe hydronephrosis will have oliguria, enlarged kidney(s), and abdominal distension. With the lower urinary tract obstruction, a distended and palpable bladder may be noted. A poor urinary stream is almost definitive of posterior urethral valves in male infants.

- Other possible clinical signs would be proteinuria, hematuria, leukocyturia (UTI), increased BUN, and increased creatinine. There is also an increase in other associated anomalies and a thorough assessment must be completed.

- Diagnosis of hydronephrosis can be made with a renal ultrasound (before or after birth) or by a renal scan.

- A VCUG is usually done to rule out obstruction, especially with VUR or PUV. An intravenous pyelogram (IVP) can also be done to view obstructions in the urinary tract. Both of these tests involve the use of contrast media and radiation (Bates & Schwaderer, 2018; Maguire, 2021; McEwen & Vogt, 2020; Merguerian & Rowe, 2018; Samuels et al., 2017; Vogt & Springel, 2020).

MANAGEMENT AND OUTCOME

- Management of hydronephrosis involves getting rid of the obstruction and facilitating urine passage through the urinary tract, mainly with surgical correction.
  - Pyeloplasty is a surgical correction of the obstruction seen at the ureteropelvic junction (UPJ).
  - Management of PUV is to catheterize the infant, relieving the obstruction of the "valves" or membranes in the urethra. Direct transurethral ablation surgery can also be used to relieve the obstruction as a more permanent solution.
  - Surgical repair with antibiotic prophylaxis for prevention of UTI is the treatment of choice for VUR and for UPJO if it does not resolve spontaneously.

- The outcome of hydronephrosis depends on the extent of kidney damage and whether there is any pulmonary involvement causing respiratory distress or lung hypoplasia. Prompt treatment improves the prognosis with many infants, and the outcome with prenatally diagnosed hydronephrosis often results in spontaneous resolution.

- Infants with PUV usually do well, with some incontinence in about half of the infants, which improves with age; others may develop some renal insufficiency and chronic or progressive renal disease.

- If surgery is not successful, the infant may require a kidney transplant (Maguire, 2021; Merguerian & Rowe, 2018; Samuels et al., 2017; Vogt & Springel, 2020).

▶ PRUNE BELLY SYNDROME (EAGLE-BARRETT SYNDROME)

DEFINITION AND PATHOPHYSIOLOGY

- Prune belly syndrome is also called Eagle-Barrett syndrome and includes a triad of three abnormalities: (a) lack of abdominal wall muscles, causing wrinkled, abdominal skin with a "prune-like" appearance; (b) hydronephrosis with a dilated bladder without obstruction; and (c) bilateral cryptorchidism.

- Causes of the prune belly association include obstructive uropathy or mesenchymal dysplasia, and often with dysplastic kidneys; although there is no genetic abnormality noted, there may be some variations in genetic phenotype presentations in the infant.

- The incidence of prune belly syndrome is approximately 1 in 35,000 to 50,000 live births, with a definitive, male predominance (Blackburn, 2018; Bradshaw, 2021; Cavaliere, 2019; Engen & Hingorani, 2018; Maguire, 2021; Merguerian & Rowe, 2018; Vogt & Springel, 2020).

DIAGNOSIS

- Infants born with prune belly syndrome are first noted to have wrinkled skin on the abdomen with the appearance of a "prune." The abdomen appears large and distended. The bladder is often noted to be enlarged or distended on physical exam, associated with other urinary tract abnormalities. Infant boys will exhibit undescended testes. Gastrointestinal (GI) abnormalities with obstruction and distension of the gut may also be present.
- Diagnosis is initially by observation. An ultrasound and/or VCUG can be used to evaluate the urinary tract, although there are some controversies in the use of VCUG.
- CT and nuclear scan are also possible methods of evaluating the urinary tract (Bates & Schwaderer, 2018; Bradshaw, 2021; Cavaliere, 2019).

MANAGEMENT AND OUTCOME

- Possible management plans depend on the extent of the abnormality and renal/respiratory symptoms. Management may include vesicostomy, self-catheterization, surgery on the abdominal wall or urinary tract, bilateral orchiopexy, and dialysis or renal transplant if needed.
- Infants with prune belly syndrome may develop an enlargement of the bladder from the hydronephrosis and renal dysplasia, distension of the intestines from an obstruction, and renal failure.
- If the infant has dysplastic kidneys, the infant may die in infancy. Many infants survive into adulthood after urinary tract and abdomen reconstruction and repair are completed (Bradshaw, 2021; Cavaliere, 2019; Merguerian & Rowe, 2018).

▶ RENAL VEIN THROMBOSIS

DEFINITION AND PATHOPHYSIOLOGY

- Most deep vein thromboses in neonates are associated with the use of a central venous or arterial catheter (umbilical artery catheter [UAC], umbilical venous catheterization [UVC], percutaneously inserted central catheter [PICC], or Broviac catheter).
- Renal vein thrombosis (RVT) is the most common cause of thrombosis in newborns unrelated to catheter placement. The thrombosis usually occurs during the first week of life, is usually unilateral, and occurs slightly more often on the left side.
- Prenatal conditions include maternal diabetes (infant of a diabetic mother [IDM]), maternal preeclampsia/eclampsia, or perinatal asphyxia. There are many disorders or treatments that may contribute to RVT, including a high hematocrit at birth with or without maternal diabetes.
- Blood clots are more prevalent with polycythemia and/or hyperviscosity of the blood. Blood clots can result from the use of UVC or from abnormal coagulation factors or disseminated intravascular coagulation (DIC). Since premature infants have low levels of clotting factors, they are more at risk of clot formation.
  - Severe dehydration can also cause thicker blood. Cyanotic congenital heart disease can result in polycythemia because of the low oxygen level to the tissues.
  - Hypovolemia or low blood volume leads to low blood pressure (hypotension).
  - Clots can start in the smaller renal veins and extend into the major renal vein and the IVC.
- About 1% to 2% of neonatal deaths are the result of RVT and they occur in about 2.4 per 1,000 neonatal admissions to the NICU or 2.2 cases per 100,000 live births, with most associated with the use of umbilical catheters.
- There is a slight male predominance, with other authors stating no sexual preference. Most infants with RVT are term and large for gestational age (LGA; Askenazi et al., 2018; Cadnapaphornchai et al., 2021; Letterio & Ahuja, 2020; Letterio et al., 2020; Samuels et al., 2017; Sparger & Gupta, 2017; Vogt & Springel, 2020).

DIAGNOSIS

- Infants with RVT usually present with an abdominal flank mass (larger than normal kidneys), either unilateral or bilateral, with possible abdominal distension, but with significant hematuria and thrombocytopenia.
- If clots occur with umbilical venous catheters, they often occur in the IVC, and edema distal to the clot can be the result.
- RVT is usually diagnosed by renal ultrasound (with or without color Doppler flow studies).
- Contrast angiography has been the gold standard for diagnosis, but radiation exposure makes it dangerous to newborns (Bates & Schwaderer, 2018; Cadnapaphornchai et al., 2021; Letterio & Ahuja, 2020; Letterio, et al., 2020; Letterio & Ahuja, 2020; Merguerian & Rowe, 2018; Samuels et al., 2017; Vogt & Springel, 2020).

MANAGEMENT AND OUTCOME

- Treatment of the underlying cause is most important with this diagnosis.
  - Treatment of RVT is supportive care only if the thrombi are unilateral and not a large clot. Removal of the catheter is usually essential and may resolve the clot.
  - If clots are bilateral or in the IVC, then heparin or tissue plasminogen activator (t-PA) is used to try to

- break up the clot and reestablish circulation from the lower part of the body.
  - The use of low-dose heparin (e.g., 0.5–1 unit/mL) in umbilical catheters can prevent the development of thrombi.
  - Surgical excision of the clot is considered if (a) renal failure is apparent, (b) the thrombosis was the result of a UVC, or (c) the thrombosis is bilateral and resistant to heparin or t-PA.
- RVT can result in renal tubular dysfunction, leading to renal failure and atrophy of the kidney. Prolonged lack of blood flow to the lower extremities with an IVC thrombosis can result in hypertension, distal clots, loss of toes or limbs, adrenal hemorrhage, chronic renal insufficiency, and death.
- Many of the kidneys of infants with an RVT will atrophy, becoming smaller, and infants may develop hypertension due to damage to the kidney. Death rarely occurs, with a mortality rate of about 3% (Askenazi et al., 2018; Cadnapaphornchai et al., 2021; Letterio & Ahuja, 2020; Letterio et al.; Merguerian & Rowe, 2018; Samuels et al., 2017; Sparger & Gupta, 2017; Vogt & Springel, 2020).

▶ RENAL ARTERY THROMBOSIS

DEFINITION AND PATHOPHYSIOLOGY

- Renal artery thrombosis (RAT) is the result of a clot in the renal artery, blocking blood flow to the kidneys.
- RATs frequently occur after or during the use of a UAC. The thromboses can also occur with coagulation disorders or severe hypotension (Letterio et al., 2020; Samuels et al., 2017).

DIAGNOSIS

- Infants with RAT can be asymptomatic or present with systemic hypertension, hematuria, thrombocytopenia, oliguria, or anuria, as well as lack of blood flow to the lower abdomen and the lower extremities.
- Magnetic resonance (MR) angiography and renal ultrasound with color Doppler flow studies are both used to diagnose an arterial thrombosis (Bates & Schwaderer, 2018; Letterio et al., 2020).

MANAGEMENT AND OUTCOME

- Management of RAT initially involves removal of the arterial catheter, and then can involve removal of the clot, thrombolytic agents (heparin or t-PA), or supportive care with antihypertensives, especially if affecting only one kidney or a unilateral clot. Peritoneal dialysis with a possible transplant may become necessary if kidney failure becomes permanent.

- The overall mortality rate with aortic and renal arterial thrombosis is between 9% and 20%, with mortality being higher with major aortic and renal arterial thrombosis.
- Renovascular hypertension is the most common long-term complication of renal arterial thrombosis. Another consequence of renal arterial thrombosis is chronic renal insufficiency caused by irreversible renal parenchymal damage; this is seen less frequently (Askenazi et al., 2018; Letterio et al., 2020; McEwen & Vogt, 2020; Samuels et al., 2017).

▶ URINARY TRACT INFECTIONS

DEFINITION AND PATHOPHYSIOLOGY

- A UTI is an infection of the urinary tract with a bacteria, virus, or fungus.
- The cause of a UTI can be an abnormality of the urinary tract, which facilitates colonization or infection due to either reflux or an obstruction.
- Some of the main bacteria causing UTI are the following: *Escherichia coli* is the most common bacteria causing a UTI; *Klebsiella* species (gram-negative bacilli) can also be a contributing bacterium. Some gram-positive bacteria are also seen in neonates (e.g., coagulase-negative *Staphylococcus* or group B beta-hemolytic *Streptococcus* [GBS]).
- Risk factors for a UTI are uncircumcised males, a maternal history of UTI, or VUR.
- In the United States, up to 1% of infants will develop a UTI during the first 3 days of life, but the rates are higher in premature infants and in male infants. After 1 year of age, female infants will have more UTI than male infants. There is also a prevalence rate of 5% to 20% in children under 2 months of age with a fever and no other known source of infection (Cadnapaphornchai et al., 2021; Esper, 2020; Ramachandra, 2020; Samuels et al., 2017; Wang et al., 2018).

DIAGNOSIS

- Infants with a UTI can be asymptomatic or have very nonspecific signs of sepsis. Infants may have poor feeding, respiratory distress, or lethargy. It is rare for infants to have a UTI before 48 hours of life. A fever with UTI results in an increased incidence of bacteremia, so a blood culture MUST be obtained. Approximately 33% of infants with a UTI would also have a positive blood culture.
- The definitive diagnostic test is a positive urine culture (obtained by sterile bladder tap or catheterization) or a Gram stain with a high colony count. A renal ultrasound showing urinary tract abnormalities would assist with the diagnosis of a continuing UTI.

A VCUG is used to diagnose a possible VUR (Bates & Schwaderer, 2018; Esper, 2020; Ramachandra, 2020; Samuels et al., 2017; Vergales, 2020; Wang et al., 2018).

MANAGEMENT AND OUTCOME

- Antibiotics should be given for a minimum of 10 to 14 days, depending on the symptoms and resolution of the urine culture. Follow-up of urine cultures is required after antibiotics are discontinued. Supportive care is essential, which may include continuous antibiotic prophylaxis.
- Infants with a UTI can have renal scarring, a reoccurrence of the UTI, systemic sepsis, or meningitis.
- There are excellent outcomes for infants with a UTI if they are treated promptly and adequately (Cadnapaphornchai et al., 2021; Esper, 2020; Ramachandra, 2020; Wang et al., 2018).

▶ PATENT URACHUS

DEFINITION AND PATHOPHYSIOLOGY

- The urachus is a prenatal communication between the bladder and the umbilicus which usually regenerates but can remain patent after birth.
- The cause of this defect is failure of the normal closing of the urachal tube during fetal development (Blackburn, 2018; Goodwin, 2019; Ledbetter et al., 2018; Merguerian & Rowe, 2018).

DIAGNOSIS

- The appearance of urine or clear fluid from the umbilicus at birth or in the newborn period is one of the first signs of a patent urachus. The umbilicus can appear "wet," and the wetness can cause a delay in cord separation from the stump for greater than 14 days.
- Confirmed diagnosis is made after analysis of fluid for urea and creatinine to confirm urine. Abdominal ultrasound may show the defect, but a VCUG is definitive (Bates & Schwaderer, 2018; Cavaliere, 2019; Merguerian & Rowe, 2018).

MANAGEMENT AND OUTCOME

- Infants with a patent urachus are given supportive care. Surgical closure will occur after 1 year of age if spontaneous closure does not occur.
- Most infants will have a good outcome with few if any complications. Infants with patent urachus can develop an infection (e.g., UTI) or excoriation of the skin after exposure to the urine (Cavaliere, 2019; Ledbetter et al., 2018; Merguerian & Rowe, 2018).

▶ HYPOSPADIAS AND EPISPADIAS

DEFINITION AND PATHOPHYSIOLOGY

- These two defects occur when the urethral meatus is located on the ventral surface of the penis (hypospadias) or located on the dorsal surface of the penis (epispadias) rather than on the tip.
- The most probable cause of abnormal urethral placement is due to a multifactorial mode of inheritance and therefore related to a delay or arrest of the normal sequence of urethral development due to lack of testosterone or androgens in utero.
- The incidence is about 1 per 250 to 300 live male births and may be increasing in the United States (Maguire, 2022; Merguerian & Rowe, 2018; Sorbara & Wherritt, 2020).

DIAGNOSIS

- The hypospadias is visually apparent on the underside of the penis, especially during voiding. The urinary stream comes from the underside of the penis with hypospadias and from the top with epispadias.
- Observation or a physical exam is necessary for diagnosis by identifying the location of the meatus or opening. Incomplete formation of the prepuce often occurs with hypospadias, so the first indication of hypospadias could be what is sometimes called a "natural circumcision" on a male infant. Chordee often occurs with downward curving of the penis and results in a deviation of stream during voiding.
- Hypospadias was classified based on the location of the meatus; however, this classification was not sufficient to encompass the complexity of this defect. A new scoring system called the GMS score (glans, meatus, shaft) has been used. This scale includes a scale of 1 to 4 for each component, with higher scores indicating unfavorable characteristics (Maguire, 2021; Merguerian & Rowe, 2018).

MANAGEMENT AND OUTCOME

- Infants with hypospadias or epispadias should not be circumcised because the foreskin will be used for surgical repair and correction of the defect, which is usually completed between 6 and 18 months of age.
- More severe cases will be delayed and repaired after the age of 1 year. Testosterone therapy may be given to increase phallic size if necessary (Merguerian & Rowe, 2018 Sorbara & Wherritt, 2020).

▶ EXSTROPHY OF THE BLADDER

DEFINITION AND PATHOPHYSIOLOGY

- Exstrophy of the bladder is defined as an exposed bladder through the lower anterior abdominal wall. The umbilicus can be displaced downward, and most are associated with epispadias and separation of the symphysis pubis.
- The etiology is essentially unknown, but may be due to abnormal development of the cloacal membrane with rupture and a possible genetic influence.
- The incidence of bladder exstrophy is about 1 in 10,000 to 60,000 live births, with a male predominance (Ledbetter et al., 2018; Maguire, 2021; Merguerian & Rowe, 2018; Ringer & Hansen, 2017; Vogt & Springel, 2020).

DIAGNOSIS

- Diagnosis is made by prenatal ultrasound or by observation after birth. An ultrasound and flat plate x-ray of the abdomen should be done to rule out any other urinary tract or bone anomalies.
- Infants present with an external bladder (outside the lower abdominal wall), usually with epispadias (male) or bifid clitoris (female), and anterior displacement of the anal opening, and may also present with undescended testes, inguinal hernia, or umbilical hernia (Ledbetter et al., 2018; Merguerian & Rowe, 2018; Vogt & Springel, 2020).

MANAGEMENT AND OUTCOME

- Early management would include providing a cover to the exposed bladder with clear plastic or saline dressing to permit drainage but also to protect the bladder. Later management includes surgical closure, reconstruction of the bladder with antispasmodics, analgesics, and antibiotics.
- Infections, postoperative hydronephrosis, or anal incontinence may occur after surgery. A malignancy of renal tissue may occur in childhood or adulthood. Good bladder control is likely with proper management (Ledbetter et al., 2018; Merguerian & Rowe, 2018).

▶ TESTICULAR TORSION

DEFINITION AND PATHOPHYSIOLOGY

- A testicular torsion is caused by an incomplete attachment of the testes allowing it to twist, causing the blood flow to the testes to be cut off, resulting in necrosis.
- Most torsions of the testes occur prenatally rather than during the neonatal period, although they are diagnosed after birth (Cavaliere, 2019; Maguire, 2021; Ringer & Hansen, 2017).

DIAGNOSIS

- Infants with testicular torsion will present with swelling of the testes in the scrotum and discoloration of the testes/scrotum—the scrotum appears bruised or "dusky" and bluish—and the testes will be painful to palpation if it is a recent strangulation; necrotic testes are not painful to palpation.
- Diagnosis of testicular torsion is by observation. Upon assessment, there is no cremasteric reflex noted and the testes tests negative to transillumination. The testis and blood flow may be seen by ultrasound (Cavaliere, 2019; Maguire, 2021; Merguerian & Rowe, 2018; Ringer & Hansen, 2017).

MANAGEMENT AND OUTCOME

- Emergent surgery for detorsion should occur within 4 to 6 hours and will include a contralateral orchiopexy to protect the nonaffected testes.
- Most infants with testicular torsion noted will already have a loss of function of the testes and necrosis will occur. Oligospermia is the main complication of testicular torsion. Testicular prostheses can be used for cosmetic purposes (Cavaliere, 2019; Maguire, 2021; Merguerian & Rowe, 2018; Ringer & Hansen, 2017).

▶ INGUINAL HERNIA

DEFINITION AND PATHOPHYSIOLOGY

- Inguinal hernia is failure of the proximal part of the processus vaginalis to close at birth, producing a hernia sac.
- It affects about 5% of infants under 1,500 g at birth and about 30% of infants under 1,000 g at birth. It is more frequent in males, premature infants, and small-for-gestational-age (SGA) infants (Cavaliere, 2019; Ledbetter et al., 2018; Ringer & Hansen, 2017).

DIAGNOSIS

- An inguinal hernia will present as a swelling, lump, or bump in the inguinal area (groin) of female infants or in the scrotal sac(s) of male infants. Cryptorchidism may be present with inguinal hernia.
- Diagnosis is made by observation of the swelling/ lump and by palpation of the herniated bowel or abdominal organs through the skin with the ability to manually reduce the herniation (Cavaliere, 2019; Ledbetter et al., 2018).

MANAGEMENT AND OUTCOME

- Treatment for unilateral or bilateral inguinal hernia is herniorrhaphy, usually just prior to discharge in a premature infant. Incarceration of the hernia (inability to manually reduce the hernia), ischemic injury, and venous infection are serious complications.
- Prognosis for full recovery is excellent. Recurrence risk is very small (Cavaliere, 2019; Ledbetter et al., 2018; Ringer & Hansen, 2017).

▶ CRYPTORCHIDISM

DEFINITION AND PATHOPHYSIOLOGY

- *Cryptorchidism* is defined as undescended testicles. The testes (one or both) are not in the scrotal sac or scrotum.
- There are three possible causes of cryptorchidism: (a) endocrine dysfunction of the hypothalamic–pituitary–gonadal axis, (b) abnormal epididymal development without testicular descent into the scrotum, or (c) an anatomic abnormality preventing the descent of the testes into the scrotum.
- The incidence of undescended testes is about 1% to 7% in full-term infants, up to as much as 45% in premature infants, and may go as high as 100% in the very premature infant, with most being unilateral (about 70%). Most spontaneous descent occurs within 6 to 10 weeks after birth, but usually by 6 to 9 months of age (Merguerian & Rowe, 2018; Sorbara & Wherrett, 2020; Swartz & Chan, 2017).

DIAGNOSIS

- There is an absence of testes in the scrotum. Types may include:
  - *Abdominal:* Testes are located inside the internal inguinal ring, therefore remaining in the abdomen.
  - *Canalicular:* Testes are located between the internal and external inguinal rings, and remain within the canal.
  - *Ectopic:* Testes are located between the abdominal cavity and the scrotum, but outside the inguinal canal.
  - *Retractile:* Testes are fully descended but move between the scrotum and the groin.
- The following syndromes have all been associated with undescended testes: Down, Klinefelter, Noonan, Prader–Willi, Smith–Lemli–Opitz, and fetal hydantoin syndrome, as well as other genetic, neurologic, or renal abnormalities.
- Ultrasound and/or CT scan are both used for diagnosis (Bates & Schwaderer, 2018; Cavaliere, 2019; Sorbara & Wherrett, 2020; Swartz & Chan, 2017).

MANAGEMENT AND OUTCOME

- Infants with undescended testes will usually have an orchiopexy between 6 and 24 months of age. Hormonal treatment with human chorionic gonadotropin can also be attempted but is usually not recommended due to side effects.
- Testicular torsion, inguinal hernia, testicular cancer, and potential infertility have all been associated with persistent undescended testes, although the overall outcome is very good (Merguerian & Rowe, 2018; Sorbara & Wherrett, 2020; Swartz & Chan, 2017).

▶ CONCLUSION

The kidney is a vital organ which is essential to the infant's survival; therefore, renal function must be considered when discussing any neonatal therapies. This chapter serves as a brief review of the anatomy and physiology of the kidney, outlining accompanying pathologies which may be congenital or develop during an infant's hospitalization, as well as guidelines for the assessment of the infant with suspected renal dysfunction, in addition to potential interventions ranging from benign to invasive.

1. The fractional excretion of sodium (FENa) reflects the balance of sodium between:

   A. Glomerular filtration and tubular reabsorption
   B. Major and minor calyces and Bowman's capsule
   C. Renal vein and the intraparenchymal pyramids

2. A medication which, if administered to the mother during pregnancy, can cause structural and/or functional anomalies of the fetal kidney is:

   A. Dexamethasone (Decadron)
   B. Indomethacin (Indocin)
   C. Magnesium sulfate ($MgSO_4$)

3. The neonatal nurse practitioner (NNP) notes a newborn male infant has testicular swelling and discoloration of the testes/scrotum. The scrotum appears bruised or "dusky" and bluish and painful to palpation. The correct next action for the NNP to take is to:

   A. Consult a pediatric surgeon
   B. Order a CT scan
   C. Test the urine for presence of infection

4. Reabsorption is defined as the movement of substances from the:

   A. Peritubular capillaries across the tubular epithelium into the renal tubules
   B. Renal tubule into the peritubular capillaries
   C. Vascular space into the Bowen's capsule forming a filtrate

5. A finding on the physical exam of a neonate that would prompt the neonatal nurse practitioner (NNP) to further evaluate the renal/urinary tract would be a/an:

   A. Abdominal mass
   B. Inguinal hernia
   C. Testicular hydrocele

6. A differential diagnosis includes prerenal kidney injury; therefore, the neonatal nurse practitioner (NNP) orders which of the following interventions as part of a diagnostic workup?

   A. Fluid challenge
   B. Peritoneal dialysis
   C. Renal ultrasound

7. The neonatal nurse practitioner (NNP) is called to evaluate an infant with facial dysmorphia and notes the infant has a blunted nose with a depressed nasal bridge, micrognathia, wide-spaced eyes, epicanthal folds, and low-set, malformed ears. The NNP becomes suspicious the infant may have:

   A. Acute kidney injury
   B. Bilateral renal agenesis
   C. Renal tubular acidosis

1. A) Glomerular filtration and tubular reabsorption

FENa reflects the balance between glomerular filtration and tubular reabsorption of sodium. A level of <1% indicates prerenal factors that may decrease renal blood flow leading to prerenal azotemia. A level of 2.5% is seen with an intrinsic cause of acute kidney injury (AKI). It is not a useful diagnostic test in preterm infants <32 weeks' gestation due to renal immaturity (Doherty, 2017).

2. B) Indomethacin (Indocin)

Indomethacin is a nonsteroidal anti-inflammatory drug that if taken during pregnancy has been associated with both structural and/or functional alterations in the newborn kidney due to decreased glomerular capillary pressure and glomerular filtration rate (GFR) that can lead to acute kidney injury (AKI; Samuels et al., 2017). Neither dexamethasone nor magnesium sulfate causes such alterations.

3. A) Consult a pediatric surgeon

Testicular torsion is identified by swelling of testes in the scrotum and discoloration of the testes/scrotum, and the scrotum appears bruised or "dusky" and bluish. This is a surgical emergency and can result in loss of testicular function and/or fertility if untreated. Surgery is needed to assess the viability of the testis that is twisted, but also to ensure that the second testis does not become twisted also (Merguerian & Rowe, 2018). A CT scan or urinalysis will not offer pertinent information to the situation and will only delay diagnosis and treatment.

4. B) Renal tubule into the peritubular capillaries

Reabsorption is the movement of substances from the renal tubules across the tubular epithelium into the peritubular capillaries (Maguire, 2021).

5. A) Abdominal mass

Palpable abdominal masses, particularly flank masses, in neonates most often originate from the urinary tract and are commonly cystic or obstructive (Bates & Schwaderer, 2018; Engen & Hingorani, 2018; Samuels et al., 2017). Inguinal hernias and testicular hydroceles are not associated with congenital renal anomalies.

6. A) Fluid challenge

The initial management for prerenal kidney injury is a fluid challenge with an isotonic solution such as normal saline 10 to 20 mL/kg over 30 minutes to replace intravascular volume and determine intravascular fluid loss (Askenazi et al., 2018; Cadnapaphornchai et al., 2021; Gomella, 2020; Kogon & Truong, 2020; Vogt & Springel 2020). Renal ultrasounds are useful for assessing the presence of urine in the bladder and the presence of an obstruction. Dialysis is a last resort intervention for significant renal dysfunction.

7. B) Bilateral renal agenesis

Potter facies (or "squished face") is a unique appearance of the face and body of the fetus/infant due to fetal compression in utero. The infant has a flat face and a "pushed-in" or blunted nose with a depressed nasal bridge. These infants may have micrognathia or receded chin, with wide-spaced eyes, epicanthal folds, low-set or malformed ears, and wrinkled skin. The diagnosis of bilateral renal agenesis can be accomplished by renal ultrasound either prenatally or after birth (Bates & Schwaderer, 2018; Engen & Hingorani, 2018; Samuels et al., 2017; Vogt & Springel, 2020). Infants with renal tubular acidosis (RTA) will have signs of polyuria and weight loss despite adequate caloric intake. Acute kidney injury (AKI) is characterized by an abrupt decline in renal function, which manifests as deranged fluid and electrolyte homeostasis.

The Hematopoietic System

Kimberly Horns

INTRODUCTION

The neonatal hematologic system is a complex interaction between multiple organ systems to support growth and function of blood cells within the serous fluids of the body. This chapter covers the basics of hematopoiesis and alterations which affect blood cells' volume, content, and efficiency. Anemias, platelet disorders, coagulopathies, and maternal–fetal ABO and Rh compatibilities are covered. Common forms of neonatal hyperbilirubinemia and common management of types of hyperbilirubinemia are discussed. Finally, current transfusion recommendations and interventions when physiologic systems cannot maintain hemostasis are summarized.

FETAL HEMATOPOIETIC DEVELOPMENT

- Hematopoiesis is responsible for the formation, production, and maintenance of blood cells. This process development begins with delineation of pluripotent stem cells into different blood cells. Hematopoiesis begins in the yolk sac as early as 2 weeks' gestation and results in red blood cells (RBCs) and macrophages.
  - Hematopoietic stem cells' primordial development starts in the mesoderm and later they are found in organs such as the yolk sac, liver, and bone marrow. The liver becomes the main source of hematopoiesis by 6 weeks' gestation and remains the major site of hematopoiesis until the 16th week of gestation.
- By 24 weeks' gestation, the bone marrow becomes the primary site of hematopoiesis. From late gestation to the end of the first postnatal year, RBCs gradually shift from the production of fetal hemoglobin (HgF) to the production of adult hemoglobin (HgA).
  - Figure 23.1 describes the stem cell differentiation. Pluripotent hematopoiesis infers that the "mother (progenitor) cell" can develop into different cell likes, namely RBCs, granulocytes, monocytes, eosinophils, basophils, megakaryocytes/platelets, B- and T-lymphocytes, and osteoclasts (Blackburn, 2018b; Diehl-Jones & Fraser, 2021; Juul & Christensen, 2018; Letterio et al., 2020).

ERYTHROPOIESIS

- Fetal erythropoiesis, the process of RBC production, is controlled in the fetus by the protein erythropoietin (EPO). EPO is the primary factor that stimulates the growth and development of erythrocytes and is regulated by mechanisms in the fetal liver and kidney. This feedback loop ultimately drives the erythropoietic system using hypoxia-based oxygen concentrations of tissue and oxygen saturation of hemoglobin.
- The bone marrow becomes the primary site for erythropoiesis from 22 weeks' gestation and continues postnatally.
  - Once the bone marrow becomes the primary site of RBC production, extramedullary erythropoiesis can occur during periods of hemolysis, common with congenital infections. The major organs of fetal extramedullary hematopoiesis are the liver, spleen, and yolk sac.
  - When extramedullary erythropoiesis (organs outside the bone marrow) occurs in the skin, the characteristic "blueberry muffin rash" associated with congenital cytomegalovirus (CMV) infection can be seen.
- Postnatally, EPO is produced in the kidneys. As RBCs mature, they become very dependent on EPO's regulation.
  - The EPO concentration in the neonate decreases rapidly in response to the relatively hyperoxic extrauterine environment.
  - EPO levels reach their nadir by 1 month of life in normal, term newborns. Then, following a physiologic decrease in RBCs, EPO levels increase to their peak at 2 months of life, then gradually decline to adult levels.
- EPO levels increase in response to anemia and in the presence of hypoxemia. Other disorders where EPO levels increase include Down syndrome or intrauterine growth restriction, as well as infants born to mothers with diabetes or pregnancy-induced hypertension. EPO levels decrease after transfusion of packed RBCs (Blackburn, 2018b; Diehl-Jones & Fraser, 2021; Juul & Christensen, 2018; Letterio & Ahuja, 2020; Letterio et al., 2020).

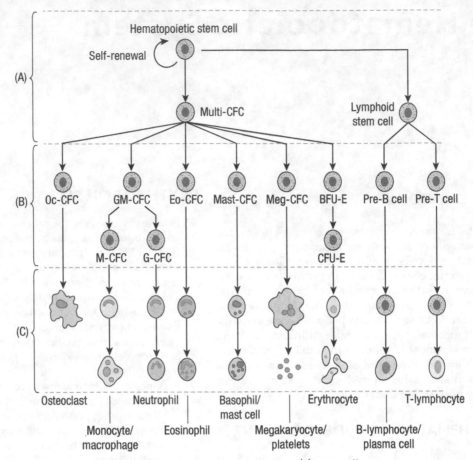

Figure 23.1 Stem cell differentiation: (a) stem cells,
(b) committed progenitors, and (c) mature cells.

BFU-E, burst-forming units, erythroid; CFC, colony forming cells; CFU-E, colony-forming unit, erythroid; Eo-CFC, eosinophil colony-forming cells; G-CFC, granulocyte colony-forming cells; GM-CFC, granulocyte-macrophage colony-forming cells; M-CFC, macrophage colony-forming cells; Meg-CFC, megakaryocyte colony-forming cells; Oc-CFC, osteoclast colony-forming cells.
Source: Adapted from Letterio, J., Pateva, I., Petrosiute, A., & Ahuja, S. (2020). Hematologic and oncologic problems in the fetus and neonate. In R. J. Martin, A. A. Fanaroff, & M. C. Walsh (Eds.), *Fanaroff & Martin's neonatal-perinatal medicine: Diseases of the fetus and infant* (11th ed., pp. 11416–1475). Elsevier.

HEMOGLOBIN SYNTHESIS

■ The primary purposes of mature RBCs are to carry oxygen to the body's tissues, maintain adequate adenosine triphosphate (ATP) stores, produce substances that act as antioxidants, and produce 2,3-diphosphoglycerate (2,3 DPG), which modifies the oxygen affinity of hemoglobin.

■ A mature hemoglobin molecule has four globin chains, two alpha chains, and two beta chains. The synthesis of HgF begins around the 14th day of embryonic development. The transition from production of HgF to HgA begins near term or at the end of fetal life.

  ● RBCs contain approximately 70% to 90% of HgF at birth. A delay in this transition can occur in certain situations, including maternal hypoxia or fetal growth restriction and in infants of diabetic mothers.

■ The reticulocyte count can be a useful measure of erythrocyte production. High reticulocyte levels reflect active erythropoiesis, while low values indicate reduced levels of erythropoiesis. Immediately after delivery, reticulocyte values tend to be higher in

preterm infants when compared with term newborns (Blackburn, 2018b; Diehl-Jones & Fraser, 2021; Juul & Christensen, 2018; Letterio & Ahuja, 2020; Letterio et al., 2020).

▶ ANEMIA

■ *Anemia* is defined as hemoglobin level of 2 *SD* below the mean for age, or when the hemoglobin, hematocrit, or RBC count is below the fifth percentile lower reference level for gestational and postnatal age.

■ Hematocrit values increase immediately after delivery and then decline during the first week of life. The normal mean hematocrit in healthy term infants is 53% (range 52%–58%). In the absence of any stress and while in the bone marrow, reticulocytes mature in approximately 1 to 2 days and then another day in circulation before maturing into erythrocytes.

■ The average life span of the RBC is related and proportional to the gestational age of the infant, with an average of 35 to 50 days among premature infants and 60 to 70 days in term infants. Fetal RBCs have a much shorter life span in contrast to adult RBCs, who have an average RBC life span of 100 to 120 days (Juul & Christensen, 2018; Letterio et al., 2020).

PHYSIOLOGIC ANEMIA

Definition and Pathophysiology

- In utero, a low fetal partial pressure of oxygen in arterial blood (PaO_2) stimulates EPO production, resulting in erythropoiesis. The relatively hyperoxic extrauterine environment results in suppression of EPO production until 6 to 8 weeks of life. The result is an expected decline in a normal term infant's hemoglobin levels over the first 2 to 3 months of life, with a nadir at 6 to 12 weeks of life. Physiologic anemia is the expected, asymptomatic decline in erythropoiesis seen in term and preterm infants following birth as a result of postnatal EPO suppression.
- The decline in hemoglobin, and thus oxygen-carrying capacity, is offset by the gradual right shift of the oxygen–hemoglobin dissociation curve.
  - A right shift of the oxygen–hemoglobin dissociation curve increases oxygen availability to the tissue (Figure 23.2). Eventually, a continued decline in hemoglobin levels results in a decrease in oxygen delivery to the tissue, stimulating EPO production.
  - By 10 to 12 weeks of life, EPO levels in infants are like those of adults. By 4 to 6 months of life, physiologic anemia has resolved and normal levels of hemoglobin are once again present.
- Once hemoglobin synthesis restarts following the physiologic nadir, iron stored from the reticuloendothelial system is released. Term infants have sufficient iron stores to last for approximately

6 to 12 weeks; subsequently, without adequate iron availability (approximately 1 mg/kg/d), hemoglobin production will decrease.
  - Infants who have received an exchange *RBC* transfusion or multiple RBC transfusions may experience a later hemoglobin nadir. Blood used in *RBC* transfusions results in increased HgA in these neonates and thus in increased oxygen availability to tissue, resulting in suppression of EPO production.
  - Infants with hemolysis due to isoimmunization may experience a late, severe anemia due to the continued presence of maternal antibodies that cause continued hemolysis. Physiologic anemia of infancy can be exaggerated in the sick or premature infant by frequent blood sampling: The smaller the infant, the proportionally greater the volume of blood that is withdrawn for laboratory testing.
- Infants with hemolytic disorders due to isoimmunizations may experience a late and often severe anemia that is not physiologic but the result of continued hemolysis.
- The normal hemoglobin decrease after birth is often not seen in infants with cyanotic heart disease, who maintain higher EPO levels due to their low PaO_2 levels and thus higher hemoglobin levels (Blackburn, 2018b; Letterio et al., 2020).

Clinical Presentation

- Physiologic anemia is usually well tolerated without any clinical indications.
  - The method to determine hematocrit can significantly affect the value. Capillary hematocrit measurements are highly subject to variations in blood flow, which may produce an artificially high hematocrit value. Prewarming does minimize the artifactual increase in the sample. There may be as much as 20% difference between the value obtained from a capillary sample and the hematocrit value obtained from a central (venous or arterial) sample.
- In extremely low birth weight (ELBW) infants whose nadir falls below 7 g/dL, clinical signs of anemia include pallor, tachypnea, tachycardia, poor feeding, and poor weight gain. Other causes of blood loss and suppression of erythropoiesis in the ill neonate can contribute to more severe and earlier anemia (Blackburn, 2018b; Letterio et al., 2020).

Management and Outcome

- Physiologically lower levels of EPO in neonates provided the rationale for the pharmacologic use of recombinant human EPO (r-HuEPO) to treat symptomatic anemia or as prophylactic therapy to reduce the volume and risks of blood transfusions.
  - Supplementation of between 1 and 10 mg/kg/d elemental iron has been used to lessen the risk of iron deficiency.

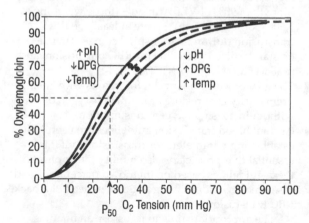

Figure 23.2 Oxygen-hemoglobin dissociation curve.

DPG, Diphosphoglycerate.

Source: Reproduced with permission from Letterio, J., Pateva, I., Petrosiute, A., & Ahuja, S. (2020). Hematologic and oncologic problems in the fetus and neonate. In R. J. Martin, A. A. Fanaroff, & M. C. Walsh (Eds.), *Fanaroff & Martin's neonatal-perinatal medicine: Diseases of the fetus and infant* (11th ed., pp. 11416–1475). Elsevier.

■ Therapy with r-HuEPO and iron stimulates erythropoiesis and increases reticulocyte counts.
■ Two approaches to EPO therapy have been systematically reviewed in neonates:
  ● The early approach, defined by the use of r-HuEPO before day 8 of life, has been shown to reduce (but not eliminate) RBC transfusions, volume of RBC transfusions, and donor exposures, but did not impact morbidity and mortality measures.
  ● Later use of r-HuEPO (on day 8 of life or after) resulted in a reduction in the number of blood transfusions, but not the total volume of blood, per infant, so that meaningful clinical outcomes were not affected by the use of r-HuEPO (Blackburn, 2018b; Diehl-Jones & Fraser, 2021; Letterio et al., 2020).

ANEMIA OF PREMATURITY

Definition and Pathophysiology

■ Anemia of prematurity is thought to be principally a direct consequence of delivery before placental iron transport and fetal erythropoiesis are complete, and is exaggerated by various factors, including blood losses associated with phlebotomy to obtain samples for laboratory testing, low plasma levels of EPO as a result of both diminished production and accelerated catabolism, rapid body growth, and the need for commensurate increases in RBC volume and mass, and disorders causing RBC losses as a result of bleeding and/or hemolysis.
■ Because preterm infants have more HgF and the life span of HgF is shorter than that of HgA, physiologic anemia of preterm neonates occurs earlier and is more pronounced. This normocytic normochromic anemia is characterized by low EPO levels.
■ Preterm infants, especially those born prior to 32 gestational weeks, experience lower nadir and lower hemoglobin levels for a longer period of time.
  ● For these preterm infants, hemoglobin levels may reach the lowest point by about 4 to 6 weeks of life and remain low for 3 to 6 months of life. The more preterm the infant, the lower the nadir.
■ Once RBC production resumes, iron stores are quickly depleted by 2 to 3 months of life. As a result, adequate iron intake is necessary for continued erythropoiesis.
■ Rates of decline and nadir are inversely proportional to gestational age.
  ● Low birth weight (LBW) infants are at high risk for late-onset anemia of prematurity due to the low endogenous production of EPO and frequent laboratory sampling.
  ● The precipitous drop in hematocrit may be exacerbated in sick infants who have repeated blood draws. Additionally, preterm infants do not readily increase serum EPO levels in the presence

of hypoxia (Blackburn, 2018b; Diehl-Jones & Fraser, 2021; Letterio & Ahuja, 2020; McKinney et al., 2021).

Clinical Presentation

■ Infants with anemia of prematurity may be symptomatic or asymptomatic. Clinical signs of anemia include the following: tachycardia, tachypnea, poor feeding or fatigue with feeding, poor weight gain, pallor, increased lactate levels, increased oxygen requirement, or apnea and bradycardia.
■ If levels drop below a tolerable point, the infant may display decreased activity, poor growth, tachypnea, and tachycardia (Blackburn, 2018b; Diehl-Jones & Fraser, 2021; Letterio et al., 2020; McKinney et al., 2021).

Management and Outcome

DELAYED CORD CLAMPING

■ Delayed clamping of the umbilical cord by 30 to 90 seconds has been reported as a successful variation of autologous transfusion. Delayed cord clamping (DCC) has been shown to decrease the need for transfusions among very low birth weight (VLBW) infants and is another strategy to decrease the need for RBC transfusion and improve outcomes. A DCC protocol should be considered as part of an institutional transfusion protocol.
■ Two recent randomized clinical trials have disproven the concern regarding DCC leading to polycythemia. There was no increased incidence of polycythemia or hyperbilirubinemia (Diehl-Jones & Fraser, 2021; Jacquot et al., 2020; Letterio et al., 2020; McKinney et al., 2021; Patel & Josephson, 2018).

RED BLOOD CELL TRANSFUSION THERAPY

■ Small, premature infants often undergo RBC transfusions because they are critically ill and have the highest blood sampling loss in relation to their weight. More than 90% of VLBW infants (those weighing 1,500 g or less at birth) receive at least one RBC transfusion during their hospital course. There is no standardized guideline for RBC transfusion, and practices vary among NICUs.
■ The goal of RBC transfusion for infants with anemia of prematurity is to restore or maintain oxygen delivery without increasing oxygen consumption.
■ Current blood transfusion guidelines are useful in establishing parameters for transfusion, but it is essential that physicians also modify the application of these guidelines based on their own perceptions and assessments in identifying patients in need of a packed RBC transfusion.
  ● The appropriate time to transfuse an infant is controversial since there are no clinical signs which are consistently useful or predictive alone or when in a group. Current *RBC* transfusion recommendations are published for critically ill children, but not neonates. There is consensus to

transfuse critically ill children with a hemoglobin of <5 g/dL. Advantages of *RBC* transfusion must be weighed against the risks and in consideration of gestational and postnatal age, intravascular volume, and coexisting cardiac, pulmonary, or vascular conditions.

- Potential complications of red cell blood transfusions may include:
  - *Acute hemolytic reactions:* These types of reactions usually occur secondary to an incompatibility of the donor's RBCs with antibodies in the infant's plasma.
  - *Volume overload:* This condition may occur with large-volume *RBC* transfusions, greater than 20 mL/kg. Infants with chronic anemia are more vulnerable to volume overload. Congestive heart failure and pulmonary edema are consequences of fluid volume overload.
- Several studies have suggested an association between RBC transfusion and necrotizing enterocolitis (NEC) in premature neonates. Withholding feeds during transfusion has never been clearly demonstrated to be beneficial but may have a protective effect against the development of NEC (Blackburn, 2018b; Diehl-Jones & Fraser, 2021; Jacquot et al., 2020; Letterio & Ahuja, 2020; Patel & Josephson, 2018).

ERYTHROPOIETIN

- Multiple studies have reported favorable use of r-HuEPO and long-acting EPO (darbepoetin), thus decreasing the severity of anemia of prematurity and use of blood transfusions, especially in smaller, premature infants. Large multicenter trials have demonstrated that administration of r-HuEPO plus iron supplementation cannot prevent early transfusions, particularly in VLBW newborns and in infants with severe neonatal diseases. However, this approach may be effective in preventing late transfusions.
- Multiple randomized controlled trials have shown that treatment of extremely preterm infants with r-HuEPO during the period when their endogenous EPO system is inactive stimulates erythropoiesis, maintains a higher hematocrit, and reduces the need for transfusions (Diehl-Jones & Fraser, 2021; Letterio & Ahuja, 2020).

SUPPLEMENTAL IRON

- Because placental iron (Fe) transport is incomplete in the preterm infant, these babies require supplemental iron to mount an effective erythroid response.
- The American Academy of Pediatrics (AAP) recommends 2 to 4 mg/kg/d of elemental iron for preterm infants; however, higher doses for prevention of iron deficiency may be associated with improved outcomes. Additionally, it has been found that there is a positive correlation with use of enteral iron supplementation and neurodevelopmental outcomes

(Blackburn, 2018b; Diehl-Jones & Fraser, 2021; McKinney et al., 2021; Sloan, 2017).

OUTCOMES

- The use of restrictive RBC transfusion guidelines appears to have similar results in terms of numbers of transfusion compared with the use of r-HuEPO. Concerns have been raised that RBC transfusion guidelines which are too restrictive may increase the risk of neurologic injury and alter neurodevelopmental outcomes.
- Iron deficiency with or without accompanying anemia has been associated with cognitive and behavioral deficits.
- In preterm infants 24 to 28 weeks' gestational age, the rates of common neonatal morbidities at follow-up (2 years), such as chronic lung disease, NEC, severe neurodevelopmental impairment, retinopathy of prematurity, sepsis, and intraventricular hemorrhage, were found to be similar in control and experimental (r-HuEPO) groups (Blackburn, 2018b; McKinney et al., 2021).

▶ **POLYCYTHEMIA**

DEFINITION AND PATHOPHYSIOLOGY

- Several conditions are associated with polycythemia in utero. These include chronic hypoxia as a result of maternal toxemia and placental insufficiency, placental insufficiency with postmaturity syndrome, pregnancy at high altitudes, pregnancy in a diabetic patient, and trisomy 21.
- *Polycythemia* is defined as a peripheral venous hemoglobin and hematocrit of more than 2 *SD* above the mean. This is equivalent to a venous hematocrit of 65% or greater or a hemoglobin of 22 mg/dL or greater.
  - Hematocrit values vary greatly based on several factors, including sample site, with some capillary hematocrits higher than 20% that of venous samples.
  - Capillary sampling can be used as a screening test, but a central venous sample should be analyzed to confirm polycythemia. Polycythemia should be confirmed by measuring the venous blood hematocrit because capillary values correlate poorly with the central venous hematocrit (capillary hematocrits are generally higher).
- The diagnosis of polycythemia is not based solely on hematocrit because there is no precise hematocrit at which symptoms appear in all infants. This is partly attributed to the fact that other factors affect viscosity in addition to hematocrit. Although symptoms are more common when the venous hematocrit exceeds 66%, signs of organ dysfunction may develop in some infants with lower hematocrits.

- Box 23.1 summarizes the potential causes of polycythemia.
- Polycythemia is estimated to occur anywhere from 1% to 5% of term infants. The incidence is increased in infants who are growth-restricted, small for gestational age, or postterm.
- Maternal–fetal risk factors such as insulin-dependent diabetes, hypertension and heart disease, cigarette smoking, and living at high altitudes should be identified (Blackburn, 2018b; Diehl-Jones & Fraser, 2021; Letterio & Ahuja, 2020; Letterio et al., 2020; Mancho-Johnson et al.; O'Reilly, 2017).

Box 23.1 Causes of Polycythemia

Causes or Etiologic Factors
- Placental transfusion
  - Holding the infant below the mother at delivery
  - Maternal-to-fetal transfusion
  - Twin-to-twin transfusion
- Placental insufficiency
  - Small for gestational age
  - Intrauterine growth restriction
  - Maternal hypertension syndromes, such as preeclampsia and renal disease
  - Maternal diabetes
  - Maternal smoking
  - Cyanotic heart disease or pulmonary disease in the mother
  - Postterm infants or large-for-gestational-age infants
  - High-altitude pregnancies
- Fetal factors
  - Trisomy 13, 18, and 21
  - Hyperthyroidism
  - Neonatal thyrotoxicosis
  - Congenital adrenal hyperplasia
  - Beckwith–Wiedemann syndrome
- Other conditions
  - Certain maternal medications, such as propranolol
  - Neonatal dehydration
  - Sepsis

Source: Data from Blackburn, S. (2018b). Hematologic and hemostatic systems. In S. Blackburn (Ed.), *Maternal, fetal, & neonatal physiology: A clinical perspective* (5th ed., pp. 216–251). Elsevier.

Hyperviscosity

- It is important to recognize that polycythemia is not synonymous with hyperviscosity and that not every neonate with polycythemia also has hyperviscosity. The viscosity of blood increases linearly with hematocrit up to 60%, then increases exponentially. Viscosity cannot easily be measured directly, so hematocrit is often used as a surrogate for viscosity.
  - Viscosity is the property of the liquid to resist changes in shape; for example, honey is more viscous than water.
  - When whole blood viscosity testing is not convenient, hyperviscosity can be inferred when a neonate with polycythemia has signs of hyperviscosity.
- Blood viscosity increases with hematocrits greater than 65% or when venous hemoglobin is greater than 22 g/dL. Hyperviscosity leads to reduction of blood flow to the organs (Blackburn, 2018b; Christensen, 2018; Diehl-Jones & Fraser, 2021; McKinney et al., 2021).

CLINICAL PRESENTATION

- The clinical manifestations are distinct in each organ system. Skin manifestations include plethora and delayed capillary filling. Renal symptoms include proteinuria and hematuria, and in extreme conditions renal disease can be indistinguishable from renal vein thrombosis. Babies with polycythemia are at increased risk of NEC. The central nervous system manifestations of polycythemia may be mild, including poor feeding, irritability, and an abnormal cry; more concerning cases are those manifesting apnea, seizures, and cerebral infarction.
- Most polycythemic infants have no clinical signs, particularly if the polycythemia becomes apparent only on routine neonatal screening. Infants are often asymptomatic. Clinical signs tend to appear at or after 2 hours of life, when the hematocrit is at its highest value. In some infants, especially those with excessive extracellular fluid losses, clinical signs may not be apparent until day 2 or 3 of life. These clinical signs are typically transient.
- Clinical signs, when present, are usually attributable to hyperviscosity and poor tissue perfusion characterized by impaired circulation occurring from an increased resistance to blood flow, or to associated metabolic abnormalities such as hypoglycemia and hypocalcemia.
- The clinical manifestations associated with polycythemia and hyperviscosity are common to many neonatal conditions and may include:
  - Central nervous abnormalities, such as lethargy or irritability, jitteriness, hypotonia, apnea, seizures, and cerebral venous thrombosis
  - Respiratory distress, including tachypnea, pulmonary edema, and pulmonary hemorrhage, and persistent pulmonary hypertension of the newborn; there may be prominent vascular markings on chest radiograph
  - Cardiac compromise, including cyanosis, tachycardia, congestive heart failure, heart murmur, cardiomegaly, and elevated pulmonary vascular resistance
  - Renal manifestations, such as renal vein thrombosis, hematuria, and proteinuria
  - Gastrointestinal signs, including behaviors associated with poor feeding, such as poor nippling and emesis, decreased bowel sounds, abdominal distention; increased RBC load also contributes to

hyperbilirubinemia (Christensen, 2018; Letterio & Ahuja, 2020; Letterio et al., 2020; McKinney et al., 2021; O'Reilly, 2017).

MANAGEMENT AND OUTCOME

- Management of polycythemia should be based on the presence of clinical manifestations that are consistent with hyperviscosity and not laboratory values alone.
- Asymptomatic infants with a hematocrit between 60% and 70% can be managed by increasing the total fluid intake and repeating the hematocrit 4 to 6 hours later.
  - Supportive care includes insertion of a peripheral intravenous catheter (PIC) and initiation of IV fluids and of phototherapy to treat hyperbilirubinemia.
  - A normal saline bolus of 10 mL/kg can be given to asymptomatic infants whose hematocrit is greater than 70% or in infants who demonstrate clinical manifestations of polycythemia with a hematocrit between 65% and 70%.
- Symptomatic infants may require an exchange or partial exchange transfusion to dilute the circulating blood volume and improve perfusion to vulnerable areas. Blood is removed from the infant via the umbilical cord and replaced (also through the cord) with normal saline. The total volume exchanged is usually 15 to 20 mL/kg of body weight; however, this will depend on the infant's body weight.
- Hyperviscosity syndrome is associated with development of vascular thrombosis (renal cerebral, mesenteric), neurologic sequelae, fine motor abnormalities, and speech delays.
- The long-term neurologic outcomes in infants with asymptomatic polycythemia and/or hyperviscosity remain controversial. A partial exchange transfusion has not shown to improve neurodevelopmental outcomes in infants with asymptomatic polycythemia.
- Newborns with a diagnosis of hyperviscosity are at greater risk of adverse neurologic outcomes. The presence of adverse neurologic outcomes may be related to the underlying risk factors as opposed to polycythemia alone (Diehl-Jones & Fraser, 2021; Jacquot et al., 2020; Letterio et al., 2020; McKinney et al., 2021; O'Reilly, 2017; Patel & Josephson, 2018).

▶ NEONATAL PLATELET DISORDERS

THROMBOCYTOSIS

Definition and Pathophysiology

- Platelets are small, nonnucleated, disc-shaped cells that aid in hemostasis, coagulation, and thrombus formation. They are derived from megakaryocytes in the bone marrow. Any disruption in the endothelium stimulates platelet plug formation and initiates hemostasis.

- In term and healthy preterm infants, platelet counts are similar to those in adults, ranging from 150,000 to 450,000/mm³. Preterm infants tend to have values slightly lower than term infants but still within the normal range.
- *Thrombocytosis* (i.e., thrombocythemia) is defined as a platelet count that is moderately elevated, ranging from 450,000 to 600,000/mL.
  - Primary (essential) thrombocytosis is extremely rare in infants and children and is often caused by monoclonal antibodies or other etiologies which may lead to an uncontrollable production of platelets.
  - Secondary (reactive) thrombocytosis tends to occur more often in infants and neonates. Following the interruption of platelet consumption by thrombus, after successful anticoagulation, infants may manifest thrombocytosis from increased bone marrow production.
- The most common causes of reactive thrombocytosis in neonates and children are infections, tissue damage (surgeries, trauma, burns), vitamin D deficiency, and anemia (frequently, iron deficiency). Reactive thrombocytosis has also been described in association with medications (e.g., corticosteroids), maternal exposure to methadone or psychopharmaceutical drugs, and metabolic diseases, myopathies, or neurofibromatosis (Blackburn, 2018b; Deschmann & Sola-Visner, 2018; Diehl-Jones & Fraser, 2021; McKinney et al., 2021).

Clinical Presentation

- Based on severity, thrombocytosis has been traditionally classified as mild (platelet counts between 500 and 700 × 10⁹/L), moderate (700–900 × 10⁹/L), severe (900–1,000 × 10⁹/L), or extreme (>1,000 × 10⁹/L; Deschmann & Sola-Visner, 2018).

Management and Outcome

- Reactive thrombocytosis usually does not lead to thromboembolic or hemorrhagic complications, and for this reason therapy with anticoagulants or platelet function inhibitors (e.g., aspirin) is usually not indicated in asymptomatic children. Individually tailored thrombosis prophylaxis should be considered only in neonates with additional thrombotic risk factors, such as maternal antiphospholipid syndrome or cardiac malformation.
- No long-term complications from thrombocytosis have been studied (Deschmann & Sola-Visner, 2018).

THROMBOCYTOPENIA

Definition and Pathophysiology

- Platelets are small, nonnucleated cells which are derived from megakaryocytes in the bone marrow. After release into the bloodstream, they will circulate for 7 to 10 days before being removed by the spleen. They are hypoactive in the first few days after birth, which protects the infant against thrombosis but may increase the risk of bleeding.

■ *Thrombocytopenia* is defined as a decreased number of platelets in the infant's blood. It is traditionally defined as a platelet count of less than 150×10^9/L. A normal platelet count in healthy newborn infants regardless of gestational age is 150,000 to 450,000.

■ Neonatal thrombocytopenia is the most common acquired hematologic condition in the infant, occurring in approximately 1% to 5% of healthy term infants at birth and up to 35% of critically ill neonates.

■ Infants predisposed to thrombocytopenia include those who are exposed to maternal antibodies or whose fetal platelets contain an antigen lacking in the mother. Congenital or acquired infections may cause thrombocytopenia. Infants born with hemangiomas such as Kasabach–Merritt syndrome will demonstrate thrombocytopenia, as will some infants born with trisomy 13 or 18.

■ Causes of thrombocytopenia can be classified into those leading to increased platelet destruction (including consumption), those resulting in decreased platelet production, and those involving both. Classification can also be based on whether the thrombocytopenia was caused by maternal factors (Blackburn, 2018b; Deschmann et al., 2017; Diehl-Jones & Fraser, 2021; Letterio & Ahuja, 2020; Letterio et al., 2020; McKinney et al., 2021).

Clinical Presentation

■ Thrombocytopenia presenting during fetal life is most commonly caused by an alloimmune reaction, congenital infection, or aneuploidy. Immune thrombocytopenia occurs because of the passive transfer of antibodies from the maternal to the fetal circulation. There are two distinct types of immune-mediated thrombocytopenia:

● In neonatal alloimmune thrombocytopenia (NAIT), the antibody is produced in the mother against a specific human platelet antigen (HPA) present in the fetus but absent in the mother.

● Autoimmune thrombocytopenia should be considered in any neonate who has early-onset thrombocytopenia and a maternal history of either immune thrombocytopenic purpura (ITP) or an autoimmune disease. Neonatal thrombocytopenia secondary to maternal ITP may last for weeks to months (unlike NAIT, which usually resolves within 2 weeks) and requires long-term monitoring.

■ Thrombocytopenia presenting within 72 hours of birth (early-onset neonatal thrombocytopenia) mostly affects preterm neonates born after pregnancies characterized by impaired placental function. Neonatal alloimmune or autoimmune thrombocytopenia is common as well.

● The most frequent cause of early-onset thrombocytopenia in a well-appearing neonate is placental insufficiency, seen in infants born to mothers with pregnancy-induced hypertension/ preeclampsia and in those with intrauterine growth restriction. The thrombocytopenia is usually mild to moderate and resolves within 72 hours.

■ Thrombocytopenia presenting in infants in the NICU after the first 72 hours of life (late-onset neonatal thrombocytopenia) can result from late-onset sepsis or NEC.

■ Thrombocytopenia can be the first presenting sign of these processes and can precede clinical deterioration. If bacterial/fungal sepsis and NEC are ruled out, viral infections such as herpes simplex virus (HSV), CMV, or enterovirus should be considered. Other less common causes of late-onset thrombocytopenia include inborn errors of metabolism and Fanconi anemia (rare).

■ Patients with platelet function disorders present with bleeding signs including mucocutaneous bleeding (nose, mouth, gastrointestinal tract, genitourinary tract) and bruising. The extent, location, and nature of the bruises are generally related to birth trauma and invasive procedures (e.g., IV starts, heel sticks, or endotracheal suctioning). They also show platelet-type bleeding such as petechiae, purpura, and epistaxis. If delivered vaginally, the infant will have a cephalohematoma (Deschmann et al., 2017; Deschmann & Sola-Visner, 2018; Diehl-Jones & Fraser, 2021; Letterio & Ahuja, 2020; Letterio et al., 2020).

Management and Outcome

■ The decision to administer a prophylactic platelet transfusion should be made on the basis of many factors, including the platelet count, the mechanism responsible for the thrombocytopenia, the medications administered, and the condition of the patient. Usually such decisions are institution-driven, "best-guess" estimates.

● Patients qualifying for a platelet transfusion should initially receive 10 to 15 mL/kg of CMV-negative standard platelet suspension, prepared from a fresh unit of whole blood or by platelet pheresis.

● Administration of prophylactic platelet transfusions at trigger thresholds of up to 50 $\times 10^9$/L is generally considered to represent acceptable and safe clinical practice.

■ Random donor platelet transfusions are now considered the first line of therapy for infants with suspected NAIT, although they rarely result in sustained increase due to antibody destruction.

● If able, obtain HPA testing on the infant, and in the absence of neonatal HPA the use of maternal platelets is recommended.

■ First-line therapy for autoimmune thrombocytopenia is IV immunoglobin Ig (IVIG), with the addition of random donor platelets for infants with active bleeding.

- Management of late-onset thrombocytopenia includes treatment appropriate to the suspected etiology (e.g., antibiotics, supportive respiratory and cardiovascular care, bowel rest in case of NEC, and surgery in case of surgical NEC). The platelet count usually improves in 1 to 2 weeks, although in some infants the thrombocytopenia persists for several weeks for unclear reasons.
- The outcomes for patients with thrombocytopenia are variable and depend on the specific disorders (Deschmann & Sola-Visner, 2018; Diehl-Jones & Fraser, 2021; Letterio & Ahuja, 2020).

▶ COAGULOPATHIES

VITAMIN K DEFICIENCY

Definition and Pathophysiology

- Newborns are deficient in all vitamin K-dependent factors: II, VII, IX, and X. In the absence of vitamin K, these proteins are dysfunctional and are released into the circulation as proteins induced by vitamin K absence (PIVKA). Previously termed *hemorrhagic disease of the newborn*, the newer term *vitamin K-dependent bleeding* (VKDB) is thought to describe the link more accurately between vitamin K deficiency and spontaneous bleeding.
- The etiology of vitamin K-dependent factor deficiency is twofold: Vitamin K is poorly transferred through the placenta to the fetus during pregnancy, and the newborn intestine lacks colonization of bacteria normally responsible for producing vitamin K.
- Risk factors are related to three forms of VKDB:
  - *Early onset (within 24 hours):* can occur in infants of mothers who are taking certain anticonvulsants (e.g., phenytoin) and vitamin K antagonists such as warfarin (Coumadin)
  - *Classic onset (2–6 days):* occurs due to a physiologic deficiency in vitamin K at birth combined with a sole breast milk diet or inadequate feeding
  - *Late onset (2–12 weeks of age):* occurs in infants who did not receive vitamin K at birth and are receiving an inadequate dose (e.g., breastfeeding) or in infants with hepatobiliary disease (Blackburn, 2018b; Croteau, 2017; Diehl-Jones & Fraser, 2021; Letterio & Ahuja, 2020; Letterio et al., 2020; McKinney et al., 2021; Saxonhouse, 2018)

Clinical Presentation

- Early hemolytic disease of the newborn (HDN) develops in the first 24 hours of life and is linked to maternal use of specific medications that interfere with vitamin K stores or function, such as some anticonvulsants. Bleeding can be in the form of intracranial hemorrhage (ICH), gastrointestinal bleeding, or cephalohematomas. Late HDN occurs between weeks 2 and 8 of life and is linked to disorders

that compromise ongoing vitamin K supply, such as cystic fibrosis, alpha-1 antitrypsin deficiency, biliary atresia (BA), and celiac disease.
- In general, oozing occurs, which may be localized or diffuse, and frequently gastrointestinal (hematemesis, melena) or from puncture sites, the umbilical cord, or postcircumcision. There may also be diffuse ecchymosis and/or petechiae.
- Laboratory assessment shows elevated prothrombin time (PT) and partial thromboplastin time (PTT), low levels of vitamin K-dependent clotting factors, and high PIVKA levels (Croteau, 2017; Diehl-Jones & Fraser, 2021; Letterio & Ahuja, 2020; Saxonhouse, 2018).

Management and Outcome

- Prophylactic therapy has mostly eliminated VKDB. When intramuscular (IM) vitamin K prophylaxis is provided, the incidence of late VKDB decreases to 0.24 to 3.2 per 100,000 live births.
- If VKDB occurs, transfusions of blood products (RBCs, fresh frozen plasma [FFP]) and repeated doses of vitamin K may be indicated (Croteau, 2017; Diehl-Jones & Fraser, 2021; Letterio et al., 2020; Saxonhouse, 2018).

DISSEMINATED INTRAVASCULAR COAGULATION

Definition and Pathophysiology

- Disseminated intravascular coagulation (DIC) is a complex process that is characterized by systemic activation of coagulation and fibrinolysis, consumption of platelets and coagulation factors, and generation of fibrin clots that can lead to ischemic organ damage or failure.
  - This dysregulation of the coagulation and inflammatory systems results in massive thrombin generation with widespread fibrin deposition and consumption of coagulation proteins and platelets, ultimately leading to multiorgan damage.
- In DIC, activation of blood clotting proteins is initiated by tissue factor from bacterial products (endotoxin) or inflammation. The activation of clotting proteins leads to a hypercoagulable state and thromboses form, especially in the small vessels of the liver, spleen, brain, lungs, kidneys, and adrenal glands. The bone marrow releases platelets; however, the system which regulates coagulation is immature and the ability to neutralize activated clotting proteins is quickly overwhelmed. This results in deficiency of platelets and clotting factors and is called *consumptive coagulopathy*.
- DIC always occurs as a secondary event and can be triggered by a variety of pathologic conditions. These include birth asphyxia, respiratory distress syndrome, meconium aspiration syndrome, infection, NEC, hypothermia, severe placental insufficiency, and thrombosis.

■ Neonatal precipitating factors include infection (bacterial, viral, fungal); conditions causing hypoxia, acidosis, and shock; severe Rh incompatibility; and tissue injury (traumatic birth or NEC; Diehl-Jones & Fraser, 2021; Letterio & Ahuja, 2020; Letterio et al., 2020; McKinney et al., 2021; Saxonhouse, 2018).

Clinical Presentation

■ The cardinal manifestations of overt DIC are caused by excessive bleeding and microvascular thrombosis. Hemorrhagic clinical signs include petechiae and bruising, oozing from venipuncture sites, bleeding from traumatic and surgical wounds, and in severe cases bleeding involving internal organs, and organ and tissue ischemia. Microvascular thrombosis causes potential ischemia and necrosis of any organ, particularly the kidney. Multisystem organ failure can result as end-stage failure.

■ The diagnosis of DIC, particularly in the early stages, can be problematic because there is no single laboratory test that can establish or rule out DIC. Hence, the diagnosis is often made on the basis of an appropriate clinical suspicion supported by laboratory evidence of procoagulant, and fibrinolytic system activation coupled with anticoagulant consumption and diffuse clinical bleeding.

● Laboratory abnormalities seen in DIC include thrombocytopenia, elevated fibrin degradation products (FDP) or D-dimers, prolonged PT, prolonged activated partial thromboplastin time (aPTT), prolonged thrombin clotting time, and a low fibrinogen (Diehl-Jones & Fraser, 2021; Letterio et al., 2020).

Management and Outcome

■ The most important aspect of treatment for DIC is to treat the underlying disorder. Successful treatment of DIC relies largely on reversal of the underlying condition and supporting adequate blood flow and oxygen delivery.

■ The focus of acute management in the neonate is to support adequate hemostasis to reduce the risk of spontaneous hemorrhage. This is usually achieved with platelet transfusions, FFP, or cryoprecipitate.

● Blood component transfusions (platelets, FFP, and cryoprecipitate) are an important part of supportive treatment in DIC. In cases of DIC in which thrombosis predominates, such as arterial or venous thromboembolism or severe purpura fulminans, therapeutic anticoagulation with unfractionated heparin may be considered.

■ Outcomes are related to the prognosis of the underlying disease and the severity of DIC (Croteau, 2017; Diehl-Jones & Fraser, 2021; Letterio et al., 2020; Saxonhouse, 2018).

▶ IMMUNE-MEDIATED HEMOLYTIC DISEASE

■ Immune-mediated disorders are the most common cause of hemolysis in neonates and should be suspected when there is a heterospecific mother–infant pair where the infant expresses a red cell antigen(s) foreign to the mother, the presence of a maternal antibody directed to the infant RBC antigen, and/or a positive direct Coombs test in the neonate indicating maternal antibody bound to the infant RBC (Watchko, 2018).

RH DISEASE

Definition and Pathophysiology

■ *Isoimmune hemolytic disease*, HDN, and *erythroblastosis fetalis* are all terms for a disorder caused by transplacental passage of maternal immunoglobulin G (IgG) antibody that reacts with antigens on the fetal RBC and leads to cell lysis.

■ Several Rho antigens are recognized, each of which is detected by specific antibodies. The most clinically relevant of the membrane Rh proteins to neonatal hemolytic disease is the Rho(D) antigen, since the D antigen is most implicated in maternal–fetal incompatibility.

■ At birth, quantities of fetal blood may enter the maternal circulation; if the fetus is Rho(D)-positive, this will stimulate the formation of both anti-D antibodies and memory cells in the mother.

■ Rh-positive RBCs are those that possess the D antigen. A lowercase *d* is used to denote the absence of the D antigen, or Rh-negative status.

■ The hallmark of isoimmunization is a positive direct antiglobulin test (DAT; also known as the direct Coombs test). This indicates a maternally produced antibody that has traversed the placenta and is now found within the fetus.

● The test is termed *direct* if the antiglobulin is adhered to the RBCs.

● An *indirect* test refers to the antibody being detected in the maternal serum.

■ Rh isoimmunization is of particular concern because the D antigen is strongly expressed in large amounts early in gestation. Additionally, the D antigen stimulates the production of maternal IgG and memory cells in the mother. Following exposure to the D antigen on the fetal RBCs, the mother's immune system responds by forming anti-D IgG antibodies. The IgG then crosses the placenta and adheres to fetal RBCs containing the D antigen. The subsequent antigen–antibody interaction leads to hemolysis and anemia.

● Isoimmune hemolytic disease, HDN, and erythroblastosis fetalis are synonymous with the disorder by which maternal IgG antibodies cross into the fetal circulation.

- Rh hemolytic disease is rare during the first pregnancy involving an Rh-positive fetus, but the risk increases with each subsequent pregnancy. This is because small volumes of fetal RBCs enter the maternal circulation throughout gestation, although the major fetomaternal bleeding responsible for sensitization occurs during delivery. Once sensitization has occurred, reexposure to Rh(D) RBCs in subsequent pregnancies leads to an exaggerated response, with an increase in the maternal anti-D titer.
- Rh-negative mothers are unlikely to have anti-D antibodies unless they have been exposed to D antigen in a previous pregnancy or have received a mismatched blood transfusion. Significant hemolysis occurring in the first pregnancy indicates previous maternal exposure to Rh-positive RBCs. On occasion, the sensitization is a consequence of an earlier transfusion in which Rh-positive RBCs were administered by mistake or in which some other blood components (e.g., platelets) containing Rh(D) RBCs were transfused. Even a tiny amount of Rh-positive fetal blood is enough to cause anti-D antibody formation and memory cell production in the mother.
- A prior pregnancy with a Rho(D)-positive fetus increases the risk in subsequent pregnancies. The formation of memory cells results in permanent immunization. During subsequent pregnancies, even a very small amount of blood from a rho(d)-positive fetus entering the mother's system may be enough to trigger memory cells to produce antibodies against the d antigen on the fetal RBC (Blackburn, 2018c; Christensen, 2018; Kaplan et al., 2020).

Clinical Presentation

- The infant may present with pathologic hyperbilirubinemia, and in severe cases severe anemia, congestive heart failure, and death.
- The infant of a mother who received Rh immune globulin (RhIG) prophylaxis within 12 weeks may have a weakly positive direct Coombs test due to the placental transfer of RhIG antibodies (Blackburn, 2018c).

Management and Outcome

- Management first requires the identification of those fetuses at risk. An increase in the maternal anti-D titer in a previously sensitized Rh-negative woman is a good serologic measure of a fetus in potential jeopardy. A history of neonatal hemolytic disease resulting from anti-D antibodies suggests that the current fetus may also be at risk.
- RhIG (RhoGAM) is a concentrated form of anti-D antibodies given to Rh-negative women at various points antepartum and postpartum to prevent HDN. RhIG works by destroying fetal Rh-positive RBCs in the maternal circulation before the D antigen is recognized by the maternal circulation so that antibodies and memory cells are not made.
  - RhIG is administered at 28 weeks' gestation prophylactically, and within 72 hours of delivery of an Rh-positive newborn, or after any other event that may increase the risk of maternal–fetal blood mixing, including after an abortion, amniocentesis, or with significant bleeding during pregnancy.
- It is important to note that RhD-positive infants delivered to RhD-negative mothers during the first isoimmunized pregnancy (conversion from negative to positive maternal antibody titer in that pregnancy) are at an approximately 20% risk of developing HDN. An infant born of a pregnancy during which maternal antibody conversion occurs will by definition carry the foreign antigen and may have a positive direct Coombs test. Such infants are at risk of hemolytic diseases and should be monitored closely for severe hyperbilirubinemia with serial serum total bilirubin (TSB) measurements. These infants should not be discharged early from the birth hospital as they will likely require treatment, including the possibility of an exchange transfusion.
- The sibling of an infant with hemolytic disease will be at increased risk for the same. It is important that parents feel empowered to ask questions about hyperbilirubinemia and its symptoms so that they can bring any concerns to the attention of healthcare providers (Blackburn, 2018c; Christensen, 2018; Kamath-Rayne et al., 2021; Watchko, 2018).

ABO INCOMPATIBILITY

Definition and Pathophysiology

- With the reduction of the incidence of Rh isoimmunization by immune prophylaxis, DAT-positive ABO incompatibility is now the single most prominent cause of immune hemolytic disease in the neonate.
  - Although ABO incompatibility is much more common than Rh disease, it is less severe than Rh incompatibility. Mechanisms responsible for Rh isoimmunization, such as previous exposure and immunization, are not needed with ABO incompatibility because the mother has naturally occurring antibodies to fetal ABO antigens.
- In mothers with type A or type B blood, naturally occurring anti-B and anti-A isoantibodies are typically IgM antibodies and consequently do not cross the placenta to affect fetal RBCs. In contrast, the anti-A and anti-B alloantibodies present in mothers with type O blood typically also include IgG antibodies that can cross the placenta and affect the fetal erythrocytes. For this reason, ABO hemolytic disease of the fetus and newborn is largely limited to type O mothers carrying type A or type B fetuses.

- The most common situation in which ABO incompatibility occurs is with a type O mother and a type A, or less frequently type B, infant. The A antigen seems to be more antigenic than the B antigen. The type O mother has naturally occurring anti-A and anti-B antibodies in their serum that can react with the fetal RBCs.
- ABO incompatibility could also occur with a type AB infant but never with a type O infant (Blackburn, 2018c; Christensen, 2018; Kaplan et al., 2020).

Clinical Presentation

- A priority in evaluating every newborn is knowledge of the maternal blood type and the maternal antibody screen routinely performed at maternal registration upon pregnancy diagnosis to identify non-ABO alloantibodies in the maternal serum that may pose a risk of hemolytic disease in the newborn.
  - Although about one of every three groups A or B infants born to a group O mother have anti-A or anti-B antibodies attached to their red cells (as indexed by a positive DAT), only one in five of those develop a modest to significant degree of hyperbilirubinemia.
- The resulting hyperbilirubinemia in the newborn is highly variable and generally milder than that seen with Rh incompatibility. Although some 15% of pregnancies are a "set-up" for ABO incompatibility (mother O, baby A or B), only 33% of these infants show a positive DAT and only 15% of these have clinically significant hemolysis and hyperbilirubinemia. If the DAT is negative, these infants, as a group, do not have an increased incidence of significant hyperbilirubinemia compared with non–ABO-incompatible infants.
- The diagnosis of ABO hemolytic disease as opposed to ABO incompatibility should generally be reserved for infants who have a positive DAT finding *and* clinical jaundice within the first 12 to 24 hours of life. Reticulocytosis and the presence of microspherocytes on the smear support the diagnosis (Kamath-Rayne et al., 2021; Watchko, 2018; Watchko & Maisels, 2020).

Management and Outcome

- Close observation of any newborn born to a blood group O mother is important, as well as performing a transcutaneous bilirubinometry (TcB) or serum total bilirubin (TB) measurement at the first appearance of jaundice. Routine blood group and DAT determination on umbilical cord blood is an option and may allow for additional risk determination.
- ABO hemolytic disease is often detected within the first 12 to 24 hours of life ("icterus praecox").
- In most cases, pallor and jaundice are minimal. Hepatosplenomegaly is uncommon. Laboratory evidence includes minimal to moderate hyperbilirubinemia, and occasionally some degree of anemia. The DAT is sometimes negative.

- Symptomatic ABO hemolytic disease should be considered in infants who develop marked jaundice in the context of ABO incompatibility that is generally accompanied by a positive direct Coombs test and prominent microspherocytosis on red cell smear.
  - In suspected cases of ABO incompatibility, it is essential to exclude other antibodies and other nonimmune causes of hemolysis, such as glucose-6-phosphate dehydrogenase (G6PD) deficiency or hereditary spherocytosis.
- Severe cases are generally treated effectively with phototherapy, occasionally with an exchange transfusion in which group O Rh-compatible RBCs are used. Additional follow-up at 2 to 3 weeks of age to check for anemia in these infants is essential.
- Signs and symptoms of jaundice should be explained in a manner that is understandable and meaningful for parents, emphasizing that neonatal hyperbilirubinemia is usually a transient condition and one to which all infants must adapt after birth.
- The use of phototherapy can be distressing for parents and should be explained to them before they see their infant under phototherapy lights for the first time. In addition, incubators, bili-masks, and phototherapy lights can all contribute to a sense of separation between the parents and their infant by creating a physical and emotional barrier (Christensen, 2018; Kamath-Rayne et al., 2021; Kaplan et al., 2020; Watchko, 2018).

▶ NEONATAL JAUNDICE AND LIVER DISEASE

BILIARY ATRESIA

Definition and Pathophysiology

- BA is a condition in infants that is characterized by inflammation and fibrosis of the bile ducts. The hepatic biliary ducts become scarred, and as the disease progresses there is complete obliteration of the bile ducts. As the bile builds up in the liver, damage to this organ occurs.
  - BA is one of the more common causes of chronic liver disease in infants, with an incidence of approximately 0.5 to 3.2 per 10,000 live births. This reported incidence varies based on geographic location and ethnicity.
- BA is characterized by the anatomy of extrahepatic biliary obstruction. Two clinical phenotypes exist:
  - "Classical" BA, which is not associated with extrahepatic congenital anomalies
  - "BA with splenic malformation," which presents with other congenital anomalies such as situs inversus, polysplenia or asplenia, vascular and cardiac malformations, and intestinal malrotation (Kaplan et al., 2020; Lane et al., 2018)

Clinical Presentation

- Infants with BA typically present between 2 and 5 weeks of life with clinical signs including:
  - Acholic stools, which can appear after the onset of jaundice
  - Cholestatic or prolonged jaundice; cholestatic jaundice may not be recognized as new, which highlights the importance of evaluating any prolonged or new jaundice in infants
  - Ascites, which may present later in the disease course
  - Inadequate weight gain related to malabsorption that occurs secondary to chronic inflammation and cholestasis (Lane et al., 2018)

Management and Outcome

- Expedient differentiation of BA from other causes of neonatal cholestasis is critical, as surgical intervention before 2 months of age has been shown to improve surgical success and outcome. The immediate goal of surgical correction is the reestablishment of bile drainage, which is now achieved in most neonates when operated on before 3 months of age.
- BA may be suspected based on clinical manifestations. The following are part of the workup to confirm a diagnosis of BA:
  - Conjugated hyperbilirubinemia, which is often between 2 and 7 mg/dL
  - Total serum bilirubin levels, which may be between 5 and 12 mg/dL
  - Elevated alanine aminotransferase (ALT), alkaline phosphatase (ALP), and gamma-glutamyl transferase (GGT)
- Abdominal ultrasound (US) should be performed if BA is present. US will demonstrate absence of the gallbladder or a fibrotic remnant of the extrahepatic bile duct. There may also be the "triangle cord sign," which is a triangular or tubular echogenic cord of fibrous tissue that represents the biliary remnant.
- Hepatobiliary iminodiacetic acid (HIDA) scan should also be performed. In infants with BA, there is lack of excretion of bile into the bowel of the radioactive tracer that is injected into the infant. Oral phenobarbital can be administered at 5 mg/kg/d to the infant for 5 days prior to the procedure to enhance sensitivity of the scan.
- Once a diagnosis is confirmed, surgery is done with a Kasai hepatic portoenterostomy, which attempts to restore the normal flow of the bile. This may prevent or delay progression of the disease as well as worsening of fibrosis and the development of end-stage liver disease.
- Without rapid intervention, the natural history of BA is uniform fatality by 2 years of age. Unrelieved by surgery, the defect inevitably leads to death from biliary cirrhosis in the first 2 to 3 years of life.
- Even with surgery intervention with the Kasai portoenterostomy, many infants tend to go on to develop cirrhosis and portal hypertension with the need

for a liver transplant (Juul & Christensen, 2018; Kaplan et al., 2020; Lane et al., 2018).

HYPERBILIRUBINEMIA

Normal Physiology

- In order to understand bilirubin pathology, an understanding of natural physiology is necessary. The pathway of bilirubin synthesis, transport, and metabolism is summarized in Figure 23.3.
- *Bilirubin production* in the newborn is as high as 8 to 10 mg/kg/24 hours, which when compared with adults is 2 to 2.5 times faster.
- A majority of bilirubin (75%–85%) production occurs from the breakdown of hemoglobin from RBCs or ineffective erythropoiesis, a process that is accelerated in infants.
  - Each gram of hemoglobin produces 35 mg of bilirubin.
- The remaining 15% to 25% of bilirubin is derived from the breakdown of other forms of heme in the body. This form of hemoglobin includes heme in the liver, such as in cytochromes and in muscle myoglobin. Ineffective erythropoiesis in the bone marrow also contributes to the production of bilirubin.
- Bilirubin metabolism occurs in the reticuloendothelial system, primarily in the liver and spleen as old or abnormal RBCs are removed from the circulation. The breakdown of RBCs is a normal process that destroys red cells that are aging, immature, or malformed.
  - The enzyme heme oxygenase acts on heme to produce biliverdin. Biliverdin reductase will then convert biliverdin into bilirubin.
- Once converted to bilirubin by biliverdin reductase, the unconjugated bilirubin is released into the bloodstream. There it must be bound to a carrier for *transport to the liver*. Albumin is this carrier which rapidly and tightly binds with bilirubin.
  - Each molecule of adult albumin can bind with at least two molecules of bilirubin, with the first molecule being more tightly bound than the second.
- Infants have a reduced capacity to bind albumin with bilirubin when compared with adults and older children secondary to reduced concentrations of albumin.
- Bilirubin is removed from albumin prior to entering the cells in the liver and is then *transported into the hepatocyte* by intracellular carrier proteins. Once in the liver, unconjugated bilirubin is bound to glutathione-S-transferase A, also known as ligandin or with B-ligandin (Y protein). To a lesser degree, unconjugated bilirubin may also bind with Z protein, another hepatic carrier.
- *Conjugation of bilirubin* occurs within the smooth endoplasmic reticulum of the liver cell, converting unconjugated bilirubin to a more polar, water-soluble substance in order for bilirubin to be excreted in bile.

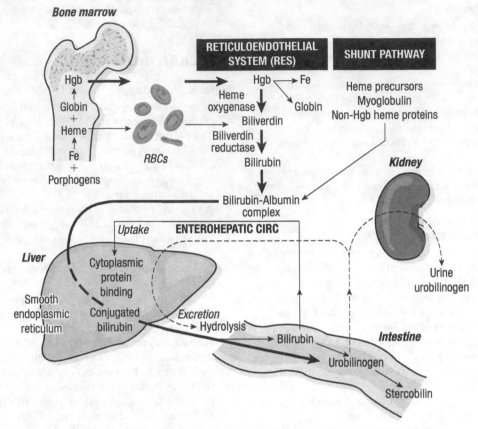

Figure 23.3 Pathways of bilirubin synthesis, transport, and metabolism.

Fe, iron; Hgb, hemoglobin; RBC, red blood cells.
Source: Reproduced with permission from Assali, N. S. (1972). *Pathophysiology of gestation.* Academic Press.

- In the liver, conjugation of bilirubin occurs by another enzyme, *uridine diphosphate glucuronosyltransferase* (UGT-1A1), which leads to the formation of water-soluble compounds called *bilirubin glucuronides.*
- Conjugated bilirubin can now be *actively secreted in the bile* and into the small intestine.
- *Enterohepatic circulation* is the reabsorption and recycling of the unconjugated form of bilirubin back into the circulation. Enterohepatic reabsorption of bilirubin that is excreted into the intestine is enhanced in infants. This increases their risk for hyperbilirubinemia.
  - Conjugated bilirubin can be spontaneously or enzymatically converted back to unconjugated bilirubin. Typically, the more unstable forms of conjugated bilirubin are reverted back to unconjugated bilirubin, such as the mono- and diglucuronides of bilirubin.
  - Reverted unconjugated bilirubin can now readily cross the intestinal mucosa and contribute to the circulating pool of unconjugated bilirubin through the enterohepatic circulation.
  - Additional factors that play a role in enterohepatic circulation include a mildly alkaline pH of the

duodenum and jejunum and a lack of intestinal flora, the latter of which reduces bilirubin to urobilinogen. High concentrations of bilirubin are also found in meconium.
- Bilirubin levels may be affected by several issues, including:
  - There is delayed passage of meconium as meconium contains a substantial amount of bilirubin.
  - There is a reduction in UGT activity.
  - *Albumin levels:* An increase in the amount of albumin limits the amount of unbound, unconjugated bilirubin that is available to cross the blood–brain barrier to cause neuronal damage.
  - *Decreased life span of the RBC:* The life span of the RBC is shorter at 70 to 90 days in newborns, thereby increasing bilirubin load.
  - An accelerated breakdown of RBCs results in more bilirubin production/load in newborns.
  - Diminished hepatic uptake of bilirubin may be related to inadequate perfusion of the sinusoids in the liver or a deficiency of the carrier proteins Y and Z (Blackburn, 2018a; Kamath-Rayne et al., 2021; Kaplan et al., 2020; Watchko, 2018; Watchko & Maisels, 2020).

Unconjugated (Indirect) Nonpathologic "Physiologic" Hyperbilirubinemia

DEFINITION AND PATHOPHYSIOLOGY

- Bilirubin is a weak acid that is not water-soluble or easily excreted from the body. In order to be excreted from the body, it must be conjugated to glucuronic acid.
- A majority of fetal bilirubin is in the unconjugated form, which can be found in amniotic fluid as early as 12 weeks' gestation. The fetus begins producing bile acids and pigments early in pregnancy, the majority of which are biliverdin and bilirubin.
  - Bilirubin levels in the amniotic fluid usually rise, followed by a plateau between 16 and 25 weeks, before decreasing and disappearing by 36 weeks' gestation.
- Bile acids and bilirubin levels are low in the fetus, related to enzymes and transport systems that encourage the removal of these potentially harmful substances.
  - Bilirubin in the unconjugated state occurs for many reasons, including liver and intestinal immaturity. The ductus venous also shunts some placental blood away from the liver, thereby decreasing blood flow to this organ. Additionally, bilirubin is recirculated by the enterohepatic shunt. All these processes allow bilirubin to remain in the unconjugated form.
- There is evidence to suggest that bilirubin may not only be toxic but beneficial as well in infants. Unconjugated bilirubin can diffuse into any cell and might be helpful in times of stress, and at lower levels bilirubin acts as an antioxidant. As an antioxidant, bilirubin limits cellular damage by binding to the membrane to prevent peroxidation and scavenging of reactive oxygen species.
- Unconjugated hyperbilirubinemia is the most common condition in the neonatal period that requires evaluation and treatment; however, for most newborns, it is a benign condition without clinical significance. Physiologic hyperbilirubinemia is the most common reason for readmission to the hospital during the first week of life.
- Jaundice is a self-limiting process, with bilirubin levels typically returning to normal, defined as less than 1 mg/dL, by 12 days of life.
- Physiologic jaundice occurs in approximately 85% of infants during the first several days after delivery. Almost all term infants will have a bilirubin level greater than 2 mg/dL during the first week of life. Approximately 60% to 80% of normal newborns will appear jaundiced during the first week of life.
  - In a minority of healthy infants, approximately 6%, bilirubin levels increase to 12 mg/dL, while about 3% of healthy newborns will have bilirubin levels that exceed 15 mg/dL.
- It occurs in term infants and is characterized by progressive increase in total bilirubin concentration and peaks between 3 and 4 days of life in White and African American infants. This is followed by a rapid decline in bilirubin levels to approximately 3 mg/dL by the fifth day of life in White and African American infants and by the seventh day on Asian American infants.
- Physiologic jaundice in premature infants tends to be more severe when compared with term neonates, with peak total bilirubin concentrations in larger preterm newborn that may reach 10 to 12 mg/dL by the fifth day of life.
- Some infants are at greater risk for hyperbilirubinemia when compared with other neonates. Risk factors for hyperbilirubinemia can be divided into three categories and are listed in Box 23.2 (Blackburn, 2018a; Dragoo, 2017; Kamath-Rayne et al., 2021; Kaplan et al., 2020; Watchko, 2018).

Box 23.2 Risk Factors for Hyperbilirubinemia in the Newborn

Major Risk Factors
- A serum or transcutaneous bilirubin level in the high-risk zone prior to discharge
- Jaundice observed within the first 24 hours of life
- Blood group incompatibility with positive direct antiglobulin test, other known hemolytic disease (such as G6PD deficiency)
- Late preterm infant of 35 to 36 weeks' gestation
- Previous sibling who received phototherapy
- Cephalohematoma or significant bruising
- Exclusive breastfeeding, especially if breastfeeding is not going well and weight loss is excessive
- East Asian race

Minor Risk Factors
- A serum or transcutaneous bilirubin level in the high intermediate-risk zone prior to discharge
- Gestational age of 37 to 38 weeks
- Jaundice observed prior to discharge
- Previous sibling who received phototherapy
- Macrosomic infant of a diabetic mother
- Maternal age greater than 25 years
- Male gender

Decreased Risk
- A serum or transcutaneous bilirubin level in the low-risk zone prior to discharge
- Gestational age greater than 41 weeks
- African American race
- Discharge after 72 hours of age

G6PD, glucose-6-phosphate dehydrogenase.
Source: Data from Kamath-Rayne, B. D., Froese, P. A., & Thilo, E. H. (2021). Neonatal hyperbilirubinemia. In S. L. Gardner, B. S. Carter, M. Enzman-Hines, & S. Niermeyer (Eds.), *Merenstein & Gardner's handbook of neonatal intensive care nursing: An interprofessional approach* (9th ed., pp. 662–691). Elsevier.

CLINICAL PRESENTATION

- When serum bilirubin levels are elevated, jaundice becomes visible in the skin. Jaundice does not become visible in infants until levels exceed 5.0 to 7.0 mg/dL.
  - Visual inspection for jaundice should be performed in a well-lit room with natural lighting or daylight at least every 8 hours when hyperbilirubinemia is suspected.
  - Jaundice initially becomes apparent on the face and progresses in a cephalocaudal fashion; therefore, assessment for jaundice includes blanching the skin with pressure using the fingers on the forehead, sternum, or knee to reveal the underlying color or tone.
  - Inspecting the skin of the infant is helpful in identifying jaundice but is not an accurate method to determine bilirubin levels. Because accuracy of identifying jaundice varies with clinician experience and neonatal skin differences, it is very important to obtain bilirubin levels for all newborns who appear jaundiced with either serum or transcutaneous bilirubin measurement.
- Bilirubin levels can be measured within the blood sera or through the skin using a transcutaneous device.
  - Serum bilirubin measurement is most commonly obtained through heel-stick puncture sampling. Serum measurement is the most accurate way to determine a bilirubin level but also the most painful for the infant. Total serum bilirubin is the most recommended method on which to make clinical decisions.
  - TcB is a noninvasive method that uses reflectance photometry or transcutaneous colorimetry to estimate bilirubin level. Several studies have demonstrated that using a handheld TcB device can accurately determine TSB levels in term and late preterm infants of different ethnic groups to within 2 to 3 mg/dL when the TSB is less than 15 mg/dL.
  - One limitation of using the TcB device is that it often underestimates the bilirubin level when total serum levels are greater than 15 mg/dL. The recommendation is that all bilirubin levels greater than 15 and above the 75th percentile be confirmed with serum bilirubin levels.
- All bilirubin level concentrations must be interpreted based on the infant's age in hours. Using the nomogram developed by Bhutani and colleagues for infants greater than 35 weeks' gestation, the newborn's TSB should be plotted and interpreted based on age in hours to determine the risk of hyperbilirubinemia and need for additional testing. Once plotted, the nomogram will suggest whether the infant is at high, intermediate, or low risk for requiring further intervention for hyperbilirubinemia, based on total serum bilirubin concentration (Dragoo, 2017; Kamath-Rayne et al., 2021; Kaplan et al., 2020; Watchko, 2018; Watchko & Maisels, 2020).

MANAGEMENT WITH PHOTOTHERAPY

- Phototherapy was initially introduced in 1958. Phototherapy is the most common and effective form of therapy to treat unconjugated hyperbilirubinemia. Phototherapy is the mainstay of treatment for indirect hyperbilirubinemia.
- The use of phototherapy reduces the increase in total bilirubin concentration, regardless of gestational age, the presence or absence of hemolysis, and the degree of skin pigmentation.
- The widespread use of phototherapy to treat hyperbilirubinemia has greatly reduced the need for exchange transfusions in infants. Additionally, the incidence of kernicterus and long-term neurobehavioral performance in children is greatly decreased in infants treated with phototherapy. There has been no documentation of adverse long-term outcomes in infants who received phototherapy in the neonatal period.
- Phototherapy *mechanism of action* creates a photochemical reaction that transforms the unconjugated bilirubin in the capillaries and interstitial spaces of the skin and subcutaneous tissue into photoisomers that can be excreted from the body in the bile and urine without conjugation.
  - During phototherapy, bilirubin absorbs the light so that photochemical reactions occur. These photochemical reactions, photoisomerization and photo-oxidization, facilitate changing the structure and shape of bilirubin and converting it to photoproducts that can be excreted from the body in bile and urine without conjugation.
  - Photoisomerization, which is responsible for more than 80% of the bilirubin that is eliminated with the use of phototherapy, converts indirect bilirubin that is poorly soluble into a water-soluble reversible configurational or an irreversible structural photoisomer. The photoisomers can then be excreted into the bile without conjugation.
- Lumirubin is the major pathway through which bilirubin is eliminated with phototherapy use. It is a stable, nonreversible structural photoisomer that does not require conjugation and is formed slowly but is excreted very rapidly in both bile and to a lesser extent in urine, with a serum half-life of 2 hours.
  - The production of lumirubin is dose-dependent with the amount of irradiance.
  - The photoisomers are unlikely to cross the blood–brain barrier because they are polar and need transporters in order to reach neurons. For this reason, they do not enter the brain to cause kernicterus.
- The breakdown of bilirubin in the presence of phototherapy occurs primarily in the superficial capillaries and in the intestinal spaces. Configurational isomers are formed very rapidly but are excreted very slowly in bile. They have a serum half-life of 12 to 21 hours. After 6 to 12 hours of phototherapy, approximately 20% of the total serum bilirubin has

been converted to configurational isomers. Because these isomers are unstable and the process reversible, they may be reverted back to unconjugated bilirubin in the intestines and recirculated by way of enterohepatic shunting.

- *Special blue fluorescent lights* are the most effective phototherapy available because they deliver light in the blue-green spectrum and have more irradiance at 450 nm. They provide maximal absorption and adequate skin penetration.
  - There are many types of fluorescent lights, including daylight, white, and blue lamps. Although widely used, these types of lights are less effective than special blue fluorescent tubes, which provide significantly more irradiance in the blue spectrum.
- Fiberoptic blankets use a tungsten–halogen lamp as the light source for use as a spotlight. This type of system is a convenient way of delivering phototherapy above and below the infant simultaneously. They generate little heat and provide higher irradiance when compared with fluorescent lights. Because they are small, they cover only a small surface area, which significantly reduces the achieved spectral power. For this reason, they are rarely effective when used alone in term infants.
- Another method of delivering phototherapy is with the use of blue light-emitting diodes (LEDs), which allows a higher level of irradiance to be delivered to the infant with minimal generation of heat. An LED unit is a low-weight, low-voltage, low-power device that has been shown to be an effective and safe alternative to other modes of phototherapy. They are available as either overhead or underneath devices.
- The *AAP issued comprehensive guidelines for the initiation of phototherapy* in infants 35 weeks or greater. The guidelines are based on limited evidence and the levels for initiation of treatment are estimates. The guidelines by the AAP do not apply to premature infants born less than 35 weeks' gestation.
  - Additional online applications, such as the BiliTool, have been endorsed and recommended by the AAP to aid in the decision-making process regarding the treatment of jaundice in infants.
- There is no single serum bilirubin level at which phototherapy should be initiated. Instead, each infant needs to be evaluated individually with consideration of the bilirubin level and the infant's level of risk for hyperbilirubinemia.
- When discontinuing phototherapy, the level must be considered in combination with the overall clinical presentation and risk factors of the infant. A rebound bilirubin level should be obtained for at least 24 hours in infants less than 37 weeks, have a positive DAT, and those treated at or before 72 hours of age. A rebound total serum bilirubin level of 1 to 2 mg/dL or more can occur after phototherapy has been discontinued.
- There are many *factors that influence the efficacy of phototherapy*, including variations among light sources,

the spectrum of light that is delivered, the intensity of the energy output or irradiance, the peak wavelength of the light that is delivered, the surface area of skin exposed to the light, and the transmission of the light through the infant's skin.

- The amount of body surface exposed to phototherapy light also determines the effectiveness of therapy. Under ideal circumstances, the infant should be naked when under phototherapy. However, a diaper is often in place and folded back to expose as much surface area as possible.
- The use of several phototherapy lamps positioned around the infant or a combination of a phototherapy mattress with overhead lights can increase the intensity and effectiveness of therapy.
- Using a reflective surface, such as a white sheet, around the incubator or open crib can encourage more light to be transmitted to the skin, especially onto relatively underexposed areas, thus increasing the light irradiance.
- Although *complications associated with the use of phototherapy* are rare, several may occur. There have been no studies suggesting that there is an increase in mortality or morbidity with the use of phototherapy. Some complications may include the following:
  - *Intestinal hypermotility:* Stools may be loose and diarrhea-looking in appearance. Infants may have more frequent stools.
  - *Temperature instability:* Phototherapy may potentially cause an increase in body and environmental temperature.
  - *Increased insensible water losses:* With the use of phototherapy, increased insensible and intestinal water losses can occur and need to be taken into consideration with fluid management. The overall fluid intake may need to be increased by as much as 25% above the estimated fluid needs without phototherapy. The use of fiberoptic phototherapy seems to result in insensible water losses that are lower and therefore less need for an increase in maintenance fluids.
  - *Retinal degeneration:* This condition can occur after several days using phototherapy. For this reason, the eyes must be covered with adequate layers to protect against the possibility of damage. The use of fiberoptic phototherapy does not eliminate the need to protect the infant's eyes.
  - *Bronze baby syndrome:* Bronze baby syndrome is characterized by a brown-black (bronze) color appearance of the serum, urine, and skin that appears several hours or more after initiation of phototherapy lights, especially if the serum conjugated bilirubin is elevated. A majority of reported infants with this condition have recovered without sequelae.
  - *Psychobehavioral issues:* These include a lack of sensory experiences, behavioral and activity changes, and alterations in state organization and biologic rhythms. Parental stress has also

been documented with the use of phototherapy. Maternal separation with the potential for interference with parental bonding may occur (Blackburn, 2018a; Dragoo, 2017; Kamath-Rayne et al., 2021; Kaplan et al., 2020; Watchko & Maisels, 2020).

OUTCOMES

■ There is no single TB concentration that can be regarded as safe or categorically dangerous. The TB level, although used clinically to determine the need for phototherapy and exchange transfusion, is a poor predictor of subsequent neurodevelopmental outcomes.

■ It is important to understand that bilirubin metabolism is a dynamic process influenced by many factors. An isolated TB level obtained at one point in time is inadequate to fully assess the risk of sequelae for a particular neonate. Many other factors, including gestational age and relative health of the newborn, need to be carefully evaluated.

■ The recognition that unconjugated bilirubin may penetrate the brain cell under certain circumstances and its association with neuronal dysfunction and death is a reason to carefully manage newborn infants with significant hyperbilirubinemia.

■ Recent studies have raised concerns that both conventional and intensive phototherapy are associated with DNA damage that could result in adverse long-term outcomes and that the duration of phototherapy was positively correlated with markers of genotoxicity (Kamath-Rayne et al., 2021; Kaplan et al., 2020).

BREAST MILK JAUNDICE

Definition and Pathophysiology

■ Breast milk jaundice differs from physiologic jaundice because in the former bilirubin levels begin to rise during the second week of life when physiologic jaundice is beginning to improve.

■ Breast milk jaundice is often a benign condition that occurs during the first weeks of life in newborns receiving mother's own milk (MOM). These infants have exaggerated unconjugated bilirubin levels that can persist through the end of the first week of life. They are three times more likely to have a TSB level greater than 12 mg/dL, with levels reaching as high as 25 to 30 mg/dL.

● Breast milk jaundice typically may be prolonged, occurring after the first 3 to 5 days of life and persisting into the third week of life or beyond. Peak bilirubin levels tend to occur at 4 weeks of life and last up to 12 weeks of age.

■ Infants with breast milk jaundice are well-appearing. They appear healthy with normal weight gain, stooling patterns, and urine output. The physical examination of these infants is normal. There is no evidence of

hemolysis in infants with breastfeeding-associated jaundice.

■ Breast milk jaundice typically resolves without the need for intervention (Dragoo, 2017; Kamath-Rayne et al., 2021; Kaplan et al., 2020).

■ *Breast milk jaundice can occur in two forms or phases.* Breastfeeding-associated jaundice that occurs early is the more common form, while late breast milk jaundice is less prevalent. These phases can overlap and may not be distinguishable from one another.

● Phase 1 is the phase historically associated with breastfeeding-associated jaundice. A major factor that increases the risk of breastfeeding-associated jaundice is increased enterohepatic shunting. Increased enterohepatic shunting occurs in infants exclusively breastfeeding because these infants have a reduced fluid and caloric intake and less frequent feedings and stooling patterns. In the presence of decreased caloric intake, there is an increase in the breakdown of fat, which is needed for energy.

❑ Additionally, infants who are fed breast milk produce lower weight stools and their stool output is initially lower when compared with newborns fed formula. The stools of breastfed infants contain less bilirubin than formula-fed neonates. This occurs because more conjugated direct bilirubin is switched back to indirect bilirubin by beta-glucuronidase, which has a greater affinity in breastfed infants.

● Breast milk jaundice that occurs during phase 2 occurs later and is characterized by increasing bilirubin levels after 3 to 5 days of life, with peak levels of 5 to 10 mg/dL by 2 weeks of life. These levels eventually decrease to more normal levels over the next 3 to 12 weeks of life.

● This phase of jaundice is thought to be related to the properties of breast milk that interferes with normal conjugation and excretion (Blackburn, 2018a; Kaplan et al., 2020).

■ Risk factors for breast milk jaundice include:

● Decreased fluid and/or poor caloric intake due to delay in lactation or lactation failure

● Large amount of weight loss; infants who lose more than 7% of their birth weight are at greater risk for significant dehydration and subsequent jaundice

● Delayed passage of meconium

● The type of number of bacteria in the intestine of breastfed infants

● Breastfeeding failure jaundice; the intricates of breastfeeding (poor technique, cracked nipples, fatigue) may be difficult, especially with first-time mothers (Dragoo, 2017; Watchko, 2018)

Clinical Presentation

■ Other than jaundice, the neonates appear healthy (Kaplan et al., 2020).

Management and Outcome

- Jaundice occurring in breastfed infants can be minimized by preventive measures. Frequent feeding with breast milk, as often as eight or nine times within a 24-hour period during the first 3 days of life, is encouraged. Frequent feeding stimulates intestinal activity and the passage of meconium, allowing for less availability of bilirubin for enzymes to convert back to the indirect form. Frequent feedings also reduce the risk of enterohepatic shunting and facilitate stimulation of breast milk production. Continued and frequent breast milk feedings also increase intestinal motility and can act as a laxative to encourage the passage of meconium. This removes conjugated bilirubin from the small intestine, thereby decreasing the tendency that this bilirubin will be deconjugated and recirculated by the enterohepatic shunt.
- Replacing breast milk with formula may be warranted at a bilirubin level greater than 25 mg/dL even while undergoing intensive phototherapy. Also consider formula if the infant's weight loss from birth is greater than 12% or if there is clinical evidence of dehydration.
- Although not recommended unless hyperbilirubinemia levels reach levels that might be of danger to the infant, interruption of nursing and substitution with formula feeding for 1 to 3 days usually cause a prompt decline in the bilirubin level to about half or less of the original level. On resumption of nursing, the bilirubin level does not usually increase substantially (Blackburn, 2018a; Kaplan et al., 2020; Stark & Bhutani, 2017).

KERNICTERUS/CHRONIC BILIRUBIN ENCEPHALOPATHY

Definition and Pathophysiology

- The term *kernicterus* is derived from bilirubin staining of the "kern" or the nuclear region of the brain. Kernicterus is an irreversible condition that causes devastating injury to the brain. It is also known as *chronic bilirubin encephalopathy* (CBE).
- CBE defines the permanent clinical sequelae of bilirubin toxicity that become evident in the first year of life. Sequelae are distinguished by remarkably selective involvement of the globus pallidus, subthalamic nucleus, sectors of the hippocampus, the reticular portion of the substantia nigra, the red nuclei, the dentate nuclei and Purkinje cells of the cerebellum, and select brainstem nuclei.
- The blood–brain barrier is normally intact and with tight junctions between the endothelial cells of the cerebral blood vessels. These junctions are permeable to lipid-soluble substances and impermeable to water-soluble substances, proteins, and other large molecules.
  - Unconjugated bilirubin is fat-soluble. Under normal conditions, the blood–brain barrier is impermeable to bilirubin that is bound to albumin.

However, when this barrier becomes damaged, reversible alterations or "openings" occur, which allows the entry of albumin-bound bilirubin into the brain. There may also be an increased movement of unbound bilirubin across a blood–brain barrier that is damaged.

- It is not exactly known how bilirubin exerts its toxic effects in the brain. It is thought that bilirubin enters the brain through several different mechanisms.
  - Bilirubin can enter the brain when there is a significant increase in the amount of unbound bilirubin in the bloodstream. In the presence of an increased amount of unbound bilirubin, the normal buffering capacity of the blood and tissues becomes overwhelmed, and bilirubin enters the brain.
  - Alterations in the bilirubin-binding capacity of albumin and other proteins can lead to increased levels of unconjugated bilirubin in the bloodstream. Even when bound to albumin, bilirubin can enter the brain when the blood–brain barrier is disrupted. Disruption of the blood–brain barrier increases the permeability of the central nervous system to bilirubin.
- Conditions that can potentially damage the blood–brain barrier include infection, dehydration, severe respiratory acidosis, hypoxemia, or other injury. Additionally, the ability of bilirubin to bind to albumin is decreased in sick term and preterm infants and the serum albumin concentration lower in this population. These factors can increase the risk of kernicterus at lower serum bilirubin levels in the sick term or preterm infant when compared with the term newborn.
- Other areas of the brain at risk for bilirubin toxicity include the hippocampal cortex, subthalamic nuclei, and cerebellum. The cerebral cortex is generally spared and not affected by elevated levels of unconjugated bilirubin.
- The incidence of kernicterus varies among countries as well as between industrialized countries and those with developing medical systems. It is estimated that kernicterus occurs between 0.4 and 2 per 100,000 children. CBE as a consequence in infants born in developing countries is a serious *endemic* problem; for example, in Nigeria approximately 3% of neonatal hospital admissions evidence bilirubin encephalopathy.
- A diagnosis of kernicterus tends to occur more often in infants born term or late preterm. The most important determinant of brain injury caused by hyperbilirubinemia is the concentration of unconjugated bilirubin and free (unbound) bilirubin.
- Although rare in preterm infants, it can occur in this population due to an immature central nervous system and clinical conditions that potentiate bilirubin neurotoxicity.
- Additional risk factors for kernicterus, especially at lower bilirubin levels, include prematurity, respiratory distress syndrome, G6PD deficiency, hypoxia,

asphyxia, hypercapnia, and acidosis (Blackburn, 2018a; Kamath-Rayne et al., 2021; Kaplan et al., 2020; Watchko, 2018).

Clinical Manifestations

■ Clinical signs of bilirubin toxicity do not become clinically apparent until serum bilirubin levels are elevated for several hours. The infant passes through several stages of bilirubin encephalopathy, characterized by abnormal clinical signs that are progressive in severity.
  ● The initial phase of acute bilirubin encephalopathy (ABE), which is reversible in its early stages, is characterized by clinical signs of poor sucking, progressive lethargy, vomiting, temperature instability, and hypotonia.
  ● If left untreated, pathology advances to the intermediate stage. Infants may demonstrate alternating hypotonia and hypertonia of the extensor muscles and a high-pitched cry. Hypertonia is characterized by backward arching of the neck (retrocollis) and a high-pitched cry.
■ Clinical signs of advanced kernicterus (*ABE*) include ataxia, opisthotonos, choreoathetoid movements (rapid, highly complex, involuntary, spasmodic movements), extrapyramidal disturbances, auditory abnormalities with sensorineural hearing loss, and oculomotor paresis. At this stage, permanent damage to the brain has occurred (Blackburn, 2018a; Kaplan et al., 2020; Watchko, 2018).

Management and Outcome

■ The central nervous system sequelae reflect the regional topography of bilirubin-induced neuronal damage. These include the extrapyramidal movement disorders of dystonia and/or choreoathetosis, hearing loss caused by auditory neuropathy spectrum disorders, and the eye movement abnormality of paresis of upward gaze.
■ Although there is overwhelming evidence to suggest that infants with advanced clinical manifestations of CBE have permanent central nervous damage, recent studies have challenged this notion. There are few reports in the literature that some infants who present with advanced clinical signs of CBE may have no neurologic sequelae if treated aggressively (Watchko, 2018).

▶ CONCLUSION

A thorough understanding of the neonatal hematopoietic system and the process of erythropoiesis is important in the evaluation of and decision for intervention in the neonate. The role and importance of red cells, platelets, and coagulation factors cannot be overstated, and the neonatal nurse practitioner (NNP) must recognize the pathophysiology involved in order to intervene appropriately. Recognition and appropriate management of infants at risk of hyperbilirubinemia will prevent long-term sequelae. Overall, the hematologic system is vital to the continued healthy growth and development of the neonate.

1. In the clinical case of an immune-mediated thrombocytopenia, when an antibody is produced in the mother against a specific human platelet antigen (HPA) and can be found in the fetus, this is known as neonatal:

   A. Alloimmune thrombocytopenia
   B. Autoimmune thrombocytopenia
   C. Congenital amegakaryocytic thrombocytopenia

2. Suppression of the normal erythropoietin (EPO) response occurs physiologically by:

   A. Adequate iron stores
   B. Postnatal hyperoxia
   C. Signaling from gut flora

3. An infant at 30 weeks' corrected gestational age is now 1-hour postsurgical repair of a bowel perforation secondary to necrotizing enterocolitis (NEC). The surgery resulted in 20 cm of small bowel loss and included the ileocecal valve. The blood culture is positive for *Escherichia coli*. Laboratory results reveal a platelet count of 28,000/mm³. Prior to surgery, this value was 160,000/mm³. The finding which indicates the infant is at high risk for disseminated intravascular coagulation (DIC) is the:

   A. Bowel loss from NEC
   B. Decreased platelet count
   C. Positive blood culture

4. The manager of the NICU asks the neonatal nurse practitioner (NNP) to help write a protocol for transcutaneous (TcB) bilirubin screening. The review of the literature reveals that TcB levels are generally:

   A. Accurate compared with serum levels
   B. Higher compared with serum levels
   C. Lower compared with serum levels

5. The neonatal nurse practitioner (NNP) admits a term 3.6-kg infant for hyperbilirubinemia. The infant is 5 days old and has been exclusively breastfed. The serum bilirubin level is 19.9 mg/dL. In addition to phototherapy, the NNP orders:

   A. Continued breastfeeding on demand and supplements as necessary
   B. Discontinuation of breastfeeding and the use of term formula
   C. The infant NPO and begins parenteral nutrition at 150 mL/kg/d

6. Prior to beginning phototherapy, the neonatal nurse practitioner (NNP) considers an infant's individual:

   A. Blood type compared with the mother's type
   B. Current bilirubin level and the level of risk
   C. Hours of age and anticipated rate of increase

7. The neonatal nurse practitioner (NNP) understands that an infant with polycythemia will also:

   A. Be at high risk for hyperviscosity
   B. Have confirmed hyperviscosity
   C. Require treatment of hyperviscosity

1. A) Alloimmune thrombocytopenia

Neonatal alloimmune thrombocytopenia (NAIT) occurs when an antibody is produced in the mother against a specific HPA present in the fetus but absent in the mother. Autoimmune thrombocytopenia results from maternal immune thrombocytopenic purpura (ITP) during pregnancy. Congenital amegakaryocytic thrombocytopenia is an inherited thrombocytopenic syndrome rather than a condition acquired during gestation (Deschmann et al., 2017; Deschmann & Sola-Visner, 2018; Diehl-Jones & Fraswer, 2021; Letterio et al., 2020).

2. B) Postnatal hyperoxia

In utero, a low fetal PaO_2 stimulates EPO production, resulting in erythropoiesis. The relatively hyperoxic extrauterine environment results in suppression of EPO production until 6 to 8 weeks of life. The result is an expected decline in normal term infant's hemoglobin levels over the first 2 to 3 months of life, with a nadir at 6 to 12 weeks of life. Physiologic anemia is the expected, asymptomatic decline in erythropoiesis seen in term and preterm infants following birth due to postnatal EPO suppression (Blackburn, 2013a). Iron stores or gut flora do not stimulate erythropoiesis.

3. B) Decreased platelet count

It is impossible to make a diagnosis of DIC in a neonate unless thrombocytopenia or a falling platelet count is detected in the 50,000 to 100,000 mL range. Hence, the diagnosis is often made on the basis of an appropriate clinical suspicion supported by laboratory evidence of procoagulant and fibrinolytic system activation coupled with anticoagulant consumption and diffuse clinical bleeding. Laboratory abnormalities seen in DIC include thrombocytopenia, elevated fibrin degradation products (FDP) or D-dimers, prolonged prothrombin time (PT), prolonged activated partial thromboplastin time (aPTT), prolonged thrombin clotting time, and a low fibrinogen (Diehl-Jones & Fraser, 2021).

4. C) Lower compared with serum levels

One limitation of using the TcB device is that it often underestimates the bilirubin level when total serum levels are greater than 15 mg/dL. The recommendation is that all bilirubin levels greater than 15 and above the 75th percentile be confirmed with serum bilirubin levels (Dragoo, 2017; Kaplan et al., 2020).

5. A) Continued breastfeeding on demand and supplements as necessary

Frequent feedings reduce the risk of enterohepatic shunting and facilitate stimulation of breast milk production. Continued and frequent breast milk feedings also increase intestinal motility and can act as a laxative to encourage the passage of meconium. This removes conjugated bilirubin from the small intestine, thereby decreasing the tendency that this bilirubin will be deconjugated and recirculated by the enterohepatic shunt (Blackburn, 2013c; Stark & Bhutani, 2017). Replacing breast milk with formula may be warranted at a bilirubin level greater than 25 mg/dL even while undergoing intensive phototherapy. Also consider formula if the infant's weight loss from birth is greater than 12% or if there is clinical evidence of dehydration (Blackburn, 2013c).

6. B) Current bilirubin level and the level of risk

There is no single serum bilirubin level at which phototherapy should be initiated. Instead, each infant needs to be evaluated individually with consideration of the bilirubin level and the infant's level of risk for hyperbilirubinemia (Kaplan et al., 2020; Dragoo, 2017).

7. A) Be at high risk for hyperviscosity

It is important to recognize that polycythemia is not synonymous with hyperviscosity and that not every neonate with polycythemia also has hyperviscosity (Christensen, 2018). The viscosity of blood increases linearly with hematocrit up to 60%, then increases exponentially. Viscosity cannot easily be measured directly, so hematocrit is often used as a surrogate for viscosity (McKinney et al., 2021)).

Neonatal Infectious Diseases

Debra Armbruster and Alexandra Medoro

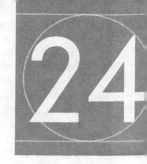

▶ INTRODUCTION

Of any age group, newborns and infants are at the highest risk of infection-induced morbidity and mortality. The unique functions of fetal, neonatal, and maternal immunity reflect adaptation to developmental challenges, such as preservation of fetal well-being as an allogeneic graft versus adequate immunologic protection in the extrauterine environment. There are differences in immunologic responsiveness between newborns and adults, which are highly regulated ontogenic differences that facilitate transitions between distinct age-specific challenges (Weitkamp et al., 2018).

This chapter provides a basic review of developmental immunity and infections of concern in the neonatal period. Overall risk factors, incidence, and organisms, as well as treatment recommendations, are discussed. Pharmacology related to the treatment of sepsis is reviewed in a separate chapter (Chapter 14).

▶ IMMUNE SYSTEM/DEVELOPMENTAL IMMUNITY

- In general, the immunologic system comprises two major defense mechanisms: innate-nonspecific immune response and acquired-specific immune response. Defense mechanisms that operate effectively without prior exposure to a microorganism or its antigens are *innate-nonspecific immune responses*. This includes physical barriers—skin and mucous membranes; and chemical barriers—gastric acid and digestive enzymes.
- An *acquired-specific immune response* describes the development of a protective response to a specific foreign antigen that has been processed and presented by the innate immune system, and the establishment of an immunologic memory of responses. It includes cell-mediated (T-lymphocyte) and humoral (B-lymphocyte and immunoglobulin [Ig]) responses (Benjamin & Maheshwari, 2020; Blackburn, 2018).

INNATE IMMUNITY

Polymorphonuclear Neutrophils

- Phagocytic cells including polymorphonuclear neutrophils (PMNs), monocytes, and macrophages ingest and kill bacteria and other microorganisms. Natural killer (NK) cells kill invading pathogens by nonphagocytic mechanisms.
- Pathogens are more efficiently eliminated from the host when opsonized, or coated, by complement components and other soluble proteins of the innate immune system. Equally, nonphagocytic methods such as lysis of infected cells by NK cells, PMNs, and monocytes are augmented in the presence of specific antibody to the target organism.
- Progenitor cells that are committed to maturation along the granulocyte or macrophage cell lineages (granulocyte–macrophage colony-forming units) are detectable in the human liver between 6 and 12 weeks. Human fetal blood has detectable granulocyte–macrophage colony-forming units from 12 weeks' gestation to term. Cells committed to phagocyte maturation are seen in the human fetal liver by 6 weeks and the peripheral fetal blood by 15 weeks' gestation. In the human fetus, granulocytopoiesis takes place almost exclusively in the bone marrow.
- Mature PMNs are first identified in the fetal bone marrow at approximately 14 weeks of gestation. By 22 to 23 weeks' gestation, the circulating PMN count has increased but remains lower than in term infants. At midgestation, the neutrophil storage pool (NSP) for the fetus is very small and can be readily exhausted during sepsis. The neutrophil proliferating pool (NPP) is also small. PMNs of term and preterm infants are limited in chemotactic, phagocytic, and microbicidal activities. Circulating PMNs increase dramatically at birth, peak at 12 to 24 hours, and decline slowly by 72 hours to remain stable during the rest of the neonatal period.
- The PMN is qualitatively and quantitatively the most effective killing phagocyte of the host defense. The influx of mononuclear phagocytes to sites of

inflammation is delayed and attenuated in newborns. This defect is most likely related to the impaired chemotactic activity by the peripheral blood monocytes of these infants. Phagocytosis and microbicidal activity seem equivalent to the level displayed by mononuclear phagocytes of adults.

■ When searching for the cause of neutropenia (<1,500 PMNs/mm³) in infants, a strong suspicion of infection is warranted, although maternal preeclampsia, premature birth, birth depression, intravascular hemorrhage, and hemolytic disease may also result in low peripheral PMN counts (Benjamin & Maheshwari, 2020; Weitkamp et al., 2018).

Monocytes

■ The first monocytes in circulation are not seen until about the fifth month of gestation and remain uncommon until bone marrow becomes the predominant site of hematopoiesis.

■ In neonates, monocytosis has been associated with lower birth weight (BW) and gestational age (GA), multiple transfusions, albumin infusions, and theophylline therapy.

■ The ability of fetal monocytes to kill a variety of pathogens, including *Staphylococcus aureus*, *S. epidermidis*, *Escherichia coli*, and *Candida albicans*, appears to be equivalent to that of adults.

■ Impaired migration in response to chemoattractants may be a primary factor in the delayed influx of monocytes at inflammatory sites during the neonatal period. Impaired monocyte function in neonates may be partially responsible for poorer cytokine responses of neonatal T-cells.

■ Generally, mononuclear phagocyte recruitment and accumulation lag behind the brisk PMN influx by 6 to 12 hours, but the former process persists for several days.

Macrophages

■ Resident macrophages are often the first phagocytic cells of the innate immune system to encounter invading pathogens. These cells serve important host defense functions through phagocytosis and also as sentinel cells that regulate local inflammatory responses by producing various cytokines and chemokines.

■ During resolution of inflammation, the macrophage populations switch from a proinflammatory to an anti-inflammatory phenotype.

■ Newborn monocytes, macrophages, and dendritic cells (DCs) demonstrate reduced chemotaxis and phagocytosis, as well as anti-inflammatory cytokine production (Benjamin & Maheshwari, 2020; Weitkamp et al., 2018).

Natural Killer Cells

■ NK cells are relatively normal in number in the neonatal period, but surface membrane expression of certain antigens is altered compared with adult NK cells. NK cell cytolytic activity against target cells in vitro is diminished during the neonatal period. The role of NK cell immaturity in contributing to the increased susceptibility of newborns to viral infection remains unknown.

■ NK progenitor cells have been identified in the fetal thymus, bone marrow, and liver as early as 6 weeks' gestation. In the human neonate, the NK cell population is immature, but expresses decreased cytolytic activity (Benjamin & Maheshwari, 2020; Weitkamp et al., 2018).

■ Table 24.1 lists, compares, and contrasts the innate and adaptive immune systems.

The Complement System

■ Its major function is to facilitate the neutralization of foreign substances either in the circulation or on mucous membranes. Complement proteins are synthesized early in gestation.

■ *The classical pathway* of complement activation requires the presence of specific antibodies against a particular antigen and the formation of immune complexes.
  ● Newborns have a limited spectrum of antibody transmitted across the placenta; they receive immunoglobulin G (IgG) and no immunoglobulin M (IgM).
  ● The classical pathway has relatively little value at and shortly after birth.
  ● Therefore, it follows that in the absence of specific antibody, activation of the biologically active fragments and complexes of the complement system through the alternative or lectin pathways becomes an extremely important defense mechanism for neonates during the first encounter with bacteria.

■ In contrast, *the alternative pathway* may be activated by bacterial or mammalian cell surfaces in the absence of specific antibodies.
  ● Activation of the alternative pathway or lectin pathway enables opsonization of invading organisms without specific IgG recognition.
  ● For preterm infants or those without organism-specific maternal IgG, alternative or lectin pathway activation provides a critical mechanism for engaging complement effector functions.
  ● Proteins in the lectin pathways are also lower in neonates compared with adults and are decreased in preterm compared with term infants.
    ❑ Defects in the complement system, and the alternative pathway in particular, likely play a role in susceptibility to infection, especially in preterm infants.

Table 24.1 Comparison of Innate and Adaptive Immunity

	Innate Immunity	Adaptive Immunity
Function	■ Includes inflammation, lysis of an antigen cell membrane, and phagocytosis ■ Activation of adaptive immune response	■ Development of a protective response to a specific foreign antigen that has been processed and presented by the innate immune system and establishment of an immunologic memory of responses
Mechanism of response	■ First line of defense following exposure to antigen ■ No long-term memory, with repeat exposures producing same response	■ Includes both humoral-mediated and antibody-mediated (B-lymphocytes) responses ■ Cell-mediated (T-lymphocytes) ■ Long-term memory with repeat exposures producing heightened response

Key characteristics	■ Involves nonspecific inborn responses to foreign antigen activated the first time an antigen is encountered
	■ Important characteristics:
	  ● Prior exposure not required
	  ● Repeated exposures to an antigen will not alter response
	  ● Ability to recognize molecular patterns shared by groups
		■ Six characteristics:
		  ● *Specificity:* ability to respond to distinct antigen or part of an antigen
		  ● *Diversity:* ability to respond to a wide variety of antigens
		  ● *Memory:* repeated exposures to an antigen elicit more vigorous responses
		  ● *Specialization:* optimizing immune responses against different antigens
		  ● *Self-limiting:* ability to return to homeostasis
		  ● Nonreactive to self-defend foreign antigens while not harming the human's own cells

Effector cells	■ Polymorphonuclear neutrophils, macrophages, monocytes, mast cells, and natural killer cells ■ *TLRs:* on cell surfaces are responsible for recognizing molecular patterns of microbials ■ Endothelial cells, circulating factors (complement and acute-phase proteins, like CRP) as well as cytokines and chemokines (secreted by macrophages; mediate the innate immune response)	■ T-lymphocytes, B-lymphocytes ■ *APCs:* dendritic cells, monocytes, macrophages ■ *Effector cells:* mononuclear phagocytes

Activation	■ TLRs sense molecular patterns of pathogens; induce expression of cytokines and chemokines to activate defensive cells
	■ Pattern recognition receptors on cell surfaces, intracellular vesicles, and cytoplasm recognize damaging molecular patterns (cytokines, intracellular proteins, substances released from damaged cells, and pathogen associated with molecular patterns)
	■ Pathogens bind to TLR and other receptors on monocytes, macrophages, initiate a complement cascade with release of prostaglandin
	■ Transcription factor NK-κB is released, which stimulates synthesis and release of both proinflammatory (IL-1B, IL-6, TNF-α) and anti-inflammatory (IL-1, IL-10) cytokines
		■ *Primary antibody response:* activation, proliferation, and differentiation of naive B-lymphocytes into antibody-secreting cells or memory cells
		■ *Secondary antibody response:* memory B-lymphocytes that are activated to produce increasing amounts of antibodies
		■ *Cell-mediated response* by T-lymphocytes:
		  ● Presentation of antigen by histocompatibility glycoprotein complexes (MCHs) on the surface of APC or B-lymphocyte
		  ● Cell-associated antigen recognition by naive T-cells
		  ● Activation of T-cells to produce cytokines
		  ● T-cell proliferation and clonal expansion
		  ● Differentiation of naive T-cells into effector or memory cells
		  ● Inhibition of response by suppressor or regulatory T-cells when control or elimination foreign antigen is complete

APCs, antigen-presenting cells; CRP, C-reactive protein; IL, interleukin; MCH, major histocompatibility complexes; NK-kB, natural killer kappa B; TLR, toll-like receptors; TNF-α, tumor necrosis factor alpha.
Source: Data from Blackburn, S. T. (2018). *Maternal, fetal, & neonatal physiology: A clinical perspective* (5th ed.). Elsevier.

- The components of the classical and alternative complement systems and their functional activity in full-term neonates are generally lower than in normal adults.
- Serum alternative complement component values reach adult levels by 6 to 18 months.
- In most neonates, functional deficiencies in these pathways, in conjunction with impaired functioning PMNs, are likely clinically relevant (as suggested by lower levels of mannose-binding lectins [MBL] and ficolin lectins in neonates with culture-proven sepsis; Benjamin & Maheshwari et al., 2020; Weitkamp et al., 2018).

Neonatal Complement System Function

- These cytokines and chemokines are responsible for the generation of the immune response and differentiation of a wide variety of immune and nonimmune cells. A network of regulatory glycoproteins and phospholipids that mediate the interactions between cells controls the responses.
- The infant's ability to generate the right balance of proinflammatory and anti-inflammatory cytokines when challenged with an infectious agent allows recovery from the encounter with minimal residua.
  - Circulating concentrations of fibronectin are decreased in the neonatal period and are directly correlated with GA (lower GA = lower levels). Even lower plasma concentrations are measured in infants who are ill.
- Plasma fibronectin increases phagocyte function in vitro. The role of fibronectin in host immune defense in neonates remains uncertain, but in vitro data suggest a potential role as an enhancer of phagocyte function.
  - Antigen-presenting cells (APCs) of the innate immune system (e.g., macrophages, NK cells, neutrophils, mucosal epithelial cells, endothelial cells, and DCs) play pivotal roles in the initiation of an inflammatory response to invading pathogens.
  - Activated, macrophages synthesize and secrete a cascade of proinflammatory cytokines, chemokines, and mediators. Some of these cytokines activate neutrophils to release proteases and free radicals that have the capacity to damage endothelium and promote capillary leak.
  - The proinflammatory cascade is interrupted by the initiation of counterregulatory mechanisms.
    - ❏ The concentration of anti-inflammatory substances (e.g., interleukin [IL]-1ra and soluble receptors) increases substantially with time and has been termed *compensatory anti-inflammatory response syndrome*. This is a response of the host to limit the toxicity of proinflammatory substances (Benjamin & Maheshwari, 2020).

NEONATAL-ACQUIRED IMMUNITY FUNCTION

- The ability to mount cell-mediated or antibody-mediated immune responses to specific antigens is acquired sequentially during the course of embryonic development.
  - Early in gestation, fetuses can respond to certain antigens, whereas other antigens elicit antibody production or cell-mediated immune responses only after birth.
- Fetuses and newborns do not respond to some antigens (e.g., pneumococcal polysaccharide), and the antibody responses to other antigens (e.g., rubella, cytomegalovirus [CMV], *Toxoplasma*) are predominately of the IgM type.
- B-cells of newborns differentiate predominantly into IgM-secreting plasma cells, whereas activated adult B-cells produce IgG- and immunoglobulin A (IgA)-secreting plasma cells. This adult pattern of differentiation develops over the first year of life.
- T-lymphocytes are less experienced in neonates and tend to suppress rather than stimulate B-cell differentiation.
  - Cord blood T-cells have reduced ability to proliferate and synthesize cytokines such as IL-2, interferon gamma (IFN-γ), IL-4, and granulocyte–macrophage colony-stimulating factor (GM-CSF). Both CD4+ and CD8+ lymphocytes decrease with GA and are lower at birth in preterm compared with term infants.
- Neonatal T-cells are impaired in producing a robust Th1 response and produce less IFN-γ and tumor necrosis factor (TNF) under conditions of physiologic stimulation, including in response to the multichain T-cell receptor/CD3 complex (TCR-CD3) stimulation, although adult-level cytokine production can be elicited in human neonatal T-cells by increasing the magnitude of Th1 promoting costimulatory signals.
  - However, neonatal cytotoxic T-lymphocytes are capable of generating long-lasting memory effectors against several viral infections, including CMV (and Rous sarcoma virus).
  - Qualitative differences in neonatal T-cells and APCs compared with adult cells might contribute to these deficient T-cell-mediated responses of neonates (Benjamin & Maheshwari, 2020).

PASSIVE IMMUNITY

- Maternal transfer of IgG antibodies across the placenta provides a newborn with a measure of immune protection.
- Both protective and potentially damaging maternal antibodies cross the placenta. Maternal IgG antibodies are the only ones to cross in significant amounts. Maternal antibody has multiple functions in the fetus and neonate, including passive immunity against pathogens, epigenetic inheritance of immunologic memory, immunologic imprinting, suppression

of immunoglobulin E (IgE) responsiveness, and suppression of tumor development.

■ Fetal levels of IgG are low until 20 to 22 weeks' gestation, when passive and active transfer of IgG across the placenta increases. All four IgG subclasses cross, although IgG_1 and IgG_3 subclasses predominate and are transferred more efficiently. Active transfer allows for movement of IgG to the fetus even when maternal levels are low. IgG_1 is the primary immunoglobulin before 28 weeks. IgG_3 crosses later and does not reach maternal levels until after 32 to 33 weeks' gestation. In most infants, IgG levels near term are higher than maternal levels.

● Depending on the maternal antibody complement, the newborn may have passive immunity against tetanus, diphtheria, polio, measles, mumps, group B *Streptococcus* (GBS), *E. coli*, hepatitis B virus (HBV), *Salmonella enterica*, and others.

● Antibodies to viral agents, diphtheria, and tetanus antitoxins, which are usually of the IgG class, are efficiently transported across the placenta and attain protective levels in the fetus.

● However, antibodies to agents that evoke primarily IgA or IgM antibody responses are poorly transported across the placenta, thereby leaving the neonate unprotected against those organisms. *Infants are not protected against agents to which the mother has not made significant amounts of antibody.*

■ Most viruses and many bacteria are capable of being transferred across the placenta, although relatively few are actually transferred. Immune factors that prevent maternal rejection of the fetus also protect the placenta from infectious agents.

● The organisms that most commonly cross the maternal–placental barrier are *Listeria monocytogenes*, *Treponema pallidum*, HIV, parvovirus B19, rubella, *Toxoplasma gondii*, and CMV.

● Amniotic fluid also protects the fetus through antibacterial and other substances found in maternal milk, including transferrin, beta-lysin, peroxidase, fatty acids, IgG and IgA immunoglobulins, and lysozyme (Benjamin & Maheshwari, 2020; Blackburn, 2018).

▶ **NEONATAL SEPSIS**

■ Sepsis is a common cause of death in infants born <1,500 g. Failure to identify early signs of sepsis contributes to morbidity, mortality, and increased healthcare costs.

● An infection occurs when a susceptible host comes in contact with a potentially pathogenic organism. *When the encountered organism proliferates and overcomes the host defenses, infection results.*

■ Epidemiologically, neonatal sepsis is divided into the following categories: early-onset sepsis (EOS), late-onset sepsis (LOS), and very late-onset sepsis (also sometimes termed *hospital-acquired infection* [*HAI*]).

The age of onset of sepsis reflects the likely mode of acquisition, microbiologic features, mortality rate, and presentation of infection (Table 24.2).

■ Sources of infection in a newborn can be divided into three categories: transplacental acquisition, perinatal acquisition, and postnatal acquisition.

■ Definitive therapy should be completed with the narrowest spectrum of appropriate antimicrobial. Consider consultation with infectious disease specialists when sepsis is complicated by meningitis or resistant or unusual etiologic agents (Desai & Leonard, 2020; Esper, 2020; Pammi et al., 2021; Rudd, 2021).

RISK FACTORS FOR NEONATAL SEPSIS

■ Newborns are extremely susceptible to infection. The immature immune system of the neonate is characterized by immature activation and function of the immune system responses, making newborns more susceptible to infections, with a frequency and an intensity greater than any other period of life.

● Susceptibility stems from maternal risk factors, obstetrical complications, the postnatal environment, and the immature host defenses of the newborn (Desai & Leonard, 2020; Esper, 2020; Rudd, 2021).

Maternal Risk Factors

■ Risk factors include inadequate prenatal care, inadequate nutrition, low socioeconomic status, recurrent abortion, substance abuse, history of maternal sexually transmitted diseases (STDs), maternal urinary tract infections (UTIs), and premature rupture of membranes (PROM).

■ Other factors include PROM (>12–18 hours) prior to labor/delivery, GBS colonization, chorioamnionitis, uterine tenderness, purulent amniotic fluid, foul-smelling amniotic fluid, maternal fever (>101°F/38.3°C), prolonged or difficult labor, premature birth, maternal UTI, invasive intrapartum procedures (internal fetal monitoring), elevated maternal heart rate (HR; >100 beats per minute [bpm]), and elevated fetal HR (>180 bpm).

Neonatal Risk Factors

■ Risk factors include prematurity, low birth weight (LBW), difficult birth, birth asphyxia, meconium staining, resuscitation, low Apgar score (<6 at 5 minutes), congenital anomalies, breach of skin integrity, and multiple births.

● Importantly, the risk of EOS in infants born to women with chorioamnionitis is inversely correlated with GA; therefore, it remains prudent to empirically treat chorioamnionitis-exposed preterm infants.

■ Other factors include hospital admission and length of stay; invasive procedures such as peripheral intravenous catheter (PIV), intubation, umbilical venous/arterial catheters (UVC/UAC), central venous catheters (CVC), peripherally inserted central catheters (PICCs), chest tubes, and other surgical interventions;

Table 24.2 Comparison of Early-Onset and Late-Onset Sepsis

	Early-Onset Sepsis	Late-Onset Sepsis
Definition	■ Occurs before 72 hours of life, with 90% of infants symptomatic by 24 hours of age ■ Vertical acquisition from the infant's environment ■ Infants colonized with pathogenic bacteria ubiquitous to their physical environment, including flora of the caregivers	■ Commonly occurs after the first week of life (7 days) but may occur as early as 3 days, in the continuously hospitalized infant ■ Described as CAI or HAI ■ Horizontal acquisition during birth
Risk factors	*Maternal factors:* ■ Premature rupture of membranes, prolonged rupture of membranes (>18 hours), chorioamnionitis, fever (>100.4°F/38°C), GBS status, and maternal UTI *Neonatal factors:* ■ Prematurity, gestational age (<37 weeks), and low BW (<2,500 g); these factors may be altered with administration of intrapartum antibiotics	*Neonatal factors:* ■ Prematurity, inversely related to gestational age, and low BW *Need for NICU devices:* ■ Intubation, mechanical ventilation, OG/NG tube insertion, and central lines (CLABSI, most common HAI) *Need for high-risk medications:* ■ Broad-spectrum antibiotics (increase bacterial colonization), parenteral nutrition, antacids, H2 blockers, and proton pump inhibitors
Presentation	■ Clinical signs and symptoms are variable and nonspecific. ■ Common signs include respiratory distress (most common), hemodynamic instability with poor perfusion or shock, and temperature instability. ■ It may present as fulminant onset of respiratory symptoms, due to pneumonia, shock, or poor perfusion, resulting in a systemic, multiorgan disease. ■ Clinical signs and symptoms may reflect noninfectious etiologies.	■ Presentation may be slow and progressive or fulminant. ■ Common signs include poor feeding, temperature instability, and lethargy. ■ Focal disease is common: UTI, osteoarthritis, or soft tissue infection. ■ Meningitis is common. ■ GBS LOS is more often complicated by meningitis (primarily caused by polysaccharide serotype strains).
Etiology	■ It is most commonly acquired before delivery via vertical transmission either through ascending amniotic fluid infection or through acquisition of bacterial flora from the mother's anogenital tract during vaginal delivery, and reflects maternal genitourinary and gastrointestinal colonization.	■ It is most commonly acquired from the infant's postnatal environment. ■ Prematurity is the most significant factor; invasive procedures performed on a neonate (intubation, catheterization, and surgery) increase the risk of bacterial infection. ■ CLABSIs are a prominent concern in the NICU setting. ■ VAP is the second most common HAI in the NICU, associated with aspiration of secretions, colonization, and use of contaminated equipment.

Incidence	■ Incidence in the United States is estimated to be 0.77 per 1,000 live births overall.
	  ● BW <1,500 g 10 to 15 cases per 1,000 live births
	  ● BW 1,500–2,500 g 1.38 per 1,000 live births
	■ Universal antenatal screening for GBS colonization with antibiotic prophylaxis for women colonized with GBS has significantly reduced the rate of early-onset GBS sepsis.
	■ Increases in non-GBS EOS and ampicillin-resistant EOS are reported among VLBW infants.
		■ Incidence is 0.27 cases per 1,000 live births (2013 data).
		■ Approximately 50% of cases occur in infants born <37 weeks.
		■ Rates of LOS are most common in LBW infants and inversely associated with BW.
		■ IAP has no impact on LOS GBS.

(continued)

Table 24.2 Comparisons of Early Onset Sepsis and Late-Onset Sepsis (continue)

	Early-Onset Sepsis	Late-Onset Sepsis
Microorganisms	■ The most common organisms include group B *Streptococcus*, *E. coli*, and *Listeria monocytogenes*. ■ Less common organisms include *Staphylococcus aureus*, viridans group streptococci, enterococci, group A streptococci, *L. monocytogenes*, *Haemophili*, and other gram-negative bacteria such as *Klebsiella*, *Enterobacter*, *Citrobacter*, *Acinetobacter*, and *Pseudomonas*. ■ Fungal species can cause EOS primarily in preterm infants. ■ Since IAP for GBS began, predominance of gram-negative organisms has been noted in infants weighing less than 1,500 g at birth.	■ Gram-positive organisms predominate in LOS in VLBW and premature infants, CONS, and *S. aureus*, as well as invasive candidiasis. ■ Approximately 50% of LOS cases are caused by CONS. ■ Gram-negative organisms account for about one-third of LOS cases in VLBW infants. ■ GBS and *E. coli* are common organisms—*E. coli* is a frequent cause of urosepsis in young infants. ■ Common community LOS organisms include GBS, *E. coli*, or *Klebsiella*; less common organisms include *Streptococcus pneumoniae* and *Neisseria meningitides*. ■ Very LOS disease includes GBS, gram-negative bacilli, and *Streptococcus pneumoniae*.
Evaluation	■ Blood culture, CBC, and LP (routine urine unlikely to yield results in EOS)	■ Blood culture, CBC, LP, and urine culture
Treatment	■ The appropriate empiric regimen for most infants is ampicillin and gentamicin. ■ The use of broad-spectrum antibiotics is associated with increased antibiotic resistance and invasive fungal infections and thus should be reserved for critically ill neonates. ■ Antibiotic regimens should cover GBS, gram-negative bacilli, and *L. monocytogenes*.	■ Empiric therapy usually consists of vancomycin and an aminoglycoside, providing coverage for CONS, *S. aureus*, and gram-negative organisms. ■ The antibiotic therapy in LOS and very LOS is not definitively in favor of any one regimen. ■ Nafcillin is the appropriate coverage for MSSA. ■ Vancomycin is the first-line coverage for MRSA. ■ Consider empiric antifungal coverage for invasive candidiasis. ■ Local variation in microbiology of LOS is important in considering empiric antibiotic therapy. ■ The regimen for an infant admitted from the community should include coverage for GBS, *E. coli*, and *Streptococcus pneumoniae*.
Mortality and morbidity	■ Mortality may be as high as 30% to 50%, GBS 38%, *E. coli* 24%. ■ Mortality rate for early preterm infants is as high as 30% to 54%. ■ Mortality rates are inversely proportional to gestational age.	■ Mortality is lower than EOS but may still be 20%–40%. ■ Mortality from GBS LOS is low at 1%–2% and 5%–6% in term and preterm infants, respectively. ■ The sequelae in survivors of GBS meningitis can be severe.

BW, birth weight; CAI, community-acquired infection; CBC, complete blood count; CLABSI, central-line bloodstream infection; CONS, coagulase-negative *Staphylococcus*; EOS, early-onset sepsis; GBS, group B *Streptococcus*; HAI, hospital-acquired infection; IAP, intrapartum antibiotic prophylaxis; LBW, low birth weight; LOS, late-onset sepsis; LP, lumbar puncture; MRSA, methicillin-resistant *S. aureus*; MSSA, methicillin-susceptible *S. aureus*; NG, nasogastric tube; OG, orogastric; UTI, urinary tract infection; VAP, ventilator-associated pneumonia; VLBW, very low birth weight.

Sources: Data from Desai, A. P., & Leonard, E. G. (2020). Infections in the neonate. In A. Fanaroff & J. Fanaroff (Eds.), *Klaus and Fanaroff's care of the high-risk neonate* (7th ed., pp. 275–295). Elsevier; Esper, F. (2020). Postnatal bacterial infections. In R. Martin, A. Fanaroff, & M. Walsh (Eds.), *Fanaroff & Martin's neonatal-perinatal medicine: Diseases of the fetus and infant* (11th ed., pp. 789–808). Elsevier; Pammi, M., Brand, M. C., & Weisman, L. (2021). Infection in the neonate. In S. Gardner, B. Carter, M. Hines, & J. Hernandez (Eds.), *Merenstein & Gardner's handbook of neonatal intensive care* (9th ed., pp. 692–727). Elsevier; Puopolo, K. M. (2017). Bacterial and fungal infections. In E. Eichenwald, A. Hansen, C. Martin, & A. Stark (Eds.), *Cloherty and Stark's manual of neonatal care* (8th ed., pp. 691–718). Wolters Kluwer.

use of broad-spectrum antibiotics; and use of humidification systems in ventilation and incubators (Polin & Randis, 2020; Rudd, 2021).

INCIDENCE OF NEONATAL SEPSIS

■ The overall incidence of neonatal sepsis in the United States is estimated to be 0.77 per 1,000 cases, with a

fatality rate of 10.9%, although the incidence is twice as high among moderately premature infants compared with term infants and highest among very low birth weight (VLBW; <1,500 g) infants. The most important risk factors for neonatal sepsis are prematurity and low BW and the incidence is inversely proportional to GA or BW.

■ Other risk factors include compromised immune function, exposure to invasive procedures, hypoxia, metabolic acidosis, hypothermia, and low socioeconomic status, all of which are factors associated with prematurity and low BW.

- Neonatal sepsis is twice as common in Black infants than White infants. African American preterm infants remain at considerably greater risk than White preterm infants and both Black and White term infants. Males have higher incidence, but not a higher risk. Sepsis is more common in firstborn twins.
- Infants with a diagnosis of galactosemia are more likely to become infected with gram-negative organisms, particularly *E. coli* (Desai & Leonard, 2020; Pammi et al., 2021; Puopolo, 2017; Rudd, 2021).

CLINICAL SIGNS AND SYMPTOMS

- Detection of neonatal sepsis requires a high index of suspicion as clinical signs may be nonspecific and nonlocalizing.
  - Familiarity with epidemiology risk factors is crucial to determining the threshold index of suspicion because most neonates are asymptomatic without correlation with positive cultures.
  - Lethargy or poor feeding may be the only symptoms initially, although the most common clinical sign is respiratory distress.
  - Other less specific signs of sepsis include irritability, lethargy, temperature instability, poor perfusion, and hypotension, but disseminated intravascular coagulation (DIC) with purpura and petechiae can occur in more severe septic shock. However, lethargy, irritability, and seizures can all occur secondary to electrolyte, metabolic, or hormonal disturbances.
- Metabolic manifestations may include hyperglycemia or hypoglycemia, acidosis, and jaundice.
- Noninfectious etiologies that mimic neonatal sepsis include transient tachypnea of the newborn (TTNB), pulmonary hypertension, cardiogenic pulmonary edema, surfactant deficiency, noninfectious metabolic acidosis, and meconium aspiration syndrome (MAS; Esper, 2020; Pammi et al., 2021; Puopolo, 2017).

DIAGNOSIS

- Definitive diagnosis is the isolation of an organism from a sterile body site, such as blood, cerebrospinal fluid (CSF), or urine.
- Blood culture volume should be at least 1 mL for improved recovery, particularly in bacteremia with low colony count. A blood culture may be falsely negative if the mother received antibiotics, the infant has been exposed to multiple courses of antibiotics, or due to inadequate blood volume.
- A lumbar puncture (LP) should be considered in any infant with suspected sepsis.

- There is a poor correlation between the results of neonatal blood cultures and CSF cultures (underscores the need for LP). Up to 15% of neonates with bacteremia will develop meningitis.
- A study among VLBW infants with meningitis showed that one-third had corresponding negative blood cultures; therefore, failure to perform an LP may result in a missed diagnosis.
- *92% of cultures are positive by 24 hours.* If positive culture is obtained from blood or CSF, a follow-up culture should be obtained to document sterility.
- Contaminants usually take longer time to grow (>2–3 days), although if the infant is symptomatic an infection should be presumed.
- Gram-positive bacteria can be detected after up to 36 hours of antimicrobial therapy, and some gram-negative organisms can be detected for several days in CSF (Desai & Leonard, 2020; Esper, 2020; Rudd, 2021).

INDIRECT MARKERS OF SEPSIS

- Indirect indices of infection include the following: white blood cells (WBC), absolute neutrophil count (ANC), C-reactive protein (CRP), procalcitonin level, and various cytokines; however, none are specific or sensitive enough to confirm or exclude sepsis.
- Other nonspecific laboratory abnormalities that may accompany neonatal sepsis include hyperglycemia, hypoglycemia, and unexplained metabolic acidosis (Desai & Leonard, 2020; Pammi et al., 2021).

White Blood Cells

- There is a roller-coaster shape of WBC and ANC and immature-to-total neutrophil ratio (I:T) curves in the first 72 hours of life.
  - It is recommended to wait for 6 to 12 hours after birth for WBC evaluation as later counts are more likely to be abnormal and reflect an inflammatory response of the neonate compared with those obtained at birth.
  - Optimal interpretation of WBC data to predict EOS should account for the natural rise and fall in WBC during this period.
- The WBC and ANC are most predictive of infection when these values are low (WBC <5,000 and ANC <1,000).
  - Calculation of ANC: %WBCs × (%Immature neutrophils +%Mature neutrophils) × 0.01
- I:T is most informative if measured between 1 and 4 hours after birth.
  - Calculation of I:T:
  $$\frac{\% \text{ Bands} + \% \text{ Immature forms}}{\% \text{ Mature} + \% \text{ Bands} + \% \text{ Immature forms}}$$
- I:T is best used for negative predictive value: If I:T is normal, infection is unlikely, with 99% predictive value.

- The combination of low ANC and elevated I:T is the most predictive combination of WBC indices for EOS.
- The WBC and its components may be of more value in the VLBW infant and/or in the evaluation of LOS infection, especially if interpreted in relation to values obtained prior to the concern for infection.
- Studies have shown that leukopenia and high percentage of immature to total WBCs are associated with EOS. LOS has been associated with both low and high WBC, high ANC, and high percentage of immature to total WBCs (Esper, 2020; Puopolo, 2017; Rudd, 2021).

C-Reactive Protein

- CRP is a nonspecific marker of inflammation. It is one of the most rapidly responsive acute-phase proteins, with increases of 100- to 1,000-fold (in adults) in the serum concentration detectable during an infection. CRP is produced by both the fetus and the newborn.
  - Elevated cord blood CRP levels are associated with chorioamnionitis with prolonged rupture of membranes (ROMs).
  - An elevated neonatal CRP may be found in bacterial sepsis and meningitis. It may also be present in an infant delivered through meconium-stained amniotic fluid or one with a significant caput.
- CRP levels increase within 6 to 8 hours and peak after 24 hours. CRP sensitivity is lowest early, and sensitivity increases with serial values 24 to 48 hours after onset of symptoms. Serial levels may be useful in identifying infants who do not have a bacterial infection or in monitoring response to treatment of infected infants.
- A single determination of CRP at birth lacks both sensitivity and specificity for infection, although serial CRP determinations at the time of blood culture, 12 to 24 hours and 48 hours later, have been used to manage infants at risk of LOS and can be helpful in excluding serious infection.
  - Serial CRP patterns have been found to be useful to follow resolution of infection and guide antibiotic therapy (Benjamin & Maheshwari, 2020; Esper, 2020; Pammi et al., 2021; Puopolo, 2017; Rudd, 2021).

Procalcitonin

- Procalcitonin is an acute-phase reactant that is elevated in response to bacterial toxins.
- Procalcitonin concentrations peak 12 hours after infection (physiologic increase 24 hours after birth). Increases can be seen in noninfectious causes, such as respiratory distress syndrome (RDS).
  - Procalcitonin appears to have better sensitivity but less specificity than CRP in identifying neonatal sepsis. The most important information guiding clinical decisions continues to be the patient's overall clinical status and culture data (Esper, 2020).

NEONATAL SEPSIS RISK CALCULATOR

- This model estimates an infant's risk of EOS by using the infant's clinical data and physical exam findings within the first 6 hours of birth in infants born ≥34 weeks' gestation.
- This calculator has definitions for clinical status, including clinical illness, equivocal symptoms, and well-appearing.
- By combining an infant's clinical risk and maternal risk factors, a numerical estimate of the risk of sepsis and recommendations for management and monitoring are provided. The results are most accurate when the local incidence data on EOS are used in the calculation.
- This calculator has been shown to reduce the number of neonatal sepsis workups, thus decreasing the days of antibiotic exposure without an increase in adverse effects (Ferrieri & Wallen, 2018; Pammi et al., 2021; Puolpolo, 2017).

TREATMENT RECOMMENDATIONS

- Once a pathogen is identified, therapy should be tailored to the species and antimicrobial susceptibilities. Duration of therapy is determined by the site of infection and the patient's clinical response. The most targeted antibiotic or antibiotic combination should be continued for an appropriate period by a suitable route.
- Antibiotics are not the entire solution to treating the infected newborn; meticulous attention to the treatment of associated conditions (shock, hypoxemia, thermal abnormalities, electrolyte, or acid–base imbalance, inadequate nutrition, anemia, or presence of pus or foreign bodies) is as important as choosing an antibiotic.
- Supportive treatments for sepsis include mechanical ventilation, exogenous surfactant therapy for pneumonia and RDS, volume and pressor support for hypotension, sodium bicarbonate for metabolic acidosis, and anticonvulsants for seizures.
- Adjunct therapies for neonatal sepsis including double-volume exchange transfusions, granulocyte infusions, and intravenous immunoglobulin G (IVIG) have been studied with variable results.
- Decision on length of therapy should be made based on current evidence and/or in collaboration with infectious disease experts (Esper, 2020; Pammi et al., 2021; Puopolo, 2017).

SEPSIS PREVENTION STRATEGIES

- Intrapartum antibiotic prophylaxis (IAP) has been highly effective in reducing GBS EOS, although there has been no direct effect on LOS GBS. Table 24.3 lists the recommended maternal IAP for GBS.

Table 24.3 Recommended Maternal Intrapartum Antibiotic Prophylaxis

Prophylaxis	No Prophylaxis
■ Women with positive GBS culture results ■ Women with history of GBS bacteremia during current pregnancy ■ Women with a history of an infant with invasive GBS disease ■ Pregnant women in preterm labor, if <37 weeks, unknown GBS status, IAP recommended if fever >100.4°F/38°C occurs, or ROM >18 hours prior to delivery	■ Women with intact membranes and planned Cesarean delivery ■ Women with negative GBS prenatal culture results

GBS, group B *Streptococcus*; IAP, intrapartum antibiotic prophylaxis; ROM, rupture of membranes.

Sources: Data from Esper, F. (2020). Postnatal bacterial infections. In R. Martin, A. Fanaroff, & M. Walsh (Eds.), *Fanaroff & Martin's neonatal-perinatal medicine: Diseases of the fetus and infant* (11th ed., pp. 789–808). Elsevier; Puopolo, K. M. (2017). Bacterial and fungal infections. In E. Eichenwald, A. Hansen, C. Martin, & A. Stark (Eds.), *Cloherty and Stark's manual of neonatal care* (8th ed., pp. 684–719). Lippincott Williams & Wilkins.

- Preventive efforts to reduce the risk of LOS focus on infection control/hand hygiene, proper management of CVCs, appropriate use of antibiotics, and limited use of H2 blockers or proton pump inhibitors.
- A systematic and multidisciplinary approach to reducing central-line bloodstream infections (CLABSIs) should be included in the infection control policies of every NICU.
- Prevention of healthcare-associated infections:
  - Two-tiered approach recommended by the Centers for Disease Control and Prevention (CDC):
    - Standard precautions, which are used in all patients; universal precautions
    - Transmission-based precautions
  - Hand hygiene (Esper, 2020; Pammi et al., 2021; Rudd, 2021)

▶ SEPTIC SHOCK

- *Shock* is defined as a state of cellular energy failure resulting from an inability of tissue oxygen delivery to satisfy tissue oxygen demand. When the tissue oxygen demand cannot be met, the organs begin to fail and without corrective measures will progress to irreversible damage, end-organ failure, and death.
- In septic distributive shock, there is insufficient perfusion, oxygenation, and delivery of nutrients to satisfy tissue requirements, resulting in cellular dysfunction and ultimately cell destruction.
- There are three phases of shock: the compensated phase, the uncompensated phase, and the irreversible phase.
  - During the *compensated* phase, blood flow to nonvital organs is sacrificed in order to

continue to perfuse vital organs such as the brain and heart. This is accomplished with vasoconstriction to the former and vasodilation to the latter. During this phase, blood pressure is maintained in the normal range but HR increases. Additionally, signs of nonvital organ compromise begin to appear along with evidence of overall poor perfusion. If untreated or inadequately treated, the infant will progress to uncompensated shock.

- In *uncompensated* shock, perfusion to the vital organs can no longer be maintained and blood pressure falls. Cardiac output and systemic perfusion decrease, and lactic acidosis develops.
- Without correction and treatment, the infant progresses to *irreversible shock*, where permanent damage to organ systems occurs and death is imminent without reversal of the infant's condition.

- Limited data are available on the exact hemodynamics of neonatal septic shock. Two patterns have been identified in older patients, warm and cold shock, with cold shock being well described in neonates.
  - Cold shock is characterized by increased vascular tone, low systemic blood flow, and eventually falling blood pressure.
  - Warm shock, which is characterized by loss of vascular tone, increased systemic blood flow, and low blood pressure, is more difficult to clinically recognize. Recent studies have described high cardiac output, low systemic vascular resistance, and increased left ventricular output consistent with neonatal warm shock.
    - The mediators of neonatal warm septic shock remain unclear; however, if similarity to the adult pathogenesis is assumed, the dysregulated cytokine release and the upregulated nitric oxide production combined with the deficiency of vasopressin production could have relevance to vasopressor-resistant hypotension in preterm infants (Noori et al., 2018; Rudd, 2021).
- Rapid identification and treatment is paramount in preventing the progression of septic shock and death. Clinical presentation includes:
  - Respiratory distress progressing to respiratory insufficiency and failure; progresses to persistent pulmonary hypertension (PPHN) with decreased oxygenation
  - Myocardial complications, arrhythmias, and eventually cardiac arrest, tachycardia or bradycardia, and poor perfusion; hypotension with resulting decreased urinary output, organ dysfunction, and ileus
  - Other findings include metabolic acidosis and other electrolyte disorders, coagulopathy, oozing, or bleeding which can progress to DIC, and generalized edema due to capillary leak
- Treatment of septic shock is centered around supporting body systems and function, with the goal

of restoring adequate tissue perfusion to improve outcomes. This includes:

- Adequate respiratory support should be provided.
- Close watch must be kept on cardiac function and arrhythmias with echocardiograms and EKGs. Inotropic agents, typically dopamine or epinephrine, or hydrocortisone, may be required to support blood pressure.
- Hypovolemia should be managed with normal saline, lactated Ringer's, or blood products. The infant may need any combination of red blood cells (RBCs), platelets, fresh frozen plasma, and/or cryoprecipitate to manage blood loss and DIC.
- Electrolyte imbalances and metabolic acidosis need to be corrected while providing adequate nutrition and euglycemia.
- The underlying infection must be treated with tailored antimicrobial therapy (Rudd, 2021).

▶ MENINGITIS

- Meningitis is diagnosed by isolation of a pathogen in the CSF, regardless of CSF count or chemistries, and can occur independently or as a sequela of bacteremia. The incidence of bacterial meningitis is less than 1 per 1,000 live births, but occurs more often in preterm and LBW infants.
- Meningitis can manifest in EOS or LOS with either vertical or horizontal transmission. EOS is vertically transmitted from the maternal genital tract and occurs within the first week of life, while LOS can be either vertically transmitted from maternal flora or horizontally transmitted from colonized caregivers.
  - Within the first week of life, GBS or *E. coli* causes 70% of cases. After the first week of life coagulase-negative *Staphylococcus* (CONS) is more commonly isolated in the hospitalized infant. Other less common causative organisms include *Klebsiella, Enterobacter, Citrobacter,* and *Serratia*.
- The clinical presentation of meningitis is difficult to distinguish from sepsis. Nonneurologic symptoms include temperature instability, poor feeding, respiratory distress, apnea, and diarrhea. Neurologic signs include irritability, lethargy, poor tone, seizures, and later a full or bulging fontanel. Seizures are more common in gram-negative meningitis and are usually focal.
- Diagnosis of meningitis requires a full septic workup and must include an LP for CSF cell count, glucose, protein, Gram stain, and culture. The WBC count and protein levels in the CSF can be difficult to interpret as they vary with gestational and postnatal age.
  - Generally, CSF glucose will be low and WBC and protein levels high, although up to 10% of infants have normal CSF analysis, leaving culture and Gram stain as the gold standard.

- Treatment of meningitis requires a tailored antibiotic regimen with repeat CSF cultures to verify sterility. Gram-positive organisms will usually clear within 24 to 48 hours, but gram-negative organisms may persist.
  - Infants are frequently very ill and require supportive therapy with any combination of mechanical ventilation, complex fluid management, vasopressor support, and cardiopulmonary monitoring. Length of treatment depends on the organism and the quickness of CSF clearance, usually 2 weeks after sterilization of gram-positive bacteria and 3 weeks after clearance of gram-negative organisms.
- Gram-negative bacilli are responsible for 3.6% of the cases of meningitis in infants and are the fifth most common cause. Overall mortality of gram-positive disease is about 10%.
  - Of the survivors, 40% to 50% have some evidence of neurologic damage due to complications from hydrocephalus, multicystic encephalomalacia, porencephaly, white matter atrophy, abscesses, subdural effusions, and ventriculitis, manifesting as developmental delays, late-onset seizures, cerebral palsy, hearing loss, and blindness (Desai & Leonard, 2020; Esper, 2020; Ferrieri & Wallen, 2018; Hostetter & Gleason, 2018; Puopolo, 2017; Rudd, 2021).

▶ OSTEOMYELITIS

- Osteomyelitis is an infection of the bone that is uncommon and difficult to diagnose in neonates due to the delayed onset of symptoms. Neonates are susceptible in part due to their immature immune responses, resulting in vulnerability to organisms not ordinarily virulent. The most common sites of infection are the femur, humerus, tibia, radius, and maxilla.
- There are three causative mechanisms associated with osteomyelitis: bacteremia or hematogenous spread, direct inoculation from a puncture wound, and a contiguous spread from an adjacent infection. The most common of these is hematogenous spread, with the metaphysis the most common site.
- The structure and circulation of bone during the neonatal period predispose infants to infection. In the first 12 to 18 months of life, the epiphysis and metaphysis are not separated by a formed physis; consequently, their blood supply is linked because the barrier created by the formed physis (growth plate) has yet to completely develop. This allows bacteria and infection to spread from one to the other and to cross and touch the physeal area.
  - Additionally, blood vessels enter the bone centrally and ascend to the metaphysis, making a 180-degree turn when they reach the physis and emptying into the venous sinusoids. The 180-degree turn creates

an area of sluggish blood flow where bacteria can become trapped and proliferate.

■ The most common organism responsible for osteomyelitis is *S. aureus*, with methicillin-resistant *S. aureus* (MRSA) being particularly destructive. Other common offenders include GBS and *E. coli*, with some cases caused by *Neisseria gonorrhoeae*, *Candida*, other enteric gram-negative bacteria, and group A *Streptococcus*.

■ The signs and symptoms of osteomyelitis are subtle, vary with age, and can mimic sepsis, with severity of presentation directly correlated with the health of the infant prior to infection.

   ● In term, previously healthy neonates' symptoms usually occur in the first 2 weeks of life, with limited spontaneous movement and pseudoparalysis of the involved extremity, local tenderness, erythema, swelling, and increased warmth.

   ● Premature neonates in the NICU commonly present with systemic illness and require prolonged hospitalization. Infants most at risk are those with a history of multiple peripheral and central vascular catheters and repetitive percutaneous arterial blood sampling.

■ Evaluation of osteomyelitis should initially mimic a septic workup with blood, CSF, and urine cultures, along with culture of any purulent skin lesions. Radiographic testing along with ultrasound and bone aspiration can aid diagnosis. MRI and nuclear scintigraphy may be used. Fluid collection from bone aspirations is positive majority of the time.

   ● Early radiographs may be normal, with soft tissue swelling presenting by 3 days and bone changes at 7 to 10 days. More advanced films will show deep edema; joint effusion, separation, and dislocation; and even bone destruction.

   ● Ultrasound can be a useful method for diagnosis and evaluation as it detects joint effusions, deep edema, and subperiosteal and soft tissue fluid collection, and can guide aspiration.

   ● MRI and nuclear scintigraphy are both highly sensitive and can be considered.

   ● Fluid collection in the soft tissue and bone should be aspirated and sent for culture and Gram stain. Aspiration should be done over the point of maximal swelling, bone tenderness, and fluctuation.

■ Treatment of uncomplicated osteomyelitis requires antimicrobial therapy for at least 3 weeks. If there is abscess formation in the bone or soft tissue or septic arthritis, surgical drainage and debridement are required, followed by immobilization of the affected limb. If the infant is unresponsive to the initial treatment of an isolated infection, suspect that an abscess has formed.

■ Due to the previously described physiology of neonatal bone, osteomyelitis can lead to epiphyseal and physeal damage, chronic infection and joint infection, or secondary septic arthritis. Damage to the physis and articular cartilage can cause growth disturbances, limb shortening, angular deformity, physeal closure, loss of motion, and precocious arthritis (Esper, 2020; Gilmore & Thompson, 2020; Puopolo, 2017; White et al., 2018).

▶ NEONATAL INFECTIOUS CAUSES: BACTERIAL

ENTEROCOCCUS

■ *Enterococcus faecalis* and *E. faecium* can be associated with LOS and infections associated with indwelling central line catheters. These organisms resemble CONS organisms in their ability to produce a biofilm and slime and adhere to catheter surfaces.

■ Approximately 3% of NICU bloodstream infections (BSIs) are attributable to these bacteria, but *Enterococcus* spp. may also be associated with meningitis, UTIs, and necrotizing enterocolitis (NEC), but with low overall mortality.

   ● Gram-positive organisms such as *Enterococcus*, CONS, *S. aureus*, *L. monocytogenes*, and beta-hemolytic *Streptococcus* contribute to a minority of cases of meningitis. As a gram-positive coccus, *Enterococcus* is the third most common organism responsible for UTIs in the neonate.

■ Enterococci are among the common fecal organisms found in preterm infants, along with Enterobacteriaceae, *E. coli*, *Staphylococcus*, *Streptococcus*, *Clostridium* species, and *Bacteroides* species. The colonization of these pathogenic bacteria lasts longer in preterm infants than in term infants, and this abnormal colonization of the preterm gut is thought to contribute to the pathogenesis of NEC (McElory et al., 2018; Puopolo, 2017; Rudd, 2021; Srinivasan & Evans, 2018; Wang et al., 2018).

VANCOMYCIN-RESISTANT ENTEROCOCCI

■ Widespread use of antibiotics has led to the development of vancomycin-resistant enterococci (VRE). VRE has been seen in some NICUs and is difficult to treat. Treatment for VRE should be discussed and decided on in consultation with infectious disease experts and will also require infection control measures such as isolation, barrier precautions, and cohorting of patients (Puopolo, 2017; Srinivasan & Evans, 2018).

ESCHERICHIA COLI

- *E. coli* are aerobic gram-negative rods that are found universally in human intestinal tract, human vagina, and urinary tract. It is the organism most commonly implicated in neonatal UTI (LOS).
- EOS *E. coli* infections, particularly those complicated by meningitis, are primarily due to strains with the K1-type polysaccharide capsule. Strains with complete lipopolysaccharides (LPS) and/or K antigen polysaccharide capsule (designated K2) have been shown to specifically evade both complement-mediated bacteriolysis and neutrophil-mediated killing. There is usually little protective maternal antibody of K1 strain available to infants (Pammi et al., 2021; Puopolo, 2017).

GROUP B *STREPTOCOCCUS*

- GBS or *Streptococcus agalactiae* are gram-positive diplococcus encapsulated bacterium and have been the principal GBS pathogen for over 50 years. GBS is the most common cause of vertically transmitted neonatal invasive bacterial disease.
  - Factors for GBS can be modified by IAP at least 4 hours prior to delivery. The primary mode of transmission is following ROM and during passage through the birth canal. High genital inoculum at delivery increases the likelihood of transmission and the consequential rate of GBS EOS.
  - Virulence has been associated with a polysaccharide capsule, although surface-localized GBS proteins may also be factors.
- GBS disease accounts for 95% of EOS and more than 90% of LOS in neonates in the United States today. Neonatal GBS infection is acquired in utero or during passage through the birth canal. Nearly 50% of infants who pass through colonized birth canal become colonized; however, only 1% to 2% will develop invasive disease. Documented maternal colonization of GBS is the strongest predictor of GBS EOS.
- GBS or *Streptococcus agalactiae* are a significant cause of maternal bacteriuria and endometritis and a major cause of serious bacterial infection in infants up to 3 months of age.
  - Maternal factors predictive of GBS disease include documented maternal GBS colonization, intrapartum fever (>38°C), or prolonged ROM (>18 hours). The primary risk factor is intrapartum maternal colonization of the genitourinary or gastrointestinal tract disease acquired vertically during passage through the birth canal.
  - Neonatal risk factors include prematurity (<37 weeks' gestation) and LBW (<2,500 g).
    - ❑ Lack of maternally derived, protective capsular polysaccharide-specific antibody is associated with the development of GBS invasive disease (Desai & Leonard, 2020; Esper, 2020; Ferrieri & Wallen, 2018; Puopolo, 2017; Rudd, 2021).

Maternal Evaluation and Intrapartum Antibiotic Prophylaxis

- The 2010 CDC guidelines for maternal surveillance of GBS include rectal and vaginal screening at 35 to 37 weeks' gestation for all women, except those with bacteremia during the current pregnancy and those with a history of an infant with GBS invasive disease, as these women should receive IAP regardless of GBS culture results. *Adequate IAP* includes administration of penicillin, ampicillin, or cefazolin at least 4 hours prior to delivery.
  - Maternal IAP has reduced neonatal EOS GBS disease; however, despite implementation of IAP, GBS remains the leading cause of EOS in term infants. Neither maternal IAP nor neonatal antibiotic administration prevents the development of primary-onset GBS disease infection ≥7 days of life (LOS GBS disease). Infants whose mothers received IAP are less likely to have sepsis, need mechanical ventilation, or have documented GBS bacteremia.
  - Of cases of GBS LOS, 50% are attributed to vertical transmission at birth or horizontal transmission in household or community settings.
    - ❑ One-quarter of all GBS EOS occur among infants >37 weeks; most GBS EOS occur with negative antepartum screens, although surveillance testing remains standard.
    - ❑ African American infants are at twice the risk for GBS EOS disease than non-African American infants as well as infants born to mothers who are less than 20 years of age, although the exact etiology is unclear (Esper, 2020; Puopolo, 2017; Rudd, 2021).

Neonatal Evaluation and Treatment

- Table 24.4 describes the evaluation of an infant for GBS disease.
- Penicillin remains the preferred agent and is the narrowest spectrum agent, with ampicillin an acceptable alternative. Other acceptable alternatives include first- or second-generation cephalosporin and vancomycin.
- Mortality from GBS disease is highest in preterm infants or LBW infants (Desai & Leonard, 2020; Esper, 2020; Rudd, 2021).

Klebsiella Species

- Gram-negative organisms such as *Klebsiella* spp. and *E. coli* are the leading causes of LOS and nosocomial infections and are important causes of BSIs, meningitis, and pneumonia. These bacteria are responsible for 15% of NICU infections and are associated with up to a 3.5-fold higher risk of death as opposed to gram-positive bacteria.
- With the introduction of intrapartum prophylaxis of GBS, gram-negative enteric bacteria-like *Klebsiella* is increasingly responsible for EOS in term and preterm

Table 24.4 Evaluation of Infant for Group B *Streptococcus* Disease

Asymptomatic Infant	Symptomatic Infant
▪ If signs/symptoms of maternal chorioamnionitis present: ▪ Limited evaluation recommended and includes: ▪ CBC with differential ▪ Blood cultures ▪ Empiric antibiotic therapy ▪ Inadequate IAP (<4 hours prior to delivery)	▪ Full diagnostic evaluation includes: ▪ CBC with differential ▪ Blood culture ▪ Lumbar puncture including CSF culture ▪ Chest radiograph ▪ Empiric antibiotic therapy

CBC, complete blood count; CSF, cerebrospinal fluid; IAP, intrapartum antibiotic prophylaxis.
Source: Data from Puopolo, K. M. (2017). Bacterial and fungal infections. In E. Eichenwald, A. Hansen, C. Martin, & A. Stark (Eds.), *Cloherty and Stark's manual of neonatal care* (8th ed., pp. 641–650, 691–718). Wolters Kluwer.

infants. *Klebsiella* is a common cause of early-onset neonatal pneumonia and can result in lung injury, abscess formation, empyema, and pneumatoceles.

▪ *Klebsiella* can also be the offending organism in UTIs and omphalitis.
  ● Neonatal UTIs are commonly caused by gram-negative rods, with *E. coli* and *Klebsiella* species responsible for over 80% of cases. In addition, *Klebsiella pneumoniae* has a higher incidence in neonates with vesicular urethral reflux (VUR) presenting with UTI compared with those without VUR.
  ● Omphalitis is a bacterial infection of the umbilical stump that presents around day 3 of life. It is commonly caused by *S. aureus*, *S. epidermidis*, *Streptococcus* spp., *E. coli*, *Clostridium difficile*, *Klebsiella*, and *Pseudomonas* (Boos & Sidbury, 2018; Esper, 2020; Puopolo, 2017; Srinivasan & Evans, 2018; Wang et al., 2018).

Pseudomonas Species

▪ *Pseudomonas* is noted as a cause of EOS and LOS, specifically BSIs, meningitis, omphalitis, UTIs, and pneumonia. In preterm infants, *Pseudomonas*, along with other gram-negative enteric bacteria, is a leading cause of EOS. Of particular interest is the species *Pseudomonas aeruginosa*, which can be quite wide-reaching and virulent.
▪ *Pseudomonas* thrives in moist environments, such as respiratory equipment, and can lead to colonization of the respiratory tract. *P. aeruginosa* pneumonia can cause pneumatoceles.
▪ *P. aeruginosa* is particularly virulent in LBW babies, with a mortality rate as high as 75%. This is due to its bacterial factors: a lipopolysaccharide outer membrane (endotoxin), mucoid capsule, adhesins, invasins, and toxins, specifically exotoxin A.

● Nosocomial acquisition and IV antibiotic exposure lead to overcolonization of this bacteria in the preterm gut. This is due in part to *Pseudomonas'* resistance to most common antibiotics. A severe illness during or after prolonged exposure to common antibiotics should trigger suspicion for *Pseudomonas*-induced LOS.
● Gram-negative bacteria *P. aeruginosa* is a less common cause of meningitis. *P. aeruginosa* can cause a rare and devastating form of bacterial conjunctivitis, requiring IV antibiotics.
▪ *Pseudomonas* causes LOS and nosocomial infections, specifically BSIs, meningitis, and pneumonia. In these instances, it is frequently resistant to beta-lactam antibiotics. *Pseudomonas* is particularly virulent among the enteric bacteria.
▪ As opposed to simple UTIs commonly caused by *E. coli* and *Klebsiella*, UTIs that are associated with VUR have distinctly different bacterial etiology, including *P. aeruginosa*.
  ● *Pseudomonas* can cause omphalitis, an infection of the umbilical stump (Boos & Sidbury, 2018; Esper, 2020; Puopolo, 2017; Rudd, 2021; Srinivasan & Evans, 2018; Wang et al., 2018).

COAGULASE-NEGATIVE *STAPHYLOCOCCUS*

▪ CONS is a facultative, anaerobic, gram-positive organism frequently found in the respiratory tract and on the skin. *S. epidermidis* is the most common species of CONS recovered from human skin and mucous membranes and is a primary cause of NICU disease.
  ● Most infants are colonized within the first week of life from passage through the birth canal and repeated exposure from colonized caregivers.
  ● BSIs caused by CONS are much more prevalent than bacteremia caused by *S. aureus* and are most commonly associated with umbilical or central venous lines.
    ❑ Believed to first colonize central catheter surfaces, polysaccharide surface adhesion (PSA) results in adherence to catheter surfaces. Production of a biofilm and slime subsequently inhibit host defenses and significantly decrease the hosts' abilities to eliminate the organisms.
▪ Infants may present with systemic instability, temporary cessation of enteral feeding, and escalated respiratory support. It is associated with prolonged hospitalizations and poorer neurodevelopmental outcomes. Typically, infants present without localizing signs, such as fever, new-onset respiratory distress, or deterioration in respiratory status. Other common nonspecific signs include apnea, bradycardia, poikilothermia, poor perfusion, poor feeding, irritability, and lethargy.

■ It is rarely fatal and rarely causes meningitis or site-specific disease. Indolent disease is more common than fulminant disease. However, CONS is a major source of morbidity leading to increased antibiotic exposure, length of stay, and hospital costs (Desai & Leonard, 2020; Esper, 2020; Puopolo, 2017).

STAPHYLOCOCCUS AUREUS

■ S. aureus is an encapsulated gram-positive organism that may result in multiple adhesions, produce virulence-associated enzymes, and/or release toxins to cause a wide range of systemic dysfunctions, including bacteremia, meningitis, cellulitis, omphalitis, osteomyelitis, and arthritis.

■ S. aureus differs from CONS by the production of coagulase and the presence of protein A, which is a component of the cell wall that contributes to virulence by binding to a portion of the IgG antibody and blocks the body's ability to break down the bacteria; however, S. aureus is identical to CONS under light microscopy.
  ● S. aureus is considered part of normal skin flora; however, it can cause a much wider and potentially more invasive disease than CONS through production of numerous toxins, enzymes, and binding proteins that facilitate its ability to establish possible life-threatening pyogenic infection.
  ● Neonatal infection may be associated with maternal infection: mastitis, cellulitis, or Cesarean section wound infection.

■ Symptoms of S. aureus disease begin after the first week of life. They are frequently complicated with focal site infections: soft tissue, bone/joint infections, and marked by persistent bacteremia despite antibiotic administration. LOS caused by S. aureus can result in significant morbidity.
  ● Small-inoculum colonization or infection can cause catastrophic, toxin-mediated disease—that is, scalded skin syndrome or toxic shock.

■ The most effective treatment includes systemic antibiotics and removal of foreign body. Empiric therapy is vancomycin. Most bacteria are resistant to penicillin, semisynthetic penicillins, and gentamicin. Nafcillin is appropriate for methicillin-susceptible S. aureus (MSSA); however, vancomycin is the preferred treatment for MRSA in neonates.
  ● Clindamycin or linezolid can be used as alternative to vancomycin; however, it should be noted that clindamycin is bacteriostatic, not bactericidal, and should not be used for bacteremia or severe infection.

■ Infants who clinically improve and have a negative blood culture or CSF culture can be switched to oral therapy. Infants with systemic symptoms (especially preterm infants and LBW infants) should be treated with parenteral antibiotics (Desai & Leonard, 2020; Esper, 2020; Puopolo, 2017).

METHICILLIN-RESISTANT STAPHYLOCOCCUS AUREUS

■ Methicillin-resistant *Staphylococcus aureus* (MRSA) isolates are categorized as hospital-associated (HA-MRSA) or community-associated (CA-MRSA) and can be rapidly spread in the NICU by nosocomial transmission on the hands of caregivers. methicillin-resistant *S. aureus* (MRSA) is a problem in all ages and is increasingly a recognized pathogen in the NICU.
  ● Community MRSA has developed an additional virulence factor which results in a significant increase in pyogenic infection. MRSA may present in previously healthy neonates who may develop pustulosis, cellulitis, skin abscess, bacteremia, UTI, pneumonia, or musculoskeletal infections. Infection of MRSA can be complicated with deep tissue involvement and persistent bacteremia which may require surgical debridement for resolution.
  ● Routine surveillance, cohorting, and isolation of colonized infants may be required to prevent spread and persistence of organism.
  ● Rifampin can be used as adjunctive therapy for persistent MRSA infection, but not as a single agent. Consultation with an infectious disease specialist is recommended for persistent MRSA infection (Bany-Mohammed, 2020d; Desai & Leonard, 2020; Esper, 2020; Puopolo, 2017).

▶ **NEONATAL INFECTIOUS CAUSES: VIRAL**

HEPATITIS B VIRUS

■ HBV has a spherical structure with a double shell. HBV concentrates in the hepatic parenchymal cells and circulates in the blood. An outer surface lipoprotein layer (hepatitis B surface antigen [HBsAg]) and an inner core nucleocapsid layer (hepatitis B core antigen [HBcAg]), a regulatory X protein, and viral polymerase soluble antigen (hepatitis B e antigen [HBeAg]) are also present.
  ● For neonates born to mothers who are HBsAg-positive and HBeAg-positive, the risk of acquiring HBV is higher than if HBsAg-positive alone. HBsAg has been found in the breast milk of HBsAg-positive mothers, but transmission has not been documented. With use of appropriate immunoprophylaxis, breastfeeding is safe.

■ Transmission is by the following mechanisms:
  ● *Transplacental:* either during pregnancy or at the time of delivery secondary to placental leaks; rarely do the viral antigens cross the placenta; occurrence more likely if the mother is HBeAg-positive
  ● *Natal transmission:* by exposure during labor and delivery to HBV in amniotic fluid, vaginal secretions, or maternal blood

- *Postnatal transmission:* may be by fecal–oral spread, blood transfusion, or other means
- Age at the time of acute infection is the primary determinant of risk of progression to chronic hepatitis B infection.
- Neonates with an HBV infection are usually asymptomatic at birth. Without appropriate immunoprophylaxis, a percentage will become HBsAg-positive within 4 to 12 weeks, placing them at risk of chronic infection, with potential sequelae of chronic hepatitis, cirrhosis, or hepatocellular carcinoma as an adult.
- The diagnosis of HBV is made by specific serologies with detection of viral antigens and antibodies, as described in the following:
  - HBsAg is a protein on the surface of the HBV, usually found 1 to 2 months after exposure and lasts a variable period. Any patient positive for HBsAg is potentially infectious.
  - Hepatitis B surface antibody (anti-HBs or HBsAb) appears after resolution of infection or immunization and indicates immunity.
  - HBcAg assists in differentiating between natural immunity from disease and immunity from vaccination.
  - Hepatitis B core antibody (anti-HBc or HBcAb) is present with all HBV infections and lasts for an indefinite period of time.
  - IgM antibody to hepatitis B core antigen (anti-HBc IgM) appears early in infection, is detectable for 4 to 6 months after infection, and is a good marker of acute or recent infection.
  - HBeAg is present in both acute and chronic infections and correlates with viral replication and high infectivity.
  - Hepatitis B e antibody (anti-HBeAg or HBeAb) develops with resolution of viral replication and indicates resolving infection (Permar, 2017).
  - Hepatitis B DNA (HBV DNA) is measured by polymerase chain reaction (PCR) and the concentration correlates with the amount of virus present.
- An HBV DNA PCR may assist in confirming the diagnosis, but also to assess viral load and monitor response to therapy.
- Baseline and follow-up of the infant's liver function, including aspartate aminotransferase (AST), alanine transaminase (ALT), and bilirubin levels, should be done.
- There are two types of products available for hepatitis B immunoprophylaxis: Hepatitis B vaccine is used for preexposure and postexposure protection and provides long-term protection. The vaccine is safe and effective. Hepatitis B immune globulin (HBIG) provides short-term protection from 3 to 6 months, indicated in postexposure circumstance.
- Neonatal therapy is based on maternal status:
  - Infants born to HBsAg-positive mothers:
    - Infants should receive both active and passive immunization within 12 hours of birth.
    - Infants should be followed up with hepatitis B serologies at 9 and 12 months of age.
  - Therapy for infants born to mothers with unknown maternal HBV status:
    - The mother's status should be checked immediately.
    - The infants should receive the first dose of the HBV within 12 hours of birth. HBIG should be given if maternal status remains unknown, with time frame based on BW.
- Of infants born to HbeAg-positive mothers, regardless of appropriate immunoprophylaxis, 5% to 10% progress to become chronic HBV carriers.
- If a neonate progresses to fulminant hepatitis disease, the mortality is around 67% (Greenberg et al., 2019; Pammi et al., 2021; Permar, 2017; Rudd, 2021; Schleis & Martin, 2018).

RESPIRATORY SYNCYTIAL VIRUS

- Respiratory syncytial virus (RSV) is an RNA virus of Paramyxovirus. There is only one identified serotype; however, multiple strains may affect virulence and susceptibility with two major strains: group A and group B. The virus replicates in the nasopharynx and spreads to the small bronchiolar epithelium.
- The majority of infants infected with RSV experience upper respiratory tract symptoms, but 20% to 30% will go on to develop lower respiratory tract disease and 1% to 3% of these will be hospitalized due to RSV lower respiratory tract disease. Most hospitalizations occur between 30 and 60 days of age.
- RSV is one of the most common diseases in early childhood. Most children are affected during their first 2 years of life. Humans are the only source of infection, and the transmission is through respiratory droplets or fomites. The incubation period ranges from 2 to 8 days and viral shedding may take from 3 days to weeks, especially in immunocompromised infants. There is no lifelong immunity.
  - In the NICU, RSV is a common nosocomial infection. Most commonly, RSV is spread via the hands of healthcare workers or family members.
  - Neonates at the highest risk include the following:
    - Infants less than 6 months of age, especially those born prematurely and who developed lung disease
    - Infants <2 years of age with heart disease
    - Infants who were the product of multiple-birth pregnancies
    - Infants with school-age siblings or those who attend day care
    - Neonates less than 1 month of age and are formula-fed
    - Male infants and male or female infants who are immunocompromised
    - Regular exposure to secondhand smoke or air pollution and/or family history of asthma

■ Symptoms of RSV may be nonspecific, such as poor feeding, lethargy, apnea, and irritability. Other symptoms that manifest include cough, wheezing, tachypnea, rales, rhonchi, retractions, nasal flaring, use of accessory muscles to breathe, pneumonia, cyanosis, and pulmonary infiltrates.

■ Rapid diagnosis is made by PCR or immunofluorescent antigen testing of respiratory secretions (95% sensitivity, with good specificity). Respiratory viral cultures will not produce results until 3 to 5 days.

■ Isolation precautions are necessary if the infant/child requires hospitalization. Supportive care with hydration, supplemental oxygen, and mechanical ventilation is as needed.

 ● Ribavirin is an antiviral with activity against RSV but should be considered on a case-by-case basis in cases of severe infection in conjunction with an infectious disease specialist.

■ *Passive immunization:*Palivizumab (Synagis) provides passive immunity and may be given monthly to high-risk infants during the RSV season. Guidelines should be reviewed seasonally to evaluate infants for dosing (Permar, 2017; Rudd, 2021; Schleis & Marsh, 2018).

▶ NEONATAL INFECTIOUS CAUSES: FUNGAL

■ Invasive fungal infection occurs in approximately 2% of all infants admitted to U.S. NICUs. *Candida* spp. are the third most common cause of LOS in the NICU.

■ The most important risk factor for fungal infection is GA. Apart from colonization and GA, other host factors that contribute to the susceptibility of the NICU neonate to fungal infection include a 5-minute Apgar score of less than 5 and an age-dependent immunocompromised state.

 ● Concomitants of NICU care that are thought to increase the risk of fungal infections include length of stay greater than 1 week, indwelling CVCs, abdominal surgery, parenteral nutrition, intralipids, H2 blockers, endotracheal intubation, and prolonged use of broad-spectrum antimicrobials, especially third-generation cephalosporins.

 ● One of the primary factors is the prolonged and frequent use of broad-spectrum antibiotics that suppress the growth of bacteria in the gastrointestinal tract and consequently allow candidal overgrowth. In particular, the use of third-generation cephalosporins seems to increase the risk of gastrointestinal colonization and subsequent candidemia.

■ *C. albicans* and *C. parapsilosis* account for 80% to 90% of invasive *Candida* infections (ICI).

 ● ICI in neonates include congenital cutaneous candidiasis (CCC) and late-onset cutaneous candidiasis, BSIs, UTIs, meningitis, peritonitis, and infection of other sterile sites (bone and joint infections).

■ Congenital candidiasis, a very rare entity, manifests as a deeply erythematous skin rash in the setting of pronounced neutrophilia, with WBC counts often rising to 50,000 mm^3 or more.

■ Local infections with *Candida* species include diaper dermatitis, funisitis (infection of the umbilical cord), UTI, and peritonitis as a result of bowel perforation.

■ Clinical signs and symptoms of candidemia are similar to bacteremia. Systemic infection is associated with a variety of nonspecific clinical findings, including respiratory decompensation, feeding intolerance, temperature instability, or mild thrombocytopenia.

■ The slow-growing nature of *Candida* facilitates its ability to progress from colonization to dissemination into the bloodstream and body tissues before clinical signs and symptoms of infection become apparent. Any *Candida* spp. isolated from a blood culture should never be regarded as a contaminant and should prompt an immediate search for evidence of dissemination, which occurs in approximately 10% of premature newborns with candidemia.

 ● Four major steps can be identified in infected infants after exposure to *Candida* spp.: (a) adhesion, (b) colonization, (c) dissemination, and (d) abscess formation.

■ A thorough evaluation for colonization includes ophthalmologic examination and ultrasonography of the heart, venous system, and abdomen. Most commonly, with BSIs, an initial end-organ dissemination (EOD) screen including an echocardiogram, liver and renal ultrasound, cranial ultrasound, and ophthalmologic examination should be performed.

 ● If candidemia persists, EOD is even more likely, and surveillance after 5 to 7 days should also include (a) ultrasound at the location of the tip of any previous or current central catheters for infected thrombus, (b) complete abdominal ultrasound for abscesses (laparotomy is sometimes considered if there is high clinical suspicion), and (c) cranial ultrasound/MRI to detect brain dissemination. Abscesses that are amenable to drainage should be drained.

■ Amphotericin B is the "gold standard" antifungal agent for treatment of systemic neonatal fungal infection. Fluconazole is the most frequently used azole medication.

 ● The Red Book 2015 released guidelines regarding antifungal prophylaxis for preterm infants less than 1,000 g (1 kg). The finding that prophylactic fluconazole reduces the incidence of invasive fungal infection must be interpreted "with caution," although current guidelines from the Infectious Diseases Society of America recommend IV or oral fluconazole twice weekly for 6 weeks in neonates with BW less than 1,000 g in nurseries with high rates (>10%) of invasive candidiasis.

■ ICI may lead to significant neurodevelopmental impairment even in the absence of documented fungal meningitis. In infants less than 1,000 g with ICI, these rates range from an attributable mortality of 13% to 20% to overall mortality rates of 23% to 66% (Bohannon et al., 2020c; Desai & Leonard, 2020; Hostetter & Gleason, 2018; Kaufman & Manzoni, 2020; Pammi et al., 2021; Puopolo, 2017; Rudd, 2021).

▶ NEONATAL INFECTIOUS CONCERNS SECONDARY TO SEXUALLY TRANSMITTED INFECTIONS

CHLAMYDIA

■ *Chlamydia trachomatis* is an obligate intracellular organism that can cause ophthalmia neonatorum and pneumonia in the infant and neonate. It is the most common cause of sexually transmitted genital infections.

● Infants born to infected mothers have a 50% chance of acquiring an infection, primarily transmitted through infected genital secretions, although transmission through intact membranes has been reported in infants delivered by Cesarean section.

● *C. trachomatis* is the leading cause of ophthalmia neonatorum in the United States due to its prevalence in the population. Infected infants have a 25% to 50% chance of developing conjunctivitis and a 5% to 20% chance of developing pneumonia.

■ Usual presentation of symptoms occurs between 5 and 14 days of life, with a spectrum ranging from mild eyelid edema to mucopurulent discharge, with significant swelling and redness.

■ The infection is diagnosed with culture which must contain epithelial cells due to the intracellular nature of the organism. If positive, infants should also be evaluated for pneumonia.

● Systemic treatment along with follow-up retesting is necessary, with up to 20% of infants requiring a second course of therapy.

● If untreated, symptoms of the infection can last up to 1 year and result in conjunctival scarring, micropannus formation, and less frequently corneal scarring.

■ *C. trachomatis* can cause pneumonia in the presence or absence of conjunctivitis, with approximately half of pneumonia cases having a conjunctival history. *C. trachomatis* pneumonia usually presents between 2 and 4 weeks of life but can present as early as week 1 through the first 4 months of life.

■ Pneumonia can present from 2 to 19 weeks of age. Initially, the infant experiences a period of 1 to 2 weeks of rhinorrhea, a persistent staccato cough, tachypnea, and nasal congestion without fever. There is a gradual increase in symptoms over several weeks. Approximately one-third of infants will have accompanying otitis media.

■ Diagnoses are largely clinical, but culture of the organism is the gold standard for diagnosis. Nucleic acid amplification tests are also available. Chest radiographs usually show bilateral interstitial infiltrates with hyperinflation. Some infected infants will have a positive nasopharyngeal swab, although a negative swab does not exclude the disease. *C. trachomatis* IgM titers do elevate, with a 1:32 or greater titer being diagnostic.

■ As with *C. trachomatis* conjunctivitis, systemic treatment and rescreening are required with pneumonia (Bany-Mohammed, 2020a; Desai & Leonard, 2020; Esper, 2020; Puopolo, 2017).

GONORRHEA

■ Gonorrhea is a sexually transmitted infection (STI) caused by a bacterial infection with *N. gonorrhoeae* (a gram-negative, oxidase-positive diplococcus). *N. gonorrhoeae* primarily affects the endocervical canal of the mother, and the infant may become infected during passage or by contact with contaminated amniotic fluid.

■ The most common manifestation of *N. gonorrhoeae* in neonates is ophthalmia neonatorum, with rare dissemination to bacteremia, osteomyelitis, septic arthritis, and meningitis. In the United States, most systemically infected infants do not have ocular disease due to universal prophylaxis at birth.

● Infection of mucosal surfaces can occur along with scalp abscesses when fetal electrode monitoring is used.

■ Ophthalmia neonatorum or bacterial conjunctivitis typically presents within 1 to 5 days of life with profuse and purulent drainage, bilateral eyelid edema, and chemosis. Without treatment, it can progress to clouding and damage of the cornea and panophthalmitis and loss of vision.

■ Gram stain of any exudate should be performed for diagnosis. The material may be obtained by swabbing the eye, pharynx, or anorectal areas.

■ An infant born to a mother with a known gonococcal infection should be evaluated for other STDs and hospitalized for treatment and testing for invasive disease. Like *C. trachomatis*, systemic treatment is required for gonococcal conjunctivitis (Bany-Mohammed, 2020b; Desai & Leonard, 2020; Esper, 2020; Puopolo, 2017).

SYPHILIS

- Congenital syphilis (CS) infection is caused by the *T. pallidum* organism, a hematogenous and sexually transmitted, corkscrew-shaped spirochete that is extremely fastidious, surviving only briefly outside the host. Treponemes are able to cross the placenta at any time during pregnancy and may infect the fetus. There is an increase in risk as the pregnancy progresses. Syphilis can cause stillbirth, preterm delivery, congenital infection, or neonatal death.

- It is transmitted to the fetus transplacentally in utero or during delivery via contact with a maternal genital lesion. Vertical transmission is highest during a recent maternal infection in either the primary and the secondary stage of syphilis. For the untreated mother, the primary or secondary stage of syphilis has a transmission rate of nearly 100% and decreases to between 10% and 30% during the latent stages.

- Symptoms are difficult to differentiate from other neonatal infections. Infants with "snuffles" (nasal stuffiness without copious discharge) are rarely seen in today's nurseries, but if noted are highly contagious. Maternal data, a thorough infant exam, and appropriate laboratory testing are essential.
  - The skin lesions or pemphigus syphiliticus are vesicles or bullous lesions unique to infants. These appear on the palms and soles and may be associated with desquamation. Lesions are highly contagious after rupture.

- More than 50% of infants with CS will be asymptomatic at birth. Symptoms of early-onset syphilis may develop in the first 2 years of life and late-onset syphilis after 2 years of life.
  - Chronic granulomatous inflammation of untreated syphilis leads to deformities that most often involved the bones, joints, teeth, eyes, and nervous system. The Hutchinson triad denotes a combination of findings: blunted upper incisors, interstitial keratitis, and eighth nerve deafness.

- Classifications for evaluating infants for CS are available in the literature.

- Box 24.1 lists the clinical findings of CS in the neonatal period.
  - Evaluation includes maternal history, physical examination, and laboratory testing. The laboratory testing of an infant should be identical to maternal testing for comparison.
  - Laboratory tests are grouped into two distinctive categories: nonspecific nontreponemal antibody (NTA) tests and specific treponemal antibody (STA) tests.
  - Table 24.5 lists the laboratory testing for *T. pallidum*.

Box 24.1 Clinical Findings of Congenital Syphilis in the Neonatal Period

Most Common
- Hepatitis
- Hepatomegaly with or without splenomegaly
- Radiographic bone changes (periostitis, osteochondritis)
- Rash involving the palms and soles
- Oval and maculopapular rash that becomes copper-colored with desquamation
- Condylomata lata
- Mucocutaneous lesions
- Jaundice, both direct and indirect hyperbilirubinemia
- Bone marrow failure, anemia, and/or thrombocytopenia with petechiae or purpura

Less Common to Rare
- Lymphadenopathy
- Pemphigus syphiliticus
- Respiratory distress due to pneumonia or pneumonitis
- Myocarditis
- Meningitis or other central nervous symptom findings (leptomeningitis, cranial nerve palsies, cerebral infarction, seizures, hypopituitarism)
- Nephrotic syndrome
- Rhinitis (snuffles)
- Pseudoparalysis of an extremity, pseudoparalysis of Parrot
- Fever
- Small for gestational age
- Nonimmune hydrops

Sources: Data from Desai, A. P., & Leonard, E. G. (2020). Infections in the neonate. In A. Fanaroff & J. Fanaroff (Eds.), *Klaus and Fanaroff's care of the high-risk neonate* (7th ed., pp. 275–295). Elsevier; Heresi, G. (2017). Syphilis. In E. Eichenwald, A. Hansen, C. Martin, & A. Stark (Eds.), *Cloherty and Stark's manual of neonatal care* (8th ed., pp. 788–737). Wolters Kluwer; Michaels, M. G., Sanchez, P., & Lin, L. (2018). Congenital toxoplasmosis, syphilis, malaria, and tuberculosis. In C. Gleason & S. Juul (Eds.), *Avery's diseases of the newborn* (10th ed., pp. 527–552.e6). Elsevier; Pammi, M., Brand, M. C., & Weisman, L. (2021). Infection in the neonate. In S. Gardner, B. Carter, M. Hines, & J. Hernandez (Eds.), *Merenstein & Gardner's handbook of neonatal intensive care* (9th ed., pp. 692–727). Elsevier.

- Infants should be treated for CS when proven or probable disease is suspected.
  - Aqueous penicillin G is the only acceptable antimicrobial treatment for syphilis in both the mother and the infant.

- Manifestations of untreated CS may develop after 2 years of age whether or not the baby had clinical symptoms during infancy. Long-term complications include impairments of the bones, central nervous system (CNS), eyes, joints, and teeth (Bany-Mohammed, 2020f; Desai & Leonard, 2020; Greenberg et al., 2019; Heresi, 2017; Michaels et al., 2018; Pammi et al., 2021).

Table 24.5 Laboratory Testing for *Treponema pallidum*

Diagnostic Test Category	Specific Diagnostic Test	Testing Information
■ Nonspecific NTA tests	■ VDRL ■ RPR	■ Screening tools ■ Allows quantitative monitoring ■ Follow serially to evaluate therapy effectiveness ■ A normal result in either test equates to a negative result ■ Any positive test should be followed with a (STA) test ■ VDRL is the test to use on CSF fluid (not RPR)
■ STA tests— not used for quantitative findings	■ FTA-ABS	■ Verify presence of the antibody, indicating current or past infection ■ If positive, remains positive always ■ May be used for testing CSF
	■ MHA-TP	
	■ TP-EIA	■ Used for screening in some institutions (instead of NTA)

CSF, cerebrospinal fluid; FTA-ABS, fluorescent treponemal antibody absorption; MHA-TP, microhemagglutination test for antibodies to *T. pallidum*; NTA, nontreponemal antibody; RPR, rapid plasma reagin; STA, specific treponemal antibody; TP-EIA, *T. pallidum* enzyme immunoassay; VDRL, venereal disease research laboratory.
Source: Reproduced with permission from Heresi, G. (2017). Syphilis. In E. Eichenwald, A. Hansen, C. Martin, & A. Stark (Eds.), *Cloherty and Stark's manual of neonatal care* (8th ed., pp. 788–737). Wolters Kluwer.

NEONATAL IMPLICATIONS OF TORCH INFECTIONS

■ TORCH is an acronym that denotes a chronic nonbacterial perinatal infection. It stands for **T**oxoplasmosis, **O**ther infections, **R**ubella virus, **C**ytomegalovirus, and **H**erpes simplex virus (HSV). A Zika virus (ZIKV) infection during pregnancy results in a congenital infection syndrome in the fetus and the newborn similar to other TORCH infections; thus, it has been suggested that **Z**IKV be added to the TORCH acronym to become TORCHZ.

■ Another acronym noted in the literature is TORCHES CLAP. This has been suggested to be more inclusive of other well-described pathogens acquired congenitally and in the neonatal period. It stands for **To**xoplasmosis, **R**ubella virus and respiratory syncytial virus, **C**ytomegalovirus, **H**erpes simplex virus and hepatitis B virus, **E**nteroviruses, **S**yphilis, **C**hickenpox, **L**yme disease, **A**cquired immunodeficiency syndrome/HIV, and **P**arvovirus B19 (Bany-Mohammed, 2020g; Rudd, 2021).

Toxoplasmosis (*TORCH*)

■ Toxoplasmosis is caused by *T. gondii*, a protozoan and obligate intracellular parasite capable of causing intrauterine infection.

■ The incidence of congenital toxoplasmosis in the United States is estimated between 500 and 5,000 infants each year. Toxoplasmosis is caused by *T. gondii*, an intracellular parasitic protozoan that is found most places in nature.

■ Risk factors include lower socioeconomic status, lower level of education, and having at least three or more kittens. Cats are the host where *T. gondii* is shed by oocysts in the cat's intestinal tract. The oocysts enter the cat's feces and are left in the soil.
  ● Risk is higher in those who work with raw meats. Additional food risk factors include eating undercooked or raw meats, including oysters and clams. There is high risk of transmission when consuming unwashed raw fruits and vegetables, drinking unpasteurized goat's milk, or drinking water from an untreated well.

■ A congenital toxoplasmosis infection results when a maternal primary infection during pregnancy spreads to the placenta and fetus. A reactivated infection does not predispose the infant to infection.
  ● The severity of the infection is greater in the first trimester, but the transmission rate is lower.

■ Postnatal transmission can occur from blood product or bone marrow transfusion via a seropositive donor with a latent infection. There is no documentation of transmission through breastfeeding.

■ There are four recognized patterns of presentation for congenital toxoplasmosis:
  ● *Subclinical/asymptomatic infection:* Most infants fall into this category (79%–90%) and do not have clinical symptoms at birth. If untreated, a large population will later demonstrate visual and CNS deficits, including hearing impairment, learning disabilities, or mental retardation several months to years later.
  ● *Neonatal symptomatic disease:* Signs of congenital disease at birth include maculopapular rash, lymphadenopathy, hepatosplenomegaly, jaundice, petechiae, and thrombocytopenia.
  ● *Delayed onset:* This is most often seen in premature infants and usually occurs within the first 3 months of age. It can behave like neonatal symptomatic disease. Chorioretinitis is the most common late manifestation.
  ● *Sequelae or relapse in infancy through adolescence of a previously untreated infection:* Chorioretinitis develops in up to 85% of adolescents/young adults with previously untreated congenital infection.
  ● Table 24.6 offers a summation of clinical symptoms of congenital toxoplasmosis.

■ Laboratory tools for the diagnosis of *T. gondii* infection include serologic tests, such as the *Toxoplasma* IgG, IgM, IgA, IgE, or IgG avidity and differential agglutination (AC/HS) tests; PCR assays; and

Table 24.6 Clinical Symptoms of Congenital Toxoplasmosis

Prenatal Presentation on Ultrasound	Postnatal Presentation	
	One-third present with generalized symptoms	Two-thirds present mostly with CNS symptoms, which is the hallmark of congenital *Toxoplasma gondii* infection
■ Intracranial hyperechogenic foci ■ Ventricular dilation ■ Anemia ■ Hydrops ■ Ascites ■ Brain, splenic, and hepatic calcifications ■ Hepatosplenomegaly	■ IUGR ■ Temperature instability ■ Hepatosplenomegaly, jaundice ■ Pneumonitis ■ Generalized lymphadenopathy ■ Maculopapular rash, petechiae ■ Chorioretinitis ■ Anemia, thrombocytopenia, and eosinophilia	*Classic triad of congenital toxoplasmosis:* ■ Chorioretinitis ■ Diffuse intracranial calcifications ■ Obstructive hydrocephalus *Other CNS symptoms:* ■ Pleocytosis (elevated WBC in CSF) ■ Elevated protein count in CSF ■ Microcephaly ■ Hyper/hypothermia related to hypothalamic involvement ■ Seizures ■ Direct hyperbilirubinemia ■ Meningoencephalitis

CNS, central nervous system; CSF, cerebrospinal fluid; IUGR, intrauterine growth restriction; WBC, white blood cell.

Sources: Data from Holzmann-Pazgal, G. (2017). Congenital toxoplasmosis. In E. Eichenwald, A. Hansen, C. Martin, & A. Stark (Eds.), *Cloherty and Stark's manual of neonatal care* (8th ed., pp. 720–727). Wolters Kluwer; Michaels, M. G., Sanchez, P., & Lin, L. (2018). Congenital toxoplasmosis, syphilis, malaria, and tuberculosis. In C. Gleason & S. Juul (Eds.), *Avery's diseases of the newborn* (10th ed., pp. 527–552.e6). Elsevier; Pammi, M., Brand, M. C., & Weisman, L. (2021). Infection in the neonate. In S. Gardner, B. Carter, M. Hines, & J. Hernandez (Eds.), *Merenstein & Gardner's handbook of neonatal Intensive care* (9th ed., pp. 692–727). Elsevier.

histologic and cytologic examinations of tissue and body fluids.

- Persistence of positive *Toxoplasma* IgG in the child beyond 12 months of age is considered the gold standard for diagnosis of congenital toxoplasmosis. Positive PCR assay results from peripheral blood, CSF, urine, or other body fluid in symptomatic patients are also diagnostic.
■ Prevention of congenital toxoplasmosis is through avoidance of high-risk behaviors. If exposed to cats, avoid changing cat litter, or change cat litter daily as the oocysts are not infective during the first 1 to 2 days after passage.
- Gardening and other outdoor work should be performed wearing gloves and with appropriate handwashing.
■ The pregnant mother with known toxoplasmosis infection and the neonate with a confirmed or probable diagnosis are treated with the same medications. Antiparasitic therapy is indicated for infants in whom congenital toxoplasmosis is confirmed or probable based on serology. Treatment of infants with toxoplasmosis infections can reduce the risk of sensorineural hearing loss (SNHL) and visual and neurodevelopmental morbidities. Treatment of diagnosed toxoplasmosis is long term and requires treatment for no less than 1 year with pyrimethamine, sulfadiazine, and folinic acid.
■ Congenital infection with *T. gondii* has a mortality rate as high as 12%. Morbidities may include ophthalmologic, neurodevelopmental, and audiologic impairments, including mental retardation, seizures, spasticity and palsies, and deafness, which may occur in subclinical infections

(Bany-Mohammed, 2020h; Holzmann-Pazgal, 2017; Michaels et al., 2018; Rudd, 2021).

Other Infections (TORCH)

HUMAN IMMUNODEFICIENCY VIRUS

■ HIV is a cytopathic RNA virus of the *Lentivirus* genus, which belongs to the Retroviridae family. HIV results in a broad spectrum of disease, with AIDS representing the most severe end of the clinical spectrum.
■ HIV is particularly tropic for CD4+ T-cells and cells of monocyte or macrophage lineage. After infection of the cell, viral RNA is uncoated and a double-stranded DNA transcript is made (through the activity of a viral enzyme, reverse transcriptase [RT]). This DNA then moves to the nucleus and integrates into the host genome DNA where it persists as a provirus. There is eventual destruction of both the cellular and humoral arms of the immune system.
■ There are two types of HIV viruses: HIV-1 and HIV-2.
- HIV-1 is the most prevalent in the United States and is the most pathogenetic of the two types.
- HIV-1 enters the immune system, especially the CD4+ T-lymphocytes, where it incorporates itself through the RNA to the host's DNA and becomes part of the genome, where it replicates.
- HIV-2 is mostly found in West Africa and is associated with a milder disease course, which takes longer time to develop.
■ HIV is transmitted by three primary modes: sexual contact, parenteral inoculation, and perinatal transfer. HIV is found in the blood, semen, vaginal secretions, and breast milk.

- The rate of transmission of HIV is highest in the late third trimester or at delivery. If untreated, the infant's transmission rate has been estimated to be between 15% and 40%. Infection risk increases with ROMs and assistive techniques.
  - ❏ Other factors that increase maternal–neonatal transmission are low maternal CD4+ counts, maternal IV drug use, no antiviral treatment during pregnancy, premature birth, and breastfeeding (particularly nonexclusive breastfeeding).
- Infants are generally asymptomatic at birth. Early symptoms could be missed since they are nonspecific and consistent with other more common viruses. Infants who are infected in utero may present with growth restriction, hepatosplenomegaly, and/or recurrent candidiasis.
  - Breastfeeding is the predominant means of postnatal HIV transmission to infants. Risk correlated with the degree of viremia and breast milk HIV DNA/RNA levels.
- Most neonates with untreated HIV infection present with acute illness during the first 2 to 4 weeks of life. Infants may present with any of the following symptoms, which may develop, persist, or recur during the first year of life: unexplained fevers, opportunistic infections (viral and bacterial), chronic diarrhea, failure to thrive, generalized lymphadenopathy, hepatosplenomegaly, parotitis, hepatitis, nephropathy, cardiomyopathy, and recurrent oral and diaper candidiasis; or encephalopathy, neurologic disease that is either delayed or progressive.
- Do not use cord blood for neonatal testing as there may be maternal blood present. The preferred test to diagnose HIV infection in infants and young children is HIV DNA or RNA PCR as this is highly sensitive and specific by 2 weeks of age. The HIV DNA PCR assay is the preferred diagnostic tool. This assay detects plasma (cell-free) viral RNA by PCR amplification. A number of commercially rapid tests are available but still require confirmation. Serial testing is recommended in HIV-exposed infants at 2 to 3 weeks of age, 1 to 2 months of age, and 4 to 6 months of age.
  - Two positive samples from two different time points represent HIV infection.
  - Infants at high risk of perinatal acquisition (no prenatal care, no antepartum or intrapartum antiretrovirals, late initiation of antiretroviral therapy (ART), detectable maternal viral load) should also be tested at birth and at 8 to 10 weeks of age. Transplacental transfer of maternal antibodies occurs in all deliveries; therefore, do not use antibody-based assays (enzyme-linked immunosorbent assay [ELISA] or western blot) to diagnose neonatal HIV.
- Because HIV recommendations and therapies change over time, consultation with an infectious disease specialist is recommended when managing neonatal HIV. The most recent recommendations can also be found online through the CDC or the National Institutes of Health (NIH).
- Due to unproven ability of prophylaxis to be completely protective against mother-to-child transmission (MTCT) of HIV, in countries where safe alternative sources are available, such as the United States, HIV-infected women should be counseled not to breastfeed their infants or to donate to human milk banks.
  - If a mother still chooses to breastfeed, it is vital that an appropriate plan of management be developed, including encouraging prolonged use of ART in both the mother and the infant while breastfeeding.
  - Caregivers should remain vigilant on the risk of opportunistic infections such as pneumonia. The HIV-positive infant should receive all recommended childhood immunizations.
- With the prevention and treatment protocols and subsequent interruption of vertical transmission, the number of infected children has been greatly reduced. HIV infection in untreated infants has a mortality rate of 10% to 20% by 4 years of age as the virus spreads more rapidly in infants and children due to their immature immune and organ systems.
  - Without appropriate treatment, infants would progress quickly to having HIV-related complications, including AIDS, *Pneumocystis jirovecii* pneumonia, and other bacterial and viral opportunistic infections (Bany-Mohammed, 2020c; Desai & Leonard, 2020; Greenberg et al., 2019; Pammi et al., 2021; Permar, 2017; Rudd, 2021; Schleis & Marsh, 2018).
- Table 24.7 describes the plan of care for maternal HIV in correlation with neonatal treatment and monitoring.

VARICELLA ZOSTER VIRUS

- Varicella zoster virus (VZV) is a member of the Herpesviridae family which affects neurons and can lie dormant to reactivate at a later time. A primary varicella infection is *chickenpox*, whereas reactivation of a latent virus is *zoster* or *shingles*. Reactivation infection does not result in fetal infection. Individuals are contagious 1 to 2 days before onset of lesions and until all lesions are crusted.
- The incidence of congenital varicella syndrome (CVS) among infants born to mothers who experience varicella during pregnancy is approximately 2% when infection occurs between 8 and 20 weeks of gestation. Rarely, cases of CVS have been reported in infants of women infected after 20 weeks of pregnancy.
- Maternal infection during the first or second trimester can be devastating to the fetus, resulting in limb, skin, and CNS abnormalities, and death. Transmission during the first two trimesters of pregnancy holds an increased risk of teratogenic effects to the fetus (CVS). Maternal infection in the third trimester is not associated with CVS. Transmission occurs through direct contact with

Table 24.7 Plan of Care for Maternal HIV

Scenario	Maternal Treatment/Monitoring	Neonatal Treatment/Monitoring

High-risk perinatal HIV exposure: mother is HIV-positive with any of the following high-risk criteria:
■ No ART or concerns regarding adherence
■ HIV RNA load greater than 50 copies/mL or unknown viral load
■ Primary HIV infection during pregnancy
	Mother to continue ART during and after pregnancy
	■ IV ZDV 3 hours prior to delivery or as soon as possible
	  ● *Monitoring:*
	    ❑ Viral resistance testing
	    ❑ HIV RNA PCR for viral load
	  ● *Delivery:*
	    ❑ Plan for c/s delivery at 38 weeks
	    ❑ Avoid artificial rupture of membranes, invasive fetal monitoring, and use of forceps or vacuum-assisted delivery as these will increase the risk of maternal–child transmission
		Therapy:
		■ ART started within 6–12 hours of birth for the first 4–6 weeks
		■ No breastfeeding if resides in country where safe feeding alternatives are readily available
		Evaluation:
		■ HIV DNA PCR at birth, 2–3 weeks, 1–2 months, 8–10 weeks, and 4–6 months
		■ Baseline CBC and differential (at risk for anemia)

Mother is HIV-positive not meeting the high-risk criteria above	Mother to continue cART during and after pregnancy ■ Including a minimum of three antiretroviral treatments regardless of CD4 count or viral load ■ IV zidovudine not indicated ■ Individualized decision for c/s	*Therapy:* ■ ART for the first 4–6 weeks *Monitoring:* ■ HIV DNA PCR at 2–3 weeks, 1–2 and 4–6 months ■ No breastfeeding if resides in a country where safe feeding alternatives are readily available

ART, antiretroviral therapy; cART, combination antiretroviral therapy; CBC, complete blood count; c/s, Cesarean section; PCR, polymerase chain reaction; ZDV, zidovudine.

Sources: Data from Desai, A. P., & Leonard, E. G. (2020). Infections in the neonate. In A. Fanaroff & J. Fanaroff (Eds.), *Klaus and Fanaroff's care of the high-risk neonate* (7th ed., pp. 275–295). Elsevier; Pammi, M., Brand, M. C., & Weisman, L. (2021). Infection in the neonate. In S. Gardner, B. Carter, M. Hines, & J. Hernandez (Eds.), *Merenstein & Gardner's handbook of neonatal intensive care* (9th ed., pp. 692–727). Elsevier; Schleis, M. R., & Marsh, K. J. (2018). Viral infections of the fetus and newborn. In C. Gleason & S. Juul (Eds.), *Avery's diseases of the newborn* (10th ed., pp. 482–526.c18). Elsevier.

individuals who have vesicular lesions or respiratory tract secretions.

● Varicella infection has a high fatality rate in infants when the mother develops varicella from 5 days before to 2 days after delivery because there is inadequate time for the development and transfer of maternal antibody across the placenta.

● When varicella develops in a mother more than 5 days before delivery and the GA is 28 weeks or more, the severity of disease in the newborn infant is modified by transplacental transfer of VZV-specific maternal IgG antibody.

■ There are three forms of varicella zoster infections involving the fetus and the neonate: fetal, congenital (early neonatal), and postnatal.

● Fetal varicella syndrome (FVS) occurs when VZV crosses the placenta and results in a pattern of congenital malformation called *FVS*.

● Congenital (early neonatal) varicella infection occurs when the pregnant woman suffers from chicken pox during the last 3 weeks of pregnancy. Disease begins in the neonate just before delivery or within the first 10 to 12 days of age.

● The postnatal form presents after the 12th day of age and does not represent transplacental infection, but rather results from droplet transmission.

■ Skin lesions appear to be the major source of transmissible VZV. Person-to-person transmission occurs either from direct contact with VZV lesions from varicella or herpes zoster or from airborne spread. Patients are contagious from 1 to 2 days before onset of the rash until all lesions have crusted.

■ Diagnosis is via PCR assay of vesicular fluid, scab, saliva, or buccal swabs, and via tissue culture of vesicles, CSF, or biopsy. PCR has lower yield in congenital viral infection compared with acquired infection.

■ Full-term healthy infants who acquire varicella postnatally only require routine supportive care.

● Acyclovir is recommended when a full-term infant acquires a congenital infection or an infection becomes systemic, even in a full-term healthy infant.

● Varicella zoster immune globulin (VariZIG) should be administered when a neonate is exposed to a maternal infection between 5 days prior to and 2 days after delivery. Immunoprophylaxis should be given within 96 hours of exposure. IVIG may be given when VariZIG is not available.

● Infants treated with immunoglobulins need to be in respiratory isolation for 28 days following treatment (Bany-Mohammed, 2020i; Permar, 2017; Rudd, 2021; Schleis & Marsh, 2018).

● Table 24.8 summarizes the stages of varicella exposure, clinical findings, and suggested therapies.

Table 24.8 Congenital Varicella Exposure, Clinical Findings, and Treatment

Stage	Exposure to VZV	Clinical Findings	Treatment
FVS	■ In utero transmission ■ Mother exposed during the first half of pregnancy	■ Skin lesions may scar, with skin loss ■ *Profound neurologic impairment:* microcephaly, seizures, encephalitis, cortical atrophy, and cerebral calcifications ■ *Ocular abnormalities:* microphthalmia, chorioretinitis, and/or cataracts ■ Limb hypoplasia and other skeletal defects ■ Prematurity and IUGR	■ Provide supportive care. ■ Acyclovir therapy may be beneficial to prevent progressive complications. ■ Isolation is not indicated.
CVS	■ Active maternal VZV in the last 3 weeks of pregnancy or within the first few days postpartum ■ Transmitted transplacentally or via ascending infection through the birth canal ■ Active VZV begins in the neonate before delivery or within 10 to 12 days, after birth ■ Infant mortality increases with maternal infection within 5 days to 2 days after delivery	■ A generalized pruritic, vesicular, or centripetal rash; potential superinfection of skin lesions ■ Low-grade fever ■ Pneumonia ■ Thrombocytopenia ■ Glomerulonephritis, hepatitis, and arthritis ■ Latent infection may occur ■ Infection after vaccination may also occur	■ Administer VZIG or VariZIG within 96 hours of exposure. ■ If VZIG not available, then administer IVIG. ■ Strict respiratory isolation is required for 28 days. ■ Acyclovir may be prescribed as adjunct therapy. ■ Antibiotics may be prescribed for secondary skin infections. ■ Prognosis is good if maternal infection occurs more than 5 days prior to delivery.
Postnatal chickenpox	■ Not transmitted transplacentally	■ Presents between 12 and 28 days of life ■ May see a typical chickenpox rash: erythematous macular rash to vesicular rash occurring in multiple stages	■ If acquired postnatally, disease is usually mild.

CVS, congenital (early neonatal) varicella syndrome; FVS, fetal varicella syndrome; IUGR, intrauterine growth restriction; IVIG, intravenous immunoglobulin G; VZIG or VariZIG, varicella zoster immune globulin; VZV, varicella zoster virus.

Sources: Data from Permar, S. R. (2017). Bacterial and fungal infections. In E. Eichenwald, A. Hansen, C. Martin, & A. Stark (Eds.), *Cloherty and Stark's manual of neonatal care* (8th ed., pp. 641–650). Wolters Kluwer; Schleis, M. R., & Marsh, K. J. (2018). Viral infections of the fetus and newborn. In C. Gleason & S. Juul (Eds.), *Avery's diseases of the newborn* (10th ed., pp. 482–526.e18). Elsevier; Rudd, K. M. (2021). Infectious diseases in the neonate. In T. Verklan & M. Walden (Eds.), *Core curriculum for neonatal intensive care nursing* (6th ed., pp. 588–616). Elsevier.

Rubella (TORCH)

■ Rubella virus is an enveloped, positive-stranded RNA virus classified as a rubivirus in the Togaviridae family. It is capable of causing chronic intrauterine infection and damage to the developing fetus (congenital rubella syndrome [CRS]).
  ● Of childbearing women, 92% are estimated to be seropositive (rubella immune). Endemic transmission of rubella was declared eliminated from the Americas in 2015. However, rubella continues to be endemic in other parts of the world. It is estimated that >100,000 infants worldwide are born with CRS each year.
■ Virus is spread by respiratory secretions and also from stool, urine, and cervical secretions. Maternal viremia is a prerequisite to placental infection, which may or may not spread to the fetus.
■ Rubella infection can have catastrophic effects on the developing fetus, resulting in spontaneous abortion, fetal infection, stillbirth, or intrauterine growth restriction. The fetal infection rate varies according to the timing of maternal infection during pregnancy.

■ Congenital rubella infection has a wide spectrum of presentations, ranging from asymptomatic infection to acute disseminated infection, to deficits not evident at birth.
  ● Systemic transient manifestations include LBW, hepatosplenomegaly, meningoencephalitis, thrombocytopenia with or without purpura, and bony radiolucencies.
  ● Systemic permanent manifestations include heart defects (e.g., patent ductus arteriosus [PDA], pulmonary artery stenosis, or hypoplasia), eye defects (e.g., cataracts, iris hypoplasia, microphthalmos, and retinopathy), CNS problems (e.g., intellectual disability and psychomotor developmental delay, speech and language delay), microcephaly, and sensorineural deafness (unilateral or bilateral).
■ Timely diagnosis of congenital rubella infection is important both for management of the individual patient and for prevention of secondary infection because these infants may remain infectious for 1 year.

- Serologic studies are the mainstay of rubella diagnosis. CRS is diagnosed by detection of rubella-specific IgM in serum or oral fluid taken before 3 months of age. The virus can be cultured for up to 1 year despite measurable antibody titer. The best specimens for viral recovery are from nasopharyngeal swabs, conjunctival scrapings, urine, and CSF, in decreasing order of usefulness.
- CRS may also be diagnosed by detection of viral RNA by nested RT-PCR in nasopharyngeal swabs, urine, oral fluid, CSF, lens aspirate, and ethylenediaminetetraacetic acid (EDTA) blood.
- All newborns who fail hearing screening and born to mothers who are rubella nonimmune should undergo evaluation for rubella (measurement of rubella-specific IgM antibodies) and other intrauterine infections.
- Children with congenital rubella should be considered contagious until they are at least 1 year of age, unless two cultures of clinical specimens (nasopharyngeal and urine cultures) obtained 1 month apart are negative for rubella virus after 3 months of age (Bany-Mohammed, 2020e).

Cytomegalovirus (TORCH)

- CMV is a member of the herpes virus family. The hallmark of the virus is the histologic presence of large cells with generous amounts of cytoplasm (cytomegaly) and "inclusion-bearing" cells in both the nucleus and the cytoplasm. The virus may be found in body fluids such as saliva, urine, blood and blood products, breast milk, and genital fluids (cervical and seminal secretions).
  - It is the most common cause of congenital infection in the United States. Infants are at high risk for brain damage and birth defects. The incidence of CMV is 0.5% to 2% of live births or about 40,000 infants born in the United States.
  - It is transmitted horizontally and vertically. Horizontal transmission results from person-to-person contact with virus-containing secretions.
- Most severe sequelae are associated with a primary or acute infection during the first trimester of pregnancy. Primary CMV infection during pregnancy carries a neonatal transmission rate of 30% to 40%.
  - Only 10% to 15% of neonates with congenital CMV will have symptomatic CMV infection. Of infants with congenital CMV, 90% are asymptomatic at birth; however, they may have SNHL later in childhood.
- Testing using PCR can be done on blood, urine, or saliva by viral isolation in tissue culture from the infant's urine or saliva, and by spin-enhanced culture. Urine is considered the ideal specimen.
  - Testing of CMV should be completed within 2 to 3 weeks after birth to differentiate congenital infection from perinatal or postnatal infection.
  - Testing completed after 3 weeks of age may represent a perinatal or postnatal infection.
  - Table 24.9 presents the clinical findings of congenital CMV infection.
- Due to limited evidence of efficacy as well as concerns of possible toxicities, which include neutropenia, antiviral therapies are only recommended for neonates with CNS involvement started within the first month of life. Ganciclovir or valganciclovir is the antiviral of choice for congenital CMV infection with proven CNS involvement (Desai & Leonard, 2020; Pammi et al., 2021; Permar, 2017; Rudd, 2021; Schleis & Marsh, 2018).

Table 24.9 Clinical Findings of Congenital Cytomegalovirus Infection

Timing of Presentation	Clinical Findings
Prenatal signs of CMV infection	■ Amniotic fluid abnormalities ■ Placental enlargement ■ Fetal growth restriction ■ Cerebral periventricular echogenicity or calcifications or ventriculomegaly ■ Microcephaly, polymicrogyria, or cerebellar hypoplasia ■ Hyperechogenic fetal bowel, hepatosplenomegaly ■ Ascites and/or pleural effusions
Symptoms present at birth: 1. Fulminant infection (congenital symptomatic CMV infection) 2. Non–life-threatening infection	■ IUGR ■ Severe central nervous system involvement, neurologic complications (microcephaly, intracerebral calcifications, chorioretinitis), sensorineural hearing loss ■ Hepatosplenomegaly with jaundice, abnormal LFTs ■ Thrombocytopenia with or without purpura ■ Hemolytic anemia ■ Pneumonitis
Asymptomatic at birth: late or subclinical disease	■ Developmental abnormalities, acquired microcephaly ■ Neurodevelopmental impairment, seizures, hearing loss, visual impairment ■ Motor spasticity

CMV, cytomegalovirus; IUGR, intrauterine growth restriction; LFT, liver function test.
Source: Data from Permar, S. R. (2017). Bacterial and fungal infections. In E. Eichenwald, A. Hansen, C. Martin, & A. Stark (Eds.), *Cloherty and Stark's manual of neonatal care* (8th ed., pp. 641–650). Wolters Kluwer.

Herpes Simplex Virus (TORCH)

- HSV is a double-stranded DNA virus with the ability to enter a latent state and produce a lifelong infection. It consists of a viral DNA core surrounded by a protein capsid, which is surrounded by an envelope of proteins. There are two distinct types: HSV-1 and HSV-2. Both types induce perinatal infections that are clinically identical.
  - In the past, clinicians concluded that HSV-1 affected the person above the waist (face and skin) and that HSV-2 involved the area below the waist (genitals). It is now accepted that both viruses can affect any part of the body and the neonate, although 75% of congenital HSV are due to HSV-2.
- Perinatal transmission of HSV to the fetus is highest if the mother has a primary infection at or near the time of delivery. During the first trimester, the transmission rate is less than 2%, whereas near the end of pregnancy it increases to 25% to 60%.
  - Most mothers of severely affected infants have no known history of HSV or lesion present at the time of delivery; therefore, a negative maternal history should not deter the practitioner from evaluating the infant with HSV symptoms.
- *Prevention is key in reducing the mortality and morbidity in neonates and infants.* Neonatal infection can occur through contact with the hands or mouth of a care provider or from breast lesions during breastfeeding.
- Table 24.10 outlines the categories of HSV in correlation with presentation, evaluation, and suggested treatment.

Table 24.10 Herpes Simplex Virus Presentation, Evaluation, and Suggested Treatment

Category of HSV	Presentation	Diagnostics/Evaluation	Treatment
Asymptomatic infants born to mothers with suspected or proven primary infection with active lesions at delivery	■ Asymptomatic	■ Thorough physical assessment ■ CBC ■ Surface PCR or culture at 24 hours of age ■ Blood PCR	■ Dependent on maternal history and infant virology testing ■ Pending diagnostic results may treat with IV acyclovir versus routine follow-up
Localized SEM disease	■ Symptoms present by 7–14 days of life ■ Skin lesions (in <30%) ■ Lesions localized to the mouth and eyes	■ Culture or PCR of vesicular fluid, blood, CSF ■ Evaluation should include ■ ophthalmologic examination, brain imaging, EEG, and audiologic testing	■ Oral acyclovir is not adequate therapy ■ Recommendation includes 14 days of IV acyclovir therapy
Localized CNS disease (encephalitis)	■ Symptoms present by 14–21 days of life ■ May have skin lesions ■ Lethargic, irritable, and tremors ■ Meningoencephalitis ■ Seizures ■ Microcephaly	■ The indicated diagnostic tests stated above	■ IV acyclovir as oral therapy is not adequate ■ Minimum 21 days of IV acyclovir therapy ■ Obtain a CSF PCR at the end of treatment; if positive continue treatment
Disseminated disease	■ Initially, asymptomatic ■ Skin lesions (in <30%) ■ Present at 7–14 days of life ■ CNS involvement ■ Fever/temperature instability ■ Pneumonia ■ Severe liver dysfunction ■ Abnormal CSF findings ■ Seizures ■ Profound sepsis with septic shock ■ Microcephaly	■ The indicated diagnostic tests stated above	■ IV acyclovir as oral therapy is not adequate ■ Minimum 21 days of IV acyclovir therapy ■ Obtain a CSF PCR at the end of treatment; if positive continue treatment

CBC, complete blood count; CSF, cerebrospinal fluid; CNS, central nervous system; HSV, herpes simplex virus; PCR, polymerase chain reaction; SEM, skin, eyes, and mouth.

Sources: Data from Desai, A. P., & Leonard, E. G. (2020). Infections in the neonate. In A. Fanaroff & J. Fanaroff (Eds.), *Klaus and Fanaroff's care of the high-risk neonate* (7th ed., pp. 275–295). Elsevier; Greenberg, J. M., Haberman, B., Narendran, V., Nathan, V., & Schibler, K. R. (2019). Neonatal morbidities of prenatal and perinatal origin. In R. Resnik, R. K. Creasy, J. D. Iams, C. J. Lockwood, T. Moore, & M. F. Greene (Eds.), *Creasy and Resnik's maternal-fetal medicine: Principles and practice* (8th ed., pp. 1309–1333.e8). Elsevier; Pammi, M., Brand, M. C., & Weisman, L. (2021). Infection in the neonate. In S. Gardner, B. Carter, M. Hines, & J. Hernandez (Eds.), *Merenstein & Gardner's handbook of neonatal intensive care* (9th ed., pp. 692–727). Elsevier; Schleis, M. R., & Marsh, K. J. (2018). Viral infections of the fetus and newborn. In C. Gleason & S. Juul (Eds.), *Avery's diseases of the newborn* (10th ed., pp. 482–526.e18). Elsevier; Rudd, K. M. (2021). Infectious diseases in the neonate. In T. Verklan & M. Walden (Eds.), *Core curriculum for neonatal intensive care nursing* (6th ed., pp. 588–616). Elsevier.

- Treatment with IV acyclovir has decreased the mortality rate of disseminated disease and neurologic sequelae of surviving infants. Infants with CNS disease have a higher mortality rate.
- Infants who develop interstitial pneumonia, hemorrhagic pneumonia, or NEC with pneumonitis intestinalis have the highest mortality rate of over 80% if untreated and as high as 30% with appropriate treatment (Desai & Leonard, 2020; Greenberg et al., 2019; Permar, 2017; Rudd, 2021; Schleis & Marsh, 2018).

▶ UNIVERSAL PRECAUTIONS/INFECTION CONTROL

- All healthcare providers are responsible for following infection control practices and staying informed and educated on the latest guidelines and practices to help prevent HAIs.
- Standard precautions should be used with all patient contacts regardless of the underlying diagnosis or infectious status. These precautions consist of:
  - *Universal precautions:* designed to prevent blood and body fluid contamination
  - *Body substance precautions:* designed to prevent contamination with moist substances
  - *Transmission-based precautions:* necessary when a patient is infected with a known or suspected pathogen that is associated with a high risk of contamination via airborne or droplet transmission or contact with the skin or contaminated surfaces
- Core components of universal precautions include:
  - Use gloves when touching blood, body fluids, mucous membranes, or nonintact skin, and when handling items or surfaces soiled with blood or body fluids. All human blood and certain human body fluids are treated as if known to be infectious for HIV, HBV, and other blood-borne pathogens.
  - Use mask and eye protection during procedures that might generate splashing or droplets in the air.
  - Use a gown or a plastic apron when splashing of blood or body fluid is likely.
  - Perform careful handwashing if contaminated with blood or body fluids.
  - Take extraordinary care when handling needles and other sharp objects.
- The CDC provides the following surveillance definition for HAI: illness associated with a pathogen or its toxins that is not present or incubating at the time of admission. HAIs are a potentially highly modifiable contributor to a spectrum of adverse outcomes, across all gestational and postnatal ages, but especially in the most immature infants.
  - These are a major cause of morbidity and mortality in infants and children. The CDC estimates

approximately 5% to 10% of hospitalized patients in the United States develop HAIs.
  - HAIs have been shown to significantly and independently impact neonatal outcomes, including death, short-term and long-term morbidities, hospital length of stay, and healthcare costs. The estimated cost for each central line-associated infection is $46,000.
- Each NICU must establish reasonable guidelines for restriction of assignments based on the employee's potential to transmit a disease and the potential risk of acquiring a disease. Transmission of disease among patients and employees can occur bidirectionally. Clinicians can minimize HAIs by consistently and reliably following best practices for infection prevention and minimizing invasive procedures to the extent possible.
- Handwashing is the most important procedure for controlling infection in the NICU.
  - Hand hygiene techniques are effective in decreasing the colonization rate of resident and transient flora and have been shown to reduce cross-contamination among patients. These guidelines will be effective only if every healthcare provider performs hand hygiene before and after every patient contact.
  - Alcohol-based hand rubs are the most effective products for reducing the number of pathogenic microorganisms on the hands of healthcare providers.
    - The CDC recommends at least 15 seconds of rubbing the solution on the hands, paying particular attention to the areas between the fingers, thumb, and little finger.
  - In addition to hospital personnel, parents and visitors should also be taught to adhere to strict hand hygiene as nosocomial infections can also be spread by family members.
  - Gloves are not an alternative to hand hygiene. Gloves are not completely impermeable to microorganisms, and the warm, wet skin surface under the gloves offers an ideal environment for bacterial multiplication.
- Overcrowding in the NICU increases the risk of cross-contamination.
- Cohorting is an important infection control measure used primarily during outbreaks or epidemics in the NICU. The object of cohorting is to limit the number of contacts of one infant with other infants and personnel.
- Medical devices facilitate infections. The presence of indwelling intravascular or transmucosal medical devices has also been identified as one of the greatest risk factors for HAIs. The most common invasive devices used in the nursery are intravascular catheters, mechanical ventilators, ventriculoperitoneal shunts, and urinary catheters. In general, risk increases as the duration of exposure lengthens.
- The CDC has published guidelines and recommendations for prevention of HAIs, including

isolation precautions, guidelines for protecting healthcare workers, and guidelines for prevention of postoperative and device-related infections. These guidelines can be found on the CDC website (Choi, 2020; Esper, 2020; Pammi et al., 2021; Ringer, 2017; Rudd, 2021; Srinivasan & Evans, 2018).

▶ CONCLUSION

Throughout pregnancy, the fetus is protected to an extent by the chorioamniotic membranes, the placenta, and various antimicrobial factors in the amniotic fluid, many mechanisms of which remain incompletely understood.

Even with these protections, congenital and perinatal bacterial and viral infections may occur and have long-term impact on the neonate's growth and development. Understanding the implications of an immature immune system and the common bacterial and viral risks facing the neonate will allow the neonatal nurse practitioner (NNP) to make clinically appropriate decisions in the evaluation and treatment of neonatal infections.

1. Embryology, Physiology, Pathophysiology & Systems Management Infectious Disease Recall A 17-day-old preterm infant with a central line in place presents with lethargy and feeding intolerance. What is the most common organism associated with bacteremia and an indwelling central venous line?

    A. Coagulase-negative *Staphylococcus* spp.
    B. *Escherichia coli*
    C. *Staphylococcus aureus*

2. Definitive diagnosis of neonatal sepsis is achieved by:

    A. Elevated serial C-reactive protein serum levels
    B. Isolation of an organism from a sterile body site
    C. Shifted immature-to-total ratio on the complete blood count

3. Intrapartum antibiotic prophylaxis (IAP) has been highly effective in reducing:

    A. *Escherichia coli* early-onset sepsis disease
    B. Group B streptococcal early-onset sepsis disease
    C. Group B streptococcal late-onset sepsis disease

4. Methicillin-resistant *Staphylococcus aureus* (MRSA) is a resistant bacterial organism which can be easily spread through horizontal transmission in the NICU. The neonatal nurse practitioner (NNP) should follow the recommendations for:

    A. All parents and caregivers to wear sterile gowns for contact
    B. Cohorting and isolation of colonized infants
    C. Prophylactic use of rifampin as a single agent

5. Chronic infection with which of the following viruses has been associated with hepatic carcinoma?

    A. Hepatitis B virus
    B. Human cytomegalovirus
    C. Human enterovirus

6. For which of the following infants should palivizumab be considered to prevent severe disease from respiratory syncytial virus (RSV)?

    A. Infant born at 26 weeks' gestation with no home-going oxygen requirement during the first year of life
    B. Infant born at 28 weeks' gestation with a home oxygen requirement of 0.2 L during the second year of life
    C. Infant born at 33 weeks' gestation with a home oxygen requirement of 0.2 L during the first year of life

7. The neonatal nurse practitioner (NNP) reviews the laboratory results presented here and calculates the absolute neutrophil count (ANC) and immature-to-total ratio (I:T).

White blood cells	5
Hemoglobin (Hgb)	18
Hematocrit (Hct)	53
Platelets	173
Neutrophils (or segs or polys)	10
Bands (or stabs)	8
Lymphs	10
Monos	22
Eosinophils	5
Metas	0
Myelos	0
Promyelos	0

Based on the findings, the NNP has a:
A. High concern for infection
B. Low concern for infection
C. Moderate concern for infection

8. The neonatal nurse practitioner (NNP) reviews the laboratory results presented here and calculates the immature-to-total ratio (I:T) as:

White blood cells	13
Hgb	18
Hct	53
Platelets	259
Neutrophils (or segs or polys)	55
Bands (or stabs)	2
Lymphs	28
Monos	18
Eosinophils	3
Metas	0
Myelos	0
Promyelos	0

A. 0.04
B. 0.08
C. 0.12

(See answers next page.) 449

1. A) Coagulase-negative *Staphylococcus* spp.

Bloodstream infections caused by coagulase-negative *Staphylococcus* (CONS) are much more prevalent than bacteremia caused by *S. aureus* (Desai & Leonard, 2020) and are most commonly associated with umbilical or central venous lines (Esper, 2020). *E. coli* and *S. aureus* are not associated with line infections.

2. B) Isolation of an organism from a sterile body site

Definitive diagnosis is the isolation of an organism from a sterile body site, such as blood, cerebrospinal fluid (CSF), or urine. Indirect indices of infection include the following: white blood cells (WBC), absolute neutrophil count (ANC), C-reactive protein (CRP), procalcitonin level, and various cytokines; however, none are specific or sensitive enough to confirm or exclude sepsis. The immature-to-total ratio (I:T) is most informative if measured between 1 and 4 hours after birth. I:T is best used for negative predictive value: If I:T is normal, infection is unlikely, with 99% predictive value (Desai & Leonard, 2020; Esper, 2020; Rudd, 2021).

3. B) Group B streptococcal early-onset sepsis disease

IAP has been highly effective in reducing group B *Streptococcus* (GBS) early-onset sepsis (EOS), although there has been no direct effect on late-onset sepsis (LOS) GBS. The relationship between *E. coli* early-onset neonatal sepsis as an untoward side effect of IAP is controversial (Esper, 2020; Puopolo, 2017).

4. B) Cohorting and isolation of colonized infants

MRSA isolates are categorized as hospital-associated (HA-MRSA) or community-associated (CA-MRSA) and can be rapidly spread in the NICU by nosocomial transmission on the hands of caregivers. Routine surveillance, cohorting, and isolation of colonized infants may be required to prevent spread and persistence of organisms. The use of sterile gowns during contact with infants is extreme and the cost not justified by resultant decreases in infection. Rifampin can be used as adjunctive therapy for persistent MRSA infection, but not as a single agent (Desai & Leonard, 2020; Puopolo, 2017).

5. A) Hepatitis B virus

Chronic infection with hepatitis B virus is associated with cirrhosis and hepatic carcinoma. Enterovirus and cytomegalovirus do not have this association (Permar, 2017; Schleis & Marsh, 2018).

6. A) Infant born at 26 weeks' gestation with no home-going oxygen requirement during the first year of life

Palivizumab can be considered for the infant born at 26 weeks' gestation, regardless of diagnosis of chronic lung disease, during the first year of life. An infant born at 28 weeks' gestation with an oxygen requirement could receive palivizumab in the first year of life but not the second. An infant born at 33 weeks would not qualify regardless of diagnosis of chronic lung disease during either the first or second year of life (Rudd, 2021).

7. A) High concern for infection

There is a high concern for infection as both the ANC and I:T ratio are abnormal. The ANC is 1,000 and the I:T ratio is 0.2. Calculations: I:T ratio = 8/8 + 10 + 0 + 0 = 8/18 = 0.44; ANC = (8 +1 0) × (5 × 10) = 900.

8. A) 0.04

Calculation of I:T ratio = bands/total neutrophils; total neutrophils = bands + segs + metas + myelos
2/2 + 55 + 0 + 0 = 2/55 = 0.04

The Musculoskeletal System

Chandler Williams and Brooke Murdock

▶ INTRODUCTION

Complete understanding of the development and abnormalities throughout the musculoskeletal system is crucial to prompt diagnosis and treatment of abnormalities and congenital syndromes.

▶ MUSCULOSKELETAL DEVELOPMENT

EMBRYOLOGIC DEVELOPMENT

- The embryologic development of the musculoskeletal system stems from both the mesoderm and the neural crest, as the musculoskeletal system requires both functional tissue and innervation to function properly.
- Development and differentiation of both the mesoderm and the neural crest occur in weeks 3 to 4.
  - The innervation of the musculoskeletal system rises from the notochord, a tubular column of cells formed cephalocaudally on the long axis of the embryo.
- The extremities develop from the limb buds beginning in week 4 and continue in a proximal–distal pattern until week 8.
  - During this time, cells forming connective tissue differentiate from the mesoderm into three segments:
    - ❑ Dermatomes, which become the skin
    - ❑ Myotomes, which become the muscle cells
    - ❑ Sclerotomes, which become the cartilage and bone
- Differentiation of the spinal cord begins in the fourth week of embryologic development, beginning with somites which create mesodermal tissue that migrates dorsally and anterolaterally to give rise to the trunk structures and limbs.
- The first cervical vertebra, the atlas, differs physically from other vertebrae as it only has a narrow anterior arch which does not ossify nor is visible until 1 year of age.
- Teratogens and genetic abnormalities in the embryologic period affecting the musculoskeletal system result in malformations of the extremities and spine or can impair growth and development of the musculoskeletal system.
  - Teratogens include irradiation, industrial chemicals, therapeutic drugs, and maternal infections such as rubella, congenital syphilis, cytomegalic inclusion disease, and congenital herpes.
  - Genetic disorders are classified as either Mendelian, chromosomal, or multifactorial (see Chapter 15 for the definition of inheritance patterns).
  - Congenital limb malformations vary in their presentation and are classified according to the primarily affected embryologic failure, including failure of formation of parts, failure of differentiation, duplication, overgrowth, undergrowth, congenital constriction band syndrome, and generalized skeletal abnormalities (Liu & Thompson, 2020).

FETAL DEVELOPMENT

- After the embryologic foundation is laid, skeletal development continues throughout gestation, the postnatal period, and through the end of adolescence. Primary skeletal ossification centers are present in the long bones near the end of the first trimester, and growth occurs from the ends of the long bones (i.e., humerus, radius, ulna, metacarpals, phalanges, femur, tibia, fibula, metatarsals).
- In utero fetal movements strengthen and develop the muscular system. Muscle cells (myocytes) continue to differentiate and mature, with full maturation present at 38 weeks' postmenstrual age. Myocytes grow primarily by hypertrophy, with little myogenesis occurring after birth.
- Muscle tone develops in a caudocephalad and distal–proximal patterns, and active tone develops prior to passive tone (Blackburn, 2018; Liu & Thompson, 2020; Tappero, 2019).

▶ CONGENITAL SYNDROMES AFFECTING THE MUSCULOSKELETAL SYSTEM

APERT SYNDROME

- Apert syndrome occurs in approximately 1 in 55,000 births and is typically described as a sporadic mutation involving the *FGFR2* gene.
- It is characterized by craniosynostosis involving the coronal sutures, and a wide anterior fontanel and metopic suture, micrognathia or maxillary hypoplasia, hypertelorism with downward slanting palpebral fissures, and symmetric syndactyly of the hands and feet (Tomei & Smith, 2020).

Presentation

- Presentation includes congenital craniosynostosis of the coronal sutures, wide anterior fontanel and metopic suture, micrognathia, short-beaked nose, and symmetric syndactyly of the hands and feet (Tomei & Smith, 2020).

Interventions and Outcomes

- Respiratory distress should be routinely managed.
- Consider cranial ultrasound and neurosurgical consult if ventriculomegaly is present. Ventriculomegaly and/or hydrocephalus do not appear to affect intellectual functions (Tomei & Smith, 2020).

CROUZON

- The incidence of Crouzon is approximately 1 in 25,000 live births. Approximately 50% of Crouzon cases are familial; the other half have been linked to mutations of the *FGFR2* gene.
- Crouzon syndrome is characterized by craniosynostosis not usually present at birth, bulging and wide-set eyes due to shallow eye sockets, micrognathia, fusion of cervical vertebrae, and ankylosis of the elbows which becomes more emphasized as the infant grows (Tomei & Smith, 2020).

Presentation

- Presentation includes craniosynostosis not usually present at birth, bulging and wide-set eyes due to shallow eye sockets, micrognathia, beaked nose, small nasopharynx, fusion of cervical vertebrae, and ankylosis of the elbows which becomes more emphasized as the infant grows.
- It may initially present as respiratory distress due to malformed nasal structures.
- Subluxation of the eyes may occur.
- Hydrocephalus may occur (Tomei & Smith, 2020).

Interventions and Outcomes

- Respiratory distress should be routinely managed.
- Consider cranial ultrasound and neurosurgical consult if ventriculomegaly is present, although hydrocephalus does not appear to affect intellectual functions.
- Ophthalmology follow-up may be indicated if exophthalmos is severe (Tomei & Smith, 2020).

CONGENITAL MYOTONIC DYSTROPHY

- Congenital myotonic dystrophy (CMD) is an autosomal dominant disease that affects 1 in 3,500 live births and is caused by genetic mutations of chromosome 19q13.3. It is typically inherited from the mother who is also affected but typically to a lesser degree. CMD is a genetic disorder characterized by muscular dystrophy and hypotonia (Bass, 2020).

Presentation

- Prenatal history of polyhydramnios and decreased fetal movement are common. In addition, mothers may experience prolonged labor due to poor uterine contractions related to their own myotonic dystrophy.
- CMD ranges in severity but presents as respiratory distress accompanied by profound generalized hypotonia, diminished or absent deep tendon reflexes, and facial diplegia with ptosis.
- Generalized hypotonia with weak suck–swallow coordination may lead to feeding aspiration (Bass, 2020).

Interventions and Outcomes

- Upon suspicion of CMD, clinical and electromyographic exams of the mother should be performed, as well as genetic studies, including molecular genetic analysis.
- Routine management of respiratory distress depends on the degree of severity.
- Infants may require ancillary services such as physical, occupational, and speech therapies.
- Mortality of neonates with CMD is high, despite intensive care. Mortality is increased in infants requiring mechanical ventilation for greater than 30 days. Of infants who survive without comorbidities of prematurity, such as cerebral palsy, most walk by age 3. However, significant learning disabilities develop with maturation (Bass, 2020).

▶ ABNORMALITIES OF THE EXTREMITIES

SYNDACTYLY

- Syndactyly is a fusion of digits that can occur as a normal variant but also may be associated with genetic syndromes (see Box 25.1). Syndactyly is the most common congenital abnormality involving the upper extremities and is a result of failure of separation between the fifth to eighth week of gestation.

Box 25.1 Congenital Syndromes Associated With Syndactyly and Polydactyly

- **Syndactyly**
  - Apert syndrome
  - Streeter's dysplasia
- **Polydactyly**
  - Trisomy 13
  - Trisomy 21
  - Meckel–Gruber syndrome
  - Other skeletal malformations in White infants with postaxial polydactyly

Sources: Data from Son-Hing, J., & Thompson, G. (2020). Congenital abnormalities of the upper and lower extremities and spine. In R. Martin, A. Fanaroff, & M. Walsh (Eds.), *Fanaroff & Martin's neonatal–perinatal medicine: Diseases of the fetus and infant* (11th ed., pp. 1995–2015). Elsevier; Tappero, E. (2019). Musculoskeletal system assessment. In E. P. Tappero & M. E. Honeyfield (Eds.), *Physical assessment of the newborn* (6th ed., pp. 139–166). Springer Publishing Company.

- Syndactyly occurs in 1 in 2,000 to 3,000 live births, is more common in males than females, and occurs more frequently in White infants than infants of African descent.
- Most cases (approximately 80%) are spontaneous without genetic inheritance. It may be an incidental, familial finding, or associated with several congenital syndromes (Son-Hing & Thompson, 2020; Tappero, 2019).

Presentation

- Severity of syndactyly ranges from mild webbing to complete fusion, with bone structure involvement. It may be present on the fingers, toes, or both (Son-Hing & Thompson, 2020; Tappero, 2019).

Interventions and Outcomes

- Intervention of syndactyly is not routine but may be requested by parents. Treatment depends on the severity of the webbing, bony structure, and vascular involvement. When encountered, consultation with pediatric orthopedic and plastic surgery is recommended to determine the course of treatment for function and cosmetic appearance.
- Syndactyly of the toes does not affect function.
- Near-equal-length digits typically do not need separation until 2 to 3 years of age. Syndactyly of unequal lengths, that is, the thumb and the index finger fused, can cause tethering and deformity of the longer digit. Earlier intervention is recommended (Son-Hing & Thompson, 2020; Tappero, 2019).

POLYDACTYLY

- Polydactyly is a duplication of digits, and is most commonly an incidental, familial finding, but may also be associated with several congenital syndromes.
- Polydactyly also occurs commonly, approximately 1 in 300 Black live births and 1 in 3,000 White live births.
  - Radial polydactyly rates are similar in Black and White infants. Ulnar polydactyly is more common in Black infants and associated anomalies are *not* usually present.
  - In White infants, ulnar polydactyly is less common and often *is* associated with other skeletal anomalies, that is, syndactyly, coalescence of carpal bones, radioulnar synostosis, tibia and fibula hypoplasia and/or aplasia, hemivertebrae, and dwarfism (Kasser, 2017; Son-Hing & Thompson, 2020; Tappero, 2019).

Presentation

- There is presence of extra digits on the radial or ulnar aspect of the hand or the medial or lateral aspect of the foot, and may be present unilaterally or bilaterally.
- Severity ranges from bulbous formation to complete skeletal and vascular formation of the digit (Kasser, 2017; Son-Hing & Thompson, 2020; Tappero, 2019).

Interventions and Outcomes

- Treatment may or may not be necessary and outcome depends on the severity of the defect and presence of associated syndromes. Decisions to treat also depend on the degree of development of the digit; some less severe tags can be tied off, whereas digits with bony structures and complete vasculature may require more complex surgical intervention. Surgical intervention is usually completed between 6 and 18 months of age.
- Ligation of extra radial digits should not be routinely performed by the neonatal nurse practitioner (NNP) due to risk of incomplete arterial ligation, resulting in subsequent venous congestion and pain. Instead, consultation with a pediatric hand specialist should be completed (Kasser, 2017; Son-Hing & Thompson, 2020; Tappero, 2019).

DEVELOPMENTAL DYSPLASIA OF THE HIP

- Developmental dysplasia of the hip (DDH) is the presence of a dislocatable femoral head from the acetabulum present at birth, which may be unilateral or bilateral and ranges in severity from hip laxity to complete, irreducible dislocation.
- DDH is classified as typical when the infant has normal neurologic findings, or it may be classified as teratogenic when the infant has other neuromuscular abnormalities. Typical DDH is a multifactorial condition involving genetic predisposition, physiology, and mechanical factors. See Box 25.2 for risk factors for DDH.

Box 25.2 Risk Factors for Developmental Dysplasia of the Hip

- **Genetic Factors**
  - Family history of DDH
  - Inherited ligamentous laxity
- **Physiologic Factors**
  - Female
  - Maternal estrogen and other hormones related to pelvic relaxation during labor
- **Mechanical Factors**
  - Primigravida
  - Breech presentation
  - Postnatal positioning, including adduction and extension of lower extremities

DDH, developmental dysplasia of the hip.
Sources: Data from Lubbers, L. A. (2021) Congenital anomalies. In M. T. Verklan, M. Walden, & S. Forest (Eds.), *Core curriculum for neonatal intensive care nursing* (6th ed., pp. 654–677). Elsevier; Son-Hing, J., & Thompson, G. (2020). Congenital abnormalities of the upper and lower extremities and spine. In R. Martin, A. Fanaroff, & M. Walsh (Eds.), *Fanaroff & Martin's neonatal–perinatal medicine: Diseases of the fetus and infant* (11th ed., pp. 1980–2015). Elsevier; Tappero, E. (2019). Musculoskeletal system assessment. In E. P. Tappero & M. E. Honeyfield (Eds.), *Physical assessment of the newborn* (6th ed., pp. 139–166). Springer Publishing Company.

- DDH of ranging severity occurs in 11.5 per 1,000 live births and frank dislocations occur in 2 per 1,000 live births in the United States. It occurs more commonly in females than males, and in Native American and Eastern European ethnicities.
- The most common risk factors resulting in DDH are firstborn and breech presentation. Breech position results in extreme flexion and decreased motion, causing increased instability (Lubbers, 2021; Son-Hing & Thompson, 2020; Tappero, 2019).

Presentation

- DDH diagnosis is highly suspected with positive Barlow and Ortolani tests, asymmetric thigh and gluteal skin folds, uneven knee levels (Allis or Galeazzi sign), and absence of normal knee flexion contractures (Son-Hing & Thompson, 2020; Tappero, 2019).

Interventions and Outcomes

- Interventions include accurate and early diagnosis, use of Pavlik harness, and orthopedic referral. If spontaneous reduction or recurrent dislocation occurs, surgical closed reduction may be necessary.
- Imaging includes hip ultrasound, and radiographs may be performed to confirm diagnosis.
- Decreased motion results in decreased stimulation and growth of the acetabulum cartilage (Kasser, 2017; Lubbers, 2021; Son-Hing & Thompson, 2020; Tappero, 2019; White et al., 2018).

TALIPES EQUINOVARUS (CLUBFOOT)

- Talipes equinovarus (TE) is characterized as adduction of the forefoot, pronounced varus, foot and toes in downward pointing position, equinus position, and atrophy of the affected lower extremity. TE may be unilateral or bilateral.
- It is the most common neonatal foot abnormality occurring in 1 to 2 per 1,000 live births.
- There are three classifications: congenital, teratologic, and positional.
  - Congenital TE is generally an isolated abnormality and the etiology is unknown; however, there is thought to be a familial component.
  - Teratologic TE is associated with neuromuscular disorders such as myelodysplasia or arthrogryposis.
  - Positional TE occurs in utero when a normal foot has been held in the equinovarus position (Kasser, 2017; Son-Hing & Thompson, 2020; Tappero, 2019; White et al., 2018).

Presentation

- When manipulated, the foot is unable to be passively positioned midline; this differentiates clubfoot from metatarsus adductus (Kasser, 2017; Son-Hing & Thompson, 2020; Tappero, 2019; White et al., 2018).

Interventions and Outcomes

- Intervention includes range-of-motion exercises to be started in the nursery, followed by pediatric orthopedic and physical therapy referrals. The Ponseti method of positioning and serial casting is the common form of treatment; occasionally surgical intervention is necessary for severe deformities or when nonoperative treatments are unsuccessful.
- Successful treatment using nonoperative methods has been achieved when treatment begins prior to 1 year of age. Nonoperative treatment is a lengthy process that can take several years to fully correct TE (Kasser, 2017; Son-Hing & Thompson, 2020; Tappero, 2019; White et al., 2018).

METATARSUS ADDUCTUS

- Metatarsus adductus is the medial positioning of the forefoot without pathologic structural changes to the metatarsals. It is the most common foot anomaly in neonates. Approximately 10% of children with metatarsus adductus have DDH.
- The etiology is unclear; however, it is suspected that intrauterine positioning is a contributing factor (Son-Hing & Thompson, 2020; Tappero, 2019).

Presentation

- Presentation includes adduction of the forefoot with occasional supination. Infants will have normal ankle dorsiflexion and plantar flexion.
- The degree of flexibility of the foot determines the severity of malformation; however, the foot should be able to be positioned midline (Kasser, 2017; Son-Hing & Thompson, 2020; White et al., 2018).

Interventions and Outcomes

- It typically corrects without intervention by age 3. Imaging is unnecessary initially, but weight-bearing radiographs may be necessary to diagnose rigid versus moderate deformities.
- Intervention includes parental reassurance and routine pediatric follow-up (Kasser, 2017; Son-Hing & Thompson, 2020; White et al., 2018).

▶ SKELETAL DYSPLASIA

ACHONDROPLASIA

- Achondroplasia is a form of dwarfism characterized by frontal bossing and shortened lower limbs.
- It is estimated that achondroplasia occurs in 1 in 15,000 to 1 in 40,000 live births. Achondroplasia is caused by a mutation in the gene that controls fibroblast growth factor receptor 3 (FGFR3), causing disturbances in bone growth in early development. In achondroplasia, mutations of FGFR3 cause an overproduction of the protein responsible for converting cartilage to bone. This occurs in an autosomal dominant inheritance pattern (Son-Hing & Thompson, 2020; Tappero, 2019).

Presentation

- Characteristics include frontal bossing, flattened nasal bridge, shortened arms and thighs, and average torso length with protruding abdomen. The knees and hands may be hyperextendable. The hands may be short and broad, with widely spaced long and ring fingers, forming a "trident hand." There is generally some degree of genu varum. Mild to moderate hypotonia is also common in newborns (Son-Hing & Thompson, 2020; Tappero, 2019).

Interventions and Outcomes

- The infant should receive routine care unless other concerns are noted, and if so consultation with neurology, genetics, and orthopedics should be considered.
- Homozygous achondroplasia is a lethal defect due to respiratory insufficiency related to rib cage hypoplasia.
- Infants with heterozygous achondroplasia have a normal life expectancy. However, these children are at high risk for motor milestone delays as well as middle ear infections and unresolving genu varum (Son-Hing & Thompson, 2020; Tappero, 2019).

ARTHROGRYPOSIS MULTIPLEX CONGENITA

- Arthrogryposis multiplex congenita (AMC) is a syndrome classified by the presence of multiple joint contractures at birth.
- AMC occurs in approximately 1 in 8,000 live births and the cause is attributed to intrinsic and extrinsic factors.
  - Intrinsic factors include neurologic, muscular, and joint problems, with neurologic problems being the most common.
  - Extrinsic factors include fetal crowding or intrauterine constraint (Bennett & Meier, 2019; Son-Hing & Thompson, 2020).

Presentation

- Infants present with multiple contractures, fixed or limited mobility limb extensions, and joint dislocations at birth (Bennett & Meier, 2019; Son-Hing & Thompson, 2020).

Interventions and Outcomes

- The infant should be evaluated for the degree of contracture and the presence of scoliosis, which may include radiographs.
- Given the cause of AMC, referral to pediatric neurology and orthopedics should be considered, and neonates may require physical therapy and serial casting to correct clubfoot and other contractures.
- Outcomes depend on the cause of AMC and the severity of contractures. In some cases, surgical interventions are necessary to aid in range of motion, but this is not typically done in the neonatal period (Son-Hing & Thompson, 2020).

▶ SPINAL ABNORMALITIES

CONGENITAL SCOLIOSIS AND KYPHOSIS

- Congenital scoliosis is a lateral curvature of the spine resulting from an embryologic failure of spinal formation or segmentation.
- Congenital kyphosis is the failure of formation of all or part of the vertebral body with preservation of the posterior elements, as well as the failure of anterior segmentation of the spine.
- Congenital spinal deformities, including scoliosis, kyphosis, or a combination of the two, occur in 0.5 to 1 in 1,000 live births. Neither is inherited or chromosomal, but typically results from embryologic failure of formation or segmentation of the vertebrae. Congenital scoliosis is more common in females

than males and may be accompanied by cardiac or genitourinary anomalies.

■ Congenital spinal anomalies can occur in Klippel–Feil and VACTERL/VATER syndromes (Kasser, 2017; Son-Hing & Thompson, 2020; Tappero, 2019; White et al., 2018).

Presentation

■ Both scoliosis and kyphosis may be difficult to detect at birth; however, early detection is critical to prevent severe deformities and maintain neurologic function (Kasser, 2017; Son-Hing & Thompson, 2020; Tappero, 2019; White et al., 2018).

Interventions and Outcomes

■ Evaluation includes radiographic evaluation of spine, echocardiogram, renal ultrasound, and orthopedic follow-up.

■ Outcomes depend on the severity and location of the deformity, as well as the presence of multiple anomalies at multiple levels such as hemivertebrae. Progressive kyphosis in the thoracic region can result in paraplegia (Kasser, 2017; Son-Hing & Thompson, 2020; Tappero, 2019; White et al., 2018).

SACRAL AGENESIS

■ Sacral agenesis is the complete absence of the sacrum; with lower lumbar spine involvement, it is termed *lumbosacral agenesis*.

■ Sacral agenesis is a rare disorder, occurring in 1 in 25,000 live births. The etiology is unknown; however, it tends to be associated with maternal diabetes (Son-Hing & Thompson, 2020).

Presentation

■ Presentation is variable, but in most severe forms includes a small pelvis, pterygia (webbing) of the hips and knees, and bilateral foot deformities.

■ Spinopelvic instability may be present.

■ Neurologic exam tends to show no motor function below the last complete vertebrae; however, innervation and sensation may be present (Son-Hing & Thompson, 2020).

Interventions and Outcomes

■ Observation is appropriate in patients with partial agenesis and stable spinopelvic exam. Depending on the degree of agenesis, ambulation may be possible with proper orthopedic consultation and orthotic use.

■ Orthopedic and neurosurgical consultation should be included in the plan of care in case patients with complete agenesis or unstable spinopelvic exam require spinal fusion during childhood.
  ● Spinal fusion can enhance sitting balance and improve upper extremity function (Son-Hing & Thompson, 2020).

▶ MUSCULOSKELETAL BIRTH INJURIES

FRACTURES

■ Most fractures occur during delivery secondary to birth trauma from fetal malpositioning or difficult delivery. Fractures of the neonatal period most commonly occur in the upper extremities. Lower extremity fractures may be associated with an underlying neuromuscular disorder or bone disorder (Liu & Thompson, 2020).

Clavicular Fractures

■ Clavicle fractures are among the most common birth injuries and are typically associated with shoulder dystocia and difficult delivery.

■ Intervention includes pinning the sleeve of the infant's shirt to the front as a means to immobilize the extremity for 7 to 10 days (Abdulhayoglu, 2017; Tappero, 2019; White et al., 2018).

Humeral Fractures

■ Humeral fractures are second to clavicle fractures and are also associated with difficult delivery.

■ Intervention includes immobilization via plaster splint or elastic bandage (Abdulhayoglu, 2017; Tappero, 2019; White et al., 2018).

Femoral Fractures

■ Femoral fractures are less common and associated with breech delivery.

■ Intervention includes immobilization via simple plaster splint or Pavlik harness.
  ● Splinting may be discontinued when callus formation is evident on radiograph (Abdulhayoglu, 2017; Tappero, 2019; White et al., 2018).

BRACHIAL PLEXUS INJURIES

■ Brachial plexus injury, also known as brachial palsy, is paralysis of the muscles involving the upper extremity following trauma during birth to the spinal roots of the fifth cervical through the first thoracic nerves. These include both Erb and Klumpke palsy. The incidence is 0.1% to 0.3% of live births. Risk factors include macrosomia, prolonged labor, shoulder dystocia, breech presentation, high maternal body mass index, and fetal asphyxia. On average, recovery takes approximately 5 years. Shoulder contracture and osseous deformity are possible if recovery does not start within the first 3 weeks of life (Liu & Thompson, 2020).

Erb Palsy

■ Erb palsy is caused by injury to the fifth and sixth cervical nerve roots.

- Defining characteristics of the affected arm include adducted, internally rotated, and extended at the elbow with flexion of the wrist with an intact grasp, known as the "waiter's tip" position. The infant may have normal grasp with absent Moro reflex.
- Intervention includes gentle handling of the affected arm and gentle passive range of motion to prevent contractures of the shoulder, elbow, forearm, and hand.
- Outcomes depend on nerve root involvement; most infants achieve functional improvement by 3 months of age. If improvement is not seen by 3 months, surgical intervention may be necessary (Abdulhayoglu, 2017; Tappero, 2019; White et al., 2018).

Klumpke Palsy

- Klumpke palsy is caused by injury to the eighth cervical and first thoracic nerve roots.
- Defining characteristics include upper arm mobility, with complete lower arm paralysis with absent grasp. This is a less common birth injury compared with Erb palsy.
- Intervention includes gentle handling of the affected arm and gentle passive range of motion to prevent contractures of the shoulder, elbow, forearm, and hand (Abdulhayoglu, 2017; Tappero, 2019; White et al., 2018).

Torticollis

- Torticollis is caused by injury to the sternocleidomastoid (SCM) muscle, likely due to intrauterine positioning or birth trauma.
- Defining characteristics include firm, immobile circumscribed mass on SCM present at birth to 14 days of age, and tilting of the head toward the affected side, with inability to passively move to neutral position.
- Intervention includes early physical therapy; if torticollis persists greater than 4 years, possible surgical interventions may be necessary.
  - If undiagnosed, torticollis may go unnoticed until plagiocephaly is evident (Kasser, 2017; Tappero, 2019; White et al., 2018).

▶ CONCLUSION

Musculoskeletal development spans from infancy through adolescence. A thorough understanding of fetal and neonatal musculoskeletal development and associated pathologies is vital to provide quick and accurate diagnosis of a variety of birth-related injuries, anomalies, and associated genetic disorders.

1. The neonatal nurse practitioner (NNP) notes that an infant has asymmetric abduction of the hips. The NNP places the infant in a supine position and flexes the hips and knees to a 90-degree angle and determines the knees are unequal in height. The NNP has elicited the:

   A. Barlow sign
   B. Galeazzi sign
   C. Ortolani sign

2. The neonatal nurse practitioner (NNP) notes that a neonate has bilateral postaxial polydactyly of the hands. The NNP will tell the parents this finding is a/an:

   A. Concern for which they will see a specialist
   B. Element identified from the prenatal ultrasound
   C. Known, benign familial inheritance trait

3. The neonatal nurse practitioner (NNP) is called to the delivery of a 39-week gestational age, large-for-gestational-age (LGA) infant who was a difficult extraction. Upon initial assessment, the NNP notes that the infant moves the right upper extremity freely but has no movement of the left upper extremity. The NNP diagnoses this decreased or absent movement of an extremity as a/an:

   A. Deformation
   B. Fracture
   C. Tumor

4. The most common neonatal fracture site is the:

   A. Clavicle
   B. Femur
   C. Humerus

5. The neonatal nurse practitioner (NNP) attends the delivery of a small-for-gestational-age, 38 weeks' gestational age infant. The prenatal history is significant for oligohydramnios and maternal bicornuate uterus. The NNP notes on the initial exam that the left foot is adducted and pointed downward and cannot be positioned midline. The NNP correctly documents the finding in the chart as:

   A. Metatarsus abduction
   B. Talipes equinovarus
   C. Varus adductus

1. B) Galeazzi sign

A positive Galeazzi sign is noted when knees are determined to be of unequal height when infants are placed in a supine position and the hips and knees are flexed into a 90-degree angle. The Ortolani sign is positive when the femoral head is felt to slip out of the acetabulum when infants are placed in supine position and the hips and knees are flexed into a 90-degree angle. The Barlow sign is positive when the femoral head is palpated to slip out of the acetabulum with maneuvering (White et al., 2018).

2. C) Known, benign familial inheritance trait

Postaxial (ulnar) digits are most common and are typically not associated with other anomalies. Typically, other family members have also been born with postaxial digits of either one or both hands (Son-Hing & Thompson, 2020; Tappero, 2019). Although a specialist may eventually be consulted, it is not an emergency. Polydactyly generally is not visible on prenatal ultrasound.

3. B) Fracture

LGA babies are at greater risk for birth trauma. Infants with clavicle or humerus fractures may have pseudoparalysis of the affected upper extremity. Deformations occur in utero and lead to anomalous development of the limb, while a tumor would be visible to the NNP (White et al., 2018).

4. A) Clavicle

Clavicle fractures are among the most common birth fractures and are associated with shoulder dystocia and difficult delivery. Neither the humerus nor femur is susceptible to fracture except in extreme rare cases of significant malpositioning (Abdulhayoglu, 2017; Song-Hing & Thompson, 2015; Tappero, 2019; White et al., 2018).

5. B) Talipes equinovarus

Talipes equinovarus (TE) is characterized as adduction of the forefoot, pronounced varus, foot, and toes in downward pointing position, equinus position, and atrophy of the affected lower extremity. TE may be unilateral or bilateral. Metatarsus adductus, also known as metatarsus varus, is the medial positioning of the forefoot without pathologic structural changes to the metatarsals (Kasser, 2017; Son-Hing & Thompson, 2015; Tappero, 2019; White et al., 2018).

The Integumentary System

Rebecca Chuffo Davila

INTRODUCTION

Neonatal nurse practitioners (NNPs) need to be familiar with newborn skin development, skin care, and common skin disorders of the integumentary system. The skin is the largest organ in the body and is responsible for many functions, including protection, metabolic functions, sensation, and thermoregulation. Understanding of skin variations can alert the NNP to a benign versus a life-threatening disease process. This chapter addresses skin development, newborn skin care, and common skin disorders in neonates.

SKIN DEVELOPMENT

- The *epidermis* develops around 5 to 8 weeks' gestation. By 30 to 40 days, two layers can be identified: the inner basal layer and the outer periderm.
  - The inner basal layer develops into the true epidermis.
  - The periderm is an embryonic layer that is gone by the second half of gestation. It is protective of the embryo and the fetus, forms part of the vernix caseosa, and acts as a nutrient interface between the embryo and the amniotic fluid.
- By 60 days, the epidermis has three layers: the basal layer (where melanocytes are found), an intermediate layer, and the superficial periderm.
- At term, the *epidermis* consists of an outer stratum corneum, stratum granulosum, and the stratum germinativum, which consists of the stratum spinosum, the stratum basale. The basal layer contains the melanocytes and keratinocytes. Keratinocytes are the major cells of the epidermis.
- The *dermis* lies beneath the epidermis and comprises the connective tissue, nerves, blood vessels, and lymphatic vessels. It also contains mast cells, histiocytes, and neutrophils. The dermis provides mechanical strength, protection, and elasticity to the skin. The dermis contains nerves and blood vessels and carries sensations from the skin to the brain.
- The intermediate layer of the integumentary system becomes more complex by the end of the fourth month when the epidermis has stratified.
- The *subcutaneous layer* is composed of fatty connective tissue that provides insulation and caloric storage (Blackburn, 2018; Douma et al., 2017; Lund & Durand, 2021; Narendran, 2020).

EPIDERMAL APPENDAGES

- Glands, the hair, and the nails are considered epidermal appendages.
  - Sebaceous glands are formed from epidermal cells around 4 weeks' gestation and are complete around 8 to 16 weeks. They are only found where hair grows.
  - Eccrine and apocrine are two types of sweat glands located within the dermal layer.
  - Mammary glands are adapted sweat glands seen at 4 weeks of gestation.
- Hair originates in the dermis and projects up through the epidermis. Hairs are first seen at 10 to 12 weeks. The hair that appears along the embryo's body is called *lanugo*.
- Fingernails and toenails develop as thickenings in the epidermal layer appearing around the 10th week (Lund & Durand, 2021; Narendran, 2020).

FULL- AND PRETERM INFANT SKIN

- In full- and preterm infants, the skin is an organ that comprises at least 13% of the total body weight, in contrast to only 3% of body weight in adults.
- The term infant has fewer problems with thermoregulation, fluid, and electrolyte management, and is able to use calories for growth.
- Transfer from the intrauterine amniotic fluid environment to the external air environment results in accelerated maturation of skin function in preterm infants; however, these infants still have many more issues related to electrolyte disturbances and fluid shifts.
  - Immature skin is very thin and fragile and may be gelatinous due to the underdeveloped stratum corneum. The organization of the epidermis has been compared to a brick wall, with the

corneocytes being the brick and the lipid matrix the mortar.

- The lipid matrix acts as a barrier to transepidermal water loss (TEWL). Because the matrix is less well developed in immature infants and the corneocytes are arranged in a disorganized fashion, an extremely low birth weight (ELBW) infant can have water losses 10 times higher than term infants. As a result, fluid losses equivalent to 30% of their total body weight can occur.
- Due to the thinner stratum corneum, higher water content, and increased permeability of the skin in preterm infants, TEWL is greatly increased, especially in the first 2 to 3 weeks after birth, and remains higher than term infants for up to a month.

■ Although both term and preterm infants are at risk of developing infections, preterm infants are at higher risk due to fewer layers of stratum corneum for protection (Blackburn, 2018; Douma et al., 2017; Lund & Durand, 2021; Narendran, 2020).

RISK FACTORS FOR SKIN INJURY

■ Gestational age <32 weeks
■ Edema
■ Use of paralytic agents and vasopressors
■ Multiple tubes and lines
■ Numerous monitors
■ Surgical wounds
■ Ostomies
■ Technologies that limit movement, such as high-frequency oscillatory ventilation (HFOV) and extracorporeal membrane oxygenation (ECMO; Douma et al., 2017; Lund & Durand, 2021)

▶ SKIN CARE

■ Understanding the physiology of skin development is important to understanding how to care for the skin of term and preterm infants. The next section discusses skin care for both term and preterm neonates.

ADHESIVE REMOVAL

■ There is a risk of damage to the skin in all the infants we care for in the NICU. Damage that can occur from adhesive removal includes epidermal stripping, tearing of the skin, maceration, tension blisters, chemical irritation, sensitization, and folliculitis.
■ Hydrocolloid barriers may be helpful in securing tubes and lines to the skin. They can aid in preventing permanent damage and scarring of the skin. Use of adhesives, solvents, and bonding agents should be minimized.
■ Silicone tapes are very gentle on the skin but do not adhere well to plastics. They should not be used

when securing critical, life-sustaining tubes and appliances (Douma et al., 2017; Lund & Durand, 2021; Narendran, 2020).

BATHING

■ Immersion bathing for physiologically stable term and preterm infants has been shown to be beneficial. It can be more soothing and less stressful than sponge bathing.
■ The Neonatal Skin Care Guideline recommends using warm tap water with or without a mild cleansing bar or liquid cleanser that has a neutral or slightly acidic pH to assist in the removal of blood and meconium.
- For premature infants <32 weeks, warm water only during the first week of life is the recommendation. In an effort to reduce alterations in skin pH, dryness, and irritation in premature infants less than 32 weeks, cleanse with warm water baths during the first week using soft cotton cloths, cotton balls, or the caregiver's hands.
■ Bathing two to three times per week with cleansing products compared with water alone has been shown to have little or no difference in skin pH (Douma et al., 2017; Lund & Durand, 2021; Witt, 2021).

CIRCUMCISION CARE

■ Male infants should be carefully examined for any penile anomalies prior to circumcision. Premature infants should not have circumcision until they are healthy and working toward discharge.
■ Maintain dressing with petroleum gauze for the first 24 hours and up to 3 days after the procedure to avoid adhesion of the glans to the infant's diaper. Check the circumcision site with every diaper change and wipe the area gently with soap and water during diaper changes as needed.
■ Check the circumcision site and make sure there is no significant bleeding for at least 2 hours before discharge from the hospital. Normal healing will include slight swelling and the formation of a crust on the glans. Cleansing gently with water (and soap, if soiled) is all that is necessary to keep the penis clean (Busenhart, 2017; Cheffer & Rannalli, 2016; Douma et al., 2017; Kanter, 2020).

EMOLLIENTS

■ Maintaining the hydration of the stratum corneum is essential for intact skin and normal barrier function. If emollients are used, they should be free of dyes and perfumes. They should be single patient use tubes or jars and not shared between infants (Douma et al., 2017; Lund & Durand, 2021).

SKIN DISINFECTANTS

- Skin decontamination is necessary prior to procedures in the NICU. Which product and when to use a disinfectant are common issues in the NICU and influenced by institutional availability and provider choice. Povidone-iodine is widely used. Whichever skin disinfectant is used, it should be completely removed from the infant's skin once the procedure is finished (Douma et al., 2017; Lund & Durand, 2021).

INTRAVENOUS EXTRAVASATIONS

- Once the extravasation is identified, the IV should be removed and the extremity involved should be elevated. The use of heat or cold is *not* recommended because the tissue is susceptible to extended injury from these extreme temperatures.
- Hyaluronidase can be helpful in preventing tissue necrosis if given within 1 hour of the extravasation. Phentolamine should be used in the event of extravasation by a vasoconstrictive drug, such as dopamine (Douma et al., 2017; Lund & Durand, 2021).

UMBILICAL CORD CARE

- Evidence suggests that dry cord care, defined as keeping the cord clean and leaving it exposed to air or loosely covered by a clean cloth, is effective and is the recommended, evidence-based practice. Cord separation time was significantly decreased for infants having dry cord care compared with those cleaned with 95% isopropyl alcohol.
- Recommendations for umbilical cord care include washing hands before handling the cord, and, if the cord becomes soiled with urine or stool, cleansing with water, drying with absorbent gauze, and keeping the diaper folded down and away from the umbilical stump to prevent contamination (Bowe, 2020; Douma et al., 2017; Lund & Durand, 2021; Witt, 2021).

▶ TERMS TO DESCRIBE SKIN LESIONS/ DISORDERS

- *Bulla:* a fluid-filled lesion larger than 1 cm (e.g., sucking blisters, epidermolysis bullosa, and bullous impetigo)
- *Ecchymosis:* a large area of subepidermal hemorrhage
- *Macule:* pigmented, flat spot that is visible but not palpable; if >1 cm in diameter, may be referred to as a patch (clinical examples include café-au-lait spots and capillary ectasias)
- *Nodule:* a solid lesion that is elevated with depth and up to 2 cm in size (e.g., neuroblastoma)
- *Papule:* a solid, elevated, palpable lesion with distinct borders and <1 cm in diameter (e.g., milia)
- *Petechiae:* subepidermal hemorrhages and are pinpoint in size; do not blanch with pressure
- *Plaque:* a solid, elevated, palpable lesion with distinct borders that is >1 cm in diameter (e.g., nevus sebaceous)
- *Pustule:* a vesicle filled with cloudy or purulent fluid (e.g., neonatal pustular melanosis, erythema toxicum neonatorum, infantile acropustulosis)
- *Tumor:* a solid lesion that is elevated with depth and greater than 2 cm in size (e.g., hemangioma and rhabdomyosarcoma)
- *Vesicle:* an elevated lesion or blister filled with serous fluid less than 1 cm in diameter (e.g., herpes simplex virus [HSV], varicella zoster virus, and miliaria crystalline)
- *Wheal:* area of edema in the upper dermis, creating a palpable, slightly raised lesion (e.g., urticaria, bite reactions, and drug eruptions)
- *Ulcer:* erosion of skin with damage of the epidermis into the dermis; leaves a scar after healing (e.g., ulcerated hemangiomas and aplasia cutis congenita; Bowe, 2020; Narendran, 2020; Witt, 2021)

▶ NORMAL SKIN FINDINGS AND VARIATIONS

ACCESSORY TRAGUS (PREAURICULAR TAGS)

- Accessory tragi are a relatively common congenital malformation of the external ear. They are present at birth and can be multiple and/or bilateral.
- Association between deafness and renal abnormalities is controversial.
- Removal by tying off of the tragi should not be done and could lead to complications (Gupta & Sidbury, 2018).

ASH LEAF MACULES

- Ash leaf macules are small, oval areas of hypopigmentation. They are one of the few congenital markers for infants with tuberous sclerosis (TS). TS is a hereditary disorder characterized by cutaneous and central nervous system (CNS) tumors resulting in seizures, developmental delays, and behavioral problems (Bowe, 2020; Gupta & Sidbury, 2018; Narendran, 2020; Witt, 2019).

CAFÉ-AU-LAIT MACULES

- Café-au-lait macules are well-demarcated oval or round, light brown macules in White patients and dark brown in Black patients which may differ in size.
- Six or more of these macules measuring 0.5 cm or greater in diameter should alert the practitioner to a possible diagnosis of neurofibromatosis type 1 (NF-1; Bowe, 2020; Douma et al., 2017; Gupta & Sidbury, 2018; Narendran, 2020).

CAPILLARY MALFORMATION: PORT-WINE STAIN

- A port-wine stain is a flat, pink, or reddish-purple lesion.
- Lesions on the face may follow a pattern similar to that of the trigeminal nerve and may be associated with a diagnosis of Sturge–Weber Syndrome (SWS; Bowe, 2020; Douma et al., 2017; Gupta & Sidbury, 2018; Witt, 2021).

ECCHYMOSIS

- Ecchymosis is a hemorrhagic blotching due to the pooling of blood under the skin or mucous membrane. It also does not blanch with pressure.
- Ecchymosis in newborns is most commonly caused by birth, in particular if assistive devices are used, such as midforceps or vacuum extraction. Infants, especially large ones, who are delivered vaginally in breech position may demonstrate ecchymosis from birth. The ecchymosis is transient and will fade away in a few days (Cavaliere, 2019; Prazad et al., 2020; Witt, 2021).

ERYTHEMA TOXICUM

- Lesions may be firm, 1 to 3 mm in diameter, pale yellow to white, and manifest as papules or pustules that sit on an erythematous base. It is most commonly seen on the trunk but may be seen on any area of the body, but only rarely on the palms and soles.
- It presents in the first 1 to 3 days of life, and is more common among term than premature infants.
- If examined microscopically, it would reveal a large number of *eosinophils*.
- No treatment is required (Bowe, 2020; Douma et al., 2017; Khorsand & Sidbury, 2018; Narendran, 2020).

HARLEQUIN CHANGES

- Seen only during the newborn period, harlequin color changes appear to be more common in the low-birth weight infant. It has been attributed to immature autonomic vasomotor control. When the newborn is lying on one side, a sharply demarcated red color is seen in the dependent half of the body, with the superior half appearing pale. If the newborn is rotated to the other side, the color reverses.
- This phenomenon occurs in both healthy and ill newborns and is of no pathologic significance. No treatment is required; however, recognition and education are important as the occurrence can be alarming for parents (Khorsand & Sidbury, 2018; Narendran, 2020; Whitt, 2019).

HYPERPIGMENTED MACULE (DERMAL MELANOCYTOSIS; PREVIOUSLY MONGOLIAN SPOT)

- It is caused by an excessive number of dermal melanocytes and is seen mostly on the buttocks and lower back.
- The characteristic "bluish-grey" color is due to the Tyndall effect, which is light reflection off the dermal-based melanocytes. It lacks a sharp border and may span a diameter of 10 cm or more.
- This common skin finding is seen mainly in infants of Black, Asian, and Hispanic descent. They fade over time and approximately 42% disappear by 1 year of age (Bowe, 2020; Douma et al., 2017; Khorsand & Sidbury, 2018; Narendran, 2020).

MILIA

- Milia are tiny inclusion cysts that form in the epidermis and present as tiny, white monomorphic papules with a smooth surface. They are commonly seen on the forehead, cheeks, and chin, and are common in up to 40% to 50% of newborns.
- No treatment is necessary, and they will resolve spontaneously over several months (Douma et al., 2017; Khorsand & Sidbury, 2018; Narendran, 2020).

MILIARIA

- Miliaria, also known as heat rash, is a benign rash due to obstruction of the eccrine ducts. There are three types of known miliaria:
  - *Miliaria crystallina:* Eccrine ducts within or below the stratum corneum are blocked, causing small, clear vesicles that can be wiped away.
  - *Miliaria rubra:* This is blockage of the eccrine duct at the level of the epidermis and is thought to be related to overheating.
  - *Miliaria profunda (pustulosis):* This is blockage of the eccrine ducts at or below the dermal–epidermal junction. It resembles a papular eruption that is rarely seen in newborns.
- Miliaria occur in the first 1 to 2 weeks of life, with rapid resolution within days (Bowe, 2020; Khorsand & Sidbury, 2018; Narendran, 2020; Witt, 2019).

PETECHIAE/PURPURA

- Petechiae are pinpoint, flat, round, red spots under the skin surface caused by intradermal hemorrhage. They will *not* blanch when compressed.
- They can commonly be seen right after birth, especially on the presenting part.

- If the infant is delivered vaginally following rapid labor, presented in a vertex position, or had a tight nuchal cord, petechiae may be present.
- Petechiae may be benign or an indication of severe platelet malfunction; further evaluation should be done if the infant is symptomatic (e.g., prolonged bleeding from heel sticks; Bowe, 2020; Prazad et al., 2020; Verklan, 2021a; Witt, 2021).

SUCKING BLISTERS

- A vesicle or bulla may appear on the lip, finger, or hand of a newborn as a result of vigorous sucking, either in utero or after birth. These lesions appear to result from repetitive vigorous sucking in utero at one particular site. Often, when the neonate is presented after birth with the affected extremity, they will immediately demonstrate sucking behavior on that area.
  - Sucking blisters on the extremities may be mistaken for other serious disorders such as herpes simplex, but their solitary, asymmetric nature and characteristic location should help establish the correct diagnosis. A sucking blister may be intact or ruptured and requires no treatment (Witt, 2019).

TRANSIENT NEONATAL PUSTULAR MELANOSIS

- Transient neonatal pustular melanosis is a distinctive eruption that consists of three types of lesions:
  - *First stage:* consists of lesions that are small, superficial vesiculopustules with little or no surrounding erythema
  - *Second stage:* consists of fine collarettes of scale or scale crust surrounding the resolving pustule
  - *Third stage:* hyperpigmented brown macules develop at the site of the previous pustules
- The lesions may be profuse or sparse and occur on any body surface, including the palms, soles, and scalp. Sites of predilection are the forehead, submental area and anterior neck, and lower back. Examination would reveal a predominance of *neutrophils*.
- No therapy is required as this skin condition is benign and transient. The residual hyperpigmentation may take months to resolve (Khorsand & Sidbury, 2018; Narendran, 2020).

▶ COMMON DERMATOLOGIC DISORDERS

INFANTILE HEMANGIOMAS

Incidence and Etiology

- Infantile hemangiomas (IHs) are the most common skin anomaly of infancy and occur in up to 10% of newborns, more commonly in females and premature infants.

- Risk factors for developing IHs include prematurity, multiple gestation, preeclampsia, placental abnormalities, advanced maternal age, and in vitro fertilization. It is hypothesized that formation of IHs is linked to hypoxia (Bowe, 2020; Douma et al., 2017; Gupta & Sidbury, 2018; Narendran, 2020; Witt, 2019).

Findings

- Hemangiomas are clinically heterogeneous. Superficial hemangiomas are located in the upper dermis and present as elevated bright red, well-demarcated papules or plaques which sometimes are referred to as *strawberry hemangiomas*. It is soft and compressible, with sharply demarcated margins. The tumor may also occur in the throat (deep), causing airway obstruction. (Gupta & Sidbury, 2018; Narendran, 2020; Witt, 2019).

Treatment and Outcomes

- Hemangiomas that require immediate attention are those that are in the airway and those involved in the hepatic and parotid areas. Laser therapy and surgical excision have been used. The preferred treatment is one that allows natural spontaneous regression.
- Most IHs (80%) have completed their growth by 3 months of age and 90% regress by 4 years of age. Up to 40% can cause permanent skin changes, including disfigurement. Complications include: ulceration, those located around the eyes could cause visual impairment, and those around the ears could cause hearing deficits (Gupta & Sidbury, 2018; Narendran, 2020; Witt, 2019).

HERPES SIMPLEX VIRUS

Incidence and Etiology

- Despite a high prevalence of HSV infections in adults, neonatal herpes is relatively uncommon. Neonatal herpes is one of the most serious viral infections in the newborn, with a mortality rate of up to 40% in newborns with disseminated disease.
- Neonatal HSV infection is classified based on the extent of involvement: skin, eye, and/or mouth (SEM) disease (Boos & Sidbury, 2018; Witt, 2019).

Findings

- Infants infected in utero (congenital HSV infection) have a distinct clinical presentation. Skin lesions are almost always present at birth and include widespread erosions and bullae, scars, hyperpigmentation, hypopigmentation, and aplasia cutis.
- Of newborns with neonatal herpes, 50% to 70% eventually develop this characteristic rash, but not always before they exhibit other clinical signs. The absence of vesicles does not rule out the presence of the disease.
- The rash appears as vesicles or pustules on an erythematous base. Clusters of lesions are common.

The lesions ulcerate and crust over rapidly. Characteristic cutaneous lesions begin as erythema that quickly evolves into isolated or grouped vesicles on an erythematous base. Continued evolution may result in pustules, crusts, or erosions. Vesiculation typically occurs at sites of trauma, including the presenting part and sites of fetal electrode placement.

■ Precautions for blood and body secretions must be observed (Boos & Sidbury, 2018; Witt, 2019).

Treatment and Outcomes

■ Birth via Cesarean delivery for women with active lesions or prodromal symptoms has been shown to reduce the risk of neonatal HSV infection.

■ Early treatment with antiviral agents is critical in decreasing the risk of serious complications and death. All cases of presumptive neonatal HSV infection should be treated with IV antiviral agent such as acyclovir. Topical ophthalmic antiviral therapy should be used if there is ocular involvement. Other signs, such as seizures, should be treated as they occur (Boos & Sidbury, 2018; Witt, 2019).

ICHTHYOSIS

Incidence and Etiology

■ This is a rare disorder. X-linked ichthyosis is the most common form of ichthyosis in the newborn period, affecting approximately 1 in 2,500 male babies. The term *ichthyosis* derives from the similarity of the skin condition to the scales of a fish. Ichthyosis is caused by excessive production of stratum corneum cells or faulty appropriate shedding of the stratum corneum.

Findings

■ There are four types of ichthyoses:
  ● Ichthyosis vulgaris is an autosomal dominant disorder and usually appears after 3 months of age. It presents as fine white scales and excessively dry skin. It is the most common and most benign of the four types.
  ● X-linked ichthyosis appears at birth or during the first year of life. There are large thick, brown scales over the entire body, excluding the palms and soles. This form only occurs in males.
  ● Lamellar ichthyosis is an autosomal recessive disorder that is manifested at birth as bright red erythema and desquamation. Scales are large, flat, and coarse, and there may be eversion of the lips and eyelids.

● Bullous ichthyosis is an autosomal dominant disorder characterized by recurrent bullous lesions. There is excessive dryness and peeling (Narendran, 2020; Witt, 2021).

Treatment and Outcomes

■ A skin biopsy is necessary to determine the subtype of ichthyosis. Reduce dryness of the skin and protect the skin from infection. Prevention of infection is key as there is no definitive cure for ichthyosis.

SUBCUTANEOUS FAT NECROSIS

Incidence and Etiology

■ Subcutaneous fat necrosis is a skin lesion caused secondarily by some form of intrauterine or perinatal trauma. It is reported in some infants undergoing therapeutic hypothermia (Narendran, 2020; Witt, 2019).

Findings

■ Subcutaneous fat necrosis (SFN) is characterized by subcutaneous nodule or nodules that are hard, nonpitting, and sharply circumscribed.

■ They may be red or purplish in color.

■ Lesions are located in areas with fat pads, such as the buttocks, thighs, arms, face, and shoulders (Prazad et al., 2020; Witt, 2019).

Treatment and Outcomes

■ Intervention with fluids, calcium-wasting diuretics, and glucocorticoids may be necessary.

■ Nodules may grow slightly larger over several days, but then resolve on their own after several weeks to months.

■ Calcification can occur and be associated with hypercalcemia. Hypercalcemia may occur up to 6 months after presentation of the initial nodule.

■ Serum calcium levels should be monitored (Bowe, 2020; Khorsand & Sidbury, 2018; Narendran, 2020; Witt, 2019).

▶ CONCLUSION

Knowing the physiology of skin development and careful physical assessment of the newborn skin are of utmost importance for NNPs. Thorough examinations and understanding of the skin allow insight into the health and well-being of the newborn. Being able to distinguish between benign and life-threatening skin conditions is imperative.

1. The neonatal nurse practitioner (NNP) manages the care of a 1-day-old infant and notes the presence of superficial vesiculopustules, some with scales surrounding a hyperpigmented macule. Microscopic examination of the fluid content shows a predominance of neutrophils; therefore, the NNP is confident in a diagnosis of:

   A. Herpes simplex virus (HSV)
   B. Miliaria crystallina toxicum
   C. Transient pustular melanosis

2. On exam, a newborn term infant is noted to have a unilateral ear tag. The neonatal nurse practitioner (NNP) counsels the parents that the presence of accessory tragi is:

   A. Diagnostic of hearing loss
   B. Easily remedied by excision
   C. Relatively common in neonates

3. The neonatal nurse practitioner (NNP) manages the care of an infant with epidermolysis bullosa (EB) and understands that one of the primary management goals is to prevent the occurrence of:

   A. Nonfocal clonic seizures
   B. Pathologic hyperbilirubinemia
   C. Secondary infections

4. During a physical exam, the neonatal nurse practitioner (NNP) notes on the infant's skin the presence of seven, light brown, oval macules. Three of these macules measure greater than 0.5 cm in diameter. These findings should prompt the NNP to evaluate the infant for a diagnosis of:

   A. Erythema toxicum
   B. Neurofibromatosis
   C. Tuberous sclerosis

5. The neonatal nurse practitioner (NNP) counsels the parents of an infant who has a small strawberry infantile hemangioma (IH) located on the scalp and focuses the discussion on the fact that the IH will:

   A. Increase in size over the next few months before it regresses
   B. Necessitate the use of topical antibiotic prophylactic therapy
   C. Require surgical removal in order to allow normal hair growth

6. The neonatal nurse practitioner (NNP) manages a preterm infant born at 30 weeks' gestation who weighs 1,200 g, and as part of a skincare protocol the NNP orders the most appropriate intervention for this infant by choosing the plan to:

   A. Offer immersive bathing two to three times per week if the infant is stable
   B. Sponge-bath the infant daily with a washcloth and warm water
   C. Use alcohol to remove routinely any adhesive from monitor leads

7. An infant with a history of seizures and glaucoma is also noted to have a flat, reddish-purple lesion on the face, and the neonatal nurse practitioner (NNP) identifies the most likely diagnosis as:

   A. Klippel–Trénaunay syndrome
   B. Proteus syndrome
   C. Sturge–Weber syndrome (SWS)

1. C) Transient pustular melanosis

Transient neonatal pustular melanosis is a distinctive eruption that when examined reveals a predominance of neutrophils. Neither HSV nor miliaria will demonstrate neutrophils on microscopic exam (Khorsand & Sidbury, 2018).

2. C) Relatively common in neonates

Accessory tragi (preauricular tags) are a relatively common congenital malformation of the external ear. They are present at birth and can be multiple and/or bilateral. Removal by tying off the tragi should not be done and could lead to complications. Association between deafness and renal abnormalities is controversial and unproven (Gupta & Sidbury, 2018).

3. C) Secondary infections

EB is a group of inherited diseases that are characterized by blistering lesions. Treatment aims are preventing trauma to the skin, providing wound healing dressings, maximizing nutrition, and preventing secondary infections. Neither seizures nor pathologic hyperbilirubinemia is associated with EB (Witt, 2021).

4. B) Neurofibromatosis

Café-au-lait macules are well-demarcated, oval or round, light brown macules in Caucasians and dark brown in African Americans which may differ in size. Six or more of these macules measuring 0.5 cm or greater in diameter should alert the practitioner to a possible diagnosis of neurofibromatosis type 1 (NF-1). Ash leaf macules (small, oval areas of hypopigmentation) are congenital markers for infants with tuberous sclerosis (TS). Erythema toxicum is a common neonatal finding and not indicative of more overt disease (Gupta & Sidbury, 2018).

5. A) Increase in size over the next few months before it regresses

Most IHs (80%) have completed their growth by 3 months of age and 90% regress by 4 years of age. They are not bacterial in origin and therefore do not require topical therapy. Surgical removal is unwarranted except in cases of physiologic compromise (e.g., airway compromise; Gupta & Sidbury, 2018).

6. A) Offer immersive bathing two to three times per week if the infant is stable

Immersion bathing for stable term and preterm infants has been shown to be beneficial. They can be more soothing and less stressful than sponge bathing. Only nonabrasive objects such as cotton balls or the caregiver's hands should be used in order to not abrade the skin. Routine use of alcohol can cause damage to the skin and underlying layers and is not recommended (Lund & Durand, 2021).

7. C) Sturge–Weber syndrome (SWS)

Infants with SWS can have seizures, hemiparesis, developmental delays, and ophthalmologic abnormalities, most commonly glaucoma. Lesions on the face may follow a pattern similar to that of the trigeminal nerve and may be associated with a diagnosis of SWS. Infants with Klippel–Trénaunay syndrome or Proteus syndrome will have the additional finding of overgrowth of soft tissues and bones, fatty tissues, and internal organs (Gupta & Sidbury, 2018; Witt, 2016).

Evidence-Based Practice and Quality Improvement

Patricia E. Thomas

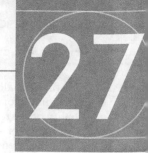

▶ INTRODUCTION

This chapter provides an overview and history of evidence-based practice (EBP) in healthcare. The relationship between EBP and research is described. The process of EBP is outlined and resources for developing EBP projects are provided. Quality improvement (QI) is then described with strategies for improving the quality of care for newborns.

▶ DEFINITION AND EVOLUTION OF EVIDENCE-BASED PRACTICE

■ The process of EBP is the utilization of the best available evidence for care with the integration of nursing expertise and consideration of the individual needs and values of each patient.

■ EBP is an important strategy to improve the quality and safety of patient care. Large variations in practice exist, clinicians may lack competency in critically appraising research findings, and there is often a delay of years or even decades in integrating research findings into practice.

■ At its core, EBP is an application of *critical thinking*, which is defined as the ability to apply higher order cognitive skills (conceptualization, analysis, evaluation) and the disposition to be deliberate about thinking (being open-minded or intellectually honest), leading to action that is logical and appropriate instead of accepting established practices. The clinician should be able to ask appropriate questions and modify their practice based on new/emerging evidence.

■ With their nursing expertise and educational preparation, nurse practitioners are in an excellent position to lead and participate in EBP projects. In the most recent version of their essential competencies for nursing education, the American Association of Colleges of Nursing identified translation of evidence from science as well as the synthesis of emerging evidence for advanced-level nursing education programs (www.aacnnursing.org; Ligappan &

Gautham, 2022; Lopez & Tyson, 2020; Melnyk & Fineout-Overholt, 2019; Polit & Beck, 2018; Profit et al., 2020; Tuuli & Macones, 2019).

RELATIONSHIP BETWEEN RESEARCH AND EVIDENCE-BASED PRACTICE

■ *Research* is the generation of new knowledge through systemic inquiry or investigation, conducted to expand knowledge and increase understanding. This new knowledge is then used to guide EBP. The EBP process includes taking knowledge gleaned from research and incorporating nursing expertise and patient values to establish best practices (Table 27.1).

■ All nurses are consumers of research in their practice when they identify a problem in patients under their care and then research the evidence for solutions. This application of research findings, regardless of research method, is the first step toward reducing the gap between research and practice (Hill, 2021; Melnyk & Fineout-Overholt, 2019; O'Mathúna, 2019).

Table 27.1 Processes of "Doing" and "Using" Research in Nursing

Research	Evidence-Based Practice
Formulate a question or hypothesis.	Specify a clinical problem.
Choose study design.	Conduct literature review.
Plan study methods and procedures.	Gather evidence.
Collect data.	Critically appraise evidence.
Analyze data and generate findings.	Develop practice guideline.
Disseminate results.	Apply the practice change.
Translate findings into practice.	Evaluate patient/family outcomes and share results.

Source: Data from Hill, A. (2021). Foundations of neonatal research. In M. T. Verklan, M. Walden, & S. Forest (Eds.), *Core curriculum for neonatal intensive care nursing* (6th ed., pp. 705–713). Elsevier.

LEVELS OF EVIDENCE

■ One of the challenging aspects of selecting research appropriate for use as evidence lies in determining the quality of the research. Although sources vary in their designation of specific levels for each type of study, all reflect the strength of evidence found in meta-analyses of randomized controlled trials (RCT), such as those published in the Cochrane Database of Systematic Reviews.

■ The levels presented in Table 27.2 enable consumers of research to compare the strength of different types of evidence (Polit & Beck, 2018).

Table 27.2 Levels of Evidence

Level	Evidence Type
I	Meta-analysis and/or systematic review of RCT
II	Single RCT
III	Quasi-experiment (nonrandomized)
IV	Nonexperimental study (case–control, cohort, correlational)
V	Systematic reviews of descriptive studies or qualitative studies
VI	Single qualitative study or cross-sectional study (survey)
VII	Expert opinion, case reports, committee reports

RCT, randomized controlled trials.
Source: Data from Polit, D. F., & Beck, C. T. (2018). *Essentials of nursing research: Appraising evidence for nursing practice* (9th ed.). Wolters Kluwer.

RESOURCES FOR EVIDENCE-BASED PRACTICE

■ Preappraised sources of evidence are readily available for clinicians to use, including systematic reviews and clinical practice guidelines.
  ● Systematic reviews are critical appraisals of existing research data on a selected topic using clear criteria. Systematic reviews are rich sources of evidence which can be found in the Cochrane Database of Systematic Reviews as well as in professional journals. The international Cochrane Collaboration is a collection of independent evidence that can be used by providers to inform practice (Polit & Beck, 2018).
  ● Clinical practice guidelines are another source of preappraised evidence. They include recommendations for practice based on a systematic review of evidence with the goal of improving patient care and patient outcomes. Examples of neonatal clinical practice guidelines are those for skin care, pain management, and peripherally inserted central catheters developed

by the National Association of Neonatal Nurses (https://nann.org).

■ For those looking to improve care within their own healthcare system, frameworks exist to guide in the design and implementation of EBP projects. One of the most popular EBP models is the Iowa Model Revised: Evidence-Based Practice to Promote Excellence in Healthcare. Others include the Advancing Research and Clinical Practice Through Close Collaboration (ARCC) model, the Johns Hopkins Nursing Evidence-Based Practice model, and the Promoting Action on Research implementation in Health Services (PARiHS) model (Dang et al., 2019; Grinspun et al., 2019; Polit & Beck, 2018).

THE PROCESS OF EVIDENCE-BASED PRACTICE

■ The process of EBP begins when a clinician identifies a question in their clinical practice. The clinician then searches for available evidence in the literature that could solve the clinical problem. Once the available research on the topic has been retrieved, the clinician appraises and synthesizes the evidence to determine which potential solutions are in line with their prior experience and potential relevance to their practice site. Prior to utilizing the new intervention, the clinician will consider its appropriateness to the individual patient based on the patient's and the family's beliefs and values. After initiating the new intervention, the clinician will then evaluate its effectiveness (Ligappan & Gautham, 2022; Polit & Beck, 2018).

POSING THE QUESTION

■ Once a clinician has identified an issue in their clinical practice for which there may be solutions within the current body of research, the clinician must formulate the question in a way that will yield results from a literature search.

■ *PICO question:* The essential elements of the PICO question must identify the patient population (**P**), intervention (**I**), and outcome (**O**) of interest. An intervention of interest may be included as the comparison (**C**) treatment, which will result in a PICO question.

■ *PICOT question:* Another component which can be added to the PICO question includes that of time frame (**T**) of the proposed intervention, resulting in a PICOT question (Ligappan & Gautham, 2022; Polit & Beck, 2018).
  ● Examples of PICO and PICOT questions:
    ❏ An example of a *PICO* question is: "Are premature babies who receive Curosurf less likely to develop bronchopulmonary dysplasia than those who receive Infasurf?" In this

example, the patient population (P) is premature babies. The intervention (I) is Curosurf. The comparison (C) is Infasurf and the outcome (O) is bronchopulmonary dysplasia.

❏ An example of a *PICOT* question is: "Do term newborns who are given glucose gel prior to a heel stick have lower pain scores on the NIPS than babies who are only swaddled?" The patient population (P) in this example is term babies. The intervention (I) is glucose gel with a comparison (C) of swaddling. The timing (T) of the intervention is prior to heel stick and the outcome (O) is pain score on the Neonatal Infant Pain Scale (NIPS).

SEARCHING FOR EVIDENCE

■ The plethora of available evidence means that the search for relevant evidence can be the most time-consuming part of the EBP process. Both primary research reports and systematic reviews can be found in the MEDLINE database, which can be searched using PubMed. The Clinical Queries page of PubMed includes predefined filters that allow users to narrow their search and more quickly retrieve desired results. Users can retrieve systematic reviews from the Cochrane Library by searching PubMed using the descriptor for the topic plus the words "and" and "Cochrane" (Ligappan & Gautham, 2022; Lopez & Tyson, 2020).

■ Although MEDLINE contains millions of articles, it may still not contain all the relevant articles, and if an exhaustive search is essential other databases such as CINAHL (an index of journal articles in nursing, allied health, biomedicine, and healthcare) and EMBASE (a biomedical and pharmacologic database of published literature) should also be searched.

■ The search is typically performed by entering keywords and using Boolean operators ("OR," "AND," and "NOT") to restrict the results to the most relevant articles. Custom search filters can be used to narrow the search by criteria, such as study type, publication period, or type of journal.

■ Collaboration with a medical librarian can ensure that the search is efficient, comprehensive, and identifies all key published articles, abstracts, and reviews (Ligappan & Gautham, 2022).

APPRAISING THE EVIDENCE

■ A rapid critical appraisal (RCA) of the evidence involves answering questions regarding the validity, reliability, and applicability of the information pertinent to the clinical question.

● *Validity* asks if the study was conducted using the best research methods possible and whether the results are as close to the truth as possible.

● *Reliability* asks if the research approach fits the purpose of the study and if clinicians could expect similar results in their own practice.

● *Applicability* addresses the question of whether the study findings could be applied to the practitioner's own patient population (Melnyk & Fineout-Overholt, 2019).

■ Determining the quality (certainty) of evidence requires each article or abstract to be critically appraised. To do this, the clinician should be aware of the strengths and weaknesses of different study designs (Ligappan & Gautham, 2022).

■ When evaluating individual sources of evidence, the level of the evidence can be determined from Table 27.2. For single studies, an RCT provides the strongest evidence for practice as randomization of patients to treatment groups is the best way to assess the effect of the treatment (O'Mathúna & Fineout-Overholt, 2019; Polit & Beck, 2018).

INTEGRATING EVIDENCE IN EVIDENCE-BASED PRACTICE

■ Once the practitioner identifies relevant evidence in the literature to answer the PICO or PICOT question, the next step is to integrate those findings into the individual's setting and experience. Each practitioner views evidence for practice through the lens of their own clinical experience; considering the local context (policy and work culture) is an integral part of making EBP happen. In addition, the practitioner has knowledge of the clinical setting which must be considered when utilizing research findings for practice. The process of EBP must include consideration of patient values and preferences, which also supports the goal of patient-centered care. Engaging stakeholders (leadership, bedside nurses, respiratory therapists) is important, and it may entail education and training of all the team members involved in patient care before the research knowledge can be translated to clinical practice (Fineout-Overholt et al., 2019; Ligappan & Gautham, 2022; Polit & Beck, 2018).

IMPLEMENTING EVIDENCE AND EVALUATING OUTCOMES

■ After completing the steps outlined above, the practitioner is ready to make an evidence-based decision for the patient's care. The final step in the process is evaluation. The question must be asked: Did the action that was made based on the EBP process improve the patient outcome as expected? The question can be challenging to answer as an individual. Some EBP questions are better answered within a group, such as the organization in which care is provided (Polit & Beck, 2018).

▶ PROMOTING EVIDENCE-BASED PRACTICE WITHIN ORGANIZATIONS

■ For EBP projects within an organization, Polit and Beck (2018) recommend that a model of EBP, such as the Iowa Model, be used to ensure that a proper site-specific assessment is made prior to the project and that strategies are developed to ensure staff support with the proposed practice change. Also, training of staff on the new intervention and an evaluation plan are crucial to the success of an organizational EBP project (Polit & Beck, 2018).

▶ QUALITY IMPROVEMENT

■ Medical and nursing providers of healthcare must work together to ensure the quality and safety of their patients through the process of continuous quality improvement (CQI). Hospital performance on quality indicators is increasingly important as results are shared publicly and with accrediting organizations. Patient outcomes vary in NICUs across the world (Profit et al., 2020).

■ QI initiatives are often designed to improve patient safety, such as those aimed at reducing the rates of medical errors and healthcare-associated infection. Quality-of-care issues may include the overuse, underuse, and/or misuse of interventions. The systematic use of QI can be used to improve the quality and safety of the care delivered to babies in the NICU (Profit et al., 2020).

ASSESSING AND MONITORING THE QUALITY OF CARE

■ The choice of quality indicators to be monitored depends on the individual NICU's priorities, practice patterns, and resources including access to databases on patient outcomes. Clinicians utilize outcome data on quality indicators from databases such as the Vermont Oxford Network (VON) and the California Perinatal Quality Care Collaborative (CPQCC) to benchmark their own unit's performance.

TEAM APPROACH

■ Unlike EBP, which can be used by any individual practitioner, QI requires a multidisciplinary team approach. Members of the team for each QI initiative can serve as champions for the project as well as contributors to a culture of improvement in their NICU. The inclusion of parental input into the unit's QI work can be valuable as well (Profit et al., 2020).

IDENTIFYING AIMS

■ The first step of any QI project is to determine the aim, or focus, of the project. Profit et al. (2020) recommend using the SMART Aim framework to ensure that the aim is phrased in a way that is "specific, measurable, achievable, realistic, and time-bound" (pp. 74–75). Examples of patient outcomes that are often of interest to NICU QI teams include bronchopulmonary dysplasia, intraventricular hemorrhage, and retinopathy of prematurity (Profit et al., 2020).

MEASUREMENT

■ Effective QI projects rely on measurement of care delivery processes and patient outcomes. The QI process begins with measurement of the outcome of interest prior to initiation of any changes to establish a baseline or retrieval of patient outcome data from an existing data set. This baseline can be compared with benchmark data retrieved from a neonatal database, such as the VON, to determine priorities for the individual NICU. The next step involves process mapping, where the steps of a care intervention are broken down to determine which factors may be affecting the patient outcome of interest. Then members of the team search for available evidence on interventions which could improve the outcome of interest in their patients (Profit et al., 2020).

PLAN–DO–STUDY–ACT CYCLES

■ Once the aim of the project has been determined and a potentially better change in practice identified, the QI team will often use a Plan–Do–Study–Act (PDSA) cycle to test if the change in practice produced the desired patient outcome. The steps of the PDSA cycle include: change in practice is planned (Plan), change is implemented (Do), patient outcome data are collected and analyzed (Study), and the need to refine the change (Act) is determined (Fineout-Overholt & Stevens).

OVERCOMING BARRIERS

■ With the focus on QI from accrediting bodies, it is essential for every NICU to embody the culture of CQI. While this culture must include all levels of caregivers, the commitment of leadership to CQI is essential to the success of any QI project. Close communication between clinicians in the NICU and hospital leadership can help ensure that unit quality initiatives are in line with leadership priorities and assist in gaining resources needed for the team (Profit et al., 2020).

▶ CONCLUSION

EBP is the integration of the best available research into clinical practice while giving consideration of the patients' and the organizations' values. QI and EBP begin with the identification of important clinical questions and determining the focus of the project. Clinical questions are then formulated, and relevant evidence is evaluated for use. Models exist to help formulate and implement EBP projects within organizations. A multidisciplinary QI approach intertwined with evidence gathered during the EBP activities offers the highest probability of successfully implementing change to improve patient care.

1. Evidence-based practice (EBP) is informed by research with the integration of provider expertise and:

   A. Patient beliefs and values
   B. Patient educational preparation
   C. Provider time and availability

2. In the hierarchy of levels of evidence, an individual randomized controlled trial is an example of which level of evidence?

   A. Level I
   B. Level II
   C. Level III

3. The neonatal nurse practitioner (NNP) questions best actions to manage infant diaper dermatitis and begins to search the literature. This is an example of the NNP performing a/an:

   A. Investigative prioritizing
   B. Original research
   C. Systematic review

4. The neonatal nurse practitioner (NNP) drafts the following clinical question in the PICO format to address an issue they see in their practice: Do premature babies with respiratory distress syndrome who are extubated to bubble continuous positive airway pressure (CPAP) have lower oxygen needs than those extubated to a nasal cannula? Which of the following elements represents the O in the PICO question?

   A. Oxygen need
   B. Premature babies
   C. Respiratory distress syndrome

5. In the NICU, the primary purpose of continuous quality improvement (QI) is to:

   A. Improve communication among hospital departments
   B. Improve practices and processes which affect the safety of patient care
   C. Retrieve data on patient outcomes to share with accrediting agencies

(See answers next page.)

1. A) Patient beliefs and values

The process of EBP is the utilization of the best available evidence for care with the integration of nursing expertise and consideration of the individual needs and values of each patient (Polit & Beck, 2018).

2. B) Level II

At the top of the hierarchy of levels of evidence (level I) is the systematic review of randomized controlled trials, whereas a single randomized controlled trial provides level II evidence. Level III evidence is a quasi-experiment (nonrandomized; Polit & Beck, 2018).

3. C) Systematic review

The evidence-based practice (EBP) process includes taking knowledge gleaned from research in the literature and incorporating nursing expertise and patient values in order to establish best practices. Original research is the generation of new knowledge. This new knowledge can be used to guide EBP. Prioritizing investigation in patient care is determined generally by the setting and unit culture (Melnyk & Fineout-Overholt, 2019).

4. A) Oxygen need

The PICO question format must identify the patient population (**P**), intervention (**I**), the comparison (**C**) treatment, and outcome (**O**) of interest. Oxygen need is the outcome of interest, while premature babies with respiratory distress syndrome are the population of interest (Polit & Beck, 2018).

5. B) Improve practices and processes which affect the safety of patient care

The primary purpose of QI is to improve the quality and safety of patient care. A secondary benefit of QI is having the improvement data available to share with accrediting agencies (Profit et al., 2020).

Legal and Ethical Principles

Rebecca Chuffo Davila

▶ INTRODUCTION

Professional, ethical, and legal issues are important concepts for all neonatal nurse practitioners (NNPs). Knowing and understanding key concepts related to ethics and the law will only enhance the NNP's practice. This chapter explores ethical theories and frameworks as they relate to nursing. Key legal concepts such as tort law, malpractice, and liability are addressed. Other topics include the consent process, the importance of accurate documentation, and privacy rights. Finally, the topic of staffing and safety issues related to NNP practice is reviewed.

▶ PROFESSIONAL ISSUES

ETHICAL FOUNDATIONS OF HEALTHCARE AND NURSING PRACTICE

- *Ethics* comes from the Greek word *ethos*, meaning "custom" or "character," established by Socrates. The Socratic discipline deals with what is good or bad and with moral duty and obligation.
- *Medical ethics* involves the systematic, reasoned evaluation and justification of the "right" action in pursuit of human good or well-being in the context of medical practice. It involves a critical examination of the concepts and assumptions underlying medical and moral decision-making, and may include a critical examination of the kind of person a physician should be.
- *Ethical issues* may be experienced as moral dilemmas, moral uncertainty, or moral distress.
  - A *moral dilemma* is present when the physician believes there is an obligation to pursue two (or more) conflicting courses of action.
  - *Moral uncertainty* arises when the presenting issue is unclear.
  - *Moral distress* arises when the decision-maker feels certain about the morally right thing to do. Still, this perceived "right" course of action is precluded for numerous reasons, including the caregiver's

lack of decision-making authority or institutional or financial constraints.
  - ❏ *Moral residue* is that which each of us carries with us from those times in our lives when, in the face of moral distress, we have seriously compromised ourselves or allowed ourselves to be compromised.
- *Shared moral work* implies that individual healthcare practitioners are aware of their professional values and the need to work collaboratively, build understanding, and work toward a resolution with other professionals, particularly when different perspectives threaten team function (Drago & Mercurio, 2022; Laventhal & Fanaroff, 2020; Stephenson, 2016).

ETHICAL DECISION-MAKING FRAMEWORKS

- Ethical discussion in medicine has been highly influenced by the ideas of principlism, which describes four overriding principles that must be considered when making ethical decisions for patients. These principles are beneficence, nonmaleficence, respect for autonomy, and justice.
- The principles of autonomy, beneficence, nonmaleficence, and justice are summarized in Table 28.1.
- Ethical decision-making frameworks can help guide one in resolving ethical dilemmas. Various models for ethical decision-making typically have 5 to 14 ordered steps that begin with fully comprehending the ethical dilemmas and conclude with evaluation of the implemented decision (Beals, 2020; Guido, 2020; Placencia & Cummings, 2017).

PROFESSIONAL CODE OF ETHICS

- The professional code of ethics enumerates standards of integrity, professionalism, and ethical norms for members of a given discipline.
  - *Bioethics* is a subdivision of ethics that determine the most morally desirable course of action in healthcare when there are conflicting values inherent in varying treatment options.

Table 28.1 Four Key Principles Needed to Examine Ethical Issues

Beneficence	This ethical principle is derived from the Hippocratic Oath, which states a duty to help others and to balance good and harm. Some people, however, may have difficulty deciding what is "good" for others. A moral and legal *standard of judgment* helps establish the primacy of duties to infants, ensuring they be regarded as fully human individuals with interests, even when clearly unable to express their own value system.
Nonmaleficence	This ethical principle is also derived from the Hippocratic Oath. It is an obligation to "first do no harm." A person must avoid intentional harm. The critical aspect of this principle is the intent of the healthcare provider's actions. Nonmaleficence requires that no initiation or continuation of treatment be considered without consideration of whether the therapy is overly burdensome or harmful.
Autonomy	Autonomy addresses personal freedom. There are four essential concepts of autonomy: liberty, self-determination, independence, and agency. Liberty is the freedom to choose without coercion. Self-determination is the ability to access information and then act upon it with the understanding of that information. Independence is the ability to act, reason, and decide for oneself. Agency is the power to be in command and responsible for one's actions. The term *parental autonomy* is often used interchangeably with *parental authority*. However, most argue *parental authority* is the correct term when referring to the role of parents in decision-making for their newborn infants.
Justice	This ethical principle is derived from Aristotle. It is the obligation to treat individuals equally or comparably and to distribute benefits and burdens equally throughout society. Justice is how we determine how social benefits, such as healthcare, and burdens, such as research risks, are distributed. Concepts of justice range from the broader utilitarian calculus to promote the greatest good for the greatest number in underwriting the distribution of resources (macroallocation) to a more narrowly focused equality of opportunity for each individual (microallocation).

Sources: Original table compiled from Beals, D. A. (2020). Neonatal bioethics. In T. L. Gomella, F. G. Eyal, & F. Bany-Mohammed (Eds.), *Gomella's neonatology. Management, procedures, on-call problems, diseases, and drugs* (8th ed., pp. 290). McGraw-Hill Education; Guido, G. W. (2020). *Legal & ethical issues in nursing* (7th ed., pp. 36–37). Pearson Education; Laventhal, N. T., & Fanaroff, J. M. (2020). Medical ethics in neonatal care. In R. J. Martin, A. A. Fanaroff, & M. C. Walsh (Eds.), *Fanaroff and Martin's neonatal-perinatal medicine* (11th ed., pp. 26–28). Elsevier; Stephenson, C. (2016). Ethics. In S. Mattson & J. Smith (Eds.), *Core curriculum for maternal-newborn nursing* (5th ed., pp. 664–665). Elsevier; Sudia, T., & Catlin, A. (2021). Ethical issues. In M. T. Verklan, M. Walden, & S. Forest (Eds.), *Core curriculum for neonatal intensive care nursing* (6th ed., pp. 715–716). Elsevier.

- *Metaethics* is the division of ethics where professional ethicists or philosophers attempt to analyze the reasons behind the ethical principles.
- *Descriptive ethics* is where sociologists, anthropologists, psychologists, historians, and others describe or attempt to explain moral behaviors and why humans are moral.
- *Normative ethics* are moral standards based on the fundamental principle that determines right or wrong.
- *Consequentialism* or *goal outcomes ethics* explains that the rightness or wrongness of an act depends on its utility, usefulness, or outcome. Right consists of actions that have good consequences, and wrong consists of actions that have bad consequences.
- *Principle-based ethics* attempts to identify the fundamental principles that form the foundation of ethical deliberation.
- *Virtue ethics* is based on character and therefore identifies moral aspects rather than applied principles.
- *Narrative ethics* uses the narrative of the story itself as the method of clinical reasoning.
- ■ The American Nurses Association (ANA) first published a code for nurses in 1950, most recently revised in 2001. The Code of Ethics for Nurses with Interpretive Statements has nine provisions regarding the professional practice of nursing and gives direction for those entering the nursing profession about their ethical accountability, sets a nursing standard for ethical practice, and informs the consumer about nursing's ethical standards.
  - For the NICU nurse, primary professional guidance is provided through the ANA Code of Ethics for Nurses with Interpretive Statements, the ANA Position Statements on Ethics and Human Rights.
- ■ Neonatal nurses utilize the ethical guidance established by professional nursing organizations, such as the ANA Code of Ethics (2015) and the National Association of Neonatal Nurses (2021) Position Statement on NICU Nurse Involvement in Ethical Decisions. These essential documents provide the foundation for ethical practice in the NICU.
- ■ The NICU NNP plays a critical role in the direct care of the neonate and support for the parents. Parents will need help coping and understanding all the intricacies of the NICU. They will also need support to learn how to care for their infant. NNPs, along with other members of the healthcare team, have an obligation to keep the parents thoroughly informed of the infant's condition and honestly outline the risks and benefits of that care (Guido, 2020; Stephenson, 2016; Sudia & Catlin, 2021; Swaney et al., 2021).

▶ NEONATAL NURSE PRACTITIONERS' PROFESSIONAL REGULATION AND PRACTICE

- Credentials are the practitioner's proof of qualifications. Nursing credentials are those of licensure and certification. NNPs, like all other APRNs, require licensure and certification.
- The legal description of the NNP's scope of practice according to state law is vital to establish the NNP as a professional entity and allows them to perform at their level of education and training. By doing so, the NNP avoids any charges of practicing medicine without a license; however, it will allow for reimbursement for physician services when provided by an NNP. Accountability for benefits and harm to patients is placed squarely on the NNP.
  - Each state has its own set of nurse practice acts. Some conditions are more restrictive than others when it comes to APRNs. However, with more autonomy of practice also comes increased responsibility. Advanced practice providers have a legal obligation to their patients.
- *A standard of care* is the minimum criteria by which proficiency is defined in the clinical arena. Five basic types of evidence are used to establish the legal standard of care. These are state and federal regulations, institutional policies, procedures and protocols, testimony from expert witnesses, and standards of professional organizations and current professional literature.
  - State and federal regulations establish NNPs' care and scope of practice. Hospital policies, procedures, and protocols are fundamental to acknowledge and outline the standard of care for that particular institution. Standards are also outlined by NNPs' various professional organizations. Therefore, it is essential for practitioners to utilize the most up-to-date evidence and keep current with practice guidelines.
  - Professional decision-making should be based on standards of care and ethical concepts of duty, beneficence, and nonmaleficence. Treatment goals for NICU infants should include contributions by both healthcare professionals and parents, respecting parental autonomy so that there is a joint plan (Guido, 2020; Stephenson, 2016; Verklan, 2021).

▶ LEGAL ISSUES

- Although each state has its practice act, some things ring true for any state where NNPs practice. With the increasing scope of practice, autonomy, and authority, there is an increased risk of greater exposure to liability situations. APRNs are held to a higher standard than RNs regarding legal liability.

All NNPs should be familiar with legal terms and precedence.
- Tort law is the most commonly seen classification of law in healthcare settings. A tort is a civil wrong committed against a person or the person's property. Tort law is based on fault and is applicable to situations where a professional either failed to meet their responsibility or performed the act below the allowable standard of care. Torts are civil wrongs based on personal transgressions rather than contracts (Guido, 2020).
- *Negligence* is a general term that denotes conduct lacking in due care and equates with carelessness. A person commits negligence when deviating from actions a reasonable person would use in a particular set of circumstances. The reverse is also true in that negligence may also denote a person acting in a manner that the reasonable and prudent person would *not* act.
  - To clarify, a *mistake in judgment* is not evidence of negligence if the nurse possesses reasonable and ordinary skills akin to professional colleagues. The nurse will not be liable for negligence even if the decision is subsequently proven incorrect.
- *Malpractice,* or *professional negligence,* is a more specific term that addresses a professional standard of care. Malpractice has routinely been defined by the courts as any professional misconduct, or unreasonable lack of skill or fidelity, in professional duties resulting in injury, unnecessary suffering, or death to the injured party. There must be a clear precedent of ignorance, carelessness, want of proper professional skill, disregard of established rules and principles, neglect, or malicious or criminal intent.
  - In a more modern definition, *malpractice* is the failure of a professional person to act according to the prevailing professional standards or to foresee consequences that a professional person, having the necessary skills and education, should foresee.
  - To be liable for malpractice, the tortfeasor (person committing the civil wrong) must be a professional, such as a nurse, an NPP, or a physician (Guido, 2020; Verklan, 2021).

Elements of Malpractice or Negligence

- To be successful in a court case involving malpractice or negligence, the plaintiff (injured party) must prove the following four elements in a malpractice case; a malpractice suit cannot be won if all four elements are not present:
  - A duty was owed to the patient. An individual is under a legal duty to act as an ordinary, prudent, reasonable person would act given the same set of circumstances, including taking precautions against the risk of injury to other persons.
  - There was a breach of that duty.
  - Harm or damage occurred to the patient.
  - Breach of the duty resulted in harm (proximal cause). This involves showing a deviation from the standard

Box 28.1 Other Legal Pitfalls for Neonatal Nurse Practitioners to Avoid

- Neglecting to make safety a high priority
- Failing to spot and report possible violence
- Not following institutional policies and procedures
- Neglecting to use due care in physical procedures
- Not checking equipment
- Assuming that someone else is responsible for their duties
- Assuming or not assuming responsibility for informed consent
- Failing to act like a professional
- Failing to communicate
- Failing to monitor and assess
- Failing to listen to information provided by the family
- Wrongfully disclosing confidential information

Source: Data from Verklan, M. T. (2021). Legal issues. In M. T. Verklan, M. Walden, & S. Forest (Eds.), *Core curriculum for neonatal intensive care nursing* (6th ed., pp. 720–733). Elsevier.

of care owed to the patient—that is, something was done that should not have been done, or nothing was done when it should have been done (Guido, 2020; Verklan, 2021).

- NNPs should practice without fear of legal ramifications. Common sense and understanding of patients and their families are important. Being empathetic and genuine is a desirable trait in the medical profession. NNPs are rarely sued but do need to be aware of malpractice law. Examples of other legal pitfalls to avoid are summarized in Box 28.1.

▶ LIABILITY

- Nurses and NNPs are recognized as professionals who are responsible and accountable for the care they give to their patients. If the nurse/NNP is liable to the patient due to negligent conduct, that nurse/NNP can be held legally responsible for the harm incurred by the patient. As advanced practice registered nurses (APRNs), NNPs are held to a higher standard than RNs due to the necessary training and education to become an NNP. The standard of care expected of the APRN is the degree of care expected of any reasonable and prudent APRN who practices in the same specialty.
- The most common areas in which APRNs have incurred liability are the following:
  - Conduct exceeding their scope of expertise or exceeding physician-delegated authority, resulting in damages
  - Practicing independently in a state that mandates a sponsoring physician
  - Failure to correctly diagnose or to refer
- The costs of liability when a neonate is involved are high for three reasons: (a) the costs of healthcare for a damaged infant with a normal life expectancy are high; (b) there is a longer statute of limitations for minors; and (c) sympathy toward the family.

- Essentially four types of damages may be compensated:
  - General damages are inherent to the injury itself.
  - Special damages account for all losses and expenses incurred as a result of the injury.
  - Emotional damages may be compensated if there is apparent physical harm as well.
  - Punitive or exemplary damages may be awarded if there is malicious, willful, or wanton misconduct (Guido, 2020; Verklan, 2021).

▶ CONSENT

- *Informed consent* is enshrined as a foundational cornerstone of the ethical practice of protecting human subjects from research risk. In getting consent for procedures and consent for research studies, one must be sure that the patient or the patient's legal representative understands fully and does not feel coerced in any way.
- The four domains within informed consent are (a) disclosure of information, (b) understanding, (c) competence or capacity, and (d) voluntariness or freedom to choose.
  - Informed consent is the voluntary authorization by a patient or the patient's legal representative to do something to the patient. The key to true and valid consent is patient (or legal representative) comprehension.
  - *Expressed consent* is consent given by direct words, written or oral. *Implied consent* refers to the patient's conduct or what may be perceived in an emergent situation. For emergency consent, the patient must not be able to make their wishes known and a delay in providing care could have devastating outcomes that may lead to death.
- To satisfy the definition of informed consent, the consent must be authorized by someone with the legal capacity to give such consent. In most cases, this is the patient or the patient's legal representative.
  - The person giving the consent must fully comprehend the procedure to be done and who will be doing it; the risks involved; the expected or desired outcomes; any complications or side effects; and alternative therapies, including none at all.
  - Our society has designated parents as the patient's legal representative, with the right to make decisions about their children; however, there are a variety of reasons why a social worker or a state-appointed guardian may be designated the patient's legal representative.
- The right of consent also involves the right of refusal. For *informed refusal*, the patient or the patient's legal representative must fully understand what the consequences are to them (or their child) by their refusal of treatment or diagnostic tests.

- Courts recognize the following four exceptions to the need for informed consent in circumstances in which consent is required:
  - Emergency situations give rise to implied consent.
  - *Therapeutic privileges* describe the situation where caregivers are allowed to withhold information based on the emotional stability of the recipient, and that could potentially cause significant harm to the recipient.
  - *Patient waiver* is used when the patient or the patient's legal representative does not wish to know about the potential complications or risks. This is the only situation in which the patient or the patient's legal representative may initiate a consent waiver; medical personnel are not allowed to initiate the conversation.
  - *Prior patient knowledge* waiver is in effect when the procedure has been explained to the patient or the patient's legal representative with a previous procedure. The consent process does not need to be repeated.
- The physician or the NNP is responsible for obtaining informed consent on procedures for which they are responsible.
- Professionals have an ethical and legal obligation to inform parents of facts regarding the care of their neonate. The NNP and/or physician should update parents on their infant's diagnosis and what interventions are available given the infant's overall condition. Being truthful regarding the outcomes, risks, and benefits of certain procedures is imperative (Guido, 2020; Laventhal & Fanaroff, 2020; Polit & Beck, 2018; Stephenson, 2016; Verklan, 2021,).

▶ DOCUMENTATION

- The most important purpose of documentation is communication.
- Documentation is a professional responsibility. Attorneys use medical records to provide evidence in legal proceedings.
  - For proper documentation, all entries must be signed with a name and proper credentials. Proper documentation also includes avoiding inappropriate comments, making corrections to charting appropriately, documenting events accurately and concisely, and documenting objectively and promptly.

- Effective documentation includes an entry for every observation in clear and objective language that is factual and realistic. Chart only your observations, chart refusal of care, and chart all patient education.
  - Never alter the medical record at someone else's request.
  - The use of standardized checklists, daily notes, and procedure notes may help in preventing liability (Guido, 2020; Verklan, 2021).

▶ CONFIDENTIALITY/RIGHT TO PRIVACY (HEALTH INSURANCE PORTABILITY AND ACCOUNTABILITY ACT AND PROTECTED HEALTH INFORMATION)

- NNPs have the duty to maintain and protect patients' and their families' confidentiality of their medical records. The right to privacy should always be maintained.
  - In August 1996, President Bill Clinton signed the Health Insurance Portability and Accountability Act (HIPAA) into law. This act provides for the portability of healthcare coverage through the streamlining of the transfer of patient information between insurers and providers, an antifraud and abuse program, tax incentives toward the acquisition of health insurance and accelerated benefits, and the establishment of the federal government as a national healthcare regulator.
- HIPAA also protects patients' protected health information (PHI). Information such as name, phone number, Social Security number, and other unique identifiers is a PHI. One should only know pertinent information needed to care for their patients. Violations of HIPAA could result in termination and loss of license (Guido, 2020; Polit & Beck, 2018).

▶ CONCLUSION

Understanding of ethical and legal issues is critical for all NNPs. As NNPs, we cannot practice fully unless we have knowledge of these key concepts. NNPs who have proper training and education should not have to practice in fear of legal ramifications, but having an understanding of the law and ways to prevent negligence and malpractice is so critical. Understanding ethical concepts will not only help in your practice day to day but will guide you through many tough situations personally and professionally.

1. The standard of care expected of the neonatal APRN is the degree of care expected of any:

   A. Clinical APRN whose practice exceeds their scope of expertise

   B. Reasonable and prudent APRN who practices in the same specialty

   C. Supervising medical professional with whom the APRN collaborates

2. The neonatal nurse practitioner (NNP) recognizes that the primary purpose for all documentation within a patient's medical record is for:

   A. Avoidance of the appearance of impropriety

   B. Communication with other team members

   C. Providing proof of care for billing purposes

3. An example of an action the neonatal nurse practitioner (NNP) could take in an attempt to avoid a malpractice claim is to:

   A. Document according to standards and not what happened

   B. Encourage parents to engage a lawyer during hospitalization

   C. Unite with and support their professional organizations

4. Actions deemed to be lacking in due care and equated with carelessness are termed:

   A. Civil tort

   B. Malpractice

   C. Negligence

5. A neonatal APRN overlooks a cranial ultrasound report of a grade 3 intraventricular hemorrhage (IVH), resulting in an extended delay in neurology and neurosurgical consultations. The APRN has incurred a:

   A. Dilemma

   B. Liability

   C. Near miss

(See answers next page.)

1. B) Reasonable and prudent APRN who practices in the same specialty

APRNs are held to a higher standard than RNs due to the training and education that is necessary to become an APRN. The standard of care expected of the APRN is the degree of care expected of any reasonable and prudent APRN who practices in the same specialty (Verklan, 2021). Any practice exceeding the scope of practice should be discouraged, and medical professionals are held to standards different from those governing an APRN.

2. B) Communication with other team members

The most important purpose of documentation is communication (Guido, 2020, p. 154). While the other answer options offered may be pertinent, they are not the overarching primary goal of documentation in a medical record.

3. C) Unite with and support their professional organizations

NNPs should practice without fear of legal ramifications. Common sense and understanding of the patients and their families are important. Being empathetic and genuine is a trait that is desirable in the medical profession. NNPs are rarely sued but do need to be aware of malpractice law and follow a few basic recommendations: Always be honest and respectful with the patients and their families. Know relevant law and legal doctrine. (Just saying "I didn't know" is not a defense!) Be a lifelong learner. Join and support your professional organizations. Know and understand that many malpractice claims occur from a lack of knowledge of patient education and discharge planning issues (Guido, 2020). Documentation should reflect actual events even in the event of an error or mishap, and NNPs should not advise parents as to any potential legal actions.

4. C) Negligence

Negligence is a general term that denotes conduct lacking in due care and equates with carelessness. A person commits negligence when deviating from actions a reasonable person would use in a particular set of circumstances (Guido, 2020; Verklan, 2021). Malpractice is the failure of a professional person to act according to the prevailing professional standards or to foresee consequences that a professional person, having the necessary skills and education, should foresee. A tort is a civil wrong committed against a person or the person's property.

5. B) Liability

The most common areas in which APRNs have incurred liability are the following: Conduct exceeding their scope of expertise or exceeding physician-delegated authority, resulting in damages; practicing independently in a state that mandates a sponsoring physician; and failure to correctly diagnose or to refer (Guido, 2020; Verklan, 2021). Dilemmas arise when there is a perceived obligation to pursue two or more conflicting courses of action. A near miss describes errors detected before they reach the patient.

Patient Safety in the NICU

Amy R. Koehn

▶ INTRODUCTION

Since 1999, patient safety has become a national priority. That year, the Institute of Medicine (IOM), now the National Academy of Medicine, issued two landmark reports that challenged all levels of healthcare professionals to improve the safety and quality of care for all patients and families. Medically fragile NICU patients are at a great risk for medical errors that lead to adverse events due to the fast-paced and complex environment. In the NICU, care is around the clock, with multiple team members and many handoffs, high-technology equipment, weight-based medication, and neonates who have limited physiologic capacity to defend themselves against adverse events and who are nonverbal, which adds to the risk of medical errors. There are many agencies and resources available to assist with identifying risk and applying quality improvement processes to help prevent errors.

▶ KEY CONCEPTS IN PATIENT SAFETY

- *Patient safety* is defined by the National Academy of Medicine as the prevention of harm to patients by placing emphasis on the system in which that care is delivered. Safety is the foundation on which all other aspects of quality are built (Gautham & Shafer, 2022; Pettker & Grobman, 2019; Profit et al., 2020; Tyler & Napoli, 2019).
- A culture of safety involves understanding the limitations of human abilities, anticipating and planning for the unexpected, and actively modeling a nonpunitive learning environment. This comprehensive approach, using human factors science, can improve system processes and structure.
  - Identifying and eliminating sources of patient harm or potential harm are critical to the delivery of safe and quality care in nursing and all other healthcare disciplines (Pettker & Grobman, 2019; Smith & Donze, 2021; Tyler & Napoli, 2019).
- A culture of safety uses a comprehensive approach based on human factors science to improve system processes and structures in a nonpunitive environment.
  - Traditional practice is for organizations to respond to errors by naming and blaming individuals. This is known as a *person-centered approach.*
  - A *systems approach* recognizes the complexity of a system and that most errors are based on flawed systems in which the individuals work (Smith & Donze, 2021).
    - ❑ Potential for errors within systems are generally related to either:
      - ○ *Active failures*, which are unsafe acts committed by a person or persons who are in direct contact with the patient or system
      - ○ *Latent conditions*, which are flaws within the system caused by failures in design (Tyler & Napoli, 2019)
  - A *just culture* recognizes that individuals should not be held responsible for system failures and that even the most competent professionals can be prone to errors (Pettker & Grobman, 2019; Smith & Donze, 2021; Tyler & Napoli, 2019).
- In 1999, the concepts, theories, and attributes of high-reliability organizations (HROs) was applied to clinical practice. HROs share similar characteristics, such as a preoccupation with failure, a reluctance to simplify interpretations, a sensitivity to operations, commitment to resilience, and deference to expertise. HROs operate highly complex and hazardous technological systems essentially without mistakes over long periods of time.
- Safety events are generally classified in four ways:
  - *Near misses:* These errors are detected before they reach the patient, usually through skillful nursing assessment and intervention.
  - *Precursor events:* These errors reach the patient but result in no detectable or only minimal harm.
  - *Serious safety issues:* These are any error that reaches the patient and results in moderate to severe harm, including death. They may also be called a "sentinel" event.

- ❑ It has been suggested that for every serious safety issue, there are potentially tens of precursor safety events and hundreds of near misses. Reporting these less severe errors may prevent the occurrence of a serious safety issue.
- *"Never" events:* These are errors that are unambiguous (clearly identifiable and measurable), serious (usually resulting in death), and considered universally preventable (Pettker & Grobam, 2019; Simpson, 2021; Smith & Donze, 2021; Tyler & Napoli, 2019).

▶ SAFETY BEHAVIORS

- ■ All members involved in patient care need to engage in the *culture of safety*, including hospital administrators, all healthcare team members, and families. Safety is the number one priority and takes precedence over institution and provider convenience, production issues, and costs. Safety guides all unit operations and clinical actions. Safety is created through accountability based on standardization, simplification, and clarity, as supported by the principles of safety science (Pettker & Grobman, 2019; Simpson, 2021; Smith & Donze, 2021; Suresh & Raghavan, 2017).
- ■ Safety behaviors should be promoted throughout the organizational culture, and means to incorporate safety behaviors should be viewed as a positive intervention rather than punitive action. Examples of these actions are:
  - *Cross-checking:* involves confirmation of information from two separate sources to verify the accuracy
  - *Speaking up for safety:* involves the use of key phrases that focus on system concern and not an individual
  - *Coaching:* modeling the safety behaviors and encouraging their use by others (Tyler & Napoli, 2019)
- ■ Systemwide approaches that may both initiate and continue conversations about safety concerns may include safety huddles, daily check-ins, executive rounds, and performance management concepts (Smith & Donze, 2021; Tyler & Napoli, 2019).
- ■ Transparency and full disclosure are also important concepts in the development and maintenance of a culture of safety. Transparency is a process in which errors are fully disclosed to the patients and/or the families, including details before, during, and after the error.
  - All healthcare providers find these to be very difficult conversations, although research routinely supports the expressed desire of the patient/family to be informed of an error. Literature reviews also confirm providers are less likely to be sued if an error is fully disclosed in a timely manner rather than hidden from the patient/family (Smith & Donze, 2021).
- ■ Organizational approaches used in developing and sustaining a culture of safety include both technological and nontechnological improvements:

- Nontechnological improvements:
  - ❑ The five rights are right patient, right drug, right dose, right route, and right time.
  - ❑ Forcing functions guide the user to the next appropriate action/decision.
  - ❑ Medication reconciliation processes create the most accurate list of medications a patient is taking.
  - ❑ Read-backs require the repetition of a message one has received in order to acknowledge its correctness.
  - ❑ Time-outs are a preprocedure pause that allows all members involved to identify the correct patient and procedure.
  - ❑ Executive walk-arounds occur when healthcare leaders visit each unit/department to show the organization prioritizes patient safety and to learn from the healthcare team about near misses, errors, or challenges to patient safety.
  - ❑ Storytelling is intended to open dialogue among healthcare providers who may be able to prevent similar occurrences.
  - ❑ Safety briefings allow information to be shared among staff both to increase safety awareness among staff and to cement the principles of a culture of safety into the daily routine (Smith & Donze, 2021; Suresh & Raghavan, 2017).
- Technological improvements:
  - ❑ Health information technology (HIT) has proven effective in reducing human errors in industries such as aviation and banking. HIT systems enable a more reliable, effective means of communication between and across healthcare settings and improve accessibility to patient information at the time of care.
    - ○ Technology eliminates duplicate work, improves caregivers' decision-making through automated menus, places evidence-based clinical guidelines within easy access, and removes the dangers of illegible handwriting.
    - ○ Some technologies that improve medication administration are electronic medical records (EMR), computerized provider order entry (CPOE), bar coding medications, smart infusion pumps, and automated dispensing units (ADUs).
    - ○ If the HIT is not well-integrated into the workflow of the organization, it may become more dangerous than valuable. HIT may also be costly to acquire, implement, train staff on, and "go live" over time. Culture barriers may also exist which challenge the implementation of a new or different HIT (Smith & Donze, 2021; Tyler & Napoli, 2019).

▶ TEAMWORK AND COMMUNICATION

- A healthy work environment is critical to promoting patient safety, and the work environment is enhanced through effective communication and teamwork from all disciplines. These will create and sustain a culture of safety.
- The Joint Commission records that more than two-thirds of serious safety issues were caused primarily by breakdown in communication. Other data cite the root cause of an error as poor communication (72%), with 55% of cases involving an organizational culture that prevented effective teamwork and communication (Pettker & Grobman, 2019; Smith & Donze, 2021; Tyler & Napoli, 2019).

METHODS TO IMPROVE COMMUNICATION

- Respectful communication is highly valued and rewarded. Team members in HROs do not wait until there is an adverse outcome to evaluate operations and practices. Evaluation is ongoing through use of established measurement processes (Simpson, 2021).
- Crew resource management (CRM):
  - Each team member is empowered within their role and responsibilities to alert on safety concerns. In fact, assertions of safety concerns are not only encouraged, but are also promoted as an expectation and part of the role of team members (Pettker & Grobman, 2019; Tyler & Napoli, 2019).
- Team Strategies and Tools to Enhance Performance and Patient Safety (TeamSTEPPS):
  - This is a three-step process developed by the Agency for Healthcare Research and Quality (AHRQ) founded on four core competencies: leadership, situation monitoring, mutual support, and communication. TeamSTEPPS is designed to provide hospitals a systematic approach to integrating teamwork into everyday practices of healthcare workers to improve quality, safety, and efficiency of care (Profit et al., 2020; Smith & Donze, 2021; Tyler & Napoli, 2019).
- Situation, Background, Assessment, and Recommendation (SBAR):
  - This is a tool used to help prevent omission of information through standardization of presentation. It is also used to ensure consistency in methods of communication between team members during critical time periods, such as shift change, team reports, and patient transfers (Pettker & Grobman, 2019; Smith & Donze, 2021; Tyler & Napoli, 2019).
- Communication among team members must flow freely regardless of their authority gradient. Patient care decision-making should be shared among all members of the healthcare team.
  - Respectful, collegial interactions between nurses and physicians and with patients are the bedrock of the unit culture. The *different but equal* contribution of nurses to clinical outcomes should be recognized and valued.
  - Aggressive or disruptive behavior (e.g., throwing items, intimidation, angry outbursts, making demeaning comments to team members and/or patients, or using profanity) should not be tolerated within the system, regardless of with whom the provider is involved. Competent clinical practice is a basic expectation and cannot be substituted for irresponsible, inappropriate, dysfunctional, or abusive behavior (Simpson, 2021).
- Examples of other structured communication processes are summarized in Table 29.1.

Table 29.1 Structured Communication Processes

SBAR	Provides a framework for communicating information that requires a clinician's immediate attention and action in a specific, structured format
DESC	A method of conflict resolution
"Two-challenge rule"	A patient safety concern must be raised a second time if it has gone unacknowledged and/or uncorrected. A quick conflict resolution technique by which a team member may question an action two times and if a sufficient answer is not provided may halt that action
"Check backs"	Require the receiver of an order or instruction to repeat it back to the sender to ensure it was clearly transmitted and understood
"Callouts"	Critical steps in a procedure are announced to team members so everyone is clear where they are in a given situation and so the next step can be anticipated, and it identifies who is in charge
"Stop the line"	A coded expression is chosen by the team to be used in front of a patient and understood by all team members to indicate a patient safety concern

DESC, Describe, Explain, Share/Specify, Compromise/Consequence; SBAR, Situation, Background, Assessment, Recommendation.
Sources: Data from Pettker, C., & Grobman, W. (2019). Patient safety and quality improvement in obstetrics. In R. Resnik, C. Lockwood, T. Moore, M. Greene, J. Copel, & R. Silver (Eds.), *Creasy and Resnik's maternal–fetal medicine: Principles and practice* (8th ed., p. 842). Elsevier; Simpson, K. (2021). Perinatal patient safety and professional liability issues. In K. R. Simpson, P. A. Creehan, N. O'Brien-Abel, C. Roth, & A. J. Rohan (Eds.), *Awhonn's perinatal nursing* (5th ed., pp. 1–17). Lippincott Williams & Wilkins.

Box 29.1 Factors That Increase Risk of Adverse Reactions in Neonatal Patients

- Greater pharmacokinetic variability
- Dependence on individualized dosage calculations
- Lack of appropriate pediatric dosage forms
- Lack of Food and Drug Administration-approved pediatric labeling
- Dependence on precise measurement and delivery devices
- Inability of neonatal patients to communicate adverse drug effects directly to providers

Sources: Data from Hanff, L. (2021). Medication errors in children. In J. V. Aranda & J. N. Van Den Anker, (Eds.), *Yaffe and Aranda's neonatal and pediatric therapeutic principles in practice* (5th ed., pp. 943). Lippincott Williams & Wilkins; Pettker, C., & Grobman, W. (2019). *Patient safety and quality improvement in obstetrics.* In R. Resnik, C. Lockwood, T. Moore, M. Greene, J. Copel, & R. Silver (Eds.), *Creasy and Resnik's maternal–fetal medicine: Principles and practice* (8th ed., pp. 848). Elsevier; Profit, J., Lee, H. C., Gould, J. B., & Horbar, J. D. (2020). Evaluating and improving the quality and safety of neonatal intensive care. In R. J. Martin, A. A. Fanaroff, & M. C. Walsh (Eds.), *Neonatal–perinatal medicine: Diseases of the fetus and infant* (11th ed., pp. 69). Elsevier Saunders.

▶ ERRORS IN THE NEONATAL INTENSIVE CARE UNIT

- NICU data have demonstrated that 47% of errors were medication-related, 11% were related to patient misidentification, 7% were from delay or errors in diagnosis, and 14% involved errors in the administration or methods of using a treatment (Profit et al., 2020; Smith & Donze, 2021; Tyler & Napoli, 2019). See Box 29.1 for factors that increase the risk of adverse events in neonatal patients.

COMMON ERRORS

- A *medication error* is defined as any preventable event that may cause or lead to inappropriate medication use or patient harm while the medication is in the control of the healthcare professional, patient, or consumer (Hanff, 2021).
- Medication errors are those that occur during the process of administrating medication. Approximately 47% of medical errors in the hospital are related to medication. Although establishing the frequency of medication errors in the NICU is difficult, published studies indicate that medication errors in the NICU are common, ranging from 13 to 91 medication errors per 100 NICU admissions.

- The five steps in the process of medication use where medication errors may occur are prescription, transcription, preparation/dispensing, administration, and effects. Incorrect dosing prescription is the most common medication error.
- NICU patients are more likely to experience a medication error than other hospital patients and to experience more harm when a medication error occurs (Hanff, 2021; Profit et al., 2020; Smith & Donze, 2021).
- Patient misidentification can happen more easily in the NICU since the patients cannot self-identify. In order to avoid this, patient barcode identifiers and a time-out prior to procedures are encouraged to avoid patient misidentification.
- Errors in administration of breast milk or blood products are also common. Multiple steps are involved with both processes and therefore there are multiple places in which the process can go badly. The wrong patient may receive the wrong product, or, in cases of blood products, incompatibility errors may be overlooked. Either substance may inadvertently be mishandled or incorrectly stored.
- Healthcare-associated infections occur in patients during the course of receiving treatment in a healthcare setting. Of particular concern are central-line-associated bloodstream infections (CLABSIs) and ventilator-associated pneumonias (VAPs). The risk of either or both can be minimized through the use of standardized guidelines and practice bundles.
- Unplanned extubations may be accidental or caused by the patient. Unplanned endotracheal extubations requiring reintubation generally rank within the top five adverse events in the NICU (Smith & Donze, 2021).

▶ CONCLUSION

Due to the emphasis on creating a culture of safety and transparency, neonatal units across the country are making progress to provide consistent, safe, and evidence-based care. The goal remains to identify, report, and learn from near misses, precursor events, and serious safety issues. This will allow healthcare systems to evolve into HROs with patient safety being at the forefront. The Joint Commission stresses new patient safety goals each year for which healthcare organizations strive toward to provide the safest care to our patients.

1. The overarching distinction between active failures and latent conditions is that active failures focus on:

   A. Competent professionals who cause errors
   B. Flaws in the system caused by failures in design
   C. Unsafe acts committed by a person or persons

2. Simulation in conjunction with debriefing is an effective method that allows team members to become aware of:

   A. How others can cause errors without thought
   B. Language to include to avoid future lawsuits
   C. Their role in error occurrence and/or prevention

3. A neonatal nurse reports a medication error to the neonatal nurse practitioner (NNP). In the report, the nurse focuses on issues of staffing and computer access as contributors to the medication error. These actions are examples of:

   A. Positive safety behaviors
   B. Professional competence
   C. Remedial actions

4. Patient safety is defined by the National Academy of Medicine as the prevention of harm to patients by placing emphasis on the:

   A. Fiduciary practices of a healthcare facility
   B. Person who is responsible for the error
   C. System in which that care is delivered

5. The neonatal nurse practitioner (NNP) orders a dose of gentamicin (Garamycin) but is unable to complete the order in the computerized system. An automated message informs the NNP of an error in the medication's dose. This is an example of a:

   A. Computerized glitch
   B. Forcing function
   C. Provider obstacle

1. C) Unsafe acts committed by a person or persons

Active failures are unsafe acts committed by a person or persons who are in direct contact with the patient or system. Latent conditions are flaws within the system caused by failures in design. A *just culture* recognizes that individuals should not be held responsible for system failures and that even the most competent professionals can be prone to errors (Tyler & Napoli, 2019).

2. C) Their role in error occurrence and/or prevention

Debriefing after a simulation provides the opportunity for teams to critique performances and learn lessons as to how, when, and where errors occurred and could be prevented in a real-life situation. Simulation in conjunction with debriefing is an effective method that allows team members to become aware of their role in error occurrence and/or prevention (Pettker & Grobman, 2019; Smith & Donze, 2021).

3. A) Positive safety behaviors

Safety behaviors should be promoted throughout the organizational culture, and means to incorporate safety behaviors should be viewed as a positive intervention rather than a punitive action. Examples of these actions are cross-checking, which involves confirmation of information from two separate sources to verify the accuracy; speaking up for safety, which involves the use of key phrases that focus on system concern and not an individual; and coaching, which means modeling the safety behaviors and encouraging their use by others. Even the most competent professionals can be prone to errors (Tyler & Napoli, 2019).

4. C) System in which that care is delivered

Patient safety is defined by the National Academy of Medicine as the prevention of harm to patients by placing emphasis on the system in which that care is delivered. Safety is the foundation on which all other aspects of quality are built (Gautham & Shafer, 2022; Pettker & Grobman, 2019; Profit et al., 2020; Suresh & Raghavan, 2017; Tyler & Napoli, 2019).

5. A) Computerized glitch

Forcing functions guide the user to the next appropriate action/decision. An obstacle, such as a computer glitch, should not be dismissed out-of-hand as an unworthy finding when in fact it is an attempt to steer the provider correctly (Smith & Donze, 2021; Suresh & Raghavan, 2017).

Practice Test

1. An example of a non-Mendelian pattern of inheritance is a/an:

   A. Autosomal dominant pattern
   B. Mitochondrial DNA pattern
   C. Sex-linked inheritance pattern

2. The neonatal nurse practitioner (NNP) is caring for a 4-day-old infant who was admitted to the NICU for hypocalcemia. The infant required multiple boluses and a daily supplement to maintain low normal serum levels. On exam on the fifth day, the infant exhibits some cyanosis, requires oxygen, and has a new murmur. The NNP considers evaluating the infant for:

   A. 11p15 methylation association
   B. 17q21.1 COL1A1 mutations
   C. 22q11.2 deletion syndrome

3. The neonatal nurse practitioner (NNP) is called to speak to an infant's parents who are concerned as to the appearance of tiny, white papules on the infant's forehead. The NNP explains these papules:

   A. Are common in infants and do not require treatment
   B. Should soon be assessed by a pediatric dermatologist
   C. Will spread down the neck and torso before resolving

4. A 3-week-old infant has tearing of one eye that has worsened over the past week. There is no sign of purulence or conjunctivitis; therefore, the neonatal nurse practitioner (NNP) recognizes the most appropriate initial management for this infant is to:

   A. Administer intravenous ampicillin (Omnipen)
   B. Dilate surgically the lacrimal duct
   C. Initiate routine lacrimal duct massages

5. A term infant of a diabetic mother (IDM), with a birth weight of 4.5 kg, is admitted to the NICU with hypoglycemia. The probable physiology responsible for this problem related to neonatal insulin production is:

   A. Less than it was in utero
   B. More than it was in utero
   C. The same as it was in utero

6. The neonatal nurse practitioner (NNP) distinguishes the type of hearing loss which involves pathology of the inner hair cells and eighth cranial nerve with intact outer hair cells as:

   A. Conductive loss
   B. Neural loss
   C. Sensorineural loss

7. An infant delivered at 39 weeks' gestational age is small for gestational age. The mother had good prenatal care and had no health problems. The neonatal nurse practitioner (NNP) should query the mother as to their use of:

   A. Herbal supplements
   B. Nutritional shakes
   C. Tobacco

8. The neonatal nurse practitioner (NNP) has the highest suspicion for meningitis in an infant who is:

   A. 3 days old with *Staphylococcus epidermidis* bacteremia
   B. 6 weeks old with late-onset group B *Streptococcus* (GBS) bacteremia
   C. Less than 1 month old with *Escherichia coli* bacteremia

9. The neonatal nurse practitioner (NNP) calculates the sodium (Na) delivery for a 0.82-kg infant who is receiving normal sodium acetate (NaAce) at 1 mL/hr via an umbilical arterial line at:

   A. 2.9 mEq/kg/d
   B. 3.6 mEq/kg/d
   C. 4.4 mEq/kg/d

10. A neonate is diagnosed with a defect in the neural tube in which the vertebral canal does not close. However, there is no herniation through the opening and the defect can be hidden. These are characteristics of:

    A. Spina bifida
    B. Spina bifida cystica
    C. Spina bifida occulta

11. A neonate is assessed by a neonatal nurse practitioner (NNP) after a nurse reports that the infant did not pass a hearing screen. The pregnancy was complicated by intrauterine growth restriction. The NNP is concerned about the congenital cytomegalovirus (CMV) infection of this infant. Which of the following is most accurate regarding this diagnosis?

   A. Antiviral therapy is universally indicated for infants with congenital CMV infection
   B. Diagnosis is made by polymerase chain reaction (PCR) testing of urine shortly after birth
   C. Most infants with congenital CMV infection are symptomatic

12. The neonatal nurse practitioner (NNP) notes that an African American neonate has bilateral postaxial polydactyly of the hands. The NNP will ask the parents if this finding is a/an:

   A. Concern for which they will see a specialist
   B. Element noted on the prenatal ultrasound
   C. Known, benign familial inheritance trait

13. The neonatal nurse practitioner (NNP) is informed by the RN of a discrepancy between a medication dosage order and the amount of medication delivered from the pharmacy. The difference was logged before the medication was given. This is an example of a/an:

   A. Near miss
   B. Precursor event
   C. Serious issue

14. Treatment of early-onset pneumonia includes the use of:

   A. Ampicillin and gentamicin
   B. Cefotaxime and gentamicin
   C. Vancomycin and gentamicin

15. The bedside RN pages the neonatal nurse practitioner (NNP) to report an infant who has a rectal temperature of 37.9°C (100.2°F). The first step the NNP should direct the bedside RN to perform is to:

   A. Add a cooling blanket to the infant's incubator
   B. Perform an evaluation for sepsis on the infant's blood
   C. Remove external heat sources from the infant

16. Supraventricular tachycardia (SVT) is a neonatal medical emergency because sinus tachycardia leads to:

   A. Delayed cardiac afterload
   B. Poor myocardial oxygenation
   C. Reduced diastolic filling time

17. Following a traumatic delivery, a neonate develops seizure activity at 2 days of age with no other abnormal signs. The neonatal nurse practitioner (NNP) identifies the most likely cause is bleeding into the:

   A. Cerebellum
   B. Intraventricular space
   C. Subarachnoid space

18. The neonatal nurse practitioner (NNP) understands that the absence of which expected change to the respiratory system during pregnancy could result in significant fetal compromise?

   A. Carbon dioxide excretion
   B. Minute ventilation
   C. Residual lung volume

19. The neonatal nurse practitioner (NNP) knows that the efficacy of omeprazole (Prilosec) in neonates will be altered by any condition which reduces:

   A. Fundal size and thereby tightens the cardiac notch
   B. Gastric motility and emptying into the duodenum
   C. Hydrogen ion secretion by the parietal cells

20. The anticoagulant preferred by the neonatal nurse practitioner (NNP) due to its predictable pharmacokinetics and ease of monitoring is:

   A. Low-molecular-weight heparin (LMWH)
   B. Protein-induced vitamin K absence (PIVKA)
   C. Unfractionated formulated heparin (UFH)

21. Autoregulation of blood flow in the cerebral vascular bed is the mechanism by which:

   A. Blood flow into the brain is controlled in a steady manner
   B. Pressure-passive gradients allow overflow into brain tissues
   C. Venous blood is removed from the ventricular spaces

22. The neonatal nurse practitioner (NNP) is called to attend the delivery of a premature female infant who is small for gestational age (SGA). The infant has respiratory distress after birth and requires intubation. The intubation is difficult due to the size of the mouth, but the procedure is successful. On brief exam after resuscitation, the NNP noted the infant has clenched hands and rocker bottom feet, and radial dysplasia. The NNP becomes concerned the infant has trisomy:

   A. 13
   B. 18
   C. 21

23. A laboratory assessment appropriate to evaluate the structure and banding pattern of chromosomes is called:

    A. Chromosomal microarray (CMA)
    B. Fluorescence in situ hybridization (FISH)
    C. Karyotyping (K)

24. Knowing that preterm infants are more likely to develop iron deficiency, the neonatal nurse practitioner (NNP) orders daily supplements in order to avoid which can have a negative impact on:

    A. Brain development
    B. Cardiac development
    C. Renal development

25. The neonatal nurse practitioner (NNP) identifies that the diagnostic test to confirm Hirschsprung disease is a/an:

    A. Abdominal radiograph
    B. Contrast enema
    C. Suction rectal biopsy

26. A female term newborn infant rooming with the mother is noted to have a systolic ejection murmur at 6 hours of age and an echocardiography performed at 10 hours of age for the diagnosis of critical aortic stenosis. The neonatal nurse practitioner (NNP) formulates an appropriate management plan for this baby including:

    A. Administration of sodium bicarbonate to counter acidosis
    B. Consideration of initiating prostaglandin E2 (alprostadil) infusion
    C. Ordering diuretic therapy to reduce cardiac afterload

27. The neonatal nurse practitioner (NNP) understands that for an infant with a ductal-dependent congenital heart defect (CHD), a continuous infusion of prostaglandin E2 (Alprostadil) will maximize systemic oxygenation by a resultant improvement in:

    A. Opening of the aortic tract
    B. Oxygen-carrying capacity
    C. Pulmonary blood flow

28. After performing a lumbar puncture, red blood cells and protein counts are elevated in the cerebral spinal fluid (CSF). The neonatal nurse practitioner (NNP) recognizes this finding is consistent with:

    A. Grade 1 intraventricular hemorrhage
    B. Subarachnoid hemorrhage
    C. Subdural hemorrhage

29. The neonatal nurse practitioner (NNP) understands the etiology of complications following preterm delivery in the presence of chorioamnionitis is related to fetal systemic:

    A. Cytokines
    B. Inflammation
    C. Leukocytes

30. The fetus of a mother with clinically significant anemia adapts to the environment by:

    A. Increasing growth of myocardial fibers
    B. Redistributing blood within the fetal organs
    C. Suppressing red blood cell production

31. Thermoregulation for a neonate is defined as a/an:

    A. Innate ability to balance heat production and heat loss
    B. Manipulation of the neonate's external environment
    C. Warming device to maintain an infant's temperature

32. The finding of aplasia cutis congenita on the admission exam of a newborn leads the neonatal nurse practitioner (NNP) to further evaluate for:

    A. DiGeorge syndrome
    B. Trisomy 13 duplication
    C. Urea cycle disorder

33. A 26-week preterm infant is intubated due to respiratory distress and respiratory acidosis. During the intubation procedure, a small amount of pink-tinged fluid is noted in the upper airway. What is the most likely diagnosis and what are the contributory risk factors?

    A. Pulmonary hemorrhage; PDA, prematurity, surfactant administration
    B. Sepsis; prematurity, sex, age
    C. Surfactant insufficiency; age, prematurity, respiratory failure

34. In what phases of lung development do many pulmonary developmental anomalies occur?

    A. Canalicular and embryonic
    B. Embryonic and pseudoglandular
    C. Saccular and alveolar

35. An infant with a proximal bowel obstruction will likely have a/an:

    A. Abdomen that is distended
    B. Late onset of recurrent emesis
    C. Scaphoid abdomen

36. Identifying variable decelerations on a fetal monitoring strip, the neonatal nurse practitioner (NNP) understands that these decelerations result from:

A. Change in pressure
B. Restricted blood flow
C. Significant fetal hypoxia

37. The neonatal nurse practitioner (NNP) is planning discharge for an infant who was born at 25 weeks' gestational age and is now 112 days old. As part of anticipatory guidance, the NNP discusses with the mother that, as the infant moves into toddler stage, alterations in pain processing will cause the child's perception of pain to be:

A. Destroyed
B. Exaggerated
C. Suppressed

38. An infant experiences an IV infiltration of dopamine (Intropin) and the neonatal nurse practitioner (NNP) correctly selects the most appropriate medication for therapy by choosing:

A. Epinephrine (Adrenalin)
B. Hyaluronidase (Wydase)
C. Phentolamine (Regitine)

39. When observing normal neonatal transition following birth, the neonatal nurse practitioner (NNP) recalls a newborn may require:

A. 1 hour for their feet and hands to become pink
B. No more than 5 minutes after birth to achieve oxygen saturation above 80%
C. Up to 10 minutes after birth to achieve oxygen saturation above 90%

40. The neonatal nurse practitioner (NNP) is concerned an infant has congenital adrenal hyperplasia (CAH). Routine labs included serum Na = 128 mEq/L. A physical finding that may support the diagnosis is:

A. Bilateral hydroceles
B. Increased pigmentation of the genitalia
C. Micropenis

41. The RN questions the neonatal nurse practitioner (NNP) as to why an infant is receiving caffeine (Cafcit) while on mechanical ventilation. The NNP answers based on the knowledge that caffeine (Cafcit) may serve as a/an:

A. Inotropic effect suppressor
B. Neuroprotective therapy
C. Pulmonary bronchodilator

42. The neonatal nurse practitioner (NNP) incorporates into discharge teaching an anticipated timeline for follow-up evaluations and relates to the parents that the earliest age at which a fairly reliable evaluation of neurodevelopmental outcomes can be performed is at:

A. 2 years of age
B. 4 years of age
C. 7 years of age

43. The neonatal nurse practitioner (NNP) elects to perform a lumbar puncture (LP) on an infant with bacteriemia based on the knowledge that:

A. Both bodily fluids must be tested for legal coverage
B. Clinical signs of meningitis may be delayed 4 to 7 days
C. Meningitis with bacteremia may be asymptomatic

44. A 1-week-old infant is preparing for discharge when the neonatal nurse practitioner (NNP) notes the infant is unable to turn their head to the right and a mass is palpated on the left side of the neck. The NNP plans for outpatient physical therapy for the infant, explaining to the mother that the infant likely has:

A. Clavicular fracture
B. Erb palsy
C. SCM torticollis

45. An example of tachyphylaxis is:

A. Hypocapnia that resolves following intubation and mechanical ventilation
B. Hypoperfusion during continuous infusion
C. Hypotension no longer responsive to dopamine

46. The neonatal nurse practitioner (NNP) is called to attend a Cesarean delivery that is a result of a failed induction, meaning the attempts to induce labor resulted in:

A. Inadequate pharmacologic stimulation of the uterine wall
B. Rupture of membranes greater than 18 hours of length
C. Scant mechanical dilation of the cervix membrane

47. The neonatal nurse practitioner (NNP) advocates for standardized feeding guidelines based on the knowledge that the protocols guiding the use of expressed breast milk, donor breast milk, and infant formulas have been shown to decrease the overall incidence of:

A. Necrotizing enterocolitis
B. Neurodevelopmental delays
C. Oral aversion

48. A mother with primary immune thrombocytopenia (idiopathic thrombocytopenic purpura) is scheduled to deliver and their platelet count is 30,000/mcL. The neonatal nurse practitioner (NNP) knows precautions to be taken by the newborn delivery team should include:

A. Large-volume fluid boluses to counter neonatal acidemia

B. Nothing additional as the mother's count is adequate

C. Preparation to treat neonatal hemorrhage complications

49. The neonatal nurse practitioner (NNP) informs non–English-speaking parents via an interpreter the need for their infant to undergo an invasive procedure. The parents verbally agree and then sign the form that is written in English. The NNP has violated the standard of:

A. Expressed consent

B. Implied consent

C. Informed consent

50. Starter or stock parenteral nutrition (PN; premade amino acid solution with dextrose) is recommended for preterm infants within the first 24 hours of postnatal life to compensate for:

A. Blunted glucose production

B. Low caloric intake

C. Negative nitrogen balance

51. A term infant is admitted to the NICU with obtundation after breastfeeding well for 2 days. A blood gas revealed severe metabolic acidosis; therefore, the neonatal nurse practitioner (NNP) recognizes the need to begin intravenous fluids and:

A. Administer bicarbonate

B. Provide intralipids

C. Stop enteral feedings

52. What mode of high-frequency ventilation (HFV) employs active inspiration and expiration?

A. High-frequency flow interruption (HFFI)

B. High-frequency jet ventilation (HFJV)

C. High-frequency oscillation ventilation (HFOV)

53. The neonatal nurse practitioner (NNP) recognizes a maternal cardiac complication considered high risk in combination with pregnancy is:

A. DiGeorge syndrome

B. Marfan syndrome

C. Turner syndrome

54. A mother reports their 1-month-old son has excessive tearing of both eyes and seems to be sensitive to bright light. On exam, red reflexes are not present and the infant has cloudy corneas and corneal and eye enlargement (buphthalmos). The neonatal nurse practitioner (NNP) identifies the best method for diagnosing this condition is:

A. Blood sampling for genetic testing

B. Examination using a slit lamp

C. Measurement of intraocular pressure

55. The mathematical relationship between drug dose and blood levels over time is termed:

A. Bioavailability

B. Metabolism

C. Pharmacokinetics

56. A 3-day-old infant is admitted to the NICU from the ED with a rash, decreased urine output, vomiting, and seizure activity. Laboratory results reveal a base excess of −15 mmol/L, serum lactate of 9 mmol/L, and serum ammonia level of 180 µmol/L. Which subspecialist may be helpful to contact to evaluate for the diagnosis?

A. Dermatologist

B. Geneticist

C. Nephrologist

57. A 37-week gestational age infant is transferred to the NICU at 40 hours of age due to lethargy and poor feeding after initially breastfeeding well. The neonatal nurse practitioner (NNP) suspects a metabolic or endocrine disorder. Following lab draws, the findings which may confirm the diagnosis of an aminoacidopathy is:

A. Arterial pH of 7.52

B. Base deficit of −18 mmol/L

C. Carbon dioxide of 22 mmHg

58. The best approach to improving ventilation for an infant on synchronized intermittent mandatory ventilation (SIMV) or high-frequency oscillatory ventilation (HFOV) is to adjust the:

A. Expiratory time

B. Peak inspiratory pressure (PIP)

C. Tidal volume or amplitude

59. The neonatal nurse practitioner (NNP) demonstrates proper infant handling techniques to parents and praises their attempts, pointing out the positive infant responses. The NNP's actions serve to facilitate long-term parental:

A. Ambiguity

B. Confidence

C. Protectiveness

60. Prior to ordering or obtaining a laboratory sample, the neonatal nurse practitioner (NNP) reflects on the:

    A. Necessity of documenting a numerical value
    B. Risk of laboratory error causing harm
    C. Substantive value of the lab result

61. The neonatal nurse practitioner (NNP) is preparing to discharge a 72-hour-old, well, term infant who has a positive Ortolani test on the discharge exam. The NNP includes in the discharge summary a reminder for the primary care provider to recheck the Ortolani sign after the usual age of spontaneous resolution, which occurs between:

    A. 2 and 9 weeks of age
    B. 3 and 6 months of age
    C. 30 and 60 days of age

62. Radiographic overexposure will result in images which are:

    A. Bright, light, and hazy
    B. Dark and lacking contrast
    C. Positionally rotated to supine

63. The neonatal nurse practitioner (NNP) counsels the parents of infants with confirmed hearing loss that the infants should be enrolled postdischarge in an early intervention program by the time they are:

    A. 3 months of age
    B. 6 months of age
    C. 9 months of age

64. A leading risk factor for retinopathy of prematurity (ROP) is:

    A. Assisted ventilation
    B. Extreme prematurity
    C. Intraventricular hemorrhage

65. Cross-checking, speaking up, and coaching are actions regarded as:

    A. Injurious to patient safety
    B. Positive safety behaviors
    C. Remedial or punitive actions

66. The neonatal nurse practitioner (NNP) distinguishes between histamine 2 (H2) receptor antagonists and proton pump inhibitors (PPIs) by noting that PPIs have a/an:

    A. Longer duration of action
    B. Minimal complication rate
    C. Shorter half-life elimination

67. A laboring mother known to be HIV-positive presents to the hospital. They have been maintained on antiretroviral therapy and at the time of delivery had an undetectable HIV viral load. What is the most appropriate delivery and postnatal plan for this mother–infant dyad?

    A. The mother should continue their antiretroviral therapy after pregnancy. The delivery method should be an individualized decision. Breastfeeding is contraindicated. The infant should be started on antiretroviral therapy within 6 to 12 hours of birth.
    B. The mother should undergo Cesarean section and continue their antiretroviral therapy after pregnancy. Breastfeeding is contraindicated. The infant should be started on antiretroviral therapy within 6 to 12 hours of birth.
    C. The mother should undergo Cesarean section and continue their antiretroviral therapy after pregnancy. Breastfeeding is contraindicated. The infant should be tested for HIV by HIV DNA PCR. If this test is negative, no antiretroviral therapy is indicated.

68. Physical and physiologic factors that predispose a neonate to atelectasis include:

    A. Narrow shape of the chest, rib orientation, compliant chest wall, and noncompliant lungs
    B. Shape of the chest, rib orientation, compliant upper airway, noncompliant lungs, and excess alveoli
    C. Wide shape of the chest, rib orientation, compliant lungs, and noncompliant chest wall

69. A 28-week gestational age neonate requires intubation and mechanical ventilation. At 1 day of age, an arterial blood gas reveals a pH of 7.29, partial pressure of carbon dioxide in arterial blood ($PaCO_2$) of 44 mmHg, partial pressure of oxygen in arterial blood (PaO_2) of 38 mmHg, and concentration of bicarbonate in arterial blood (HCO_3) of 7 mmol/L. The correct action for the neonatal nurse practitioner (NNP) is to:

    A. Decrease the tidal volume to improve mean airway pressure and ventilation
    B. Increase the peak inspiratory pressure (PIP) to improve mean airway pressure and oxygenation
    C. Increase the positive end-expiratory pressure (PEEP) to improve ventilation

70. The nurse calls the neonatal nurse practitioner (NNP) to report an infant having a large bilious emesis after having no instances of feeding intolerance. On exam, the infant does appear to have abdominal tenderness and mild abdominal distention. The NNP identifies the most appropriate diagnostic study for this infant is:

    A. Abdominal flat-plate radiograph
    B. Contrast enema with Gastrografin
    C. Upper gastrointestinal tract study

71. The neonatal nurse practitioner (NNP) correctly interprets a positive, indirect Coombs test to mean a maternal antibody is found in the infant's:

    A. Blood sera
    B. Progenitor cells
    C. Red blood cells

72. The neonatal nurse practitioner (NNP) understands the necessity of supplying the very low birth weight infant with protein soon after birth due to the knowledge that poor postnatal growth is strongly associated with:

    A. Adverse neurodevelopmental outcomes
    B. Increased risk of septicemia/meningitis
    C. Lower IQ scores at adjusted age of 5

73. The neonatal nurse practitioner (NNP) initiates parenteral nutrition as soon as possible after birth in order to:

    A. Deliver protein for renal filtration
    B. Increase weight above birth weight
    C. Preserve existing nutritional stores

74. While doing a daily physical exam on an infant who underwent cooling therapy for hypoxic–ischemic encephalopathy (HIE), the neonatal nurse practitioner (NNP) notes a subcutaneous nodule that is hard, non-pitting, and sharply circumscribed. The NNP suspects this nodule is secondary to a subcutaneous collection of:

    A. Calcium
    B. Potassium
    C. Sodium

75. The neonatal nurse practitioner (NNP) pursues a second-line laboratory test of a metabolic disorder by ordering a/an:

    A. Arterial blood oxygen level
    B. Spinal fluid glycine level
    C. Whole blood serum lactate level

76. An infant is born to a mother with a 10-year history of treatment for genital herpes type 2. The mother states they have not had an outbreak in several years; therefore, the neonatal nurse practitioner (NNP) understands the risk of transmission of herpes to this baby is:

    A. High regardless of the time since the last outbreak
    B. Less than during a primary outbreak
    C. Negligible since the mother was treated

77. The neonatal nurse practitioner (NNP) recognizes that of the following cardiac disorders a disorder associated with the clinical findings of decreased or absent pulses is:

    A. Hypoplastic left heart (HLH)
    B. Patent ductus arteriosus (PDA)
    C. Truncus arteriosus (TA)

78. The neonatal nurse practitioner (NNP) notes on an infant's initial exam that the left foot is adducted and pointed downward, and the NNP is unable to move the foot to a midline position. The NNP correctly documents the finding as:

    A. Metatarsus adductus
    B. Streeter dysplasia
    C. Talipes equinovarus

79. The typical distance for a newborn to focus on an object is between:

    A. 6 and 8 in.
    B. 10 and 12 in.
    C. 18 and 24 in.

80. Infants born at 24 weeks' gestational age are at high risk for infections primarily due to the:

    A. Fewer layers of stratum corneum
    B. Immature dermis and other layers
    C. Thinner layers of subcutaneous fat

81. A full-term male infant born by emergency Cesarean required intubation immediately after birth. The Apgar scores were 1, 2, and 5 at 1, 5, and 10 minutes, respectively. On admission examination, the infant is difficult to arouse, limp, and has nonreactive pupils. The neonatal nurse practitioner (NNP) categorizes the patient's physical exam as Sarnat stage:

    A. 1
    B. 2
    C. 3

82. An infant with intrauterine growth restriction (IUGR) presents with a coloboma, a ventricular septal defect (VSD), choanal atresia, genital anomalies, and preauricular skin tags. The neonatal nurse practitioner (NNP) should include in the differential diagnosis:

    A. Beckwith–Wiedemann syndrome
    B. CHARGE syndrome
    C. Cornelia de Lange syndrome

83. The neonatal nurse practitioner (NNP) is rounding on this week in January NICU discharges. The NNP knows which of the following babies will qualify for Synagis prophylaxis?

    A. Baby born at 30 weeks, now 40 weeks, who spent 7 weeks on continuous positive airway pressure (CPAP) and is now going home on 0.2 L nasal cannula (NC)/100% fraction of inspired oxygen (FiO_2)

    B. Baby born at 31 weeks, now 38 weeks, going home in room air

    C. Baby born at 33 weeks, now 42 weeks, with a history of apnea and is a poor feeder

84. To manage primary atrial tachycardias or reciprocating tachycardias, the neonatal nurse practitioner (NNP) chooses:

    A. Adenosine (Adenosine)

    B. Atenolol (Tenoretic)

    C. Procainamide (Pronestyl)

85. The neonatal nurse practitioner (NNP) recognizes an increase in the serum carbon dioxide (CO_2) level following administration of sodium bicarbonate is a result of the:

    A. Accumulation of bicarbonate within the lungs

    B. Dissociation of bicarbonate into H_2O and CO_2

    C. Inefficient excretion of bicarbonate by the kidneys

86. The neonatal nurse practitioner (NNP) is called to assess a 10-minute-old infant. Of the following, an abnormal exam finding would be to encounter an infant who experienced:

    A. Acrocyanosis

    B. Stridor

    C. Tremors

87. The neonatal nurse practitioner (NNP) notes that an infant has asymmetric abduction of the hips. The NNP places the infant in a supine position and flexes the hips and knees into a 90-degree angle and determines the knees are unequal in height. The NNP has elicited the:

    A. Barlow sign

    B. Galeazzi sign

    C. Ortolani sign

88. The minimum criteria by which proficiency is defined in the clinical arena is termed a/an:

    A. Clinical guideline

    B. Practice protocol

    C. Standard of care

89. The neonatal nurse practitioner (NNP) recognizes that the efficacy of indomethacin (Indocin) is inversely related to an infant's advancing postnatal age due to the change in ductal smooth muscle:

    A. Hypoxic–ischemic constriction

    B. Metabolism of cyclooxygenases

    C. Prostaglandin (PGE2) signaling

90. A 4-day-old, 27-week preterm infant remains on stable respiratory support but the RN calls to report a 3-cm increase in the infant's abdominal girth since the previous feeding, with the abdominal wall being firm and discolored. The x-ray shows a large pneumoperitoneum outlining the entire abdominal cavity. There is no pneumatosis, no portal venous gas, and nonspecific gaseous distention, with air visible to the rectum. The neonatal nurse practitioner (NNP) identifies the most likely diagnosis for this infant is:

    A. Distal bowel obstruction (DBO)

    B. Necrotizing enterocolitis (NEC)

    C. Spontaneous ileal perforation (SIP)

91. The neonatal nurse practitioner (NNP) manages an infant who has had progressive abdominal distention, increased lethargy, increased apnea and bradycardia events, and developed metabolic acidosis on capillary blood gas. Radiographs demonstrate extensive pneumatosis and pneumoperitoneum. The NNP identifies the infant at Bell stage:

    A. 2B

    B. 3A

    C. 3B

92. Maternal breast milk is the optimal primary nutritional source for premature neonates because evidence has shown that it:

    A. Increases rate of growth compared with formula-fed infants

    B. Meets the nutritional requirements of preterm infants

    C. Reduces the risk of necrotizing enterocolitis

93. An advantage of the use of amplitude-integrated EEG (aEEG) includes the:

    A. Availability to bring to the bedside

    B. Detection of low-amplitude seizures

    C. Resistance to artifact interference

94. The neonatal nurse practitioner (NNP) notes on physical exam that an infant's anterior fontanel is closed and has a palpable coronal suture ridging. The NNP recognizes this infant will require surgical correction of the synostosis:

    A. At 6 to 12 months of age

    B. At 18 to 24 months of age

    C. Within the first 30 days of age

95. The evidence-based practice (EBP) process involves an assessment of the validity, reliability, and applicability of the evidence in a process known as:

A. Random control inquiry (RCI)

B. Rapid critical appraisal (RCA)

C. Root source analysis (RSA)

96. The neonatal nurse practitioner (NNP) is preparing for the delivery of an infant who has been prenatally diagnosed with achondroplasia. The NNP knows to expect an infant who will have:

A. Frontal bossing and "trident hands"

B. Large but deformed cranium

C. Stenothorax and dark-blue sclerae

97. The neonatal nurse practitioner (NNP) recognizes an infant with an omphalocele that has a ruptured sac should:

A. Be positioned supine in order not to compromise mesenteric bowel blood flow

B. Have a sterile gauze dressing placed over the defect until it is surgically repaired

C. Have their torso and lower body placed in a bowel bag due to insensible water losses

98. A 3-day-old term infant is admitted to the NICU with hypoglycemia, metabolic acidosis, and direct hyperbilirubinemia. The liver edge is palpable at 5 cm below the right costal margin, and the infant exudes a sweet-smelling odor. The infant overall is very lethargic, minimally responsive to painful stimuli. The neonatal nurse practitioner (NNP) recognizes that the symptom that is suspicious for a disorder of protein metabolism is:

A. Hepatosplenomegaly

B. Overall lethargy

C. Sweet-smelling odor

99. An asymmetric startle reflex is noted in the presence of a/an:

A. Brachial plexus injury

B. Brainstem injury

C. Metatarsal injury

100. The neonatal nurse practitioner (NNP) diagnoses an infant who has abdominal contents, including the intestines and other organs such as the liver, herniated into the umbilical cord as having:

A. Gastroschisis

B. Omphalocele

C. Patent urachus

101. The neonatal nurse practitioner (NNP) identifies a contraindication to starting trophic enteral feedings is:

A. Gastric residuals

B. Hemodynamic instability

C. Less than 24 hours of age

102. Which of the following lists presents the correct sequence of emergent pharmacologic therapy for symptomatic hyperkalemia?

A. Dilution and intracellular shifting of K^+, stabilization of the conductive tissue, and facilitating K^+ excretion

B. Facilitating K^+ excretion, stabilization of the conductive tissue, and dilution and intracellular shifting of K^+

C. Stabilization of the conductive tissue, dilution and intracellular shifting of K^+, and facilitating K^+ excretion

103. As a component of intravenous nutrition, anions are provided as:

A. Chloride

B. Gluconate

C. Phosphorus

104. The neonatal nurse practitioner (NNP) targets a delivery of carbohydrates to supply what percent of an infant's total caloric intake?

A. 25% to 35%

B. 40% to 50%

C. 60% to 70%

105. Infants who are born at less than 34 weeks' gestational age have a low glomerular filtration rate due to:

A. Immature response of the alpha receptors in the kidney

B. Limited autoregulation of renal blood flow

C. Partial or unfinished nephrogenesis

106. In order to obtain real-time dynamic images, the neonatal nurse practitioner (NNP) selects evaluation of the neonate by:

A. Fluoroscopy

B. Radiography

C. Ultrasonography

107. The neonatal nurse practitioner (NNP) orders a study of neonatal blood using a direct antiglobulin test (DAT) in order to assess for the presence of:

A. Fetal hemoglobulin

B. Maternal IgG antibodies

C. Occult blood in feces

108. The neonatal nurse practitioner (NNP) includes in a preterm infant's discharge summary the recommendation to continue the use of premature infant formula until the postnatal age of:

A. 6 months
B. 9 months
C. 12 months

109. The neonatal nurse practitioner (NNP) selects the correct test to differentiate swallowed maternal blood from neonatal blood by selecting the:

A. Apt test
B. DAT test
C. ERT test

110. The neonatal nurse practitioner (NNP) identifies the most common cause of seizures in the early neonatal period is:

A. Benign myoclonus of early infancy
B. Hypoxic–ischemic encephalopathy (HIE)
C. Systemic infectious meningitis

111. An antibiotic which poses particular risk of damaging the neonate's kidney if given in high doses or over a prolonged period of time is:

A. Ampicillin (Omnipen)
B. Cefotaxime (Claforan)
C. Gentamicin (Garamycin)

112. The neonatal nurse practitioner (NNP) recognizes a medication class routinely used in the treatment of hypertensive disorders in pregnancy is:

A. Angiotensin inhibitors
B. Beta-blockers
C. Corticoid antagonists

113. When evaluating an intubated preterm neonate, the neonatal nurse practitioner (NNP) understands that factors indicating extubation readiness, from a volume guarantee mode of ventilation, include:

A. Breath initiated receives a fully supported breath at the set pressure
B. Peak pressure needed to achieve the set volume indicates improved compliance
C. Peak pressure set to a maximum of 18 mmHg and the breath rate below 20 breaths per minute

114. The neonatal nurse practitioner (NNP) is called to the delivery of a 39-week gestational age, large-for-gestational-age (LGA) infant who was a difficult extraction. Upon initial assessment, the NNP notes that the infant moves the right upper extremity freely but has no movement of the left upper extremity. The NNP knows the mostly likely reason for decreased or absent movement of an extremity is a/an:

A. Deformation
B. Fracture
C. Tumor

115. With this genetic pattern, a phenotype usually appears in every generation, and each affected person has an affected parent. This genetic pattern is termed:

A. Autosomal dominant
B. Autosomal recessive
C. Sex-linked

116. The methods by which inotropic/vasopressive agents increase cardiac output include increasing the cardiac:

A. Contraction, rhythm, and atrial size
B. Preload, contraction, and afterload
C. Rate, contraction, and vascular tone

117. Evaluation of osteomyelitis should include:

A. Blood culture and culture of any purulent skin lesions
B. Blood culture, CSF, and culture of any purulent skin lesions
C. Blood culture, CSF, and urine cultures, along with culture of any purulent skin lesions

118. A mother presents for delivery with urine toxicology positive for cocaine and fentanyl. After delivery, the mother asks if they can put the baby to breast. The neonatal nurse practitioner (NNP) best replies by discussing the:

A. Necessity of the mother stopping medications immediately
B. Option to delay breastfeeding until medication is metabolized
C. Risks of passing substances to the baby through the breast milk

119. The neonatal nurse practitioner (NNP) endorses the practice of delayed cord clamping (DCC) for the neonate in order to:

   A. Delay innate erythropoiesis
   B. Improve physiologic stability
   C. Minimize maternal antibodies

120. The neonatal nurse practitioner (NNP) is managing an infant with refractory hypotension and recognizes the need to add natural glucocorticoid replacement therapy in the form of:

   A. Fludrocortisone (Florinef)
   B. Hydrocortisone (Cortef)
   C. Prednisone (Pediapred)

121. The Ballard gestational age examination is most accurate for the extremely preterm infant when done within:

   A. 8 to 12 hours after birth
   B. 24 to 30 hours after birth
   C. 36 to 48 hours after birth

122. Inborn errors of metabolism are genetic, biochemical disorders in which the function, structure, or volume is altered for a key pathway in the synthesis of:

   A. Carbohydrates
   B. Fatty acids
   C. Proteins

123. Interpretation of any neonatal radiographic image begins with a/an:

   A. Established baseline of disease process
   B. Systematic approach to interpretation
   C. Theory of anticipated findings

124. The term *dysmorphism* indicates a/an:

   A. Anomalous external physical feature
   B. Friction force pulling on a tissue group
   C. Malformed morphogenesis of tissue

125. An infant is born with a lack of abdominal wall muscles, hydronephrosis with a dilated bladder, and cryptorchidism. The most likely diagnosis is:

   A. Bardet–Biedl syndrome
   B. Churg–Strauss syndrome
   C. Eagle–Barrett syndrome

126. The neonatal nurse practitioner (NNP) recognizes that family-centered care (FCC) approach requires a change from:

   A. Acute care to chronic care model of neonatal follow-up
   B. Paternalistic to holistic framework of collaboration
   C. Task-oriented to relationship-based model of care

127. The neonatal nurse practitioner (NNP) recognizes the mechanism of action of hydrocortisone (Hydrocort) may be related to an infant's:

   A. Paucity of alpha-1-adrenergic receptors
   B. Relative adrenal insufficiency
   C. Unresponsive hypothalamus

128. Which of the following statements regarding neonatal herpes simplex virus (HSV) disease is most accurate?

   A. If the mother has no history of HSV lesions, no evaluation for neonatal HSV is needed for this infant
   B. Maternal primary infection at or near the time of delivery carries a higher risk of neonatal infection than remote maternal primary infection
   C. The infant should be given intravenous ganciclovir for presumed HSV infection while testing is pending

129. The neonatal nurse practitioner (NNP) identifies on physical exam a grade 2/6 systolic murmur, +3 right brachial pulse, +1 right femoral pulse, and capillary refill of 5 seconds in the lower extremities. These findings prompt additional evaluation for:

   A. Coarctation of the aorta
   B. Ductus arteriosus
   C. Tetralogy of Fallot

130. In preparation for discharge, the neonatal nurse practitioner (NNP) provides anticipatory guidance to the family on topics such as:

   A. Expectations of parent–child relationship
   B. The family budget for food and supplies
   C. When to place the infant in a day care

131. Failure of complete recanalization of the esophagus results in esophageal atresia and is known to occur during the:

   A. 4th week of gestation
   B. 6th week of gestation
   C. 8th week of gestation

132. The neonatal nurse practitioner (NNP) attends a scheduled Cesarean delivery of a mother placed under routine general anesthesia and knows that, after delivery, the neonate will be:

   A. Affected by meconium and will need treatment for meconium aspiration
   B. Heavily sedated and require manual positive pressure ventilation
   C. Stable as long as delivery occurs at 1.5 to 2 minutes after uterine incision

133. The form of renal failure associated with ischemic damage resulting in functional compromise to the glomerulus, tubules, and/or collecting system is called:

    A. Intrinsic
    B. Postrenal
    C. Prerenal

134. The neonatal nurse practitioner (NNP) is notified that an infant's lab results revealed a serum triglyceride level of 378 mg/dL. The most appropriate action for the NNP in response to this is to:

    A. Ask the RN to repeat the lab
    B. Discontinue the current intralipid infusion
    C. Obtain a serum bilirubin level

135. The neonatal nurse practitioner (NNP) identifies the risk factors for infantile hemangiomas (IHs) include:

    A. Euploidy
    B. Hypoxia
    C. Postmaturity

136. Brushfield spots can be found on an infant's:

    A. Eyes
    B. Palate
    C. Skin

137. The neonatal nurse practitioner (NNP) analyzes the lean mass growth of a neonate by following changes in the baby's:

    A. Body length
    B. Dry weight
    C. Head circumference

138. A newly born infant is diagnosed with congenital glaucoma, and the neonatal nurse practitioner (NNP) recognizes that a disorder associated with congenital glaucoma is:

    A. Beckwith–Wiedemann syndrome
    B. Sturge–Weber syndrome
    C. Trisomy 21 syndrome

139. Differentiating critical congenital heart disease (CCHD) from persistent pulmonary hypertension (PPHN) is best determined by performing a/an:

    A. Doppler flow study
    B. Echocardiogram
    C. Hyperoxia test

140. An expected change to the maternal cardiovascular system in pregnancy and whose absence would result in significant fetal compromise is an increase in the mother's:

    A. Diastolic blood pressure
    B. Ejection fraction
    C. Total blood volume

141. The neonatal nurse practitioner (NNP) is called to evaluate an infant who is noted to be intermittently cyanotic. The cyanosis appears to be more intense at rest and improves when the baby is crying, which led the NNP to suspect a/an:

    A. Cardiac anomaly, such as total anomalous pulmonary venous return
    B. Developmental obstructive disorder, such as choanal atresia of the airway
    C. Respiratory disorder, such as persistent pulmonary hypertension of the newborn

142. The neonatal nurse practitioner (NNP) attends the vaginal delivery of a 38-week male with a significant maternal history of uncontrolled type 1 diabetes. The large-for-gestational-age (LGA) infant is vigorous with a lusty cry at delivery; however, upon exam, there is asymmetrical movement of the upper extremities, with the right more flaccid than the left. The right hand exhibits a positive grasp reflex; therefore, the NNP recognizes the asymmetry is likely related to:

    A. Barlow maneuver
    B. Erb palsy
    C. Klumpke palsy

143. Dobutamine (Dobutrex) primarily exerts its actions to increase blood pressure by causing a/an:

    A. Decrease in pulmonary artery to aortic pressure gradient
    B. Escalation in myocardial contractility
    C. Increase in contractility and peripheral vascular resistance

144. The embryonic closure of the neural tube is complete by:

    A. 2 weeks of gestation
    B. 3 weeks of gestation
    C. 4 weeks of gestation

145. An echocardiogram done on an infant with congenital heart disease (CHD) reveals poor cardiac output secondary to poor contractility. The correct pharmacologic approach to these findings would be for the neonatal nurse practitioner (NNP) to order a continuous infusion of:

    A. Dobutamine (Dobutrex)
    B. Dopamine (Intropin)
    C. Epinephrine (Adrenalin)

146. The neonatal nurse practitioner (NNP) recalls that, within the renin–angiotensin–aldosterone–ADH system, angiotensin II acts primarily to:

    A. Constrict blood vessels
    B. Convert aldosterone
    C. Dilate blood vessels

147. An infant has been nothing by mouth (NPO) for an extended period of time due to impaired biliary excretion. Regarding the delivery of parenteral nutrition (PN), the neonatal nurse practitioner (NNP) follows the recommendation to reduce or omit:

A. Chromium
B. Manganese
C. Selenium

148. A 39-week gestational age infant with a birth weight of 3.26 kg is transferred to the NICU for hypoglycemia. The infant requires an umbilical venous catheter due to the high glucose infusion rate to maintain normal blood sugar levels. The neonatal nurse practitioner (NNP) recognizes it is also appropriate to order as part of the laboratory evaluation a/an:

A. Insulin level
B. Lactate level
C. Thyroid hormone level

149. The neonatal nurse practitioner (NNP) is caring for a 24-week, now 3-day-old infant and knows to adjust the cysteine content in the parenteral nutrition due to the risk of inducing:

A. Electrolyte abnormalities
B. Increased triglycerides
C. Metabolic acidosis

150. The neonatal nurse practitioner (NNP) manages the care of an infant with a diagnosis of collodion and counsels the parents as to the need to observe the infant closely for:

A. Anemia
B. Dehydration
C. Hyperthermia

151. An asymptomatic infant is noted to have a soft cardiac murmur. Echocardiography discovers a restrictive ventricular septal defect (VSD). The neonatal nurse practitioner's (NNP's) discussion with the parents centers on the fact that:

A. Many VSDs resolve spontaneously by 1 year of age
B. Signs and symptoms of the defect will worsen as the neonate ages
C. The neonate will need urgent surgery to redirect blood flow

152. The neonatal nurse practitioner (NNP) recognizes a priority when initially caring for an infant with an omphalocele in the delivery room and upon admission to the NICU includes:

A. Adequate blood pressures
B. Surgical correction
C. Thermoregulation

153. After a prolonged labor and vaginal delivery, the nurse notes the infant has a large ecchymotic swelling over the presenting portion of the scalp that crosses the suture lines, and identifies this as:

A. Caput succedaneum
B. Cephalohematoma
C. Subgaleal hemorrhage

154. The neonatal nurse practitioner (NNP) orders a skin scraping of an infant's undetermined rash and the report reveals a large number of eosinophils. The NNP recognizes this is indicative of:

A. Erythema toxicum
B. Lamellar ichthyosis
C. Scalded skin syndrome

155. An encephalocele arises from a failed closure of part of the rostral neural tube and most commonly occurs in the:

A. Frontonasal region
B. Occipital region
C. Parietal region

156. What radiologic findings would the neonatal nurse practitioner (NNP) expect to find in an infant with meconium-stained amniotic fluid presenting with respiratory distress?

A. Diffuse, asymmetrical patchy infiltrates, areas of atelectasis with areas of alveolar hyperaeration
B. Ground-glass, hazy appearance, low lung volumes, and air bronchograms
C. Hyperlucent or opacified collection of air inside the pleural cavity, accompanied by a shift of mediastinal structures

157. The neonatal nurse practitioner (NNP) recognizes features of vulnerable child syndrome occur when the infant or child is:

A. Acutely unwell during the prolonged ICU stay
B. Engaging in repeated high-risk behaviors with parent support
C. Overprotected by the parent or parents to an extreme degree

158. An infant with biliary atresia (BA) may demonstrate which of the following at 24 hours of age?

A. Hyperbilirubinemia
B. Loose, yellow seedy stools
C. No apparent clinical signs

159. The neonatal nurse practitioner (NNP) reviews data for a preterm infant born at 26 weeks, now 2 days old. The 24-hour urine output was 185 mL and the infant's weight decreased from a birth weight (BW) of 1,279 to 1,008 g. The NNP recognizes these numbers reflect a/an:

   A. Appropriate amount of both urine output and weight loss
   B. Elevated urine output and rapid weight loss
   C. Low urine output but normal expected weight loss

160. Which of the following is true concerning the role of the mature kidney in acid–base regulation?

   A. Collecting tubules retain sodium if serum chloride is low
   B. Renal tubules reabsorb bicarbonate ions in the presence of acidosis
   C. Renal tubules secrete bicarbonate ions in the presence of hypochloremia

161. The neonatal nurse practitioner (NNP) understands the difference between a diagnosis of gestational hypertension and a diagnosis of preeclampsia is the presence or absence of maternal:

   A. Albuminemia
   B. Hematochezia
   C. Proteinuria

162. The neonatal nurse practitioner (NNP) should observe an infant who is undergoing the rewarming process for signs/symptoms of:

   A. Apnea
   B. Hyperglycemia
   C. Hypotension

163. An infant is born at 34 weeks' gestation and after the initial steps of resuscitation remains apneic. The neonatal nurse practitioner (NNP) initiated the correct next appropriate steps by:

   A. Beginning positive pressure ventilation (PPV), placing the pulse oximeter probe on the right hand or wrist, and evaluating the heart rate
   B. Stimulating the infant, initiating the heart rate
   C. Suctioning the airway, initiating PPV and placing the pulse oximeter probe on the right hand

164. A true statement about cardiac monitoring during newborn resuscitation is that EKG leads:

   A. Should be placed when compressions are begun
   B. Are not as accurate as use of a stethoscope
   C. Depend on adequate circulation for accuracy

165. The neonatal nurse practitioner (NNP) orders 2.5 g/kg/d of 20% intralipids (ILs) for a 1.8-kg preterm infant and calculates the infusion rate over 24 hours as:

   A. 0.74 mL/hr
   B. 0.84 mL/hr
   C. 0.94 mL/hr

166. The neonatal nurse practitioner (NNP) observes bilateral leukocoria (white pupils) in a term infant. There is also a clinical history of severe hearing impairment. The NNP is concerned about a congenital infectious etiology, specifically:

   A. Cytomegalovirus (CMV)
   B. Rubella
   C. Toxoplasmosis

167. The neonatal nurse practitioner (NNP) recognizes a primary risk factor for the development of neonatal early-onset sepsis (EOS) in the presence of maternal chorioamnionitis is the infant's:

   A. Fetal weight
   B. Gestational age
   C. Previous exposure

168. The neonatal nurse practitioner (NNP) recognizes the need to closely monitor an infant following an initial dose of captopril (Capoten) due to the risk of acute:

   A. Arrhythmias
   B. Hypotension
   C. Tachycardia

169. The neonatal nurse practitioner (NNP) correctly selects medications which promote gastrointestinal motility by choosing:

   A. Cimetidine (Tagamet) and famotidine (Pepcid)
   B. Metoclopramide (Reglan) and erythromycin ethylsuccinate (EES)
   C. Pantoprazole (Protonix) and rabeprazole (Aciphex)

170. The process which is responsible for the formation, production, and maintenance of pluripotent stem cells as they delineate into segregated blood cells is:

   A. Erythropoiesis
   B. Hematopoiesis
   C. Monopoiesis

171. The neonatal nurse practitioner (NNP) correctly chooses an indication for home monitoring in the event of a/an:

   A. History of sibling death from sudden infant death syndrome (SIDS)
   B. Infant discharged at 46 weeks' postmenstrual age (PMA)
   C. Request by the parent of a term infant

172. A male infant is born with congenital ichthyosis and the neonatal nurse practitioner (NNP) discusses with the parents the origins of this disorder, citing that it is a/an:

A. Error in zinc production
B. Genetic disorder
C. Infectious process

173. The major source of nonprotein energy for the growing preterm infants is:

A. Fat
B. Glucose
C. Minerals

174. The neonatal nurse practitioner (NNP) manages an infant with acute, symptomatic hypertension and understands the best control of the rate and optimal therapy results are achieved by using:

A. Intramuscular injection
B. Intravenous infusion
C. Oral loading dose

175. The neonatal nurse practitioner (NNP) recognizes a primary means to assess the adequacy of nutritional delivery is through the use of:

A. Behavioral maturation scores
B. Biochemical testing of blood
C. Bone density scanning with x-ray

Answers

1. **B. Mitochondrial DNA pattern**

   Mitochondrial DNA (mtDNA) is located only in the mitochondria of a cell and inherited entirely from the maternal side. More than 100 different mutations in mtDNA have been identified to cause disease in humans. Most of these involve the central nervous system or musculoskeletal system. Autosomal dominant and sex-linked patterns of inheritance are Mendelian (Bajaj & Gross, 2015)

2. **C. 22q11.2 deletion syndrome**

   Most patients with a deletion receive the diagnosis of 22q11.2 deletion syndrome (DiGeorge syndrome) following identification of significant cardiovascular malformations, conotruncal cardiac anomaly. With further evaluation, often aplasia or hypoplasia of the thymus and parathyroid glands is noted, along with functional T-cell abnormalities and hypocalcemia. Hypocalcemia occurs in 60% of neonates; severe cases will cause seizures. 11p15 methylation association is with Beckwith–Wiedemann syndrome, which does not involve issues with hypocalcemia, but rather hypoglycemia. 17q21.1 COL1A1 mutations are associated with osteogenesis imperfecta and have distinctive skeletal presentations not mentioned in the scenario (Haldeman-Englert et al., 2018; Sterk, 2015).

3. **A. Are common in infants and do not require treatment**

   Milia present as tiny, white monomorphic papules with a smooth surface. They are commonly seen on the forehead, cheeks, and chin. They are tiny inclusion cysts that form in the epidermis. No treatment is necessary and they will resolve spontaneously over several months (Khorsand & Sidbury, 2018).

4. **C. Initiate routine lacrimal duct massages**

   Nasolacrimal duct obstruction (NLDO) presents with epiphora (excess tearing). A simple NLDO usually requires conservative management. This consists of digital massage downward from the lacrimal sac over the nasolacrimal duct on the side of the nose. The massage empties the sac, reducing the opportunity for bacterial growth. Antibiotics and invasive procedures should be reserved for proven, complicated infection and are not appropriate as initial management (Campomanes & Binenbaum, 2018; Örge, 2020).

5. **C. The same as it was in utero**

   Neonatal hypoglycemia in IDMs is most likely due to hyperinsulinism. Despite high energy stores, after birth, the amount of insulin production remains the same, with less neonatal glucose supply, so the neonate has hypoglycemia in the first few hours of life, which may persist for several days. Less production would result in normal glucose levels, while increased (more) production would result in refractory hypoglycemia (Brown & Chang, 2018; Werny et al., 2018).

6. **B. Neural loss**

   Neural hearing loss occurs with the pathology of the inner hair cells and eighth cranial nerve with intact outer hair cells. Failure of sound transmission within the cochlea, outer and inner hair cells, and eighth cranial nerve is a manifestation of sensorineural hearing loss. Conductive loss occurs secondary to blockage(s) in the middle ear (Vohr, 2020).

7. **C. Tobacco**

   Nicotine has the most adverse effects on perinatal outcomes and readily crosses the placenta and the blood–brain barrier during pregnancy. Nicotine use in pregnancy is associated with intrauterine growth restriction (IUGR). There is no published information regarding the effects of herbal supplements or nutritional shakes on fetal growth (Blackburn, 2018; Wallen & Gleason, 2018).

8. **C. Less than 1 month old with *Escherichia coli* bacteremia**

   Meningitis can manifest in early-onset sepsis (EOS) or late-onset sepsis (LOS) with either vertical or horizontal transmission. EOS is vertically transmitted from the maternal genital tract and occurs within the first week of life, while LOS can be either vertically transmitted from maternal flora or horizontally transmitted from colonized caregivers. Within the first week of life, GBS or *E. coli* cause 70% of cases. After the first week of life, coagulase-negative staphylococci are more commonly isolated in the hospitalized infant. Other less common causative organisms include *Klebsiella*, *Enterobacter*, *Citrobacter*, and *Serratia* (Desai & Leonard, 2019; Esper, 2020; Ferrieri & Wallen, 2015; Hostetter & Gleason, 2018; Puopolo, 2017; Rudd, 2021).

9. **C. 4.4 mEq/kg/d**

Normal saline (using either chloride or acetate) equates to 15 mEq of Na per 100 mL of fluid.
Infant receiving 24 mL/d of fluid:
15 mEq × 24 mL/d = 360 mEq/mL/d
360 mEq/mL/d divided by 100 mL = 3.6 mEq/d
3.6 mEq/d divided by 082 kg = 4.4 mEq/kg/d Na delivery

10. **C. Spina bifida occulta**

Spina bifida occulta is the mildest form of spina bifida and is due to one or more vertebrae remaining open at the level of the spinous process; however, the spinal cord remains intact. Spina bifida presents with protruding meninges, except in the case of spina bifida cystica which presents with a fluid-filled transparent sac (cyst; Hills & Tomei, 2020).

11. **B. Diagnosis is made by polymerase chain reaction (PCR) testing of urine shortly after birth**

The diagnosis of congenital CMV infection is made through PCR testing (ideally urine) shortly after birth. It is difficult to differentiate acquired from congenital infection beyond 3 weeks of age. Most infants with congenital CMV infection are asymptomatic. Antiviral therapy is currently only recommended for symptomatic infants with central nervous system (CNS) involvement (Rudd, 2021).

12. **C. Known, benign familial inheritance trait**

Postaxial (ulnar) digits are most common among African Americans and are typically not associated with other anomalies. Typically, other family members have also been born with postaxial digits of either one or both hands. Polydactyly is not easily visualized on prenatal ultrasound. The involvement or not of specialists would need to be discussed with the family and the medical team together (Son-Hing & Thompson, 2015; Tappero, 2016).

13. **A. Near miss**

Safety events are generally classified in four ways: near misses, these errors are detected before they reach the patient; precursor events, these errors reach the patient but result in no detectable or only minimal harm; and serious safety issues, any error that reaches the patient and results in moderate to severe harm, including death. It may also be called a "sentinel" event (Pettker & Grobam, 2019; Simpson, 2021; Smith & Donze, 2021; Tyler & Napoli, 2019).

14. **A. Ampicillin and gentamicin**

Suspected early-onset pneumonia is usually treated with ampicillin and gentamicin. Late-onset pneumonia is treated with vancomycin and gentamicin. Cefotaxime is not an appropriate respiratory therapy (Rudd, 2019).

15. **C. Remove external heat sources from the infant**

The most common causes of neonatal hyperthermia are iatrogenic and environmental in nature. High room temperatures, improperly set heating controls (e.g., radiant warmer left in manual control mode or excessive servo control temperature setting), malpositioned temperature probes, excessive swaddling, and conditions that alter heat control, such as phototherapy use and incubator sun exposure, have been linked to neonatal hyperthermia. Until the potential iatrogenic and environmental causes of hyperthermia are removed as a first step and the infant's temperature reevaluated, no acute interventions should be performed (Chatson, 2017; Gardner & Cammack, 2021; Gardner & Snell).

16. **C. Reduced diastolic filling time**

SVT shortens diastole and compromises cardiac output, resulting in congestive heart failure. Cardiac afterload is not delayed due to the rapid heart rate with SVT. Reduced myocardial oxygenation is a secondary effect of reduced diastolic filling time (Tappero & Honeyfield, 2019).

17. **C. Subarachnoid space**

Subarachnoid hemorrhage is often silent, with seizures that can occur in term infants and with onset most commonly on day 2 of life. Massive hemorrhage with catastrophic deterioration is very rare but can occur. Usually, these infants have sustained severe perinatal asphyxia or an element of trauma. Intraventricular hemorrhages are only rarely associated with traumatic delivery, and bleeding into the cerebellum causes atrophy of tissues but not seizures (Inder et al., 2018).

18. **B. Minute ventilation**

Pregnancy causes increased minute ventilation. Other changes in the pulmonary system include increased minute ventilation, alveolar ventilation, tidal volume, and oxygen consumption, elevated pAO_2 and arterial pH, as well as decreased functional residual capacity, residual volume, and pCO_2. Respiratory rate does not change in pregnancy (Whitty & Dombrowski, 2019).

19. C. Hydrogen ion secretion by the parietal cells

Proton pump inhibitors (PPIs) are effective only if converted to their respective active moieties in the parietal cell canaliculi where active H⁺ ion secretion is taking place. Consequently, any condition or circumstance (e.g., administration of food, concomitant medications) that reduces H⁺ ion secretion (and raises pH) by the parietal cell will prolong the time of onset of effect consequent to delayed prodrug activation. Neither the fundal size nor the rate of gastric emptying affects the efficacy of omeprazole (Bohannon et al., 2020b; Domonoske, 2017; Taketomo, 2021).

20. A. Low-molecular-weight heparin (LMWH)

The most frequently used LMWH in pediatrics is enoxaparin. In neonates, LMWH (enoxaparin) has replaced UFH as the anticoagulant of choice in the initial treatment of thromboembolism because of the more predictable pharmacokinetics and ease of administration and monitoring. LMWH is also the preferred agent for long-term anticoagulation in neonates. PIVKA and UFH require more frequent monitoring and are less predictable in their actions (Bohannon et al., 2020b; Domonoske, 2017; Taketomo, 2021).

21. A. Blood flow into the brain is controlled in a steady manner

A factor that puts premature infants at higher risk for hemorrhage is the inability to autoregulate their cerebral blood flow. This concept refers to local control of blood flow in the brain. Sustaining consistent blood flow to the brain is vital in regulating pressure in these fragile vessels. Without autoregulation, the cerebral blood flow is in a pressure-passive state, unprotected from wide swings or changes. The more premature the infant, the more time spent in a pressure-passive state. Lack of autoregulation results in pressure-passive gradients. Venous blood is removed from ventricular spaces through normal circulatory patterns and is not dependent or associated with the autoregulation phenomena (Neil & Volpe, 2018).

22. B. 18

There is a 4:1 preponderance of females to males. Physical findings in Edwards syndrome (trisomy 18) include prenatal and postnatal growth deficiency, micrognathia, overlapping digits, complex congenital heart disease, low-set ears, rocker bottom clubfeet, and generalized hypertonicity. Associated anomalies include tracheoesophageal fistula or esophageal atresia, hemivertebrae, omphalocele, myelomeningocele, and radial dysplasia. Trisomy 13 physical findings include orofacial clefts, microphthalmia or absence of the eyes, low-set ears, moderate microcephaly, and scalp cutis aplasia. Down syndrome (trisomy 21) principal features include hypotonia, poor or absent Moro reflex, hyperextensibility of joints, excess skin at the nape of the neck, flat facial profile, low-set ears, slanted palpebral fissures, and single transverse palmar (simian) creases (Haldeman-Englert et al., 2018; Schiefelbein, 2015; Sterk, 2015).

23. C. Karyotyping (K)

A karyotype is the standard pictorial arrangement of chromosome pairs. The pairs are organized according to size and then evaluated for overall structure and banding pattern. CMA analysis allows for detection of chromosomal deletions and duplications too small to be seen in a high-resolution analysis. FISH uses DNA probe labeled with a fluorochrome, and the fluorescent signal is visible with microscopy. Some chromosomal structural abnormalities may be missed as the test detects genetic sequence, not its location (Matthews & Robin, 2021; Powell-Hamilton, 2020).

24. A. Brain development

Preterm infants are more likely to develop iron deficiency, which can have a negative impact on brain development (Poindexter & Martin, 2020).

25. C. Suction rectal biopsy

True confirmation of Hirschsprung disease is a rectal biopsy that demonstrates absence of ganglion cell and hypertrophic nonmyelinated axons in the nerve plexus. A contrast enema that demonstrates a transition zone is highly suggestive of Hirschsprung disease as there is delayed emptying of barium; however, it is not definitive. An abdominal radiograph is not specific enough to diagnose Hirschsprung disease (Bradshaw, 2021; Flynn-O'Brien et al., 2018; Gallagher et al., 2021; Ringer & Hansen, 2017).

26. B. Consideration of initiating prostaglandin E2 (alprostadil) infusion

The initiation of prostaglandin E2 (PGE2) is appropriate to manage clinical symptoms and prevent deterioration until a thorough diagnostic assessment can be done in order to determine the severity of aortic stenosis. Chest x-ray, EKG, and echocardiography are needed to assist in the diagnosis of stenosis severity or ventricular dysfunction. No indication of acidosis was given; therefore, sodium bicarbonate is unnecessary. Diuretic therapy is not applicable due to the low-volume (rather than high-volume) circulation induced by an aortic blockage (Fanaroff, 2020).

27. C. Pulmonary blood flow

Prostaglandin E by continuous infusion will improve oxygenation of babies with cyanotic heart disease due to decreased pulmonary blood flow (tetralogy of Fallot, truncus arteriosus, transposition of the great vessels, and tricuspid valve abnormalities). The same dose of prostaglandin E will open the ductus and facilitate right ventricular blood flow, which benefits the systemic circulation of babies presenting with decreased peripheral pulses and acidosis (critical aortic stenosis, coarctation of the aorta, and hypoplastic left heart syndrome [HLHS]). Prostaglandin does not affect the oxygen-carrying capacity nor the patency of the aorta (Gomella 2020).

28. B. Subarachnoid hemorrhage

Primary subarachnoid hemorrhage is blood within the subarachnoid space that is not a secondary extension from hemorrhage anywhere else within the skull (subdural, intraventricular, cerebellar, pia arachnoid). This includes any time elevated red blood cells and elevated protein counts are found in the CSF. Grade 1 intraventricular hemorrhage (IVH) does not involve bleeding into the CSF, while the subdural space is outside the CSF system (Hall & Reavey, 2021; Heaberlin, 2019; Inder et al., 2018; Soul, 2017).

29. A. Cytokines

The unifying hypothesis for these varying morbidities is that intraamniotic infection leads to fetal infection and to an excessive fetal production of cytokines, which in turn leads to pulmonary and central nervous system (CNS) damage. Inflammation is an incomplete answer as it is specifically cytokines, and leukocytes are only one component of the inflammatory system (Costantine et al., 2020; Duff, 2019; Polin & Randis, 2020).

30. B. Redistributing blood within the fetal organs

Infant adaptations to maternal anemia include redistribution of blood within the fetal organs, increased red blood cell production (not decrease) to increase oxygen-carrying capacity, and increased placental blood flow. Decreased growth and increased mortality are complications of maternal anemia as opposed to adaptations. Myocardial fibers will not grow in the absence of adequate oxygen and nutrition delivery (Blackburn, 2018).

31. A. Innate ability to balance heat production and heat loss

Thermoregulation is defined as the means by which the neonate's body temperature is maintained by balancing heat generation and heat loss in a changing environment and is a critical component in the physiologic adaptation to extrauterine life. Manipulation of the environment, sometimes by the use of warming devices, is an action taken in response to the neonates' innate thermoregulation ability or lack thereof (Cheffer & Rannalli, 2016).

32. B. Trisomy 13 duplication

Trisomy 13 is associated with midline malformations including congenital heart disease, cleft palate, holoprosencephaly, renal anomalies, and postaxial polydactyly. Eye anomalies and scalp defects can suggest the diagnosis. Aplasia cutis congenita is a congenital absence of skin involving the scalp. Cutis aplasia is not associated with DiGeorge syndrome or urea cycle disorder (Skert, 2015).

33. A. Pulmonary hemorrhage; PDA, prematurity, surfactant administration

Predisposing factors linked to pulmonary hemorrhage (PH) include patent ductus arteriosus (PDA), exogenous surfactant administration, sepsis, severe systemic illness, extreme prematurity, coagulopathy, intraventricular hemorrhage (IVH), heart disease, perinatal asphyxia, hypothermia, male sex, and multiple birth. It is rarely an isolated condition and is typically exhibited by the clinical presence of hemorrhagic fluid (pink or red frothy fluid) in the trachea. PH incidence is not related to sepsis, prematurity, sex, or age (Crowley, 2022; Fraser, 2021; Hansen & Levin, 2019; Jensen et al., 2022; Plosa, 2017).

34. B. Embryonic and pseudoglandular

The earliest phases of lung development establish the framework for the respiratory system, hence developmental aberrations resulting in anomalies occur more commonly in these phases. The embryonic phase occurs between 3 and 6 weeks. Abnormal development during this period can result in tracheal agenesis, tracheal stenosis, tracheoesophageal fistula (TEF), and pulmonary sequestration. The pseudoglandular period of lung development occurs between weeks 6 and 16. Abnormal development during this phase can result in congenital diaphragmatic hernia, bronchogenic cysts, and congenital lobar emphysema. Later stages are marked by evolution of the relationships between the air spaces, capillaries. The canalicular phase is marked by completion of the conducting airways through the level of the terminal bronchioles and the development of the rudimentary gas exchange units that are no longer invested with cartilaginous support. The saccular phase of lung development (24–38 weeks of human gestation) are when alveolar type I and type II cells are readily identified. True alveoli become evident as early as 36 weeks of gestation in the human fetus, initiating the alveolar phase of lung development (Joyner, 2019; Kallapur & Jobe, 2022; Keszler & Abubakar, 2022).

35. C. Scaphoid abdomen

The more proximal the obstruction, the more likely the infant will have an early onset of feeding intolerance/

emesis, with a more scaphoid abdomen due to the obstruction occurring high in the intestinal tract. The more distal the obstruction, the lower in the intestinal tract the obstruction occurs, allowing more intestines to have buildup of air with increased distention, and the later the onset of emesis will occur (Bradshaw, 2021; Gallagher et al., 2021; Gomella, 2020).

36. A. Change in pressure

The theorized physiology of variable decelerations is the following: Partial compression of the umbilical cord results first in hypotension secondary to umbilical vein compression that causes a chemoreceptor-stimulated bradycardia. Restrictions to blood flow that indicate fetal hypoxia are evidenced by "late" decelerations.

37. B. Exaggerated

With repeated exposure to pain, infants may lose discriminatory ability and develop hypersensitive states for long periods. This hypersensitivity persists even if nonnoxious stimuli are introduced. Chronic pain may alter perception, causing nonnoxious events to be perceived as painful, leading to a chronic pain response. Suppressed or destroyed pain responses are the opposite of what happens as a result of the hypersensitive state brought on by chronic pain.

38. C. Phentolamine (Regitine)

Phentolamine should be used in the event of extravasation by a vasoconstrictive drug such as dopamine. Hyaluronidase is indicated for infiltration caused by total parenteral nutrition. Epinephrine is not indicated for use in extravasations (Lund & Durand, 2016).

39. C. Up to 10 minutes after birth to achieve oxygen saturation above 90%

Preductal oxygen levels generally should be above 85% to 95% after 10 minutes. Newborns should become pink by 2 to 5 minutes of age (Heideric & Leone, 2020; Katheria & Finer, 2018; Niermeyer & Clarke, 2021; Owen et al., 2022; Papps & Robey, 2021; Ringer, 2017).

40. B. Increased pigmentation of the genitalia

The most common cause of CAH is 21-hydroxylase enzyme deficiency, accounting for more than 95% of all cases. Unprovoked hyponatremia may be an indication of CAH when paired with other findings. Both female and males may have increased pigmentation of the genitalia. Micropenis is associated with other congenital anomalies. Hydroceles are unrelated to genetic anomalies (Sorbara & Wherrett, 2020; Swartz & Chan, 2017).

41. B. Neuroprotective therapy

Prolonged treatment with caffeine reduces hypoxemia events in premature infants, the severity and duration of which are probably associated with adverse neurodevelopmental outcomes. Caffeine has a positive inotropic effect (rather than suppresses it) and does not act as a pulmonary vasodilator (Bohannon et al., 2020b; Domonoske, 2017; Taketomo, 2021).

42. A. 2 years of age

Two years is the earliest age to obtain a fairly reliable assessment of neurodevelopmental outcome. At age 4 to 5 years, cognitive function and language can be better measured, and follow-up at age 7 to 9 years allows an assessment of subtle neurologic and behavioral dysfunction and school academic performance (Wilson-Costello & Payne, 2020a).

43. C. Meningitis with bacteremia may be asymptomatic

An LP should be considered in any infant with suspected sepsis. Up to 15% of neonates with bacteremia will develop meningitis. Failure to perform an LP may result in a missed diagnosis (Desai, & Leonard, 2019; Esper, 2020; Rudd, 2021).

44. C. SCM torticollis

Torticollis may be caused by injury to the SCM) muscle, likely due to intrauterine positioning or birth trauma. Defining characteristics include firm, immobile circumscribed mass on SCM present at birth to 14 days of age and tilting of the head toward the affected side with inability to passively move to neutral position. Intervention includes early physical therapy. Neither Erb palsy nor a fractured clavicle prevents the infant from turning the head side-to-side (Kasser, 2015; Son-Hing, 2015; Tappero, 2019; White & Goldberg, 2018).

45. C. Hypotension no longer responsive to dopamine

Prolonged administration of sympathomimetic amines may result in diminished clinical efficacy secondary to diminished responses of alpha- and beta-receptors, referred to as tachyphylaxis. Hypoperfusion and hypocapnia are not part of the definition of tachyphylaxis (Domonoske, 2021).

46. A. Inadequate pharmacologic stimulation of the uterine wall

Whether induction is elective or indicated, adequate stimulation of uterine contractions is important in reducing the incidence of failed induction of labor. A minimum of 12 hours of oxytocin stimulation after membrane rupture is necessary before failed labor induction is diagnosed. As induction relates to stimulation of uterine contractions, cervical dilation is not a considered factor (Thorp, & Grantz, 2019).

47. A. Necrotizing enterocolitis

Standardized feeding guidelines have shown improved nutritional outcomes with optimized growth, reduced duration of parenteral nutrition (PN), and decreased incidence of necrotizing enterocolitis (NEC). Reduction of NEC and its comorbidities may in turn impact neurodevelopmental outcomes, but no consistent practice has demonstrated a tangible outcome. Development of an oral aversion is related to previous hospital experiences (e.g., an endotracheal tube [ETT]) and readiness to orally feed based on developmental assessments (Poindexter & Martin, 2020).

48. C. Preparation to treat neonatal hemorrhage complications

The goal for the mother's platelet count at delivery is greater than 50,000/mcL at the end of pregnancy. There is a risk of thrombocytopenia to the fetus due to maternal antiplatelet immunoglobulin G (IgG) crossing the placenta. This can lead to hemorrhage, and the delivery should be attended to by a team who can treat possible hemorrhage complications. Platelets, fresh frozen plasma, and IV immunoglobulin should be available. Acidemia secondary to hemorrhage is dependent on volume loss and is a later finding not addressed by the immediate newborn delivery team (Rodgers & Silver, 2019).

49. C. Informed consent

The key to true and valid consent is patient (or legal representative) comprehension. Informed consent is the voluntary authorization by a patient or the patient's legal representative to do something to the patient. Expressed consent is consent given by direct words, written or oral. Implied consent refers to the patient's conduct or what may be perceived in an emergency situation (Guido, 2013).

50. C. Negative nitrogen balance

Starter or stock PN (premade amino acid solution with dextrose) is recommended for preterm infants within the first 24 hours of postnatal life to compensate for high protein losses, even if providing a lower caloric intake. Blunted glucose productions and low caloric intake could be managed with dextrose-only solution but would not replace the protein losses which are critical to maintain positive nitrogen balance and prevent wasting (Poindexter & Martin, 2020; Denne, 2018).

51. C. Stop enteral feedings

The goal of acute management of metabolic or endocrine problems is to stop further decompensation and buildup of toxic metabolites. This may be accomplished through reducing or eliminating any food or drug that cannot be metabolized properly; replacing missing or inactive enzymes or other chemicals if possible; and removing toxic products of metabolism that accumulate due to the metabolic disorder. Bicarbonate will worsen metabolic acidosis. If fat oxidation defects are excluded after a metabolic evaluation, then lipids may be considered (Cederbaum, 2018; El-Hattab & Sutton, 2017; Konczal & Zinn, 2020; Swartz & Chan, 2017; Wassner & Belfort, 2017).

52. C. High-frequency oscillation ventilation (HFOV)

The defining difference among these three modes of HFV is the mechanism of action during inspiration and expiration. HFOV is the only one of these modes that uses an electromagnetically operated piston to generate oscillations in a push–pull method that achieves both active inspiration and expiration. The mechanism of action for expiration during HFJV and HFFI occurs as a result of passive lung recoil (Donn & Attar, 2020; Keszler et al., 2022).

53. B. Marfan syndrome

Six cardiac complications are classified as high risk by the World Health Organization (WHO). These are aortic valve stenosis, coarctation of the aorta, Marfan syndrome, peripartum cardiomyopathy, severe pulmonary hypertension, and tetralogy of Fallot (TOF; Blanchard & Daniels, 2019).

54. C. Measurement of intraocular pressure

Symptoms of congenital glaucoma can be apparent at birth or weeks to months later and include tearing, light sensitivity, blepharospasm (blinking), Haab striae (tears in the Descemet membrane, seen as lines in the red reflex), or lack of a red reflex. With acute glaucoma, high intraocular pressure is painful enough to manifest as crying, irritability, grimacing, poor feeding, or emesis in an infant. Slit lamps are used to examine the posterior segments of the eye. Genetic testing will not address the immediate problem (Campomanes & Binenbaum, 2018; Örge, 2020).

55. C. Pharmacokinetics

Pharmacokinetics is the mathematical relationship between drug dose and blood levels over time. Pharmacokinetic processes include absorption, distribution, metabolism (biotransformation), and excretion. Bioavailability is defined as the amount of drug administered that reaches the circulation or the amount of drug delivered to the site of action. Drug metabolism is the biotransformation of drug into inactive and active metabolites (Allegaert et al., 2018; Blackburn, 2018; Wade, 2020).

56. B. Geneticist

When physical examination findings or laboratory test results are abnormal (e.g., a metabolic acidosis combined with significantly elevated serum lactate and ammonia levels), then this may be the appropriate time to ask for a consult from a pediatric subspecialist. Depending on the case and stability of the infant, it may be appropriate to request a consult from a pediatric endocrinologist or geneticist. When an inborn error of metabolism is suspected, a geneticist is the appropriate initial consultation. There are no dermatologic findings noted, so this specialist consult would not be necessary. A nephrologist would not be appropriate to consult because there is no mention of intrinsic or extrinsic renal disease that led to these lab findings (Cederbaum, 2018; El-Hattab & Sutton, 2017; Swartz & Chan, 2017; Wassner & Belfort, 2017).

57. B. Base deficit of −18 mmol/L

Small molecule disorders include aminoacidopathies, including phenylketonuria (PKU), organic acidurias, urea cycle defects, and sugar intolerances, and result from the accumulation of toxic compounds before the blockage in the metabolic pathway or process. The infant may be symptom-free initially, then demonstrate acute or progressive intoxication after the metabolite accumulates. The accumulation leads to metabolic acidosis, demonstrated by a negative base deficit lab. A pH of 7.52 indicates an alkalosis, while a carbon dioxide of 22 mmHg is within the normal range (Merritt & Gallagher, 2018).

58. C. Tidal volume or amplitude

Ventilation refers to the removal of carbon dioxide (CO_2). In conventional ventilation strategies, CO_2 removal is most affected by tidal volume (amplitude of the breath defined by PIP minus positive end expiratory pressure [PEEP]) and frequency. In high-frequency ventilation (HFV) strategies, CO_2 removal is the product of the frequency and the square of the tidal volume (amplitude; Donn & Attar, 2020).

59. B. Confidence

Prior studies have demonstrated that when parents experience less stress, they are able to form early attachments to their sick infants. Mothers with greater stress have fewer positive attitudes and interactions with their infants than those with less stress. This lack of parenting confidence has been associated with lower levels of child competence, poorer developmental outcomes, and altered relationships with children into adulthood, and it affects multigenerational familial relationships. Conversely, multiple studies have shown that positive attitudes and parental confidence are associated with secure infant attachments, which lead to increased competence and better developmental outcomes (Gardner & Voos, 2021).

60. C. Substantive value of the lab result

There are questions the NNP should consider prior to ordering or obtaining a laboratory sample, which will assist in refining critical thinking skills and aid in the selective use of lab work. Does the patient require the laboratory test? Will the laboratory test request answer the "so what" question? If the laboratory sample is inadequate, faulty, or "lost," is it necessary to redraw it? (Scheans, 2022).

61. A. 2 and 9 weeks of age

When a positive Ortolani or Barlow test is present at birth and persists beyond the usual age of spontaneous resolution (2–9 weeks), the infant should be referred to an orthopedist for management. However, if the positive Ortolani or Barlow test disappears, then age-appropriate imaging (ultrasonography at 6 weeks or radiograph by 6 months) is warranted. If the baby has positive risk factors, such as breech positioning at birth or a family history but with stable hip examination findings, then age-appropriate imaging is recommended (ultrasonography at 6 weeks or radiograph at 6 months).

62. A. Bright, light, and hazy

Radiographic exposure denotes the amount of radiation used. With underexposure/underpenetration, images appear light and hazy. It is particularly difficult to view the vertebral bodies and/or any line placement due to the radiograph's brightness. With overexposure/overpenetration, images are dark and lack contrast. Positional rotation is not related to exposure (Trotter, 2022).

63. A. 3 months of age

The Joint Committee on Infant Hearing's 1-3-6 recommendation is that all infants should be screened for hearing loss no later than 1 month of age and that those who do not pass the screen should have a comprehensive evaluation by an audiologist no later than 3 months of age for confirmation of hearing status. Infants with confirmed hearing loss should receive appropriate intervention no later than 6 months of age from professionals with expertise in hearing loss and deafness in infants and young children (Carter & Carter, 2021; Stewart et al., 2017; Vohr, 2018, 2020).

64. B. Extreme prematurity

The incidence of ROP decreases with increasing gestational age. Over 80% of infants born at less than 26 weeks' gestation will develop some form of ROP compared with only 50% at 29 weeks. Assisted ventilation itself is not a risk factor, but the supplemental oxygen which may be delivered by devices is. Intraventricular hemorrhage is not related to ROP except in terms of each are more prevalent in lower gestational ages (Campomanes & Binenbaum, 2018; Fraser & Diehl-Jones, 2021; Sun et al., 2020).

65. B. Positive safety behaviors

Safety behaviors should be promoted throughout the organizational culture, and means to incorporate safety behaviors should be viewed as a positive intervention rather than punitive action. Examples of these actions are cross-checking, which involves confirmation of information from two separate sources to verify the accuracy; speaking up for safety, which involves the use of key phrases that focus on the system concern and not an individual; and coaching, modeling the safety behaviors and encouraging their use by others. The actions detailed here are not considered injurious or remedial (Tyler & Napoli, 2019).

66. A. Longer duration of action

PPIs decrease acid secretion by blocking the hydrogen/potassium (H^+/K^+) ATPase on the gastric parietal cell. Compared with H2 receptor antagonists, PPIs are more potent by directly blocking acid secretion and have a resultant increase in pH higher than 4 for a longer period of time (Bohannon et al., 2020b; Domonoske, 2017; Taketomo, 2021).

67. A. The mother should continue their antiretroviral therapy after pregnancy. The delivery method should be an individualized decision. Breastfeeding is contraindicated. The infant should be started on antiretroviral therapy within 6 to 12 hours of birth.

This mother is HIV-positive but has been on antiretroviral therapy throughout pregnancy and has a low viral load. Therefore, the decision for Cesarean section can be individualized. The infant should be started on antiretroviral therapy within 6 to 12 hours of birth. A mother who had not been on antiretroviral therapy or with an HIV RNA viral load greater than 1,000 copies/mL should have a scheduled Cesarean section. Breastfeeding is contraindicated if this woman resides in a country where safe feeding alternatives are regularly available. For mother–infant dyads at high risk of perinatal transmission, HIV DNA polymerase chain reaction (PCR) testing may be performed at the time of delivery; however, a negative result does not eliminate the possibility of perinatal transmission (American Academy of Pediatrics, 2021).

68. A. Narrow shape of the chest, rib orientation, compliant chest wall, and noncompliant lungs

The neonatal chest is more cylindrical compared with the elliptical shape of the adult. Neonatal ribs have a more horizontal orientation resulting in a relative shortening of the intercostal muscles. The compliant neonatal chest wall, in combination with noncompliant lungs, fewer interalveolar communications, less alveoli, and minimal surfactant production, can lead to chest wall collapse on expiration and atelectasis. This results in an increase in work of breathing (WOB; intercostal/subcostal retractions) and exaggerated abdominal breathing (Keszler & Abubakar, 2022).

69. B. Increase the peak inspiratory pressure (PIP) to improve mean airway pressure and oxygenation

This arterial blood gas demonstrates a low oxygen concentration in the blood. Poor oxygenation can be addressed by increasing the mean airway of mechanical ventilation. Mean airway pressure (P_{aw}) is the average pressure applied to the lungs during the respiratory cycle. P_{aw} is affected by PEEP, PIP, inspiratory time, frequency, and gas flow. In conventional ventilation strategies, carbon dioxide (CO_2) removal is most affected by tidal volume (amplitude of the breath defined by PIP minus PEEP) and frequency. Decreasing the tidal volume would increase CO_2 retention but would not affect oxygenation. Increasing the PEEP alone will increase the P_{aw} but also increase CO_2 retention, ultimately worsening respiratory acidosis (Donn & Attar, 2020).

70. C. Upper gastrointestinal tract study

The sudden onset in an infant that has been well-appearing, feeding with no issues, and with normal stooling must be considered a malrotation with volvulus until proven otherwise. The best diagnostic study for this infant is an upper gastrointestinal (GI) study. While it is always imperative to rule out a pneumoperitoneum prior to any contrast study, it is routine for this to be evaluated prior to administration of contrast by the radiologist. The upper GI will demonstrate absent or abnormal position of the ligament of Treitz. An abdominal flat-plate radiograph will not provide the positional details an upper GI would. A contrast enema would not focus on the area of concern (Bradshaw, 2021; Dingeldein, 2020a; Gallagher et al., 2021; Ringer & Hansen, 2017; Trotter, 2021).

71. A. Blood sera

The hallmark of isoimmunization is a positive direct antiglobulin test (DAT; also known as the Coombs test). This is indicative of maternally produced antibody that has traversed the placenta and is now found within the fetus. An indirect test refers to the antibody being detected in the serum. The test is termed direct if the antiglobulin is adhered to the red blood cells (RBCs). Progenitor cells do not adhere to maternal antibodies (Kaplan, 2015).

72. A. Adverse neurodevelopmental outcomes

Of particular concern is the association between suboptimal postnatal growth and adverse neurodevelopmental outcomes. There is increasing evidence that the amount of protein intake early in life correlates with improved neurodevelopmental outcomes. There is growing evidence that malnutrition during this critical period of central nervous system development results in irreversible long-term neurologic deficits (Demauro & Hintz, 2018; Poindexter & Martin, 2021).

73. C. Preserve existing nutritional stores

The initial goal of parenteral nutrition is to minimize losses and preserve existing body stores; this is particularly important for protein. Protein losses are significant in all neonates in the absence of amino acid intake, and these losses are the highest in the most immature neonates. Infants are provided with no amino acid supply; they lose over 1.5% of their body protein per day when they should be accumulating protein at a rate of 2% per day. Renal filtration is not dependent on the presence or absence of parenteral nutrition. Weight loss is expected and desired in the first few days after birth; therefore, no goal to artificially increase birth weight is appropriate (Denne, 2018).

74. A. Calcium

Subcutaneous nodule or nodules that are hard, non-pitting, and sharply circumscribed. Nodules may grow slightly larger over several days, then resolve on their own after several weeks to months. Calcification can occur and be associated with hypercalcemia. Neither sodium nor potassium is associated with SFN (Khorsand & Sidbury, 2018; Witt, 2018).

75. B. Spinal fluid glycine level

Second-line investigations may include urine, cerebral spinal fluid, or serum samples for metabolites or markers, such as urine succinylacetone, cerebral spinal fluid glycine, serum acylcarnitines, and other markers or metabolites. Arterial blood oxygen and whole blood serum lactate are considered first-line investigations (Cederbaum, 2018; El-Hattab & Sutton, 2017; Kim et al., 2018; Swartz & Chan, 2017; Wassner & Belfort, 2017).

76. B. Less than during a primary outbreak

The risk of neonatal transmission is lower in women with recurrent infections. The highest risk is associated with primary infection late in pregnancy (Bayley & Gonzalez, 2020; Duff, 2019; Schleiss & Marsh, 2018).

77. A. Hypoplastic left heart (HLH)

PDA and TA are considered aortic runoff lesions and are associated with bounding pulses. Left-side obstructive lesions such as HLH syndrome are associated with decreased or absent pulses (Tappero & Honeyfield, 2019).

78. C. Talipes equinovarus

Talipes equinovarus (TE) is characterized as adduction of the forefoot, pronounced varus, foot and toes in downward pointing position, equinus position, and atrophy of the affected lower extremity. TE may be unilateral or bilateral. When manipulated, the foot is unable to be passively positioned midline; this differentiates clubfoot from metatarsus adductus. Metatarsus adductus is a descriptive term for malpositioning of the toe(s). Streeter dysplasia is another term for amniotic band syndrome (Kasser, 2017; Son-Hing & Thompson, 2020; Tappero, 2019; White et al., 2018).

79. B. 10 and 12 in.

The newborn visual field is narrow and they are able to focus on objects at a distance of 10 to 12 in. (Tappero & Honeyfield).

80. A. Fewer layers of stratum corneum

Although both term and preterm infants are at risk of developing infections, preterm infants are at higher risk due to fewer layers of stratum corneum for protection. The stratum corneum constitutes the first line of defense against infection. The immature dermis or the thinner layers of subcutaneous fats play a secondary role of lesser import (Lund & Durand, 2016).

81. C. 3

Sarnat stage 3 (severe encephalopathy) is characterized by the following difficult to arouse or comatose with flaccid tone, intermittent decerebrate posturing (rare), absent reflexes (suck, gag, and Moro), and poorly reactive pupils. EEG has infrequent periodic discharges or is isoelectric. Stage 1 is mild encephalopathy in which the infant has normal activity and tone but with a weak suck. Stage 2 indicates moderate encephalopathy demonstrated by lethargy, hypotonia, and a weak or absent Moro reflex (Groenendaal & De Vries, 2020; Inder & Volpe, 2018; McAdams & Traudt, 2018).

82. B. CHARGE syndrome

There are numerous ocular abnormalities and systemic findings associated with colobomas, including more than 200 syndromes such as CHARGE syndrome. Choanal atresia occurs in approximately 1 in 5,000 to 7,000 live births. Congenital anomalies are present in approximately 50% of cases, CHARGE syndrome being a main one. Preauricular and auricular skin tags are sometimes associated with other dysmorphic features or syndromes (e.g., CHARGE).

Colobomas are not present in Beckwith–Wiedemann syndrome or Cornelia de Lange syndrome (Arnold, 2015; Bennett & Meier, 2018; Campomanes & Binenbaum, 2018; Lissauer & Hansen, 2020; Örge, 2020; Otteson & Wang, 2020).

83. **A. Baby born at 30 weeks, now 40 weeks, who spent 7 weeks on continuous positive airway pressure (CPAP) and is now going home on 0.2 L NC/100% FiO_2**

Respiratory syncytial virus (RSV) prophylaxis palivizumab (Synagis) is recommended for all high-risk infants and young children by the American Academy of Pediatrics (AAP). The criteria for RSV prophylaxis have not changed since 2014 and include but are not limited to infants born before 29 0/7 weeks of gestation; infants born before 32 0/7 weeks of gestation with chronic lung disease; infants with a persistent need for respiratory medical intervention into the second year of age; and other infants with compromised cardiopulmonary, neuromuscular, or respiratory system. Shots should begin before discharge into the community setting during the RSV season. These shots are administered monthly from November through March (Carter & Carter, 2021; Demauro & Hintz, 2018; Hummel & Naber, 2021).

84. **C. Procainamide (Pronestyl)**

Procainamide is indicated for treatment of supraventricular tachycardia (SVTs), such as atrial, reentrant, junctional, or ventricular tachycardia. Adenosine and procainamide are not indicated for treatment of SVT (Bohannon et al., 2020b; Domonoske, 2017; Taketomo, 2021).

85. **B. Dissociation of bicarbonate into H_2O and CO_2**

The major buffer, HCO_3^-, teams with H^+ to form carbonic acid, which dissociates into water and CO_2 to be eliminated. Bicarbonate does not accumulate within the lungs; kidneys govern bicarbonate. Immature or ill kidneys will overly excrete bicarbonate rather than retain it (Bell, 2021).

86. **B. Stridor**

Stridor is an abnormal finding at any age. Crackles can be heard as lung fluid is expelled after birth. Acrocyanosis is normal during transition (Tappero & Honeyfield).

87. **B. Galeazzi sign**

The Galeazzi sign is identified by placing the infant in a supine position and flexing the hips and knees into a 90-degree angle. If the knees are unequal in height, the infant is positive for Galeazzi sign. Ortolani sign is identified by placing fingers on the trochanter and the thumb on the femur while the femur is lifted forward as the thighs are abducted. If the femur head was dislocated, it can be felt to reduce. The Barlow sign is identified by adducting the thighs; if the femur head dislocates, it will be both felt and seen as it jerks suddenly over the acetabulum (White et al., 2018).

88. **C. Standard of care**

A standard of care is the minimum criteria by which proficiency is defined in the clinical arena. Clinical guidelines or practice protocols are unique to individual healthcare environments and do not define national standards (Verklan, 2015).

89. **C. Prostaglandin (PGE2) signaling**

With advancing postnatal age, dilator prostaglandins play less of a role in maintaining ductus patency. Hypoxic–ischemic constriction and metabolism of cyclooxygenases are not dependent on gestational age (Bohannon et al., 2020b; Domonoske, 2017; Taketomo, 2021).

90. **C. Spontaneous ileal perforation (SIP)**

The clinical presentation and x-ray are most likely related to an SIP; SIP typically presents early, in the first 1 to 2 weeks of life, with acute abdominal distention as a result of a focal perforation in the intestinal mucosa resulting in air in the abdominal cavity (pneumoperitoneum). Air being visible to the rectum rules out a bowel obstruction. Lack of pneumatosis and portal venous gas rules out NEC (Bradshaw, 2021; Dingeldein, 2020a; Gomella, 2020; Javid et al., 2018; Weitkamp et al., 2017).

91. **C. 3B**

Stage 3B best describes this infant due to presence of pneumoperitoneum. Stage 2B describes an infant with x-ray findings of pneumatosis and/or portal venous gas with systemic clinical signs. Stage 3A describes an infant with x-ray findings of pneumatosis and/or portal venous gas and is now critically ill with concerns of impending perforation (Caplan, 2020, 2021; Javid et al., 2018; Weitkamp et al., 2017).

92. **C. Reduces the risk of necrotizing enterocolitis**

There are multiple bioactive factors in human milk that influence host immunity, inflammation, and mucosal protection. Preterm infants exclusively fed with expressed human milk are at decreased risk of developing necrotizing enterocolitis (NEC). Both maternal milk and formulas are capable of meeting the nutritional requirements of growing infants (Kudin & Neu, 2020; Weitkamp et al., 2017).

93. **A. Availability to bring to the bedside**

Advantages of aEEG include bedside availability and interpretation, as well as reduced cost, as compared with continuous EEG monitoring. Disadvantages of aEEG include an inability to detect brief or low-amplitude seizures, or seizures that may occur in other parts of the brain not monitored by the two or four probes. aEEG does not detect low-amplitude seizures nor is it resistant to interference (Inder, 2020; Natarajan & Gospe, 2018).

94. **A. At 6 to 12 months of age**

Although the specific timing of the surgical treatment may differ between teams, it is generally accepted that individuals with synostosis should undergo cranial surgery in the first year of life. Delay past this point may impact (restrict) overall cranial development (Evans et al., 2018).

95. **B. Rapid critical appraisal (RCA)**

An RCA of the evidence involves answering questions as the validity, reliability, and applicability of the information the clinical question. RSA and RCI are not processes used in EBP (Ligappan & Gautham, 2022).

96. **A. Frontal bossing and "trident hands"**

Achondroplasia is a form of dwarfism characterized by frontal bossing, flattened nasal bridge, shortened arms and thighs, and average torso length with protruding abdomen. Knees and hands may be hyperextendable. Hands may be short and broad with widely spaced long and ring fingers, forming a "trident hand." There is generally some degree of genu varum. Mild to moderate hypotonia is also common in newborns. Dark-blue sclerae are indicative of osteogenesis imperfecta. A large but deformed cranium is not a typical finding within musculoskeletal disorders (Son-Hing & Thompson, 2020; Tappero, 2019).

97. **B. Have their torso and lower body placed in a bowel bag due to insensible water losses**

An infant with an omphalocele that has a ruptured sac is very similar to an infant with gastroschisis; both are at high risk for infection and increased evaporative and heat losses due to lack of covering of the intestinal contents. An infant with a omphalocele should be positioned on the side to prevent kinking of the viscera leading to vascular compromise. The dressing surrounding the defect should be clean but will not be able to remain sterile until or if it is surgically repaired (Bradshaw, 2021; Gallagher et al., 2021; Ledbetter et al., 2018).

98. **C. Sweet-smelling odor**

An infant with a disorder in protein metabolism may present with hypoglycemia, poor feeding, vomiting, unusual odor (including a "sweet" smell), hypothermia, respiratory distress, hyperammonemia, azotemia, metabolic acidosis, ketosis, cholestasis, hepatosplenomegaly, lymphadenopathy, or hematologic problems. Hepatosplenomegaly and lethargy are common presentation of a variety of disorders and not particular to disorders of protein metabolism (El-Hattab & Sutton, 2017; Konczal & Zinn, 2020).

99. **A. Brachial plexus injury**

A startle reflex (Moro reflex) that happens only on one side of the body (asymmetrical) may be due to an injury, such as damage to a nerve or spinal cord, or a fracture to the collarbone. A metatarsal injury affects the hand, and a brainstem injury would present with devastating whole-body dysfunction (Tappero & Honeyfield).

100. **B. Omphalocele**

An omphalocele will be covered by a sac contiguous with the umbilical cord. Gastroschisis typically occurs to the right of midline and is not enclosed in the cord, while patent urachus is a persistent embryonic connection between the bladder and the umbilicus (Martin et al., 2020).

101. **B. Hemodynamic instability**

Contraindications to trophic feedings include, but are not limited to, severe hemodynamic instability, medical treatment for patent ductus arteriosus, indications of ileus or clinical signs of intestinal pathology, or suspected or confirmed necrotizing enterocolitis (NEC). Less than 24 hours of age is not a contraindication to feedings of a healthy infant. Gastric residuals have been shown to be an unreliable indicator of feeding tolerance and should not be the sole rationale for feeding decisions (Anderson et al., 2017).

102. **C. Stabilization of the conductive tissue, dilution and intracellular shifting of K^+, and facilitating K^+ excretion**

Each of the steps in the sequence may be required depending on the severity of the symptoms; however, the first step is to ensure stabilization of the conductive tissue, which may include the administration of Ca^{2+}. Once the cardiac function is stable, the focus should shift to dilution with fluids, if indicated, and shifting K^+ into the intracellular space through the use of insulin/glucose drips, altering pH with sodium bicarbonate, or use of beta-2-adrenergic (such as albuterol). The last step is the facilitation of K^+ excretion, which may be accomplished by using Lasix to increase renal K^+ excretion, cation exchange resins, or double-volume blood exchange (Doherty, 2017).

103. A. Chloride

Anions are provided as either acetate or chloride (ions that are negatively charged). Cations are positively charged. Gluconate is a form of gluconic acid, while phosphate may be an anion or cation depending on the element with which it is paired (Denne, 2018).

104. B. 40% to 50%

Carbohydrates are the principal source of energy for the brain and heart and should supply 40% to 50% of an infant's total caloric intake (Anderson et al., 2017).

105. A. Immature response of the alpha receptors in the kidney

Differences in premature glomerular filtration rate and renal function in the premature infant 34 weeks' gestation are due primarily to incomplete nephrogenesis. Principle in nephrogenesis is the development of alpha receptors; therefore, immature alpha receptor responses lead to low glomerular filtration in the premature infant. Autoregulation of renal blood flow is accomplished through vasorelaxation and vasoconstriction of the afferent and efferent arterioles to maintain a constant blood supply to the kidneys, despite variations in systemic blood pressure (hypotension or hypertension). Nephrogenesis, the process of nephron formation, is complete by about 34 to 36 weeks of gestation (McAleer, 2018).

106. A. Fluoroscopy

Fluoroscopy is the most commonly used in neonates and infants due to the real-time dynamic images using rapid, sequential x-rays to image the gastrointestinal (GI) and genitourinary tracts. Benefits include real-time evaluation of motion, such as swallowing function, GI peristalsis, and diaphragmatic motion. Ultrasonography and radiography obtain one-time, static images singular to the point in time in which the images are taken and do not reflect changes over time, which can be captured with fluoroscopy (Abdulhayoglu, 2017; Crisci, 2020; Jensen et al., 2022; Weinman et al., 2021).

107. B. Maternal IgG antibodies

A positive result on DAT/Coombs test indicates the presence of maternal immunoglobulin G (IgG) antibodies in an infant's red blood cells (RBCs). Fetal hemoglobin in maternal blood is tested for using the Kleihauer–Betke test. Hemoccult testing does not involve the positive or negative state of the DAT (Diehl-Jones & Fraser, 2022; McKinney et al., 2021).

108. B. 9 months

Currently, the American Academy of Pediatrics (AAP) concurs that the use of postdischarge formulas to a postnatal age of 9 months results in greater linear growth, weight gain, and bone mineral content compared with the use of term infant formula. The AAP states that because these formulas are iron- and vitamin-fortified, no other supplements are needed. However, the average preterm infant taking 150 mL/kg/d may benefit from an additional 1 mg/kg/d iron until 12 months of age.

109. A. Apt test

The Apt test (alkali denaturation test) is based on the alkali resistance of fetal hemoglobin (HbF) to differentiate swallowed maternal blood with neonatal blood. Direct antiglobulin test (DAT) indicates the presence of maternal immunoglobulin G (IgG). Erythrocyte rosette test (ERT) for fetomaternal hemorrhage is the identification of HbF in maternal blood circulation specifically in Rh-negative women (Barry et al., 2021; Cadnapaphornchai et al., 2021; McKinney et al., 2021; Vogt & Springer, 2020).

110. B. Hypoxic–ischemic encephalopathy (HIE)

HIE is the most common cause of seizures in the neonatal period. Myoclonic events are not seizure-related, while meningitis is not a common etiology (McAdams & Traudt, 2020).

111. C. Gentamicin (Garamycin)

Gentamicin, an aminoglycoside, is the one antibiotic frequently given to infants that can cause kidney damage in high doses. Ampicillin and cefotaxime do not pose the same risk in the absence of intrinsic renal disease (Askenazi, 2018).

112. B. Beta-blockers

Medications used to treat hypertension include labetalol (beta-blockers), hydralazine (vasodilator), and methyldopa (antiadrenergics). The following classes of drugs are avoided due to risk of fetal damage: angiotensin-converting enzyme inhibitors, angiotensin receptor blockers, renin inhibitors, and mineralocorticoid receptor antagonists (Burgess, 2021; Harper et al., 2019; Jeyabalan, 2020; Moore, 2018).

113. B. Peak pressure needed to achieve the set volume indicates improved compliance

In the volume guarantee mode of ventilation, the NNP should recognize that improving lung compliance is demonstrated by a decrease in the peak inspiratory pressures necessary to achieve the desired tidal volume. The volume guarantee mode of ventilation sets a desired tidal volume and an acceptable peak pressure limit needed and allowing the patient's lung compliance to determine peak pressure for each breath. In this mode, there is no set pressure goal for each breath to achieve, as is seen in assist control/pressure control, nor would the peak pressure be set for a predetermined number of breaths, as is seen in synchronized intermittent mandatory ventilation (SIMV; Donn & Attar, 2020; Keszler & Abubakar, 2022).

114. **B. Fracture**

LGA babies are at greater risk for birth trauma. Infants with clavicle or humerus fractures may have pseudoparalysis of the affected upper extremity. A deformation occurs due to in utero pressures on normal tissues. A tumor would be a very rare finding (White et al., 2018).

115. **A. Autosomal dominant**

Approximately half of Mendelian disorders are inherited in an autosomal dominant fashion. This indicates that the phenotype usually appears in every generation, with each affected person having an affected parent. For each offspring of an affected parent, the risk of inheriting the mutated allele is 50% if there is only one parent with the gene. If both parents carry the gene, it will be inherited in all offspring. An autosomal recessive condition occurs when an individual possesses two mutant alleles that were inherited from heterozygous parents. Disorders of genes located on the X chromosome have a characteristic pattern of inheritance that is affected by sex (Bennett & Meier, 2019; Gross & Gheorghe, 2020; Lubbers, 2021; Powell-Hamilton, 2020).

116. **C. Rate, contraction, and vascular tone**

Inotropic/vasopressive agents include a broad range of medications that act to improve cardiac output by increasing the heart rate (chronotropic effect), the force of myocardial contraction (inotropic effect), and the vascular tone. They are used both for cardiovascular resuscitation and long-term support of the myocardium (Domonoske, 2021).

117. **C. Blood culture, CSF, and urine cultures, along with culture of any purulent skin lesions**

Evaluation of osteomyelitis should initially mimic a septic workup with blood, cerebrospinal fluid (CSF), and urine cultures, along with culture of any purulent skin lesions. Radiographic testing along with ultrasound and bone aspiration can aid diagnosis. Fluid collection from bone aspirations is positive 70% of the time and blood cultures are positive 60% of the

time (Gilmore & Thompson, 2020; Puopolo, 2017; White et al., 2018).

118. **C. Risks of passing substances to the baby through the breast milk**

Breastfeeding when a mother is not in recovery from substance use disorder is contraindicated due to the risk of passing substances to the baby through the breast milk. A person with substance use disorder should not be counseled to stop their intake immediately due to the risk of withdrawal. Individual metabolism processes are too varied to accurately predict when the medication will no longer transfer to the fetus or neonate (Prasad & Jones, 2019).

119. **B. Improve physiologic stability**

Benefits of delayed cord clamping for both term and preterm infants include an increase in blood volume and improvement in physiologic stability. DCC also increases lung-fluid absorption and oxygen-carrying capacity to tissues. A delay in erythropoiesis or a quantitative measurement of maternal antibodies has not been reported in infants who receive DCC (Goldsmith, 2020; Heideric & Leone, 2020; Katheria & Finer, 2018; Katheria et al., 2020; Niemeyer & Clarke, 2021; Papps & Robey, 2021).

120. **B. Hydrocortisone (Cortef)**

In critically ill preterm and term infants with vasopressor-resistant hypotension, steroid administration also serves as hormone substitution therapy. Hydrocortisone in preterm and term infants with vasopressor-resistant hypotension increases blood pressure within 2 hours of initiation of treatment. Fludrocortisone is a mineralocorticoid, while prednisone is a synthetic glucocorticoid (Bohannon et al., 2020b; Domonoske, 2017; Taketomo, 2021).

121. **A. 8 to 12 hours after birth**

Examination at a postnatal age of less than 12 hours of birth ensures validity of the examination in extremely premature infants (Tappero and Honeyfield). Delaying the exam to 24 hours or more lessens the exam's accuracy.

122. **C. Proteins**

Inborn errors of metabolism are genetic biochemical disorders in which the function of a protein is compromised, resulting in alteration of the structure or amount of protein synthesized. Fatty acids and carbohydrates do not have key functions in metabolism pathways (Sterk, 2015).

123. **B. Systematic approach to interpretation**

It is important to develop a systematic approach and order, as well as identify any anatomic and pathologic changes when assessing a film, including the lung fields, mediastinum, skeletal system, and catheters. Use the alphabetic approach: airway, bones, cardiac structures, diaphragm, effusions, fields and fissures, gastric fundus, and hilum and mediastinum. Preconceptions regarding disease or findings may cause anomalies to be overlooked (Jensen et al., 2022; Trotter, 2022).

124. **A. Anomalous external physical feature**

Anomalous external physical features are called dysmorphisms (Parikh & Mitchell, 2015). An abnormal mechanical force acting on otherwise normal tissues is a deformation.

125. **C. Eagle–Barrett syndrome**

Eagle–Barrett syndrome or prune belly syndrome results in a lack of abdominal musculature, hydronephrosis (dilated but unobstructed urinary tract) with dilated bladder, and bilateral cryptorchidism. This is the only disorder that presents in this manner. The lack of abdominal wall muscles, "prune-belly" presentation, is singular to Eagle–Barrett syndrome and therefore is not found in other syndromes (Maguire, 2021).

126. **C. Task-oriented to relationship-based model of care**

FCC demands a change from task-oriented, healthcare provider-centered care to a collaborative, relationship-based model of family advocacy and empowerment. The FCC principles stress that parents are the most important persons in their infant's life, that they have expertise in caring for the infant, and that their values and beliefs should be central during NICU care. FCC is applicable to either the acute or chronic care setting for either inpatient or outpatient follow-up (Gardner & Voos, 2021).

127. **B. Relative adrenal insufficiency**

Hydrocortisone induces the final enzyme in the transformation of norepinephrine to epinephrine in the adrenal gland and may therefore upregulate the release of epinephrine into circulation if these enzyme systems have matured sufficiently to be active. It is important to understand the rationale for hydrocortisone administration; because of the role of glucocorticoids in the physiologic regulation of adrenergic receptor expression, the emergence of vasopressor resistance may indicate a state of relative adrenal insufficiency. Hydrocortisone does not act on alpha-1-adrenergic receptors or on the hypothalamus (Bohannon et al., 2020b; Domonoske, 2017; Taketomo, 2021).

128. **B. Maternal primary infection at or near the time of delivery carries a higher risk of neonatal infection than remote maternal primary infection**

Maternal primary infection at or near the time of delivery carries the highest risk for neonatal HSV disease. Most mothers of affected infants have no known history of HSV or lesions present at the time of delivery; therefore, a negative maternal history should not deter practitioners from evaluating infants with HSV symptoms. Antiviral therapy should not be administered without evidence (laboratory or clinical) of disease (Greenberg et al., 2019; Schleis & Marsh, 2018).

129. **A. Coarctation of the aorta**

Aortic arch abnormalities such as coarctation of the aorta and interrupted aortic arch present with decreased perfusion distal to the area of the lesion. A ductus arteriosus or tetralogy of Fallot (TOF) will not present with a discrepancy between the upper and lower extremities (Martin et al., 2020).

130. **A. Expectations of parent–child relationship**

Anticipatory guidance describes the provision of information about what to expect from themselves and others. This term may be applied to the situation of a family taking their less-than-perfect infant home from the NICU. Knowledge of potential issues once at home can give parents confidence and aid in the transition (e.g., where they are in the grief process, issues with attachment, the risk for postpartum depression). Infant behaviors, parent–child relationship, safe-sleep practices. A family budget is a private matter not all families may wish to share; instead, actions should focus on determining available resources to assist the family with day-to-day expenses. Decisions regarding when or whether to place the infant in day care should be made collaboratively between the family and their primary care provider (Gardner & Carter, 2021; Reinhart & Gardner, 2017).

131. **C. 8th week of gestation**

Failure of the esophagus to recanalize during the 8th week results in esophageal atresia (Ditzenberger, 2018).

132. **C. Stable as long as delivery occurs at 1.5 to 2 minutes after uterine incision**

Benefits of general anesthesia include the establishment of a secure airway and ability to control ventilation. The process is rapid and has reliable onset, and there is potential for less hemodynamic instability. General anesthesia administration requires prompt delivery of the infant. Delivery of the infant within 90 to 120 seconds after making the uterine incision reduces the risk of fetal hypoxemia from altered uteroplacental and umbilical blood flow. Fetal sedation occurs with prolonged maternal anesthesia, and meconium aspiration can occur with either Cesarean or vaginal delivery independent of the type of anesthesia (Hoyt, 2020; Rollins & Rosen, 2018; Thorp & Gtrantz, 2019).

133. A. Intrinsic

Intrinsic renal failure may result from prolongation of hypovolemia, ischemic damage, or injury as a result of obstructive renal injury. Prerenal azotemia occurs in response to decreased renal blood flow (RBF). Postrenal acute kidney injury (AKI) is primarily due to obstructive kidney dysfunction occurring in utero secondary to congenital malformations (Askenazi et al., 2018).

134. B. Discontinue the current intralipid infusion

Debates on lipids are primarily centered on the acute metabolic effects of potentially adverse effects, such as chronic lung disease and bilirubin toxicity. Lipids should be infused to maintain serum triglycerides at less than 200 mg/dL. The lab may be repeated, but the infusion discontinued first. Bilirubin level is only necessary in the setting of hyperbilirubinemia (Poindexter & Martin, 2020).

135. B. Hypoxia

IHs are the most common skin anomaly of infancy. Risk factors for developing IHs include prematurity, multiple gestation, preeclampsia, placental abnormalities, advanced maternal age, and in vitro fertilization. It is hypothesized that the formation of IHs is linked to hypoxia. Euploidy and postmaturity are not associated with IHs (Gupta & Sidbury, 2018).

136. A. Eyes

Brushfield spots are white spots visualized around the iris. They may be a normal variant; however, they are a frequent finding in infants with trisomy 21. Brushfield spots do not occur on the palate or skin (Martin et al., 2020).

137. A. Body length

Lean mass growth is represented by an increase in length. Prolonged periods of inadequate nutrition can affect linear growth. Head circumference measures can be an indicator of brain growth but not overall growth. Dry weight can relate to an infant's perfusion and/or kidney function rather than growth (Brown et al., 2021).

138. B. Sturge–Weber syndrome

Congenital glaucoma can occur as a primary disease or secondary to numerous other ocular conditions or systemic syndromes, such as aniridia, congenital rubella, Hallermann–Streiff syndrome, Lowe syndrome, Axenfeld or Rieger syndrome, Sturge–Weber syndrome, and neurofibromatosis. It is not associated with Beckwith–Wiedemann or trisomy 21 (Őrge, 2020).

139. B. Echocardiogram

Echocardiography provides the most definitive diagnosis of CCHD. A hyperoxia test is a useful, quick screening which is helpful in the investigation of cyanotic congenital heart disease etiologies. Murmurs are also helpful but may be entirely absent in the presence of cyanotic congenital heart disease. A Doppler flow study cannot be performed on a neonatal chest (Gomella, 2020).

140. C. Total blood volume

Expected changes in pregnancy include increased total blood volume, plasma volume, red blood cell volume, cardiac output, heart rate, and myocardial contractility. Decreases in diastolic blood pressure, systemic vascular resistance, and pulmonary circulation are also seen. The following aspects do not change as a result of pregnancy: systolic blood pressure, central venous pressure, pulmonary capillary wedge pressure, ejection fraction, and left ventricular stroke work index (Blackburn, 2018; Blanchard & Daniels, 2019; Simpson & Creehan, 2021).

141. B. Developmental obstructive disorder, such as choanal atresia of the airway

Cyanosis at rest indicates that the newborn airway, which relies on obligate nose breathing, is obstructed. Choanal atresia is characterized by a blockage or narrowing of the nasal passage either bilaterally or unilaterally. While congenital heart disease and respiratory compromise are at the top of any differential diagnosis, the scenario presented here with the contrast between cyanosis at rest and relieved with crying should trigger thoughts of an airway obstruction (Dasgupta et al., 2016).

142. B. Erb palsy

Erb palsy is caused by injury to the fifth and sixth cervical nerve roots. Defining characteristics of the affected arm include adducted, internally rotated, and extended at the elbow with flexion of the wrist, with an intact grasp, known as the "waiter's tip" position. The infant may have a normal grasp with absent Moro reflex. Klumpke palsy results in complete lower arm paralysis with absent grip. The Barlow maneuver refers to hip stability rather than shoulder (Abdulhayoglu, 2017; Manguten et al., 2015; Tappero, 2019; White & Goldberg, 2018).

143. **B. Escalation in myocardial contractility**

Dobutamine is a synthetic catecholamine that promotes direct stimulation of myocardial adrenergic receptors. The resultant net hemodynamic effect is increased inotropy and chronotropy with either no effect or a decrease in systemic vascular resistance (SVR). Dobutamine increases myocardial contractility exclusively through the direct stimulation of myocardial adrenergic receptors. Increase in contractility and peripheral vascular resistance is the primary action of dopamine rather than dobutamine. Vasopressors in general act to increase the pulmonary artery to aortic pressure gradient (Bohannon et al., 2020b; Domonoske, 2017; Taketomo, 2021).

144. **C. 4 weeks of gestation**

Closure of the neural tube is complete by approximately the 26th day of gestation (Gressens et al., 2020).

145. **A. Dobutamine (Dobutrex)**

Dobutamine is a direct beta-2 agonist that increases myocardial contractility, oxygen delivery, and oxygen consumption. Dobutamine has a more prominent effect on cardiac output than dopamine. In comparison, dopamine has less impact on blood pressure. Epinephrine infusion results in peripheral vasoconstriction, which will increase the heart's workload (Gomella).

146. **A. Constrict blood vessels**

Angiotensin II is a potent vasoconstrictor of the peripheral blood vessels and the efferent arteriole. It also stimulates the release of aldosterone (rather than conversion of), thereby increasing sodium, chloride, and water reabsorption, increasing intravascular volume (Maguire, 2021).

147. **B. Manganese**

It is recommended to reduce or omit copper and manganese from PN in patients with impaired biliary excretion and/or liver disease because they are excreted in the bile. Chromium and selenium are excreted from the kidneys (Anderson et al., 2017).

148. **A. Insulin level**

Hyperinsulinemia will be diagnosed with measurement of glucose, insulin, cortisol, beta-hydroxybutyrate, and free fatty acid levels. Neither thyroid nor lactate levels will contribute pertinent information to manage the hypoglycemia (Burris, 2017).

149. **C. Metabolic acidosis**

It is important to note that cysteine hydrochloride supplements can produce metabolic acidosis unless appropriately buffered with acetate. Cysteine hydrochloride can result in metabolic acidosis, but this possibility can be appropriately countered by the use of acetate in the parenteral nutrition solution as a buffer. The presence or absence of cysteine does not affect electrolyte or triglyceride levels (Demauro & Hintz, 2018; Poindexter & Martin, 2021).

150. **B. Dehydration**

Because collodion causes infants to have an abnormal epidermal barrier, the practitioner needs to follow closely for complications such as dehydration, electrolyte imbalance, temperature instability, and infection. Hyperthermia is unlikely due to the compromised skin integrity, while anemia could happen independent of the skin condition (Witt, 2015).

151. **A. Many VSDs resolve spontaneously by 1 year of age**

In asymptomatic newborns, 45% of VSDs remain asymptomatic and spontaneously close during the first year of life. The infant will be monitored for signs of compromise but will not need emergent surgical intervention (Fanaroff, 2020).

152. **C. Thermoregulation**

It is important to next place a clear plastic bag over the exposed (omphalocele) as a temporary covering to minimize evaporative heat and fluid loss in the entire lower body. Surgical correction comes later in the plan of care, and adequate blood pressures are a priority regardless of accompanying abdominal wall defects (Ledbetter et al., 2018).

153. **A. Caput succedaneum**

Caput succedaneum is caused by edema (subcutaneous, extraperiosteal fluid) from the birth process. Findings include maximum swelling noted at birth, which may include ecchymosis, petechiae, or purpura; poorly defined edges; crosses the suture lines; occurs over the presenting portion of the scalp; and usually presents with molding. Cephalohematomas are confined to within the suture lines, and a subgaleal hemorrhage collection will extend posteriorly down the neck (Abdulhayoglu, 2017; Johnson, 2019; Tappero, 2021; Vargo, 2019).

154. **A. Erythema toxicum**

Erythema toxicum neonatorum is a benign, inflammatory condition in the newborn period. If examined microscopically, it would reveal a large number of eosinophils. No treatment is required. Lamellar ichthyosis or scalded skin syndrome does not demonstrate eosinophils (Khorsand & Sidbury, 2018).

155. **B. Occipital region**

Encephalocele arises from a failed closure of part of the rostral neural tube and most commonly occurs in the occipital region (70%–80%), with a sac protruding at the base of the skull or top of the neck. The remaining 20% to 30% are in the parietal, frontonasal, intranasal, or nasopharyngeal region (Huang & Doherty, 2018).

156. **A. Diffuse, asymmetrical patchy infiltrates, areas of atelectasis with areas of alveolar hyperaeration**

Classic findings of meconium aspiration syndrome (MAS) on chest radiography include diffuse, asymmetrical patchy infiltrates, areas of consolidation mixed with areas of atelectasis, alveolar hyperaeration, as well as a flattened diaphragm. Hyperaeration is due to air trapping from meconium debris. Ground-glass, hazy, low-volume lung fields with air bronchograms and atelectasis on chest x-ray are consistent with respiratory distress syndrome (RDS). Air leaks can occur in MAS due to overdistension and rupture of alveoli. A hyperlucent collection of air inside the pleural cavity, sometimes accompanied by a shift of mediastinal structures, is indicative of a pneumothorax or pulmonary air leak (Blackburn, 2018; Fraser, 2021; Guttentag, 2017; Hansen & Levin, 2019; Jensen et al., 2022; Shepherd & Nelin, 2022; Trotter, 2021).

157. **C. Overprotected by the parent or parents to an extreme degree**

Children may become victims of the vulnerable child syndrome, a condition in which a child is overprotected by their parents and treated as if they had a medical problem when it is no longer the case. Prolonged hospitalization, diagnosis of a chronic health condition, being a medically fragile survivor of a complicated neonatal hospital course or multiple pregnancy, and in some instances even a non–life-threatening, self-limited condition can predispose the child to vulnerable child syndrome. Parental reactions to their child's illness or perceived vulnerability can have long-term psychological consequences, with deleterious effects to the child and the family. Vulnerable child syndrome focuses on parental actions toward the child rather than the child's behaviors, high-risk or otherwise (Gardner & Voos, 2021).

158. **C. No apparent clinical signs**

Infants with BA typically present between 2 and 5 weeks of life with clinical signs. BA is associated with cholestatic rather than physiologic jaundice. An infant with BA will have acholic stools rather than yellow (Lane et al., 2018).

159. **B. Elevated urine output and rapid weight loss**

Fluid balance in the first few days after birth is associated with a urine output of 1 to 3 mL/kg/hr and a weight loss of 5% to 10% in term infants and 10% to 15% in preterm infants.

Weight loss calculation:

1,008 g divided by 1,279 g = 0.78

0.78 × 100 = 78% of BW = a 21% weight loss, which rapidly exceeds the expected losses

Urine output calculation:

185 mL/d divided by 1,279 kg = 144.64 mL/kg/d divided by 24 hours per day = 6 mL/kg/hr, which is elevated above usual expectations (Wright et al., 2018)

160. **B. Renal tubules reabsorb bicarbonate ions in the presence of acidosis**

In the presence of metabolic acidosis, the kidneys will release hydrogen ions in the urine and reabsorb bicarbonate ions from the filtrate in the tubules. Reabsorption of sodium is variable and dependent on the presence of aldosterone (Maguire, 2021).

161. **C. Proteinuria**

Gestational hypertension is defined as new-onset blood pressure elevations in the absence of proteinuria. Preeclampsia is defined as new-onset blood pressure elevations accompanied by proteinuria in pregnancy. Albuminemia and hematochezia are not associated with gestational hypertension or preeclampsia.

162. **C. Hypotension**

During the rewarming process, the hypothermic infant should be observed for hypotension as vasodilation occurs. Hypoglycemia, not hyperglycemia, may occur as a result of increased metabolic demand as an infant is rewarmed. Apnea is unrelated to the rewarming process (Gardner & Cammack, 2021).

163. **A. Beginning positive pressure ventilation (PPV), placing the pulse oximeter probe on the right hand or wrist, and evaluating the heart rate**

Begin PPV, after the initial steps, if the infant is without respiratory effort (apnea) or has gasping respirations despite tactile stimulation. The lack of respiratory effort increases the partial pressure of carbon dioxide ($PaCO_2$), lowering blood pH and causing metabolic acidosis. Suctioning and stimulation are actions that should have already been completed as part of the initial steps of resuscitation (Heiderich & Leone, 2020; Katheria & Finer, 2018; Niermeyer, Clarke, 2021; Pappas & Robey, 2021; Ringer, 2017).

164. A. Should be placed when compressions are begun

EKG leads should be placed when compressions are anticipated or begun. Cardiac monitoring is more accurate than pulse oximetry in determining the infant's response to resuscitation. Pulse oximetry relies on circulation, which may be poor, and cardiac monitor measures the heart's electrical activity (Goldsmith, 2020; Katheria & Finer, 2018; Niermeyer & Clarke, 2021; Owen et al., 2022).

165. C. 0.94 mL/hr

Determine g/kg/d of IV lipids needed (2.5 g/kg/d). Calculate g/d of IV lipids: weight of infant × desired g/kg/d = g/d, or 1.8 kg × 2.5 = 4.5 g/d. Convert g/kg into mL/kg/d: g/kg/d 0.2 (20% IV lipid solution) = mL/kg/d, or 4.5 g/d ÷ 0.2 = 22.5 mL/kg/d of IV lipids. Calculate mL/hr of IV lipids: mL/d 24 = mL/hr, 22.5 ÷ 24 = 0.94 mL/hr.

166. B. Rubella

Congenital cataracts are present in 30% of newborn infants with congenital rubella syndrome. Cataracts present as white pupils (leukocoria) that can be dense, milky white opacities in the lens. Cataracts are not associated with CMV or toxoplasmosis infections (Campomanes & Binenbaum, 2018; Fraser & Diehl-Jones, 2021; Órge, 2020).

167. B. Gestational age

Importantly, the risk of EOS in infants born to women with chorioamnionitis is inversely correlated with gestational age; therefore, it remains prudent to empirically treat chorioamnionitis-exposed preterm infants. Fetal weight and previous exposure to infectious processes are not primary risk factors (Polin & Randis, 2020; Rudd, 2021).

168. B. Hypotension

Angiotensin-converting enzyme (ACE) inhibitors are considered the drug of choice for adults and children with renal forms of hypertension (HTN), and although there is a long history of their use in neonatal HTN many neonatologists and pediatric nephrologists have serious concerns about potential major side effects, such as excessive hypotension. Arrhythmias, including tachycardia, are not potential effects of captopril (Bohannon et al., 2020b; Domonoske, 2017; Taketomo, 2021).

169. B. Metoclopramide (Reglan) and erythromycin ethylsuccinate (EES)

Drugs that promote gastrointestinal motility are thought to decrease gastroesophageal reflux (GER) by increasing gastric emptying or by improving esophageal motility and lower esophageal sphincter tone. The primary motility agents currently available in the United States are metoclopramide and erythromycin. Cimetidine and famotidine are histamine receptor agonists. Pantoprazole and rabeprazole are proton pump inhibitors (Bohannon et al., 2020b; Taketomo, 2021).

170. B. Hematopoiesis

Hematopoiesis is responsible for the formation, production, and maintenance of blood cells. It is the process of pluripotent stem cells delineation into segregated blood cells. Erythropoiesis is the process of red blood cell (RBC) production. Monopoiesis is the process of formation or production of monocytes (Blackburn, 2013a; Diab & Luchtman-Jones, 2015; Diehl-Jones & Fraser, 2015; Juul & Christensen, 2018).

171. A. History of sibling death from sudden infant death syndrome (SIDS)

Home monitoring is indicated in the following: premature infant with symptoms of idiopathic apnea of prematurity who is otherwise ready for hospital discharge; a survivor of an apparent life-threatening event defined as apnea, cyanosis, altered muscle tone, choking, or gagging; sibling death due to SIDS; tracheostomy, mechanically supported ventilation; a sleep apnea syndrome caused by a neurologic disorder, periodic breathing, upper airway abnormality, or idiopathic syndromes; and other conditions of ill or high-risk infants, as determined on an individual basis. Home monitoring is not indicated in the prevention of SIDS in symptom-free, healthy infants. In 80% of infants, apnea of prematurity will cease between 40 and 44 weeks of postmenstrual age; in asymptomatic infants, home monitoring can be stopped at 45 weeks of postmenstrual age.

172. B. Genetic disorder

Congenital ichthyosis is a rare disorder; X-linked ichthyosis is the most common form of ichthyosis in the newborn period, affecting approximately 1 in 2,500 male babies. Ichthyosis is not infectious and is not dependent on zinc production (Witt, 2015).

173. A. Fat

Fat provides the major source of nonprotein energy for growing preterm infants, which should include approximately 50% of the postnatal caloric intake. Glucose provides carbohydrate energy, while minerals are not sources of energy (Bell, 2021; Poindexter & Martin, 2020).

174. B. Intravenous infusion

Critically ill infants should be treated with an intravenous agent administered by continuous infusion, as this allows the greatest control of the rate and magnitude. Oral or intramuscular dosing routes are less reliable in terms of absorption and action (Allegaert et al., 2018; Domonoske, 2021).

175. B. Biochemical testing of blood

Measurements of chemical substances in the body reflect metabolic processes, disease states, and chemical activity or state. These measurements are useful in the diagnosis, planning of care, monitoring of therapy, screening, and determining the severity of disease and response to treatment. Biochemical testing also provides information for assessing nutritional adequacy or medication toxicity (Bell, 2022; Scheans, 2022).

References

Abbott, K. L., Kendrick, D. E., Chen, X., Krumm, A. E., Jones, A. T., & George, B. C. (2021). How many attempts are needed to achieve general surgery board certification? *Journal of Surgical Education, 78*(3), 885–888. https://doi.org/10.1016/j.jsurg.2020.08.047

Abdulhayoglu, E. (2017). Birth trauma. In E. Eichenwald, A. Hansen, C. Martin, & A. Stark (Eds.), *Cloherty and Stark's manual of neonatal care* (8th ed., pp. 64–75). Lippincott Williams & Wilkins.

Abend, N., Jense, F., Inder, T., & Volpe, J. (2018). Neonatal seizures. In J. Volpe, T. Inder, B. Darras, L. deVries, A. Plessis, & J. Perlman (Eds.), *Volpe's neurology of the newborn* (6th ed., pp. 275–321.e14). Elsevier.

Abrams, S. A. (2017a). Abnormalities of serum calcium and magnesium. In E. Eichenwald, A. R. Hansen, C. R. Martin, & A. R. Stark. (Eds.), *Cloherty and Stark's manual of neonatal care* (8th ed., pp. 326–334). Lippincott Williams & Wilkins.

Abrams, S. A. (2017b). Osteopenia (metabolic bone disease) of prematurity. In E. Eichenwald, A. Hansen, C. Martin, & A. Stark (Eds.), *Cloherty and Stark's manual of neonatal care* (8th ed., pp. 853–858). Lippincott Williams & Wilkins.

Abrams, S. A., & Tiosano, D. (2020). Disorders of calcium, phosphorus, and magnesium metabolism in the neonate. In R. J. Martin, A. A. Fanaroff, & M. C. Walsh (Eds.), *Fanaroff and Martin's neonatal-perinatal medicine: Diseases of the fetus and infant* (11th ed., pp. 1611–1642). Elsevier.

Abubakar, M. K. (2020a). Cardiorespiratory monitoring. In J. Ramasethu & S. Seo (Eds.), *MacDonald's atlas of procedures in neonatology* (6th ed., pp. 73–80). Wolters Kluwer.

Abubakar, M. K. (2020b). Continuous blood gas monitoring. In J. Ramasethu & S. Seo (Eds.), *MacDonald's atlas of procedures in neonatology* (6th ed., pp. 91–100). Wolters Kluwer.

Abubakar, M. K. (2020c). End-tidal carbon dioxide monitoring. In J. Ramasethu & S. Seo (Eds.), *MacDonald's atlas of procedures in neonatology* (6th ed., pp. 101–104). Wolters Kluwer.

Adamkin, D. H., & Radmacher, P. G. (2020). Nutrition and selected disorders of the gastrointestinal tract. Part one: Nutrition for the high-risk infant. In A. Fanaroff & J. Fanaroff (Eds.), *Klaus and Fanaroff's care of the high-risk neonate* (7th ed., pp. 80–120). Elsevier.

Adams, E. D. (2021). Antenatal care. In K. Simpson, P. A. Creehan, N. O'Brien-Abel, C. K. Roth, & A. J. Rohan (Eds.), *AWHONN's perinatal nursing* (5th ed., pp. 66–98). Lippincott Williams & Wilkins.

Ades, A., & Johnston, L. C. (2020). Endotracheal intubation. In J. Ramasethu & S. Seo (Eds.), *MacDonald's atlas of procedures in neonatology* (6th ed., pp. 281–293). Wolters Kluwer.

Agren, J. (2020). Thermal environment of the intensive care nursery. In R. J. Martin, A. A. Fanaroff, & M. C. Walsh (Eds.), *Fanaroff & Martin's neonatal-perinatal medicine: Diseases of the fetus and infant* (11th ed., pp. 566–576). Elsevier.

Ahmad, I. (2020a). Necrotizing enterocolitis. In T. L. Gomella, F. G. Eyal, & F. Bany-Mohammed (Eds.), *Gomella's neonatology: Management, procedures, on-call problems, diseases, and drugs* (8th ed., pp. 991–997). McGraw-Hill Education.

Ahmad, I. (2020b). Spontaneous intestinal perforation. In T. L. Gomella, F. G. Eyal, & F. Bany-Mohammed (Eds.), *Gomella's neonatology: Management, procedures, on-call problems, diseases, and drugs* (8th ed., pp. 1067–1069). McGraw-Hill Education.

Ali, N., & Sawyer, T. (2020). Resuscitation of the newborn. In T. L. Gomella, F. G. Eyal, & F. Bany-Mohammed (Eds.), *Gomella's neonatology: Management, procedures, on-call problems, diseases, and drugs* (8th ed., pp. 19–30). McGraw-Hill Education.

Allegaert, K., Smits, A., & van den Anker, J. N. (2021). Aminoglycosides. In S. J. Yaffe & J. V. Aranda (Eds.), *Yaffe and Aranda's neonatal and pediatric therapeutic principles in practice* (5th ed., pp. 310–320). Lippincott Williams & Wilkins.

Allegaert, K., Ward, R. M., & Van Den Anker, J. N. (2018). Neonatal pharmacology. In C. A. Gleason & S. E. Juul (Eds.), *Avery's diseases of the newborn* (10th ed., pp. 419–431). Elsevier.

Alpan, G. (2020a). Infant of a mother with substance use disorder. In T. L. Gomella, F. G. Eyal, & F. Bany-Mohammed (Eds.), *Gomella's neonatology: Management, procedures, on-call problems, diseases, and drugs* (8th ed., pp. 945–954). McGraw-Hill Education.

Alpan, G. (2020b). Patent ductus arteriosus. In T. L. Gomella, F. G. Eyal, & F. Bany-Mohammed (Eds.), *Gomella's neonatology: Management, procedures, on-call problems, diseases, and drugs* (8th ed., pp. 1027–1031). McGraw-Hill Education.

American Association of Collages of Nursing. (2021). *The essentials: Core competencies for professional nursing education.* https://www.aacnnursing.org/Portals/42/AcademicNursing/pdf/Essentials-2021.pdf

American Nurses Association. (2015). *Code of ethics for nurses with interpretive statements.* https://www.nursingworld

.org/practice-policy/nursing-excellence/ethics/code-of-ethics-for-nurses/coe-view-only/

Anderson, D. M., Poindexter, B. B., & Martin, C. R. (2017). Nutrition. In E. C. Eichenwald, A. R. Hansen, C. R. Marin, & A. R. Stark (Eds.), *Cloherty and Stark's manual of neonatal care* (pp. 248–284). Lippincott Williams & Wilkins.

Anderson, T., Ogruk, G., & Beu, T. J. (2021). Taking professional certification exams: The correlation between exam preparation techniques and strategies and exam results. *Journal of Higher Education Theory and Practice, 21*(5), 42–52. https://doi.org/10.33423/jhetp.v21i5.4267

Angelidou, A. I., & Christou, H. A. (2017). Anemia. In E. Eichenwald, A. Hansen, C. Martin, & A. Stark (Eds.), *Cloherty and Stark's manual of neonatal care* (8th ed., pp. 755–767). Lippincott Williams & Wilkins.

Anxiety and Depression Association of America. (2012). *Test anxiety*. Anxiety and Depression Association of America.

Aplan, G. (2020). Persistent pulmonary hypertension of the newborn. In T. L. Gomella, F. G. Eyal, & F. Bany-Mohammed (Eds.), *Gomella's neonatology: Management, procedures, on-call problems, diseases, and drugs* (8th ed., pp. 1032–1040). McGraw-Hill Education.

Arafeh, J. (2021). Cardiac disease in pregnancy. In K. Simpson & P. Creehan (Eds.), *Perinatal nursing* (5th ed., pp. 330–361). Lippincott Williams & Wilkins.

Arensman, R. M., Short, B., Koo, N., & Mudreac, A. (2022). Extracorporeal membrane oxygenation. In M. Keszler & K. S. Gautham (Eds.), *Goldsmith's assisted ventilation of the neonate: An evidence-based approach to newborn respiratory care* (7th ed., pp. 351–362). Elsevier.

Armentrout, D. (2021). Glucose management. In M. T. Verklan, M. Walden, & S. Forest (Eds.), *Core curriculum for neonatal intensive care nursing* (6th ed., pp. 162–171). Elsevier.

Askenazi, D., Selewski, D., Willig, L., & Warady, B. A. (2018). Acute kidney injury and chronic kidney disease. In C. A.Gleason & S. E. Juul (Eds.), *Avery's diseases of the newborn* (10th ed., pp. 1280–1300). Elsevier.

Asmar, B. I., & Abdel-Haq, N. (2021). Tetracyclines. In J. V. Aranda & J. N. Van Den Anker (Eds.), *Yaffe and Aranda's neonatal and pediatric therapeutic principles in practice* (5th ed., pp. 347–365). Lippincott Williams & Wilkins.

Attarian, S., & Rao, R. (2020). Nutritional management. In T. L. Gomella, F. G. Eyal, & F. Bany-Mohammed (Eds.), *Gomella's neonatology: Management, procedures, on-call problems, diseases, and drugs* (8th ed., pp. 125–165). McGraw-Hill Education.

Bacino, C. A. (2017). Genetic issues presenting in the nursery. In A. R. Hansen, A. R. Start, E. C. Eichenwald, & C. Martin (Eds.), *Cloherty and Stark's manual of neonatal care* (8th ed., pp. 117–130). Lippincott Williams & Wilkins.

Bahadue, F. L., & Gecsi, K. S. (2020). Antenatal and intrapartum care of the high-risk infant. In A. A. Fanaroff & J. M. Fanaroff (Eds.), *Klaus and Fanaroff's care of the high-risk neonate* (7th ed., pp. 9–47). Elsevier.

Bailey, T. C., & Maltsberger, H. L. (2021). Common invasive procedures. In T. Verklan, M. Walden, & S. Forest (Eds.), *Core curriculum for neonatal intensive care nursing* (6th ed., pp. 244–269). Elsevier.

Baley, J. E. (2020). Schedule for immunization of preterm infants. In R. Martin, A. Fanaroff, & M. Walsh (Eds.), *Fanaroff and Martin's neonatal-perinatal medicine: Diseases of the fetus and infant* (11th ed., pp. 2067–2068). Elsevier.

Baley, J., & Gonzalez, B. (2020). Perinatal viral infections. In R. Martin, A. Fanaroff, & M. Walsh (Eds.), *Fanaroff and Martin's neonatal-perinatal medicine: Diseases of the fetus and infant* (11th ed., pp. 844–911). Elsevier.

Bancalari, E., Claure, N., & Jain, D. (2018). Neonatal respiratory therapy. In C. Gleason & E. S. Juul (Eds.), *Avery's diseases of the newborn* (10th ed., pp. 636–652). Elsevier.

Bancalari, E. H., & Jain, D. (2020). Bronchopulmonary dysplasia. In R. Martin, A. A. Fanaroff, & M. C. Walsh (Eds.), *Fanaroff and Martin's neonatal-perinatal medicine: Diseases of the fetus and infant* (11th ed., pp. 1256–1269). Elsevier.

Bany-Mohammed, F. (2020a). Chlamydial infection. In T. L. Gomella, F. G. Eyal, & F. Bany-Mohammed (Eds.), *Gomella's neonatology: Management, procedures, on-call problems, diseases, and drugs* (8th ed., pp. 1115–1116). McGraw-Hill Education.

Bany-Mohammed, F. (2020b). Gonorrhea. In T. L. Gomella, F. G. Eyal, & F. Bany-Mohammed (Eds.), *Gomella's neonatology: Management, procedures, on-call problems, diseases, and drugs* (8th ed., pp. 1127–1128). McGraw-Hill Education.

Bany-Mohammed, F. (2020c). Human immunodeficiency virus. In T. L. Gomella, F. G. Eyal, & F. Bany-Mohammed (Eds.), *Gomella's neonatology: Management, procedures, on-call problems, diseases, and drugs* (8th ed., pp. 1143–1150). McGraw-Hill Education.

Bany-Mohammed, F. (2020d). Methicillin-resistant staphylococcus aureus. In T. L. Gomella, F. G. Eyal, & F. Bany-Mohammed (Eds.), *Gomella's neonatology: Management, procedures, on-call problems, diseases, and drugs* (8th ed., pp. 1157–1159). McGraw-Hill Education.

Bany-Mohammed, F. (2020e). Rubella. In T. L. Gomella, F. G. Eyal, & F. Bany-Mohammed (Eds.), *Gomella's neonatology: Management, procedures, on-call problems, diseases, and drugs* (8th ed., pp. 1171–1174). McGraw-Hill Education.

Bany-Mohammed, F. (2020f). Syphilis. In T. L. Gomella, F. G. Eyal, & F. Bany-Mohammed (Eds.), *Gomella's neonatology: Management, procedures, on-call problems, diseases, and drugs* (8th ed., pp. 1189–1196). McGraw-Hill Education.

Bany-Mohammed, F. (2020g). Toxoplasmosis. In T. L. Gomella, F. G. Eyal, & F. Bany-Mohammed (Eds.), *Gomella's neonatology: Management, procedures, on-call problems, diseases, and drugs* (8th ed., pp. 1197–1201). McGraw-Hill Education.

Bany-Mohammed, F. (2020h). Varicella-Zoster infections. In T. L. Gomella, F. G. Eyal, & F. Bany-Mohammed (Eds.), *Gomella's neonatology: Management, procedures, on-call problems, diseases, and drugs* (8th ed., pp. 1211–1215). McGraw-Hill Education.

Bany-Mohammed, F. (2020i). TORCH (TORCHZ) infections. In T. L. Gomella, F. G. Eyal, & F. Bany-Mohammed (Eds.), *Gomella's neonatology: Management, procedures, on-call problems, diseases, and drugs* (8th ed., p. 1196). McGraw-Hill Education.

Barrington, K. J., & Dempsey, E. M. (2022). Common hemodynamic problems in the neonates requiring respiratory support. In M. Keszler & K. S. Gautham (Eds.), *Goldsmith's assisted ventilation of the neonate: An evidence-based approach to newborn respiratory care* (7th ed., pp. 424–445). Elsevier.

Barry, J. S., Deacon, J., Hernandez, C., & Jones, M. D. (2021). Acid-base homeostasis and oxygenation. In S. L. Gardner, B. S. Carter, M. Enzman-Hines, & S. Niermeyer (Eds.), *Merenstein & Gardner's handbook of neonatal intensive care: An interprofessional approach* (9th ed., pp. 145–157). Elsevier.

Barton Associates. (2019). *Nurse practitioner scope of practice laws.* https://www.bartonassociates.com/locum-tenens -resources/nurse-practitioner-scope-of-practice-laws

Bass, N. (2020). Hypotonia and neuromuscular disease in the neonate. In R. Martin, A. Fanaroff, & M. Walsh (Eds.), *Fanaroff and Martin's neonatal-perinatal medicine: Diseases of the fetus and infant* (11th ed., pp. 1044–1059). Elsevier.

Basu, S., & Dobrolet, N. (2020). Congenital defects of the cardiovascular system. In R. J. Martin, A. A. Fanaroff, & M. C. Walsh (Eds.), *Fanaroff and Martin's neonatal-perinatal medicine: Diseases of the fetus and infant* (11th ed., pp. 1342–1363). Elsevier.

Bates, C. M., & Schwaderer, A. L. (2018). Clinical evaluation of renal and urinary tract disease. In C. A. Gleason & S. E. Juul (Eds.), *Avery's diseases of the newborn* (10th ed., pp. 1274–1323). Elsevier.

Beals, D. A. (2020). Neonatal bioethics. In T. L. Gomella, F. G. Eyal, & F. Bany-Mohammed (Eds.), *Gomella's neonatology: Management, procedures, on-call problems, diseases, and drugs* (8th ed., pp. 289–295). McGraw-Hill Education.

Beauduy, C. E., & Winston, L. G. (2021a). Aminoglycosides & spectinomycin. In B. G. Katzung & T. W. Vanderah (Eds.), *Basic and clinical pharmacology* (15th ed., pp. 857–865). McGraw Hill.

Beauduy, C. E., & Winston, L. G. (2021b). Beta-lactam & other cell wall-membrane-active antibiotics. In B. G. Katzung & T. W. Vanderah (Eds.), *Basic and clinical pharmacology* (15th ed., pp. 823–843). McGraw Hill.

Beauduy, C. E., & Winston, L. G. (2021c). Miscellaneous antimicrobial agents: Disinfectants, antiseptics, & sterilants. In B. G. Katzung & T. W. Vanderah (Eds.), *Basic and clinical pharmacology* (15th ed., pp. 932–940). McGraw Hill.

Beauduy, C. E., & Winston, L. G. (2021d). Tetracyclines, Macrolides, Clindamycin, chloramphenicol, streptogramins, oxazolidinones, & pleuromutilins. In B. G. Katzung, & T. W. Vanderah (Eds.), *Basic and clinical pharmacology* (15th ed., pp. 844–856). McGraw Hill.

Bell, S. G. (2021). Fluid and electrolyte management. In M. T. Verklan, M. Walden, & S. Forest (Eds.), *Core curriculum for neonatal intensive care nursing* (6th ed., pp. 131–143). Elsevier.

Benitz, W. E., & Bhombal, S. (2020). Patent ductus arteriosus. In R. J. Martin, A. A. Fanaroff, & M. C. Walsh (Eds.), *Fanaroff and Martin's neonatal-perinatal medicine: Diseases of the fetus and infant* (11th ed., pp. 1334–1341). Elsevier.

Benjamin, J. T., & Maheshwari, A. (2020). Developmental immunology. In R. J. Martin, A. A. Fanaroff, & M. C. Walsh (Eds.), *Fanaroff & Martin's neonatal-perinatal medicine: Diseases of the fetus and infant* (11th ed., pp. 752–788). Elsevier.

Bennet, M., & Meier, S. R. (2019). Assessment of the dysmorphic infant. In E. P. Tappero & M. E. Honeyfield (Eds.),

Physical assessment of the newborn (6th ed., pp. 219–237). Springer Publishing Company.

Berghella, V., & Giraldo-Isaza, M. A. (2020). Fetal assessment. In T. L. Gomella, F. G. Eyal, & F. Bany-Mohammed (Eds.), *Gomella's neonatology: Management, procedures, on-call problems, diseases, and drugs* (8th ed., pp. 1–13). McGraw-Hill Education.

Beriln, S. (2020). Diagnostic imaging of the neonate. In R. Martin, A. Fanaroff, & M. Walsh (Eds.), *Fanaroff and Martin's neonatal-perinatal medicine: Diseases of the fetus and infant* (11th ed., pp. 608–633). Elsevier.

Berlin, S. C., & Meyers, M. L. (2020). Neonatal imaging. In: A. A. Fanaroff & J. M. Fanaroff (Eds.), *Klaus and Fanaroff's care of the high-risk neonate* (7th ed., pp. 409–436.e2). Elsevier.

Black, S., & Miller, S. (2018). Brain injury in the preterm infant. In C. Gleason & S. Juul (Eds.), *Avery's diseases of the newborn* (10th ed., pp. 879–696). Elsevier.

Blackburn, S. T. (2018a). Bilirubin metabolism. In S. T. Blackburn (Ed.), *Maternal, fetal, & neonatal physiology: A clinical perspective* (5th ed., pp. 607–626). Elsevier.

Blackburn, S. T. (2018b). Cardiovascular system. In S. T. Blackburn (Ed.), *Maternal, fetal, & neonatal physiology: A clinical perspective* (5th ed., pp. 251–296). Elsevier.

Blackburn, S. T. (2018c). Gastrointestinal and hepatic systems and perinatal nutrition. In S. T. Blackburn (Ed.), *Maternal, fetal, & neonatal physiology: A clinical perspective,* (5th ed., pp. 387–434). Elsevier.

Blackburn, S. T. (2018d). Hematologic and hemostatic systems. In S. T. Blackburn (Ed.), *Maternal, fetal, & neonatal physiology: A clinical perspective* (5th ed., pp. 216–251). Elsevier.

Blackburn, S. T. (2018e). Immune system and host defense mechanisms. In S. T. Blackburn (Ed.), *Maternal, fetal, & neonatal physiology: A clinical perspective* (5th ed., pp. 443–483). Elsevier.

Blackburn, S. T. (Ed.). (2018f). The integumentary system. In S. T. Blackburn (Ed.), *Maternal, fetal, & neonatal physiology: A clinical perspective* (5th ed., pp. 484–508). Elsevier.

Blackburn, S. T. (2018g). *Maternal, fetal, & neonatal physiology: A clinical perspective* (5th ed., pp. 18–25, 551–612). Elsevier.

Blackburn, S. T. (2018h). Neurologic, muscular, and sensory systems. In S. T. Blackburn (Ed.), *Maternal, fetal, & neonatal physiology: A clinical perspective* (5th ed., pp. 497–542). Elsevier.

Blackburn, S. T. (2018i). Pharmacology and pharmacokinetics during the perinatal period. In S. T. Blackburn (Ed.), *Maternal, fetal, & neonatal physiology: A clinical perspective* (5th ed., pp. 180–214). Elsevier.

Blackburn, S. T. (2018j). Postpartum period and lactation physiology. In S. T. Blackburn (Ed.), *Maternal, fetal, & neonatal physiology: A clinical perspective,* (5th ed., pp. 142–161). Elsevier.

Blackburn, S. T. (2018k). Renal system and fluid and electrolyte homeostasis. In S. T. Blackburn (Ed.), *Maternal, fetal, & neonatal physiology: A clinical perspective* (5th ed., pp. 356–392). Elsevier.

Blackburn, S. T. (2018l). Respiratory system. In S. T. Blackburn (Ed.), *Maternal, fetal, & neonatal physiology: A clinical perspective* (5th ed., pp. 297–350). Elsevier.

Blackburn, S. T. (2018m). The prenatal period and placental physiology. In S. T. Blackburn (Ed.), *Maternal, fetal,*

& *neonatal physiology: A clinical perspective* (5th ed., pp. 61–114). Elsevier.

Blackburn, S. T. (2018n). Thermoregulation. In S. T. Blackburn (Ed.), *Maternal, fetal, & neonatal physiology: A clinical perspective* (5th ed., pp. 639–660). Elsevier.

Blackburn, S. T. (2021). Endocrine disorders. In M. T. Verklan, M. Walden, & S. Forest (Eds.), *Core curriculum for neonatal intensive care nursing* (6th ed., pp. 543–567). Elsevier.

Blanchard, D., & Daniels, L. (2019). Cardiac diseases. In R. Resnik, C. Lockwood, T. Moore, M. Greene, J. Copel, & R. Silver (Eds.), *Creasy and Resnik's maternal-fetal medicine: Principles and practice* (8th ed., pp. 920–948.e3). Elsevier.

Blickstein, I., & Hershkovich-Shporen, C. (2020). Fetal effects of auto immune disease. In R. J. Martin, A. A. Fanaroff, & M. C. Walsh (Eds.), *Fanaroff & Martin's neonatal-perinatal medicine: Diseases of the fetus and infant* (11th ed., pp. 346–354). Elsevier.

Blickstein, I., Perlman, S., Hazan, Y., Shinwell, E., & Gonzalez, B. (2020). Pregnancy complicated by diabetes mellitus. In R. Martin, A. Fanaroff, & M. Walsh (Eds.), *Fanaroff and Martin's neonatal-perinatal medicine: Diseases of the fetus and infant* (11th ed., pp. 304–311). Elsevier.

Blickstein, I., & Rimon, O. F. (2020). Post-term pregnancy. In R. Martin, A. Fanaroff, & M. Walsh (Eds.), *Fanaroff and Martin's neonatal-perinatal medicine: Diseases of the fetus and infant* (11th ed., pp. 364–370). Elsevier.

Blickstein, I., & Shinwell, E. S. (2020). Obstetric management of multiple gestation and birth. In R. Martin, A. Fanaroff, & M. Walsh (Eds.), *Fanaroff and Martin's neonatal-perinatal medicine: Diseases of the fetus and infant* (11th ed., pp. 355–363). Elsevier.

Bocks, M. L., Boe, B. A., & Galantowicz, M. E. (2020). *Neonatal management of congenital heart disease*. In R. J. Martin, A. A. Fanaroff, & M. C. Walsh (Eds.), *Fanaroff and Martin's neonatal-perinatal medicine: Diseases of the fetus and infant* (11th ed., pp. 1393–1414). Elsevier.

Bohannon, K., Gomella, T. L., Ho, P., & Nolt, V. D. (2020). Hyperkalemia. In T. L Gomella, F. G. Eyal & F. Bany-Mohammed (Eds.), *Gomella's neonatology: Management, procedures, on-call problems, diseases, and drugs* (8th ed., pp. 566–573). McGraw-Hill Education.

Bohannon, K., Ho, P., & Nolt, V. D. (2020a). Effects of drugs and substances on lactation and infants. In T. L. Gomella, F. G. Eyal, & F. Bany-Mohammed (Eds.), *Gomella's neonatology: Management, procedures, on-call problems, diseases, and drugs* (8th ed., pp. 1316–1334). McGraw-Hill Education.

Bohannon, K., Ho, P., & Nolt, V. (2020b). Medications used in the neonatal intensive care unit. In T. L. Gomella, F. G. Eyal, & F. Bany-Mohammed (Eds.), *Gomella's neonatology: Management, procedures, on-call problems, diseases, and drugs* (8th ed., pp. 1225–1316). McGraw-Hill Education.

Bohannon, K., Ho, P., & Nolt, V. D. (2020c). Hypertension. In T. L. Gomella, F. G. Eyal, & F. Bany-Mohammed (Eds.), *Gomella's neonatology: Management, procedures, on-call problems, diseases, and drugs* (8th ed., pp. 574–587). McGraw-Hill Education.

Boos, M. D., & Sidbury, R. (2018). Infections of the skin. In C. A. Gleason & S. E. Juul (Eds.), *Avery's diseases of the newborn* (10th ed., pp. 1495–1502.e2). Elsevier.

Boucher, N., Marvicsin, D., & Gardner, S. (2017). Physical examination, interventions, and referrals. In B. Snell & S. Gardner (Eds.), *Care of the well newborn* (pp. 101–134). Jones and Bartlett Learning.

Bowe, A. C. (2020). Rash and dermatologic problems. In T. L. Gomella, F. G. Eyal, & F. Bany-Mohammed (Eds.), *Gomella's neonatology: Management, procedures, on-call problems, diseases, and drugs* (8th ed., pp. 726–742). McGraw-Hill Education.

Bradshaw, W. T. (2021). Gastrointestinal disorders. In M. T. Verklan, M. Walden, & S. Forest (Eds.), *Core curriculum for neonatal intensive care nursing* (6th ed., pp. 504–542). Elsevier.

Brand, M. C., & Shippey, A. A. (2021). Thermoregulation. In M. T. Verklan, M. Walden, & S. Forest (Eds.), *Core curriculum for neonatal intensive care nursing* (6th ed., pp. 86–98). Elsevier.

Breinholt, J. P. G. (2017). Cardiac disorders. In E. Eichenwald, A. Hansen, C. Martin, & A. Stark (Eds.), *Cloherty and Stark's manual of neonatal care* (8th ed., pp. 510–575). Lippincott Williams & Wilkins.

Brown, L. D., Hendrickson, K., Evans, R., Davis, J., & Hay, W. A. (2021). Enteral nutrition. In S. L. Gardner, B. S. Carter, M. Enzman- Hines, & S. Niermeyer (Eds.), *Merenstein & Gardner's handbook of neonatal intensive care: An interprofessional approach* (9th ed., pp. 480–533). Elsevier.

Brown, Z., & Chang, J. (2018). Maternal diabetes. In C. Gleason & S. Juul (Eds.), *Avery's diseases of the newborn* (10th ed., pp. 90–103). Elsevier.

Brunkhorst, L. J., Nyp, M., Reavy, D., & Pallotto, E. K. (2021). Fluid and electrolyte management. In *Merenstein & Gardner's handbook of neonatal intensive care: An interprofessional approach* (9th ed., pp. 407–430). Elsevier.

Buhimsch, C. S., Mesiano, S. J., & Muglia, L. J. (2019). Pathogenesis of spontaneous preterm birth. In R. Resnik, C. J. Lockwood, T. R. Moore, M. F. Greene, J. A. Copel, & R. M. Silver (Eds.), *Creasy & Resnik's maternal-fetal medicine: Principles & practice* (8th ed., pp. 92–126e17). Elsevier.

Burgess, A. (2021). Hypertensive disorders of pregnancy. In K. Simpson & P. Creehan (Eds.), *Perinatal nursing* (5th ed., pp. 181–216). Lippincott Williams & Wilkins.

Burris, H. (2017). Hypoglycemia and hyperglycemia. In E. C. Eichenwald, A. R. Hansen, C. R. Martin, & A. R. Start (Eds.), *Cloherty and Stark's manual of neonatal care* (8th ed., pp. 312–325). Lippincott Williams & Wilkins.

Busenhart, C. (2017). Discharge teaching. In B. Snell & S. Gardner (Eds.), *Care of the well newborn* (pp. 235–251). Jones & Bartlett Learning.

Cadnapaphornchai, M. A., Soranno, D. E., Bisio, T. J., Woloschuk, R., & Kirkley, M. (2021). Neonatal nephrology. In S. L. Gardner, B. S. Carter, M. Enzman-Hines, & S. Niermeyer (Eds.), *Merenstein & Gardner's handbook of neonatal intensive care: An interprofessional approach* (9th ed., pp. 886–928). Elsevier.

Campomanes, A. G., & Binenbaum, G. (2018). Eye and vision disorders. In C. Gleason & S. Juul (Eds.), *Avery's diseases of the newborn* (10th ed., pp. 1536–1557). Elsevier.

Cannon, B., & Snyder, C. S. (2020). Disorders of cardiac rhythm and conduction in newborns. In R. J. Martin, A. A. Fanaroff, & M. C. Walsh (Eds.), *Fanaroff and Martin's neonatal-perinatal medicine: Diseases of the fetus and infant* (11th ed., pp. 1375–1392). Elsevier.

Caplan, M. (2020). Part 3: Necrotizing enterocolitis. In A. A. Fanaroff & J. M. Fanaroff (Eds.), *Klaus and Fanaroff's care of the high-risk neonate* (7th ed., pp. 115–117). Elsevier.

Carlo, W. (2020). Perinatal and neonatal care in developing countries. In R. Martin, A. Fanaroff, & M. Walsh (Eds.), *Fanaroff and Martin's neonatal-perinatal medicine: Diseases of the fetus and infant* (11th ed., pp. 120–139). Elsevier.

Carlo, W. A., & Ambalavanan, N. (2020). Assisted ventilation. In A. A. Fanaroff & J. M. Fanaroff (Eds.), *Klaus and Fanaroff's care of the high-risk neonate* (7th ed., pp. 211–226). Elsevier.

Carlson, C. A., & Shirland, L. (2010). *Neonatal parenteral and enteral nutrition: A resource guide for the student and novice neonatal nurse practitioner.* National Association of Neonatal Nurses. http://nann.org/uploads/Membershi p/MembersOnllyPDFS/Neonatal_Parenteral_and_Enter al_Nutrition.pdf

Carter, A., & Carter, B. S. (2021). Discharge planning and follow-up of the neonatal intensive care unit infant. In S. Gardner, B. Carter, M. Enzman-Hines, & S. Niermeyer (Eds.), *Merenstein & Gardner's handbook of neonatal intensive care* (9th ed., pp. 1141–1166). Elsevier.

Cassady, J. C., & Johnson, R. E. (2002). Cognitive test anxiety and academic performance. *Contemporary Educational Psychology, 27,* 270–295. https://doi.org/10.1006/ceps.2 001.1094

Cavaliere, T. (2019). Genitourinary assessment. In E. P. Tappero & M. E. Honeyfield (Eds.), *Physical assessment of the newborn: A comprehensive approach to the art of physical examination* (6th ed., pp. 121–137). Springer Publishing Company.

Cederbaum, S. (2018). Introduction to metabolic and biochemical genetic diseases. In C. Gleason & S. Juul (Eds.), *Avery's diseases of the newborn* (10th ed., pp. 209–229). Elsevier.

Chakkarapani, E., & Thoresen, M. (2020). Whole-body cooling. In J. Ramasethu & S. Seo. (Eds.), *MacDonald's atlas of procedures in neonatology* (6th ed., pp. 395–407). Wolters Kluwer.

Chatson, K. (2017). Temperature control. In E. Eichenwald, A. Hansen, C. Martin, & A. Stark (Eds.), *Cloherty and Stark's manual of neonatal care* (8th ed., pp. 185–191). Lippincott Williams & Wilkins.

Cheffer, N., & Rannalli, D. (2016). Transitional care of the newborn. In S. Mattson & J. Smith (Eds.), *Core curriculum for maternal-newborn nursing* (5th ed., pp. 343–362). Elsevier.

Chogi, H. Y., Rivera, A., & Chahine, A. A. (2020). Central venous catheterization. In J. Ramasethu & S. Seo (Eds.), *MacDonald's atlas of procedures in neonatology* (6th ed., pp. 233–252). Wolters Kluwer.

Choi, H. (2020). Aseptic preparation. In J. Ramasethu & S. Seo (Eds.), *McDonald's atlas of procedures in neonatology* (6th ed., pp. 51–56). Wolters Kluwer.

Choi, H. Y., Rivera, A., & Chahine, A. A. (2020). Central venous catheterization. In J. Ramasethu & S. Seo (Eds.), *MacDonald's atlas of procedures in neonatology* (6th ed., pp. 233–252). Wolters Kluwer.

Christensen, R. D. (2018). Neonatal erythrocyte disorders. In C. Gleason & S. Juul (Eds.), *Avery's diseases of the newborn* (10th ed., pp. 1152–1179e.4). Elsevier.

Chu, A., & Devaskar, S. U. (2020). Interuterine growth restriction. In R. Martin, A. Fanaroff, & M. Walsh (Eds.), *Fanaroff and Martin's neonatal-perinatal medicine: Diseases of the fetus and infant* (11th ed., pp. 260–273). Elsevier.

Chuang, J., & Gutmark-Little, I. (2020). Thyroid disorders in the neonate. In R. J. Martin, A. A. Fanaroff, & M. C. Walsh (Eds.), *Neonatal-perinatal medicine: Diseases of the fetus and infant* (11th ed., pp. 1643–1664). Elsevier.

Churchman, L. (2021). Apnea. In T. Verklan, M. Walden, & S. Forest (Eds.), *Core curriculum for neonatal intensive care nursing* (6th ed., pp. 417–424). Elsevier.

Claudette, M. (2014). Lived experiences of failure on the National Council Licensure Examination-Registered Nurse (NCLEX-RN): Perceptions of registered nurses. *Journal of International Nursing, 6*(1), 10–14. https://doi .org/10.5958/j.0974-9357.6.1.003

Claure, M., & Bancalari, E. (2022). Special techniques of respiratory support. In M. Keszler & K. S. Gautham (Eds.), *Goldsmith's assisted ventilation of the neonate: An evidence-based approach to newborn respiratory care* (7th ed., pp. 263–268). Elsevier.

Clemmens, C., Hysinger, E. B., & Piccione, J. (2022). Airway evaluation: Bronchoscopy, laryngoscopy, and tracheal aspirates. In M. Keszler & K. S. Gautham (Eds.), *Goldsmith's assisted ventilation of the neonate: An evidence-based approach to newborn respiratory care* (7th ed., pp. 144–150). Elsevier.

Clyman, R. I. (2018). Patent ductus arteriosus in the preterm infant. In C. A. Gleason & S. E. Juul (Eds.), *Avery's diseases of the newborn* (10th ed., pp. 790–800.e6). Elsevier.

Coe, K., Bradshaw, W. T., & Tanaka, D. T. (2021). Physiologic monitoring. In S. L. Gardner, B. S. Carter, M. Enzman-Hines, & S. Niermeyer (Eds.), *Merenstein & Gardner's handbook of neonatal intensive care: An interprofessional approach* (9th ed., pp. 165–185). Elsevier.

Colaizy, T. T., Demauro, S. B., McNeilis, K. M., & Poindexter, B. B. (2018). Enteral nutrition for the high-risk neonate. In C. A. Gleason & S. E. Juul (Eds.), *Avery's diseases of the newborn* (10th ed., pp. 1009–1022.e4). Elsevier.

Costantine, M. M., Saad, A., & Saade, G. (2020). Obstetric management of prematurity. In R. Martin, A. Fanaroff, & M. Walsh (Eds.), *Fanaroff and Martin's neonatal-perinatal medicine: Diseases of the fetus and infant* (11th ed., pp. 312–345). Elsevier.

Cotton, M., & Murray, J. (2018). The human genome and neonatal care. In C. Gleason & S. Juul (Eds.), *Avery's diseases of the newborn* (10th ed., pp. 180–189.e2). Elsevier.

Cottrill, C. M., & Hidestrand, P. (2020a). Congenital heart disease. In T. L. Gomella, F. G. Eyal, & F. Bany-Mohammed (Eds.), *Gomella's neonatology: Management, procedures, on-call problems, diseases, and drugs* (8th ed., pp. 862–873). McGraw-Hill Education.

Cottrill, C. M., & Hidestrand, P. (2020b). Defibrillation and cardioversion. In T. L. Gomella, F. G. Eyal, & F. Bany-Mohammed (Eds.), *Gomella's neonatology: Management, procedures, on-call problems, diseases, and drugs* (8th ed., pp. 336–339). McGraw-Hill Education.

Cottrill, C. M., & Mohan, S. (2020). Arrhythmia. In T. L. Gomella, F. G. Eyal, & F. Bany-Mohammed (Eds.), *Gomella's neonatology: Management, procedures, on-call problems, diseases, and drugs* (8th ed., pp. 459–468). McGraw-Hill Education.

Crisci, K. L. (2020). Imaging studies. In T. L. Gomella, F. G. Eyal, & F. Bany-Mohammed (Eds.), *Gomella's neonatology: Management, procedures, on-call problems, diseases, and drugs* (8th ed., pp. 167–196). McGraw-Hill Education.

Croteau, S. (2017). Bleeding. In E. Eichenwald, A. Hansen, C. Martin, & A. Stark (Eds.), *Cloherty and Stark's manual of neonatal care* (8th ed., pp. 586–594). Lippincott Williams & Wilkins.

Crotezzo, D. E., & Carter, B. S. (2018). Palliative care. In C. A. Gleason & S. E. Juul (Eds.), *Avery's diseases of the newborn* (10th ed., pp. 446–452.e1). Elsevier.

Crowley, M. A. (2015). Neonatal respiratory disorders. In: R. Martin, A. Fanaroff, & M. Walsh (Eds.), *Fanaroff and Martin's neonatal-perinatal medicine: Diseases of the fetus and infant*. (10th ed., pp. 374–390). Elsevier.

Crowley, M. A. (2020). Neonatal respiratory disorders. In R. J. Martin, A. A. Fanaroff, & M. C. Walsh (Eds.), *Fanaroff and Martin's neonatal-perinatal medicine: Diseases of the fetus and infant* (11th ed., pp. 1203–1230). Elsevier.

Crowley, M., & Martin, R. (2020). Respiratory problems. In A. Fanaroff & J. Fanaroff (Eds.), *Klaus and Fanaroff's care of the high-risk neonate* (7th ed., pp. 190–210). Elsevier.

Culjat, M. (2020). Lumbar puncture. In: J. Ramasethu & S. Seo (Eds.), *McDonald's atlas of procedures in neonatology* (6th ed., pp. 140–146). Wolters Kluwer.

Cypher, R. L. (2016). Antepartum fetal surveillance and prenatal diagnosis. In S. Mattson & J. E. Smith (Eds.), *Core curriculum for maternal-newborn nursing* (5th ed., pp. 135–158). Saunders Elsevier.

Dang, D., Melnyk, B. M., Fineout-Overholt, E., Yost, J., Cullen, L., Cvach, M., Larabee, J. H., Rycroft-Malone, J., Schultz, A. A., Stetler, C. B., & Stevens, K. R. (2019). Models to guide implementation and sustainability of evidence-based practice. In B. M. Melnyk & E. Fineout-Overholt (Eds.), *Evidence-based practice in nursing and healthcare* (4th ed., pp. 378–427). Wolters Kluwer.

D'Apolito, K. (2021). Perinatal substance abuse. In T. Verklan, M. Walden, & S. Forest (Eds.), *Core curriculum for neonatal intensive care nursing* (6th ed., pp. 38–53). Elsevier.

Darras, B., & Volpe, J. (2018a). Evaluation, special studies. In J. Volpe, T. Inder, B. Darras, L. deVries, A. Plessis, & J. Perlman (Eds.), *Volpe's neurology of the newborn* (6th ed., pp. 861–873). Elsevier.

Darras, B., & Volpe, J. (2018b). Muscle involvement and restricted disorders. In J. Volpe, T. Inder, B. Darras, L. deVries, A. Plessis, & J. Perlman (Eds.), *Volpe's neurology of the newborn* (6th ed., pp. 922–970). Elsevier.

Darras, B. T., & Volpe, J. J. (2018c). Levels above lower motor neuron to nueuromuscular junction. In J. J. Volpe, T. E. Inder, B. T. Darras, L. S. deVries, A. J. du Plessis, J. J. Neil, & J. M. Perlman (Eds.), *Volpe's neurology of the newborn* (6th ed., pp. 887–921.e11). Elsevier.

Davidson, L. N., Desai, N. S., & Shreve, K. V. (2020). Pain in the neonate. In T. L. Gomella, F. G. Eyal, & F. Bany-Mohammed (Eds.), *Gomella's neonatology: Management, procedures, on-call problems, diseases, and drugs* (8th ed., pp. 211–223). McGraw-Hill Education.

De Alba Campomanes, A. G., & Binenbaum, G. (2018). Eye and vision disorders. In C. Gleason & S. Juul (Eds.), *Avery's diseases of the newborn* (10th ed., pp. 1536–1557). Elsevier.

De Vries, L. (2020). Intracranial hemorrhage and vascular lesions of the neonate. In R. Martin, A. Fanaroff, & M. Walsh (Eds.), *Fanaroff and Martin's neonatal-perinatal medicine: Diseases of the fetus and infant* (11th ed., pp. 970–988). Elsevier.

Dees, E., & Baldwin, H. S. (2018). Developmental biology of the heart. In C. A. Gleason & S. E. Juul (Eds.), *Avery's diseases of the newborn* (10th ed., pp. 724–740.e3). Elsevier.

Dell, K. M. (2020). Fluid, electrolyte, and acid-base homeostasis. In R. J. Martin, A. A. Fanaroff, & M. C. Walsh (Eds.), *Fanaroff and Martin's neonatal perinatal medicine: Diseases of the fetus and infant* (11th ed., pp. 1854–1870). Elsevier.

Demauro, S. B., & Hintz, S. R. (2018). Risk assessment and neurodevelopmental outcomes. In C. Gleason & S. Juul (Eds.), *Avery's diseases of the newborn* (10th ed., pp. 971–990.e7). Elsevier.

Denne, S. C. (2018). Parenteral nutrition for the high-risk neonate. In C. A. Gleason & S. E. Juul (Eds.), *Avery's diseases of the newborn* (10th ed., pp. 1023–1031e2). Elsevier.

Desai, A. P., & Leonard, E. G. (2020). Infections in the neonate. In A. A. Fanaroff & J. M. Fanaroff (Eds.), *Klaus and Fanaroff's care of the high-risk neonate* (7th ed., pp. 275–295.e4). Elsevier.

Deschmann, E., Saxonhouse, M., & Sola-Visner, M. (2017). Thrombocytopenia. In E. Eichenwald, A. Hansen, C. Martin, & A. Stark (Eds.), *Cloherty and Stark's manual of neonatal care* (8th ed., pp. 630–640). Lippincott Williams & Wilkins.

Deschmann, E., & Sola-Visner, M. (2018). Neonatal platelet disorders. In C. Gleason & S. Juul (Eds.), *Avery's diseases of the newborn* (10th ed., pp. 1139–1151). Elsevier.

di Fiore, J. M. (2020). Biomedical engineering aspects of neonatal cardiorespiratory monitoring. In: R. J. Martin, A. A. Fanaroff, & M. C. Walsh (Eds.), *Fanaroff and Martin's neonatal-perinatal medicine: Diseases of the fetus and infant*. (11th ed., pp. 596–607). Elsevier.

DiBlasi, R. (2022). Respiratory care of the newborn. In M. Keszler & K. S. Gautham (Eds.), *Goldsmith's assisted ventilation of the neonate: An evidence-based approach to newborn respiratory care* (7th ed., pp. 363–383). Elsevier.

Diehl-Jones, W., & Fraser, D. (2021). Hematologic disorders. In M. T. Verklan, M. Walden, & S. Forest (Eds.), *Core curriculum for neonatal intensive care nursing* (6th ed., pp. 568–587). Elsevier.

Dillon Heaberlin, P. (2019). Neurologic assessment. In E. P. Tappero & M. E. Honeyfield (Eds.), *Physical assessment of the newborn: A comprehensive approach to the art of physical examination* (6th ed., pp. 167–192). Springer Publishing Company.

Dimmitt, R., Sellers, Z. K., & Sibley, E. (2018). Gastrointestinal tract development. In C. Gleason & S. Juul (Eds.), *Avery's diseases of the newborn* (10th ed., pp. 1032–1038). Elsevier.

Dingeldein, M. (2020a). Development of the neonatal gastrointestinal tract. In R. J. Martin, A. A. Fanaroff, & M. C. Walsh (Eds.), *Fanaroff and Martin's neonatal-perinatal medicine: Diseases of the fetus and infant* (11th ed., pp. 1506–1512). Elsevier.

Dingeldein, M. (2020b). Part two: Selected disorders of the gastrointestinal tract. In A. A. Fanaroff & J. M. Fanaroff (Eds.), *Klaus and Fanaroff's care of the high-risk neonate* (7th ed., pp. 108–115). Elsevier.

Dingeldein, M. (2020c). Selected gastrointestinal anomalies in the neonate. In R. J. Martin, A. A. Fanaroff, & M. C. Walsh (Eds.), *Fanaroff and Martin's neonatal-perinatal medicine: Diseases of the fetus and infant* (11th ed., pp. 1541–1570). Elsevier.

Ditzenberger, G. (2018). Gastrointestinal and hepatic systems and perinatal nutrition. In S. T. Blackburn (Ed.), *Maternal, fetal, & neonatal physiology: A clinical perspective* (5th ed., pp. 387–434). Elsevier.

Ditzenberger, G. R. (2021). Neurologic disorders. In M. T. Verklan, M. Walden, & S. Forest (Eds.), *Core curriculum for neonatal intensive care nursing* (6th ed., pp. 629–653). Elsevier.

Divall, S. A., & Megjaneh, L. (2018). Developmental endocrinology. In C. Gleason & S. Juul (Eds.), *Avery's diseases of the newborn* (10th ed., pp. 1224–1332). Elsevier.

Dix, D. (2016). Hypertensive disorders in pregnancy. In S. Mattson & J. E. Smith (Eds.), *Core curriculum for maternal-newborn nursing* (5th ed., pp. 435–451). Elsevier.

Doherty, E. G. (2017). Fluid and electrolyte management. In E. C. Eichenwald, A. R. Hansen, C. R. Martin, & A. R. Stark (Eds.), *Cloherty and Stark's manual of neonatal care* (8th ed., pp. 296–311). Lippincott Williams & Wilkins.

Domonoske, C. (2017). Common neonatal intensive care unit (NICU) medication guidelines. In E. Eichenwald, A. R. Hansen, C. R. Martin, & A. Stark (Eds.), *Cloherty and Stark's manual of neonatal care* (8th ed.). Lippincott Williams & Wilkins.

Domonoske, C. D. (2021). Pharmacology. In M. T. Verklan, M. Walden, & S. Forest (Eds.), *Core curriculum for neonatal intensive care nursing* (6th ed., pp. 191–206). Elsevier.

Donn, S. M., & Attar, M. A. (2020). Assisted ventilation of the neonate and its complications. In R. J. Martin, A. A. Fanaroff, & M. C. Walsh (Eds.), *Fanaroff and Martin's neonatal-perinatal medicine: Diseases of the fetus and infant* (11th ed., pp. 1174–1202). Elsevier.

Douma, C. E., Casey, D., & Greene, A. K. (2017). Skin care. In E. Eichenwald, A. N. Hansen, C. Martin, & A. Stark (Eds.), *Cloherty and Stark's manual of neonatal care* (8th ed., pp. 967–977). Lippincott Williams & Wilkins.

Downs, E., Tran, A., McMenemy, R., & Abegave, N. (2015). Exam performance and attitude toward multitasking in six, multimedia-multitasking classroom environments. *Computers & Education, 86,* 250–259. https://doi.org/10.1016/j.compedu.2015.08.008

Drago, M., & Mercurio, M. R. (2022). Ethical issues in assisted ventilation of the neonate. In M. Kessler & K. S. Gautham (Eds.), *Goldsmith's assisted ventilation of the neonate: An evidence-based approach to newborn respiratory care* (7th ed., pp. 39–46.e2). Elsevier.

Dragoo, S. (2017). Hyperbilirubinemia of the newborn born after 35 weeks' gestation. In B. J. Snell & S. Gardner (Eds.), *Care of the well newborn* (pp. 253–271). Jones & Barlett.

Draus, J. M., & Ruzic, A. (2020a). Surgical diseases of the newborn: Abdominal wall defects. In T. L. Gomella, F. G. Eyal, & F. Bany-Mohammed (Eds.), *Gomella's neonatology: Management, procedures, on-call problems, diseases, and drugs* (8th ed., pp. 1072–1076). McGraw-Hill Education.

Draus, J. M., & Ruzic, A. (2020b). Surgical diseases of the newborn: Alimentary tract obstruction. In T. L. Gomella, F. G. Eyal, & F. Bany-Mohammed (Eds.), *Gomella's neonatology: Management, procedures, on-call problems, diseases, and drugs* (8th ed., pp. 1076–1079). McGraw-Hill Education.

Draus, J. M., & Ruzic, A. (2020c). Surgical diseases of the newborn: Diseases of the airway, tracheobronchial tree, and lungs. In T. L. Gomella, F. G. Eyal, & F. Bany-Mohammed (Eds.), *Gomella's neonatology: Management, procedures, on-call problems, diseases, and drugs* (8th ed., pp. 1080–1085). McGraw-Hill Education.

du Plessis, A., Robinson, S., & Volpe, J. (2018). Congenital hydrocephalus. In J. Volpe, T. Inder, B. Darras, L. deVries, A. Plessis, & J. Perlman (Eds.), *Volpe's neurology of the newborn* (6th ed., pp. 58–72). Elsevier.

du Plessis, A., & Volpe, J. (2018a). Neural tube development. In J. Volpe, T. Inder, B. Darras, L. deVries, A. Plessis, & J. Perlman (Eds.), *Volpe's neurology of the newborn* (6th ed., pp. 3–33). Elsevier.

du Plessis, A., & Volpe, J. (2018b). Prosencephalic development. In J. Volpe, T. Inder, B. Darras, L. deVries, A. Plessis, & J. Perlman (Eds.), *Volpe's neurology of the newborn* (6th ed., pp. 34–57). Elsevier.

du Plessis, J. A., Limperopoulos, C., & Volpe, J. C. (2018). Cerebellar development. In J. Volpe, T. Inder, B. Darras, L. deVries, A. Plessis, & J. Perlman (Eds.), *Volpe's neurology of the newborn* (6th ed., pp. 73–99). Elsevier.

Duff, P. (2019). Maternal and fetal infections. In R. Resnik, C. J. Lockwood, T. R. Moore, M. F. Greene, J. A. Copel, & R. M. Silver (Eds.), *Creasy & Resnik's maternal-fetal medicine: Principles and practice* (8th ed., pp. 862–919.e8). Elsevier.

Dukhivny, S., & Wilkins-Haug, L. E. (2017). Fetal assessment and prenatal diagnosis. In E. C. Eichenwald, A. R. Hansen, C. R. Martin, & A. R. Stark (Eds.), *Cloherty and Stark's manual of neonatal care* (8th ed., pp. 1–14). Lippincott Williams & Wilkins.

Dysart, K. C. (2020). Infant of a diabetic mother. In: T. L. Gomella, F. G. Eyal, & F. Bany-Mohammed (Eds.), *Gomella's neonatology: Management, procedures, on-call problems, diseases, and drugs.* (8th ed., pp. 937–944). McGraw-Hill Education.

Eichenwald, E. C. (2017). Mechanical ventilation. In E. Eichenwald, A. Hansen, C. Martin, & A. Stark (Eds.), *Cloherty and Stark's manual of neonatal care* (8th ed., pp. 401–418). Lippincott Williams & Wilkins.

El-Hattab, A. W., & Sutton, V. R. (2017). Inborn errors of metabolism. In E. Eichenwald, A. Hansen, C. R. Martin, & A. Stark (Eds.), *Cloherty and Stark's manual of neonatal care* (8th ed., pp. 858–891). Lippincott Williams & Wilkins.

Engen, R., & Hingorani, S. (2018). Developmental abnormalities of the kidneys. In C. A. Gleason & S. E. Juul (Eds.), *Avery's diseases of the newborn* (10th ed., pp. 1250–1259). Elsevier.

Esper, F. (2020). Postnatal bacterial infections. In R. J. Martin, A. A. Fanaroff, & M. C. Walsh (Eds.), *Fanaroff and Martin's neonatal-perinatal medicine: Diseases of the fetus and infant* (11th ed., pp. 789–808). Elsevier.

Evans, K., Hing, A., & Cunningham, M. (2018). Craniofacial malformations. In C. Gleason & S. Juul (Eds.), *Avery's *diseases of the newborn* (10th ed., pp. 1417–1437.e2). Elsevier.

Eyal, F. G. (2020a). Air leak syndromes. In T. L. Gomella, F. G. Eyal, & F. Bany-Mohammed (Eds.), *Gomella's neonatology: Management, procedures, on-call problems, diseases, and drugs* (8th ed., pp. 808–814). McGraw-Hill Education.

Eyal, F. G. (2020b). Respiratory management. In T. L. Gomella, F. G. Eyal, & F. Bany-Mohammed (Eds.), *Gomella's neonatology: Management, procedures, on-call problems, diseases, and drugs* (8th ed., pp. 97–116, 838–850). McGraw-Hill Education.

Eyal, F. G. (2020c). Sedation and analgesia. In T. L. Gomella, F. G. Eyal, & F. Bany-Mohammed (Eds.), *Gomella's neonatology: Management, procedures, on-call problems, diseases, and drugs* (8th ed., pp. 743–748). McGraw-Hill Education.

Eyal, F. G. (2020d). Fluid and electrolytes. In: T. L. Gomella, F. G. Eyal& F. Bany-Mohammed (Eds.), *Gomella's neonatology: Management, procedures, on-call problems, diseases, and drugs.* (8th ed., pp. 117–124). McGraw-Hill Education.

Fanaroff, A. A., Lissauer, T., & Fanaroff, J. M. (2020). Physical growth: Physical examination of the newborn infant and the physical environment. In A. A. Fanaroff & J. M. Fanaroff (Eds.), *Klaus and Fanaroff's care of the high-risk neonate* (7th ed., pp. 58–79.e2). Elsevier.

Fechner, P. Y. (2018). Disorders of the adrenal gland. In C. Gleason & S. Juul (Eds.), *Avery's diseases of the newborn* (10th ed., pp. 1351–1364). Elsevier.

Ferrieri, P., & Wallen, L. D. (2018). Newborn sepsis and meningitis. In C. Gleason & S. Juul (Eds.), *Avery's diseases of the newborn* (10th ed., pp. 553–565.e3). Elsevier.

Fineout-Overholt, E., Long, L. E., & Gallagher-Ford, L. (2019). Integration of patient preferences and values and clinician expertise into evidence-based decision making. In B. M. Melnyk & E. Fineout-Overholt (Eds.), *Evidence-based practice in nursing and healthcare* (4th ed., pp. 219–232). Wolters Kluwer.

Fineout-Overholt, E., & Stevens, K. R. (2019). Critically appraising knowledge for clinical decision making. In B. M. Melnyk & E. Fineout-Overholt (Eds.), *Evidence-based practice in nursing and healthcare* (4th ed., pp. 109–123). Wolters Kluwer.

Fiore, J. M. (2022). Biomedical engineering aspects of neonatal cardiorespiratory monitoring. In R. J. Martin, A. A. Fanaroff, & M. C. Walsh (Eds.), *Fanaroff & Martin's neonatal-perinatal medicine: Diseases of the fetus and infant* (11th ed., pp. 596–607). Elsevier.

Flynn-O'Brien, K., Rice-Townsend, S., & Ledbetter, D. (2018). Structural anomalies of the gastrointestinal tract. In C. Gleason & S. Juul (Eds.), *Avery's diseases of the newborn* (10th ed., pp. 1039–1053). Elsevier.

Ford, S. M., Watanabe, M., & Devaney, E. J. (2020). Cardiac embryology. In R. J. Martin, A. A. Fanaroff, & M. C. Walsh (Eds.), *Fanaroff & Martin's neonatal-perinatal medicine: Diseases of the fetus and infant* (11th ed., p. 1292). Elsevier.

Fraser, D. (2019). Chest and lung assessment. In E. P. Tappero & M. E. Honeyfield (Eds.), *Physical assessment of the newborn* (6th ed., pp. 79–91). Springer Publishing Company.

Fraser, D. (2021a). Newborn adaptation to extrauterine life. In K. Simpson, P. Creehan, N. O'Brien-Able, C. Roth, & A. J. Rohan (Eds.), *AWHONN's perinatal nursing* (5th ed., pp. 564–578). Lippincott Williams & Wilkins.

Fraser, D. (2021b). Respiratory distress. In M. T. Verklan, M. Walden, & S. Forest (Eds.), *Core curriculum for neonatal intensive care nurses* (6th ed., pp. 394–416). Elsevier.

Fraser, D., & Diehl-Jones, W. (2021a). Assisted ventilation. In M. T. Verklan, M. Walden, & S. Forest (Eds.), *Core curriculum for neonatal intensive care nursing* (6th ed., pp. 425–445). Elsevier.

Fraser, D., & Diehl-Jones, W. (2021b). Ophthalmologic and auditory disorders. In M. T. Verklan, M. Walden, & S. Forest (Eds.), *Core curriculum for neonatal intensive care nursing* (6th ed., pp. 691–704). Saunders, Elsevier.

Friedman, S. H., Thomas-Salo, F., & Ballard, A. R. (2020). Support for the family. In R. J. Martin, A. A. Fanaroff, & M. C. Walsh (Eds.), *Fanaroff & Martin's neonatal-perinatal medicine: Diseases of the fetus and infant* (11th ed., pp. 690–702). Elsevier.

Furman, L., & Schanler, R. J. (2018). Breastfeeding. In C. Gleaso & S. Juul (Eds.), *Avery's diseases of the newborn*, (10th ed., pp. 991–1008). Elsevier.

Gallagher, M. E., Pocatti, A. S., Lauvorn, H. N., & Carter, B. S. (2021). Neonatal surgery. In S. L. Gardner, B. S. Carter, M. Enzman-Hines, & S. Niermeyer (Eds.), *Merenstein & Gardner's handbook of neonatal intensive care: An interprofessional approach* (9th ed., pp. 1000–1031). Elsevier.

Gardner, S. L., & Cammack, B. H. (2021). Heat balance. In S. L. Gardner, B. S. Carter, M. Enzman-Hines, & S. Niermeyer (Eds.), *Merenstein & Gardner's handbook of neonatal intensive care nursing: An interprofessional approach* (9th ed., pp. 137–164). Elsevier.

Gardner, S. L., & Carter, B. S. (2021). Grief and perinatal loss. In S. L. Gardner, B. S. Carter, M. Enzman-Hines, & S. Niermeyer (Eds.), *Merenstein & Gardner's handbook of neonatal intensive care: An interprofessional approach* (9th ed., pp. 1096–1140). Elsevier.

Gardner, S. L., Enzman-Hines, M., & Agarwal, R. (2021). Pain and pain relief. In S. L. Gardner, B. S. Carter, M. Enzman-Hines, & S. Niermeyer (Eds.), *Merenstein & Gardner's handbook of neonatal intensive care nursing: An interprofessional approach* (9th ed., pp. 273–332). Elsevier.

Gardner, S. L., Enzman-Hines, M., & Nyp, M. (2021). Respiratory diseases. In S. L. Gardner, B. S. Carter, M. Enzman-Hines, & S. Niermeyer (Eds.), *Merenstein & Gardner's handbook of neonatal intensive care nursing: An interprofessional approach* (9th ed., pp. 729–826). Elsevier.

Gardner, S. L., Lawrence, R. A., & Lawrence, R. M. (2021). Breastfeeding the neonate with special needs. In S. L. Gardner, B. S. Carter, M. Enzman-Hines, & S. Niermeyer (Eds.), *Merenstein & Gardner's handbook of neonatal intensive care nursing: An interprofessional approach* (9th ed., pp. 534–601). Elsevier.

Gardner, S. L., & Voos, K. (2021). Families in crisis: Theoretical and practical considerations. In S. L. Gardner, B. S. Carter, M. Enzman-Hines, & S. Niermeyer (Eds.), *Merenstein & Gardner's handbook of neonatal intensive care nursing: An interprofessional approach* (9th ed., pp. 1039–1095). Elsevier.

Garg, M., & Devaskar, S. U. (2020). Disorders of carbohydrate metabolism in the neonate. In R. J. Martin, A. A. Fanaroff, & M. C. Walsh (Eds.), *Fanaroff & Martin's neonatal* perinatal medicine: Diseases of the fetus and infant (11th ed., pp. 1584–1610). Elsevier.

Gauda, E. B., & Martin, R. J. (2018). Control of breathing. In C. A. Gleason & S. E. Juul (Eds.), *Avery's diseases of the newborn* (10th ed., pp. 600–617). Elsevier.

Gautham, K. S., & Shafer, G. J. (2022). Quality and safety in respiratory care. In M. Kessler & K. S. Gautham (Eds.), *Assisted ventilation of the neonate* (7th ed., pp. 56–63.e2). Elsevier.

Gautham, S. K., & Soll, R. F. (2022). Exogenous surfactant therapy. In M. Keszler & K. S. Gautham (Eds.), *Goldsmith's assisted ventilation of the neonate: An evidence-based approach to newborn respiratory care* (7th ed., pp. 172–184). Elsevier.

Genoveses, S. K. (2016). Hemorrhagic disorders. In S. Mattson & J. E. Smith (Eds.), *Core curriculum for maternal-newborn nursing* (5th ed., pp. 480–500). Elsevier.

Gilmore, A., & Thompson, G. H. (2020). Bone and joint infections in neonates. In R. J. Martin, A. A. Fanaroff, & M. C. Walsh (Eds.), *Fanaroff & Martin's neonatal-perinatal medicine: Diseases of the fetus and infant* (11th ed., pp. 1989–1994). Elsevier.

Goldsmith, J. P. (2020). Overview and initial management of delivery room resuscitation. In R. J. Martin, A. A. Fanaroff, & M. C. Walsh (Eds.), *Fanaroff & Martin's neonatal perinatal medicine: Diseases of the fetus and infant* (11th ed., pp. 516–529). Elsevier.

Goldsmith, J. P., & Raju, T. N. K. (2022). Introduction and historical aspects. In J. P. Goldsmith, F. H. Karotkin, M. Keszler, & G. K. Suresh (Eds.), *Goldsmith's assisted ventilation of the neonate: An evidence-based approach to newborn respiratory care* (7th ed., pp. 1–10). Elsevier.

Gomella, T. L. (2020). Newborn physical examination. In T. L. Gomella, F. G. Eyal, & F. Bany-Mohammed (Eds.), *Gomella's neonatology: Management, procedures, on-call problems, diseases, and drugs* (8th ed., pp. 59–91). McGraw-Hill Education.

Gomella, T. L. (2019). Abdominal assessment. In E. P. Tappero & M. E. Honeyfield (Eds.), *Physical assessment of the newborn: A comprehensive approach to the art of physical examination* (6th ed., pp. 111–120). Springer Publishing Company.

Gomella, T. L. (2020a). Abnormal blood gas. In T. L. Gomella, F. G. Eyal, & F. Bany-Mohammed (Eds.), *Gomella's neonatology: Management, procedures, on-call problems, diseases, and drugs* (8th ed., pp. 431–441). McGraw-Hill Education.

Gomella, T. L. (2020b). Apnea and bradycardia (A's and B's): On call. In T. L. Gomella, F. G. Eyal, & F. Bany-Mohammed (Eds.), *Gomella's neonatology: Management, procedures, on-call problems, diseases, and drugs* (8th ed., pp. 442–459). McGraw-Hill Education.

Gomella, T. L. (2020c). Bloody stool. In T. L. Gomella, F. G. Eyal, & F. Bany-Mohammed (Eds.), *Gomella's neonatology: Management, procedures, on-call problems, diseases, and drugs* (8th ed., pp. 468–476). McGraw-Hill Education.

Gomella, T. L. (2020d). Gestational age and birth-weight classification. In T. L. Gomella, F. G. Eyal, & F. Bany-Mohammed (Eds.), *Gomella's neonatology: Management, procedures, on-call problems, diseases, and drugs* (8th ed., pp. 42–59). McGraw-Hill Education.

Gomella, T. L. (2020e). Hyponatremia. In T. L. Gomella, F. G. Eyal, & F. Bany-Mohammed (Eds.), *Gomella's neonatology: Management, procedures, on-call problems, diseases, and drugs* (8th ed., pp. 608–616). McGraw-Hill Education.

Gomella, T. L. (2020f). No stool in 48 hours. In T. L. Gomella, F. G. Eyal, & F. Bany-Mohammed (Eds.), *Gomella's neonatology: Management, procedures, on-call problems, diseases, and drugs* (8th ed., pp. 645–655). McGraw-Hill Education.

Gomella, T. L. (2020g). No urine output in 24 hours. In T. L. Gomella, F. G. Eyal, & F. Bany-Mohammed (Eds.), *Gomella's neonatology: Management, procedures, on-call problems, diseases, and drugs* (8th ed., pp. 655–666). McGraw-Hill Education.

Gomella, T. L. (2020h). Pulmonary hemorrhage. In T. L. Gomella, F. G. Eyal, & F. Bany-Mohammed (Eds.), *Gomella's neonatology: Management, procedures, on-call problems, diseases, and drugs* (8th ed., pp. 719–725). McGraw-Hill Education.

Gomella, T. L., & Palla, M. R. (2020). Apnea. In T. L. Gomella, F. G. Eyal, & F. Bany-Mohammed (Eds.), *Gomella's neonatology: Management, procedures, on-call problems, diseases, and drugs* (8th ed., pp. 823–826). McGraw-Hill Education.

Gonzalez, L. M. (2019). Transport of infants and children. In B. K. Walsh (Ed.), *Neonatal and pediatric respiratory care* (5th ed., pp. 635–646). Elsevier.

Goodwin, M. (2019). Abdomen assessment. In E. P. Tappero & M. E. Honeyfield (Eds.), *Physical assessment of the newborn: A comprehensive approach to the art of physical examination* (6th ed., pp. 111–120). Springer Publishing Company.

Gorman, T. (2017). Neonatal effects of maternal diabetes. In E. Eichenwald, A. Hansen, C. R. Martin, & A. Start (Eds.), *Cloherty and Stark's manual of neonatal care* (8th ed., pp. 910–922). Lippincott Williams & Wilkins.

Goudreau, K. A. (2011). Editorial: LACE, APRN consensus . . . and WIIFM (what's in it for me)? *Clinical Nurse Specialist, 25*(1), 5–7. https://doi.org/10.1097/NUR.0b013e3182036221

Graeber, C., & Oatts, J. (2020). Retinopathy of prematurity. In: T. L. Gomella, F. G. Eyal & F. Bany-Mohammed (Eds.), *Gomella's neonatology: Management, procedures, on-call problems, diseases, and drugs.* (8th ed., pp. 1051–1055). McGraw-Hill Education.

Graeber, C. P. (2020). Eye disorders of the newborn. In T. L. Gomella, F. G. Eyal, & F. Bany-Mohammed (Eds.), *Gomella's neonatology: Management, procedures, on-call problems, diseases, and drugs* (8th ed., pp. 881–884). McGraw-Hill Education.

Greenberg, J. M., Haberman, B., Narendran, V., Nathan, A., & Schibler, K. (2019). Neonatal morbidities of prenatal and perinatal origin. In R. Resnik, C. J. Lockwood, T. R. Moore, M. F. Greene, J. A. Copel, & R. M. Silver (Eds.), *Creasy & Resnik's maternal-fetal medicine: Principles and practice* (8th ed., pp. 1309–1333.e8). Elsevier.

Gregory, M. L. P. G. (2017). Transient tachypnea of the newborn. In E. Eichenwald, A. Hansen, C. Martin, & A. Stark (Eds.), *Cloherty and Stark's manual of neonatal care* (8th ed., pp. 432–435). Lippincott Williams & Wilkins.

Gressens, P., Passemard, S., & Hüppi, P. (2020). Normal and abnormal brain development. In R. Martin, A. Fanaroff, & M. Walsh (Eds.), *Fanaroff & Martin's neonatal-perinatal medicine: Diseases of the fetus and infant* (11th ed., pp. 914–946). Elsevier.

Grinspun, D., Melnyk, B. M., & Fineout-Overholt, E. (2019). Advancing optimal care with robust clinical practice guidelines. In B. M. Melnyk & E. Fineout-Overholt (Eds.), *Evidence-based practice in nursing and healthcare* (4th ed., pp. 233–256). Wolters Kluwer.

Groenendaal, F., & De Vries, L. (2020). Hypoxic-ischemic encephalopathy. In R. J. Martin, A. A. Fanaroff, & M. C. Walsh (Eds.), *Fanaroff & Martin's neonatal-perinatal medicine: Diseases of the fetus and infant* (11th ed., pp. 989–1014). Elsevier.

Gross, S. J., & Gheorghe, C. P. (2020). Genetic aspects of perinatal disease and prenatal diagnosis. In R. J. Martin, A. A. Fanaroff, & M. C. Walsh (Eds.), *Fanaroff & Martin's neonatal-perinatal medicine: Diseases of the fetus and infant* (11th ed., pp. 154–173). Elsevier.

Guido, G. W. (2020). *Legal & ethical issues in nursing* (7th ed.). Pearson Education.

Gupta, A. O., & Dirnberger, D. R. (2020). Thoracostomy. In J. Ramasethu & S. Seo (Eds.), *MacDonald's atlas of procedures in neonatology* (6th ed., pp. 307–320). Wolters Kluwer.

Gupta, D., & Sidbury, R. (2018). Cutaneous congenital defects. In C. A. Gleason & S. E. Juul (Eds.), *Avery's diseases of the newborn* (10th ed., pp. 1511–1535.e4). Elsevier.

Guttentag, S. (2017). Respiratory distress syndrome. In E. Eichenwald, A. Hansen, C. Martin, & A. Stark (Eds.), *Cloherty & Stark's manual of neonatal care* (8th ed., pp. 436–445). Wolters Kluwer.

Hackney, D. N. (2020). Estimation of fetal well-being. In R. J. Martin, A. A. Fanaroff, & M. C. Walsh (Eds.), *Fanaroff & Martin's neonatal-perinatal medicine: Diseases of the fetus and infant* (11th ed., pp. 210–222). Elsevier.

Haefner, J. (2021). Self-care for health professionals during coronavirus disease 2019 crises. *The Journal for Nurse Practitioners, 17*, 279–282. https://doi.org/10.1016/j.nurpra.2020.12.015

Haldeman-Englert, C. R., Saitta, S. C., & Zackai, E. H. (2018). Chromosome disorders. In C. Gleason & S. Juul (Eds.), *Avery's diseases of the newborn* (10th ed., pp. 211–223.e2). Elsevier.

Hall, A. S., & Reavey, D. A. (2021). Neurologic disorders. In S. L. Gardner B. S. Carter M. Enzman-Hines & S. Niermeyer (Eds.), *Merenstein & Gardner's handbook of neonatal intensive care nursing: An interprofessional approach* (9th ed., pp. 929–968). Elsevier.

Hamar, B., & Hansen, A. (2019). Antenatal assessment and high-risk delivery. In B. K. Walsh (Ed.), *Neonatal and pediatric respiratory care* (5th ed., pp. 22–40). Elsevier.

Hanff, L. (2021). Medication errors in children. In J. V. Aranda & J. N. Van Den Anker (Eds.), *Yaffe and Aranda's neonatal and pediatric therapeutic principles in practice* (5th ed., pp. 941–948). Lippincott Williams & Wilkins.

Hansen, A., & Levin, J. (2019). Neonatal pulmonary disorders. In B. K. Walsh (Ed.), *Neonatal and pediatric respiratory care* (5th ed., pp. 407–452). Elsevier.

Hardy, W., D'Agata, A., & McGrath, J. (2016). The infant at risk. In S. Mattson & J. Smith (Eds.), *Core curriculum for maternal-newborn nursing* (5th ed., pp. 362–415). Elsevier.

Harper, L., Tita, A., & Karumanchi, S. (2019). Pregnancy-related hypertension. In R. Resnik, C. Lockwood, T. Moore, M. Greene, J. Copel, & R. Silver (Eds.), *Creasy and Resnik's maternal-fetal medicine: Principles and practice* (8th ed., pp. 810–838.e9). Elsevier.

Heaberlin, P. D. (2019). Neurologic assessment. In E. P. Tappero & M. E. Honeyfield (Eds.), *Physical assessment of the newborn* (6th ed., pp. 167–192). Springer Publishing Company.

Heiderich, A. E., & Leone, T. A. (2020). Resuscitation and initial stabilization. In A. A. Fanaroff & J. M. Fanaroff (Eds.), *Klaus and Fanaroff's care of the high-risk neonate* (7th ed., pp. 44–57). Elsevier.

Heresi, G. (2017). Syphilis. In E. Eichenwald, A. Hansen, C. Martin, & A. Stark (Eds.), *Cloherty and Stark's manual of neonatal care* (8th ed., pp. 728–737). Wolters Kluwer.

Hibbs, A. M. (2020). Gastroesophageal reflux and gastroesophageal reflux disease in the neonate. In: R. J. Martin, A. A. Fanaroff, & M. C. Walsh (Eds.), *Fanaroff and Martin's neonatal-perinatal medicine.* (11th ed., pp. 1513–1521). Elsevier.

Hill, A. (2021). Foundations of neonatal research. In M. T. Verklan, M. Walden, & S. Forest (Eds.), *Core curriculum for neonatal intensive care nursing* (6th ed., pp. 705–713). Elsevier.

Hills, B., & Tomei, K. (2020). Spinal dysraphisms. In R. J. Martin, A. A. Fanaroff, & M. C. Walsh (Eds.), *Fanaroff & Martin's neonatal-perinatal medicine: Diseases of the fetus and infant* (11th ed., pp. 1073–1080). Elsevier.

Hodson, A. (2018). Temperature regulation. In C. Gleason & S. Juul (Eds.), *Avery's diseases of the newborn* (10th ed., pp. 361–367). Elsevier.

Holford, N. H. G. (2021). Pharmacokinetics and pharmacodynamics: Rational dosing and the time course of drug action. In B. G. Katzung (Ed.), *Basic and clinical pharmacology* (15th ed., pp. 42–56). McGraw-Hill Education.

Holzmann-Pazgal, G. (2017). Congenital toxoplasmosis. In E. Eichenwald, A. Hansen, C. Martin, & A. Stark (Eds.), *Cloherty and Stark's manual of neonatal care* (8th ed., pp. 720–727). Lippincott Williams & Wilkins.

Honeyfield, M. E. (2009). Neonatal nurse practitioners: Past, present, and future. *Advances in Neonatal Care, 9*(3), 125–128. https://doi.org/10.1097/ANC.0b013e3181a8369f

Horns LaBronte, K. (2019). Recording and evaluating the neonatal history. In E. P. Tappero & M. E. Honeyfield (Eds.), *Physical assessment of the newborn: A comprehensive approach to the art of physical examination* (6th ed., pp. 9–21). Springer Publishing Company.

Hossain, F., & Clatty, A. (2021). Self-care strategies in response to nurses' moral injury during the COVID-19 pandemic. *Nursing Ethics, 28*(1), 23–32. https://doi.org/10.1177/0969733020961825

Hostetter, M., & Gleason, C. (2018). Fungal infections in the neonatal intensive care unit. In C. Gleason & S. Juul (Eds.), *Avery's diseases of the newborn* (10th ed., pp. 581–585.e2). Elsevier.

Hoyt, M. R. (2020). Anesthesia for labor and delivery. In R. J. Martin, A. A. Fanaroff, & M. C. Walsh (Eds.), *Fanaroff & Martin's neonatal-perinatal medicine: Diseases of the fetus and infant* (11th ed., pp. 424–439). Elsevier.

Huang, S., & Doherty, D. (2018). Congenital malformations of the central nervous system. In C. Gleason & S. Juul (Eds.), *Avery's diseases of the newborn* (10th ed., pp. 857–878.e5). Elsevier.

Hudak, M. L. (2020). Infants of substance-using mothers. In R. J. Martin, A. A. Fanaroff, & M. C. Walsh (Eds.), *Fanaroff*

& Martin's neonatal–perinatal medicine: Diseases of the fetus and infant (11th ed., pp. 735–750). Elsevier.

Hull, A. D., Resnik, R., & Silver, R. M. (2019). Placenta previa and accretea, vasa previa, subchorionic hemorrhage, and abruptio placentae. In R. Resnik, C. J. Lockwood, T. R. Moore, M. F. Greene, J. A. Copel, & R. M. Silver (Eds.), Creasy & Resnik's maternal-fetal medicine: Principles & practice (8th ed., pp. 786–797e4). Elsevier.

Hummel, P., & Naber, M. (2021). Discharge planning and transition to home. In M. T. Verklan, M. Walden, & S. Forest (Eds.), Core curriculum for neonatal intensive care nursing (6th ed., pp. 329–345). Elsevier.

Hüppi, P., & Gressens, P. (2020). White matter damage and encephalopathy of prematurity. In R. J. Martin, A. A. Fanaroff, & M. C. Walsh (Eds.), Fanaroff & Martin's neonatal-perinatal medicine: Diseases of the fetus and infant (11th ed., pp. 947–969). Elsevier.

Hutter, M. M., Kellogg, K. C., Ferguson, C. M., Abbott, W. M., & Warshaw, A. L. (2006). The impact of the 80-hour resident workweek on surgical residents and attending surgeons. Annuals of Surgery, 243(6), 864–875. https://doi.org/10.1097/01.sla.0000220042.48310.66

Inayat, M. (2020). Calcium disorders. In T. L. Gomella, F. G. Eyal, & F. Bany-Mohammed (Eds.), Gomella's neonatology: Management, procedures, on-call problems, diseases, and drugs (8th ed., pp. 833–836). McGraw-Hill Education.

Inder, T. (2020). Neonatal seizures. In R. J. Martin, A. A. Fanaroff, & M. C. Walsh (Eds.), Fanaroff & Martin's neonatal-perinatal medicine: Diseases of the fetus and infant (11th ed., pp. 1015–1043). Elsevier.

Inder, T. E., & Matthews, L. G. (2020). Neonatal brain disorders. In A. A. Fanaroff & J. M. Fanaroff (Eds.), Klaus and Fanaroff's care of the high-risk neonate (7th ed., pp. 386–408. e6). Elsevier.

Inder, T., Perlman, J., & Volpe, J. (2018). Intracranial hemorrhage: Subdural, subarachnoid, intraventricular (term infant), miscellaneous. In J. Volpe, T. Inder, B. Darras, L. deVries, A. Plessis, & J. Perlman (Eds.), Volpe's neurology of the newborn (6th ed., pp. 593–622.e7). Elsevier.

Inder, T., & Volpe, J. (2018a). Pathophysiology: General principles. In J. Volpe, T. Inder, B. Darras, L. deVries, A. Plessis, & J. Perlman (Eds.), Volpe's neurology of the newborn (6th ed., pp. 325–388.e26). Elsevier.

Inder, T., & Volpe, J. (2018b). Hypoxic-ischemic injury in the term infant: Clinical-neurological features, diagnosis, imaging, prognosis, therapy. In J. Volpe, T. Inder, B. Darras, L. deVries, A. Plessis, & J. Perlman (Eds.), Volpe's neurology of the newborn (6th ed., pp. 510–563.e7). Elsevier.

Ito, S., & Verstegen, R. (2021). Maternal medications during pregnancy and lactation. In J. V. Aranda & J. N. Van Den Anker (Eds.), Yaffe and Aranda's neonatal and pediatric therapeutic principles in practice (5th ed., pp. 135–147). Lippincott Williams & Wilkins.

Jackson, J., Knappen, B., & Olsen, S. L. (2021). Drug withdrawal in the neonate. In S. L. Gardner, B. S. Carter, M. Enzman-Hines, & S. Niermeyer (Eds.), Merenstein & Gardner's handbook of neonatal intensive care: An interprofessional approach (9th ed., pp. 250–272). Elsevier.

Jacquot, C., Mo, Y. D., & Luban, N. L. C. (2020). Blood component therapy for the neonate. In R. J. Martin, A. A. Fanaroff, & M. C. Walsh (Eds.), Fanaroff & Martin's

neonatal-perinatal medicine: Diseases of the fetus and infant (11th ed., pp. 1476–1503). Elsevier.

Javid, J., Riggle, K. M., & Smith, C. (2018). Necrotizing enterocolitis and short bowel syndrome. In C. Gleason & S. Juul (Eds.), Avery's diseases of the newborn (10th ed., pp. 1090–1097e2). Elsevier.

Jensen, E. A., Fraga, M. V., Biko, M. D., Raimondi, F., & Kirpalani, H. (2022). Imaging: Radiography, lung ultrasound, and other imaging modalities. In M. Keszler & K. S. Gautham (Eds.), Goldsmith's assisted ventilation of the neonate: An evidence-based approach to newborn respiratory care (7th ed., pp. 76–93). Elsevier.

Jerrim, J. (2022). Test anxiety: Is it associated with performance in high stakes examinations? Oxford Review of Education, 49(3), 321–341. https://doi.org/10.1080/03054985.2022.2079616

Jeyabalan, A. (2020). Hypertensive disorders of pregnancy. In R. J. Martin, A. A. Fanaroff, & M. C. Walsh (Eds.), Fanaroff & Martin's neonatal-perinatal medicine: Diseases of the fetus and infant (11th ed., pp. 288–303). Elsevier.

Jha, K., Nassar, G. N., & Makker, K. (2020). Transient tachypnea of the newborn. In T. L. Gomella, F. G. Eyal, & F. Bany-Mohammed (Eds.), Gomella's neonatology: Management, procedures, on-call problems, diseases, and drugs (8th ed., pp. 1107–1115). McGraw-Hill Education.

Johnson, C. E. (2019). Effect of inhaled lemon essential oil on cognitive test anxiety nursing students. Holistic Nursing, 33(2), 95–100. https://doi.org/10.1097/HNP.0000000000000315

Johnson, L. (2017). Assessment of the newborn history and physical examination of the newborn. In E. Eichenwald, C. Martin, A. Hansen, & A. Stark (Eds.), Cloherty and Stark's manual of neonatal care (8th ed., pp. 94–105). Lippincott Williams & Wilkins.

Johnson, P. J. (2019). Head, eyes, ears, nose, mouth, and neck assessment. In E. P. Tappero & M. E. Honeyfield (Eds.), Physical assessment of the newborn: A comprehensive approach to the art of physical examination (6th ed., pp. 61–77). Springer Publishing Company.

Joyner, R. L. (2019). Fetal lung development. In B. K. Walsh (Ed.), Neonatal and pediatric respiratory care (5th ed., pp. 1–12). Elsevier.

Juul, S. E., & Christensen, R. D. (2018). Developmental hematology. In C. Gleason & S. Juul (Eds.), Avery's diseases of the newborn (10th ed., pp. 1113–1120). Elsevier.

Juul, S., Fleiss, B., McAdams, M., & Gressens, P. (2018). Neuroprotection strategies for the newborn. In C. Gleason & S. Juul (Eds.), Avery's diseases of the newborn (10th ed., pp. 987–909.e4). Elsevier.

Kaimal, A. J. (2019). Assessment of fetal health. In R. Resnik, C. Lockwood, T. Moore, M. Greene, J. Copel, & R. Silver (Eds.), Creasy and Resnik's maternal-fetal medicine: Principles and practice (8th ed., pp. 549–563.e3). Elsevier.

Kallapur, S. G., & Jobe, A. H. (2020). Lung development and maturation. In R. J. Martin, A. A. Fanaroff, & M. C. Walsh (Eds.), Fanaroff & Martin's neonatal-perinatal medicine: Diseases of the fetus and infant (11th ed., pp. 1124–1142). Saunders.

Kamath-Rayne, B. D., Froese, P. A., & Thilo, E. H. (2021). Neonatal hyperbilirubinemia. In S. L. Gardner, B.

S. Carter, M. Enzman-Hines, & S. Niermeyer (Eds.), *Merenstein & Gardner's handbook of neonatal intensive care: An interprofessional approach* (9th ed., pp. 662–691). Elsevier.

Kandasamy, J., & Carlo, W. A. (2022). Pharmacologic therapies. In M. Keszler & K. S. Gautham (Eds.), *Goldsmith's assisted ventilation of the neonate: An evidence-based approach to newborn respiratory care* (7th ed., pp. 408–423). Elsevier.

Kanter, D. E. (2020). Is the infant ready for discharge? In T. L. Gomella, F. G. Eyal, & F. Bany-Mohammed (Eds.), *Gomella's neonatology: Management, procedures, on-call problems, diseases, and drugs* (8th ed., pp. 630–644). McGraw-Hill Education.

Kaplan, M., Wong, R. J., Burgis, J. C., Sibley, E., & Stevenson, D. K. (2020). Neonatal jaundice and liver disease. In R. J. Martin, A. A. Fanaroff, & M. C. Walsh (Eds.), *Fanaroff & Martin's neonatal-perinatal medicine: Diseases of the fetus and infant* (11th ed., pp. 1788–1852). Elsevier.

Kasser, J. (2017). Orthopedic problems. In E. Eichenwald, A. Hansen, C. Martin, & A. Stark (Eds.), *Cloherty and Stark's manual of neonatal care* (8th ed., pp. 845–852). Lippincott Williams & Wilkins.

Katheria, A. C., Erickson-Owens, D. A., & Mercer, J. S. (2020). Delayed cord clamping and cord milking. In J. Ramasethu & S. Seo (Ed.), *MacDonald's atlas of procedures in neonatology* (6th ed., pp. 362–367). Wolters Kluwer.

Katheria, A., & Finer, N. (2018). Newborn resuscitation. In C. Gleason & S. Juul (Eds.), *Avery's diseases of the newborn* (20th ed., pp. 273–288). Elsevier.

Katzung, B. G. (2020). Basic and clinical pharmacology. In J. Ramasethu & S. Seo (Eds.), *MacDonald's atlas of procedures in neonatology* (6th ed., pp. 224–232). Wolters Kluwer.

Katzung, B. G. (2021). Introduction: The nature of drugs & drug development & regulation. In: B. G. Katzung & T. W. Vanderah (Eds.), *Basic and clinical pharmacology.* (15th ed., pp. 1–20). McGraw Hill.

Kaufman, D. A., & Manzoni, P. (2020). Fungal and protozoal infections of the neonate. In R. J. Martin, A. A. Fanaroff, & M. C. Walsh (Eds.), *Fanaroff & Martin's neonatal-perinatal medicine: Diseases of the fetus and infant* (11th ed., pp. 809–843). Elsevier.

Kaushal, S., & Ramasethu, J. (2020). Phototherapy. In J. Ramasethu & S. Seo (Eds.), *MacDonald's atlas of procedures in neonatology* (6th ed., pp. 447–452). Wolters Kluwer.

Keller, B., Hirose, S., & Farmer, D. (2018). Surgical disorders of the chest and airways. In C. Gleason & S. Juul (Eds.), *Avery's diseases of the newborn* (10th ed., pp. 695–723.e9). Elsevier.

Kelly, T. F. (2018). Maternal medical disorders of fetal significance. In C. A. Gleason & S. E. Juul (Eds.), *Avery's diseases of the newborn* (10th ed., pp. 104–118.e3). Elsevier.

Kenner, C., & Boykova, M. (2021). Families in crisis. In M. T. Verklan, M. Walden, & S. Forest (Eds.), *Core curriculum for neonatal intensive care nursing* (6th ed., pp. 288–300). Elsevier.

Keszler, M. (2022). Overview of assisted ventilation. In M. Keszler & K. S. Gautham (Eds.), *Goldsmith's assisted ventilation of the neonate: An evidence-based approach to newborn respiratory care* (7th ed., pp. 221–231). Elsevier.

Keszler, M., & Abubakar, K. (2022a). Physiologic principles. In M. Keszler & K. S. Gautham (Eds.), *Goldsmith's assisted ventilation of the neonate: An evidence-based approach to newborn respiratory care* (7th ed., pp. 11–32). Elsevier.

Keszler, M., & Abubakar, K. (2022b). Volume-targeted ventilation. In M. Keszler & K. S. Gautham (Eds.), *Goldsmith's assisted ventilation of the neonate: An evidence-based approach to newborn respiratory care* (7th ed., pp. 249–262). Elsevier.

Keszler, M., & Mammel, M. C. (2022). Basic modes of synchronized ventilation. In M. Keszler & K. S. Gautham (Eds.), *Goldsmith's assisted ventilation of the neonate: An evidence-based approach to newborn respiratory care* (7th ed., pp. 232–240). Elsevier.

Keszler, M., Pillow, J. J., & Courtney, S. E. (2022). High frequency ventilation. In M. Keszler & K. S. Gautham (Eds.), *Goldsmith's assisted ventilation of the neonate: An evidence-based approach to newborn respiratory care* (7th ed., pp. 269–287). Elsevier.

Khan, A. M. (2017). Shock. In E. Eichenwald, C. Martin, A. Hansen, & A. Stark (Eds.), *Cloherty and Stark's manual of neonatal care* (8th ed., pp. 502–509). Lippincott Williams & Wilkins.

Khorsand, K., & Sidburn, R. (2018). Common newborn dermatoses. In C. A. Gleason & S. E. Juul (Eds.), *Avery's diseases of the newborn* (10th ed., pp. 1503–1510.e1). Elsevier.

Kim, G., Nandi-Munshi, D., & Diblasi, C. C. (2018). Disorders of the thyroid gland. In C. Gleason & S. Juul (Eds.), *Avery's diseases of the newborn* (10th ed., pp. 1388–1402). Elsevier.

Kleinman, M. E. (2017). Neonatal transport. In E. Eichenwald, A. Hansen, C. Martin, & A. Stark (Eds.), *Cloherty and Stark's manual of neonatal care* (8th ed., pp. 202–213). Lippincott Williams & Wilkins.

Kleinpell, R., Myers, C. R., Schorn, M. N., & Likes, W. (2021). Impact of COVID-19 pandemic on APRN practice: Results from a national survey. *Nursing Outlook, 69*(5), 783–792. https://doi.org/10.1016/j.outlook.2021.05.002

Kogon, A., & Truong, H. (2019). Management, procedures, on-call problems, diseases, and drugs. In E. P. Tappero & M. E. Honeyfield (Eds.), *Recording and evaluating the neonatal history* (6th ed., pp. 9–21). Springer Publishing Company.

Kogon, A., & Truong, H. (2020). Acute kidney injury. In T. L. Gomella, F. G. Eyal, & F. Bany-Mohammed (Eds.), *Gomella's neonatology: Management, procedures, on-call problems, diseases, and drugs* (8th ed., pp. 803–807). McGraw-Hill Education.

Kogon, A., & Truong, H. (2021). Pharmacology in neonatal care. In S. L. Gardner, B. S. Carter, M. Enzman-Hines, & S. Niermeyer (Eds.), *Merenstein & Gardner's handbook of neonatal intensive care: An interprofessional approach* (9th ed., pp. 226–249). Elsevier.

Konczal, L. L., & Zinn, A. B. (2020). Inborn errors of metabolism. In R. J. Martin, A. A. Faranoff, & M. C. Walsh (Eds.), *Neonatal-perinatal medicine: Diseases of the fetus and infant St* (11th ed., pp. 1706–1785). Elsevier.

Koo, N., Sims, T., Arensman, R. M., Srinivasan, N., Patel, S., Maheshwari, A., & Ambalavanan, A. (2022). Medical and surgical intrventions for respiratory distress and airway management. In M. Keszler & K. S. Gautham (Eds.), *Goldsmith's assisted ventilation of the neonate: An evidence-based approach to newborn respiratory care* (7th ed., pp. 473–490). Elsevier.

Koves, I. H., Ness, K. D., Nip, A. S., & Salehi, P. (2018). Disorders of calcium and phosphorus metabolism. In C. A. Gleason & S. E. Juul (Eds.), *Avery's diseases of the newborn* (10th ed., pp. 1333–1350). Elsevier.

Ku, L. C., Hornik, C., & Buschbach, D. (2021). Pharmacology in neonatal care. In: S. L. Gardner, B. S. Carter, M. Enzman-Hines & S. Niermeyer (Eds.), *Merenstein & Gardner's handbook of neonatal intensive care nursing: An interprofessional approach.* (9th ed., pp. 226–249). Elsevier.

Kudin, O., & Neu, J. (2020). Neonatal necrotizing enterocolitis. In R. J. Martin, A. A. Fanaroff, & M. C. Walsh (Eds.), *Fanaroff & Martin's neonatal-perinatal medicine: Diseases of the fetus and infant* (11th ed., pp. 1571–1581). Elsevier.

Lagoski, M., Hamvas, A., & Wambach, J. A. (2020). Respiratory distress syndrome in the neonate. In R. J. Martin, A. A. Fanaroff, & M. C. Walsh (Eds.), *Fanaroff & Martin's neonatal-perinatal medicine: Diseases of the fetus and infant* (11th ed., pp. 1159–1173). Elsevier.

Lakshminrusimha, S., & Keszler, M. (2022). Diagnosis and management of persistent pulmonary hypertension of the newborn. In M. Keszler & K. S. Gautham (Eds.), *Goldsmith's assisted ventilation of the neonate: An evidence-based approach to newborn respiratory care* (7th ed., pp. 429–445). Elsevier.

Lakshminrusimha, S., Keszler, M., & Yoder, B. A. (2022). Care of the infant with congenital diaphragmatic hernia. In M. Keszler & K. S. Gautham (Eds.), *Goldsmith's assisted ventilation of the neonate: An evidence-based approach to newborn respiratory care* (7th ed., pp. 446–457). Elsevier.

Lampiris, H. W., & Maddix, D. S. (2021). Antifungal agents. In: B. G. Katzung & T. W. Vanderah (Eds.), *Basic and clinical pharmacology.* (15th ed., pp. 887–896). McGraw Hill.

Lane, E., Chisholm, K., & Murray, K. (2018). Disorders of the liver. In C. Gleason & S. Juul (Eds.), *Avery's diseases of the newborn* (10th ed., pp. 1098–1112.e1). Elsevier.

Larson-Nath, C., Gurram, B., & Chelmisky, G. (2020). Disorders of digestion in the neonate. In R. J. Martin, A. A. Fanaroff, & M. C. Walsh (Eds.), *Fanaroff & Martin's neonatal-perinatal medicine: Diseases of the fetus and infant* (11th ed., pp. 1522–1540). Elsevier.

Laventhal, N. T., & Fanaroff, J. M. (2020). Medical ethics in neonatal care. In R. J. Martin, A. A. Fanaroff, & M. C. Walsh (Eds.), *Fanaroff & Martin's neonatal-perinatal medicine: Diseases of the fetus and infant* (11th ed., pp. 25–46). Elsevier.

Lazebnik, N., Judge, N. E., & Dar, P. (2020). Prenatal ultrasound. In R. J. Martin, A. A. Fanaroff, & M. C. Walsh (Eds.), *Fanaroff & Martin's neonatal-perinatal medicine: Diseases of the fetus and infant* (11th ed., pp. 174–209). Elsevier.

Le, J., & Bradley, J. S. (2021). Macrolides, Clindamycin, and oxazolidinones. In: J. V. Aranda & J. N. Van Den Anker (Eds.), *Yaffe and Aranda's neonatal and pediatric therapeutic porinciples in practice.* (5th ed., pp. 321–332). Lippincott Williams & Wilkins.

LeBeau, R. T., Glenn, D., Liao, B., Wittchen, H. U., Beesdo-Baum, K., Ollendick, T., & Craske, M. (2010). Specific phobia: A review of the *DSM-IV* specific phobia and preliminary recommendations for *DSM-V*. *Depression and Anxiety, 27*(2), 148–167. https://doi.org/10.1002/da.20655

Ledbetter, D. J., Chabra, S., & Javid, P. J. (2018). Abdominal wall defects. In C. A. Gleason & S. E. Juul (Eds.), *Avery's diseases of the newborn* (10th ed., pp. 1068–1078). Elsevier.

Lee, H. K., & Oh, E. (2017). Care of the well newborn. In: E. Eichenwald, A. Hansen, C. Martin, & A. Stark. (Eds) (Eds.), *Cloherty and Stark's manual of neonatal care.* (8th ed., pp. 225–243). Lippincott Williams & Wilkins.

Lee-Parritz, A. (2017). Maternal diabetes mellitus. In E. C. Eichenwald, A. R. Hansen, C. R. Martin, & A. R. Stark (Eds.), *Cloherty and Stark's manual of neonatal care* (8th ed., pp. 44–49). Lippincott Williams & Wilkins.

Leeman, K. T., & VanderVeen, D. K. (2017). Retinopathy of prematurity. In E. Eichenwald, C. Martin, A. Hansen, & A. Stark (Eds.), *Cloherty and Stark's manual of neonatal care* (8th ed., pp. 986–992). Lippincott Williams & Wilkins.

Lehr, V. T., & Williams, M. T. (2021). Anticonvulsants. In J. V. Aranda & J. N. Van Den Anker (Eds.), *Yaffe and Aranda's neonatal and pediatric therapeutic principles in practice* (5th ed., pp. 473–498). Lippincott Williams & Wilkins.

Letterio, I., Pateva, I., Petrosiute, A., & Ahuja, S. (2020). Hematologic and oncologic problems in the fetus and neonate. In R. J. Martin, A. A. Fanaroff, & M. C. Walsh (Eds.), *Fanaroff & Martin's neonatal-perinatal medicine: Diseases of the fetus and infant* (11th ed., pp. 1416–1475). Elsevier.

Letterio, J., & Ahuja, S. P. (2020). Hematologic problems. In A. A. Fanaroff & J. M. Fanaroff (Eds.), *Klaus and Fanaroff's care of the high-risk neonate* (7th ed., pp. 352–385). Elsevier.

Letterio, J., Pateva, I., Petrosiute, A., & Ahuja, S. (2020). Hematologic and oncologic problems in the fetus and neonate. In R. J. Martin, A. A. Fanaroff, & M. C. Walsh (Eds.), *Fanaroff & Martin's neonatal-perinatal medicine: Diseases of the fetus and infant?* (11th ed., pp. 1416–1475). Elsevier.

Li, L., & White, J. (2019). Pharmacology. In B. Walsh (Ed.), *Neonatal and pediatric respiratory care* (5th ed., pp. 370–394). Elsevier.

Limperopoulos, C., du Plessis, A., & Volpe, J. (2018). Cerebellar hemorrhage. In J. Volpe, T. Inder, B. Darras, L. deVries, A. Plessis, & J. Perlman (Eds.), *Volpe's neurology of the newborn* (6th ed., pp. 623–636). Elsevier.

Lingappan, K., & Gautham, K. S. (2022). Evidence-based respiratory care. In M. Kessler & K. S. Gautham (Eds.), *Goldsmith's assisted ventilation of the neonate: An evidence-based approach to newborn respiratory care* (7th ed., pp. 47–55.e1). Elsevier.

Link, D. G. (2016). Psychology of pregnancy. In S. Mattson & J. E. Smith (Eds.), *Core curriculum for maternal-newborn nursing* (5th ed., pp. 108–122). Elsevier.

Lissauer, T., & Hansen. (2020). Physical examination of the newborn. In R. J. Martin, A. A. Fanaroff, & M. C. Walsh (Eds.), *Fanaroff & Martin's neonatal–perinatal medicine: Diseases of the fetus and infant* (10th ed., pp. 440–457). Elsevier.

Liu, R., & Thompson, G. (2020). Musculoskeletal disorders in neonates. In R. J. Martin, A. A. Fanaroff, & M. C. Walsh (Eds.), *Fanaroff & Martin's neonatal–perinatal medicine: Diseases of the fetus and infant* (11th ed., pp. 1980–1988). Elsevier.

Lopez, S. M., & Tyson, J. E. (2020). Practicing evidence-based neonatal-perinatal medicine. In R. J. Martin, A. A. Fanaroff, & M. C. Walsh (Eds.), *Fanaroff & Martin's* neonatal–perinatal medicine: Diseases of the fetus and infant (11th ed., Vol. 1, pp. 113–119). Elsevier.

Lubbers, L. A. (2021). Congenital anomalies. In M. T. Verklan, M. Walden, & S. Forest (Eds.), Core curriculum for neonatal intensive care nursing (6th ed., pp. 654–677). Elsevier.

Lund, C., & Druand, D. J. (2021). Skin and skin care. In: S. L. Gardner, B. S. Carter, M. Enzman-Hines, & S. Niermeyer (Eds.), Merenstein & Gardner's handbook of neonatal intensive care nursing: An interprofessional approach. (9th ed., pp. 602–622). Elsevier.

Lüscher, C. (2021). Drugs of abuse. In B. G. Katzung & T. W. Vanderah (Eds.), Basic & clinical pharmacology (15th ed., pp. 596–612). McGraw-Hill Education.

Maddix, D. S. (2021). Antifungal agents. In: B. G. Katzung& T. W. Vanderah (Eds.), Basic and clinical pharmacology. (15th ed., pp. 887–896). McGraw Hill.

Madenci, A. L., Rice-Townsend, S. E., & Weldon, C. B. (2019). Surgical disorders in childhood that affect respiratory care. In B. K. Walsh (Ed.), Neonatal and pediatric respiratory care (5th ed., pp. 453–468). Elsevier.

Maguire, D. (2021). Renal and genitourinary disorders. In M. T. Verklan, M. Walden, & S. Forest (Eds.), Core curriculum for neonatal intensive care nursing (6th ed., pp. 617–628). Elsevier.

Malone, F., & D'Alton, M. (2019). Multiple gestation: Clinical characteristics and management. In R. Resnik, C. Lockwood, T. Moore, M. Greene, J. Copel, & R. Silver (Eds.), Creasy and Resnik's maternal-fetal medicine: Principles and practice (8th ed., pp. 654–675.e5). Elsevier.

Maltepe, E., & Penn, A. A. (2018). Development, function, and pathology of the placenta. In C. A. Gleason & S. E. Juul (Eds.), Avery's diseases of the newborn (10th ed., pp. 40–60. e8). Elsevier.

Mandy, G. T., & Suresh, G. (2020). Hypoglycemia. In T. L. Gomella, F. G. Eyal, & F. Bany-Mohammed (Eds.), Gomella's neonatology: Management, procedures, on-call problems, diseases, and drugs (8th ed., pp. 587–601). McGraw-Hill Education.

Manley, B. J., Davis, P. G., Yoder, B. A., & Owen, L. S. (2022). Noninvasive respiratory support. In M. Keszler & K. S. Gautham (Eds.), Assisted ventilation of the neonate (7th ed., pp. 201–220). Elsevier.

Markham, M. (2017). Pulmonary air leak. In E. Eichenwald, A. Hansen, C. Martin, & A. Stark (Eds.), Cloherty & Stark's manual of neonatal care (8th ed., pp. 482–490). Wolters Kluwer.

Matthews, A. L., & Robin, N. H. (2021). Genetic disorders, malformations, and inborn errors of metabolism. In S. L. Gardner, B. S. Carter, M. Enzman-Hines, & S. Niermeyer (Eds.), Merenstein & Gardner's handbook of neonatal intensive care nursing: An interprofessional approach (9th ed., pp. 969–995). Elsevier.

McAdams, R., & Traudt, C. (2018). Brain injury in the term infant. In C. Gleason & S. Juul (Eds.), Avery's diseases of the newborn (10th ed., pp. 987–909.e4). Elsevier.

McAleer, I. (2018). Renal development. In C. A. Gleason & S. E. Juul (Eds.), Avery's diseases of the newborn (10th ed., pp. 1238–1249). Elsevier.

McCandless, S. E., & Kripps, K. A. (2020a). Genetics inborn errors of metabolism and newborn screening. In A. A. Fanaroff & J. M. Fanaroff (Eds.), Klaus and Fanaroff's care of the high-risk neonate (7th ed., pp. 121–147). Elsevier.

McCandless, S. E., & Kripps, K. A. (2020b). Principles of drug use in the fetus and neonate. In R. J. Martin, A. A. Fanaroff, & M. C. Walsh (Eds.), Fanaroff & Martin's neonatal perinatal medicine: Diseases of the fetus and infant (11th ed., pp. 704–716). Elsevier.

McClary, J. D. (2020). Principles of drugs use in the fetus and neonate. In R. J. Martin, A. A. Fanaroff, & M. C. Walsh (Eds.), Fanaroff & Martin's neonatal-perinatal medicine: Diseases of the fetus and infant (11th ed., pp. 704–716). Elsevier.

McElroy, S. J., Frey, M. R., Torres, B. A., & Maheshwari, A. (2018). Innate and mucosal immunity in the developing gastrointestinal tract. In C. Gleason & S. Juul (Eds.), Avery's diseases of the newborn (10th ed., pp. 1054–1067). Elsevier.

McEwen, S. T., & Vogt, B. A. (2020). The kidney. In A. A. Fanaroff & J. M. Fanaroff (Eds.), Klaus and Fanaroff's care of the high-risk neonate (7th ed., pp. 623–661). Mosby.

McEwen, S. T., & Vogt, B. A. (2021). Newborn hematology. In S. L. Gardner, B. S. Carter, M. Enzman-Hines, & S. Niermeyer (Eds.), Merenstein & Gardner's handbook of neonatal intensive care: An interprofessional approach (9th ed., pp. 333–351.e2). Elsevier.

McKinney, ., B. B, C., Warren., & Harvey, S. (2021). Newborn h ematology. In: S. L. Gardner, B. S. Carter, M. Enzman-Hines& S. Niermeyer (Eds.), Merenstein & Gardner's handbook of neonatal intensive care nursing: An interprofessional approach. (9th ed., pp. 623–661). Elsevier.

McKinney, C., Warren, B. B., & Harvey, S. (2021). Newborn hematology. In S. L. Gardner, B. S. Carter, M. Enzman-Hines, & S. Niermeyer (Eds.), Merenstein & Gardner's handbook of neonatal intensive care nursing: An interprofessional approach (9th ed., pp. 623–661). Elsevier.

Melnyk, B. M., & Fineout-Overholt, E. (2019). Making the case for evidence-based practice and cultivating a spirit of inquiry. In B. M. Melnyk & E. Fineout-Overholt (Eds.), Evidence-based practice in nursing and healthcare (4th ed., pp. 7–32). Wolters Kluwer.

Mercer, B. M., & Chien, E. K. S. (2019). Premature rupture of membranes. In R. Resnik, C. Lockwood, T. Moore, M. Greene, J. Copel, & R. Silver (Eds.), Creasy and Resnik's maternal-fetal medicine: Principles and practice (8th ed., pp. 712–722 e5). Elsevier.

Merguerian, P. A., & Rowe, C. K. (2018). Developmental abnormalities of the genitourinary system. In C. A. Gleason & S. E. Juul (Eds.), Avery's diseases of the newborn (10th ed., pp. 1260–1273). Elsevier.

Merritt, J. L., & Gallagher, R. (2018). Inborn errors of carbohydrate, ammonia, amino acid, and organic acid metabolism. In C. Gleason & S. Juul (Eds.), Avery's diseases of the newborn (10th ed., pp. 230–252.e4). Elsevier.

Meschia, G. (2019). Placenta respiratory gas exchange and fetal oxygenation. In R. Resnik, C. J. Lockwood, T. Moore, M. F. Greene, J. Copel, & R. M. Silver (Eds.), Creasy and Resnik's maternal fetal medicine: Principles and practice (8th ed., pp. 210–222.e1). Elsevier.

Michaels, M. G., Sanchez, P., & Lin, L. (2018). Congenital toxoplasmosis, syphilis, malaria, and tuberculosis. In C. Gleason & S. Juul (Eds.), Avery's diseases of the newborn (10th ed., pp. 527–552.e6). Elsevier.

Mitchell, A. L. (2020). Congenital anomalies. In R. J. Martin, A. A. Fanaroff, & M. C. Walsh (Eds.), Fanaroff & Martin's neonatal-perinatal medicine: Diseases of the fetus and infant (11th ed., pp. 489–513). Elsevier.

Miyatsu, T., Nguyen, K., & McDaniel, M. A. (2018). Five popular study strategies: Their pitfalls and optimal implementations. *Perspectives on Psychology, 13*(3), 390–407. https://doi.org/10.1177/1745691617710510

Mizuno, T., Walson, P. D., & Vinks, A. A. (2021). Precision medicine and therapeutic drug monitoring. In J. V. Aranda & J. N. Van Den Anker (Eds.), *Yaffe and Aranda's neonatal and pediatric therapeutic principles in practice* (5th ed., pp. 95–113). Lippincott Williams & Wilkins.

Mooney, M. E. (2016). Maternal infections. In S. Mattson & J. E. Smith (Eds.), *Core curriculum for maternal-newborn nursing* (5th ed., pp. 452–479). Elsevier.

Moore, T. (2018). Hypertensive complications of pregnancy. In C. Gleason & S. Juul (Eds.), *Avery's diseases of the newborn* (10th ed., pp. 119–125.e2). Elsevier.

Moore, T., Hauguel-De Mouzon, S., & Catalano, P. (2019). Diabetes in pregnancy. In R. Resnik, C. Lockwood, T. Moore, M. Greene, J. Copel, & R. Silver (Eds.), *Creasy and Resnik's maternal-fetal medicine: Principles and practice* (8th ed., pp. 1067–1097.e5). Elsevier.

Moyer, J., Iqbal, C. W., Hirose, S., & Lee, H. (2020). Surgical treatment of the fetus. In R. J. Martin, A. A. Fanaroff, & M. C. Walsh (Eds.), *Fanaroff & Martin's neonatal-perinatal medicine: Diseases of the fetus and infant* (11th ed., pp. 223–238). Elsevier.

Nageotte, M. (2019). Intrapartum fetal surveillance. In R. Resnik, C. Lockwood, T. Moore, M. Greene, J. Copel, & R. Silver (Eds.), *Creasy and Resnik's maternal-fetal medicine: Principles and practice* (8th ed., pp. 564–582.e2). Elsevier.

Narendran, V. (2020). The skin of the neonate. In R. J. Martin, A. A. Fanaroff, & M. C. Walsh (Eds.), *Fanaroff & Martin's neonatal-perinatal medicine: Diseases of the fetus and infant* (11th ed., pp. 1898–1932). Elsevier.

Natarajan, N., & Gospe, S. (2018). Neonatal seizures. In C. Gleason & S. Juul (Eds.), *Avery's diseases of the newborn* (10th ed., pp. 961–970.e4). Elsevier.

Natarajan, N., & Ionita, C. (2018). Neonatal neuromuscular disorders. In C. Gleason & S. Juul (Eds.), *Avery's diseases of the newborn* (10th ed., pp. 952–960). Elsevier.

National Association of Neonatal Nurses. (2013). *Neonatal nurse practitioner workforce. Position statement #3058.* http://nann.org/uploads/About/PositionPDFS/NNP_Workforce_Position_Statement_01.22.13_FINAL.pdf

National Association of Neonatal Nurses. (2014). *Advanced practice registered nurse: Role, preparation, and scope of practice. Position statement #3059.* http://nann.org/uploads/Membership/NANNP_Pubs/APRN_Role_Preparation_position_stateet_FINAL.pdf

National Association of Neonatal Nurses. (2015). *Palliative and end-of-life care for newborns and infants. Position statement #3063 NANN Board of Directors.* http://nann.org/uploads/About/PositionPDFS/1.4.5_Palliative%20and%20End%20of%20Life%20Care%20for%20Newborns%20and%20Infants.pdf

National Association of Neonatal Nurses. (2021). *Position statement #3067 NICU nurse involvement in ethical decisions (Treatment of critically ill newborns).* Retrieved from https://nann.org/uploads/About/PositionPDFS/NICU%20Nurse%20Involvement%20in%20Ethical%20Decisions.pdf

National Association of Neonatal Nursing. (n.d.). *Clinical Practice Products.* https://nann.org/education/educational-products/clinical-practice-products

National Certification Corporation. (2019). *Certification examination core.* https://www.nccwebsite.org/content/documents/cms/exam-np-bc.pdf

National Certification Corporation. (2022). *2022 candidate guide neonatal nurse practitioner NNP-BC.* https://www.nccwebsite.org/content/documents/cms/NNP-Candidate_Guide.pdf

National Council for State Boards of Nursing. (2019). *APRN consensus model.* Retrieved from https://www.ncsbn.org/nursing-regulation/practice/aprn/aprn-consensus.page

Neil, J., & Inder, T. (2018). Neonatal neuroimaging. In C. Gleason & S. Juul (Eds.), *Avery's diseases of the newborn* (10th ed., pp. 922–951). Elsevier.

Neil, J., & Volpe, J. (2018a). Encephalopathy of prematurity: Clinical-neurological features, diagnosis, imaging, prognosis, therapy. In J. Volpe, T. Inder, B. Darras, L. deVries, A. Plessis, & J. Perlman (Ed.), *Volpe's neurology of the newborn* (6th ed., pp. 425–457.e11). Elsevier.

Neil, J., & Volpe, J. (2018b). Specialized neurological studies. In J. Volpe, T. Inder, B. Darras, L. deVries, A. Plessis, & J. Perlman (Eds.), *Volpe's neurology of the newborn* (6th ed., pp. 67–92). Elsevier.

Nguyen, J., Liu, A., McKenney, M., & Elkbul, A. (2021). Predictive factors for first time pass rate on the American Board of Surgery certification in general surgery exams: A systematic review. *Journal of Surgical Education, 78*(5), 1676–1691.

Niermeyer, S., & Clarke, S.B. (2021). Care at birth. In S. L. Gardner, B. S. Carter, M. Enzman-Hines, & S. Niermeyer (Eds.), *Merenstein & Gardner's handbook of neonatal intensive care nursing: an interprofessional approach* (9th ed., pp. 67–92). Elsevier.

Nomura, O., Onishi, H., Park, Y. S., Michihata, N., Kobayashi, T., Kaneko, K., & Ishiguro, A. (2021). Predictors of performance on the pediatric board certification. *BMC Medical Education, 21*(1), 122–122. https://doi.org/10.1186/s12909-021-02515-z

Noori, S., Azhibekov, T., Lee, B., & Seri, I. (2018). Cardiovascular compromise in the newborn. In C. A. Gleason & S. E. Juul (Eds.), *Avery's diseases of the newborn* (10th ed., pp. 741–767.e2). Elsevier.

Norwitz, E. R., Mahendroo, M., & Lye, S. J. (2019). Physiology of parturition. In R. Resnik, C. J. Lockwood, T. R. Moore, M. F. Greene, J. A. Copel, & R. M. Silver (Eds.), *Creasy & Resnik's maternal-fetal medicine: Principles and practice* (8th ed., pp. 81–95e6). Elsevier.

Nyp, M., Brunkhorst, J. L., Reavey, D., & Pallotio, E. K. (2021). Fluid and electrolyte management. In S. L. Gardner, B. S. Carter, M. Enzman-Hines, & S. Niermeyer (Eds.), *Merenstein & Gardner's handbook of neonatal intensive care: An interprofessional approach* (9th ed., pp. 407–430). Elsevier.

Obican, S. G., & Odibo, A. O. (2019). Invasive fetal therapy. In R. Resnik, C. J. Lockwood, T. R. Moore, M. F. Greene, J. A. Copel, & R. M. Silver (Eds.), *Creasy & Resnik's maternal-fetal medicine: Principles and practice* (8th ed., pp. 594–631.e10). Elsevier.

O'Brien-Abel, N., & Simpson, K. R. (2021). Fetal assessment during labor. In K. Simpson & P. Creehan (Eds.), *Perinatal nursing* (5th ed., pp. 412–465). Lippincott Williams & Wilkins.

Odackal, N. J., & Swanson, J. R. (2020). Abdominal distension. In T. L. Gomella, F. G. Eyal, & F. Bany-Mohammed (Eds.), *Gomella's neonatology: Management, procedures, on-call problems, diseases, and drugs* (8th ed., pp. 427–431). McGraw-Hill Education.

Olsen, S. L., Oschman, A., & Tracy, K. (2021). Total parenteral nutrition. In S. L. Gardner, B. S. Carter, M. Enzman-Hines, & S. Niermeyer (Ed.), *Merenstein & Gardner's handbook of neonatal intensive care: An interprofessional approach* (9th ed., pp. 459–479). Elsevier.

O'Mahony, L., & Woodward, G. (2018). Neonatal transport. In C. A. Gleason & S. E. Juul (Eds.), *Avery's diseases of the newborn* (10th ed., pp. 347–360). Elsevier.

O'Mathúna, D. P. (2019). Ethical considerations for evidence implementation and evidence generation. In B. M. Melnyk & E. Fineout-Overholt (Eds.), *Evidence-based practice in nursing and healthcare* (4th ed., pp. 681–699). Wolters Kluwer.

O'Mathúna, D. P., & Fineout-Overholt, E. (2019). Critically appraising quantitative evidence for clinical decision making. In B. M. Melnyk & E. Fineout-Overholt (Eds.), *Evidence-based practice in nursing and healthcare* (4th ed., pp. 124–188). Wolters Kluwer.

O'Reilly, D.(2017). Polycythemia. In E. Eichenwald, A. Hansen, C. Martin, & A. Stark (Eds.), *Cloherty and Stark's manual of neonatal care* (8th ed., pp. 624–629). Lippincott Williams & Wilkins.

Örge, F. (2020). Examination and common problems of the neonatal eye. In R. J. Martin, A. A. Fanaroff, & M. C. Walsh (Eds.), *Fanaroff & Martin's neonatal–perinatal medicine: Diseases of the fetus and infant* (11th ed., pp. 1934–1969). Elsevier.

Otteson, T. D., & Wang, T. (2020). Upper airway lesions in the neonate. In R. J. Martin, A. A. Fanaroff, & M. C. Walsh (Eds.), *Fanaroff & Martin's neonatal-perintal medicine: Diseases of the fetus and infant* (11th ed., pp. 1244–1255). Elsevier.

Owen, L. S., Weiner, G., & Davis, P. G. (2022). Delivery room stabilization, and respiratory support. In M. Keszler & K. S. Gautham (Eds.), *Goldsmith's assisted ventilation of the neonate: An evidence-based approach to newborn respiratory care* (7th ed., pp. 151–171). Elsevier.

Pammi, M., Brand, M. C., & Weisman, L. E. (2021). Infection in the neonate. In S. L. Gardner, B. S. Carter, M. I. Enzman-Hines, & S. Niermeyer (Eds.), *Merenstein & Gardner's handbook of neonatal intensive care: An interprofessional approach* (9th ed., pp. 692–727). Elsevier.

Pappas, B. E., & Robey, D. L. (2021). Neonatal delivery room resuscitation. In M. T. Verklan, M. Walden, & S. Forest (Eds.), *Core curriculum for neonatal intensive care nursing* (6th ed., pp. 69–85). Elsevier.

Parad, R. B., & Banjamin, J. (2017). Bronchopulmonary dysplasia/chronic lung disease. In E. Eichenwald, A. Hansen, C. Martin, & A. Stark (Eds.), *Cloherty and Stark's manual of neonatal care* (8th ed., pp. 446–460). Lippincott Williams & Wilkins.

Parker, L. A. (2021). Nutritional management. In M. T. Verklan, M. Walden, & S. Forest (Eds.), *Core curriculum for neonatal intensive care nursing* (6th ed., pp. 151–171). Elsevier.

Parker, T., & Kinsella, J. (2018). Respiratory disorders in the term infant. In C. Gleason & S. Juul (Eds.), *Avery's diseases of the newborn* (10th ed., pp. 668–677.e3). Elsevier.

Patel, R., & Josephson, C. (2018). Neonatal transfusion. In C. Gleason & S. Juul (Eds.), *Avery's diseases of the newborn* (10th ed., pp. 1180–1186.e3). Elsevier.

Patrick, S. (2017). Maternal drug use, infant exposure, and neonatal abstinence syndrome. In E. Eichenwald, A. Hansen, C. Martin, & A. Stark (Eds.), *Cloherty and Stark's manual of neonatal care* (8th ed., pp. 141–157). Lippincott Williams & Wilkins.

Patrinos, M. E. (2020). Neonatal apnea and the foundation of respiratory control. In R. J. Martin, A. A. Fanaroff, & M. C. Walsh (Eds.), *Fanaroff & Martin's neonatal-perinatal medicine: Diseases of the fetus and infant* (11th ed., pp. 1231–1243). Saunders.

Patterson, M. C. (2016). A naturalistic investigation of media multitasking while studying and the effects on exam performance. *The Teaching of Psychology*, 44(1), 51–57, 316677913. https://doi.org/10.1177/0098628

Peck, J. L., & Sonney, J. (2021). Exhausted and burned out: COVID-19 emerging impacts threaten the health of the pediatric advanced practice registered nursing workforce. *Journal of Pediatric Health Care*, 35(4), 414–424. https://doi.org/10.1016/j.pedhc.2021.04.012

Permar, S. R. (2017). Bacterial and fungal infections. In E. Eichenwald, A. Hansen, C. Martin, & A. Stark (Eds.), *Cloherty and Stark's manual of neonatal care* (8th ed., pp. 641–650). Lippincott Williams & Wilkins.

Pettker, C., & Grobman, W. (2019). Patient safety and quality improvement in obstetrics. In R. Resnik, C. Lockwood, T. Moore, M. Greene, J. Copel, & R. Silver (Eds.), *Creasy and Resnik's maternal-fetal medicine: Principles and practice* (8th ed., pp. 841–851.e3). Elsevier.

Pettker, C. M., & Campbell, K. H. (2018). Antepartum fetal assessment. In: C. A. Gleason & S. E. Juul (Eds.), *Avery's diseases of the newborn* (10th ed., pp. 145 – 157.e3). Elsevier.

Phelps, C. M., Thrush, P. T., & Cua, C. L. (2020). The heart. In A. A. Fanaroff & J. M. Fanaroff (Eds.), *Klaus and Fanaroff's care of the high-risk neonate* (7th ed., pp. 704–716). Elsevier.

Picciano, M., McGuire, M., & Coates, P. (2021). Nutrient supplements. In S. Yaffe & J. Aranda (Eds.), *Neonatal and pediatric pharmacology: Therapeutic principles in practice*, (5th ed., pp. 893–912). Lippincott Williams & Wilkins.

Placencia, F. X., & Cummings, C. L. (2017). Decision-making and ethical dilemmas. In E. Eichenwald, C. Martin, A. Hansen, & A. Stark (Eds.), *Cloherty and Stark's manual of neonatal care* (8th ed., pp. 435–448). Lippincott Williams & Wilkins.

Plosa, E. J. (2017a). Meconium aspiration. In E. Eichenwald, A. Hansen, C. Martin, & A. Stark (Eds.), *Cloherty and Stark's manual of neonatal care* (8th ed., pp. 461–466). Lippincott Williams & Wilkins.

Plosa, E. J. (2017b). Pulmonary hemorrhage. In E. Eichenwald, A. Hansen, C. Martin, & A. Stark (Eds.), *Cloherty and Stark's manual of neonatal care* (8th ed., pp. 478–481). Lippincott Williams & Wilkins.

Poduri, A., & Volpe, J. (2018). Neuronal migration. In J. Volpe, T. Inder, B. Darras, L. deVries, A. Plessis, & J. Perlman (Eds.), *Volpe's neurology of the newborn* (6th ed., pp. 120–144). Elsevier.

Poindexter, B. B., & Martin, C. A. (2020). Nutrient requirements/nutritional support in premature neonate. In R. J. Martin, A. A. Fanaroff, & M. C. Walsh (Eds.), *Fanaroff and Martin's neonatal perinatal medicine: Diseases of the fetus and infant* (11th ed., pp. 670–689). Elsevier.

Polin, R. A., & Adamkin, D. H. (2020). Glucose, calcium and magnesium. In A. A. Fanaroff & J. M. Fanaroff (Eds.), *Klaus and Fanaroff's care of the high-risk neonate* (7th ed., pp. 227–243.e2). Elsevier.

Polin, R., & Randis, T. (2020). Perinatal infections and chorioamnionitis. In R. J. Martin, A. A. Fanaroff, & M. C. Walsh (Eds.), *Fanaroff & Martin's neonatal-perinatal medicine: Diseases of the fetus and infant* (11th ed., pp. 404–414). Elsevier.

Polit, D. F., & Beck, C. T. (2018). *Essentials of nursing research: Appraising evidence for nursing practice* (9th ed.). Wolters Kluwer.

Poole, C. L., Kimberlin, D. W., & Whitley, R. J. (2021). Antivirals in newborns and children. In J. V. Aranda & J. N. Van Den Anker (Eds.), *Yaffe and Aranda's neonatal and pediatric therapeutic principles in practice* (5th ed., pp. 430–446). Lippincott Williams & Wilkins.

Powell-Hamilton, N. (2020). Genetic and genomic testing in the newborn period. In T. L. Gomella, F. G. Eyal, & F. Bany-Mohammed (Eds.), *Gomella's neonatology: Management, procedures, on-call problems, diseases, and drugs* (8th ed., pp. 234–238). McGraw-Hill Education.

Prasad, M., & Jones, H. (2019). Substance abuse in pregnancy. In R. Resnik, C. Lockwood, T. Moore, M. Greene, J. Copel, & R. Silver (Eds.), *Creasy and Resnik's maternal–fetal medicine: Principles and practice* (8th ed., pp. 1243–1257.e3). Elsevier.

Prazad, P. A., Rajpal, M. N., Mangurten, H., & Puppala, B. (2020). Birth injuries. In R. J. Martin, A. A. Fanaroff, & M. C. Walsh (Eds.), *Fanaroff & Martin's neonatal-perinatal medicine: Diseases of the fetus and infant* (11th ed., pp. 458–488). Elsevier.

Profit, J., Lee, H. C., Gould, J. B., & Horbar, J. D. (2020). Evaluating and improving the quality and safety of neonatal intensive care. In R. J. Martin, A. A. Fanaroff, & M. C. Walsh (Eds.), *Fanaroff & Martin's neonatal–perinatal medicine: Diseases of the fetus and infant* (11th ed., Vol. 1, pp. 67–101). Elsevier.

Puopolo, K. M. (2017). Bacterial and fungal infections. In E. Eichenwald, A. Hansen, C. Martin, & A. Stark (Eds.), *Cloherty and Stark's manual of neonatal care* (8th ed., pp. 684–719). Lippincott Williams & Wilkins.

Quinn, B. L., & Peters, A. (2017). Strategies to reduce nursing student test anxiety: A literature review. *Journal of Nursing Education, 56*(3), 145–151. https://doi.org/10.3928/01484834-20170222-05

Quinn, B., Smolinski, M., & Peters, A. B. (2018). Strategies to improve NCLEX-RN success: A review. *Teaching and Learning in Nursing, 13*, 18–26. https://doi.org/10.1016/j.teln.2017.09.0021

Ramachandra, P. (2020). Urinary tract infection. In T. L. Gomella, F. G. Eyal, & F. Bany-Mohammed (Eds.), *Gomella's neonatology: Management, procedures, on-call problems, diseases, and drugs* (8th ed., pp. 1207–1210). McGraw-Hill Education.

Rao, R. (2020). Osteopenia of prematurity (metabolic bone disease). In: T. L. Gomella, F. G. Eyal,& F. Bany-Mohammed (Eds.), *Gomella's neonatology: Management, procedures, on-call problems, diseases, and drugs*. (8th ed., pp. 1022–1026). McGraw-Hill Education.

Rao, A., & Scala, M. (2020). Maintenance of thermal homeostasis. In J. Ramasethu & S. Seo (Eds.), *MacDonald's atlas of procedures in neonatology* (6th ed., pp. 37–43). Wolters Kluwer.

Redline, R. W. (2020). Placental pathology. In R. J. Martin, A. A. Fanaroff, & M. C. Walsh (Eds.), *Fanaroff & Martin's neonatal-perinatal medicine: Disease of the fetus and infant* (11th ed., pp. 415–422). Elsevier.

Reinhart, K., & Gardner, S. (2017). Health maintenance visits in the first month of life. In B. Snell & S. Gardner (Eds.), *Care of the well newborn* (pp. 331–354). Jones & Bartlett Learning.

Reis, P., & Jnah, A. (2017). Perinatal history: Influences on newborn outcome. In B. Snell & S. Gardner (Eds.), *Care of the well newborn* (pp. 69–100). Jones & Bartlett Learning.

Rhein, L. (2022). Discharge and transition to home care. In J. P. Goldsmith, M. Keszler, & K. S Gautham (Eds.), *Assisted ventilation of the neonate* (7th ed., pp. 526–531). Elsevier.

Richards, M. K., & Goldin, A. B. (2018). Neonatal gastrointestinal reflux. In C. Gleason & S. Juul (Eds.), *Avery's diseases of the newborn* (10th ed., pp. 1079–1083e1). Elsevier.

Richardson, K., & Yonekawa, K. (2018). Glomerulonephropathies and disorders of tubular function. In C. A. Gleason & S. E. Juul (Eds.), *Avery's diseases of the newborn* (10th ed., pp. 1301–1307). Elsevier.

Ringer, S. A. (2021a). Common neonatal procedures. In E. Eichenwald, A. Hansen, C. Martin, & A. Stark (Eds.), *Cloherty and Stark's manual of neonatal care* (8th ed., pp. 1000–1021). Lippincott Williams & Wilkins.

Ringer, S. A. (2021b). Resuscitation in the delivery room. In E. Eichenwald, A. Hansen, C. Martin, & A. Stark (Eds.), *Cloherty and Stark's manual of neonatal care* (8th ed., pp. 33–63). Lippincott Williams & Wilkins.

Ringer, S. A., & Hansen, A. R. (2021a). Surgical emergencies in the newborn. In E. C. Eichenwald A. R. Hansen C. R. Martin & A. R. Stark (Eds.), *Cloherty and Stark's manual of neonatal care* (8th ed., pp. 942–966). Lippincott Williams & Wilkins.

Roarty, J. D. (2021). Ophthalmologic drugs in infants and children. In J. V. Aranda, J. N, & Van. Den. Anker (Eds.), *Yaffe and Aranda's neonatal and pediatric therapeutic principles in practice* (5th ed., pp. 271–277). Lippincott Williams & Wilkins.

Rodger, M., & Silver, R. M. (2019). Coagulation disorders in pregnancy. In R. Resnik, C. J. Lockwood, T. R. Moore, M. F. Greene, J. Copel, & R. M. Silver (Eds.), *Creasy and Resnik's maternal-fetal medicine: Principles and practice* (8th ed., pp. 949–976.e8). Elsevier.

Rodriguez, R. (2020). Selected procedures in neonatology. In A. A. Fanaroff & J. M. Fanaroff (Eds.), *Klaus and Fanaroff's care of the high-risk neonate* (7th ed., pp. 495–504). Elsevier.

Rohan, A. J. (2021). Common neonatal complications. In K. Simpson, P. Creehan, N. O'Brien-Abel, C. K. Roth, & A. J. Rohan (Eds.), *Perinatal nursing* (5th ed., pp. 651–688). Wolters Kluwer.

Rojas, M., Flaherty, A., Brown, H. F., & Rush, T. (2021). Perinatal transport and levels of care. In S. L. Gardner, B. S. Carter, M. Enzman-Hines, & S. Niemeyer. (Eds) (Eds.), *Handbook of neonatal intensive care an interprofessional approach* (9th ed., pp. 45–66). Elsevier.

Rollins, M. D., & Rosen, M. A. (2018). Obstetric analgesia and anesthesia. In C. A. Gleason & S. E. Juul (Eds.), *Avery's diseases of the newborn* (10th ed., pp. 70–179 e.2). Elsevier.

Ross, M. G., & Beall, M. H. (2019). Amniotic fluid dynamics. In R. Resnik, C. J. Lockwood, T. R. Moore, M. F. Greene, J. A. Copel, & R. M. Silver (Eds.), *Creasy & Resnik's maternal-fetal medicine: Principles & practice* (8th ed., pp. 62–67 e.3). Elsevier.

Roth, C. K. (2021). Diabetes in pregnancy. In K. Simpson & P. Creehan (Eds.), *Perinatal nursing* (5th ed., pp. 304–329). Lippincott Williams & Wilkins.

Rozance, P. J., McGowan, J. E., Price-Douglas, W., & Hay, W. W., Jr. (2021). Glucose homeostasis. In S. L. Gardner, B. S. Carter, M. E. Hines, & J. A. Hernandez (Eds.), *Merenstein & Gardner's handbook of neonatal intensive care: An interprofessional approach* (9th ed., pp. 431–458). Elsevier.

Rudd, K. M. (2021). Infectious diseases in the neonate. In M. T. Verklan, M. Walden, & S. Forest (Eds.), *Core curriculum for neonatal intensive care nursing* (6th ed., pp. 588–616). Elsevier.

Saad, L. (2020). *US ethics ratings rise for medical workers and teachers.* https://news.gallup.com/poll/328136/ethics-ratings-rise-medical-workers-teachers.aspx

Sadowski, S. L., & Verklan, M. T. (2021). Cardiovascular disorders. In T. Verklan, M. Walden, & S. Forest (Eds.), *Core curriculum for neonatal intensive care nursing* (6th ed., pp. 460–503). Elsevier.

Safrin, S. (2021). Antiviral agents. In B. G. Katzung & T. W. Vanderah (Eds.), *Basic and clinical pharmacology* (15th ed., pp. 897–931). McGraw Hill.

Sahai, I., & Levy, H. (2018). Newborn screening. In C. Gleason & S. Juul (Eds.), *Avery's diseases of the newborn* (10th ed., pp. 332–346.e3). Elsevier.

Samson, L. F. (2006). Perspectives on neonatal nursing: 1985–2005. *Journal of Perinatal and Neonatal Nursing, 20*(1), 19–26. https://doi.org/10.1097/00005237-200601000-00009

Samuels, J. A., Munoz, H., & Swinford, R. D. (2017). Neonatal kidney conditions. In E. C. Eichenwald, A. R. Hansen, C. R. Martin, & A. R. Stark (Eds.), *Cloherty and Stark's manual of neonatal care* (8th ed., pp. 366–400). Wolters Kluwer.

Sansevere, A. J., & Bergin, A. M. (2017). Neonatal seizures. In: E. Eichenwald, A. Hansen, C. Martin, & A. Stark (Eds.), *Cloherty and Stark's manual of neonatal care.* (8th ed., pp. 812–828). Lippincott Williams & Wilkins.

Savich, R., & Famuyide, M. (2020). Social and economic contributors to neonatal outcomes. In R. Martin, A. Fanaroff, & M. Walsh (Eds.), *Fanaroff and Martin's neonatal-perinatal medicine: Diseases of the fetus and infant* (11th ed., pp. 140–151). Elsevier.

Saxonhouse, M. A. (2018). Neonatal bleeding and thrombotic disorders. In C. A. Gleason & S. E. Juul (Eds.), *Avery's diseases of the newborn* (10th ed., pp. 1121–1138.e4). Elsevier.

Scheans, P. (2021). Laboratory and diagnostic test interpretation. In T. Verklan, M. Walden, & S. Forest (Eds.), *Core curriculum for neonatal intensive care nursing* (6th ed., pp. 207–218). Elsevier.

Schiefelbein, J. H. (2021). Genetics: From bench to bedside. In M. T. Verklan, M. Walden, & S. Forest (Eds.), *Core curriculum for neonatal intensive care nursing* (6th ed., pp. 346–358). Elsevier.

Schleis, M. R., & Marsh, K. J. (2018). Viral infections of the fetus and newborn. In C. Gleason & S. Juul (Eds.), *Avery's diseases of the newborn* (10th ed., pp. 482–526.). Elsevier.

Schmolzer, G., & Hummler, H. (2022). Pulmonary function and graphics. In M. Keszler & K. S. Gautham (Eds.), *Assisted ventilation of the neonate* (7th ed., pp. 124–143). Elsevier.

Scholz, T., & Reinking, B. (2018). Congenital heart disease. In C. Gleason & S. Juul (Eds.), *Avery's diseases of the newborn* (10th ed., pp. 801–827.e2). Elsevier.

Schumacher, M. A., Basbaum, A. I., & Naidu, R. K. (2021). Opioid agonists & antagonists. In: B. G. Katzung & T. W. Vanderah (Eds.), *Basic and clinical pharmacology* (15th ed., pp. 573–595). McGraw Hill.

Seo, S. (2020a). Umbilical artery catheterization. In J. Ramasethu & S. Seo (Eds.), *MacDonald's atlas of procedures in neonatology* (6th ed., pp. 199–216). Wolters Kluwer.

Seo, S. (2020b). Umbilical vein catheterization. In J. Ramasethu & S. Seo (Eds.), *MacDonald's atlas of procedures in neonatology* (6th ed., pp. 217–223). Wolters Kluwer.

Sharma, R., & Hammerschlag, M. R. (2021a). Lipoglycopeptides, Glycopeptides. In J. V. Aranda & J. N. Van Den Anker (Eds.), *Yaffe and Aranda's neonatal and pediatric therapeutic principles in practice* (5th ed., pp. 297–309). Lippincott Williams & Wilkins.

Sharma, R., & Hammerschlag, M. R. (2021b). Penicillins, Cephalosporins, and other ?-Lactams. In J. V. Aranda & J. N. Van Den Anker (Eds.), *Yaffe and Aranda's neonatal and pediatric therapeutic principles in practice* (5th ed., pp. 279–296). Lippincott Williams & Wilkins.

Shaw-Battista, J., & Gardner, S. (2017). Newborn transition: The journey from fetal to extrauterine life. In B. J. Snell & S. Gardner (Eds.), *Care of the well newborn* (pp. 69–100). Jones & Bartlett Learning.

Shepherd, E. G., & Nelin, L. D. (2022). Physical examination. In M. Keszler & K. S. Gautham (Eds.), *Assisted ventilation of the neonate* (7th ed., pp. 70–75). Elsevier.

Shnorhavorian, M., & Fechner, P. Y. (2018). Disorders of sexual differentiation. In C. Gleason & S. Juul (Eds.), *Avery's diseases of the newborn* (10th ed., pp. 1365–1387). Elsevier.

Sibai, B., & Wallace, C. (2017). Preeclampsia and related conditions. In E. C. Eichenwald, A. R. Hansen, C. R. Martin, & A. R. Stark (Eds.), *Cloherty and Stark's manual of neonatal care* (8th ed., pp. 50–61). Lippincott Williams & Wilkins.

Silaj, K. M., Schwartz, S. T., & Siegal, A. L. M. (2021). Test anxiety and metacognitive performance in the classroom. *Educational Psychology Review, 33*(4), 1809–1834. https://doi.org/10.1007/s10648-021-09598-6

Simhan, H. N., Berghella, V., & Iams, J. D. (2019). Prevention and management of preterm parturition. In R. Resnik, C. J. Lockwood, T. R. Moore, M. F. Greene, J. Copel, & R. M. Silver (Eds.), *Creasy and Resnik's maternal-fetal medicine: P les and practice* (8th ed., pp. 679–711.e10). Elsevier.

Simmons, P. M., & Magann, E. F. (2020). Amniotic fluid volume. In R. Martin, A. Fanaroff, & M. Walsh (Eds.), *Fanaroff and Martin's neonatal-perinatal medicine: Diseases of the fetus and infant* (11th ed., pp. 368–403). Elsevier.

Simons, S. H. P., van den Bosch, G., & Tibboel, D. (2021). Analgesics and sedatives. In J. V. Aranda & J. N. Van Den Anker (Eds.), *Yaffe and Aranda's neonatal and pediatric therapeutic principles in practice* (5th ed., pp. 511–529). Lippincott Williams & Wilkins.

Simpson, K. (2021). Perinatal patient safety and professional liability issues. In K. R. Simpson, P. Creehan, N. O-Brien-Abel, C. Roth, & A. J. Rohan (Eds.), *AWHONN's perinatal nursing* (5th ed., pp. 1–17). Lippincott Williams & Wilkins.

Simpson, K. R., & O'Brien-Abel, N. (2021). Labor and birth. In K. Simpson & P. Creehan (Eds.), *Perinatal nursing* (5th ed., pp. 325–412). Lippincott Williams & Wilkins.

Sloan, S. (2017). Blood products used in the newborn. In E. Eichenwald, A. Hansen, C. Martin, & A. Stark (Eds.), *Cloherty and Stark's manual of neonatal care* (8th ed., pp. 576–585). Lippincott Williams & Wilkins.

Smallwood, C. (2019). Noninvasive monitoring in the neonatal and pediatric care. In B. Walsh (Ed.), *Neonatal and pediatric respiratory care* (5th ed., pp. 135–148). Elsevier.

Smith, J. R., & Donze, A. (2021). Patient safety. In M. T. Verklan, M. Walden, & S. Forest (Eds.), *Core curriculum for neonatal intensive care nursing* (5th ed., pp. 301–328). Elsevier Saunders.

Smith, M. J., Steinback, W. J., Benjamin, D. K., & Cohen-Wolkowiez, M. (2021). Antifungal agents. In J. V. Aranda & J. N. Van Den Anker (Eds.), *Yaffe and Aranda's neonatal and pediatric therapeutic principles in practice* (5th ed., pp. 412–429). Lippincott Williams & Wilkins.

Smith, V. C. (2017). The high-risk newborn: Anticipation, evaluation, management, and outcome. In E. Eichenwald, A. Hansen, C. Martin, & A. Stark (Eds.), *Cloherty and Stark's manual of neonatal care* (8th ed., pp. 74–90). Lippincott Williams & Wilkins.

Smith, V. C., & Andrews, T. M. (2017). Neonatal intensive care unit discharge planning. In E. Eichenwald, A. Hansen, C. Martin, & A. Stark (Eds.), *Cloherty and Stark's manual of neonatal care* (8th ed., pp. 215–234). Lippincott Williams & Wilkins.

Snapp, B., & Reyna, B. (2019). Role of the nurse practitioner in the community hospital. *Advances in Neonatal Care,* *19*(5), 402–408. https://doi.org/10.1097/ANC.000000000 0000638

Snell, B. J., & Gardner, S. L. (2017). Newborn and neonatal nutrition. In B. Snell & S. Gardner (Eds.), *Care of the well newborn* (pp. 135–190). Jones & Bartlett Learning.

Son-Hing, J., & Thompson, G. (2020). Congenital abnormalities of the upper and lower extremities and spine. In R. J. Martin, A. A. Fanaroff, & M. C. Walsh (Eds.), *Fanaroff & Martin's neonatal-perinatal medicine: Diseases of the fetus and infant* (11th ed., pp. 1995–2015). Elsevier.

Sorbara, J. C., & Wherrett, D. K. (2020). Disorders of sex development. In R. J. Martin, A. A. Fanaroff, & M. C. Walsh (Eds.), *Fanaroff & Martin's neonatal-perinatal medicine: Diseases of the fetus and infant* (11th ed., pp. 1665–1705). Elsevier.

Soul, J. S. (2017). Intracranial hemorrhage and white matter injury/periventricular leukomalacia. In E. Eichenwald, A. Hansen, C. Martin, & A. Stark (Eds.), *Cloherty and Stark's manual of neonatal care* (8th ed., pp. 760–789). Lippincott Williams & Wilkins.

Sparger, K. A., & Gupta, M. (2017). Neonatal thrombosis. In E. C. Eichenwald, A. Hansen, C. Martin, & A. Stark (Eds.),

Cloherty and Stark's manual of neonatal care (8th ed., pp. 595–612). Lippincott Williams & Wilkins.

Spruill, C., & LaBrecque, M. (2017). Preventing and treating pain and stress among infants in the newborn intensive care unit. In E. Eichenwald, A. Hansen, C. Martin, & A. Stark (Eds.), *Cloherty and Stark's manual of neonatal care* (8th ed., pp. 1022–1042). Lippincott Williams & Wilkins.

Spruill, C. T. (2021). Developmental support. In M. T. Verklan, M. Walden, & S. Forest (Eds.), *Core curriculum for neonatal intensive care nursing* (6th ed., pp. 172–190). Elsevier.

Srinivasan, G. (2020). Thyroid disorders. In: T. L. Gomella, F. G. Eyal, & F. Bany-Mohammed (Eds.), *Gomella's neonatology: Management, procedures, on-call problems, diseases, and drugs* (8th ed., pp. 1096–1106). McGraw-Hill Education.

Srinivasan, L., & Evans, J. R. (2018). Health care-associated infections. In C. Gleason & S. Juul (Eds.), *Avery's diseases of the newborn* (10th ed., pp. 571–574). Elsevier.

Stark, A., & Bhutani, V. (2017). Neonatal hyperbilirubinemia. In E. Eichenwald, A. Hansen, C. Martin, & A. Stark (Eds.), *Cloherty and Stark's manual of neonatal care* (8th ed., pp. 335–352). Lippincott Williams & Wilkins.

Stark, A. R. (2017). Apnea. In E. Eichenwald, A. Hansen, C. Martin, & A. Stark (Eds.), *Cloherty and Stark's manual of neonatal care* (8th ed., pp. 426–435). Lippincott Williams & Wilkins.

Steinhorn, R. H. (2020). Pulmonary vascular development. In R. J. Martin, A. A. Fanaroff, & M. C. Walsh (Eds.), *Fanaroff & Martin's neonatal-perinatal medicine: Diseases of the fetus and infant* (11th ed., pp. 1306–1319). Elsevier.

Stephenson, C. (2016). Ethics. In S. Mattson & J. Smith (Eds.), *Core curriculum for maternal-newborn nursing* (5th ed., pp. 662–681). Elsevier.

Stewart, J. E., Hernandez, F., & Duncan, A. F. (2017). Follow up care of very preterm and very low birth weight infants. In E. Eichenwald, A. Hansen, C. Martin, & A. Stark (Eds.), *Cloherty and Stark's manual of neonatal care* (8th ed., pp. 192–201). Lippincott Williams & Wilkins.

Sturtz, W. J. (2020). Neonatal Palliative Care. In: T. L. Gomella, F. G. Eyal, & F. Bany-Mohammed (Eds.), *Gomella's neonatology: Management, procedures, on-call problems, diseases, and drugs.* (8th ed., pp. 295–300). McGraw-Hill Education.

Sudia, T., & Catlin, A. (2021). Ethical issues. In M. T. Verklan, M. Walden, & S. Forest (Eds.), *Core curriculum for neonatal intensive care nursing* (6th ed., pp. 714–719). Elsevier.

Sullivan, C. (2016). Substance abuse in pregnancy. In S. Mattson & J. Smith (Eds.), *Core curriculum for maternal-newborn nursing* (5th ed., pp. 564–579). Elsevier.

Sun, Y., Hellstrom, A., & Smith, L. (2020). Retinopathy of prematurity. In R. J. Martin, A. A. Fanaroff, & M. C. Walsh (Eds.), *Fanaroff & Martin's neonatal–perinatal medicine: Diseases of the fetus and infant* (11th ed., pp. 1970–1978). Elsevier.

Swaney, J. R., English, N. K., & Carter, B. S. (2021). Ethics, values, and palliative care in the neonatal intensive care unit. In S. L. Gardner, B. S. Carter, M. Enzman-Hines, & S. Niermeyer (Eds.), *Merenstein & Gardner's handbook of neonatal intensive care nursing: An interprofessional approach* (9th ed., pp. 1167–1190). Elsevier.

Swanson, T., & Erickson, L. (2021). Cardiovascular disease and surgical interventions. In S. L. Gardner, B. S. Carter, M. Enzman-Hines, & S. Niermeyer (Eds.), *Merenstein &*

Gardner's handbook of neonatal intensive care: An interprofessional approach (9th ed., pp. 836–887). Elsevier.

Swartz, J. M., & Chan, Y. M. (2017). Disorders of sex development. In E. Eichenwald, A. Hansen, C. Martin, & A. Start (Eds.), *Cloherty and Stark's manual of neonatal care* (8th ed., pp. 922–941). Lippincott Williams & Wilkins.

Taketomo, C., Hodding, J., & Kraus, D. (2021). *Lexicomp pediatric & neonatal dosage handbook* (28th ed.). Wolters Kluwer.

Tammela, O. (2020). Respiratory distress syndrome. In T. L. Gomella, F. G. Eyal, & F. Bany-Mohammed (Eds.), *Gomella's neonatology: Management, procedures, on-call problems, diseases, and drugs* (8th ed., pp. 1043–1050). McGraw-Hill Education.

Tappero, E. (2019). Musculoskeletal system assessment. In E. P. Tappero & M. E. Honeyfield (Eds.), *Physical assessment of the newborn* (6th ed., pp. 139–166). Springer Publishing Company.

Tappero, E. (2021). Physical assessment. In M. T. Verklan, M. Walden, & S. Forest (Eds.), *Core curriculum for neonatal intensive care nursing* (6th ed., pp. 99–130). Elsevier.

Tappero, E., & Honeyfield, M. E. (2019). Glossary of terms. In E. Tappero & M. E. Honeyfield (Eds.), *Physical assessment of the newborn* (6th ed., pp. 271–293). Springer Publishing Company.

Taylor, J. A., Wright, J. A., & Woodrum, D. (2018). Newborn nursery care. In C. A. Gleason & S. E. Juul (Eds.), *Avery's diseases of the newborn* (10th ed., pp. 312–331.e6). Elsevier.

Theda, C. (2020). Disorders of sex development. In T. L. Gomella, F. G. Eyal, & F. Bany-Mohammed (Eds.), *Gomella's neonatology: Management, procedures, on-call problems, diseases, and drugs* (8th ed., pp. 874–880). McGraw-Hill Education.

Thomas, J. A., Lam, C., & Berry, G. (2018). Lysosomal storage, peroxisomal, and glycosylation disorders and Smith–Lemli–Opitz syndrome presenting in the neonate. In C. Gleason & S. Juul (Eds.), *Avery's diseases of the newborn* (10th ed., pp. 253–272.e3). Elsevier.

Thorp, J., & Grantz, K. (2019). Clinical aspects of normal and abnormal labor. In R. Resnik, C. Lockwood, T. Moore, M. Greene, J. Copel, & R. Silver (Eds.), *Creasy and Resnik's maternal-fetal medicine: Principles and practice* (8th ed., pp. 723–757.e7). Elsevier.

Tiller, G., & Bellus, G. (2018). Skeletal dysplasias and heritable connective tissue disorders. In C. Gleason & S. Juul (Eds.), *Avery's diseases of the newborn* (10th ed., pp. 1450–1657.e2). Elsevier.

Tomei, K., & Smith, M. (2020). Intracranial and calvarial disorders. In R. J. Martin, A. A. Fanaroff, & M. C. Walsh (Eds.), *Fanaroff & Martin's neonatal-perinatal medicine: Diseases of the fetus and infant* (11th ed., pp. 1060–1074). Elsevier.

Travers, C., & Ambalavanan, N. (2022). Blood gases: Technical aspects and interpretation. In J. P. Goldsmith, M. Keszler, & K. S. Gautham (Eds.), *Goldsmith's ssisted ventilation of the neonate: An evidence-based approach to newborn respiratory care* (7th ed., pp. 94–110). Elsevier.

Trembath, A. (2020). Eipdemiology for neonatologists. In R. J. Martin, A. A. Fanaroff, & M. C. Walsh (Eds.), *Fanaroff & Martin's neonatal-perinatal medicine: Diseases of the fetus and infant* (11th ed., pp. 18–24). Elsevier.

Trevor, A. J. (2021). Sedative-hypnotic drugs. In B. G. Katzung (Ed.), *Basic and clinical pharmacology* (15th ed., pp. 395–409). McGraw-Hill Education.

Trotter, C. W. (2019). Gestational age assessment. In E. P. Tappero & M. E. Honeyfield (Eds.), *Physical assessment of the newborn: A comprehensive approach to the art of physical examination* (6th ed., pp. 23–44). Springer Publishing Company.

Trotter, C. W. (2021). Radiologic evaluation. In M. T. Verklan, M. Walden, & S. Forest (Eds.), *Core curriculum for neonatal intensive care nursing* (6th ed., pp. 219–243). Elsevier.

Tuuli, M. G., & Macones, G. A. (2019). Evidence-based practice in perinatal medicine. In R. Resnik, C. J. Lockwood, T. R. Moore, M. F. Greene, J. A. Copel, & R. M. Silver (Eds.), *Creasy & Resnik's maternal-fetal medicine: Principles and practice* (8th ed., pp. 235–247.e2). Elsevier.

Tyler, L., & Napoli, L. (2019). Quality and safety. In B. Walsh (Ed.), *Neonatal and pediatric respiratory care* (5th ed., pp. 669–687). Elsevier.

Van Kaam, A. H. (2022). Principles of lung protective ventilation. In M. Keszler & K. S. Gautham (Eds.), *Goldsmith's assisted ventilation of the neonate: An evidence-based approach to newborn respiratory care* (7th ed., pp. 241–262). Elsevier.

Van Marter, L. J., & McPherson, C. C. (2017). Persistent pulmonary hypertension. In E. Eichenwald, A. Hansen, C. Martin, & A. Stark (Eds.), *Cloherty and Stark's manual of neonatal care* (8th ed., pp. 467–477). Lippincott Williams & Wilkins.

Van Otterloo, L. R. (2016). Endocrine and metabolic disorders. In S. Mattson & J. E. Smith (Eds.), *Core curriculum for maternal-newborn nursing* (5th ed., pp. 501–532). Elsevier.

Vargo, L. (2019). Cardiovascular assessment. In E. P. Tappero & M. E. Honeyfield (Eds.), *Physical assessment of the newborn: A comprehensive approach to the art of physical examination* (6th ed., pp. 93–110). Springer Publishing Company.

Vento, M. (2022). Oxygen therapy. In J. P. Goldsmith, M. Keszler, & K. S. Gautham (Eds.), *Goldsmith's assisted ventilation of the neonate: An evidence-based approach to newborn respiratory care* (7th ed., pp. 185–195). Elsevier.

Vergales, B. D. (2020a). Bladder catheterization. In T. L. Gomella, F. G. Eyal, & F. Bany-Mohammed (Eds.), *Gomella's neonatology: Management, procedures, on-call problems, diseases, and drugs* (8th ed., pp. 325–329). McGraw-Hill Education.

Vergales, B. D. (2020b). Chest tube placement. In T. L. Gomella, F. G. Eyal, & F. Bany-Mohammed (Eds.), *Gomella's neonatology: Management, procedures, on-call problems, diseases, and drugs* (8th ed., pp. 329–332). McGraw-Hill Education.

Verklan, M. T. (2021a). Adaptation to extrauterine life. In M. T. Verklan, M. Walden, & S. Forest (Eds.), *Core curriculum for neonatal intensive care nursing* (6th ed., pp. 54–68). Elsevier.

Verklan, M. T. (2021b). Legal issues. In M. T. Verklan, M. Walden, & S. Forest (Eds.), *Core curriculum for neonatal intensive care nursing* (6th ed., pp. 720–733). Elsevier.

Vernon, M. M., & Lewin, M. B. (2018). Fetal and neonatal echocardiography. In C. A. Gleason & S. E. Juul (Eds.), *Avery's diseases of the newborn* (10th ed., pp. 779–789). Elsevier.

Vittner, D., & McGrath, J. (2019). Behavioral assessment. In E. P. Tappero & M. E. Honeyfield (Eds.), *Physical assessment of the newborn: A comprehensive approach to the art of physical examination* (6th ed., pp. 193–218). Springer Publishing Company.

Vogt, B. A., & Springel, T. (2020a). Pharmacokinetics in neonatal medicine. In R. J. Martin, A. A. Fanaroff, & M. C. Walsh (Eds.), *Fanaroff & Martin's neonatal-perinatal medicine: Diseases of the fetus and infant* (11th ed., pp. 722–734). Elsevier.

Vogt, B. A., & Springel, T. (2020b). The kidney and urinary tract of the neonate. In R. J. Martin, A. A. Fanaroff, & M. C. Walsh (Eds.), *Fanaroff & Martin's neonatal-perinatal medicine: Diseases of the fetus and infant* (11th ed., pp. 1871–1895). Elsevier.

Vohr, B. (2018). Ear and hearing disorders. In C. Gleason & S. Juul (Eds.), *Avery's diseases of the newborn* (10th ed., pp. 1558–1566.e2). Elsevier.

Vohr, B. (2020). Hearing loss in the newborn infant. In R. J. Martin, A. A. Fanaroff, & M. C. Walsh (Eds.), *Fanaroff & Martin's neonatal-perinatal medicine: Diseases of the fetus and infant* (11th ed., pp. 1081–1090). Elsevier.

Volpe, J. (2018a). Neurological examination: Normal and abnormal features. In J. Volpe, T. Inder, B. Darras, L. deVries, A. Plessis, & J. Perlman (Eds.), *Volpe's neurology of the newborn* (6th ed., pp. 191–221). Elsevier.

Volpe, J. (2018b). Hypoxic-ischemic injury in the term infant: Pathophysiology. In J. Volpe, T. Inder, B. Darras, L. deVries, A. Plessis, & J. Perlman (Eds.), *Volpe's neurology of the newborn* (6th ed., pp. 191–221). Elsevier.

von Zastrow, M. (2021). Drug receptors & pharmacodynamics. In: B. G. Katzung & T. W. Vanderah (Eds.), *Basic and clinical pharmacology.* (15th ed., pp. 21–41). McGraw Hill.

Voos, K. C., & Fanaroff, J. (2020). Care of the parents. In A. A. Fanaroff & J. M. Fanaroff (Eds.), *Klaus and Fanaroff's care of the high-risk neonate* (7th ed., pp. 148–170.e3). Elsevier.

Wade, K. D. (2020). Pharmacokinetics in neonatal medicine. In: R. J. Martin, A. A. Fanaroff, & M. C. Walsh (Eds.), *Fanaroff and Martin's neonatal-perinatal medicine.* (11th ed., pp. 722–734). Elsevier.

Walden, M. (2021). Pain assessment and management. In M. T. Verklan, M. Walden, & S. Forest (Eds.), *Core curriculum for neonatal intensive care nursing* (6th ed., pp. 270–287). Elsevier.

Walker, V. P. (2018). Newborn evaluation. In C. A. Gleason & S. E. Juul (Eds.), *Avery's diseases of the newborn* (10th ed., pp. 289–311.e1). Elsevier.

Wallen, L. D., & Gleason, C. A. (2018). Prenatal drug exposure. In C. A. Gleason & S. E. Juul (Eds.), *Avery's diseases of the newborn* (10th ed., pp. 126–144). Elsevier.

Wallman, C. (2019). Assessment of the newborn with antenatal exposure to drugs. In E. P. Tappero & M. E. Honeyfield (Eds.), *Physical assessment of the newborn: A comprehensive approach to the art of physical examination* (6th ed., pp. 255–262). Springer Publishing Company.

Walsh, B. K. (2019a). Administration of gas mixtures. In B. K. Walsh (Ed.), *Neonatal and pediatric respiratory care* (5th ed., pp. 338–347). Elsevier.

Walsh, B. K. (2019b). Neurologic and neuromuscular disorders. In B.K. Walsh (Ed.), *Neonatal and pediatric respiratory care* (5th ed., pp. 620–634). Elsevier.

Walsh, B. K. (2019c). Noninvasive mechanical ventilation and continuous positive pressure of the neonate. In B. K. Walsh (Ed.), *Neonatal and pediatric respiratory care* (5th ed., pp. 267–286). Elsevier.

Walsh, B. K. (2019d). Oxygen administration. In B. K. Walsh (Ed.), *Neonatal and pediatric respiratory care* (5th ed., pp. 149–161). Elsevier.

Walsh, B. K., & Chatburn, R. L. (2019). Invasive mechanical ventilation of the neonate and pediatric patient. In B. K. Walsh (Ed.), *Neonatal and pediatric respiratory care* (5th ed., pp. 301–337). Elsevier.

Wang, P., Djahangirian, O., & Wehbi, E. (2018). Urinary tract infections and vesicoureteral reflux. In C. A. Gleason & S. E. Juul (Eds.), *Avery's diseases of the newborn* (10th ed., pp. 1308–1313). Elsevier.

Wassner, A. J., & Belfort, M. B. (2017). Thyroid disorders. In E. Eichenwald, A. Hansen, C. R. Martin, & A. Start (Eds.), *Cloherty and Stark's manual of neonatal care* (8th ed., pp. 892–909). Lippincott Williams & Wilkins.

Watchko, J. F. (2018). Neonatal indirect hyperbilirubinemia and kernicterus. In C. A. Gleason & S. E. Juul (Eds.), *Avery's diseases of the newborn* (10th ed., pp. 1198–1218.e5). Elsevier.

Watchko, J. F., & Maisels, M. J. (2020). Neonatal hyperbilirubinemia. In A. A. Fanaroff & J. M. Fanaroff (Eds.), *Klaus and Fanaroff's care of the high-risk neonate* (7th ed., pp. 244–274. e6). Elsevier.

Watters, K., & Mancuso, T. (2019). Airway management. In B. Walsh (Ed.), *Neonatal and pediatric respiratory care* (5th ed., pp. 222–241). Elsevier.

Weinman, J. P., Bronsert, B. M., & Strain, J. D. (2021). Diagnostic imaging in the neonate. In S. L. Gardner, B. S. Carter, M. Enzman-Hines, & S. Niermeyer (Eds.), *Merenstein & Gardner's handbook of neonatal intensive care: An interprofessional approach* (9th ed., pp. 201–225). Elsevier.

Weitkamp, J. H., Lewis, D. B., & Levy, O. (2018). Immunology of the fetus and newborn. In C. Gleason & S. Juul (Eds.), *Avery's diseases of the newborn* (10th ed., pp. 453–481.e7). Elsevier.

Weitkamp, J., Premkumar, M., & Martin, C. (2017). Necrotizing enterocolitis. In E. Eichenwald, A. Hansen, C. Martin, & A. Stark (Eds.), *Cloherty and Stark's manual of neonatal care* (8th ed., pp. 353–365). Lippincott Williams & Wilkins.

Werny, D., Taplin, C., Bennett, J. T., & Pihoker, C. (2018). Disorders of carbohydrate metabolism. In C. Gleason & S. Juul (Eds.), *Avery's diseases of the newborn* (10th ed., pp. 1403–1416). Elsevier.

Wheeler, C., & Le, M. (2019). Extracorporeal membrane oxygenation. In B. K. Walsh (Ed.), *Neonatal and pediatric respiratory care* (5th ed., pp. 348–369). Elsevier.

White, K., Bouchard, M., & Goldberg, M. (2018). Common neonatal orthopedic conditions. In C. Gleason & S. Juul (Eds.), *Avery's diseases of the newborn* (10th ed., pp. 1438–1449.e3). Elsevier.

Whitmer, T. (2016). Psychology of pregnancy. In S. Mattson & J. E. Smith (Eds.), *Core curriculum for maternal-newborn nursing* (5th ed., pp. 297–313). Elsevier.

Whitty, J., & Dombrowski, M. (2019). Respiratory diseases in pregnancy. In R. Resnik, C. Lockwood, T. Moore, M.

Greene, J. Copel, & R. Silver (Eds.), *Creasy and Resnik's maternal-fetal medicine: Principles and practice* (8th ed., pp. 1043–1066.e3). Elsevier.

Wilkins-Haug, L., & Heffner, L. J. (2017). Fetal assessment and prenatal diagnosis. In E. Eichenwald, A. Hansen, C. Martin, & A. Stark (Eds.), *Cloherty and Stark's manual of neonatal care* (8th ed., pp. 1–10). Lippincott Williams & Wilkins.

Wilson-Costello, D. E., & Payne, A. H. (2020a). Early childhood neurodevelopmental outcomes of high-risk neonates. In R. J. Martin, A. A. Fanaroff, & M. C. Walsh (Eds.), *Fanaroff & Martin's neonatal-perinatal medicine: Diseases of the fetus and infant* (11th ed., pp. 1091–1109). Elsevier.

Wilson-Costello, D., & Payne, A. (2020b). The outcome of neonatal intensive care. In A. Fanaroff & J. Fanaroff (Eds.), *Klaus and Fanaroff's care of the high-risk neonate* (7th ed., pp. 437–446). Elsevier.

Wilson-Costello, D. E., & Payne, A. H. (2020a). Early childhood neurodevelopmental outcomes of high-risk neonates. In R. J. Martin, A. A. Fanaroff, & M. C. Walsh (Eds.), *Fanaroff & Martin's neonatal-perinatal medicine: Diseases of the fetus and infant* (11th ed., pp. 1018–1031). Elsevier.

Witt, C. (2019). Skin assessment. In E. P. Tappero & M. E. Honeyfield (Eds.), *Physical assessment of the newborn: A comprehensive approach to the art of physical examination* (6th ed., pp. 45–59). Springer Publishing Company.

Witt, C. L. (2021). Neonatal dermatology. In M. T. Verklan, M. Walden, & S. Forest (Eds.), *Core curriculum for neonatal intensive care nursing* (6th ed., pp. 678–690). Elsevier.

Wohlert, H. (1979). NAACOG–The first 10 years. *Journal of Obstetric, Gynecologic, and Neonatal Nursing, 8*(1), 9–22. https://doi.org/10.1111/j.1552-6909.1979.tb00793.x

Wolf, G. K., & Arnold, J. H. (2017). Extracorporeal membrane oxygenation. In E. Eichenwald, A. Hansen, C. Martin, & A. Stark (Eds.), *Cloherty and Stark's manual of neonatal care* (8th ed., pp. 491–501). Lippincott Williams & Wilkins.

Wolf, R. (2019). Abdominal imaging. In R. Resnik, C. Lockwood, T. Moore, M. Greene, J. Copel, & R. Silver (Eds.), *Creasy and Resnik's maternal-fetal medicine: Principles and practice* (8th ed., pp. 393–413.e11). Elsevier.

Woo, J., Carrington, S. M., & Ambia, A. (2021). Prenatal environment: Effect on neonatal outcome. In S. L. Gardner, B. S. Carter, M. Enzman-Hines, & S. Niermeyer (Eds.), *Merenstein & Gardner's handbook of neonatal intensive care nursing: An interprofessional approach* (9th ed., pp. 17–44). Elsevier.

Woodward, L. J., McPherson, C. C., & Volpe, J. J. (2018). Passive addiction and teratogenic effects. In J. J. Volpe, T. E. Inder, B. T. Darras, L. S. deVries, A. J. du Plessis, J. J. Neil, & J. M. Perlman (Eds.), *Volpe's neurology of the newborn* (6th ed., pp. 1149–1189.e20). Elsevier.

Wright, C., Posencheg, M., Seri, I., & Evans, J. (2018). Fluid, electrolyte and acid-base balance. In C. Gleason & S. Juul (Eds.), *Avery's diseases of the newborn* (10th ed., pp. 368–389.e4). Elsevier.

Yatczak, J., Mortier, T., & Silander, H. (2021). A study exploring student thriving in professional programs: Expanding our understanding of student success. *Journal of Higher Education Theory and Practice, 21*(1), 91–104. https://doi.org/10.33423/jhetp.v21i1.4040

Yoder, B. A., & Grubb, P. H. (2022). Mechanical ventilation: disease-specific strategies. In M. Keszler & K. S. Gautham (Eds.), *Goldsmith's assisted ventilation of the neonate: An evidence-based approach to newborn respiratory care* (7th ed., pp. 288–302). Elsevier.

Yonkers, K. A. (2019). Management of depression and psychoses in pregnancy and in the puerperium. In R. Resnik, C. Lockwood, T. Moore, M. Greene, J. Copel, & R. Silver (Eds.), *Creasy and Resnik's maternal fetal medicine: Principles and practice* (8th ed., pp. 1232–1242.e3). Elsevier.

Yuguo, L., Haiyan, P., Runjuang, Y., Xingjie, W., Jiawei, R., Xingshan, Z., & Congcong, P. (2021). The relationship between test anxiety and emotion regulation: The mediating effect of psychological resilience. *Annuals of General Psychiatry, 20*(40), 1–9. https://doi.org/10.1186/s12991-021-00360-4

Zakarija-Grkovic, I., Bosnjak, A. P., Buljan, I., Vettorazzi, R., & Smith, L. J. (2019). The IBLCE exam: Candidate experience, motivation, study strategies used and predictors of success. *International Breastfeeding Journal, 14*(2), 1–13. https://doi.org/10.1186/s13006-018-0197-2

Zanelli, S. A., & Kaufman, D. (2019). Surfactant replacement therapy. In B. K. Walsh (Ed.), *Neonatal and pediatric respiratory care* (5th ed., pp. 244–266). Elsevier.

Zayek, M. (2020). Bronchopulmonary dysplasia/chronic lung disease. In T. L. Gomella, F. G. Eyal, & F. Bany-Mohammed (Eds.), *Gomella's neonatology: Management, procedures, on-call problems, diseases, and drugs* (8th ed., pp. 826–833). McGraw-Hill Education.

Index